Editors Hans G. Beger, *Ulm*
Seiki Matsuno, *Sendai*
John L. Cameron, *Baltimore*

Co-Editors Bettina M. Rau, *Rostock*
Makoto Sunamura, *Sendai*
Richard D. Schulick, *Baltimore*

Diseases of the Pancreas

Current Surgical Therapy

Editors Hans G. Beger, *Ulm, Germany*
Seiki Matsuno, *Sendai, Japan*
John L. Cameron, *Baltimore, USA*

Diseases of the Pancreas

Current Surgical Therapy

With 680 Figures

Springer

Editors

Hans G. Beger, MD
University of Ulm
c/o University Hospital Ulm
Steinhoevelstraße 9
89075 Ulm, Germany

Seiki Matsuno, MD
Department of Surgery I
Tohoku University, Medical School
980-8574 Sendai, Japan

John L. Cameron, MD, PhD
The Johns Hopkins University
720 Rutland Avenue
Baltimore, MD 21205-2196, USA

Co-Editors

Bettina M. Rau, MD
Department of General, Thoracic, Vascular
and Transplantation Surgery
University of Rostock
Schillingallee 35
18057 Rostock, Germany

Makoto Sunamura, MD, PhD
Department of Surgery I
Tohoku University, Medical School
980-8574 Sendai, Japan

Richard D. Schulick, MD
The Johns Hopkins Hospital
The Sidney Kimmel Cancer Research Center
1650 Orleans Street
Baltimore, MD 21231-1000, USA

ISBN 978-3-540-28655-4 Springer Berlin Heidelberg New York

Library of Congress Control Number: 2005938806

Springer is a part of Springer Science+Business Media
springer.com

Printed in Germany

Editor: Gabriele M. Schröder, Heidelberg, Germany
Desk Editor: Stephanie Benko, Heidelberg, Germany
Production: LE-TEX Jelonek, Schmidt &. Vöckler GbR, Leipzig, Germany
Illustrations: Jörg Kühn, Heidelberg, Germany
Cover Design: Frido Steinen-Broo, eStudio Calamar, Spain
Typesetting and Reproduction: am-productions GmbH, Wiesloch, Germany
Printing and Binding: Stürtz GmbH, Würzburg, Germany

Printed on acid-free paper 19/3180YL – 5 4 3 2 1 0

Preface

Until recently, the pancreas has been considered the least understood organ of the human body. However, it has attracted the interest of basic researchers, gastroenterologists and surgeons because of the frequency of pathologic lesions. At the beginning of the 21st century, there were two major avenues of progress in clinical medicine and pancreatology as well. The molecular mechanisms producing the inflammatory and neoplastic lesions of the pancreas have been partially elucidated. In the field of clinical management, standardization of diagnostic measures, and medical and surgical treatment modalities have resulted in a significant reduction in early and late morbidity and in the improvement of the general outcome of patients. Clinical decision-making is increasingly directed by evidence-based data, except for ductal pancreatic cancer, a disease for which, even today, there is a poor prognosis.

The Editors hope this book will become an important reference material for the newest data regarding pancreatic diseases and the surgical management of common and rare pancreatic lesions. Internationally known clinicians, basic scientists and surgeons have provided detailed outlines and discussions on operative techniques and treatment modalities, accompanied by rationales for particular approaches advocated by the authors.

This book of current surgical treatment has been designed primarily to meet the needs of surgeons working specifically in the field of HBP diseases. In addition, general surgeons who wish to acquire more knowledge of basic and clinical concepts in the management of pancreatic diseases should find this text useful.

The major goal of this book is to present the current surgical therapy for diseases of the pancreas. These principles are presented together with advancements in technologic, molecular, cellular and biological sciences, in order to enhance the knowledge of individuals involved in the care of patients with pancreatic diseases. The topics and chapters are presented by leading experts in the field, and represent the most up-to-date information. Regarding details of surgical techniques, it contains more than 300 figures and sketches. We believe this book is not only of clinical importance to surgeons, but also to gastroenterologists, pancreatologists, and pathologists caring for patients with pancreatic disorders.

Hans G. Beger, Ulm
Seiki Matsuno, Sendai
John L. Cameron, Baltimore

Contents

Section 1
Anatomy of the Pancreas

Chapter 1
Development of the Pancreas and Response to Disease 3
D. E. Bockman

Chapter 2
Congenital Anomalies of the Pancreas and the Extrahepatic Bile Ducts 9
H. Fujii, Y. Matsumoto, K. Sudo

Chapter 3
Surgical Vascular Anatomy and Histology 19
Y. Mikami, A. Otsuka, M. Unno

Section 2
Physiology and Pathophysiology of the Pancreatic Functions

Chapter 4
Pancreatic Exocrine Secretion 31
P. Layer, J. Keller

Chapter 5
Physiology and Pathophysiology of Endocrine Pancreatic Secretion 37
B. Gallwitz, U. R. Fölsch

Chapter 6
Sphincter of Oddi Physiology and Pathophysiology 49
M. Staritz

Section 3
Clinical Standards of Diagnostic Measures

Chapter 7
Ultrasound 61
S. Tanaka

Chapter 8
Contrast-Enhanced CT and MRI 67
H.-J. Brambs

Chapter 9
Endoscopic Retrograde Cholangiopancreatography 75
H. Saisho

Chapter 10
Fine-Needle Aspiration Biopsy of the Pancreas 85
K. Yamao, H. N. Mizuno, K. Takahashi, Y. Shimizu, T. Koshikawa

Chapter 11
FDG-PET and PET/CT in Pancreatic Cancer 97
S. N. Reske

Chapter 12
Laboratory Diagnosis of Exocrine and Endocrine Dysfunctions in Inflammatory and Neoplastic Lesions 107
K. Schütte , S. Kahl, P. Malfertheiner

Chapter 13
Guidelines, Clinical Evaluation, Short Track 119
J. Mössner

Section 4
Acute Pancreatitis

Chapter 14
Etiology and Epidemiology of Acute Pancreatitis 131
P. G. Lankisch, P. Maisonneuve, A. B. Lowenfels

Chapter 15
Epidemiology and Intervention During the Clinical Course of Biliary Acute Pancreatitis 143
R. C. Carter, C. W. Imrie

Chapter 16
Pathogenesis and Pathophysiology of Acute Pancreatitis *153*
M. L. Steer, G. Perides

Chapter 17
Natural Course of Acute Pancreatitis *163*
H. G. Beger, B. M. Rau

Chapter 18
Classification of Severe Acute Pancreatitis *173*
R. Isenmann

Chapter 19.1
Biochemical Diagnosis, Staging, and Prediction *181*
B. M. Rau

Chapter 19.2
Imaging Diagnosis of Acute Pancreatitis *193*
E. J. Balthazar

Chapter 20
Nonsurgical Management of Acute Pancreatitis *203*
P. A. Banks, K. J. Mortele

Chapter 21.1
Indications for the Surgical Management of Necrotizing Pancreatitis *211*
H. G. Beger, B. M. Rau

Chapter 21.2
Debridement and Closed Packing for the Treatment of Necrotizing Pancreatitis *219*
M. Reinblatt, C. Fernandez-del-Castillo, A. L. Warshaw

Chapter 21.3
Necrosectomy and Redressing *225*
P. Götzinger

Chapter 21.4
Necrosectomy and Closed Lavage *231*
B. M. Rau, H. G. Beger

Chapter 21.5
Infected Necrosis – Minimally Invasive Necrosectomy *241*
R. Carter, A. P. Wysocki

Chapter 21.6
Benefits and Limitations of Necrosectomy *249*
O. Mann, T. Strate, E. Yekebas, J. Izbicki

Chapter 22
Surgical Management of Pancreatic Abscess *253*
R. Bittner, B. M. Rau, H. G. Beger

Chapter 23
Surgical Management of Pseudocysts after Acute Pancreatitis *259*
B. M. Rau, H. G. Beger

Chapter 24
Interventional Management of Pancreatic Fluid Collections and Abscesses *271*
T. H. Baron

Chapter 25
Pancreatic and Intestinal Fistulas *281*
G. Tsiotos, J. Tsiaoussis

Chapter 26
Late Outcome after Necrosectomy *289*
I. H. Nordback, J. Sand

Section 5
Chronic Pancreatitis

Chapter 27
Mechanisms of Pain in Chronic Pancreatitis *295*
P. Di Sebastiano, F. F. Di Mola

Chapter 28
Natural Course of Chronic Pancreatitis *301*
J. Enrique Domínguez-Muñoz

Chapter 29
Chronic Pancreatitis: Inflammatory Mass in the Head of the Pancreas – Pacemaker of Chronic Pancreatitis *311*
H. G. Beger, F. Gansauge, M. Schwarz, B. Poch

Chapter 30
Diagnosis: Functional Testing, Radiological Work-up of Chronic Pancreatitis *319*
M. Kahl, J. Keller, P. Layer

Chapter 31
Medical Management of Chronic Pancreatitis *331*
P. G. Lankisch, H. Lübbers, R. Mahlke

Chapter 32
Tropical Chronic Pancreatitis 349
H. Ramesh

Chapter 33
Hereditary Chronic Pancreatitis: Diagnosis and Management 361
N. Teich, V. Keim

Chapter 34
Endoscopic Interventional Treatment 373
R. Jakobs, J. F. Riemann

Chapter 35
Indication for Surgical Treatment in Chronic Pancreatitis 381
H. G. Beger, B. Poch

Chapter 36
Pancreatic Duct Drainage Procedures 387
R. A. Prinz, M. Gaffud, M. Edwards

Chapter 37
Duodenum-Preserving Pancreatic Head Resection 399
H. G. Beger, B. M. Rau, B. Poch

Chapter 38
Pancreaticoduodenctomy for Chronic Pancreatitis – With or Without Pylorus Preservation 413
L. W. Traverso

Chapter 39
Central Pancreatectomy 425
C. Iacono, L. Bortolasi, G. Serio

Chapter 40
Distal Pancreatectomy in Patients with Chronic Pancreatitis 441
J. Lunger, K. Mair, M. Junger, M. H. Schoenberg

Chapter 41
Total Pancreatectomy 453
I. Ihse

Chapter 42
Surgical Treatment of Pseudocysts in Chronic Pancreatitis 459
R. Grützmann, H. D. Saeger

Chapter 43
Late Outcome After Medical and Surgical Treatment of Chronic Pancreatitis 477
L. Gullo, R. Pezzilli

Section 6
Pancreatic Cancer

Chapter 44
Epidemiology of Pancreatic Cancer 489
A. B. Lowenfels, P. Maisonneuve

Chapter 45
Pathology of Pancreatic Cancer 497
R. H. Hruban, A. Maitra, N. Fukushima

Chapter 46
Genetic Pathways in Pancreatic Tumorigenesis 513
E. Gallmeier, S. E. Kern

Chapter 47
The Clinical Assessment of Pancreatic Cancer 527
E. J. Shin, M. I. Canto

Chapter 48
The Staging of Pancreatic Cancer 541
J. R. Rodríguez, C. Fernandez-del Castillo

Chapter 49
Oncological Management of Pancreatic Cancer in Advanced Stages 549
D. Laheru

Chapter 50
Indications for Resection of Pancreatic Cancer 559
O. J. Hines, H. A. Reber

Chapter 51
The Kausch-Whipple Pancreatectomy 567
C. R. Ferrone, M. F. Brennan

Chapter 52
Pylorus-Preserving Pancreatico-duodenectomy 581
R. D. Schulick, J. L. Cameron

Chapter 53
Management of Tumor Invasion/Adhesion to the Superior Mesenteric-Portal Vein During Pancreatectomy 593
F. Mosca, U. Boggi, M. Del Chiaro

Chapter 54
Margin Status Following Pancreaticoduodenectomy for Pancreatic Adenocarcinoma: Implications of R Status 611
C. P. Raut, G. Varadhachary, H. Wang, E. P. Tamm, J. B. Fleming, D. B. Evans

Chapter 55
Subtotal Left Resection for Pancreatic Cancer 625
A. Nakeeb, B. Safar

Chapter 56
Total Pancreatectomy for Pancreatic Cancer 639
J. Y. Tracey, M. Bouvet, A. R. Moossa

Chapter 57
Laparoscopic Management of Pancreatic Neoplasms 653
C. G. S. Hüscher, C. Ponzano, M. Di Paola

Chapter 58
Bypass Procedures in the Treatment of Nonresectable Carcinoma of the Head of the Pancreas 665
M. G. House, K. D. Lillemoe

Chapter 59
Resected Pancreatic Cancer 675
G. R. Varadhachary, J. L. Abbruzzese

Chapter 60
Management of Locally Advanced and Recurrent Pancreas Cancer 689
A. Jimeno, M. Hidalgo

Chapter 61
Survival After Medical and Surgical Treatment of Pancreatic Adenocarcinoma 695
J. F. Tseng, C. Fernandez-del Castillo, A. L. Warshaw

Section 7
Endocrine Tumors of the Pancreas

Chapter 62
Pancreatic Endocrine Tumors: Epidemiology, Pathology, Pathophysiology, and Diagnosis 707
C. Shibata, Y. Funayama, I. Sasaki

Chapter 63
Surgical Treatment of Insulinomas 715
M. Sunamura, S. Fukuyama

Chapter 64
Surgical Treatment of the Gastrinoma 723
M. Imamura, I. Komoto

Chapter 65
Surgical Treatment of Rare Endocrine Tumors 735
S. Egawa, M. Sunamura, S. Matsuno, M. Unno

Chapter 66
Outcome after Surgical Treatment of Endocrine Pancreatic Tumors 749
S. Fukuyama, S. Matsuno, S. Egawa, M. Sunamura

Section 8
Periampullary Tumors

Chapter 67
Histopathology of Tumors of the Papilla of Vater 755
W. Kimura

Chapter 68
Clinical Diagnosis of Adenoma of the Papilla of Vater 765
K. Shiratori

Chapter 69
Clinical Diagnosis of Periampullary Carcinoma 771
T. Kamisawa, A. Okamoto

Chapter 70
Endoscopic Management of Adenoma 779
H. Maguchi, M. Osanai, A. Katanuma, K. Takahashi

Chapter 71
Surgical Management of Adenoma 789
S. Ikeda, Y. Yasunami

Chapter 72
Surgical Treatment of Carcinoma of the Ampulla of Vater 797
K. Yamaguchi, M. Tanaka

Chapter 73
Surgical Resection of Distal Common Bile Duct Carcinoma 807
T. Rikiyama, M. Unno, S. Matsuno

Chapter 74
Cancer of the Duodenum – Surgical Treatment 817
T. Imaizumi, M. Ishii, K. Tobita, S. Douwaki, H. Makuuchi

Chapter 75
Long-Term Outcome After Resection of Periampullary Carcinoma 827
H. Amano, T. Takada

Section 9
Cystic Neoplasia of the Pancreas

Chapter 76
Cystic Neoplasms of the Pancreas – Pathological Aspects 839
T. Furukawa

Chapter 77
Clinical Diagnosis and Staging 843
M. Tanaka

Chapter 78
Surgical Treatment of Cystic Tumors of the Pancreas 849
T. Mori, N. Abe, M. Sugiyama, Y. Atomi

Section 10
Congenital Anomalies of the Pancreas

Chapter 79
Congenital Cysts: Diagnosis, Clinical Impact, and Management 873
G. Klöppel, H. D. Saeger

Chapter 80
Pancreas Divisum – Diagnosis and Endoscopic Management 881
N. Soehendra, T. L. Ang, Y. Zhong, S. Seewald

Chapter 81
Surgical Treatment of Pancreas Divisum 891
H. G. Beger, P. Poch

Chapter 82
Biliopancreatic Maljunction: Classification, Diagnosis, and Treatment 895
T. Onogawa, T. Rikiyama, M. Unno, S. Matsuno

Section 11
Pancreatic Injury

Chapter 83
Pancreatic Trauma: Diagnosis, Treatment, Complications, and Late Outcome 905
J. M. Mayer, P. Tuncyurek

Section 12
Transplantation of the Pancreas

Chapter 84
Islet Transplantation and Results 913
C. Ricordi, A. Pileggi

Chapter 85
Pancreas Transplantation 921
U. T. Hopt

Contributors

James L. Abbruzzese
The University of Texas
Anderson Cancer Center
1515 Holcombe Boulevard
Houston, Texas 77030
USA

Hodaka Amano
Teikyo University School of Medicine
Department of Surgery
Kaga 2-11-1
Itabashi-ku
Tokyo, 173-8605
Japan

Yutaka Atomi
Kyorin University
Department of Surgery
School of Medicine
6-20-2 Shinkawa
Mitaka
Tokyo, 181-8611
Japan

Emil J. Balthazar
New York University
Department of Radiology
Tisch Medical Center
New York, NY 10016
USA

Peter A. Banks
Harvard Medical School
Division of Gastroenterology
Center for Pancreatic Disease
Brigham and Women's Hospital
Boston, MA 02115-6092
USA

Todd H. Baron
Mayo Foundation
Division of Gastroenterology and Hepatology
200 First Street SW
Charlton 8A
Rochester, MN 55905
USA

Hans G. Beger
University of Ulm
c/o Universitiy Hospital Ulm
Steinhövelstrasse 9
89075 Ulm
Germany

Reinhard Bittner
Marienhospital
Stuttgart, Allg. Chirurgie
Böheimstraße 37
70199 Stuttgart
Germany

Dale E. Bockman
Medical College of Georgia
Department of Cellular Biology and Anatomy
Augusta, GA 30912-2000
USA

Ugo Boggi
Dipartimento di Chirurgia Generale e Trapianti
Ospedale di Cisanello
Via Paradisa 2
56124 Pisa
Italy

Hans-Juergen Brambs
University Hospital
Department of Diagnostic
and Interventional Radiology
89075 Ulm
Germany

Murray F. Brennan
Department of Surgery
Memorial Sloan-Kettering Cancer Center
1275 York Avenue
New York, NY 10021
USA

John L. Cameron
Johns Hopkins Medical Institutions
Department of Surgery
600 North Wolfe Street, Blalock 679
Baltimore, Maryland 21287
USA

Marcia Irene Canto
Johns Hopkins University
Division of Gastroenterology and Hepatology
Room 425, 1830 E. Monument Street
Baltimore, MD 21205
USA

Ross Carter
Department of Pancreatico-Biliary Surgery
Glasgow Royal Infirmary
Alexandra Parade
Glasgow G31 2ER
UK

Massimiliano Di Paola
Department of General and Emergency Surgery
San Carlo Borromeo Hospital
20153 Milano
Italy

Pierluigi Di Sebastiano
Department of Surgery
IRCCS Casa Sollievo della Sofferenza
Viale Cappuccini
71013 San Giovanni Rotondo
Italy

Fabio F. Di Mola
Department of Surgery
IRCCS Casa Sollievo della Sofferenza
Viale Cappuccini
San Giovanni Rotondo
Italy

J. Enrique Domínguez-Muñoz
University Hospital of Santiago de Compostela
Department of Gastroenterology
C/Choupana, s/n
15706-Santiago de Compostela
Spain

Shinichi Egawa
Tohoku University
Graduate School of Medicine
Department of Surgery
1-1 Seiryo-machi
Aoba-ku
Sendai 980-8574
Japan

Douglas B. Evans
University of Texas
Anderson Cancer Center
Department of Surgery,
Box 444
1515 Holcombe Boulevard
Houston, TX 77030
USA

Carlos Fernandez-del Castillo
Center for Clinical Effectiveness in Surgery
Harvard Medical School
Massachusetts General Hospital
Boston, MA 02115-6092
USA

Cristina R. Ferrone
Department of Surgery
Memorial Sloan-Kettering Cancer Center
1275 York Avenue
New York, NY 10021
USA

Ulrich R. Fölsch
Klinik für Allgemeine Innere Medizin
Universitätsklinikum Schleswig-Holstein
Campus Kiel
Schittenhelmstr. 12
24105 Kiel
Germany

Hideki Fujii
Faculty of Medicine
The First Department of Surgery
University of Yamanashi
110, Shimokato
Chuo
409-3898 Yamanashi
Japan

Noriyoshi Fukushima
The University of Tokyo
Department of Pathology
Tokyo
Japan

Shoji Fukuyama
Tohoku University Graduate School of Medicine
Department of Surgery
Division of Gastroenterological Surgery
1-1 Seiryo-Cho
Aobaku
Sendai
Miyagi 980-8574
Japan

Toru Furukawa
International Research and Educational Institute for Integrated Medical Sciences
Tokyo Women's Medical University
8-1 Kawada-cho
Shinjuku-ku
Tokyo 162-8666
Japan

Eike Gallmeier
The Sidney Kimmel Comprehensive Cancer Center at Johns Hopkins University School of Medicine
Department of Oncology
The Sol Goldman Pancreatic Cancer Research Center
Baltimore, MD 21231
USA

Baptist Gallwitz
Medizinische Klinik IV
Universitätsklinikum Tübingen
Otfried-Müller-Str. 10
72076 Tübingen
Germany

Peter Götzinger
University of Vienna
Department of Surgery
General Hospital Vienna
Leitstelle 21A
Waehringer Guertel 18-20
1090 Vienna
Austria

Robert Götzmann
Klinik für Viszeral-, Thorax- und Gefäßchirurgie
Universitätsklinikum Dresden
Fetscherstraße 74
01307 Dresden
Germany

Lucio Gullo
Department of Medicine and Gastroenterology
Sant'Orsola-Malpighi Hospital
Via Massarenti 9
40138 Bologna
Italy

O. Joe Hines
David Geffen School of Medicine at UCLA
Section of Gastrointestinal Surgery
10833 Le Conte Ave
Los Angeles, CA 90095-6904
USA

Manuel Hidalgo
Johns Hopkins University
Sidney Kimmel Comprehensive Cancer Center
1650 Orleans Street
Room 1M88
Baltimore, MD 21231-1000
USA

Ulrich T. Hopt
Chirurgischen Universitätsklinik
Hugstetter Str. 55
79106 Freiburg
Germany

Michael G. House
Johns Hopkins Medical Institutions
Department of Surgery
Baltimore, MD 21287
USA

Ralph H. Hruban
Department of Pathology
The Sol Goldman Pancreatic Cancer Research Center
401 North Broadway
Baltimore, MD 21231
USA

Cristiano G.S. Hüscher
Department of General and Emergency Surgery
San Carlo Borromeo Hospital
20153 Milano
Italy

Calogero Iacono
University of Verona Medical School
Department of Surgery and Gastroenterology
37126 Verona
Italy

Ingemar Ihse
Lund University Hospital
Department of Surgery and Gastroenterology
22185 Lund
Sweden

Seiyo Ikeda
Fukuoka University School of Medicine
Department of Surgery
7-45-1 Nanakuma
Jonan-ku
Fukuoka, 814-0180
Japan

Toshihide Imaizumi
Tokai University
Department of Surgery
School of Medicine
Bohseidai Isehara
Kanagawa 259-1193
Japan

Masayuki Imamura
Kyoto University Hospital
Department of Surgery
54-Shogoin Kawara-cho
Sakyo-ku
Kyoto 606-01
Japan

Clem Imrie
West of Scotland Pancreatic Unit
Glasgow Royal Infirmary
Alexandra Parade
Glasgow G31 2ER
UK

Rainer Isenmann
University of Ulm
Department of Abdominal
and Transplantation Surgery
Steinhoevelstrasse 9
89075 Ulm
Germany

Jakob R. Izbicki
University Hospital-Eppendorf
Chirurgischen Klinik
Department of Surgery
Martinistr. 52
20246 Hamburg
Germany

Antonio Jimeno
Johns Hopkins University
Department of Oncology
Baltimore, MD, 21231-1000
USA

Matthias Kahl
Medizinische Klinik
Israelitisches Krankenhaus
Orchideenstieg 14
22297 Hamburg
Germany

Terumi Kamisawa
Department of Internal Medicine
Tokyo Metropolitan Komagome Hospital
3-18-22 Honkomagome
Bunkyo-ku
Tokyo 113-8677
Japan

Volker Keim
Universitätsklinikum Leipzig
Medizinische Klinik II
Philipp Rosenthal Strasse 27
04103 Leipzig
Germany

Jutta Keller
Hamburg University
Israelitic Hospital
Academic Hospital
Orchideenstieg 14
22297 Hamburg
Germany

Scott E. Kern
The Sidney Kimmel Comprehensive Cancer Center
at Johns Hopkins University School of Medicine
The Sol Goldman Pancreatic Cancer
Research Center
Baltimore, MD 21231
USA

Wataru Kimura
Yamagata University School of Medicine
Department of Gastroenterological
and General Surgery
2-2-2 Iida-Nishi
Yamagata City
Yamagata 990-9585
Japan

Günter Klöppel
University of Kiel
Department of Pathology
Michaelisstr.11
24105 Kiel
Germany

Izumi Komoto
Kyoto University Hospital
Department of Surgery
54-Shogoin Kawara-cho
Sakyo-ku
Kyoto 606-01
Japan

Takashi Koshikawa
Aichi Prefectual College of Nursing and Health
Nagoya 464-8681
Japan

Paul G. Lankisch
Klinik für Allgemeine Innere Medizin
Medizinisches Zentrum
Boegelstrasse 1
21339 Lueneburg
Germany

Peter Layer
Hamburg University
Israelitic Hospital
Academic Hospital
Orchideenstieg 14
22297 Hamburg
Germany

Dan Laheru
The Sidney Kimmel Comprehensive Cancer Center
at Johns Hopkins
The Johns Hopkins University School of Medicine
Department of Medical Oncology
1650 Orleans Street
Bunting Blaustein Cancer Research Building
Room G89
Baltimore, MD 21231-1000
USA

Keith D. Lillemoe
Indiana University School of Medicine
Department of Surgery
545 Barnhill Drive, EH 203
Indianapolis, IN 46202
USA

Josef Lunger
Rotkreuz-Krankenhaus
Nymphenburger Straße 165
80634 München
Germany

Albert B. Lowenfels
New York Medical College
Department of Surgery
Valhalla, NY 10595
USA

Hiroyuki Maguchi
Center for Gastroenterology
Teine-Keijinkai Hospital
1-jo, 12 chome 1-40 Maeda
Teine-ku 006-8555
Sapporo
Japan

Reiner Mahlke
Klinik für Allgemeine Innere Medizin
Medizinisches Zentrum
Boegelstrasse 1
21339 Lueneburg
Germany

Patrick Maisonneuve
European Institute of Oncology
20139 Milano
Italy

Anirban Maitra
Departments of Pathology and Oncology,
and the Institute for Genomic Medicine
The Sol Goldman Pancreatic Cancer
Research Center
401 North Broadway
Baltimore, MD 21231
USA

Hiroyasu Makuuchi
Tokai University
Department of Surgery
School of Medicine
Bohseidai Isehara
Kanagawa 259-1193
Japan

Peter Malfertheiner
Universitätsklinikum
Klinik für Gastroenterologie, Hepatologie
und Infektiologie, Zentrum für Innere Medizin
Leipziger Strasse 44
39120 Magdeburg
Germany

Oliver Mann
Klinik und Poliklinik für Allgemein-, Viszeral-
und Thoraxchirurgie
Univ.-Krankenhaus Eppendorf
Martinistraße 52
20246 Hamburg
Germany

Jens M. Mayer
Abteilung für Viszeral- und
Transplantationschirurgie
Steinhövelstrasse 9
89075 Ulm
Germany

Yukio Mikami
Tohoku University
Division of Hepato-Biliary-Pancreatic Surgery
Graduate School of Medicine
Sendai
Japan

Seiki Matsuno
Tohoku University Graduate School
of Medical Science
Division of Hepato-Biliary Pancreatic Surgery
Department of Surgery
1-1, Seiryo-machi
Aoba-ku
Sendai, 980-8574
Japan

A. Rahim Moossa
University of California, San Diego
Department of Surgery
200 W. Arbor Drive
San Diego, CA 92103
USA

Toshiyuki Mori
Kyorin University
Department of Surgery
School of Medicine
6-20-2 Shinkawa
Mitaka
Tokyo, 181-8611
Japan

Koenraad J. Mortele
Department of Radiology
Brigham and Women's Hospital
Harvard Medical School
Boston, MA 02115
USA

Franco Mosca
Dipartimento di Chirurgia Generale e Trapianti
Ospedale di Cisanello
Via Paradisa 2
56124 Pisa
Italy

Joachim Mössner
Medizinische Klinik und Poliklinik II
Universitätsklinikum Leipzig AöR
Philipp-Rosenthal-Straße 27
04103 Leipzig
Germany

Attila Nakeeb
Indiana University School of Medicine
535 Barnhill Drive
Cancer Pavilion RT 130
Indianapolis, IN 46202
USA

Mizuno Nobumasa
Department of Gastrointestinal Surgery
Aichi Cancer Center Hospital
Nagoya 464-8681
Japan

Isto H. Nordback
Tampere University Hospital
Box 2000
Department of Surgery
Tampere 33521
Finland

Atsutake Okamoto
Department of Surgery
Tokyo Metropolitan Komagome Hospital
3-18-22 Honkomagome
Bunkyo-ku
Tokyo 113-8677
Japan

Tohru Onogawa
Tohoku University Graduate School
of Medical Science
Division of Hepato-Biliary Pancreatic Surgery
Department of Surgery
1-1, Seiryo-machi,
Aoba-ku
Sendai, 980-8574
Japan

Aiji Ostuka
Okayama University Graduate School
of Medicine and Dentistry
Department of Human Morphology,
Functional Physiology, Biophysiological Science
Okayama
Japan

George Perides
Boston Pancreas Group and Department of Surgery
Tufts-New England Medical Center
860 Washington St
Boston, MA 02111
USA

Raffaele Pezzilli
University of Bologna
Department of Internal Medicine
Sant'Orsola-Malpighi Hospital
40100 Bologna
Italy

Antonello Pileggi
University of Miami Miller School of Medicine
Clinical Islet Transplant Program
and Cell Transplant Center
Diabetes Research Institute
DeWitt Daughtry Family Department of Surgery
1450 NW 10th Avenue (R-134)
Miami, FL 33136
USA

Bertram Poch
Center for Oncological, Endocrinological,
and Minimal-Access Surgery
Silcherstr. 36
89231 Neu-Ulm
Germany

Richard A. Prinz
Department of General Surgery
Rush-Presbyterian-St. Luke's Medical Center
1653 West Congress
Parkway
Chicago, IL 60612
USA

Hariharan Ramesh
Digestive Diseases Center
Lakeshore Hospital and Research Center
Cochin
Kerala
India

Bettina M. Rau
Department of General, Thoracic, Vascular
and Transplantation Surgery
University of Rostock
Schillingallee 35
18057 Rostock
Germany

Chandrajit P. Raut
Brigham and Women‘s Hospital
Division of Surgical Oncology
75 Francis Street
Boston, MA 02115
USA

Howard A. Reber
Section of Gastrointestinal Surgery
David Geffen School of Medicine at UCLA
10833 Le Conte Ave
Los Angeles, CA 90095-6904
USA

Maura Reinblatt
Harvard Medical School,
Massachusetts General Hospital
White 506
55 Fruit St.
Boston, MA 02114
USA

Sven Norbert Reske
Universitätsklinikum Ulm
Klinik für Nuklearmedizin
Robert-Koch-Str. 8
89081 Ulm
Germany

Camillo Ricordi
University of Miami Miller School of Medicine
Clinical Islet Transplant Program
and Cell Transplant Center
Diabetes Research Institute
DeWitt Daughtry Family Department of Surgery
1450 NW 10th Avenue (R-134)
Miami, FL 33136
USA

Toshiki Rikiyama
Tohoku University Graduate School
of Medical Science
Division of Hepato-Biliary Pancreatic Surgery
Department of Surgery
1-1, Seiryo-machi
Aoba-ku
Sendai, 980-8574
Japan

Jürgen F. Riemann
Department of Medicine II
Klinikum Wetzlar-Braunfels
Forsthausstraße 1
35578 Wetzlar
Germany

J. Rubén Rodríguez
Harvard Medical School
Center for Clinical Effectiveness in Surgery
Massachusetts General Hospital
Boston, MA 02115
USA

Hans-Detlev Saeger
University Hospital Carl Gustav Carus
Department of Visceral, Thoracic,
and Vascular Surgery
Technical University of Dresden
01307 Dresden
Germany

Bashar Safar
Indiana University School of Medicine
535 Barnhill Drive
Cancer Pavilion RT 130
Indianapolis, IN 46202
USA

Hiromitsu Saisho
4-23-15, Nishishinjuku
Shinjuku-ku
Tokyo 160-0023
Japan

Juhani Sand
Tampere University Hospital
Box 2000
Department of Surgery
Tampere 33521
Finland

Iwao Sasaki
Tohoku University School of Medicine
Division of Biological Regulation and Oncology
Department of Surgery
1-1 Seiryo-machi
Aoba-ku
Sendai 980-8574
Japan

Richard D. Schulick
Johns Hopkins Medical Institutions
Cameron Division of Surgical Oncology
1650 Orleans Street, Room 442
Baltimore, MD 21231
USA

Michael H. Schoenberg
Chefarzt der Chirurg
Abteilung
Rotkreuz-Krankenhaus
Nymphenburger Straße 165
80634 München
Germany

Giovanni Serio
University of Verona Medical School
Department of Surgery and Gastroenterology
37126 Verona
Italy

Chikashi Shibata
Tohoku University School of Medicine
Division of Biological Regulation and Oncology
Department of Surgery
1-1 Seiryo-machi
Aoba-ku
Sendai 980-8574
Japan

Yasuhiro Shimizu
Department of Gastrointestinal Surgery
Aichi Cancer Center Hospital
Nagoya 464-8681
Japan

Eun Ji Shin
Johns Hopkins University
Division of Gastroenterology and Hepatology
Room 425, 1830 E. Monument Street
Baltimore, MD 21205
USA

Keiko Shiratori
Tokyo Women's Medical University School of Medicine
Department of Medicine and Gastroenterology
8-1, Kawada-cho
Shinjuku-ku
Tokyo 162-8666
Japan

Nib Soehendra
Chir. Universitätsklinik
Klinikum Eppendorf
Martinistraße 52
20251 Hamburg
Germany

Martin Staritz
Division of Gastroenterology/Hepatology
Department of Medicine
Schwarzwald-Baar Klinikum
Villingen-Schwenningen
Innere Medizin – Gastroenterologie
Röntgenstr. 20
78054 Villingen-Schwenningen
Germany

Michael L. Steer
Boston Pancreas Group and Department of Surgery
Tufts-New England Medical Center
860 Washington St
Boston, MA 02111
USA

Makoto Sunamura
Tohoku University, Graduate School of Medicine
Department of Surgery
1-1 Seiryo-machi
Aoba-ku
Sendai 980-8574
Japan

Tadahiro Takada
Teikyo University School of Medicine
Department of Surgery
Kaga 2-11-1
Itabashi-ku
Tokyo, 173-8605
Japan

Kuniyuki Takahashi
Department of Gastrointestinal Surgery
Aichi Cancer Center Hospital
Nagoya 464-8681
Japan

Masao Tanaka
Kyushu University
Department of Surgery and Oncology
Graduate School of Medical Sciences
Fukuoka 812-8582
Japan

Sachiko Tanaka
Department of Cancer Survey
Osaka Medical Center for Cancer and CVD
1–3–3, Nakamichi
Higashinari
Osaka 537-8511
Japan

Jacqueline Y. Tracey
University of California, San Diego
Department of Surgery
200 W. Arbor Drive
San Diego, CA 92103
USA

L. William Traverso
Department of General Surgery
100 Ninth Ave. C6-GSURG
Seattle, WA 98111
USA

Jennifer F. Tseng
University of Massachusetts Medical School
UMass Memorial Medical Center
Worcester, MA 01605
USA

John Tsiaoussis
University Hospital of Crete
Unit of Gastrointestinal Surgery
Department of General Surgery
Heraklion
Greece

Gregory Tsiotos
Department of Surgery
Metropolitan Hospital
18547 Athens
Greece

Michiaki Unno
Tohoku University, Graduate School of Medicine
Division of Hepato-Biliary Pancreatic Surgery
Department of Surgery
1-1 Seiryo-machi Aoba-ku
Sendai, 980-8574
Japan

Gauri R. Varadhachary
The University of Texas M.D. Anderson
Cancer Center
Department of Gastrointestinal Medical Oncology
Unit 426
1515 Holcombe Boulevard
Houston, TX 77030
USA

Andrew L. Warshaw
University of Massachusetts Medical School
Massachusetts General Hospital
Worcester, MA 01605
USA

A. Peter Wysocki
Department of Pancreatico-Biliary Surgery
Glasgow Royal Infirmary
Alexandra Parade
Glasgow G31 2ER
UK

Koji Yamaguchi
Kyushu University
Department of Surgery and Oncology
Graduate School of Medical Sciences
Fukuoka 812-8582
Japan

Kenji Yamao
Department of Gastroenterology
Aichi Cancer Center Hospital
Nagoya 464-8681
Japan

Yohichi Yasunami
Fukuoka University School of Medicine
Department of Surgery
7-45-1 Nanakuma
Jonan-ku
Fukuoka, 814-0180
Japan

Emre Yekebas
Klinik und Poliklinik für Allgemein-, Viszeral- und Thoraxchirurgie
Univ.-Krankenhaus Eppendorf
Martinistraße 52
20246 Hamburg
Germany

Section 1

Anatomy of the Pancreas

Chapter 1 Development of the Pancreas and Response to Disease *3*
D. E. Bockman

Chapter 2 Congenital Anomalies of the Pancreas and the Extrahepatic Bile Ducts *9*
H. Fujii, Y. Matsumoto, K. Sudo

Chapter 3 Surgical Vascular Anatomy and Histology *19*
Y. Mikami, A. Otsuka, M. Unno

D. E. Bockman

Development of the Pancreas and Response to Disease

The pancreas develops from the primitive gut, which is derived from endoderm. An interdependent series of signals is necessary to form the primitive gut prior to the first appearance of buds recognizable as the nascent pancreas. Continued complex interactions of gene products produce growth and differentiation first of the primitive tubules and subsequently of the islet cells, acinar cells, and mature ducts characteristic of the fully formed pancreas.

Essential elements, including blood vessels, lymphatics, and connective tissue, are contributed from the mesoderm-derived mesenchyme surrounding the developing pancreas. An extensive nervous system is produced in the pancreas by the entry of cells and nerve fibers from different parts of the developing general nervous system, derived from the ectodermal germ layer [1–4].

These events usually proceed properly, resulting in a pancreas that provides the necessary hormones and digestive enzymes throughout the life of the individual. On occasion, normal development fails, resulting in functional deficiencies. More often, however, a normal pancreas is produced, with pancreatic disease occurring considerably later. Pain, altered function, and threat to life can result. The changes that occur with pancreatic disease may sometimes be better understood on the background of pancreatic development. Moreover, it is possible that a better understanding of the mechanisms involved in pancreatic development will provide clues leading to a reversal of pancreatic disease. A common finding in pancreatic disease is a reversion of the elements derived from the embryonic endoderm to a more primitive state [5–7]. A significant goal is to learn how to reverse the regressive changes, restoring functional endocrine and exocrine cells in the diseased pancreas [8–10].

Early Development Depends on Interactions Between Major Embryonic Elements

In the early embryo, the notochord intervenes between and interacts directly with the neural tube and the endoderm, the latter representing the primitive gut. The dorsal aorta is paired and lies on either side (Fig. 1.1a). Mesenchyme lies adjacent to these developing elements. The paired dorsal aortae move toward the center and fuse with each other. The single aorta thus produced lies over the primitive gut, in the location previously occupied by the notochord (Fig. 1.1b). The vitelline veins develop within the mesenchyme ventral to the primitive gut. The right vitelline vein persists (Fig. 1.1b). The aorta and the vitelline vein interact directly with the primitive gut, playing an important role in the induction of the pancreatic primordia. The dorsal pancreatic primordium appears at the region of interaction with the aorta, and the ventral pancreatic primordium at the region of interaction with the vitelline vein (Fig. 1.1b).

The endoderm-derived epithelium of the dorsal and ventral pancreatic primordia proliferates and grows into the surrounding mesenchyme as primitive tubules that divide and sometimes reunite with each other (Fig. 1.2a). The primitive pancreatic tubules are initially solid. Lumens subsequently develop within them, eventually forming a continuous pathway from the secretory cells to the duodenum.

The cells making up the walls of the primitive ducts are morphologically similar at first, but with time begin changing into the varied elements of the mature pancreas [11]. Cells that will comprise the endocrine system of the pancreas differentiate from the primitive epithelial ductular cells, migrate into the mesenchyme, and aggregate into groups, producing islets of Langerhans (Fig. 1.2b). Examination of pancreas during fetal development reveals the importance of ductular cell proliferation in humans [12]. Differentiation of acinar cells from the primitive ductular cells in regions initiates the development of acini. Acinar cells remain within the original con-

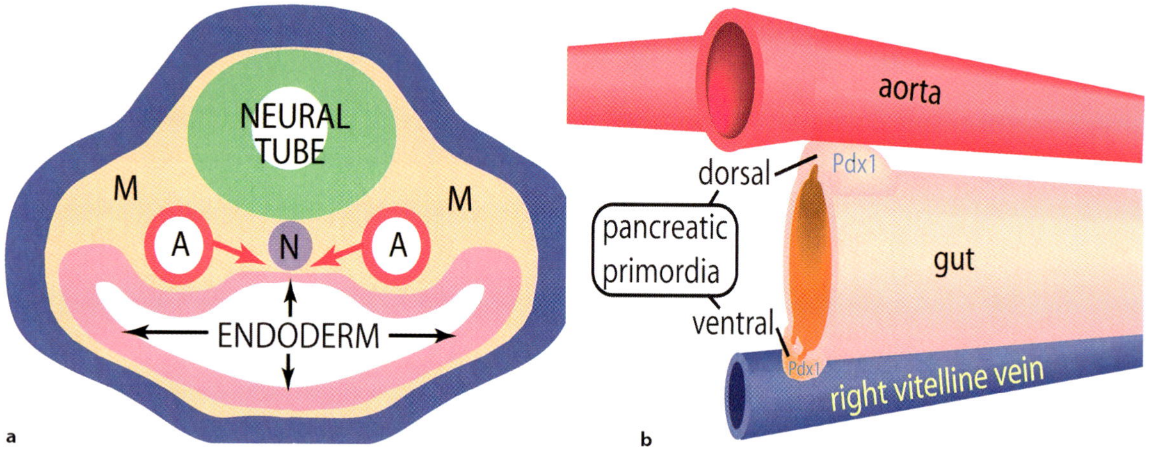

Figure 1.1

Embryonic processes leading to the induction of pancreatic primordia. a Cross section of an embryo showing the interaction between the notochord (*N*) and the neural tube and endoderm. Paired dorsal aortas (*A*) migrate between the notochord and endoderm and fuse. *M* Mesenchyme. b Induction of the pancreatic primordia (taken from Bockman [21]). The epithelial interaction between the aorta and gut produces the dorsal pancreatic bud. The originally paired aorta is single in the region of induction. Only the right vitelline vein is shown. The right vein persists to form the hepatic portal vein. Epithelial interaction between the right vitelline vein and the gut produces the ventral pancreatic primordium. *Pdx1* Homeobox gene Pdx1

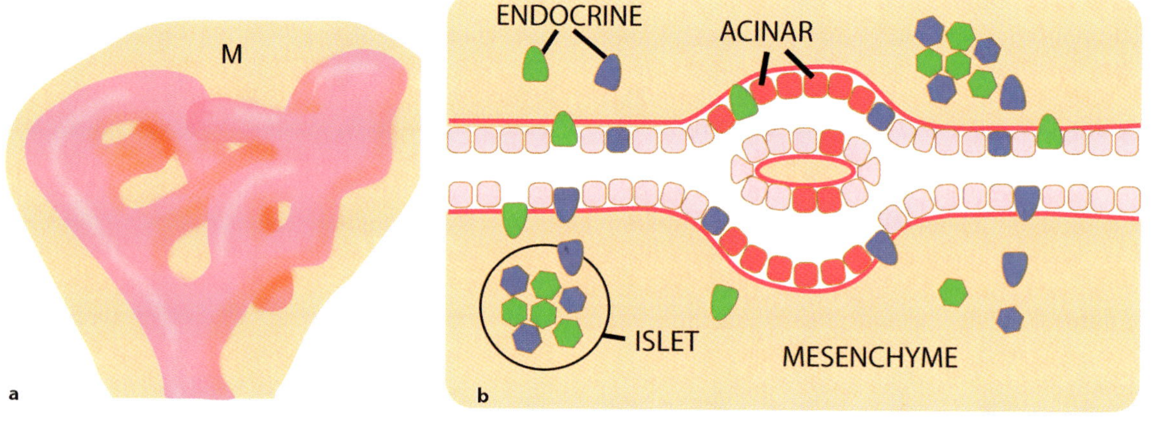

Figure 1.2

Development of pancreatic architecture and differentiation of cell types. a Pancreatic anlagen grow into the mesenchyme (*M*) as primitive tubules. Solid at first, the lumens develop within. The tubules branch, extend, and sometimes fuse with each other. b The cells forming tubules, which are derived from the endoderm, are uniform at first. Primitive ductular cells mature. Acinar cells differentiate from the primitive ductules, remaining in contact with each other, ductular cells, or centroacinar cells. Duct, ductular, and acinar cells are separated from the mesenchyme by a lamina propria (*red*). Other ductular cells differentiate, migrate into the mesenchyme, and assemble to form islets. The mature pancreas develops from these elements

fines of the primitive ductules, separated from the mesenchyme by a lamina propria (Fig. 1.2b). Differentiation of the primitive ductular cells also produces definitive ductular and ductal epithelial cells. Ductular and centroacinar cells maintain the rather nondescript morphology of primitive cells, while ductal cells and associated glands may take on the characteristics of mucous cells.

Precise Genetic Control is Necessary for Normal Pancreatic Development

The notochord, aorta, and mesenchyme all are important in producing the proliferation and differentiation inherent in achieving the fully mature and functional pancreas from small regions of cells in the primitive gut. Gene products causing stimulation and allowing responses among the involved elements are produced at the correct time and location. The products may be transient, and may rely on the presence of other, stimulative or permissive factors.

Many of the genes involved in the process of pancreatic development have been discovered relatively recently, in large as a result of animal experimentation. Nevertheless, it is likely that the same or equivalent key genes are active in human pancreatic development. Several good reviews reveal the extent and complexity of genetic controls necessary for pancreatic development and the markers convenient for assessing progress and interactions [1, 4, 8, 11].

At the time of the interaction between the notochord and the primitive gut, the notochord provides permissive signals to the endoderm [13]. The notochord secretes molecules of the transforming growth factor (TGFβ) family (activin- B) and the fibroblast growth factor (FGF) family (FGF-2). Pancreatic gene expression is activated by repressing Sonic hedgehog in the endoderm [14]. If Sonic hedgehog is not repressed, pancreatic development is inhibited. A bipotential population of precursor cells exists in the region from which the ventral pancreas originates. FGF from cardiac mesoderm induces the expression of Sonic hedgehog, inhibiting development of the pancreas, but allowing liver development [15]. The ventral pancreas develops from cells that are not affected by Sonic hedgehog expression.

A marker for induction of the pancreas is the homeobox gene Pdx1 (Fig. 1.1b). *Pdx1* expression is initiated at the point of contact between the aorta and vitelline vein, and the gut endoderm, and this interaction is necessary for appropriate pancreatic formation [16]. *Pdx1* is required for the outgrowth of gut endoderm and differentiation of the posterior foregut [17].

Mesenchyme, in addition to providing vessels and connective tissue, is essential for proper pancreatic development. Mesenchyme is required for exocrine development and seems to be necessary for the normal balance between exocrine and endocrine elements [18]. Migration of endocrine cells from ductules to form islets involves interaction with elements in the extracellular matrix.

Cells that are induced early to follow the endocrine pathway differentiate into the different definitive types: insulin-secreting β cells, glucagon-producing α cells, somatostatin (δ) cells, and PP cells, which make pancreatic polypeptide. Most of these will migrate from the duct wall to form islets in the mesenchyme. At intervals along the walls of primitive ducts and at their termination, cells proliferate and form primitive acini. Zymogen granules accumulate in the cells. Enzymes are identifiable by their immunocytochemistry. Continued development produces multiple arrangements. Acini become spheroid, elongate, or multilobed. Acinar cells may surround a lumen that follows a continuous, circular pathway. Cells of the primitive ducts show minimal morphological changes as they differentiate into definitive ductules; they are recognized mainly by their lack of zymogen granules, although distinguishing markers become detectable using immunochemical or genetic techniques. Acini that develop at the termination of primitive ducts end up with a ductule at one place, conducting secretions from each acinus. Acini that develop along the course of a primitive duct end up with a ductule that is continuous with it at two places; secretions from upstream will flow into it, secretions are added from that acinus, and the combined secretions flow out the other side. Centroacinar cells, which are differentiated from primitive ducts, are situated within acini and are in contact with acinar cells and/or ductular cells.

The Single Pancreas is Produced From Two Primordia

The precursors of the pancreas appear early in development as protrusions from the primitive gut at a stage when it is simple and quite small (Fig. 1.1b). Although the dorsal and ventral primordia are on opposite sides of the primitive gut, they are in fact very close to each other. In the ventral region, the ventral pancreatic primordium develops along with the primordia of the liver, gallbladder, and associated ducts (Fig. 1.3a). While the dorsal and ventral pancreatic primordia are expanding, the part of the primitive gut that gives rise to them is also growing and changing. The part of the primitive gut that becomes the duodenum grows more on one side than another, and rotates to the right. The result is that the ventral pancreas (primordium) comes to lie adjacent to and immediately posterior to the dorsal pancreas (primordium), and the ducts from the hepatic system and the ventral pancreas join the duodenum close to where

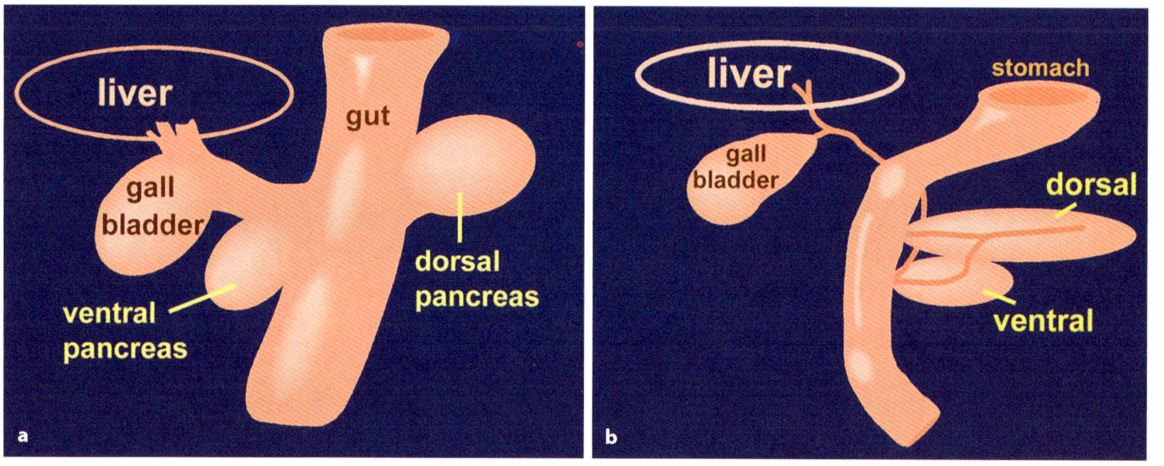

Figure 1.3

Early development of the pancreatic primordia. a The dorsal and ventral primordia grow and begin the differentiation of different cell types. The liver, gall bladder, and bile duct also develop from the ventral primordium. b Diagram of later development of the pancreatic primordia (from Bockman and Freeny [22]). The ventral pancreatic primordium swings around to the same side as the dorsal. The primordia fuse, as do their ducts. The duct from the liver and gall bladder (primitive bile duct) maintains a close association with the duct of the ventral pancreatic primordium

the duct of the dorsal pancreas joins the duodenum. The dorsal pancreas and ventral pancreas fuse. Their ducts anastomose (Fig. 1.3b). The main pancreatic duct is produced from the ventral pancreatic duct plus the distal part of the dorsal pancreatic duct. If the remainder of the dorsal pancreatic duct remains patent, it becomes the accessory pancreatic duct, emptying into the duodenum at the minor papilla. The bile duct empties into the duodenum along with the main pancreatic duct at the major papilla.

Blood Vessels Develop in the Mesenchyme

As development of the endodermally derived pancreatic epithelium continues, mesodermally derived cells in the surrounding mesenchyme differentiate into blood-vessel-forming cells. Fusion of the cells produces cysts and then elongated structures composed at first of a single layer of endothelial cells surrounding a lumen. These primitive vessels join with each other, forming a network that eventually connects with and is supplied from the aorta, as well as with the venous system draining through the hepatic portal vein. Branching and extension from the network produces the arteries, capillaries, and veins that permeate the definitive pancreas. Smooth muscle cells are derived from the mesenchyme to surround the arteries and veins. Connective tissue derived from the same source accumulates around the vessels, in greater amounts around the larger ones. The arteries that arise from the aorta and supply the mature pancreas are branches of the celiac trunk and superior mesenteric artery. It should be noted that the vessels supplying the pancreas do not originate at the duodenum and accompany the pancreatic ducts inward, but supply the organ from its periphery. This is also true for nerves.

Lymphatic vessels arise in a manner similar to that described for blood vessels. They form a network that lies in the extracellular matrix; however, their endothelial cells are not as tightly joined to each other as those of blood vessels, and they do not accumulate a coat as thick as blood vessels. Lymph nodes develop along their path, mainly external to the pancreas. The lymph carried from the pancreas eventually empties into the thoracic duct.

Nerves Connect to the Spinal Cord, Brain, and Enteric Nervous System

The nerve supply of the pancreas develops from the ectoderm and establishes itself through migration of cells as well as by extension of the nerve fibers from cells located well outside the pancreatic domain. Cells migrate from the neural crest (a population of nerve cell precursors that form dorsal to the embryonic spinal cord as its borders unite) into the developing pancreas to form intrinsic ganglia. Nerve fibers from nerve cell bodies in the brain pass through the vagus nerve and synapse on intrinsic ganglia. This combination establishes parasympathetic flow to the pancreas, with fibers extending from intrinsic ganglia to end in the extracellular matrix adjacent to acini, providing a stimulus for secretion.

Another group of neural cell precursors migrate from the neural crest to form ganglia around the celiac trunk. Nerve fibers extend from cell bodies in the intermediolateral column of the spinal cord to synapse on these celiac ganglia. Nerve fibers from the celiac ganglia enter the pancreas around arteries and provide the sympathetic stimulation for the pancreas.

A sensory nerve supply is provided through the vagus nerve by fibers extending from pancreas to nerve cell bodies in the nodose ganglion and from there into the brain. A sensory nerve supply also is provided by nerve fibers extending from pancreas through splanchnic nerves to nerve cell bodies in dorsal root ganglia and from there into the spinal cord.

In the mature normal pancreas, neural regulation of secretion and blood flow proceeds without conscious awareness. Sensation, usually pain, is a consequence of pancreatic disease.

Reorganization of the Pancreas is Associated with Disease

In the absence of disease, once the pancreas has reached its definitive state it will be maintained. So long as its blood supply and control are adequate, secretions are free to enter the duodenum, and there is no inflammation, the endocrine and exocrine divisions of the pancreas will usually function silently and efficiently. Exceptions include genetically induced diseases that involve the inability of cells to function properly. Regardless of initiating causes, known or unknown, changes in the structure and function of the pancreas are accompanied by changes in gene expression. Common changes are inadequately controlled growth of cells and loss by apoptosis or necrosis. An additional type of change is for cells to change to another type, losing normal markers and gaining markers not characteristic of their fully differentiated phenotype, frequently assuming a different morphology. Many of these changes seem to represent reversion to a previous differentiative stage.

As has already been described, primitive tubules or primitive ducts represent an early stage of differentiation of the pancreas, and several cell types stem from them. A common change associated with several pancreatic diseases is the appearance of accumulations of tubules or ductule-like structures. These have been referred to as tubular complexes.

Tubular complexes are found in the pancreas of patients with acute and chronic pancreatitis, pancreatic cancer, and cystic fibrosis. They occur with occlusion of ducts and may be produced experimentally by ligation of the pancreatic ducts. Experimental pancreatic cancer has been shown to originate through tubular complexes [6].

Tubular complexes can originate from acini [5, 19]. Similar tubules can originate from islets of Langerhans under certain conditions. Tubular complexes in the pancreas of diabetes-prone rats possess cells that display the stem cell marker nestin, *Pdx-1*, and mixed duct/endocrine and duct/acinar markers [7]. In both cases, seemingly terminally differentiated cells revert to an earlier differentiative type. In most pancreatic diseases, regressive changes are continuous, and there is little chance for reconstitution of a fully functional organ. A hope for assisting reconstitution lies in acquiring an understanding of the controlling factors that are necessary to initiate and sustain differentiation toward the mature cell type (i.e., acinar cell or endocrine cell).

When the human fetal pancreas was transplanted beneath the renal capsule of immunodeficient mice, a shift in cell types with minimal apoptosis, the presence of intermediate cell types, and an increase in endocrine cells led to the hypothesis that exocrine cells transdifferentiate into duct cells, and these eventually develop into endocrine cells [20]. Jamal et al. [10] have demonstrated a phenotypic switch of human islets to duct-like structures with markers of duct epithelium and progenitor cells; treatment of the duct-like structures with islet neogenesis-associated protein induced their reversion to islet-like structures.

The development of the pancreas from interactions between embryonic structures is quite clear and well documented. The nature of the signaling that initiates and controls these interactions is being revealed through the study of genes and their products as they occur during the developmental process. It is becoming more obvious that one of the changes that occurs with diseases of the pancreas is reversion from the definitive state to a more primitive one. Transdifferentiation of acinar and islet cells to earlier differentiative types is well established. Application of the knowledge of differentiation to the understanding of transdifferentiation may hold the key to learning how to reinitiate the formation of mature pancreatic elements from the products of pancreatic disease.

References

1. Slack JMW (1995) Developmental biology of the pancreas. Development 121:1569–1580
2. Böck P, Abdel-Monheim M, Egerbacher M (1997) Development of the pancreas. Micros Res Tech 37:374–383
3. Bockman DE (1998) Development of the pancreas and related structures. In: Beger HG, Warshaw AL, Büchler MW, Carr-Locke DL, Neoptolemos JP, Russell C, Sarr MG (eds) The Pancreas. Blackwell Science, Oxford, pp 3–10
4. Edlund H (2001) Developmental biology of the pancreas. Diabetes 50, Suppl 1:S5–S9
5. Bockman DE (1995) Toward understanding pancreatic disease: from architecture to cell signaling. Pancreas 11:324–329
6. Bockman DE, Guo J, Büchler P, Müller MW, Bergmann F, Friess H (2003) Origin and development of the precursor lesions in experimental pancreatic cancer in rats. Lab Invest 83:853–859
7. Wang G-S, Rosenberg L, Scott FW (2005) Tubular complexes as a source for islet neogenesis in the pancreas of diabetes-prone BB rats. Lab Invest 85:675–688
8. Murtaugh LC, Melton DA (2003) Genes, signals, and lineages in pancreas development. Ann Rev Cell Dev Biol 19:71–89
9. Tokoro T, Tezel E, Nagasaka T, Kaneko T, Nakao A (2003) Differentiation of acinar cells into acinoductular cells in regenerating rat pancreas. Pancreatology 3:487–496
10. Jamal A-M, Lipsett M, Sladek R, Laganiere S, Hanley S, Rosenberg L (2005) Morphogenetic plasticity of adult human pancreatic islets of Langerhans. Cell Death 12:702–712
11. Kim SK, Hebrok M (2001) Intercellular signals regulating pancreas development and function. Genes Dev 15:111–127
12. Bouwens L, Lu WG, De Krijger R (1997) Proliferation and differentiation in the human fetal endocrine pancreas. Diabetologia 40:398–404
13. Kim SK, Hebrok M, Melton DA (1997) Notochord to endoderm signaling is required for pancreas development. Development 124:4243–4252
14. Hebrok M, Kim SK, Melton DA (1998) Notochord repression of endodermal Sonic hedgehog permits pancreas development. Genes Dev 12:1705–1713
15. Deutsch G, Jung J, Zheng M, Lora J, Zaret KS (2001) A bipotential precursor population for pancreas and liver within the embryonic endoderm. Development 128:871–881
16. Lammert E, Cleaver O, Melton D (2001) Induction of pancreatic differentiation by signals from blood vessels. Science 294:564–567
17. Offield MF, Jetton TL, Labosky PA, Ray M, Stein RW, Magnuson MA, Hogan BLM, Wright CVE (1996) PDX-1 is required for pancreatic outgrowth and differentiation of the rostral duodenum. Development 122:983–985
18. Gittes GK, Galante PE, Hanahan D, Rutter WJ, Debas HT (1996) Lineage-specific morphogenesis in the developing pancreas: role of mesenchymal factors. Development 122:439–447
19. Bockman DE, Merlino G (1992) Cytological changes in the pancreas of transgenic mice overexpressing transforming growth factor alpha. Gastroenterology 103:1883–1892
20. Si Z, Tuch BE, Walsh DA (2001) Development of human fetal pancreas after transplantation into SCID mice. Cells Tissues Organs 168:147–157
21. Bockman DE (2007) Anatomy, physiology, and embryology of the pancreas. In: Yeo CJ (ed) Shackelford's Surgery of the Alimentary Tract. WB Saunders, Philadelphia pp 1287–1295
22. Bockman DE, Freeny PC (1992) Anatomy and anomalies of the biliary tree. Laparosc Surg 1:92–104

Chapter 2

H. Fujii · Y. Matsumoto · K. Suda

Congenital Anomalies of the Pancreas and the Extrahepatic Bile Ducts

Pancreaticobiliary maljunction (PBM) is frequently associated with congenital choledochal cyst, but differs with regard to its embryonic cause and clinical features. It is thought to develop as a misarrangement of the embryonic connections in the pancreaticobiliary ductal system, with the terminal bile duct joined to one of the ducts of the ventral pancreas. The clinical aspects of these anomalies of the pancreaticobiliary ductal system are intermittent abdominal pain, relapsing acute pancreatitis, jaundice, cholangitis, and gallbladder cancer. Coexistence of pancreas divisum complicates a diagnosis of pancreaticobiliary maljunction, so it is very important to understand the diagnostic criteria of pancreas divisum for correct diagnosis of pancreaticobiliary maljunction. Surgical treatment for congenital choledochal cyst with relative stricture in the upper portion of the biliary tract should be performed with care to avoid postoperative cholangitis.

Pancreaticobiliary Maljunction

Definition

PBM is a congenital anomaly in which the junction of the pancreatic duct and biliary duct is located outside the duodenal wall (Fig. 2.1a); in the normal pancreaticobiliary junction, the main pancreatic duct (MPD,

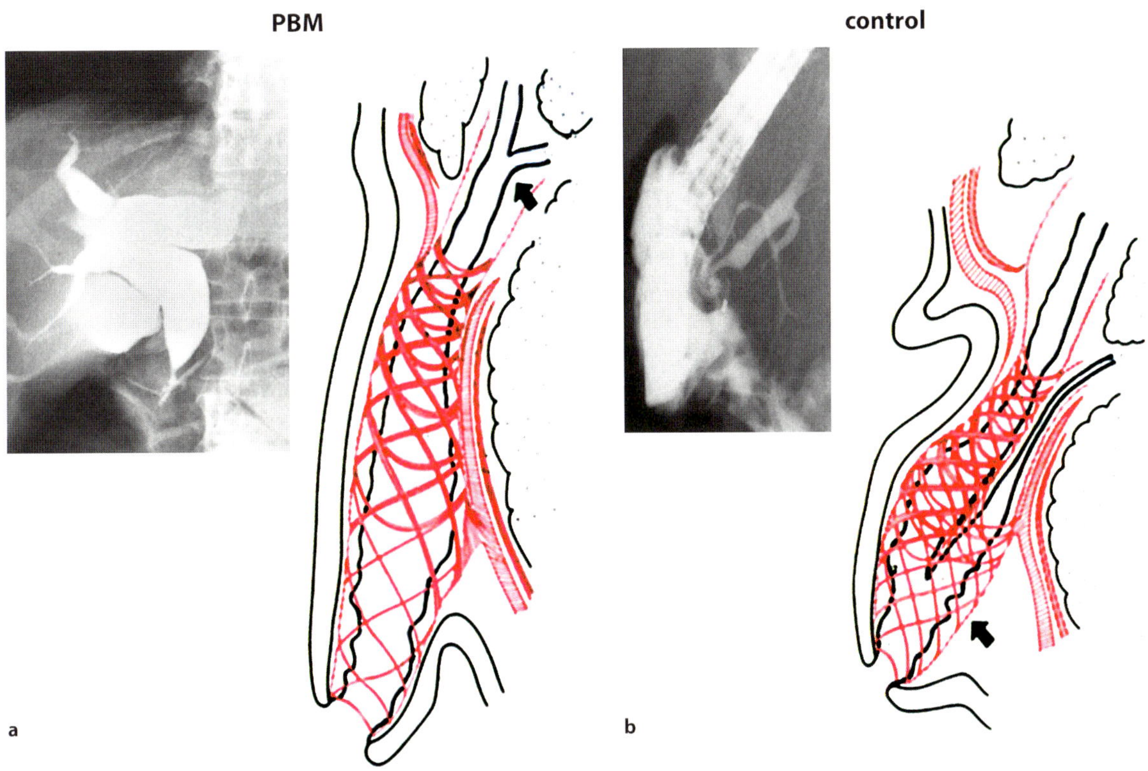

Figure 2.1

b Diagram showing the sphincter muscle at the end of the common bile duct and the main pancreatic duct in controls, and a in patients with pancreaticobiliary maljunction (PBM)

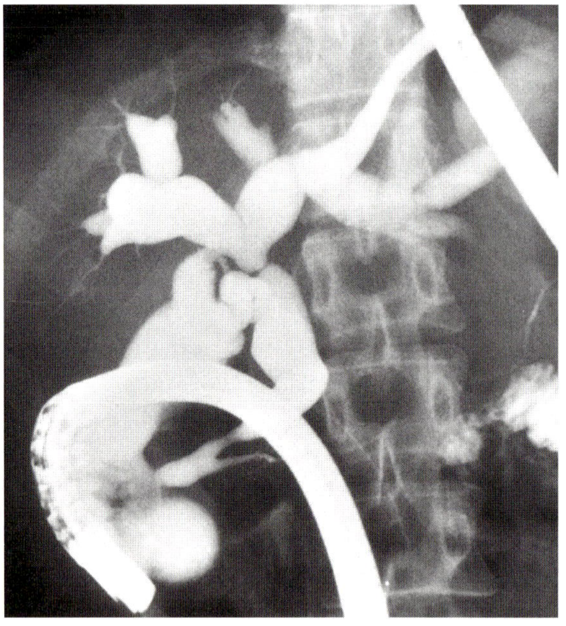

Figure 2.2

PBM is almost always seen in patients with congenital choledochal cyst or congenital biliary dilatation

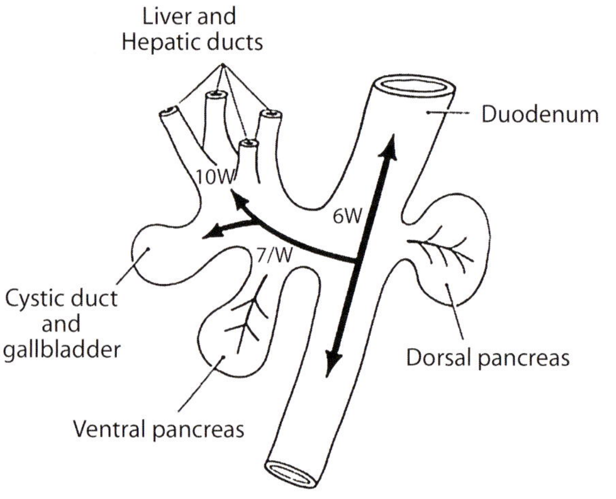

Figure 2.3

The process of normal development of hepatobiliary system and pancreas

Wirsung's duct) joins with the common bile duct (CBD) inside the muscle layer of the duodenum to form the ampulla of Vater (Fig. 2.1b). PBM is almost always seen in patients with congenital choledochal cyst or congenital biliary dilatation (Fig. 2.2). However, it may occur independently of any other developmental anomaly in the CBD.

Embryology of the Hepatobiliary System and Pancreas in Normal Human Development

Akin [1] described the process of normal development of the hepatobiliary system and pancreas (Fig. 2.3). The extrahepatic bile duct system and the ventral anlage (primordium) of the pancreas arise from the hepatic diverticulum, which is first visible on the ventral surface of the anterior intestinal portal of the embryo early in the 4th week of gestation. By late in the 4th week, the ventral anlage of the pancreas arises from the base of the hepatic diverticulum itself, and the dorsal anlage of the pancreas arises directly from the dorsal side of the duodenum almost opposite the liver primordium. By the beginning of the 5th week, the pancreatic duct, as well as the gallbladder, cystic duct, and CBD, are demarcated, and during the 5th week, the proximal portion of the hepatic diverticulum elongates but does not increase greatly in diameter, in contrast to the tremendous growth of the distal end. During this stage, the future CBD system is in an incomplete or solid cord state. By the 6th week, the ventral primordium has been carried away from the duodenum by elongation of the proximal part of the diverticulum. During the 7th week, duodenal torsion brings the two pancreatic primordia side by side, and the smaller, ventral primordium fuses with the proximal part of the dorsal pancreas. No solid stage seems to occur in the pancreatic ducts. Reestablishment of the lumen of the hepatic diverticulum commences with the CBD in the 6th week of gestation, and progress slowly to the distal portion; the lumen extends into the cystic duct by the 7th week. During the 8th week, the proximal portion of the diverticulum is usually absorbed into the intestinal wall, so that the CBD and the pancreatic duct enter the duodenum side by side. That is, the point of junction of the pancreatic duct and CBD recede to the level of the submucosa from the common bile duct orifice, with the elongation of the papilla of Vater, and with increasing thickness of the duodenal wall. The muscle fibers of the sphincter of Oddi are derived directly from the mesenchyme around the CBD during the 11th week of gestation. In short, during the normal course of development of the hepatobiliary system and the pancreas, the MPD joins to the CBD to form a "common channel" (the ampulla of Vater), and the common channel moves inside the muscle layer of the duodenum after the 12th week of gestation.

PBM Hypothesis

Alons-Lej et al. [2] and Yotuyanagi [3] described the narrowed duct segment distal to the biliary cyst as a "narrow part of the terminal bile duct" (Fig. 2.4a). Babbitt [4] described it as a long common channel that was thought to arrest the normal inward migration of the choledochopancreatic junction [5] (Fig. 2.4b), similar to the occurrence of congenital biliary atresia.

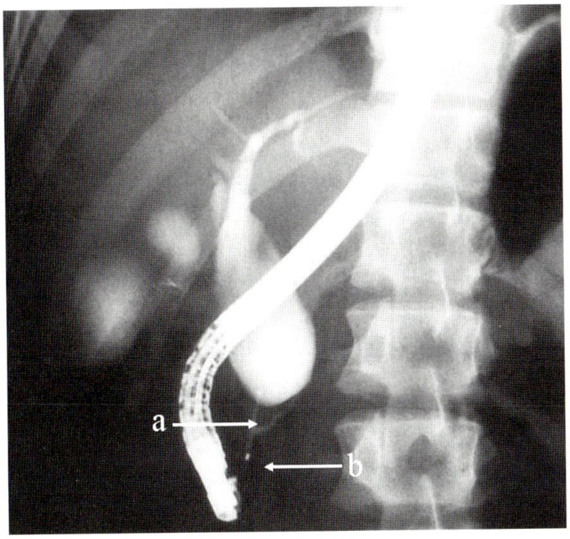

Figure 2.4

Narrow part of the terminal bile duct (a) and a long common channel (b)

We clarified that the long common channel actually represents Wirsung's duct system [6], based on a radiological and anatomical analysis of patients with PBM. Figure 2.5 shows small radicles that were thought to be branches of the pancreatic duct arising from the so-called long common channel. Figure 2.6 shows a huge choledochal cyst in a surgical specimen associated with gall bladder carcinoma that invades the duodenum; the junction of the MPD and the CBD was situated external to the muscle layer of the duodenum, a condition that is referred to as PBM, thus forming an extended common channel. Also in this case, the minute orifice was found macroscopically in the narrowed duct segment (Fig. 2.6) and was identified microscopically as a small duct from the pancreatic parenchyma; these small pancreatic ducts were derived from the ventral pancreas, based on the distribution of islets with pancreatic-polypeptide-positive (PP) cells (PP islets) [7].

In conclusion, both the long common channel and narrowed duct segment originate from pancreatic duct. Anatomical and radiological analyses of the junction of the pancreatic duct with the bile duct show that there are variations in the location of the union of the terminal bile duct with ventral pancreatic duct system, as shown in Fig. 2.7 [8].

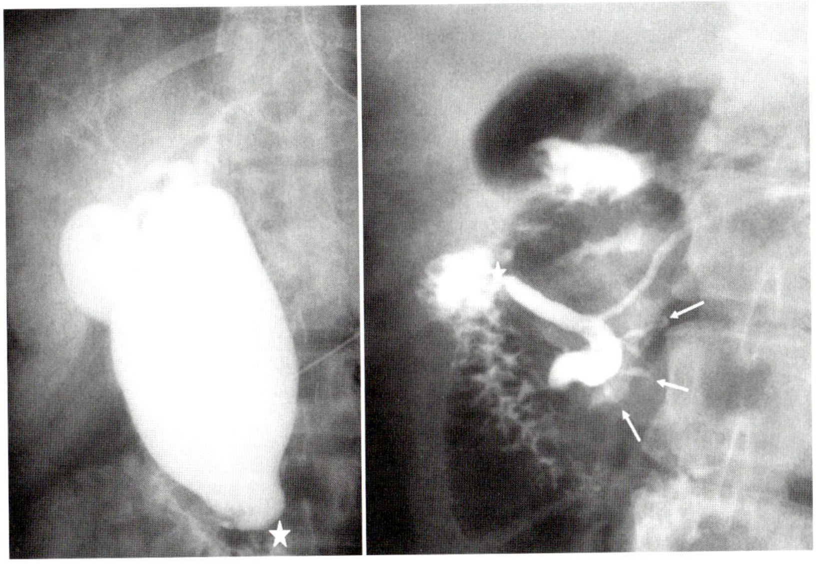

Figure 2.5

Small radicles that were thought to be branches of the pancreatic duct arise from so-called long common channels (*arrows*)

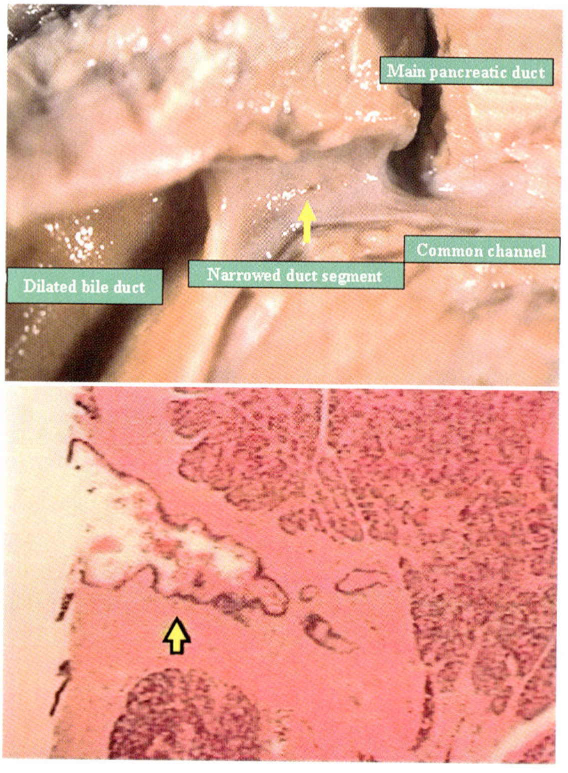

Figure 2.6

The junction of the main pancreatic duct and the common bile duct, in this case is situated external to the muscle layer of the duodenum and minute orifice, and can be found macroscopically in the narrowed duct segment and identified microscopically as a small duct from the pancreatic parenchyma

Carcinogenesis in PBM

The number of reports of biliary malignancies with PBM has recently increased. Among the 130 cases of gallbladder cancer seen in our institute in the past 20 years, 55 had concomitant PBM; the incidence is thought to be extremely high (Table 2.1). Many studies of biliary carcinogenesis in PBM have been reported, such as an assessment of the cell proliferative activity [9] and various oncogenes and tumor-suppressor genes in the epithelium of the biliary ductal system in PBM patients [10]. Kato and Mizuno [11] reported that the mixing of pancreatic juice and bile in PBM resulted in the production of various harmful substances in the biliary tract, such as activated pancreatic enzymes, lysolecitin, and some mutagens, of which mutagens in particular were thought to be involved in the development of biliary tract cancer. They identified mutagenic substances in the mixture of bile and pancreatic juice, and estimated that the substances had a molecular weight of 1500–3500 (as assessed by gel chromatography) and were complexes of low-molecular-weight stable substances containing amino acids and peptides (as assessed by gas chromatography and mass spectrometry). Accordingly, the mixture of bile and pancreatic juice due to reciprocal reflux in PBM very likely plays an important role in biliary carcinogenesis.

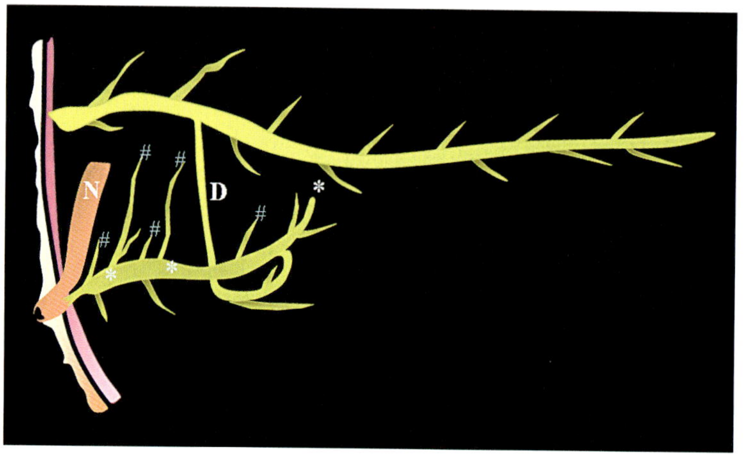

Figure 2.7

There are variations in the location of the union of the terminal bile duct with the ventral pancreatic duct system

Table 2.1. Clinical review of 250 patients with pancreaticobiliary maljunction. CCDB Congenital cystic dilatation of the common bile duct, *GB* gallbladder, *CB* common bile duct, *IHB* intrahepatic bile duct, *GBX* carcinoma of gallbladder, *CBX* carcinoma of common bile duct, *IHBX* carcinoma of intrahepatic bile duct

	Without CCDB		With CCDB			
			Infant-type cyst		Adult-type cyst	
	Men (*n*=29)	Women (*n*=64)	Men (*n*=3)	Women (*n*=9)	Men (*n*=47)	Women (*n*=98)
None (*n*=56)	8	16	3	5	11	13
Stones						
GB (*n*=44)	9	25	0	0	3	7
CB (*n*=52)	0	0	0	2	17	33
IHB (*n* =17)	0	0	0	0	5	12
Cancer						
GBX (*n* =55)	9	22	0	1	5	18
CBX (*n* =14)	3	1	0	1	2	7
IHBX (*n* =12)	0	0	0	0	4	8

Mechanism of Pancreatic Juice Reflux into the Biliary Tract in PBM

The reason why PBM is abnormal may possibly be explained more clearly by the reconstruction study of Suda et al. [12], as shown in Fig. 2.1. In the controls, the CBD and the MPD penetrate the muscle layer of the duodenum obliquely and parallel to each other, and form a junction in the submucosal layer just before opening into the duodenum. The angle of the ductal junction is therefore very sharp. The sphincter of Oddi, which surrounds both ducts and the common channel, normally consists of three sections: the sphincter choledochus, the sphincter pancreaticus, and the sphincter ampullae [13]. Of these, the sphincter muscle at the distal end of the choledochus (sphincter choledochus) is the best-developed. It regulates the outflow of bile and prevents free communication between the bile and pancreatic ducts.

In the case of PBM, however, the junction of the ducts is situated external to the muscle layer of the duodenum, thus forming an extension to the muscularis propria of the duodenum, thus forming an extended common channel [14]. The angle of the ductal junction is less sharp in these patients than in control cases. The well-developed sphincter muscle is situated in the submucosal layer, as in controls, but it mainly surrounds the common channel (sphincter ampullae); the sphincter choledochus is extremely hypoplastic. The anatomical findings suggest the possibility of the communication between the ducts in cases of PBM. As the intraductal pressure of the pancreatic duct is normally higher than that of the bile duct [15], reflux of pancreatic juice may occur into the bile duct and could lead to nonsuppurative chronic inflammation of the bile duct.

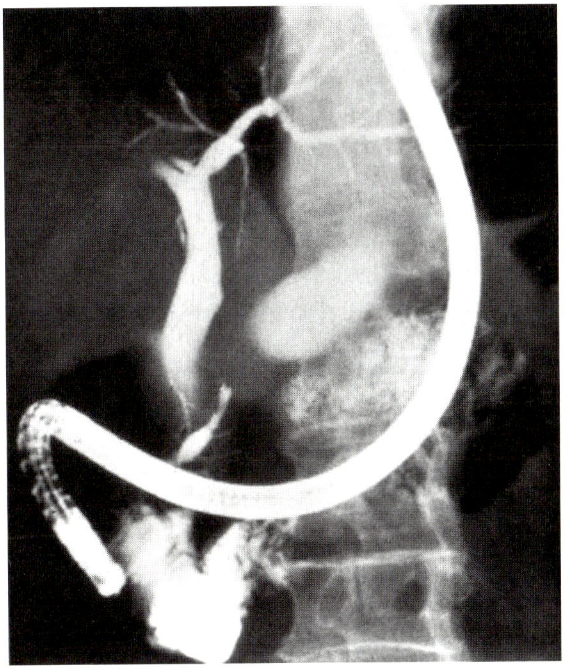

Figure 2.8

A case of isolated dorsal pancreatitis associated with pancreas divisum, the branch fusion seemed to be composed of an inferior branch of the ventral pancreatic duct and an inferior branch of the dorsal pancreatic duct

Pancreas Divisum

Definition

In the pancreas divisum, the parenchyma of the ventral pancreas and the dorsal pancreas are separated as a double pancreas. Recently, however, the term pancreas divisum has been used widely to describe two ductal systems, the ventral pancreatic duct and the dorsal pancreatic duct, which do not unite or communicate and separately drain to the two duodenal papillae [16]. In this condition, pancreatic juice from the dominant dorsal moiety flows out only through the minor papilla, in which the outlet is notably small in most cases. This raises the question of whether this variation plays a role in the development of pancreatic pain or pancreatitis. The clinical relevance of pancreas divisum has been argued repeatedly [16]. Figure 2.8 shows an example of isolated dorsal pancreatitis associated with pancreas divisum. This condition strongly suggests inadequate drainage from the minor papilla.

Branch Duct Fusion of the Ventral and Dorsal Pancreatic Ducts

A case of fusion via two so-called inferior branches between the ventral pancreatic duct and dorsal pancreatic duct was studied based on the organogenesis of the pancreas [17], as shown in Fig. 2.8. Radiologically, branch fusion seems to be composed of an inferior branch of the ventral pancreatic duct and an inferior branch of the dorsal pancreatic duct. By mapping the locations of PP islets in material obtained by pancreaticodudenectomy, however, the branch was identified as a branch of the dorsal pancreatic duct. Thus fusion between two inferior branches was not established, but was found to consist of an inferior branch of the dorsal pancreatic duct connected with the ventral pancreatic duct.

Identification of the Originating Primordium of the Pancreas

Fusion of the "ventral" and "dorsal" pancreata can be distinguished [18] according to the distribution of PP islets [19], selectively in the ventral pancreas. In some cases both pancreata can be identified macroscopically. There are two further distinct characteristic differences. One is the shape of the islets; those in the ventral pancreas, which include abundant PP cells, are irregular, in contrast to the neatly round or oval-shaped islets found in the dorsal pancreas (Fig. 2.9). The other is the distribution of fatty infiltration in the pancreas. There is more fat in the dorsal pancreas than in the ventral pancreas [18]. The ventral primordium forms the posterior part of the head of the pancreas, completely or partially surrounding the CBD and the uncinate process. However, the dorsal bud forms the remaining ventral parts of the head, the isthmus, the body, and the tail of the pancreas. The fusion line between both pancreata has no defined border, but it is the so-called "locus minoris resistantiae" and it is the easiest "pathway" for a duodenal diverticulum to penetrate the pancreas.

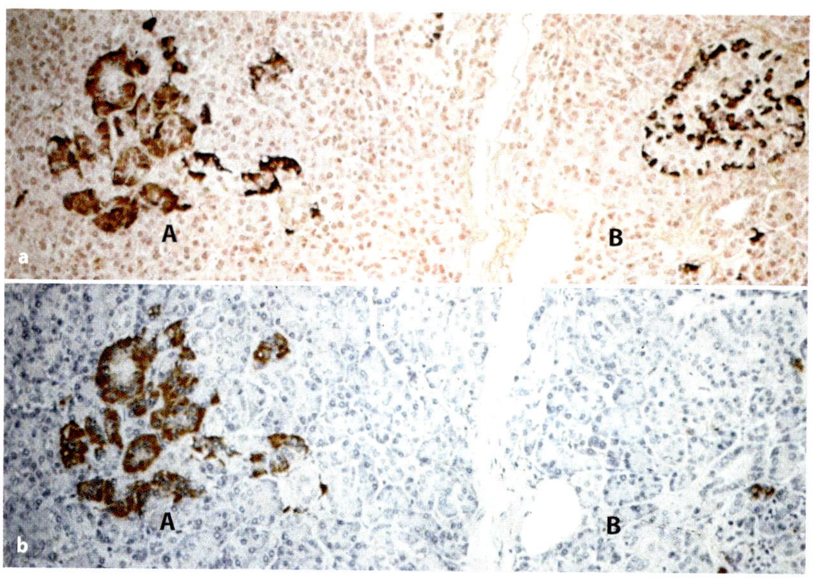

Figure 2.9

a Grimerius staining. a Irregular-shaped islet in the ventral pancreas. b Round-shaped islet in the dorsal pancreas. b Immunohistochemical staining for pancreatic polypeptide. a Islet of the ventral pancreas contains many pancreatic-polypeptide-positive (PP) cells. b Islet of the dorsal pancreas containing only a few PP cells

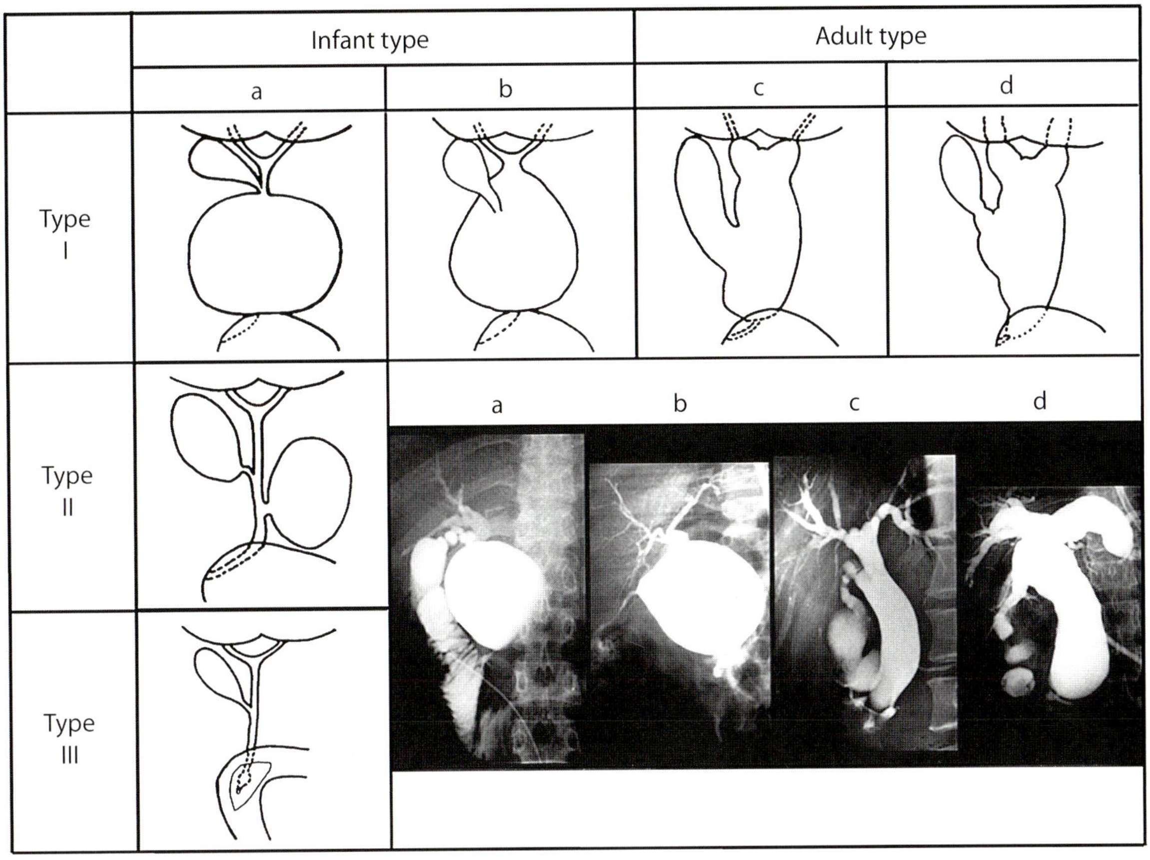

Figure 2.10

Classification of congenital cystic dilatation of the common bile duct

Congenital Cystic Dilatation of the CBD

Definition and Classification

Congenital cystic dilatation of the CBD (CCDB) has been classified into three types by Alonso-Lej et al. [2]: type I, congenital cystic dilatation of the CBD; type II, congenital diverticulum of the CBD; type III, congenital choledochocele. In addition, it was proposed that the criteria for the diagnosis of CCDB should be: (1) the intrahepatic tree is usually normal, (2) the biliary tree above the cystic dilatation of the CBD is somewhat dilated secondary to the obstructive factor in the distal choledochus, (3) the cystic dilatation of the CBD proper begins and ends sharply, and (4) the terminal CBD is frequently narrowed. However, recent advances in diagnostic techniques for biliary disease disclosed that there were many cases of choledochal cyst that dilated into the intrahepatic bile duct. We thus classified CCDB into two subtypes: "infant type" and "adult type," based on the anatomic location and clinical features [20]. Infant-type cysts are typically large cysts of the choledochus and occur most commonly in infancy and childhood. Adult-type cysts are fusiform dilatations of the biliary tract, and occur most commonly in adults (Fig. 2.10). Gallstones were seen in most of the patients with adult-type cysts.

Relative Stricture in the Upper Portion of the Biliary Tract

Definition and Classification

Stricture in the upper portion of the biliary tract is a localized reduction in the caliber of the bile duct proximal to the common hepatic duct. When biliary dilatation is present in a bile duct that continues to the strictured lesion, the caliber of the strictured portion can become larger than that of the normal bile duct; such strictures are called relative strictures.

The location of the biliary strictures is observed at the following six sites in the upper portion of the bili-

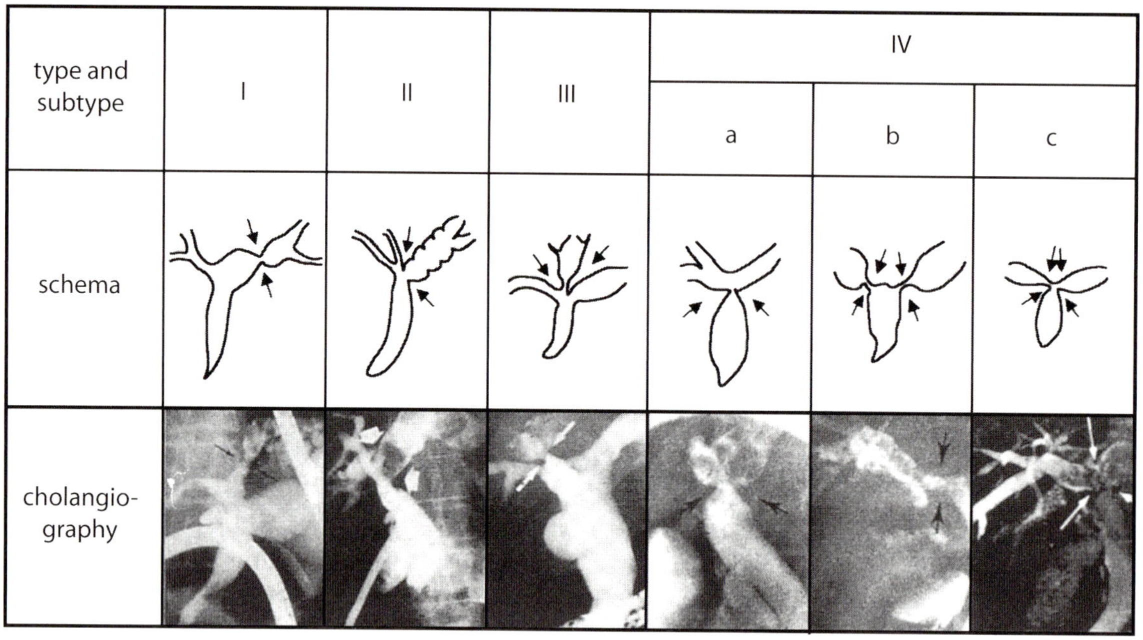

Figure 2.11

Classification of relative biliary strictures based on the anatomical location of the stricture

ary tract, and they are classified into four groups according to the anatomical location of the stricture (Fig. 2.11) [21].

1. Type I: the site of stricture is the region where the left hepatic duct enters the intrahepatic portion in the lateral segment of the liver. This type of stricture occurs with the highest frequency and is associated with intra- and extrahepatic bile duct dilatation.
2. Type II: this type of stricture is present at the root of the left hepatic duct. The liver parenchyma extends to the strictured lesion, and the entire left hepatic duct including the strictured lesion is within the liver.
3. Type III: this type of stricture is present at the region where the intrahepatic bile ducts in the anterior segment or the superior area of the anterior segment of the right hepatic lobe join the right hepatic duct. They are located immediately beneath the hepatic capsule where the bile duct enters the hepatic parenchyma. Both intra- and extrahepatic bile duct dilatations are observed in this stricture type.
4. Type IV-a: this stricture is present at the upper portion of the common hepatic duct, and dilatations in the common hepatic duct and the hepatic duct proximal to the stricture are also present.
5. Type IV-b: this stricture is present in the bilateral hepatic ducts.
6. Type IV-c: this type of stricture is located at the region encompassing the upper portion of the common hepatic duct and the confluence of the bilateral hepatic ducts.

References

1. Akin JT (1972) The liver. Anomalies of extrahepatic biliary ducts and the gall bladder. In: Gray SW, Skandalakis JE (eds) Embryology for Surgeons. W.B. Saunders, Philadelphia, London, Toronto, pp 217–262
2. Alonso-Lej F, Rever WB, Pessagno DJ (1959) Congenital choledochal cyst with a report of two and analysis of 94 cases. Intern Abstr Surg 108:1–23
3. Yotuyanagi S (1936) Contribution to aetiology and pathology of idiopathic cystic dilatation of common bile duct with report of three cases.: new aetiologic theory. Gann 30:601–650
4. Babbitt DP (1969) Congenital choledochal cyst: new etiological concept based on anomalous relationships of common bile duct and pancreatic bulb. Ann Radiol 12:231–241
5. Arey LB (1974) Developmental Anatomy: a Textbook and Laboratory Manual of Embryology, 7th edn. Saunders, Philadelphia, pp 255–262
6. Matsumoto Y, Fujii H, Itakura J, et al (2001) Pancreaticobiliary maljunction: etiologic concepts based on radiologic aspects. Gastrointest Endosc 53:614–619
7. Suda K, Matsumoto Y, Miyano T (1991) Narrowed duct segment distal to choledochal cyst. Am J Gastroenterol 86:1259–1263

8. Matsumoto Y, Fujii H, Itakura J (2002) Recent advances in pancreaticobiliary maljunction. J Hepatobiliary Pancreat Surg 9:45–54
9. Fujii H, Yang Y, Tang R, et al (1999) Epithelial cell proliferation activity of the biliary ductal system with congenital biliary maljunction. J Hepatobiliary Pancreat Surg 6:294–302
10. Hanada K, Iyoh M, Fujii K, et al (1996) K-ras and P453 mutations in stage I gall bladder carcinoma with anomalous junction of the pancreaticobiliary duct. Cancer 77:1752–1757
11. Kato T, Mizuno M (2002) Investigation of mutagenic substance in the biliary contents of patients with pancreaticobiliary maljunction. In: Koyanagi Y, Aoki T (eds) Pancreaticobiliary Maljunction. Igaku Tosyo, Tokyo, pp 93–101
12. Suda k, Miyano T, Hashimoto K (1980) The choledocho-pancreatico-ductal junction in infantile obstructive jaundice disease. Acta Pathol Jpn 30:187–194
13. Boyden EA (1996) The anatomy of the choledocho-duodenal junction in man. Surg Gynecol Obst 104:641–652
14. Frierson HF Jr (1989) The gross anatomy and histology of the gallbladder, extrahepatic bile ducts, Vaterian system, and minor papilla. Am J Surg Pathol 13:146–162
15. Parry EW, Hallenbeck GA, Grindlay JH (1955) Pressure in the pancreatic and common ducts: values during fasting, after various meals and after sphincterotomy; and experimental study. Arch Surg 70:757–765
16. Cotton PB (1980) Congenital anomaly of pancreas divisum as cause of obstructive pain and pancreatitis. Gut 21:105–114
17. Suda K, Mogaki M, Matsumoto Y, et al (1991) Gross dissection and immunohistochemical studies on branch fusion type of ventral and dorsal pancreatic ducts; a case report. Surg Radiol Anat 13:333–337
18. Suda K, Mizuguchi K, Hoshino A, et al (1981) Differences of the ventral and dorsal anlagen of pancreas after fusion. Acta Pathol Jpn 31:583–589
19. Kloppel G, Lenzen S (1984) Anatomy and physiology of the endocrine pancreas; in Kloppel G, Heitz PU (eds) Pancreatic Pathology. London, Churchill Livingstone, pp 133–153
20. Matsumoto Y, Uchida K, Nakase A, et al (1977) Clinicopathological classification of congenital cystic dilatation of the common bile duct. Am J Surg 134:569–574
21. Matsumoto Y, Fujii H, Yoshioka M, et al (1985) Biliary strictures as a cause of primary intrahepatic bile duct stones. World J Surg 10:867–875

Chapter 3

Y. Mikami · A. Otsuka · M. Unno

Surgical Vascular Anatomy and Histology

Gross anatomy

Arterial Anatomy

The pancreas receives its blood supply from branches of the celiac artery (CEA) and the superior mesenteric artery (SMA; Fig. 3.1) [1,2]. The gastroduodenal artery (GDA) generally departs from the common hepatic artery (CHA) and first gives off the posterior superior pancreaticoduodenal artery (PSPDA) near the upper border of the pancreas (Fig. 3.2). The GDA then gives off the right gastroepiploic artery (rGEA) and turns into the anterior posterior pancreaticoduodenal artery (ASPDA). The ASPDA descends on the anterior surface of the head of the pancreas to join the anterior posterior pancreaticoduodenal artery (AIPDA). The PSPDA runs in front of the common bile duct from left to right and descends on along the right side of the common bile duct on the posterior aspect of the pancreas. The PSPDA then runs behind the common bile duct from right to left to join the posterior inferior pancreaticoduodenal artery (PIPDA). The superior and inferior pancreaticoduodenal arteries (ASPDA, PSPDA, AIPDA, and PIPDA) form the anterior and posterior arterial arcades in the head of the pancreas. The ASPDA and PSPDA are consistent in origin, while the AIPDA and PIPDA arise separately or have a common trunk as the inferior pancreatoduodenal artery (IPDA) from the SMA. The IPDA also has variations, arising independently from the right side of the SMA or having a common artery composed of the IPDA and the first jejunal artery (J1A), which arises from the left side of the SMA. After branching off the J1A, the IPDA runs behind the SMA toward the right side and divides into the AIPDA and the PIPDA. These variations in the IPDA have been described in detail by Murakami and coworkers (Fig. 3.3) [3]. The IPDA was found in 80% of 125 autopsy subjects, a common artery composed of the IPDA and the J1A in 56%, and the IPDA arose in-

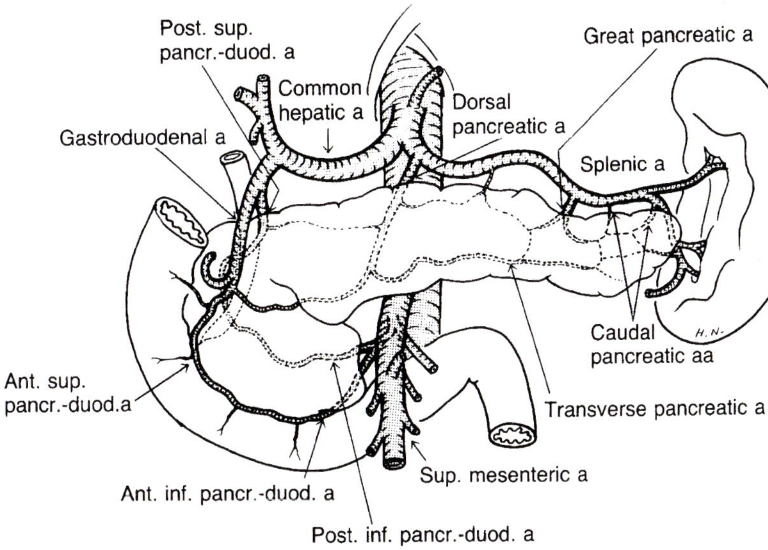

Figurge 3.1

Pancreatic arterial anatomy (with permission [6]). *a* Artery, *ant* anterior, *sup* superior, *post* posterior, *inf* inferior, *pancr.-duod a* pancreatoduodenal artery

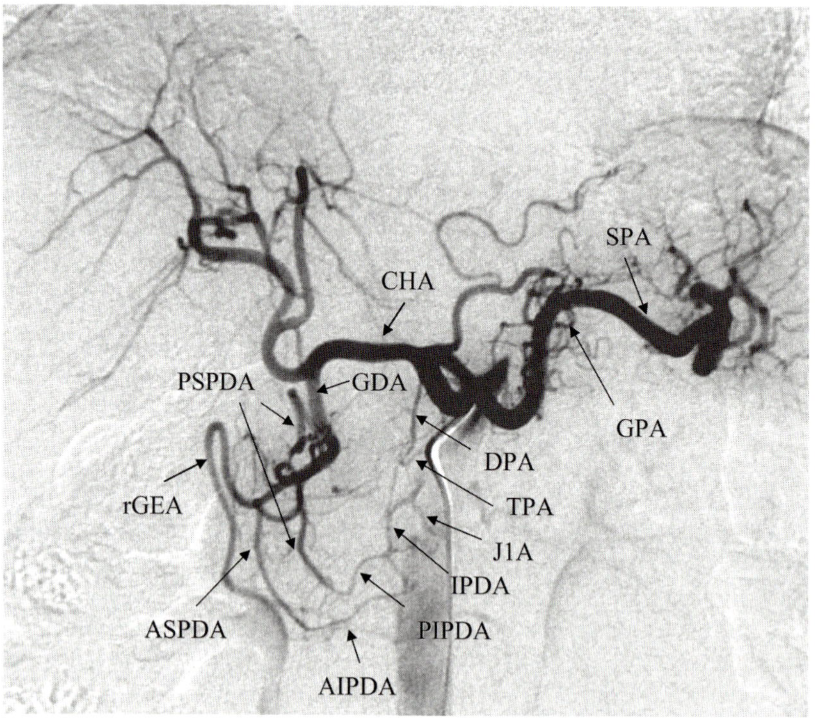

Figurge 3.2

Selective celiac arteriogram (with permission [2]). *SPA* splenic artery, *GDA* gastroduodenal artery, *CHA* common hepatic artery, *PSPDA* posterior superior pancreaticoduodenal artery, *rGEA* right gastroepiploic artery, *ASPDA* anterior posterior pancreaticoduodenal artery, *AIPDA* anterior posterior pancreaticoduodenal artery, *PIPDA* posterior inferior pancreaticoduodenal artery, *IPDA* inferior pancreatoduodenal artery, *J1A* first jejunal artery, *DPA* dorsal pancreatic artery, *TPA* transverse pancreatic artery, *GPA* great pancreatic artery

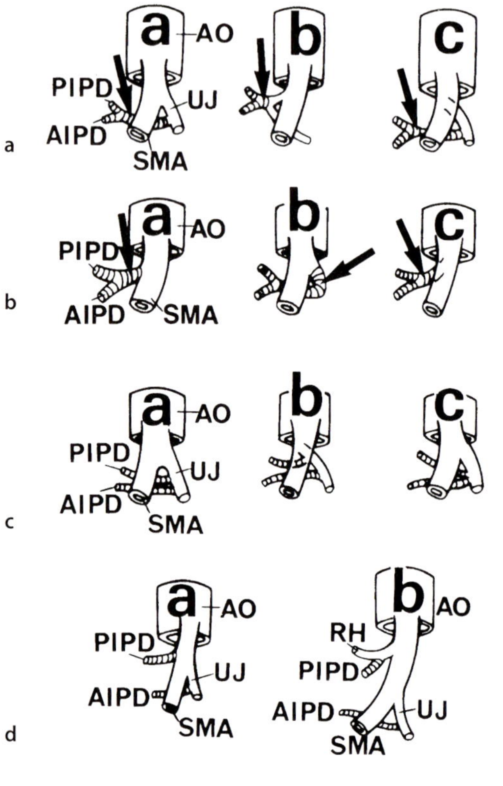

Figurge 3.3

Variations in the topographical relationships of the origin of the inferior pancreaticoduodenal arteries (with permission [3]). Anterior aspects. Four types (a, b, c, and d) and 11 subtypes (a, b, and c) were classified in 125 specimens examined. Every incidence described below was estimated in the total specimens. Type A (55.6%) has the inferior pancreaticoduodenal artery (*IPD, arrow*) arising from (and forms a common trunk with) the upper jejunal artery (*UJ*). Subtypes a (48.4%), b (6.4%), and c (0.8%) (a + b + c = A) of type A represent differences in the topographical relationships of arteries. Type B (24.2%) is a typical pattern seen in many textbooks, in which the IPD arises directly from the superior mesenteric artery (*SMA*). This type is also divided into three subtypes; a (17.8%), b (4.8%), and c (1.6%) (a + b + c = B). The AIPDA and PIPDA originate from the SMA independently in type C (3.3%) and its subtypes a (1.6%), b (0.9%), and c (0.8%) (a + b+ c = C). Type D (16.9%) consists of other patterns. In type D a (11.3%), the SMA issues the PIPDA, whereas the AIPDA arises from (and forms a common trunk with) the UJ. In type D b (5.6%), the PIPDA issues from the right (accessory) hepatic artery (*RH*) arising from the SMA. This type of RH was seen in 12.7% of the specimens examined; 44.1% of an specimens with an RH showed the type D *AO*, Aorta

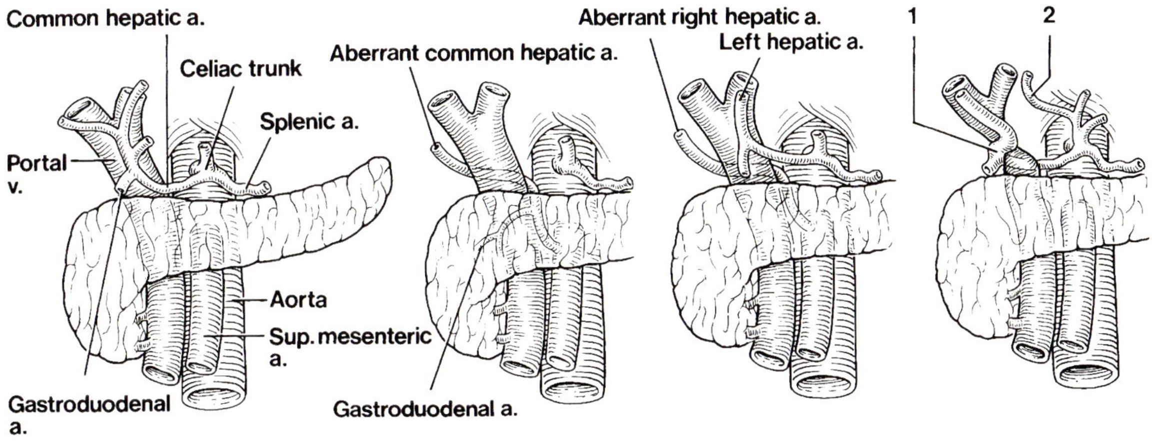

Figurge 3.4

Some variations of the hepatic arteries in relation to the pancreas (with permission [7]. a Normal configuration. b Aberrant common hepatic artery. c Aberrant right hepatic artery. d, Common hepatic artery (*1*) looping around the portal vein from behind (causing compression of the vein); aberrant left hepatic artery (*2*) arising from left gastric artery

dependently from the SMA in 24% of the subjects. The posterior arcade passes behind the common bile duct, and is farther from the duodenum and in a more cephalad position than is the anterior arcade. The head of the pancreas and duodenum are supplied with blood mainly from these arcades.

The dorsal pancreatic artery (DPA) lies behind the neck of the pancreas, arising from the splenic artery (SPA), the CEA, the CHA, or the SMA. The GDA and the DPA give off branches and form the arcade along the superior margin of the pancreas. The branch from the GDA is called the superior pancreatic branch and the branch from the DPA is called the suprapancreatic branch [4]. The DPA then runs downward to the lower border of the pancreas and divides into the left and right branches. The DPA provides the main blood supply to the neck and body of the pancreas.

The transverse pancreatic artery (TPA) has the left branch of the DPA in 90% of the cases [5], and it departs from the GDA near the point where the GDA divides into the rGEA and the ASPDA. The TPA runs along the inferior margin of the pancreas to anastomose with the great pancreatic artery (GPA) and the caudal pancreatic arteries (CPAs) to form the arcade. This arcade is called the prepancreatic arcade.

The GPA is the greatest artery among the branches of the SPA that course along the superior margin of the body and tail of the pancreas. It usually arises around the border between the body and tail of the pancreas and divides into the left and right branches to anastomoses with the TPA, the DPA, and the CPAs.

The CPAs are small branches of the SPA or the left gastroepiploic artery (lGEP). The TPA, the GPA, and the CPAs supply blood to the body and tail of the pancreas [6].

In relation to the arterial anatomy of the pancreas, it is important to understand the variations of the CHA. The CHA sometimes departs from the SMA and divides into the left and right branches in the hilus of the liver, and the right hepatic artery sometimes departs from the SMA. The CHA has other variations, as shown in Fig. 3.4 [7].

Venous Anatomy

The venous blood of the pancreas drains into the portal system around the pancreas; the splenic vein (SPV), the superior mesenteric vein (SMV), the inferior mesenteric vein (IMV), and the portal vein (PV) (Fig. 3.5). In general, the pancreatic veins run parallel to the arteries and lie superficial to them.

The SPV runs inferior to the splenic artery along the posterior aspect of the pancreas to join the SMV, which passes anterior to the inferomedial aspect of the uncinate process to form the PV behind the neck of the pancreas [6].

The anterior superior pancreaticoduodenal vein (ASPDV) generally terminates in the SMV via the gastrocolic trunk. The gastrocolic trunk is called the gastrocolic trunk of Henle or Henle's trunk, because Henle reported a common trunk of the superior right colic vein (SRCV) and the right gastroepiploic vein

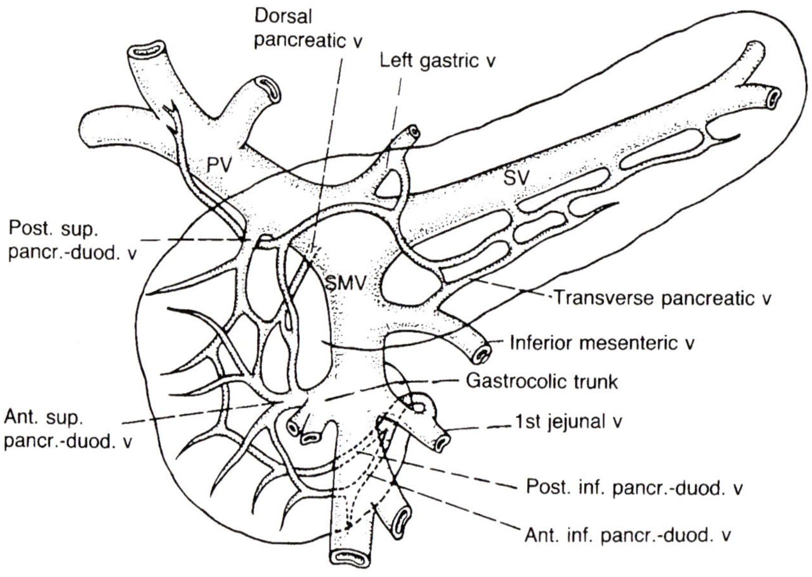

Figurge 3.5

Pancreatic venous anatomy (with permission [6]. *PV* Portal vein, *SMV* superior mesenteric vein, *SPV* splenic vein

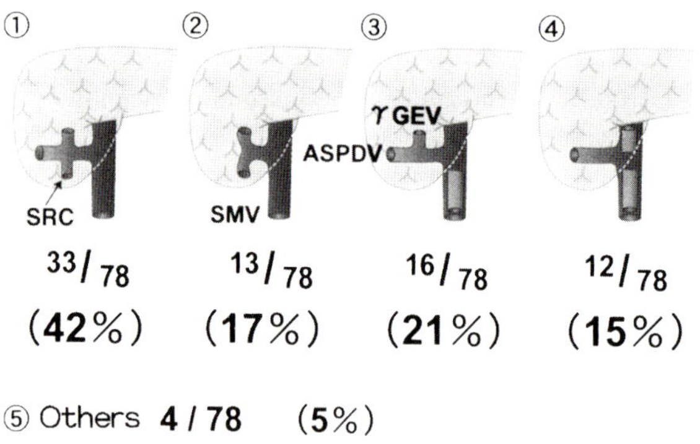

Figurge 3.6

Variations and their incidence in the gastrocolic trunk of Henle (with permission [1]). *SRC* Superior right colic vein, *GEV* gastroepiploic vein, *ASPDV* anterior superior pancreaticoduodenal vein

(rGEV) in 1868 [8]. Gillot et al. and Kimura et al. reported that a gastrocolic trunk was found in about 60% of 78 subjects (Fig. 3.6) [9].

The anterior superior pancreaticoduodenal vein (AIPDV) drains into the first jejunal vein or the SMV. The posterior superior pancreaticoduodenal vein (PSPDV) terminates in the right posterior wall of the PV. The ASPDV and the anterior inferior pancreaticoduodenal vein (AIPDV) form an arcade on the anterior surface of the pancreas. However, Takamuro et al. reported that the PSPDV and the posterior inferior pancreaticoduodenal artery (PIPDV) sometimes form arcades and at other times do not [10]. The PIPDV enters the first jejunal vein, frequently to form a common trunk with the AIPDV.

A large vein is sometimes observed running from the posterior aspect of the pancreas to the junction of the SMV and the PV; this vein is called the dorsal pancreatic vein (DPV).

The transverse pancreatic vein (TPV) branches off the small veins together with the DPV and terminates in the SMV, the IMV, or occasionally the SPV or the gastrocolic trunk. The SPV receives some short pancreatic venous branches and these branches anastomose with the TPV and drain the blood from the body and tail of the pancreas.

In relation to the venous anatomy of the pancreas, it is important to understand the variations in the IMV, SPV, and SMV. Kimura reported that the IMV joined the SV in 34% of 38 autopsy patients, the SMV in 42%, and the confluence of the SPV and the SMV in 24% [1].

Microcirculation of the pancreas

In this section, the microcirculation system of the pancreas is explained by showing the results of electron microscopic observations of vascular casts of human pancreas. These results are illustrated schematically in Fig. 3.7 [11].

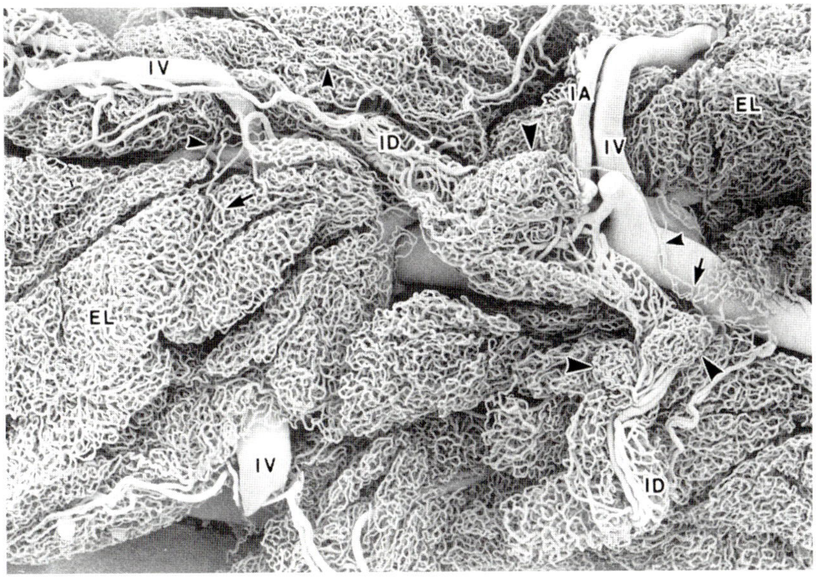

Figurge 3.7

Diagram of the vascular arrangements of the human pancreas (with permission [11]). From the top to the bottom are shown a lobule containing an islet, an extralobular (periductal) islet, and a lobule lacking in an islet. An interlobular duct is illustrated on the right side. *El* extralobular endocrine islet (islet of Langerhans) or its vascular plexus, *EL* exocrine lobule or its vascular plexus, *IA* interlobular artery, *ID* interlobular duct or its vascular bed, *II* interlobular endocrine islet or its vascular plexus, *IV* interlobular vein, *LA* lobular artery, *LD* lobular duct or its vascular bed, *LV* lobular vein, *PA* periductal artery, *PV* periductal vein, *a* afferent vessel of the islet, *e* efferent vessel of the islet, *s* surface capillary network of the extralobular islet, *v* venous efferent vessel (emissary vein) of the extralobular islet, *la* branch of the lobular artery, *lv* branch of the lobular vein

Figurge 3.8

Overview of a replicated blood vascular bed of the human pancreas (a caudal segment exposed by dissection, 25-year-old woman with permission [11]). Note that the blood vascular plexuses of the exocrine lobules (*EL*) and secretory ducts (interlobular ducts, *ID*) are thoroughly reproduced together with their connecting interlobular arteries (*IA*) and veins (*IV*), and that the exocrine lobules (*large arrowheads*) closely associated with the ducts are smaller than the other lobules. The *small arrowheads* indicate the interlobular blood vascular plexuses, some capillaries of which continue into the lobular capillaries (*arrows*). Magnification, ×40

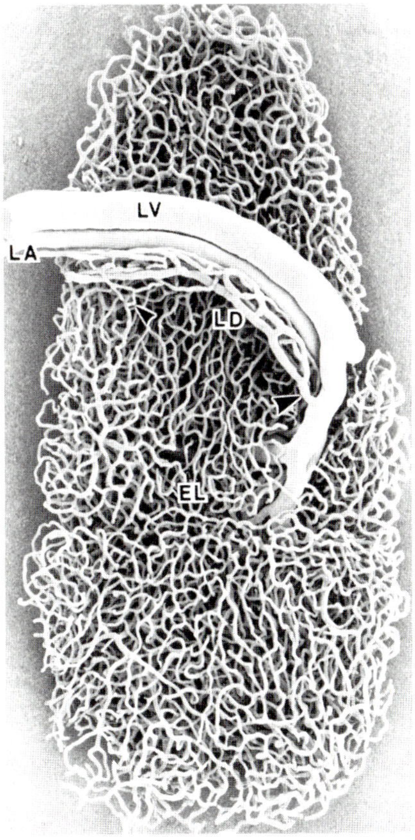

Lobular Vascular Bed

The vascular bed of the exocrine lobules (lobular plexus) consists of fine capillaries (Fig.. 3.7), which receive one or more afferent vessels (lobular arteries) from the interlobular arteries and issue one or more efferent vessels (lobular veins) continuous with the interlobular veins (Figs. 3.8 and 3.9). The lobular plexus occasionally possess insignificant fine connections with the interlobular or periductal plexus (Figs. 3.7 and 3.8).

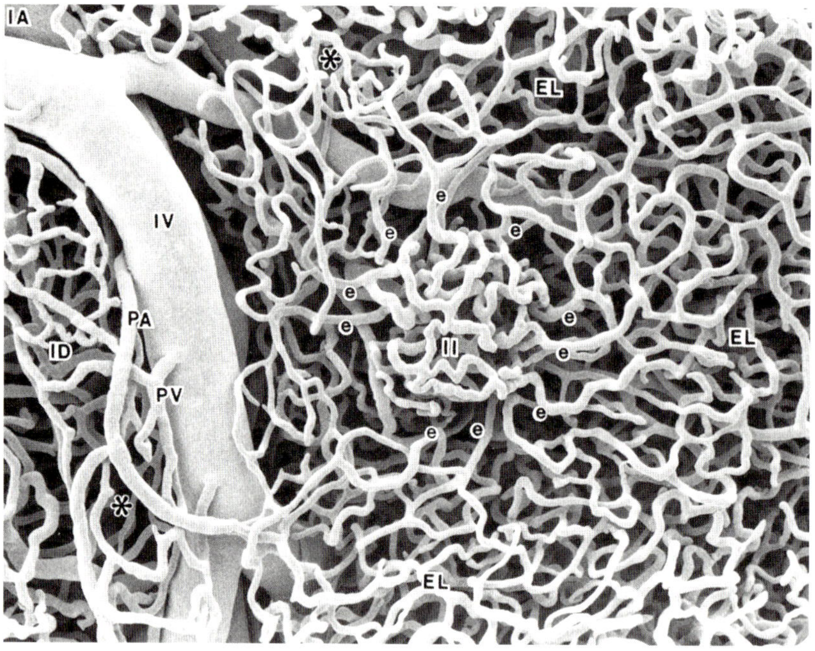

Figurge 3.9

A lobular blood vascular plexus isolated together with its connecting lobular artery, lobular vein, and ductal plexus (with permission [11]). Note that the lobule is fairly independent. The ductal plexus drains at the hilus of the lobule into a branch of the lobular vein (*large arrowhead*). The *small arrowhead* indicates a rare fine capillary connection between the lobular and ductal plexuses. Magnification, ×80

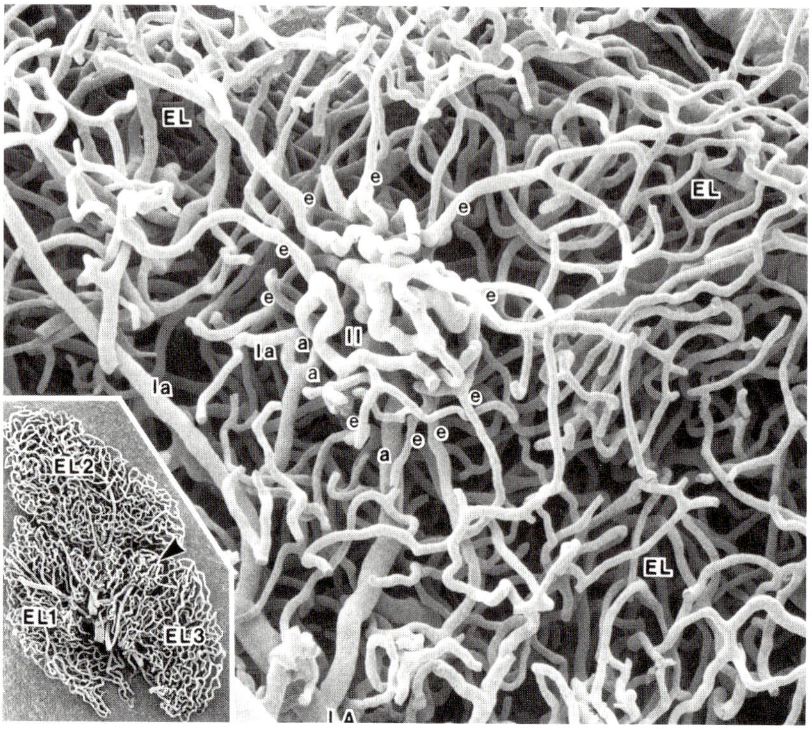

Figurge 3.10

An intralobular islet (*II*) exposed in the lobular surface (with permission [11]). Note that the islet emits marked efferent vessels (*e*), which continue, as the insuloacinar portal vessels, into adjacent lobular capillaries (*EL*). The *asterisk* indicates injection defects. Magnification, ×200

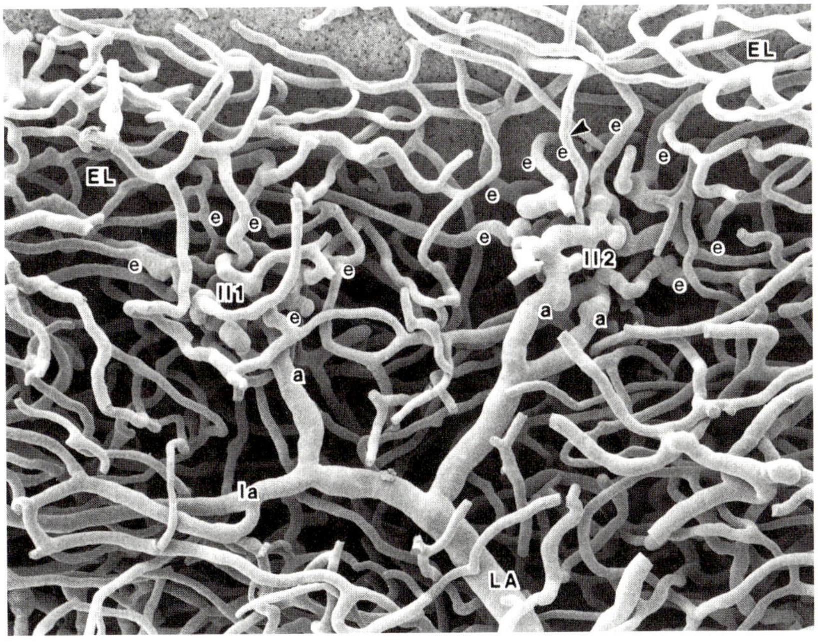

Figurge 3.11

An intralobular islet (*Il*) with three afferent vessels (*a*) (with permission [11]). The afferent vessels on the left run from the superficial aspect into the insular capillaries, while that on the right runs deep into the islet. This islet also emits many insuloacinar portal vessels (*e*) continuous with the adjacent lobular capillaries (*EL*). The *inset* shows an isolated cluster of three lobules (*EL1–EL3*). Note in this inset that only the *EL3* lobule contains an islet (*arrowhead*). Magnification, ×250; inset, ×40

The size of the lobular plexus also varies widely. Large lobules measuring more than 0.5 mm in length contain numerous fine capillaries (lobular capillaries), while small ones, 500 μm or less in length, contain a small number of lobular capillaries. Large lobules are typically located in the superficial layers of the pancreas, whereas smaller ones are typically found in the deeper layers of the organ or in close association with the interlobular ducts (Fig. 3.7).

Intralobular Islets and their Blood Vessels

The vascular network in the islets of Langerhans (insular plexus) consists of thicker (sinusoidal) capillaries conglomerated into a globular mass, measuring 30–250 μm (usually, 100–150 μm) in diameter (Figs. 3.9–3.11). The peripheral or cortical capillaries of the intralobular islets issue numerous efferent vessels that radiate into the capillary network in the surrounding exocrine tissues (Figs. 3.9–3.11). These efferent vessels of the intralobular islets are relatively long, straight, or gently winding capillaries. However, as these vessels connect the intralobular islets and the lobular capillaries covering the exocrine acini and intralobular ducts, they should therefore be described as insuloacinar portal vessels [12–14]. Some portal vessels arise deep in the islets (Fig. 3.11), others more superficially. In human, the intralobular islets issue no efferent vessels directly draining into the veins. The portal vessels are characteristically slender, being never thicker than the capillaries in the islets and as thick as or slightly thicker than the lobular capillaries (Figs. 3.9–3.11).

The number of the portal vessels varies widely among islets. In general, larger islets possess a larger number of portal vessels. Larger islets exceeding 200 μm in diameter issue 30 or more portal vessels, whereas a small islets consisting of only a few capillary loops issue 3–7 portal vessels. Usually, a part of the lobular capillary network is supplied with the portal vessels of the islets, while the remaining parts receive lobular arteries directly; both portions of the lobular capillaries are drained by the lobular veins. On rare occasions, the entire extent of the lobular capillary network is supplied by the portal vessels. In these latter cases, the lobular artery or arteries take the exclusive role as the afferent vessels of the islets.

The islets identified by this characteristic feature in the vascular casts are usually located intralobularly (Figs. 3.9–3.11), embedded in the general capillary network of the exocrine tissue (Fig. 11). Only rarely

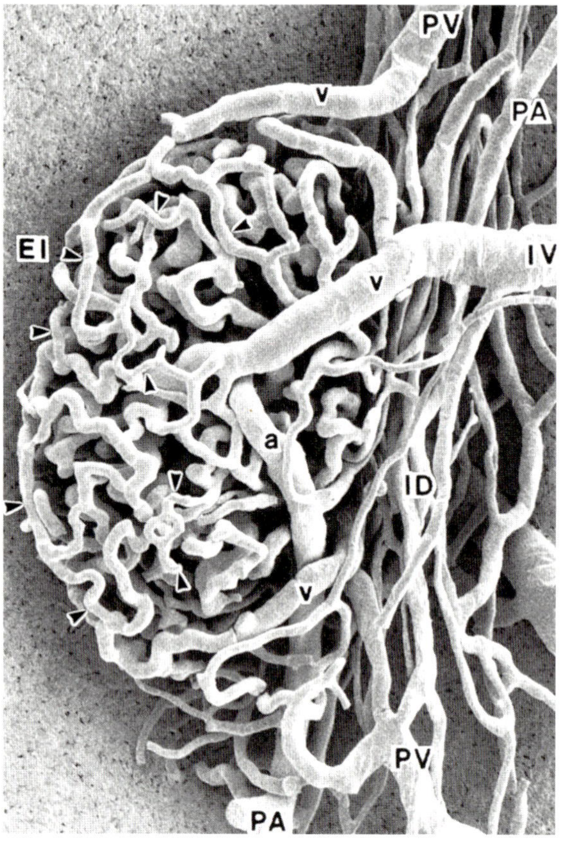

Figurge 3.12

Two intralobular islets (*Il1, Il2*) as found in the same lobule (with permission [11]). The *Il2* islet receives two afferent vessels (*a*), and one of its efferent vessels (*arrowhead*) arises deep in the islet. Even in these islets, all of the efferent vessels (*e*) (including that indicated by the *arrowhead*) continue, as the insuloacinar portal vessels, into the adjacent lobular capillaries (*EL*). Magnification, ×280

does an intralobular islet expose its body to the lobular surface (Figs. 3.9 and 3.10).

By surveying many lobules with a light microscope, a clearly definable insular plexus is able to be found in one among seven lobules (Fig. 3.10, Inset). When a lobule reveals an islet, it is usually single, but occasionally several islets can be found in a lobule (Fig. 3.12). Thicker lobules probably possess their islets more consistently. Nevertheless, it is reasonable to say that a considerable number of lobules in the human pancreas are devoid of any islets. Moreover, the range of the portal vessels is limited and rarely cover the entire exocrine lobules. It is thus suggested that in humans, insular control over the exocrine pancreas is generally valid in restricted areas of the lobule.

In humans, it is rare for an islet to be located interlobularly (extralobularly) or periductally (i.e., between the lobules or along the interlobular duct; Fig. 3.12). Species differences in this regard are conspicuous. In the mouse and rat, many islets are located interlobularly along the excretory ducts, and are drained via their surface network of fine capillaries into the interlobular or periductal veins [15,16].

The intralobular islet receives one to three afferent vessels (insular arterioles) from the lobular artery (Figs. 3.9–3.11). These afferent vessels enter deep into the islet and form a conglomeration of sinusoidal capillaries. In some other islets, the afferent vessels divide superficially on one pole of the islet and continue into the sinusoidal capillaries. In typical cases, the afferent vessels break up into superficial and deep branches, which supply the islets both from the superficial and deep aspects, respectively. When the islet receives two or more afferent vessels, one often runs deep into the insular plexus and the other splits into its superficial aspects (Fig. 3.10). In certain animal species, the pattern of insular microcirculation is known to be regular [12,13,17,18]. However, in human islets, no rule can be found as to whether afferent vessels are primarily connected to the deep or superficial portion of the islet, and A, B, and D cells are rather irregularly intermingled within the islets.

Interlobular Islets and their Vascular Connections

The human pancreas only occasionally reveals islets located in the interlobular connective tissue. The interlobular (extralobular) islets receive one or more afferent vessels from the interlobular or periductal arteries (Fig. 3.12). The afferent arterioles penetrate deep into the islets to form a conglomeration of sinusoidal capillaries. This deep capillary plexus is surrounded and drained by a thin network of fine capillaries (the outer capillary meshwork; Fig. 3.12). This marginal network, in turn, issues efferent vessels that are directly continuous with the interlobular or periductal veins (Fig. 3.12).

Periductal Vascular Plexus

The vascular networks surrounding the interlobular and lobular ducts (periductal plexuses) are supplied with periductal arteries and veins that are derived from the interlobular arteries and veins, respectively (Figs. 3.7–3.9). The terminal segments of the periductal plexus (ductal plexus surrounding the lobular ducts) consist of several capillaries that drain into the

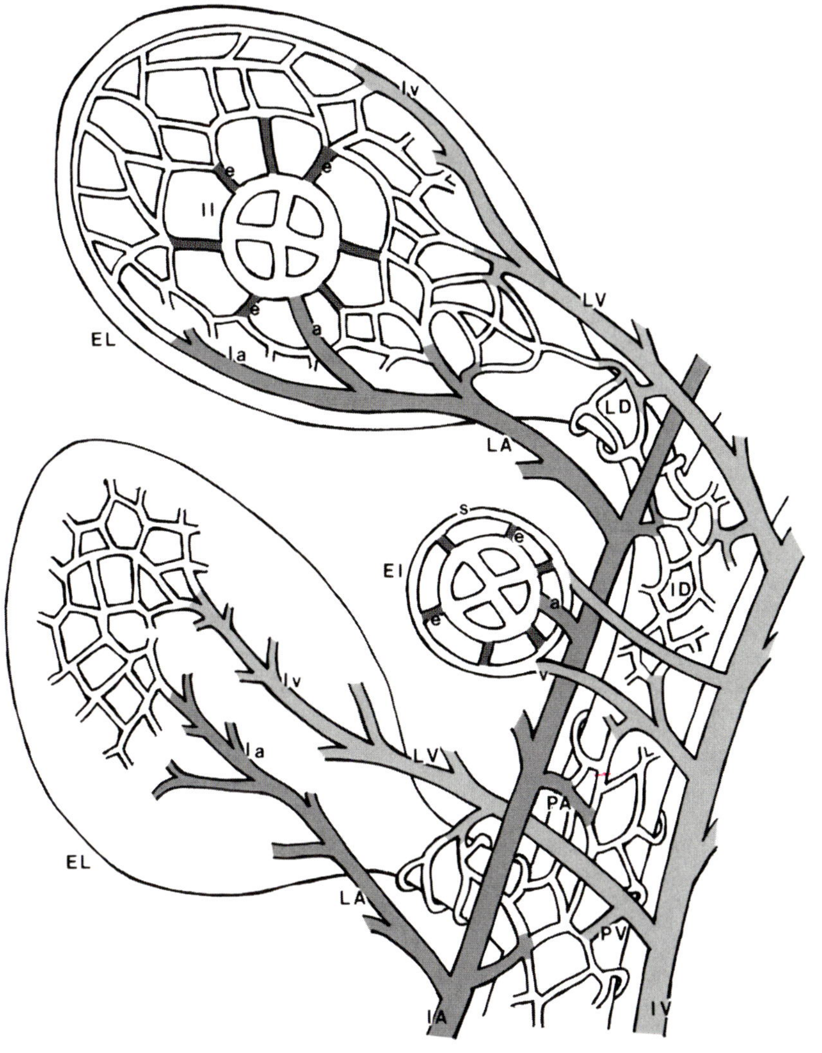

Figurge 3.13

An extralobular islet (with permission [11]). Note that this islet is provided with a set of fine capillaries (*arrowheads*), which receives the sinusoidal capillaries of the islet and confluence into the emissary veins (*v*), which are finally continuous with the PV or IV. Magnification, ×250

lobular veins in or outside the lobular plexus (Fig. 3.8). Few capillary connections can be recognized between the lobular and ductal plexuses (Fig. 3.8). This indicates that the capillary plexuses of the exocrine lobules and extralobular secretory ducts are independent of each other in terms of the blood supply. By contrast, within the lobule the exocrine acini and their connecting intercalated and intralobular secretory ducts are commonly supplied.

References

1. Kimura W (2000) Surgical anatomy of the pancreas for limited resection. J Hepatobiliary Pancreat Surg 7:473–479
2. Mikami Y, Takeda K, Matsuno S, Murakami T (2005) Vascular structure of the pancreas. In: Pour PM (ed) Toxicology of the Pancreas. Taylor and Francis, Boca Raton, Fl, pp 75–89
3. Murakami G, Hirata K, Takamuro T, Mukaiya M, Hata F, Kitagawa S (1999) Vascular anatomy of the pancreaticoduodenal region: a review. J Hepatobiliary Pancreat Surg 6:55–68
4. Bertelli E, Di Gregorio F, Bertelli L, Orazioli D, Bastianini A (1997) The arterial blood supply of the pancreas: a review. IV. The anterior inferior and posterior pancreaticoduodenal aa., and minor sources of blood supply for the head of the pancreas. An anatomical review and radiologic study. Surg Radiol Anat 19:203–212

5. Freeny PC, Lawson TL (1982) Radiology of the Pancreas. Springer Verlag, Berlin, Heidelberg, New York, pp 51–97
6. Pour PM, Konishi Y, Kloppel G, Longnecker DS (1994) Atlas of Exocrine Pancreatic Tumors – Morphology, Biology and Diagnosis with an International Guide for Tumor Classification. Springer Verlag, Berlin, Heidelberg, New York, pp 1–15
7. Trede M, Carter DC (1993) Surgery of the Pancreas. Churcill Livingstone, New York, pp23–25
8. Henle J (1868) Handbuch der systematischen Anatomie des Menschen. Druck und Verlag von Friedrich Vieweg und Sohn, Braunschweig, pp 391 (cited by Gillot et al.)
9. Gillot C, Hureau J, Aaron C, Martini R, Thaler G (1964) The superior mesenteric vein. J Int Coll Surg 41:339–369
10. Takamuro T, Oikawa I, Murakami G, Hirata K (1998) Venous drainage from the posterior aspect of the pancreatic head and duodenum. Okajimas Folia Anat Jpn 75:1–8
11. Murakami T, Fujita T, Taguchi T, Nonaka Y, Orita K (1992) The blood vascular bed of the human pancreas, with special reference to the insulo-acinar portal system. Scanning electron microscopy of corrosion casts. Arch Histol Cytol 55:381–395
12. Fujita T (1973) Insulo-acinar portal system in the horse pancreas. Arch Histol Jpn 35:161–171
13. Fujita T, Murakami T (1973) Microcirculation of monkey pancreas with special reference to the insulo-acinar portal system. A scanning electron microscope study of vascular casts. Arch Histol Jpn 35:255–263
14. Ohtani O, Fujita T (1981) Insulo-acinar portal system of the pancreas. A scanning electron microscope study of corrosion casts. Prog Clin Biol Res 59B:111–120
15. Murakami T, Fujita T, Miyake T, Ohtsuka A, Taguchi T, Kikuta A (1993) The insulo-acinar portal and insulo-venous drainage systems in the pancreas of the mouse, dog, monkey and certain other animals: a scanning electron microscopic study of corrosion casts. Arch Histol Cytol 56:127–147
16. Murakami T, Fujita T (1992) Microcirculation of the rat pancreas, with special reference to the insulo-acinar portal and insulo-venous drainage systems: a further scanning electron microscope study of corrosion casts. Arch Histol Cytol 55:453–476
17. Bonner-Weir S, Orci L (1982) New perspectives on the microvasculature of the islets of Langerhans in the rat. Diabetes 31:883–889
18. Ohtani O, Ushiki T, Kanazawa H, Fujita T (1986) Microcirculation of the pancreas in the rat and rabbit with special reference to the insulo-acinar portal system and emissary vein of the islet. Arch Histol Jpn 49:45–60

Physiology and Pathophysiology of the Pancreatic Functions

Chapter 4 Pancreatic Exocrine Secretion *31*
P. Layer, J. Keller

Chapter 5 Physiology and Pathophysiology of Endocrine Pancreatic Secretion *37*
B. Gallwitz, U. R. Fölsch

Chapter 6 Sphincter of Oddi Physiology and Pathophysiology *49*
M. Staritz

P. Layer · J. Keller

Pancreatic Exocrine Secretion

Digestion of macronutrients is required before absorption may occur, and is achieved mostly via enzymatic hydrolysis into small absorbable molecules. In this process, the pancreatic enzymes lipase, amylase, trypsin, and chymotrypsin play the most important role, although several brush-border enzymes as well as other pancreatic and extrapancreatic enzymes also participate in macronutrient digestion. The crucial importance of pancreatic exocrine function is reflected by the detrimental malabsorption that occurs in patients with untreated pancreatic exocrine insufficiency as a typical complication of chronic pancreatitis [1–4].

As a basis for optimizing enzyme treatment, comprehensive knowledge is needed about secretion and luminal fate of pancreatic enzymes and their effects on nutrient digestion under physiologic circumstances.

Pancreatic Exocrine Function in Healthy Humans

Depending on nutrient intake, the human pancreas secretes about 3 l of alkaline juice per day. Pancreatic juice contains hydrolytic enzymes (or respective zymogens that need to be activated within the intestinal lumen) for the digestion of complex carbohydrates, proteins, and lipids. The most important ones are α-amylase, trypsin and chymotrypsin, lipase, and colipase. In addition, elastases, carboxypeptidases, phospholipase A_2, carboxylesterase lipase, and ribo- and deoxyribonucleases are also secreted. The most important inorganic components of pancreatic juice are water, potassium, chloride, and bicarbonate. The high bicarbonate content of pancreatic juice causes its alkaline pH, which serves to protect enzymes from acidic denaturation and increases the hydrolytic activity of pancreatic enzymes within the intestinal lumen. α-Amylase and lipase are secreted in an active form. By contrast, proteases are delivered into the duodenum as inactive zymogens. Within the duodenum, trypsinogen is partly converted to trypsin by the duodenal enzyme enterokinase. Subsequently, trypsin has an autocatalytic effect and also cleaves and activates the other proteases.

The healthy human pancreas adopts its exocrine secretion to nutrient ingestion. Nutrient ingestion leads to a severalfold increase in exocrine secretion compared with the fasting state. The magnitude of the digestive pancreatic exocrine response is influenced mainly by dietary composition, caloric value, and its physical and biochemical properties. Overall, in healthy individuals, 10- to 20-fold more enzymes are secreted by the pancreas than are required to prevent malabsorption.

Pancreatic Exocrine Secretion During Fasting

In the fasting state, pancreatic exocrine secretion parallels cyclical changes of interdigestive intestinal motor activity during the daytime, with minimal enzyme output during phase I and maximal enzyme secretion immediately before the onset of or during phase III motility [1] (Fig. 4.1). During phase II, enzyme secretion fluctuates in concert with irregular antral motor activity [5]. As we have shown previously, the cyclical coupling between fasting motility and pancreatic secretion is preserved throughout the night in fasting humans, despite an overall decrease in motor activity [5,6]. Moreover, modulations of the fasting pancreatic enzyme pattern occur during the nighttime [7].

Postprandial Pancreatic Exocrine Secretion

Within a few minutes of ingestion of a meal, the interdigestive pattern is interrupted and postprandial secretion is induced, characterized by a rapid increase in enzyme secretion reaching maximal values within the first postprandial hour, or even within 20–30 min postprandially. Following peak output, enzyme se-

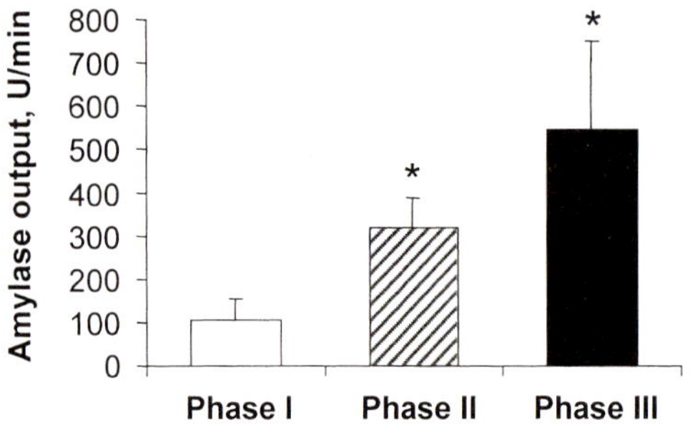

Figure 4.1

In the fasting state, pancreatic exocrine secretion parallels cyclical changes of interdigestive intestinal motor activity during the daytime, with minimal enzyme output during phase I (motor quiescence), intermediate secretory rates during phase II (irregular motor activity), and maximal enzyme secretion immediately before the onset of or during phase III motility (regular, aborally propagated contractions) [6]. *$p < 0.05$ vs phase I

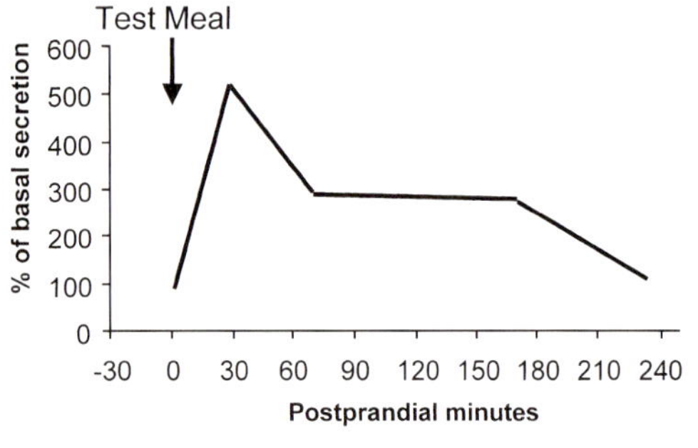

Figure 4.2

Schematic drawing of the pancreatic exocrine response to nutrients in humans. Ingestion of a meal induces a rapid increase in enzyme secretion, reaching maximal values within the first postprandial hour. Following peak output, enzyme secretion decreases to a fairly stable secretory rate before decreasing again after about 3–4 h postprandially to finally reach the interdigestive range at the end of the digestive period. The exact degree and course of pancreatic exocrine response to a meal depends mainly on its size, composition, and physical properties [7]

cretion decreases to a fairly stable secretory rate before decreasing again after about 3–4 h postprandially to finally reach the interdigestive range at the end of the digestive period (Fig. 4.2). According to several studies, maximal enzyme output may reach 3,000–6,000 U/min for lipase, 500–1,000 U/min for amylase, and 200–1,000 U/min for trypsin [7].

Influence of Nutrient Loads and Composition

Duodenal nutrient exposure is the most important stimulus for the postprandial enzyme response. Intraduodenal nutrient loads of about 1 kcal/min are required in order to convert the interdigestive secretory pattern to the fed pattern [8] Physiologically, gastric emptying rates of 2–3 kcal/min occur after ingestion of a normal meal in healthy humans [9]. With meals ranging from about 200 to 500 kcal, a positive correlation between postprandial amylase secretion and meal energy density was observed. By contrast, higher nutrient loads did not necessarily increase enzyme output [7].

However, pancreatic enzyme output is not only regulated by the caloric content of a meal, but also by acute or chronic alterations of nutrient composition. Thus, chronic ingestion of a high-fat diet is associated with higher interdigestive and postprandial enzyme outputs than an equicaloric carbohydrate-rich diet. In contrast to chronic modifications of the diet, acute changes did not alter interdigestive enzyme output, but adaptation of postprandial pancreatic enzyme secretion occurred [10].

The protein component of a meal contributes markedly to the induction of the digestive pancreatic enzyme response. However, the stimulatory effect of dietary protein on pancreatic exocrine secretion apparently depends on adequate protein digestion [11], and stimulatory potency is limited to the essential amino acids phenylalanine, valine, methionine, and tryptophan. Graded intraduodenal essential amino acid perfusion at 0, 62.25, 122.5, 225, and 450 µmol/min dose-dependently increased protease outputs (Fig. 4.3) [12]. Constant duodenal perfusion of essential amino acids at a higher dose (800 µmol/min) caused a short-lived peak trypsin output followed by a stable 50% maximal enzyme output throughout amino acid perfusion (i.e., for more than 5 h) [13].

Lipids are the strongest stimulants of pancreatic enzyme secretion; duodenal free fatty acids rather than triglycerides appear to be responsible for the release of cholecystokinin and subsequent stimulation of enzyme output in humans [14]. Again, duodenal perfusion of fatty acids at graded doses dose-dependently increased enzyme and bicarbonate output. Increasing the chain length of fatty acids delivered into the duodenum augmented pancreatic responses [7].

Carbohydrates are weaker stimulants of pancreatic exocrine secretion compared with proteins and lipids [1]. The increase in enzyme output induced by carbohydrate meals is usually short-lived [15]. A solution of 100 g glucose dissolved in 500 ml water increased

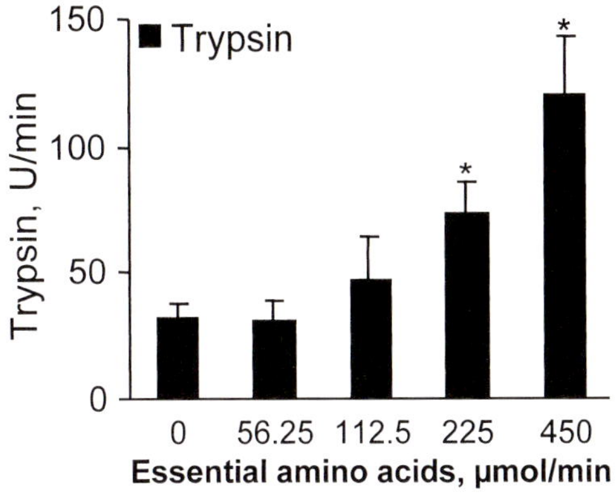

Figure 4.3

Effects of graded duodenal nutrient perfusion on protease outputs in healthy humans. Essential amino acids at doses of up to 450 µg/min dose-dependently stimulated trypsin output (*$p < 0.05$) [12]

basal lipase output (800 U/min) by about threefold (2,600 U/min). However, already 1 h postprandially, lipase output had returned to preprandial values. By contrast, a liquid mixed meal with similar caloric content increased lipase secretion for more than 2 h [15]. This may partly depend on faster gastric emptying of the carbohydrate solution compared with either fat-containing liquid test meals or solid meals.

Influence of Physical Meal Properties

Enzyme response to a solid meal is more sustained compared with an identical meal that has been homogenized. This is partly explained by slower gastric emptying of the solid compared with the homogenized meal, which leads to a prolonged stimulation of enzyme output. In addition, increased gastric acid secretion and, consequently, increased duodenal acid delivery in response to a solid meal may also cause a higher pancreatic secretory response [16].

Other physical meal properties, such as volume, osmolality, and temperature, may also influence pancreatic enzyme secretion. Thus, a stepwise increase in pancreatic amylase and bicarbonate secretion in response to duodenal perfusion with increasing flow rates of saline has been reported. Increasing osmolality of a duodenally perfused mannitol solution from 370 mOsm/kg to 520 mOsm/kg also increased enzyme secretion, but no further increase was seen with higher osmolality [17]. Moreover, Holtmann et al. observed an inverse correlation between the osmolality of duodenally perfused nutrient solutions within a much lower range (24–290 mOsm) and enzyme secretion [18]. These discrepancies still need to be clarified. Gastric emptying was found to be delayed in some but not all studies when meal temperature markedly deviated from body temperature [7]. This may indirectly reduce or postpone stimulation of pancreatic exocrine secretion by nutrients entering the duodenal lumen.

Influence of Age and Gender

It is controversial as to whether pancreatic secretion is gender-related and decreases in the elderly. Anyhow, differences in pancreatic exocrine secretion among women and men, on the one hand, and young and elderly adults, on the other hand, appear to be small and are probably clinically unimportant. Thus, even in subjects older than 80 years, a less than 30% decrease in secretion was expected, which is far from being clinically significant [7].

Initiation and Termination of Postprandial Exocrine Secretion

The sight, smell, and taste of food initiate the cephalic phase of digestive pancreatic enzyme response, which is mediated by the vagal cholinergic system and may induce about 50% of maximal enzyme secretion rates [19]. The subsequent gastric phase is quantitatively less important and is probably mediated by gastropancreatic reflexes that are activated by gastric distension. Gastric acid, free fatty acids, essential amino acids, and carbohydrates within the duodenum initiate the important intestinal phase of the digestive pancreatic exocrine response and maintain stimulation during the digestive period. However, late postprandially, pancreatic enzyme output declines to interdigestive values, despite substantial nutrient loads within the proximal small intestine. This is probably due to inhibitory factors (e.g., peptide YY and glucagon-like peptide-1) that are released from the distal intestinal mucosa in response to a meal or intraileal nutrients [20–22]. Under physiological circumstances, considerable amounts of nutrients are not absorbed during small intestinal transit but are "physiologically malabsorbed." For instance, up to 20% of a carbohydrate meal may reach the terminal ileum [23], and following ingestion of a mixed meal, intraileal lipid concentrations may reach 10 mg/ml [24–26]. Nutrients that pass the terminal ileum and the cecum release several mediators that inhibit upper gastrointestinal functions, including pancreatic exocrine secretion

[27–30]. This may contribute to the regulation of the transition from the fed to the subsequent fasting state.

Fate of Enzymes During Small Intestinal Transit

In normal individuals the activities of all major pancreatic enzymes present in postprandial chyme decrease during duodenoileal transit [31]. However, the rate of intraluminal degradation differs widely among the major enzymes due to differential stabilities against inactivating mechanisms. Following ingestion of a pure rice starch meal, only about 1%, 74%, and 22% of lipase, amylase, and trypsin, respectively, reached the terminal ileum. Thus, lipase activity is almost completely lost during small intestinal transit in the absence of its substrate. Compared with lipase activity, lipase immunoreactivity was preserved significantly longer. Conversely, trypsin activity survived small intestinal transit better than trypsin immunoreactivity. Consequently, the complete structural integrity of the molecule may not be essential for its proteolytic activity.

Following ingestion of a mixed meal or duodenal perfusion of graded doses of mixed nutrients, considerably higher amounts of lipase (20–25% of duodenal lipase) survived small intestinal transit [18,30]. This is in line with previous observations that in vitro and in vivo survival of pancreatic enzymes is enhanced by the presence of nutrients, in particular of the respective substrate. Proteases, especially chymotrypsin, are of major importance for the destruction of lipolytic activity during aboral small intestinal transit [7].

References

1. DiMagno EP, Layer P (1993) Human exocrine pancreatic enzyme secretion. In: Go VL (ed) The Pancreas: Biology, Pathobiology and Diseases. Raven, New York, pp 275–300
2. DiMagno EP, Clain JE, Layer P (1993) Chronic pancreatitis. In: Go VL (ed) The pancreas: Biology, Pathobiology and Disease. Raven, New York, pp 665–706
3. Layer P, Keller J (1999) Pancreatic enzymes: secretion and luminal nutrient digestion in health and disease. J Clin Gastroenterol 28:3–10
4. Layer P, Yamamoto H, Kalthoff L, et al (1994) The different courses of early- and late-onset idiopathic and alcoholic chronic pancreatitis. Gastroenterology 107:1481–1487
5. Layer P, Chan AT, Go VL, et al (1988) Human pancreatic secretion during phase II antral motility of the interdigestive cycle. Am J Physiol 254:G249–G253
6. Keller J, Groger G, Cherian L, et al (2001) Circadian coupling between pancreatic secretion and intestinal motility in humans. Am J Physiol 280:G273–G278
7. Keller J, Layer P (2005) Human pancreatic exocrine response to nutrients in health and disease. Gut 54 Suppl 6:vi1–28
8. Katschinski M, Dippel C, Reinshagen M, et al (1992) Induction of the fed pattern of human exocrine pancreatic secretion by nutrients: role of cholecystokinin and neurotensin. Clin Investig 70:902–908
9. Horowitz M, Edelbroek MA, Wishart JM, et al (1993) Relationship between oral glucose tolerance and gastric emptying in normal healthy subjects. Diabetologia 36:857–862
10. Boivin M, Lanspa SJ, Zinsmeister AR, et al (1990) Are diets associated with different rates of human interdigestive and postprandial pancreatic enzyme secretion? Gastroenterology 99:1763–1771
11. Thimister PW, Hopman WP, Sloots CE, et al (1996) Role of intraduodenal proteases in plasma cholecystokinin and pancreaticobiliary responses to protein and amino acids. Gastroenterology 110:567–575
12. Keller J, Daecke W, Goebell H, Layer P (1996) Integrated secretory and motor responses to submaximal endogenous stimulation by essential amino acids. Pancreas 13:442
13. Malagelada JR, Go VL, DiMagno EP, et al (1973) Interactions between intraluminal bile acids and digestive products on pancreatic and gallbladder function. J Clin Invest 52:2160–2165
14. Guimbaud R, Moreau JA, Bouisson M, et al (1997) Intraduodenal free fatty acids rather than triglycerides are responsible for the release of CCK in humans. Pancreas 14:76–82
15. Fried M, Erlacher U, Schwizer W, et al (1991) Role of cholecystokinin in the regulation of gastric emptying and pancreatic enzyme secretion in humans. Studies with the cholecystokinin-receptor antagonist loxiglumide. Gastroenterology 101:503–511
16. Malagelada JR, Go VL, Summerskill WH (1979) Different gastric, pancreatic, and biliary responses to solid-liquid or homogenized meals. Dig Dis Sci 24:101–110
17. Dooley CP, Valenzuela JE (1984) Duodenal volume and osmoreceptors in the stimulation of human pancreatic secretion. Gastroenterology 86:23–27
18. Holtmann G, Kelly DG, Sternby B, et al (1997) Survival of human pancreatic enzymes during small bowel transit: effect of nutrients, bile acids, and enzymes. Am J Physiol 273: G553–G558
19. Anagnostides A, Chadwick VS, Selden AC, et al (1984) Sham feeding and pancreatic secretion. Evidence for direct vagal stimulation of enzyme output. Gastroenterology 87:109–114
20. Adrian TE, Ferri GL, Bacarese-Hamilton AJ, et al (1985) Human distribution and release of a putative new gut hormone, peptide YY. Gastroenterology 89:1070–1077
21. Keller J, Franke A, Rippel K, Holst JJ, Goebell H, Layer P (1999) Termination of digestive pancreatic secretory and intestinal motor responses: importance of GLP-1 and PYY. Digestion 60:383
22. Layer P, Holst JJ, Grandt D, et al (1995) Ileal release of glucagon-like peptide-1 (GLP-1). Association with inhibition of gastric acid secretion in humans. Dig Dis Sci 40:1074–1082
23. Stephen AM, Haddad AC, Phillips SF (1983) Passage of carbohydrate into the colon. Direct measurements in humans. Gastroenterology 85:589–595

24. Evenepoel P, Claus D, Geypens B, et al (1999) Amount and fate of egg protein escaping assimilation in the small intestine of humans. Am J Physiol 277:G935–G943
25. Evenepoel P, Claus D, Geypens B, et al (1998) Evidence for impaired assimilation and increased colonic fermentation of protein, related to gastric acid suppression therapy. Aliment Pharmacol Ther 12:1011–1019
26. Gan KH, Geus WP, Lamers CB, et al (1997) Effect of omeprazole 40 mg once daily on intraduodenal and intragastric pH in H. pylori-negative healthy subjects. Dig Dis Sci 42:2304–2309
27. Read NW, McFarlane A, Kinsman RI, et al (1984) Effect of infusion of nutrient solutions into the ileum on gastrointestinal transit and plasma levels of neurotensin and enteroglucagon. Gastroenterology 86:274–280
28. Spiller RC, Trotman IF, Higgins BE, et al (1984) The ileal brake – inhibition of jejunal motility after ileal fat perfusion in man. Gut 25:365–374
29. Layer P, Peschel S, Schlesinger T, et al (1990) Human pancreatic secretion and intestinal motility: effects of ileal nutrient perfusion. Am J Physiol 258:G196–G201
30. Keller J, Runzi M, Goebell H, et al (1997) Duodenal and ileal nutrient deliveries regulate human intestinal motor and pancreatic responses to a meal. Am J Physiol 272:G632–G637
31. Layer P, Go VL, DiMagno EP (1986) Fate of pancreatic enzymes during small intestinal aboral transit in humans. Am J Physiol 251:G475–G480

Chapter 5

B. Gallwitz · U. R. Fölsch

Physiology and Pathophysiology of Endocrine Pancreatic Secretion

Approximately 2% of the human pancreas is comprised of the islets of Langerhans, which represent the vast majority of endocrine pancreatic tissue. In addition, small clusters of endocrine cells are dispersed within the exocrine tissue [1]. Four endocrine cell types have been identified in the islets (Fig. 5.1, Table 5.1): A-cells, which generate glucagon, B-cells, which produce insulin and islet amyloid polypeptide (IAPP, also referred to as amylin), D-cells, which synthesize somatostatin, and PP-cells, which produce pancreatic polypeptide (PP). A rapid exchange of substrates and hormones is guaranteed between the blood stream and the islets due to a higher perfusion of the islets in comparison to the exocrine pancreatic tissue and to an endothelial fenestration in the capillaries of the islets [2]. Capillaries first reach the B-cells, then the A-cells, and finally the D-cells, so that insulin may have a direct influence on the other islet cell types, whereas glucagon and somatostatin reach the B-cells via the general circulation [2]. Paracrine interaction between the different cell types, especially between D-Cells and the other endocrine cells, is also possible.

The islets of Langerhans are innervated by sympathetic and parasympathetic nerve fibers. The parasympathetic fibers originate from the vagus nerve and have their synapses in the intrapancreatic cholinergic ganglia. In addition to the classical sympathetic and parasympathetic neurotransmitters, peptidergic nerves containing vasoactive intestinal peptide (VIP), cholecystokinin (CCK), peptide histidine isoleucine (PHI), pituitary adenylate-cyclase-activating peptide (PACAP), and other neuropeptides are involved in regulating pancreatic endocrine and exocrine function. Vagal stimulation releases insulin and may play a role in the cephalic phase of insulin secretion, whereas stimulation of the sympathetic nerve fibers inhibits insulin secretion. Despite extensive research, it still remains largely unknown which physiological functions can exactly be assigned to the various types of innervation of the islets of Langerhans in man. Interestingly, the extrinsic denervation of the human pancreas, as occurs in pancreas transplantation, has only minor consequences on the endocrine function of the organ. Table 5.2 summarizes the pancreatic neuropeptides and their function in controlling pancreatic endocrine secretion [3].

Table 5.1. Endocrine cells in the islets of Langerhans and their secretory products (with permission [1]). *GRPP* Glucagon-related polypeptide, *IAPP* islet amyloid polypeptide

Cell type	Main secretion product	Secretory granules	Peptide length (number of amino acids)	Peptide size [molecular mass (Da)]	Overall abundance [%]	Minor products
A-cells	Glucagon	α	29	3,500	15–20	Major proglucagon fragment GRPP
B-cells	Insulin	β	51	5,800	70–80	C-peptide, proinsulin IAPP (amylin)
D-cells	Somatostatin 14	δ	14	1,500	5–10	–
PP-cells	Pancreatic polypeptide	–	36	1,200	15–25*	–

* Dorsal pancreas <1%; ventral pancreas 80%

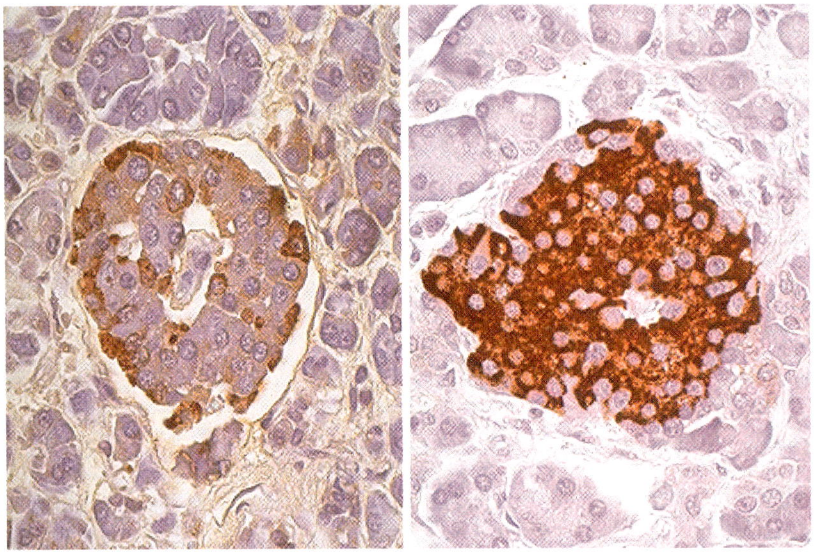

Figurge 5.1

Islets of Langerhans, microscope section. The islet is situated within the exocrine tissue (hematoxilin-eosin stain). The islet itself is presented with immunoperoxidase staining for glucagon on the left and insulin on the right. The A-cells on the left are stained brownish by peroxidase staining for glucagon; the right side of the figure shows the corresponding staining for insulin in the B-cells. Note the different distribution and number of cells, with A-cells being located at the periphery of the islet and B-cells being abundant in the center

Table 5.2. Pancreatic neuropeptides that might participate in the neural control of islet secretion (with permission, modified from [1]). *VIP* Vasoactive intestinal peptide, *PACAP* pituitary adenylate-cyclase-activating peptide, *PHI* peptide histidine isoleucine, *CCK* cholecystokinin, *GRP* gastrin-releasing peptide (mammalian bombesin), *CGRP* calcitonin gene-related peptide, *NPY* neuropeptide Y

Peptide	Pancreatic localization: Nerves	Reaching islet cells	Control by	Effect on: Insulin	Glucagon	Somatostatin
Stimulatory						
VIP	Yes (intrinsic ganglia)	Yes	Vagus	↑	↑	?
PACAP	Yes	Yes	?	↑	?	?
PHI	Yes	Yes	Vagus	↑	↑	?
Cholecystokinin (CCK 4, tetragastrin)	Yes (postganglionic fibers)	Yes	?	↑	↑	↑
GRP	Yes	?	Vagus	↑	-	↑
Substance P	Yes	?	?	↑	↑	↑
Inhibitory						
Galanin	Yes	Yes	Sympathetic nervous system	↑	↑	↑
CGRP	Yes	Yes	?	↑	-	↑
NPY	Yes	Yes	Sympathetic nervous system	↑	?	?

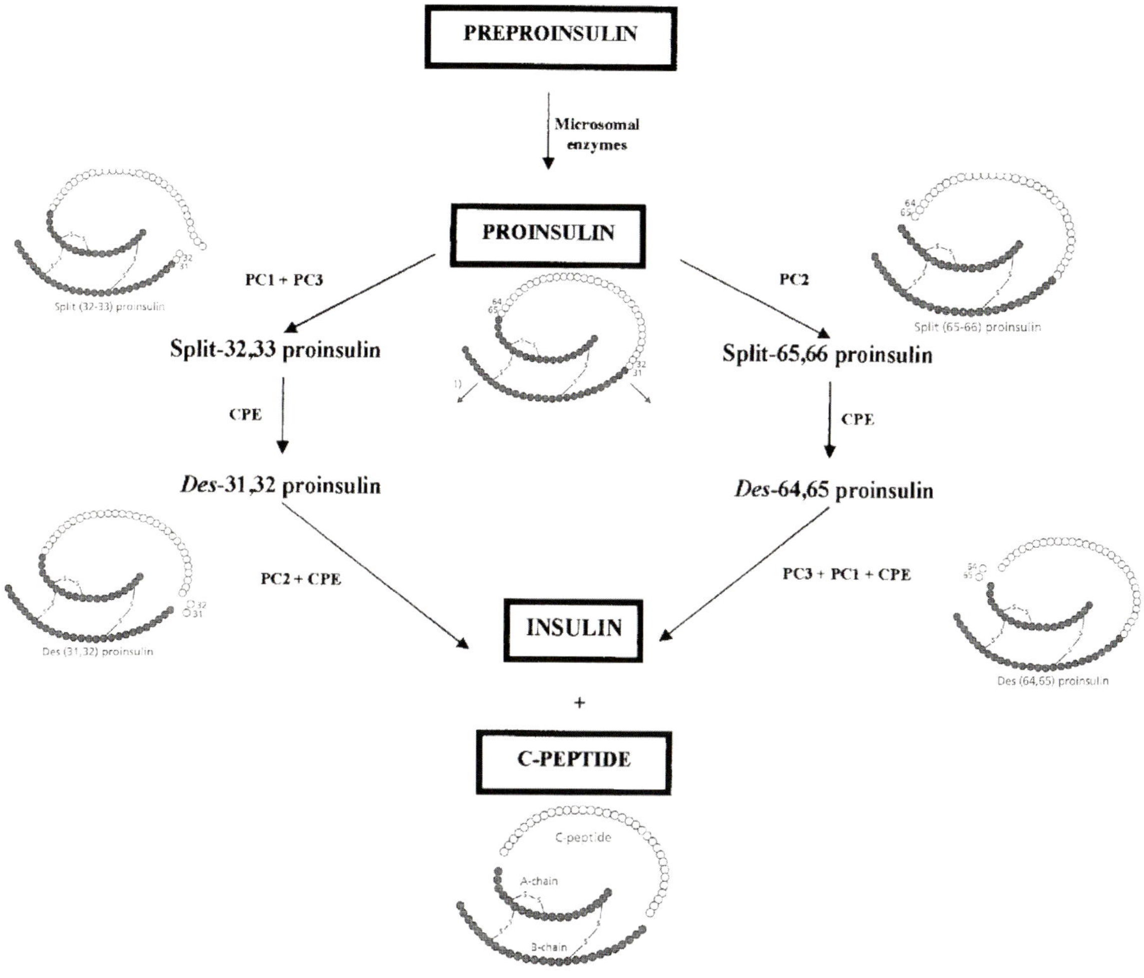

Figurge 5.2

Posttranslational processing of proinsulin (with permission, modified from [3]). Schematic diagram. Insulin is formed via conversion intermediates by the action of proprotein convertases (PC) 2 and 3 (*PC2* and *PC3*, respectively) and carboxypeptidase H (*CPE*)

The Cellular Physiology of Insulin Synthesis and Secretion

Insulin is the most important hormone of the endocrine pancreas since it is the major regulator of anabolic and metabolic processes. It is responsible for the uptake of glucose and amino acids into the peripheral tissues and for metabolic reactions leading to energy storage, such as glycogen synthesis. Generally, plasma glucose and amino acid concentrations are kept within a close range by insulin due to a very effective direction of these substrates into the respective target tissues (e.g., muscle, liver, adipose tissue) under varying metabolic situations and demands (e.g., after a meal, during physical activity). Diminished insulin secretion may lead to diabetes mellitus, whereas an inadequately high output of insulin from the B-cells causes hypoglycemia.

B-cells synthesize the larger insulin precursor molecule preproinsulin. Already in the endoplasmic reticulum, the signal sequence of the peptide is cleaved off and the resulting 86 amino acids containing proinsulin is stored in the Golgi vesicles. Proinsulin has a helical structure with two disulfide bridges connecting the C-terminal and N-terminal part of the peptide chain. In the Golgi vesicles, under acidic conditions and increased calcium concentrations, the enzymes proprotein convertase PC2 and proprotein convertase PC3 as well as carboxypeptidase H cleave the proinsulin chain along the positions 31–32 and

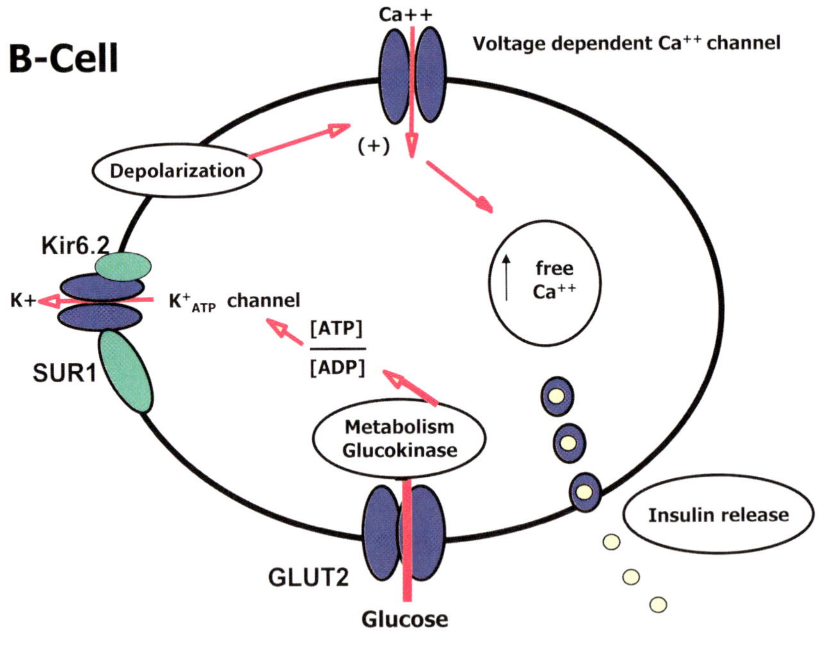

Figurge 5.3

Molecular mechanism of insulin secretion. Schematic diagram. Glucose enters the B-cell via the glucose transporter GLUT2. Intracellularly, glucose is metabolized, the first enzymatic step is phosphorylation by glucokinase. This leads to a shift in the ATP/ADP ratio and closing of the ATP-dependent K^+-channel. This channel is a hetero-octameric protein composed of the inwardly rectifying K^+ channel Kir6.2 and the sulfonylurea receptor SUR1 subunits. The B-cell consecutively depolarizes and the concentration of intracellular free Ca^{++} rises, finally leading to exocytosis of insulin granules

64–65 of the peptide chain, resulting in equimolar amounts of C-peptide and insulin. The posttranslational processing of proinsulin is shown in Fig. 5.2 [4]. Only around 5% of the proinsulin is not completely converted to C-peptide and insulin.

Mature insulin storage granules are formed independently of the actual need for insulin, so that the rate of insulin synthesis does not parallel the rate of insulin secretion, although nutrients play a role in the stimulation of both synthesis and secretion. Excess insulin is stored in the B-cells until it is released by an appropriate stimulatory signal for secretion [5].

The primary stimuli for insulin secretion are glucose and some amino acids, (predominantly arginine, lysine, leucine, and phenylalanine), which can initiate insulin secretion from B-cells at appropriate plasma concentrations [6]. Besides these primary stimuli, various modulators of insulin secretion interact with glucose-induced insulin secretion. The incretin hormones gastric inhibitory polypeptide (GIP) and glucagon-like peptide 1 (GLP-1) are important physiological modulators of insulin secretion, which in the presence of normal fasting glucose concentrations have little effect on insulin secretion, but greatly stimulate insulin release under hyperglycemic conditions [7].

Glucose-induced insulin secretion is mediated by a B-cell-specific mechanism of glucose uptake and metabolism. Glucose is taken up into the B-cell very rapidly through the fast glucose transporter GLUT-2, which is specific for B-cells and hepatocytes. Intracellularly, glucose is then immediately phosphorylated by the B-cell-specific enzyme glucokinase, a reaction that is characterized by a high Michaelis constant (K_m) toward glucose. This enzyme works as intracellular "glucose sensor," since the glucose flux through glucokinase to form glucose-6-phosphate explains the quantitative relationship of extracellular glucose concentrations and the rate of glucose-induced insulin secretion [8]. Glucose-6-phosphate is then metabolized, finally generating adenosine triphosphate (ATP). A rise in ATP closes an ATP-dependent potassium (K^+) channel (KATP) present in the plasma membrane of the B-cell. This channel belongs to a family of KATP channels that are hetero-octameric proteins composed of an inwardly rectifying K^+ channel (Kir6.x) and sulfonylurea receptor (SUR) subunits. Different combinations of Kir6.x and SUR subunits comprise KATP channels with distinct electrophysiological and pharmacological properties. In the B-cell, the predominant type of KATP channel is the

Kir6.2 type, together with the SUR1 sulfonylurea receptor. The closure of this K^+ channel leads to a depolarization of the cell membrane with a consecutive activation of a voltage-dependent L-type calcium (Ca^{2+}) channel that promotes Ca^{2+} entry into the cytoplasm. A rise in cytoplasmic Ca^{2+} finally causes exocytosis of insulin-containing secretory granules [9]. The mechanism of glucose-induced insulin secretion is demonstrated in Fig. 5.3.

Amino acids may also serve as metabolic fuels to promote ATP synthesis, like glucose, and may therefore depolarize B-cells and lead to the stimulation of insulin secretion. Arginine as a highly charged cationic amino acid may directly depolarize B-cells upon transport into the cytoplasm.

The incretin hormones GIP and GLP-1 stimulate cyclic AMP (cAMP) production via activation of the adenylate cyclase. This in turn leads to an increase in intracellular Ca^{2+} and also the phosphorylation of islet proteins, regulating the exocytosis of insulin granules [7].

Stimulation of Insulin Secretion in Man In Vivo

An intravenous infusion or injection of glucose with a rapid and large change in plasma glucose concentrations provokes a biphasic insulin secretory response in healthy subjects, with a quick, short, and pronounced first phase of insulin secretion within the first 20 min after glucose application and a slower and less pronounced second phase of insulin secretion (see Fig. 5.4). Changes in plasma glucose concentrations within physiological variations (between 80 and 150 mg/dl, corresponding to 4.4–8.3 mmol/l) release only minor amounts of insulin, indicating that there are additional stimuli for insulin secretion following a meal [10,11]. In healthy subjects, oral glucose induces dose-dependent insulin secretion with peak insulin concentrations occurring after 45–60 min postprandially (see Fig. 5.4). The stimulation of insulin secretion depends not only on B-cell characteristics, but also on other factors related to cephalic stimulation, such as taste, gastrointestinal motility such as gastric emptying, absorption of nutrients, systemic release of incretin hormones, and the sensitivity of B-cells towards the increments in glucose [3].

Insulin is not secreted steadily with continuous transitions from a low to a high secretion rate, but rather in a pulsatile manner. Pulses with different periodicity have been observed: rapid pulses, occurring at a periodicity of roughly 12–14 minutes, and slower pulses that occur approximately every 90 min. The rapid pulses originate in the islets themselves and are not initiated by extrinsic nerve stimulation, as the rapid pulses of insulin secretion are also observed in pancreatic transplants and even in transplanted islets. Pulsatile insulin secretion is biologically more effective at lowering plasma glucose than a continuous insulin secretion. Interestingly, this pulsatile insulin secretion is already lost or diminished in the very early stages of both types of diabetes mellitus, type 1 and type 2 [12].

Through a feedback-loop of insulin binding to insulin receptors on B-cells, insulin secretion is modi-

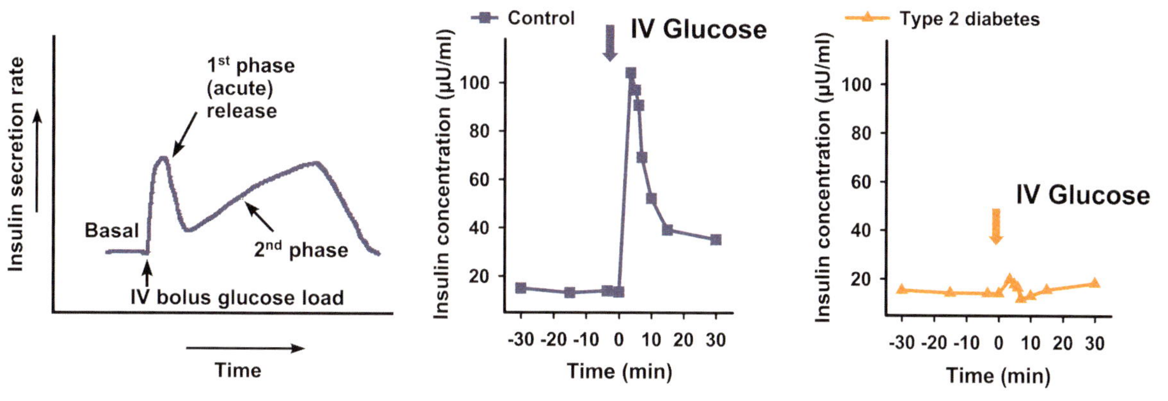

Figurge 5.4

First and second phase of insulin secretion after an intravenous (*IV*) glucose bolus (with permission, modified from [3]). On *top* is shown a schematic diagram of the first and second phase of insulin secretion. The diagram on the *left* shows the normal first phase of insulin secretion after an intravenous glucose bolus in normal subjects, the diagram on the *right* shows the loss of the first phase of insulin secretion in patients with type 2 diabetes fied by its own release in an inhibitory manner. This feedback is operative only at basal glucose concentrations. Small rises in plasma glucose already disturb this feedback loop [3].

Gastrointestinal factors stimulate insulin secretion after a meal. Physiological studies have shown that orally administered glucose evokes a greater insulin response than an intravenously administered glucose infusion calculated to lead to exactly the same serum glucose excursions. This difference in the insulin response was named the "incretin effect," and the gastrointestinal hormones stimulating insulin secretion after oral glucose ingestion, mainly GIP and GLP-1, were called "incretins". The metabolic, neural, and hormonal effects of the small intestine on the endocrine pancreas are referred to as the "enteroinsular axis". Approximately 30–60% of the C-peptide response, and 80–90% of the insulin response after an oral glucose load are conveyed by incretin hormones in nondiabetic subjects, depending on the amount of glucose [7,11].

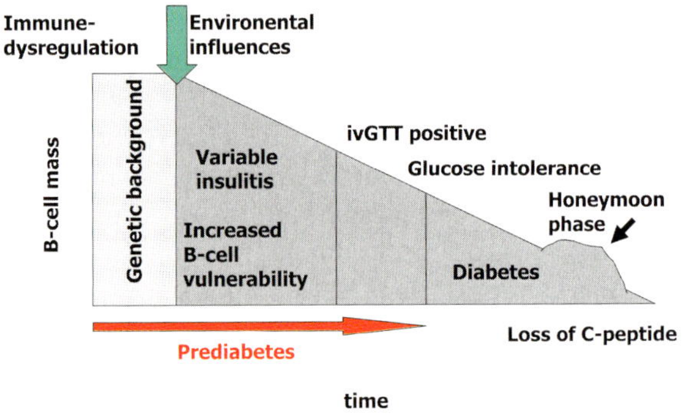

Figurge 5.5

Development of type 1 diabetes. The loss of B-cell function over time is shown along with pathological tests during that development. The environmental factors that trigger the autoimmune response leading to type 1 diabetes in genetically susceptible subjects have yet to be identified. Certain genetically determined constellations in the major histocompatibility complex (MHC-II) show a higher predisposition to type 1 diabetes and other autoimmune diseases. *ivGTT* Intravenous glucose tolerance test

Pathophysiology of Insulin Secretion

Type 1 Diabetes Mellitus

Type 1 diabetes is an autoimmune disease that leads to the destruction of B-cells. T-lymphocytes infiltrate the islets and progressively destroy the B-cells over time. Insulin deficiency is so profound that ketoacidosis – the biochemical hallmark of type 1 diabetes – will develop unless insulin replacement is given. Nevertheless, even in longstanding type 1 diabetes, some insulin-positive B-cells can still be found. Disorders of insulin secretion can be related to the progressive loss of B-cells, with the occurrence of clinically overt diabetes when approximately 80–90% of B-cells are destroyed [13]. Typical autoantibodies of type 1 diabetes (islet cell antibodies, glutamate decarboxylase antibodies, insulin autoantibodies) are often present long before an impairment of insulin secretion can be detected. The first abnormality that can be detected under investigational conditions still in the state of normal oral glucose tolerance is the deterioration of the first phase of insulin secretion after an intravenous glucose injection. This defect is highly predictive of the development of type 1 diabetes within a short time. In clinically apparent type 1 diabetes, oral glucose tolerance declines and insulin and C-peptide plasma concentrations fall. Consecutively, fasting glucose concentrations become elevated, and finally, insulin deficiency is so pronounced that lipolysis is stimulated, leading to an accumulation of ketone bodies. After initial insulin treatment, a partial recovery of insulin secretion occurs in most patients for a transient period of a few months (called the "honeymoon phase"), which allows a drastic reduction of the initial insulin doses required. In longstanding type 1 diabetes, the C-peptide concentrations (a marker of residual B-cell function) are extremely low. Nevertheless, there is evidence that in a significant proportion of patients there is still a very small amount of remaining insulin secretion that is associated with better glycemic control. Early and sufficient insulin replacement may preserve residual B-cell function [14]. A schematic of the development of type 1 diabetes is shown in Fig. 5.5.

Type 2 Diabetes

Type 2 diabetes is on the one hand characterized by insulin resistance of the peripheral tissues, mainly the muscle, the liver, and adipose tissue, and on the other hand, impaired insulin secretion also plays an important role in the pathophysiology of this disease. Obese humans with the prediabetic condition of impaired fasting glucose (IFG) or type 2 diabetes, and lean subjects with type 2 diabetes already have a significant deficit of 40–60% in relative B-cell volume compared with nondiabetic obese and lean cases, respectively. This is due to an increase in B-cell apoptosis that is

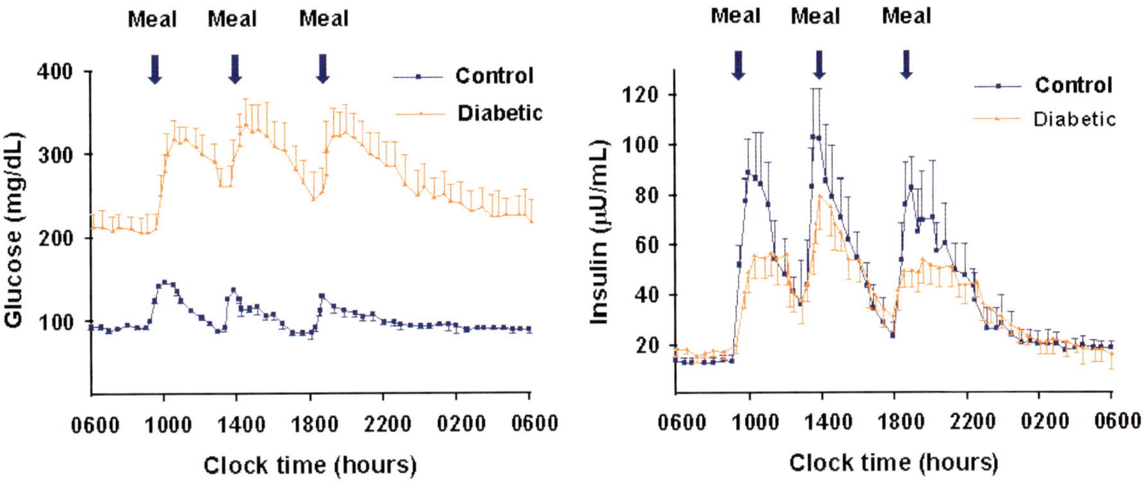

Figurge 5.6

Twenty-four-hour profiles of glucose concentrations and insulin secretion profiles in healthy subjects and patients with type 2 diabetes (with permission, modified from [16]). Note the relative decrease in prandial insulin secretion in the diabetic patients. The glucose profiles are shown in the *left* panel, the insulin secretion plasma concentrations on the *right*

tenfold in lean and threefold in obese cases of type 2 diabetes compared with their respective nondiabetic controls. New islet formation and B-cell replication are normal. The frequency of B-cell apoptosis is related to the rate of increase of islet amyloid and IAPP oligomers, but islet amyloid is not responsible for increased B-cell apoptosis. Replicating B-cells are more vulnerable to apoptosis, possibly accounting for the failure of B-cell mass to expand appropriately in response to obesity in type 2 diabetes [15].

Glucose-induced insulin secretion in patients with type 2 diabetes is diminished and sluggish. The reason is a prominent loss of the first phase of insulin secretion after a sharp rise in glucose that occurs very early in the disease. The second phase of insulin secretion is also affected and gradually deteriorates with the progression of the disease [16]. In addition, the regularity of the pulsatile release of insulin is lost early in the disease and may already be absent in first-degree relatives of patients with type 2 diabetes with normal glucose tolerance. Other stimuli of insulin secretion also show a diminished effect of varying degrees [3]. Of the incretin hormones, GLP-1 still exerts a stimulatory effect on insulin secretion under hyperglycemic conditions in pharmacological doses, making GLP-1-based "incretin mimetics" or dipeptidyl-peptidase IV (DPP IV) inhibitors preventing the degradation of endogenous GLP-1 a promising new treatment option for type 2 diabetes [7,17].

The fact that with improvement of metabolic control, type 2 diabetic B-cells partially recover, has pointed to some direct and partially reversible effects of hyperglycemia itself on B-cell function. This phenomenon, together with the influence that hyperglycemia exerts on insulin sensitivity, has been termed glucose toxicity. Also, free fatty acids, which are characteristically elevated in patients with type 2 diabetes, impair insulin secretion [18]. Figure 5.6 shows the characteristic diurnal profiles of glucose concentrations and insulin secretion rates in patients with type 2 diabetes [16].

Other Types of Diabetes in Pancreatic Disease

Maturity-onset diabetes of the young (MODY) is a genetically and clinically heterogeneous subtype of familial diabetes mellitus that is characterized by early onset, autosomal dominant inheritance and primary defects of insulin secretion. Mutations in six genes are the cause most of the MODY cases. These genes encode the enzyme glucokinase and the transcription factors hepatocyte nuclear factor 4α, hepatocyte nuclear factor 1α, insulin promoter factor-1, hepatocyte nuclear factor 1β, and neuro D1. Additional MODY genes remain to be identified. The study of families with MODY has shown that the different MODY subtypes present different metabolic and clinical profiles, most of them with a defect in insulin secretion due to a reduced activity of glucokinase and consecutive shift to the right in the glucose concentration–insulin secretory response curve. Insulin secretion to an arginine stimulus is not affected in most types of MODY [19].

Chronic pancreatitis with exocrine insufficiency is accompanied by diabetes in approximately 10% of all cases, with 30% of the patients showing an impaired glucose tolerance. The underlying cause is the increasing fibrosis of the pancreas in chronic pancreatitis and the concomitant loss of B-cells. The deterioration of endocrine function is correlated with the loss of exocrine function. There may be an accentuated loss of B-cells relative to A-cells, but clinically counter-regulation in hypoglycemia by glucagon is often impaired in patients with chronic pancreatitis [3].

Physiology of Glucagon Secretion

Glucagon is a peptide that contains 29 amino acids and is secreted by the A-cells. The main function of glucagon in humans is to modulate hepatic glucose output, which needs to be maintained during fasting states and increased energy demands (e.g., exercise). After glucagon binding to a specific G-protein-coupled receptor on the hepatocyte membrane, cAMP is generated and protein phosphorylation via protein kinase A is stimulated. Via this activation cascade, the enzymes involved in glycogenolysis and gluconeogenesis provide glucose for the organism. Hepatic ketogenesis producing β-hydroxybutyrate and acetoacetate from free fatty acids via acetyl coenzyme A is also promoted by glucagon [3].

Hypoglycemia promotes glucagon release, whereas in healthy subjects, hyperglycemia is inhibitory. Oral carbohydrate intake therefore suppresses glucagon secretion. In parallel with the aforementioned incretin effect, the suppression of glucagon secretion is more pronounced when glucose or carbohydrates are ingested by comparison to an intravenous glucose infusion. Amino acids stimulate glucagon release and are responsible for the rise in plasma glucagon concentrations after a mixed meal containing proteins. Activation of the adrenergic system by exercise, stress, or fever also leads to an increase in glucagon secretion [3,20].

Pathophysiology of Glucagon Secretion

Type 1 Diabetes

Insulin deficiency promotes hyperglucagonemia in type 1 diabetes. Since a major determinant of glucagon action is the plasma concentration of glucose in the portal blood relative to that of insulin, type 1 diabetes is characterized by a low insulin to glucagon ratio, leading to a propensity for increased hepatic glucose output. Elevated glucagon levels may also contribute to the increased lipolysis observed in type 1 diabetes and can therefore contribute to ketone-body formation and thus to the risk of developing ketoacidosis [3].

Glucagon is, along with the catecholamines, a very important hormone in first-line endocrine counter-regulation in hypoglycemia. Repeated and frequent hypoglycemia leads to a blunting of the counter-regulatory response of glucagon secretion that can only be overcome by meticulous avoidance of frequent hypoglycemia. Furthermore, with the progression of type 1 diabetes and long-term changes in islet architecture, A-cells additionally become increasingly insensitive to changes in the plasma glucose concentrations and a further defect in glucagon secretion under hypoglycemic conditions is observed [3,21].

Type 2 Diabetes

In type 2 diabetes, a relative excess of circulating glucagon is observed. Hyperglycemia does not adequately suppress glucagon release, so that plasma glucagon concentrations are normal or elevated instead of decreased. The reasons for this phenomenon are not completely clear, possible explanations could be an intrinsic defect in glucose recognition by A-cells, insulin resistance of the A-cells themselves or desensitization of the A-cells due to chronic hyperglycemia. Glucagon excess will contribute to increased hepatic glucose production and an impaired ability to suppress hepatic glucose output by insulin, resulting in a perpetuation of hyperglycemia. The incretin hormone GLP-1 is able to suppress glucagon secretion in type 2 diabetes effectively [3].

Somatostatin and Pancreatic D-cells

Somatostatin is a peptide hormone and neurotransmitter that is found ubiquitously in the hypothalamus, in the endocrine cells of the mucosa of the stomach and small intestine, and in the D-cells of the pancreas. It was first isolated from the hypothalamus, where it inhibits pituitary growth hormone secretion. There are two molecular forms, somatostatin 14, which has 14 amino acids, and the longer somatostatin 28, which are formed by alternative processing. In the D-cell, somatostatin 14 is the predominant form [22].

D-cells have long cytoplasmic processes in contact with other islets cells and capillaries, which facilitate their paracrine activities. Pancreatic somatostatin primarily inhibits insulin and glucagon secretion. The glucagon suppression in hyperglycemia is thought to be mediated by somatostatin [3].

Somatostatin from D-cells is secreted in response to elevated plasma glucose and glucagon concentrations and by insulin deficiency. In insulin deficiency, the stimulation of somatostatin release might be mediated indirectly by hyperglycemia, free fatty acids, and ketone bodies. Amino acids, peptide hormones, and various neurotransmitters (see Table 5.2) are additional secretagogues. Pancreatic somatostatin has profound effects on the secretion of other islet hormones, but it contributes only little to the circulating levels of somatostatin, which is mostly the somatostatin 28 secreted by the gut [3].

Pancreatic Polypeptide

PP is a peptide that contains 36 amino acids and is secreted by the PP-cells. Islets with a larger proportion of PP-cells are located mainly in the dorsal part of the head of the pancreas; islets in other locations of the pancreas contain only a few PP-cells. Protein and fat in meals are secretagogues for the release of PP via vagal cholinergic pathways. PP may physiologically inhibit pancreatic exocrine function and gallbladder contraction, opposing the effect of CCK, or it may have trophic effects on the pancreas. PP also has anorectic properties and has been shown to terminate feeding in animals [3]. PP does not have any stimulatory or inhibitory effect on other islet hormones.

Islet Amyloid Polypeptide (IAPP, Amylin)

Amylin, which was first discovered in 1987, is cosecreted with insulin from the B-cells. Pancreatic amylin acts as a short-term satiety hormone mainly by binding to specific binding sites in the hypothalamus. It is released during meals; exogenous amylin leads to a dose-related reduction in meal size. Amylin's anorectic effect may in part be due to reduced expression of orexigenic neuropeptides in the lateral hypothalamic area. The anorectic action of amylin is one important factor in amylin's overall role to control the influx of nutrients into the circulation. By reducing food intake and gastric acid secretion, limiting the rate of gastric emptying, and diminishing pancreatic glucagon and digestive enzyme secretion, amylin regulates nutrient disappearance and postprandial glucose concentration. Amylin seems to be a necessary and complementary factor to insulin, which regulates the rate of nutrient disappearance. In this sense, amylin and insulin are adjunct players in the control of nutrient fluxes, and amylin's role to control feeding is a pivotal factor in this regard [23].

Amylin is thus deficient in diabetic people. Amylin replacement could therefore possibly improve glycemic control in some people with diabetes. However, human amylin exhibits physicochemical properties that predispose the peptide hormone to aggregate and form amyloid fibers, which may play a part in B-cell destruction in type 2 diabetes. This obviously makes it unsuitable for pharmacological use. A stable analog, pramlintide (Symlin), which has actions and pharmacokinetic and pharmacodynamic properties similar to the native peptide, has been developed and recently approved as an adjunct therapeutic agent for patients with type 1 or type 2 diabetes treated with insulin and not achieving the desired metabolic control [24].

Pancreas and Islet Transplantation

Since 1921 and until recently, insulin by injection has been the only treatment for patients with diabetes mellitus type 1. Pancreas transplantation is currently the curative treatment for type 1 diabetes mellitus. It aims at providing physiological insulin replacement therapy for type 1 diabetes mellitus. The goal is thereby also to prevent the secondary complications of diabetes. Long-term control of glucose metabolism has only been achieved by pancreas transplantation. As a result of improvements in the surgical techniques and the efficacy of immunosuppression, the patient and graft survival rates have improved dramatically over the last two decades. As a result, pancreas transplantation, as part of simultaneous pancreas and kidney transplantation, pancreas after kidney transplantation, and exceptionally pancreas transplantation alone, has become the standard therapeutic option for patients with type 1 diabetes mellitus with end-stage renal disease [25].

After pancreas transplantation, which became possible in 1977, the next logical step to cure patients with diabetes mellitus type 1 is transplantation of the islets of Langerhans. In the last few years, the results of islet transplantation have markedly improved thanks to progress in the isolation technique of islets and better immunosuppressive protocols. In addition, the islets are infused into the portal circulation, where

Table 5.3. Enteroendocrine tumor syndromes other than carcinoid (with permission, modified from [27]). *SSTA* somatostatin analog, *WDHA* watery diarrhea-hypokalemia-achlorhydria, *ACTH* adrenocorticotropic hormone, *PTHrP* parathyroid-hormone-related peptide, *GRH* growth-hormone-releasing factor

Tumor	Syndrome	Hormone	Clinical features	Site	Percent malignant	Treatment
Insulinoma	Insulinoma	Insulin proinsulin	Hypoglycemia Weight gain	>95% Pancreas	>10	Surgery, diet intravenous dextrose, chemotherapy, diazoxide, SSTA
Gastrinoma	ZES	Gastrin	Abdominal pain, peptic ulceration, diarrhea, gastric hypersecretion	Duodenum 70%, pancreas 25%	60–90	Proton pump inhibit, surgery, SSTA, chemotherapy
VIPoma	Verner-Morrison pancreatic cholera WDHA	VIP	Secretory diarrhea hypokalemia, achlorhydria, metabolic acidosis, flushing, weight loss	90% Pancreas	>50	Intravenous fluids, surgery, SSTA, chemotherapy
Glucagonoma	Glucagonoma syndrome	Glucagon	Diabetes, necrolytic migratory erythema, deep vein thrombosis, depression	Pancreas	>50	Surgery, diet, SSTA, insulin, anticoagulant, chemotherapy
Somatostatinoma	Somatostatinoma syndrome	Somatostatin	Diabetes, gallstones, weight loss, steatorrhea	Pancreas 56%, upper intestine 44%	70–80	Surgery, insulin, pancreatic enzymes
Extremely rare tumors						
ACTHoma	Ectopic Cushing's syndrome	ACTH	Hypertension, diabetes, weakness	Pancreas 30%, lung 50%	>99	Surgery, chemotherapy, SSTA
PTHrPoma	Hyperparathyroidism	Parathyroid hormone-related peptide	Hypercalcemia, nephrolithiasis	Pancreas	>99	Surgery, chemotherapy
Neurotensinoma	?	Neurotensin	Diabetes, diarrhea, flushing, hypertension, weight loss, edema	Pancreas	?	Surgery, chemotherapy
Calcitoninoma	?	Calcitonin	?	Pancreas, lung	>80	Surgery, chemotherapy
GRFoma	Acromegaly	Growth hormone-releasing factor	Acromegaly	Pancreas, lung, thymus	30	Surgery, SSTA

they can function more physiologically than in the peripheral circulation, as in whole organ pancreatic transplants. More than 470 patients with type 1 diabetes have received islet transplants at 43 institutions worldwide in the past 5 years. High rates of insulin independence have been observed at 1 year in the leading islet transplant centers, and an international multicenter trial has demonstrated reproducible success of the approach. Loss of insulin independence by 5 years in the majority of recipients remains of concern. Ongoing problems in islet transplantation are alloimmunity, autoimmunity, and the growing shortage of donor pancreases. Alternatives to pancreas donation, be it post mortem or from a living donor, could be: xenotransplantation with the aid of pig islets, and B-cell neogenesis from embryonic stem cells or pancreatic duct cells [26].

Insulinomas and Other Endocrine Tumors of the Pancreas

Clinically significant pancreatic endocrine tumors (PET) have been reported to occur in approximately 1 per 100,000 people per year and account for only 1–2% of all pancreatic tumors. Insulinomas are the most common functioning PETs, with a 17% incidence, followed by gastrinoma (15%), PPoma (9%), VIPoma (2%), glucagonoma (1%), carcinoid (<1%), and somatostatinoma (1%); the remainder are comprised of neurotensinomas, adrenocorticotropic hormeoma (ACTHoma), GRFomas, calcitonin-producing tumors, parathyroid-hormone-related peptide tumors, and other exceedingly rare neoplasms. This whole group of very rare PETs accounts for no more than 1–2% of the group of all PETs. It must also be borne in mind that almost all of the PETs can be multiple and can arise outside of the pancreas, particularly gastrinomas (<77%), carcinoids (99%), and somatostatinomas (>40%). Nonfunctioning PETs comprise the largest group of these tumors (15–30%). Table 5.3 gives an overview on the clinical features of the most abundant PETs.

Neuroglycopenic symptoms with repeated episodes of hypoglycemia are present in almost all insulinoma patients. The symptoms are transiently relieved by the administration of carbohydrates. These symptoms are called Whipple's triad. Inappropriately high and autonomous secretion of insulin and proinsulin at rates that are not determined by metabolic needs are the cause for the recurrent hypoglycemias. Cardiovascular symptoms are the main presenting features in 17%. The most common clinical test used when a patient is suspected to have an insulinoma is prolonged fasting (for at least 48 h if hypoglycemia does not develop within shorter periods) with frequent blood sampling for the measurement of glucose, insulin, C-peptide, and if possible proinsulin. Diagnostic accuracy may be improved by using an "amended" insulin to glucose ratio with a normal value of <0.5 (mU/ml)/(mg/dl). This ratio is obtained by subtracting 30 mg/dl from the plasma glucose value, so that the glucose value may become zero or negative (with ∞ values for the ratio) when the plasma glucose falls below 30 mg/dl. Almost all insulinomas (97%) are located in the pancreas and most are small. One-half or more are undetected before surgery, but more than 90% can be localized by palpation alone or aided by intraoperative ultrasound. Surgery is the principal treatment for insulinomas. It has been noted that octreotide treatment may make hypoglycemia worse in insulinoma patients lacking the somatostatin receptor subtypes 2 (SSTr2) and 5 (SSTr5), and can therefore fail to suppress insulin production and may blunt the compensatory glucagon response. Hence, this treatment should be reserved for only the minority of insulinoma patients with positive imaging on somatostatin receptor scintigraphy (SRS) [3,27].

References

1. Klöppel G, Gepts W, In't Veld PA (1992) Morphology of the pancreas in normal and diabetic states. In: Alberti KGGM, DeFronzo RA, Kenn H, Zimmet P (eds) International Textbook of Diabetes Mellitus. John Wiley and Sons, Chichester, pp 223–259
2. Bonner-Weir S, Orci L (1982) New perspectives on the microvasculature of the islets of Langerhans in the rat. Diabetes 31:883–889
3. Nauck MA (1998) Physiology and pathophysiology of endocrine pancreatic secretion. In: Beger HG, Warshaw AL, Büchler MW, et al (eds) The Pancreas. Blackwell Science, Oxford, pp 101–137
4. Madsbad S, Hartling SG, Faber OK (1992) C-peptide and proinsulin. In: Alberti KGGM, DeFronzo RA, Kenn H, Zimmet P (eds) International Textbook of Diabetes. John Wiley and Sons, Chichester, pp 303–332
5. Hutton JC (1994) Insulin secretory granule biogenesis and the proinsulin-processing endopeptidases. Diabetologia 37 Suppl 2:S48–56
6. Malaisse WJ (1992) Insulin biosynthesis and secretion in vitro. In: Alberti KGGM, DeFronzo RA, Kenn H, Zimmet P (eds) International Textbook of Diabetes. John Wiley and Sons, Chichester, pp 261–283
7. Meier JJ, Nauck MA (2005) Glucagon-like peptide 1 (GLP-1) in biology and pathology. Diabetes Metab Res Rev 21:91–117
8. Matschinsky FM (1996) Banting Lecture 1995. A lesson in metabolic regulation inspired by the glucokinase glucose sensor paradigm. Diabetes 45:223–241

9. Minami K, Miki T, Kadowaki T, Seino S (2004) Roles of ATP-sensitive K+ channels as metabolic sensors: studies of Kir6.x null mice. Diabetes 53 Suppl 3:S176–180
10. Shapiro ET, Tillil H, Rubenstein AH, Polonsky KS (1988) Peripheral insulin parallels changes in insulin secretion more closely than C-peptide after bolus intravenous glucose administration. J Clin Endocrinol Metab 67:1094–1099
11. Creutzfeldt W (1979) The incretin concept today. Diabetologia 16:75–85
12. Porksen N, Hollingdal M, Juhl C, Butler P, Veldhuis JD, Schmitz O (2002) Pulsatile insulin secretion: detection, regulation, and role in diabetes. Diabetes 51 Suppl 1:S245–254
13. Bottazzo GF, Florin-Christensen A, Doniach D (1974) Islet-cell antibodies in diabetes mellitus with autoimmune polyendocrine deficiencies. Lancet 2:1279–1283
14. The DCCT Research Group (1987) Effects of age, duration and treatment of insulin-dependent diabetes mellitus on residual beta-cell function: observations during eligibility testing for the Diabetes Control and Complications Trial (DCCT). J Clin Endocrinol Metab 65:30–36
15. Butler AE, Janson J, Bonner-Weir S, Ritzel R, Rizza RA, Butler PC (2003) Beta-cell deficit and increased beta-cell apoptosis in humans with type 2 diabetes. Diabetes 52:102–110
16. Polonsky KS, Given BD, Hirsch LJ, et al (1988) Abnormal patterns of insulin secretion in non-insulin-dependent diabetes mellitus. N Engl J Med 318:1231–1239
17. Meier JJ, Gallwitz B, Nauck MA (2003) Glucagon-like peptide 1 and gastric inhibitory polypeptide: potential applications in type 2 diabetes mellitus. BioDrugs 17:93–102
18. Reaven GM, Hollenbeck C, Jeng CY, Wu MS, Chen YD (1988) Measurement of plasma glucose, free fatty acid, lactate, and insulin for 24 h in patients with NIDDM. Diabetes 37:1020–1024
19. Velho G, Robert JJ (2002) Maturity-onset diabetes of the young (MODY): genetic and clinical characteristics. Horm Res 57 Suppl 1:29–33
20. Jiang G, Zhang BB (2003) Glucagon and regulation of glucose metabolism. Am J Physiol Endocrinol Metab 284:E671–678
21. Mitrakou A, Ryan C, Veneman T, et al (1991) Hierarchy of glycemic thresholds for counterregulatory hormone secretion, symptoms, and cerebral dysfunction. Am J Physiol 260: E67–74
22. Reichlin S (1983) Somatostatin (parts 1 and 2). New Engl J Med 309:1495–1501; 1556–1563
23. Lutz TA (2005) Pancreatic amylin as a centrally acting satiating hormone. Curr Drug Targets 6:181–189
24. Schmitz O, Brock B, Rungby J (2004) Amylin agonists: a novel approach in the treatment of diabetes. Diabetes 53 Suppl 3:S233–238
25. Al-Shurafa HA, Jawdat MT, Bassas AF, Rogiers XC, Bechstein WO (2002) Innovations in pancreas transplantation. Saudi Med J 23:265–271
26. Shapiro AM, Lakey JR, Paty BW, Senior PA, Bigam DL, Ryan EA (2005) Strategic opportunities in clinical islet transplantation. Transplantation 79:1304–1307
27. Warner RR (2005) Enteroendocrine tumors other than carcinoid: a review of clinically significant advances. Gastroenterology 128:1668–1684

Chapter 6

M. Staritz

Sphincter of Oddi Physiology and Pathophysiology

Since its original description by Ruggero Oddi in 1887, sphincter of Oddi (SO) physiology and pathophysiology has been the subject of much studios and investigations. Its existence as a distinct anatomic and physiologic entity has been discussed with much controversy. Hence, it is not surprising that the clinical syndrome of SO dysfunction (SOD) and its therapy are controversial fields. This chapter reviews the anatomy and physiology of the SO, clinical presentations of pathophysiology, and methods of diagnosing and treating SOD.

Anatomy and Physiology

Bile Ducts, Gallbladder

The SO is located at the end of the biliary tree, which begins in the liver with canaliculi that converge to form hepatic ducts, which in turn converge to form the common hepatic duct. In these ducts there are only few small muscle cells, which are oriented circumferentially. The cystic duct also contains a thin layer of muscle that is continuous with the muscle layer of the gallbladder, with most of the cells located circumferentially. The common bile duct (CBD) has only sparse longitudinal muscle fibers, which become more prominent in the distal duct, but very few circular-oriented fibers. The gallbladder wall has a muscular layer with bundles oriented mainly along the longitudinal axis in the body and along the circular axis in the neck. Of gallbladder emptying, 20–30% actually occurs during the interdigestive period, during phase II of the migrating motor complex. It is hypothesized that this interdigestive gallbladder emptying may play housekeeping function to decrease the risk of building up gallstones. Meal-induced cholecystokinin (CCK) secretion stimulates gallbladder contraction and SO relaxation.

Sphincter of Oddi

The SO is a small complex of smooth muscles surrounding the terminal CBD, main pancreatic duct of Wirsung, and the common channel (ampulla of Vater), when present. It has both circular and longitudinal components. The high-pressure zone generated by the sphincter varies between 4 and 10 mm, in length. Its role is to regulate bile and pancreatic exocrine juice flow, to prevent duodenum-to-duct reflux, and to maintain a sterile intraductal environment. The SO possesses both a variable basal pressure and a superimposed phasic contractile activity. The former appears to be the predominant mechanism, regulating outflow of pancreaticobiliary secretion into the intestine. Although phasic SO contractions may aid in regulating bile and pancreatic juice flow, their primary role appears to be maintaining a sterile intraductal milieu. Sphincter regulation is under both neural and hormonal control. Phasic wave activity of the sphincter is closely related to the migrating motor complex of the duodenum. Innervation of the bile duct does not appear to be essential, as sphincter function has been reported to be preserved following liver transplantation [1]. Although regulatory processes vary among species, CCK and secretin appear to be most important in causing sphincter relaxation, while nonadrenergic and noncholinergic neurons, which at least in part transmit vasoactive intestinal peptide and nitric oxide, sphincter of Oddi also relax the sphincter [2]. The role of cholecystectomy in altering these neural pathways needs further definition. Luman and colleagues [3] reported that cholecystectomy suppresses the normal inhibitory effect of pharmacological doses of CCK on the SO. However, the mechanism underlying this effect is unknown.

Wedge specimens of the SO obtained at surgical sphincteroplasty from SOD patients show evidence of inflammation, muscular hypertrophy, fibrosis, or adenomyosis within the papillary zone in approximately 60% of patients [4]. In the remaining 40% with normal histology, a motor disorder is suggested. Less commonly, infections with cytomegalovirus or *Cryptosporidium*, as may occur in acquired immunodeficiency syndrome (AIDS) patients, or *Strongiloides* have caused SOD.

How does SOD cause pain? From a theoretical point of view, abnormalities of the SO may cause pain by impeding the flow of bile and pancreatic juice resulting in ductal hypertension, ischemia arising from spastic contractions, and "hypersensitivity" of the papilla. Although unproven, these mechanism may act alone or in concert to explain the genesis of pain.

Definition of SOD

SOD is a benign, noncalculous, obstructive disorder that occurs at the level of the SO. The pathogenesis of SOD relates either to passive obstruction at the SO caused by fibrosis and/or inflammation or to active obstruction caused by sphincter muscle spasm. These two mechanisms of functional obstruction at the SO are not mutually exclusive. Less precise terms for SOD in the medical literature include papillary stenosis, biliary dyskinesia, and postcholecystectomy syndrome.

SOD may be manifested clinically by pancreaticobiliary pain, pancreatitis, or deranged liver function test. It is actually made up of two entities. SO dyskinesia refers to a primary motor abnormality of the SO that may result in a hypertonic sphincter. In contrast, SO stenosis refers to a structural alteration of the sphincter, probably from an inflammatory process, with subsequent fibrosis. As it is often impossible to distinguish patients with SO dyskinesia from those with SO stenosis, the term SOD has been used to incorporate both groups of patients. In an attempt to deal with this overlap in etiology, and to determine the appropriate utilization of SO manometry (SOM), a clinical classification system has been developed for patients with suspected SOD [5] based on clinical history, laboratory results, and endoscopic retrograde cholangiopancreatography (ERCP) findings.

A variety of less accurate terms are listed in the medical literature to describe this entity, such as papillary stenosis, ampullary stenosis, biliary dyskinesia, and postcholecystectomy syndrome, even though SOD may occur with the gallbladder in situ.

Epidemiology of SOD

SOD may occur in pediatric or adult patients of any age; however, patients with SOD are typically middle-aged females [6]. A survey on functional gastrointestinal disorders confirmed that SOD affects females more frequently than males and indicated a high association with work absenteeism, disability, and healthcare use. Although SOD most commonly occurs after cholecystectomy, it may be present with the gallbladder in situ.

The Frequency of manometrically documented SOD in patients prior to cholecystectomy has received limited study. Guelrud and colleagues [4] studied 121 patients with symptomatic gallstones and a normal CBD diameter measured by transcutaneous ultrasound. Using SOM prior to cholecystectomy, an elevated basal sphincter pressure was found in 11.6%. SOD was diagnosed in 4.1% of patients with a normal serum alkaline phosphatase levels (4 of 96) and in 40% with elevated serum alkaline phosphatase levels (10 of 25).

Postcholecystectomy pain resembling the patients' preoperative biliary colic occurs in at least 10–20% of patients. The frequency of diagnosing SOD in reported series varies considerably with the patient selection criteria, the definition of SOD utilized, and the diagnostic tools employed. In a British report, SOD was diagnosed in 9% of 451 consecutive patients being evaluated for postcholecystectomy pain [7]. Robert-Thomson evaluated 431 similar patients and found SOD in 11%. In a subpopulation of such patients with a normal ERCP (except dilated ducts in 28%) and recurrent pain of more than 3 months duration, SOD was diagnosed in 68% [8]. Sherman and colleagues used SOM to evaluate 115 patients with pancreaticobiliary pain with and without liver function test abnormalities [9].

Patients with bile duct stones and tumors were excluded from analysis. Fifty-nine of 115 patients (51%) had an abnormal basal SO pressure greater than 40 mmHg. These patients were further categorized by the Hogan-Green SOD classification system. The frequency of abnormal manometry was 86%, 55%, and 28%, for type I, II, and III patients, respectively. These abnormal manometric frequencies are very similar to those reported by others for type I and type II patients [10,11]. In type III patients, the finding of an abnormal basal sphincter pressure has varied from 12 to 55% [12]. As noted, patient selection factors may be one explanation for this great variability.

Dysfunction may also occur in the pancreatic duct portion of the SO and cause recurrent pancreatitis and pancreatic-type pain. Although a pancreatic SOD classification system has been developed (similar to the biliary SOD classification system), it has not been widely utilized. Manometrically documented SOD has been reported in 15–72% of patients with recurrent pancreatitis, previously labeled as idiopathic [12–14].

Clinical Presentation

SOD is a possible cause of three clinical conditions: (1) persistent or recurrent biliary pain following cholecystectomy in the absence of structural abnormalities, (2) idiopathic recurrent pancreatitis, and (3) biliary pain in patients with intact gallbladders but without cholelithiasis. SOD also has been described in patients with previous liver transplantation, and AIDS, and in patients with hyperlipidemia.

Although SOD has been diagnosed in all age groups, it is most common in middle-aged women. The female predominance among patients varies from 75 to 90%. The pain is very often of biliary colic, mostly epigastric, or occurs in the right upper quadrant. It may radiate to the back or the right shoulder blade. The pain is usually episodic and severe, but may be continuous with episodic exacerbations. Approximately one-half of patients have abnormal liver biochemical test results, although transient elevation of serum aminotransferase levels with attacks of pain supports the diagnosis of SOD.

Diagnosis of SOD

Noninvasive Evaluation

Evaluation of patients suspected of having SOD is initiated with liver biochemical testing, serum amylase and lipase measurements, and often abdominal imaging by either ultrasonography or computed tomographic scanning. Serum aminotransferase level elevations, if present, are mild, less than three to four times the upper limit of normal. Physical examination findings are usually normal, although mild, right upper quadrant tenderness may be present. Standard evaluation and therapeutic trials for more common causes of abdominal pain, such as gastroesophageal reflux, fatty liver, and irritable bowl syndrome, are usually undertaken as well.

Diagnostic Methods (Noninvasive)

Because SOM is considered by most authorities to be the gold standard for diagnosing SOD, is difficult to perform, invasive, not widely available, and associated with a relatively high complication rate, several noninvasive and provocative tests have been designed in an attempt to identify patients with SOD.

Morphine-Prostigmin Provocative Test (Nardi Test)

Morphine has been shown to cause SO contraction. Prostigmin (Neostigmine), 1 mg, is added subcutaneously as a vigorous cholinergic secretory stimulant to morphine (10 mg subcutaneously) to make this challenge test. Historically, the morphine-prostigmin test was been used extensively to diagnose SOD. Reproduction of the patient's typical pain associated with a fourfold increase in aspartate aminotransferase, alanine aminotransferase, alkaline phosphatase, amylase, or lipase constitute a positive response. The usefulness of this test is limited by its low sensitivity and specificity in predicting the presence of SOD and its poor correlation with outcome after sphincter ablation. This test has been largely replaced by tests believed to be more sensitive.

Ultrasonographic Assessment of Extrahepatic Bile Duct and Main Pancreatic Duct Diameter After Secretory Stimulation

After a lipid-rich meal or CCK administration, the gallbladder contracts, bile flow from the hepatocytes increases, and the SO relaxes, resulting in bile entry into the duodenum. Similarly, after a lipid-rich meal or secretin administration, pancreatic exocrine juice flow is stimulated and the SO relaxes. If the SO is dysfunctional and causes obstruction to flow, the CBD or main pancreatic duct may dilate under secretory pressure. This can be monitored by transcutaneous ultrasonography. Sphincter and terminal duct obstruction from other causes (e.g., stones, tumors, strictures) may similarly cause ductal dilation and need to be excluded. Pain provocation should also be noted if present. To date, limited studies comparing these noninvasive tests with SOM or outcome after sphincter ablation show only a modest correlation [15]. Because of intestinal gas, the pancreatic duct may not be visualized on standard transcutaneous ultrasound. Despite the superiority of endoscopic ultrasound in visualizing the pancreas, it does not exceed the reported sensitivity of secretin-stimulated endoscopic ultrasound in detecting SOD (50–60%).

Quantitative Hepatobiliary Scintigraphy

Hepatobiliary scintigraphy assesses bile flow through the biliary tract. Impairment to bile flow from sphincter disease, tumors, or stones results in impaired radionuclide flow. The precise criteria for defining an abnormal study remains controversial, but a duodenal arrival time greater than 20 min and a hilum-to-duodenum time greater than 10 min are the most widely accepted. Most studies are flawed by lack of correlation with SOM or outcome after sphincter ablation.

In the absence of more definitive data, it is currently concluded that noninvasive testing for SOD has a relatively low or undefined sensitivity and specificity and therefore is not recommended for general clinical use, except in situations where more definitive testing (manometry) is unsuccessful or unavailable.

Classification of Possible SODs

Patients with suspected biliary SOD are classified into three categories, depending on the clinical data that support the diagnosis (Table 6.1). Bile duct dilation is one of these criteria, although considerable overlap in the diameter of the CBD of patients with SOD and asymptomatic postcholecystectomy patients exists, and the value of this criterion has been questioned. The common cutoff for an abnormal bile duct diameter following cholecystectomy is 12 mm, although the standard varies from 10 to 15 mm in several studies. Elevated levels of liver enzymes, especially when associated with attacks of pain, appear to be predictive of pain relief after sphincterotomy.

The Milwaukee criterion is that both serum alkaline phosphatase and aminotransferase levels should be elevated (two times the normal) on two occasions, whereas the criterion in the modified Milwaukee classification system is that any liver enzyme level be abnormal (1.1 times normal) on one occasion. Neither classification system requires that the enzyme level elevations be timed with attacks of pain, although such an association may be a predictor of response to treatment. Delayed drainage of bile into the duodenum at cholangiography (more than 45 min) is the third criterion for suspected SOD, although this criterion appears to lack specificity, because delayed drainage may occur in normal people following cholecystectomy. Additionally, few endoscopists take the time to obtain this measurement. In fact, some researchers have suggested that the Milwaukee classification should be modified further to consider only bile duct diameter and elevated serum aminotransferase levels as criteria for SOD. Despite these problems with the clinical criteria, however, these classification systems have remained useful because of their ability to predict the outcome of biliary sphincter ablation.

Table 6.1. Hogan-Geenen sphincter of Oddi classification system related to the frequency of abnormal sphincter of Oddi manometry and pain relief by biliary sphincterotomy. *SGOT* Serum glutamic oxaloacetic transaminase, *ERCP* endoscopic retrograde cholangiopancreatography, *CBD* common bile duct,

Patient group classifications	Approximate frequency of abnormal sphincter manometry	Probability of pain relief by sphincterotomy if manometry:		Manometry before sphincter ablation
		Abnormal	Normal	
Biliary I Patients with biliary-type pain Abnormal SGOT or alkaline >2 × normal documented on two or more occasions, delayed drainage of ERCP contrast from the biliary tree <45 min, and dilated CBD <12 mm diameter	75–95%	90–95%	90–95%	Unnecessary
Biliary II Patients with biliary-type pain and only one or two of the above criteria	55–65%	85%	35%	Highly recommended
Biliary III Patients with only biliary-type pain and no other abnormalities	25–60%	55–65%	<10%	Mandatory

Lehmann and colleagues [12] have devised a similar classification system for possible pancreatic SOD. Pancreatic type I patients have pancreatic-type pain, a serum amylase or lipase level of 1.1 times normal on one occasion, and pancreatic duct dilation (<6 mm in the head and <5 mm in the body); pancreatic type II patients have pain and one of the preceding criteria; type III patients have pancreatic-type pain only. Several studies have demonstrated a high frequency (60–72%) of sphincter hypertension in patients with idiopathic pancreatitis, and a 50–87% frequency in those with chronic pancreatitis. The utility of this pancreatic classification system will depend on outcome studies of the symptomatic response to pancreatic sphincter ablation.

Invasive Methods

Patients with suspected SOD have the highest complication rates for endoscopic retrograde ERCP and sphincterotomy. Rates of pancreatitis of 20% have been reported in this group. Therefore, ERCP with manometry should be reserved for persons who have severe or debilitating symptoms. Cholangiography is essential to rule out stones or tumors as the cause of biliary obstruction and associated symptoms. Alternative biliary imaging studies, such as magnetic resonance cholangiopancreatography or endoscopic ultrasonography, are safer methods than ERCP for excluding stones or tumors, although they cannot be used to diagnose SOD.

Occasionally, an intra-ampullary neoplasm may simulate SOD. If there appears to be excess tissue in the ampulla after sphincterotomy, biopsy specimens of the area should be obtained.

Sphincter Manometry: The Technique

SOM is usually performed during ERCP. All drugs that relax (nitrates, calcium channel blockers, glucagon, and anticholinergics) or stimulate (narcotics and cholinergic agents) the SO should be avoided for 12 h prior to manometry. Benzodiazepine does not affect basal sphincter pressure, and can serve as sedation. Meperidine does increase phasic wave frequency. Anecdotal evidence indicates that droperidol may also be used as a preanesthetic. Glucagon should be avoided, although some authorities use it if necessary to achieve cannulation and wait at least 8–10 min until sphincter function is restored before measuring pressures.

SOM utilizes pressure recording equipment and infusion systems similar to those used for esophageal motility studies. Important differences are that the infusion system for SOM must be sterile. The infusion rate is 0.25 ml per channel using a low-compliance pump. Performance of manometry requires a two-person approach, with one person stationed at the recorder. Triple-lumen 5-French catheters are produced by several manufactures in long-nose and short-nose types. The long-nose catheter has the advantage in the biliary duct of allowing several pull-throughs without losing cannulation, although in tortuous pancreatic ducts the nose is occasionally too long for free cannulation. The three orifices are spaced 2 mm apart and are oriented radially.

When manometry is clinically indicated, many experts begin ERCP with the manometry catheter, because the duodenum has less motility if contrast medium has not been given. The duodenal or zero pressure should be measured before cannulation and at the end of the manometry. The catheter is withdrawn across the sphincter at 1- to 2-mm intervals by using a standard station pull-through technique. Abnormalities of the basal sphincter pressure should be observed on at least two pull-throughs. Depending on the clinical indication, pancreatic SOM may then be performed by the same technique. Abnormal basal sphincter pressures are usually concordant for the two ducts but may occur in only portion of the sphincter. If the clinical indication for SOM is biliary pain, rather than idiopathic pancreatitis, and biliary SOM produces normal findings, some authorities avoid pancreatic cannulation entirely, with the goal of decreasing the frequency of pancreatitis. Other experts advise studying both ducts in all patients. It has been shown that increased basal sphincter pressure is more likely to be confined to the pancreas in patients with pancreatitis and more likely confined to the bile duct in persons with elevated levels of serum liver enzymes. When the biliary SOM result is abnormal and biliary sphincterotomy is performed, placement of a pancreatic duct stent, when there is associated pancreatic sphincter hypertension, lowers the risk of procedure-induced pancreatitis. When the clinical indication for SOM is idiopathic recurrent pancreatitis, pancreatic manometry is mandatory. After the tracings are completed, glucagon or additional meperidine may be given to facilitate subsequent contrast injection or endoscopic therapy. If a simple cholangiogram is desired, the aspirating part can be used for contrast injection.

The method of averaging interpretable trancings and the number of leads used to take these measure-

Table 6.2. Suggested standard for abnormal values for endoscopic sphincter of Oddi manometry obtained form 50 volunteers without abdominal symptoms. Values were obtained by adding 3 standard deviations to the mean (means were obtained by averaging the results on 2–3 station pull-throughs. Data combine pancreatic and biliary studies

Basal sphincter pressure[a]	>35 mmHg
Basal ductal pressure	>13 mmHg
Phasic contractions	
– Amplitude	>220 mmHg
– Duration	>8 s
– Frequency	>10/min

[a] Basal pressure determined by: (1) reading the peak basal pressure (i.e., highest single lead as obtained using a three-lumen catheter); (2) obtaining the mean of these peak pressures from multiple station pull-throughs

ments vary from center to center, although interobserver differences appear to be minimal. The standard upper limit (Table 6.2) of normal for baseline sphincter pressure is 35–40 mmHg. The reproducibility of these measurements was proven in an important study of normal volunteers by Guelrud et al. (Table 6.2) [16]. The phasic wave frequency, propagation direction of waves, and amplitude of the waves also can be determined, although the clinical significance of these measurements remains unclear. Additional pharmacologic maneuvers, such as provocation with CCK, are also of uncertain value.

SOM: Diagnostic Use

Only one controlled study of patients with suspected type II biliary SOD suggests SOM as predictive of responsiveness of pain to sphincterotomy [18]. Patients with an elevated basal SO pressure of greater than 40 mm Hg had a clinical response rate of 91% compared with a 25% rate in patients with a high basal pressure in whom a sham sphincterotomy was performed. For patients with a normal SO pressure, the response to sphincterotomy was only 42% and similar to that after the sham procedure (33%). These results were confirmed in a controlled study [19] of patients with type II SOD and elevated sphincter pressure. In this study, clinical improvement was demonstrated in 11 of 13 patients treated with sphincterotomy compared with 5 of 13 control subjects treated with sham sphincterotomy. There was no difference in pain response between sphincterotomy and sham sphincterotomy in patients with manometric abnormalities other than elevated basal SO pressure, namely, tachyoddia, increased retrograde contractions, or a paradoxical response to CCK.

Despite the findings of these studies, the use of SOM as a diagnostic tool remains somewhat controversial. Some uncontrolled studies suggest that more easily measurable criteria such as elevated liver enzyme levels or biliary dilation are superior in predicting a response to sphincter ablation.

Alternatively, manometry may be highly specific in diagnosing SOD, but may lack sensitivity. A possible explanation for the insensitivity of SOM is that short-term observation of sphincter pressure may not detect the underlying pathophysiologic process. An additional problem with manometry is the high rate of procedure-related morbidity, especially pancreatitis, which occurs in 10–25% of patients who have SOM. SOM is a difficult technique that is not widely available and has success rates of only 75–92% in experienced hands.

In biliary type III patients, SOD appears to be less common than in type II patients, and the response to sphincter ablation is only 39–60%. A response to sphincter ablation in type III patients with normal SOM findings is rare. Obviously, pain is a poor indicator of any specific regional disorder. Abnormal small-bowel interdigestive motor activity and duodenal visceral hyperalgesia in response to duodenal (but not rectal) distension have been demonstrated in SOD type III patients. As in other functional gastrointestinal disorders, somatization disorder may be more common in these patient populations than in the general population.

Other Diagnostic Methods

Placement of a pancreatic or biliary stent on a trial basis with the goal of achieving pain relief and thereby predicting a response to subsequent sphincterotomy has been suggested to be superior to manometry [20]. Although relief of pain with placement of a biliary stent is predictive of long-term relief after biliary sphincterotomy, the high rate of pancreatitis in the stented patients has dampened enthusiasm for this technique. Pancreatic duct stents are strongly discouraged as a therapeutic trial because of their propensity to cause ductal injury if left in place for more than a few days.

Injection of botulinum toxin into the SO decrease basal sphincter pressure by about 50%. Its use also has been proposed as a therapeutic trial to assess the like-

Table 6.3. Change in the mean pain score (using a 0–1, none–most severe, linear pain scale) and number of hospital days per month required for pain in patients with manometrically documented sphincter of Oddi dysfunction (SOD) randomized to endoscopic sphincterotomy (*ES*), sham sphincterotomy (*S-ES*), and surgical sphincteroplasty with or without cholecystectomy (*SSp±CCx*) [27]

Therapy	Follow-up years	Mean pain score		Hospital days/month		% patients improved
		Pre-Rx	Post-Rx	Pre-Rx	Post-Rx	
ES (*n*=19)	3.3	9.2	3.9	0.85	0.23	68%
S-ES (*n* =17)	2.2	9.4	7.2	0.87	0.89	24%
SSp±CCx (*n* =16)	3.4	9.4	3.3	0.94	0.27	69%

Table 6.4. Clinical benefit correlated with sphincter of SOD type [27]

SOD Type[a]	Patients improved/total patients ES	S-ES	SSp+/-CCx
Type II	5/6 (83%)	1/7 (14%)	8/10 (80%)
Type III	8/13 (62%)	3/10 (30%)	3/6 (50%)

[a] SOD type based on Hogan-Geenen SOD classification system

lihood of success of subsequent sphincterotomy [21]. However, because this approach requires a repeat ERCP, with its attendant risk, it has become unpopular.

Microlithiasis, or biliary crystals, has been shown to be associated with idiopathic pancreatitis. The question arises as to whether some cases of postcholecystectomy pain relate to bile duct microlithiasis, analogous to choledocholithiasis. However, detection of bile duct crystals at ERCP in postcholecystectomy patients is rare and is not associated with abnormal SOM results.

Pain after biliary injection of contrast medium at ERCP may be dramatic in some patients but unfortunately has not been shown to be predictive of SOD.

Therapy

Medical Therapy

Dietary or medical therapy for suspected or documented SOD has received limited study. A low-fat diet is recommended for reducing pancreaticobiliary stimulation. A trial of therapy with smooth muscle relaxants appears warranted. Nifedipine, nitrates, and antispasmodics lower basal SO pressure. Short-term, placebo-controlled, crossover studies showed that 75% of suspected or documented SOD patients who used oral nifedipine experienced statistically less pain. In light of the safety of medical therapy and the benign nature of SOD, medical therapy should be tried in all patients with suspected type III SOD and in patients with less severe type II SOD before invasive sphincter ablation is attempted. Type II patients with more severe pain are less likely to respond to medical therapy, and in these patients a trial of medical therapy is optional.

Sphincterotomy

Historically, surgical biliary sphincterotomy and sphincteroplasty were used successfully for sphincter ablation. Endoscopic techniques have largely replaced conventional open surgery for both biliary and pancreatic sphincter ablation. Most data on endoscopic sphincterotomy relate to biliary sphincter ablation alone.

The most common indication for SOM is biliary-type pain in a postcholecystectomy patient. If manometry findings are abnormal, relief of abdominal pain after sphincterotomy occurs in 90–95% of biliary type I patients, 85% of biliary type II patients, and 55–60% of biliary type III patients (Table 6.1) [18]. When the manometry result is normal, pain relief after sphincterotomy still occurs in 90–95% of type I patients. Because findings of manometry may be misleading in these cases (they are normal in 14–35% of type I patients), manometry is not clinically indicated. Pain relief after sphincterotomy occurs in 35–42% of patients with biliary type II pain with normal manometry results. Although this response rate is similar to that in controls, it is likely that a true clinical response occurs in a few patients. Sphincterotomy is clearly indicated in biliary type II patients with abnormal manometry findings, although it remains controversial as to whether manometry is required to justify sphincterotomy in this group. In biliary type III patients with normal manometry findings, the clinical response rate to sphincterotomy is less than 10%, and an abnormal manometry result is mandatory before sphincterotomy.

Few studies have addressed SOD in patients with biliary-type pain, intact gallbladders, and no gallstones. One possibility is to evaluate such patients for abnormal gallbladder injection fraction and fatty-meal-stimulated bile duct dilation before SOM. If there is ductal dilation it seems justified to proceed to SOM and possible sphincterotomy. If the stimulated meal does not cause duct dilation, cholecystectomy should be planed. An abnormal quantitative cholescintigraphy or SOM result is present in up to 70% of these patients. However, the response to cholecystectomy is variable. Patients with documented SOD and intact gallbladders treated with sphincterotomy first, only 43% experience long-term pain relief. Some additional patients may respond to cholecystectomy. However more information is needed on how to assess and treat this challenging group of patients.

SOD in Pancreatitis

Idiopathic Acute Recurrent Pancreatitis

SOD has been found in 25–60% of patients with idiopathic recurrent pancreatitis [22]. Recurrent attacks of pancreatitis appear to be prevented by pancreatic sphincterotomy in 60–80% of affected patients, although only pancreatic therapy carries an increased risk of complications [23]. For patients with intact gallbladders and idiopathic pancreatitis, some authors advocate either biliary sphincterotomy or treatment with ursodeoxycholic acid, with the implication that microlithiasis is the cause. Other authors report that biliary sphincterotomy alone benefits only one-third of these patients, whereas dual sphincterotomies benefit 80%, suggesting that pancreatic sphincter therapy must be included. More studies are required to select the preferred approach (biliary, pancreatic, or dual sphincterotomies) and to clarify the rates of success and complication of these approaches (Table 6.5).

Chronic Pancreatitis

SOD has been described in up to 87% of patients with chronic pancreatitis. Whether SOD is the result of the chronic inflammation or plays a role in the pathogenesis of chronic pancreatitis is not known. Endoscopic pancreatic sphincterotomy improves pain scores in 60–65% of patients. However, controlled studies are not available. In some cases pancreatic sphincterotomy may be performed to facilitate other therapeutic maneuvers, such as stone extraction and stricture dilation [24,25].

The role of sphincter manometry in patients with chronic pancreatitis remains unclear.

Failure to Respond to Biliary Sphincterotomy in SOD

There are several possible explanations (Table 6.6) for the lack of response to biliary sphincterotomy of patients with SOD. Perhaps the most likely explanation is that the pain was not of pancreatobiliary origin and was caused by altered gut motility or visceral hypersensitivity. Alternatively, the biliary sphincterotomy may have been inadequate or restenosis may have occurred. The clinical success of further biliary endoscopic treatment in such cases is unknown.

The role of residual pancreatic sphincter hypertension as a source of continuing pain is unclear. Symptomatic improvement after pancreatic sphincter ablation is reported in two-thirds of these patients. This

Table 6.5. Pancreatic sphincter dysfunction and recurrent pancreatitis: response to sphincter therapy [28]

Treatment	Patients improved/total patients
Biliary sphincterotomy alone	5/18 (28%)
Biliary sphincterotomy followed by pancreatic sphincter balloon dilation	13/24 (54%)
Biliary sphincterotomy plus pancreatic sphincterotomy at later session	10/13 (77%)
Biliary sphincterotomy and pancreatic sphincterotomy at same session	12/14 (86%)

Table 6.6. Causes for failure to achieve symptom relief after biliary sphincterotomy in SOD

1.	Residual or recurrent biliary sphincter dysfunction
2.	Pancreatic sphincter (major papilla) dysfunction
3.	Chronic pancreatitis – subtle, pancreatogram normal
4.	Other obstructive pancreatobiliary pathology (stones, strictures, tumor, pancreas divisum)
5.	Non-pancreatobiliary disease – especially gut motor disorder or irritable bowel syndrome

finding has led some experts to advocate initial dual sphincterotomies, although the outcome of this approach is unknown.

Finally, some patients with suspected SOD who have not responded to biliary sphincterotomy my have subtle chronic pancreatitis and normal pancreatographic findings. Endoscopic ultrasonography may demonstrate parenchymal changes consistent with chronic pancreatitis in these cases [26].

At the end of this chapter it should be stated that SO pathophysiology is still not sufficiently understood. More investigations and, perhaps, new approaches are required to distinguish between somatic and psychosomatic causes of biliary pain.

References

1. Richards RD, Yeaton P, Shaffer HA Jr, Pambianco, DJ, Pruett TL, Stevenson WC (1993) Human sphincter of Oddi motility and cholecystokinin response following liver transplantation. Dig Dis Sci 38:462–468
2. Becker JM, Parodi JM (1993) Basic control mechanisms of sphincter of Oddi motor function. Gastrointest Endosc Clin N Am 3:41–66
3. Luman W, Wiliams AJ, Pryde A, Smith GD, Nixon SJ, Heading RC, Palmer KR (1997) Influence of cholecystectomy on sphincter of Oddi motility. Gut 41:371–374
4. Hogan WJ, Sherman S, Pasricha P, Carr-Locke DL (1997) Sphincter of Oddi manometry. Gastrointest Endosc 45:342–348
5. Corazziari E, Shaffer EA, Hogan W, Sherman S, Toouli J (1999) Functional disorders of the biliary tract and pancreas. Gut 45:48–54
6. Guelrud M, Mendoza S, Mujica V, Uzcategui A (1993) Sphincter of Oddi (SO) motor function in patients with symptomatic gallstones. Gastroenterology 104:A361
7. Neoptolemos JP, Bailey IS, Carr-Locke DL (1988) Sphincter of Oddi dysfunction: results of treatment by endoscopic sphincterotomy. Br J Surg 75:454–459
8. Roberts-Thomson IC, Toouli, J (1985) Is endoscopic sphincterotomy for disabling biliary-type pain after cholecystectomy effective? Gastrointest Endosc 31:370–373
9. Sherman S, Troiano FP, Hawes RH, O'Connor KW, Lehman GA (1991) Frequency of abnormal sphincter of Oddi manometry compared with the clinical suspicion of sphincter of Oddi dysfunction. Am J Gastroeterol 86:586–590
10. Meshkinopous H, Mollot M (1992) Sphincter of Oddi dysfunction and unexplained abdominal pain: clinical and manometric study. Dig Dis Sci 37:257–261
11. Botoman VA, Kozarek RA, Novell LA, Patterson DJ, Ball TJ, Wechter DG, Neal LA (1994) Long term outcome after endoscopic sphincterotomy in patients with biliary colic and suspected sphincter of Oddi dysfunction. Gastrointest Endosc 40:165–170
12. Lehmann GA, Sherman S (1996) Sphincter of Oddi dysfunction. Int J Pancreatol 20:11–25
13. Eversman D, Fogel EL, Rusche M, Sherman S, Lehmann GA (1999) Frequency of abnormal pancreatic and biliary sphincter manometry compared with clinical suspicion of sphincter of Oddi dysfunction. Gastrointest Endosc 50:637–641
14. Geenen JE, Nash JA (1998) The role of sphincter of Oddi manometry and biliary microscopy in evaluating idiopathic recurrent pancreatitis. Endoscopy 30:A237–241
15. Di Francesco V, Brunori MP, Rigo L, Toouli J, Angelini G, Frulloni L (1999) Comparison of ultrasound-secretin test and sphincter of Oddi manometry in patients with recurrent acute pancreatitis. Dig Dis Sci 44:336–340
16. Catalano MF, Lahoti S, Alcocer E, Geenen JE, Hogan WJ (1998) Dynamic imaging of the pancreas using real-time endoscopic ultrasonography with secretin stimulation. Gastrointest Endosc 48:580–587
17. Guelrud M, Mendoza S, Rossiter G, Villegas MI (1990) Sphincter of Oddi manometry in healthy volunteers. Dig Dis Sci 35:38–46
18. Geenen JE, Hogan WJ, Dodds WJ, Toouli J, Venu RP (1989) The efficacy of endoscopic sphincterotomy after cholecystectomy in patients with sphincter of Oddi dysfunction. N Engl J Med 320:82–87
19. Toouli J, Roberts-Thomson IC, Kellow J, Dowsett J, Saccone GT, Evans P (2000) Manometry based randomized trial of endoscopic sphincterotomy for sphincter of Oddi dysfunction. Gut 46:98–102
20. Rolny P (1997) Endoscopic bile duct stent placement as a predictor of outcome following endoscopic sphincterotomy in patients with suspected sphincter of Oddi dysfunction. Eur J Gastroenterol Hepatol 9:467–471
21. Wehrmann T, Seifert H, Seipp M, Lembeke B, Caspary WF (1998) Endoscopic injection of botulinum toxin for biliary sphincter of Oddi dysfunction. Endoscopy 30:702–707
22. Chen JWC, Saccone GTP, Toouli J (1998) Sphincter of Oddi dysfunction and acute pancreatitis. Gut 43:305–308
23. Toouli J, Francesco V, Saccone G, Kollias J, Schloithe A, Shanks N, (1996) Division of the sphincter of Oddi for treatment of dysfunction associated with recurrent pancreatitis. Br J Surg 83:1205–1010

24. Elton E, Howell DA, Parsons WG, Qaseem T, Hanson BL (1998) Endoscopic pancreatic sphincterotomy: Indications, outcome, and a safe stentless technique. Gastrointest Endosc 47:240–249
25. Okolo PI, Pasricha PJ, Kalloo AN (2000) What are the long-term results of endoscopic pancreatic sphincterotomy? Gastrointest Endosc 52:15–19
26. Sahai AV, Mishra G, Penman ID, Williams D, Wallace MB, Hadzijahic N, Pearson A, Vanvelse A, Hoffman BJ, Hawes RH (2000) EUS to detect evidence of pancreatic disease in patients with persistent or nonspecific dyspepsia. Gastrointest Endosc 52:153–159
27. Sherman S, Lehman GA, Jamidar P, Hawes RH, Silverman W, Madura J (1994) Efficacy of endoscopic sphincterotomy and surgical sphincteroplasty for patients with sphincter of Oddi dysfunction (SOD): randomized, controlled study. Gastrointest Endosc 40:A125
28. Guelrud M, Plaz J, Mendoza S, Beker B, Rojas O, Rossiter G (1995) Endoscopic treatment in Type II pancreatic sphincter dysfunction. Gastrointest Endosc 41:A398

Section 3

Clinical Standards of Diagnostic Measures

Chapter 7 Ultrasound *61*
S. Tanaka

Chapter 8 Contrast-Enhanced CT and MRI *67*
H.-J. Brambs

Chapter 9 Endoscopic Retrograde Cholangiopancreatography *75*
H. Saisho

Chapter 10 Fine-Needle Aspiration Biopsy of the Pancreas *85*
K. Yamao, H. N. Mizuno, K. Takahashi, Y. Shimizu, T. Koshikawa

Chapter 11 FDG-PET and PET/CT in Pancreatic Cancer *97*
S. N. Reske

Chapter 12 Laboratory Diagnosis of Exocrine and Endocrine Dysfunctions in Inflammatory and Neoplastic Lesions *107*
K. Schütte, S. Kahl, P. Malfertheiner

Chapter 13 Guidelines, Clinical Evaluation, Short Track *119*
J. Mössner

Chapter 7

S. Tanaka

Ultrasound

Ultrasonography (US) is one of the most effective noninvasive imaging modalities for the pancreas. Without using irradiation or a contrast agent, detailed images of the pancreas can be visualized with US. The weak point of this method is the backyard of bone or gas in the alimentary tract [1]. Liquid intake [2–4], placing the patient in the sitting position, and/or pressing on the abdominal wall to push away the gas may increase the quality of the image (Fig. 7.1). But in some cases, the pancreas cannot be observed in its entirety by US alone, and X-ray computed tomography (CT) and/or magnetic resonance imaging (MRI) must also be performed.

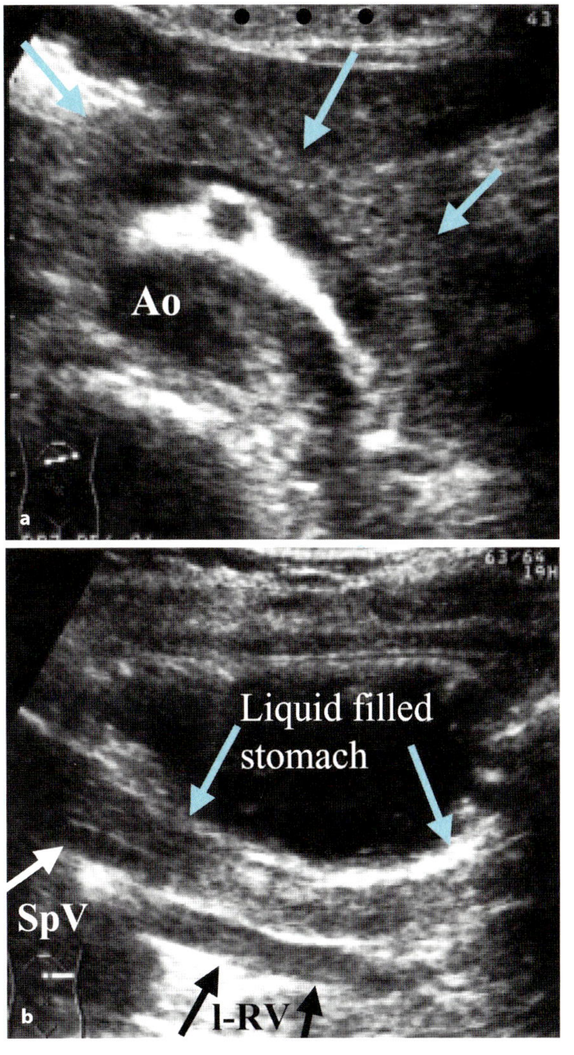

Figure 7.1

Ultrasound (US) image of the pancreas (*blue arrows*), before (a) and after (b) liquid intake. After drinking 350 ml of milk tea, the tail of the pancreas becomes entirely visualized. *Ao* Aorta, *SpV* splenic vein (*white arrows*), *l-RV* left renal vein (*black arrows*)

US Findings Associated with Pancreatic Diseases

Enlargement

The size and shape of the pancreas differ from person to person, but its maximal width is 2 or 3 cm or less in healthy subjects. Diffuse enlargement ordinarily suggests acute pancreatitis, but advanced pancreatic cancer occasionally shows overall enlargement without focal swelling.

Main Pancreatic Duct Dilatation

The diameter of the main pancreatic duct (MPD) is usually less than 2 mm at the body of the pancreas, but in the elderly, it tends to be larger [5]. When MPD dilatation is observed, it is important to search for the narrowed portion downstream. The main causes of MPD obstruction are tumor invasion, compression by a tumor, or calculus within the MPD. Diffuse, straight dilatation of the MPD is often observed in chronic pancreatitis. In patients with an intraductal papillary mucinous neoplasm, irregular dilatation of the MPD is often observed.

Common Bile Duct Dilatation

Common bile duct (CBD) dilatation is an important finding that suggests pancreatic head swelling. When the CBD is dilated, detailed observation is necessary to search for the narrowed portion downstream, particularly in the intrapancreatic part of the CBD, in order to rule out obstruction by a pancreatic tumor.

Focal Lesions in the Pancreas

Hypoechoic Lesions

Most kinds of pancreatic neoplasms, including pancreatic cancer, endocrine tumors, acinar-cell carcinoma, metastatic pancreatic cancer, and tumor-forming pancreatitis are visualized as a hypoechoic area. In patients with ductal adenocarcinoma, MPD obstruction readily occurs. In addition, the penetrating duct sign, in which the MPD passes through the tumor area, is a characteristic sign of a tumor-forming pancreatitis. In patients with metastatic cancer or an endocrine tumor, MPD obstruction is observed only when the tumor has become rather large. As for the blood flow in the lesion, pancreatic ductal adenocarcinomas are usually hypovascular, whereas endocrine tumors are hypervascular.

Hyperechoic Lesions

Small hyperechoic lesions are occasionally observed in the pancreas, but they are rarely malignant. Most of them cannot be detected by contrast-enhanced dynamic CT or MRI. Some of them are proven to be focal fat deposits by fat-saturated T1-weighted MRI, while others are surmised to be the scar of an atrophied cyst on the basis of US follow-up. But in most other cases, the origin remains unknown. Serous cyst adenomas composed of tiny multilocular cysts sometimes appear as hyperechoic lesions with low-resolution US equipment.

Cystic Lesions

Many kinds of cystic lesions are observed in the pancreas, including cystic neoplasms, retention cysts, simple cysts, and pseudocysts. Mucinous cystic neoplasms are sometimes slow-growing low-grade malignancies. A solid component in a cyst, mural nodules, and irregular thickness of the septum or wall suggest the possibility of malignancy [6].

Lymph-Node Swelling Around the Pancreas

In patients with chronic pancreatitis or recurrent acute pancreatitis, flat swelling of lymph nodes is often observed along the common hepatic artery. In advanced pancreatic cancer with lymph-node involvement, lumps of lymph nodes are observed.

Diseases of the Pancreas

Diffuse Pancreatic Disease

Acute Pancreatitis

Characteristic US findings of acute pancreatitis are diffuse enlargement and decreased echogenicity in the pancreas [7]. Fluid collection or hemorrhage is sometimes observed around the pancreas or in the retroperitoneal space. As severe complications of acute pancreatitis, portal venous thrombosis and/or arterial pseudoaneurysms may be observed. Color Doppler US is useful for evaluating the blood flow of the involved vessels or collateral vessels [8]. Differentiation of tumor embolism from thrombosis is often difficult.

Tumor-forming pancreatitis or focal pancreatitis is one of the most difficult benign focal lesions to differentiate from pancreatic cancer. Focal edema is shown as a hypoechoic area in the pancreas. The penetrating duct sign (i.e., an image of the MPD passing through the tumor without obstruction) suggests the possibility of pancreatitis. The vascularity of the tumor is rather high compared with the surrounding pancreatic tissue (Fig. 7.2). Conversely, a lesion with poor blood flow suggests pancreatic cancer. It should be noted that there are many cases with mild pancreatitis in which no abnormal US findings are shown.

Chronic Pancreatitis

The characteristic US findings of chronic pancreatitis are an atrophied pancreas with a narrow width, irregular contour, and diffusely dilated MPD. Multiple calcifications are sometimes observed within the main or branch pancreatic duct [9].

Focal Pancreatic Disease

Pancreatic Cancer

The characteristic US finding of pancreatic cancer is a hypoechoic lesion with unclear margin combined with upstream MPD dilatation. Pancreatic cancer smaller than 2 cm in diameter is usually visualized as

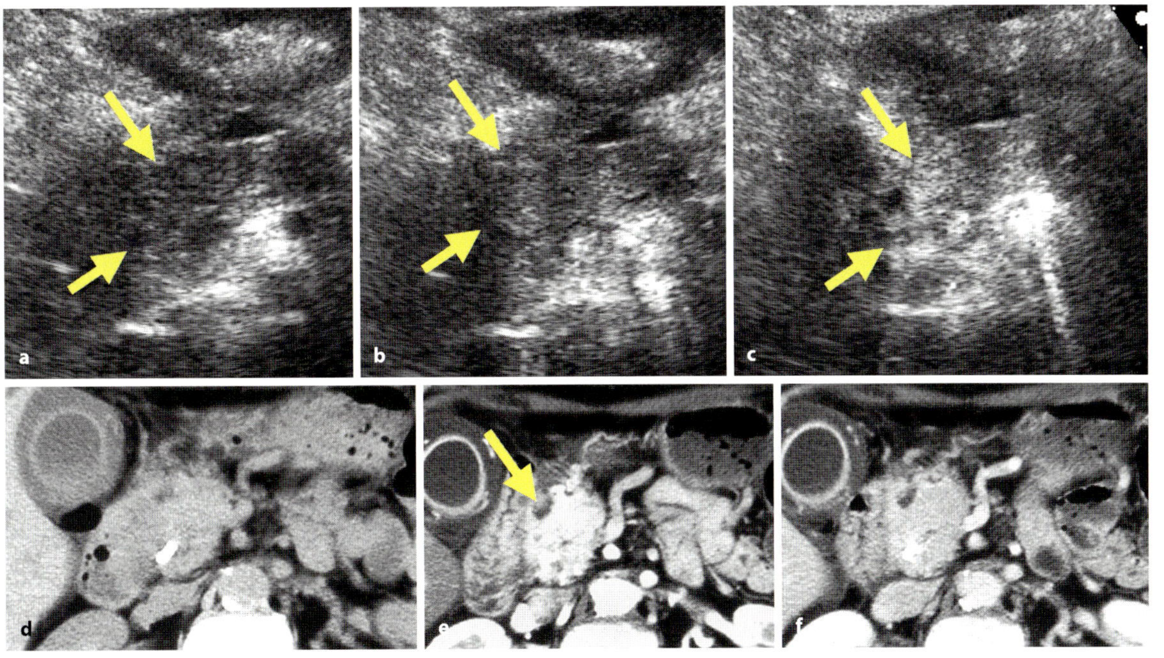

Figure 7.2

Inflammatory tumor of 40 mm in diameter (*arrow*) in the head of the pancreas a-c Contrast-enhanced dynamic US using intravenous galactose-based air microbubble contrast agent (Levovist). d-f Contrast enhanced dynamic CT. a, d Before enhancement. b, e Early phase of contrast enhancement. c, f Late phase of contrast enhancement. a Head of the pancreas is enlarged and the echo level is rather low. b-c Tumor area is gradually enhanced, and the echo level becomes similar or rather higher comparing with the body of the pancreas. d Head of the pancreas is enlarged but no focal lesion is revealed. e-f A part of the pancreatic head is strongly enhanced

a homogeneous hypoechoic lesion with or without MPD dilatation. In such early stage cases, the differentiation from focal pancreatitis or benign tumors is very difficult. Pancreatic cancer is characterized by poor blood flow compared with the surrounding pancreas (Fig. 7.3). Therefore, intravenous contrast-enhanced dynamic US or dynamic CT is effective for the differential diagnosis of small focal lesions. For the definite diagnosis of small hypoechoic and hypovascular lesion in the pancreas, pancreatic juice cytology or fine needle-biopsy is necessary.

In the case of tumors larger than 2 cm in diameter, the internal echo-pattern of the tumor becomes rough, and MPD dilatation is observed upstream of the pancreas.

Pancreatic Endocrine Tumor

The characteristic US finding of pancreatic endocrine tumor is a homogeneous hypoechoic lesion with clear margin without MPD dilatation. It is sometimes observed as a multicentric lesion in the pancreas. In the case of tumors larger than 3 cm or more, the internal echo-pattern of the tumor becomes rough, and sometimes combines with central necrosis. MPD dilatation is also observed in some cases. Different from ductal adenocarcinoma, the pancreatic endocrine tumor is hypervascular. With contrast-enhanced dynamic US or dynamic CT, tumors are well enhanced compared with the surrounding pancreas (Fig. 7.4). In many cases tumors produce endocrine hormones, such as insulin, glucagon, or gastrin. Sometimes, hypoglycemic attack caused by the hypersecretion of insulin is the primary symptom of this disease.

Other Pancreatic Tumors

There are many other kinds of primary pancreatic tumor, such as acinar cell carcinoma, squamous cell carcinoma, and adenosquamous cell carcinoma.

Metastatic Pancreatic Tumors

Metastatic cancer is not frequently observed in the pancreas. Metastasis from lung cancer, renal cell can-

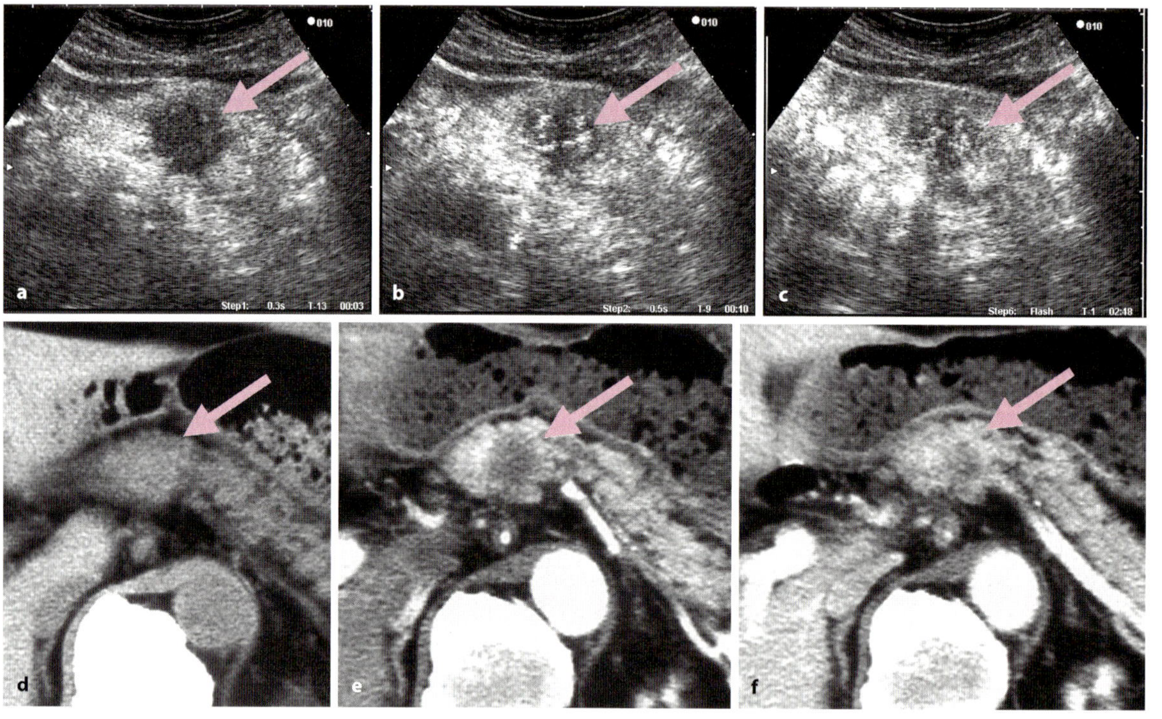

Figure 7.3

Pancreatic ductal adenocarcinoma of 27 mm in diameter (*arrow*) in the body. a-c Contrast enhanced dynamic US using intravenous galactose based air microbubble contrast agent (Levovist). d-f Contrast enhanced dynamic CT. a, d Before enhancement. b, e Early phase of contrast enhancement. c, f Late phase of contrast enhancement. a A hypoechoic lesion is observed in the body of the pancreas. b Arteries in the tumor area involved with cancer are observed as a network pattern. c Tumor is gradually enhanced from the peripheral area to the center of the tumor. The hypoechoic area is thus diminished compared with the image taken before enhancement. d No focal lesion is revealed with CT. e The enhancement effect is low in the tumor area comparing with the surrounding pancreas, so the tumor is revealed as a low-density area. f Tumor is gradually enhanced from the peripheral area to the center of the tumor

cer, or breast cancer is occasionally observed. Multiple foci and no MPD dilatation are their characteristics.

Cystic Neoplasms in the Pancreas

The classification of the cystic neoplasm in the pancreas is rather confusing. Classically, they are classified into two groups, serous cyst adenoma and cystoadenocarcinoma. The former is a microcystic tumor containing serous fluid and the latter is a macrocystic tumor containing mucus. Most malignant cystic tumors are included in the latter. A solid component in a cyst, mural nodules, and irregular thickness of the septum or wall suggest the possibility of malignancy [6]. Recently, the concept of intraductal papillary mucinous neoplasm has appeared. The definition is MPD dilatation or branch duct dilatation with mucinous pancreatic juice. This neoplasm is considered to be a low-grade malignancy.

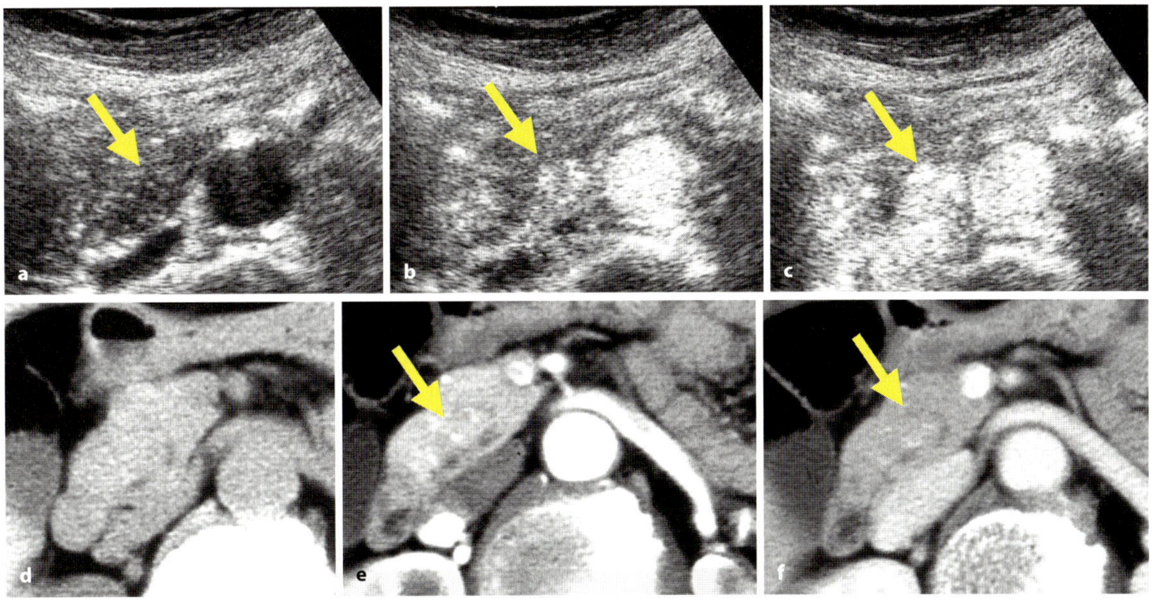

Figure 7.4

Pancreatic endocrine tumor of 17 mm in diameter (*arrow*) in the uncus. a-c Contrast enhanced dynamic US using intravenous galactose based air microbubble contrast agent (Levovist). d-f Contrast enhanced dynamic CT. a, d Before enhancement. b, e Early phase of contrast enhancement. c, f Late phase of contrast enhancement. a A hypoechoic lesion is observed in the body of the pancreas. b-c Tumor area is strongly enhanced through early phase to late phase. d No focal lesion is revealed. e-f A high-density area is observed in the early phase through late phase

Early Detection of Pancreatic Cancer with US

The prognosis of pancreatic cancer remains very poor, but it is better in patients with a small tumor without local infiltration. Screening by US can detect early stage pancreatic cancer. When indirect signs, such as MPD dilatation, CBD dilatation, or focal enlargement, are regarded as positive, the accuracy of US for the detection of pancreatic cancer is quite high. The sensitivity, specificity, and overall accuracy of routinely performed US for the evaluation of pancreatic cancer are reported to be 98%, 98%, and 96%, respectively [10].

As for the results of mass screening by US, the incidence of early stage cases in the total detected pancreatic cancer cases was reported to be rather high (TS1: 31%; Stage I: 18%), but the incidence of pancreatic cancer cases among the total screened population was low, at about 0.01% [11]. Screening US that is weighted for high-risk patients may have merit. As high-risk signs of pancreatic cancer, MPD dilatation and the presence of pancreatic cyst(s) have been reported to be particularly important [5,12]. Slight MPD dilatation (>2 mm in diameter) was observed in 65% of the precancer subject group in which pancreatic cancer was detected and surgically resected more than 4 years later. And the odds ratio compared with the control group was reported to be 32.5 [5]. Also, periodic checkups with US were performed for patients with slight dilatation of the MPD or a cyst, and the incidence of pancreatic cancer was reported to be 20 times higher than that of regional pancreatic cancer.

Contrast-Enhanced US

As noted above, blood-flow information is very important for the differential diagnosis of various pancreatic tumors [13–15]. Recent advances in the technology of US equipment and intravenous contrast agents for US have made it possible to evaluate the blood-flow information of pancreatic tumors. Intravenous contrast agents for US are composed of microbubbles, containing air or fluorocarbon gas. When ultrasound is transmitted, the microbubbles become resonant or disrupted, resulting in enhancement of the image.

Without radiation exposure, risk of iodine allergy or volume overload, differential diagnosis of pancreatic tumors can be effectively performed with contrast-enhanced dynamic US. Therefore, when a hypoechoic lesion is detected in the pancreas by screening US and the possibility of malignancy cannot be excluded, contrast-enhanced dynamic US should be the first-choice examination for characterization of the lesion. A hypoechoic, hypovascular pancreatic lesion is strongly suggestive of pancreatic cancer, even if it is not revealed by contrast-enhanced dynamic CT or MRI. The weak point of this method is related to deeply located targets or when there is gas interference. Contrast-enhanced dynamic US is thus not suited for tumors located more than 10 cm beneath the abdominal surface or when there is gas in the alimentary tract. Figures 7.2–7.4 present characteristic images of pancreatic tumors obtained with contrast-enhanced dynamic CT and US.

References

1. Jeffrey RB, Ralls PW (1995) Sonography of the Abdomen. Raven, New York
2. Pamela L, Fritz TA, Unger EC, Hunt RK, Fuller E (1992) Cellulose as a gastrointestinal US contrast agent. Radiology 185:783–788
3. Harisinghani MG, Saini S, Schima W, McNicholas M, Mueller PR (1997) Simeticone coated cellulose as an oral contrast agent for ultrasound of the upper abdomen. Clin Radiol 52:224–226
4. Tanaka S, Nakaizumi A, Ioka T, Takakura R, et al (2004) Periodic ultrasonographic checkup for the early detection of pancreatic cancer: preliminary report. Pancreas 22:268–272
5. Tanaka S, Nakaizumi A, Ioka T, et al (2002) Main pancreatic duct dilatation: a sign of high risk for pancreatic cancer. Jpn J Clin Oncol 32:407–411
6. Johnson CD, Stephens DH, Carboneau JW, et al (1998) Cystic pancreatic tumors: CT and sonographic assessment. AJR 151:1133–1138
7. Jeffrey RB Jr (1989) Sonography in acute pancreatitis. Radiol Clin North Am 27:5–17
8. Ralls PW (1990) Color Doppler sonography of the hepatic artery and portal venous system. AJR 155:517–525
9. Bolondi L, LiBassi S, Barbara L (1989) Sonography of chronic pancreatitis. Radiol Clin North Am 27:815–833
10. Tanaka S, Kitamra T, Yamamoto K, et al (1996) Evaluation of routine sonography for early detection of pancreatic cancer. Jpn J Clin Oncol 26:422–427
11. Inamoto Y, Kawamura S (1992) Nippon Shokaki-shuudan-kenshin. Gakkai-shi 96:88–94 (in Japanese)
12. Nakaizumi A, Tatsuta M, Uehara H, et al (1992) A prospective trial of early detection of pancreatic cancer by ultrasonographic examination combined with measurement of serum elastase-1. Cancer 69:936–940
13. Hollet MD, Jorgensen MJ, Jeffrey RB Jr (1995) Quantitative evaluation of pancreatic enhancement during dual-phase helical CT. Radiology 195:359–361
14. Koito K, Namieno T, Nagakawa T, Morita K (1997) Inflammatory pancreatic masses: differentiation from ductal carcinoma with contrast-enhanced sonography using carbon dioxide microbubbles. AJR 169:1263–1267
15. Oshikawa O, Tanaka S, Ioka T, et al (2002) Dynamic sonography of pancreatic tumors: comparison with dynamic CT. AJR 178:1133–1137

Chapter 8

H.-J. Brambs

Contrast-Enhanced CT and MRI

Abdominal plain films and chest radiographs play practically no more role in the work-up of pancreatic disorders. Although extensive pancreatic calcifications, which are seen frequently in patients with chronic pancreatitis, are well visualized, there is no additional information to be gained in comparison with cross-sectional imaging methods.

Since the advent and wide availability of endoscopy, the standard upper gastrointestinal series and hypotonic duodenography have also lost most of their importance. They are still required in the work-up of patients in whom significant stenoses of the duodenum due to inflammation or malignancy preclude safe passage of the endoscope.

Angiography still plays a role in the work-up of hemorrhage occurring in pancreatic disease. Otherwise, it has been completely replaced by noninvasive cross-sectional imaging methods such as computed tomography (CT) and magnetic resonance imaging (MRI). Both of these techniques have adequate capabilities for visualizing both arterial and venous vessels and for determining the involvement of these vessels in the patient's underlying inflammatory or malignant disease (Fig. 8.1).

The importance of endoscopic retrograde cholangiopancreatography (ERCP) as a diagnostic method has declined significantly with the development of ultrasound and, in particular, magnetic resonance cholangiopancreatography (MRCP). The invasive method, however, is still indicated whenever a therapeutic procedure, such as papillotomy, stone extraction, or stent implantation is contemplated.

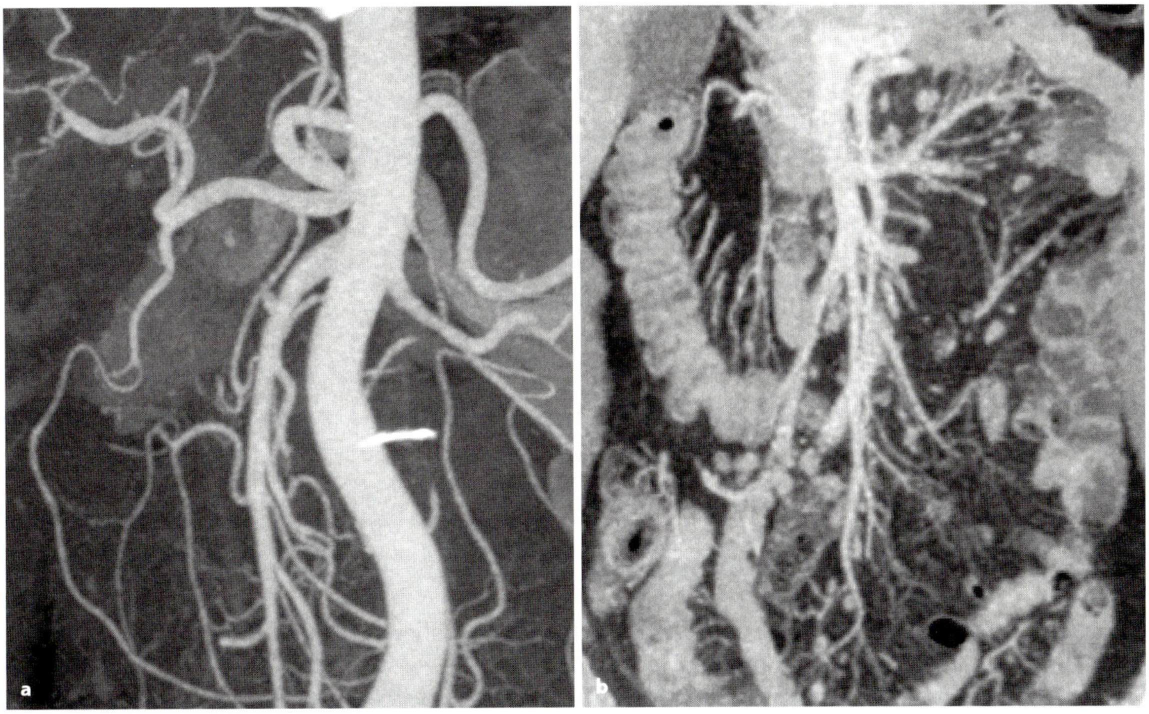

Figure 8.1 a, b

Three-dimensional volume-rendered computed tomography (CT) of the arterial and venous vessels of the abdomen

Diagnostic ultrasound has become the single most important method for visualizing the pancreas and the biliary system. This is especially true in light of the many technical refinements that have been made in recent years. Transabdominal ultrasound depends only partially on the cooperation of the patient and can be repeated rapidly and safely whenever needed. The advantages of endoscopic ultrasound (EUS) include high-resolution imaging and the capability for targeted punctures.

Spiral CT

Spiral CT, especially since the introduction of the newly developed multidetector scanners (MD-CT), has resulted in a significant improvement in resolution when imaging the pancreas [1]. In addition, it has become possible to plan contrast-enhanced studies in detail and, when required, the organ can be studied during more than one contrast medium phase (Fig. 8.2). Depending on the available technology and the clinical question, a more refined examination protocol can be devised to vary the spatial resolution, the phase of contrast enhancement, and, where needed, include more than one phase of contrast enhancement.

A further advantage of multidetector technology is the capability for reconstruction image data (Fig. 8.3). Particularly impressive are the reconstructions along duct formations (Fig. 8.4) and vessels (curved reformations and slab viewing). This can be of great importance in cases of tumor infiltration of vessels and for a more precise visualization of cystic tumors and their connection with the pancreatic duct (Fig. 8.5).

For a qualitative study, it is important that patients drink adequate amounts of liquid immediately before the examination. This helps delineate the stomach and duodenum from the pancreas and for recognizing inflammatory or malignant infiltration. The additional intravenous administration of spasmolytic agents is useful for distending the duodenum. The collapsed duodenum is often difficult to distinguish from pancreatic parenchyma.

High spatial resolution, which includes imaging of the ductal structures, the capability for very rapid reconstruction of arterial and venous structures that is comparable to angiography, and the ability to include the liver and the lungs in the same imaging session makes this method highly suitable for the diagnosis and staging of tumors. It is possible, without subjecting the patient to further studies, to make informed statements regarding the crucial issue of resectability.

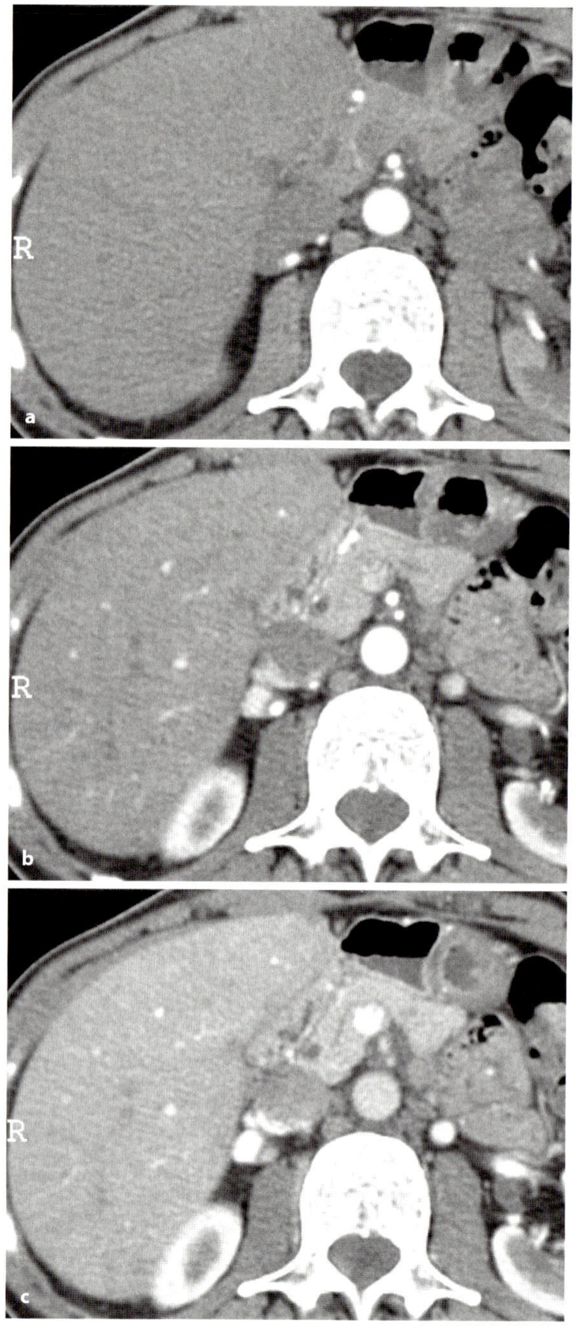

Figure 8.2 a–c

Three-phasic CT of the pancreas including an arterial, parenchymal, and portal-venous phase

The design of the examination depends on the clinical question, but the options are determined by the available technology. This latter factor is dependent on the number of detectors in modern CT units. Although modern multidetector technology allows a reduction in the required contrast medium, it is use-

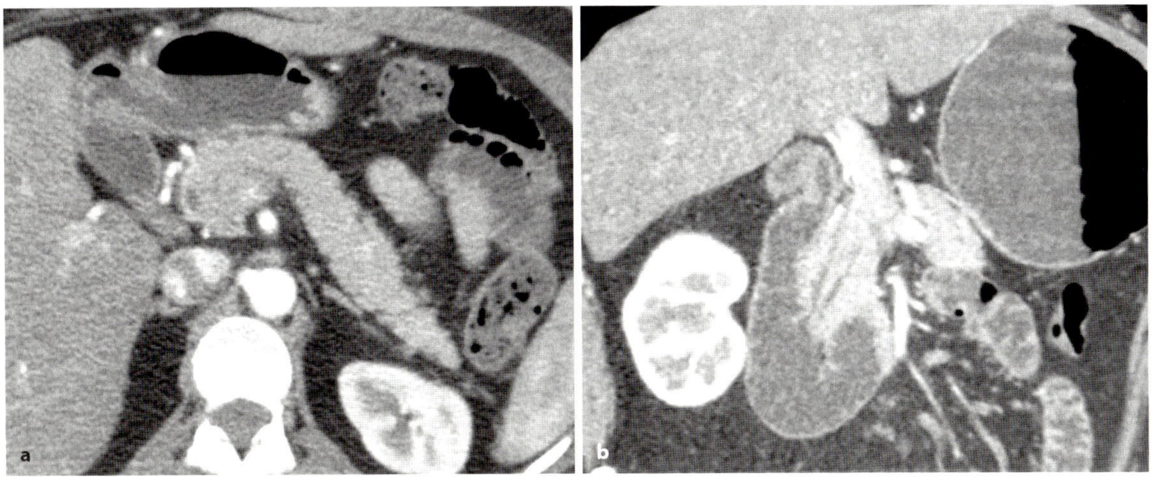

Figure 8.3 a, b

High-resolution CT of the pancreas in the axial plane (a). In the coronal reformation, the pancreatic head is well delineated from the fluid-filled duodenum, showing the normal distal bile duct and pancreatic duct

Figure 8.4

Perpendicular reconstruction along the pancreatic duct

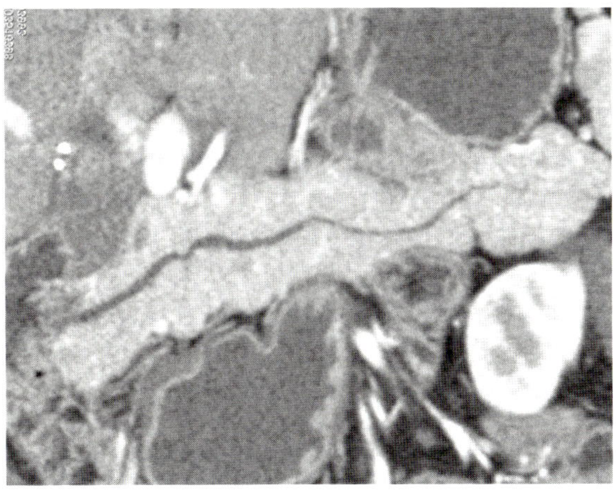

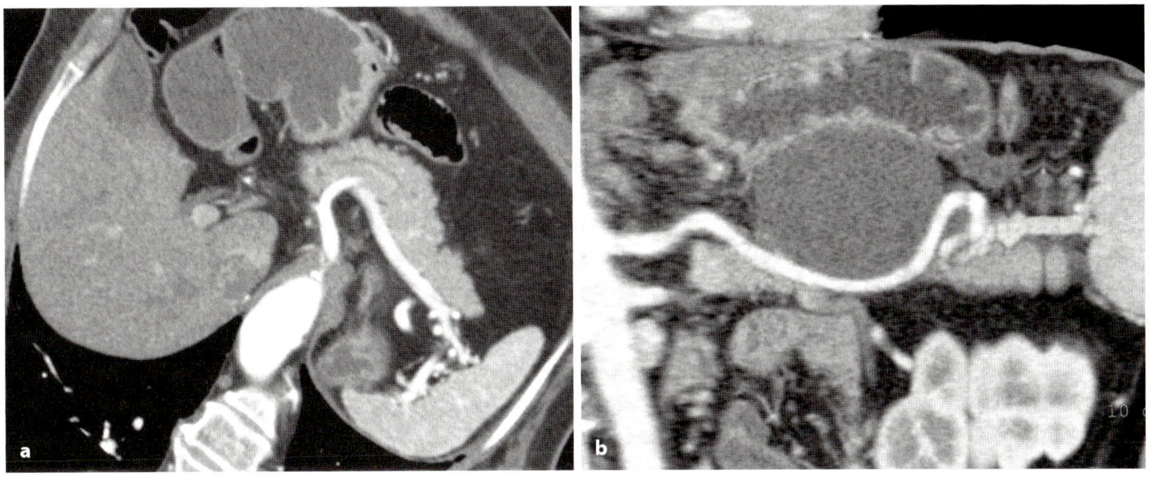

Figure 8.5 a, b

Reformation of a normal pancreas along the splenic artery (a: slab viewing), and of a pancreatic pseudocyst (b: perpendicular)

ful to increase the contrast medium concentration [2]. In most cases, a contrast medium flow of 3–4 ml/s is recommended.

Technical refinements have resulted in a sustained discussion regarding the number of contrast phases that are necessary for adequate assessment of pancreatic disorders as well as regarding which contrast phase permits optimum differentiation between normal and pathological pancreatic tissue [3,4].

The so-called arterial phase (20–25 s following the start of contrast medium injection) often occurs too soon for adequate differentiation between healthy and diseased parenchyma. It is most commonly recommended in cases of suspected endocrine tumors or when special angiographic reconstructions are desired (Fig. 8.2a).

The greatest difference in contrast uptake between normal and pathological pancreatic tissue occurs during the so-called pancreatic phase (30–70 s following start of contrast medium injection, with a maximum at 40 s). The amount and speed of injection affect this phase: larger amounts of applied contrast medium are associated with a longer duration of the phase, while a more rapid injection results in more intense contrast enhancement (Fig. 8.2b).

The portal venous phase (maximum after 60–90 s) is characterized by optimum contrast of the portal and mesenteric veins. In addition, this phase is usually best suited for the detection of hypovascular metastases of the liver (Fig. 2c).

Magnetic Resonance Imaging

MRI has enjoyed increasing acceptance in the diagnosis of pancreatic disorders. It exhibits significant advantages in the work-up of certain entities, such as cystic tumors. The method has the additional advantage that, besides the cross-sectional imaging, MRCP and angiographic sequences can be acquired, making it a well-rounded diagnostic modality that is particularly useful in the diagnosis and staging of tumors. Technical innovations such as phased-array coils have resulted in improvement in both the signal:noise ratio and spatial resolution, facilitating the imaging of the upper abdomen with rapid T1- and T2-weighted sequences in breath-hold technique [5].

In order to better distinguish the pancreas from surrounding bowel loops and the stomach, patients can, as has been recommended with CT, be asked to drink adequate amounts of water prior to the examination. Other positive and negative contrast media have been discussed favorably in the scientific literature, but have not to date gained general acceptance.

Different T1- and T2-weighted sequences in the axial and coronal plane can be used for visualization of the pancreatic parenchyma. On T1-weighted sequences, the normal pancreas shows a moderate level of signal intensity that is most frequently higher than that measured for the liver or spleen (Fig. 8.6a). This is ascribed to the high proportion of proteins in the glandular tissue, the highly developed reticuloepithelial system and the high concentration of paramagnetic ions, such as manganese. This higher signal intensity is even maintained in the presence of significant fatty degeneration of the organ, but decreases gradually with advancing age as a result of the increasing fibrosis of the gland. Signal intensity is decreased in tumors, pancreatitis, and atrophy.

The T1-weighted sequences include turbo spin echo sequences with fat suppression or gradient recalled echo sequences in breath-hold technique. Fat suppression improves visualization of many organs that, like the pancreas, are surrounded by fat tissue and are themselves characterized by a high protein content. In addition, movement artifacts are reduced, as are the so-called chemical shift artifacts that occur at the lipid–water boundary. Fat-suppressed T1-weighted images are especially useful for detecting subtle focal and diffuse changes in the pancreas; they are also suitable for excluding some pancreatic disorders (Fig. 8.6b).

As a rule, the work-up of pancreatic disorders requires intravenous contrast medium, which is administered using an MRI-compatible high-performance injector (Fig. 8.6b). Dynamic, gadolinium-enhanced sequences acquired at different perfusion phases improve the detection and characterization of pancreatic lesions less than 1 cm in diameter. In addition, they permit assessment of vascularization of pancreatic tumors and facilitate the detection and characterization of any hepatic lesions that may be simultaneously present.

T2-weighted sequences are acquired in thin-slice technique with short and long scan times in both axial and coronal planes (Fig. 8.7). Acquisition is performed either with respiratory triggering or during breath-hold. Because these sequences visualize the biliary and pancreatic ducts, they also serve as a basis of MRCP.

Application of manganese-containing contrast medium, originally conceived as a hepatobiliary contrast medium, results in a significant increase in signal intensity in healthy pancreatic parenchyma (Fig. 8.8). The use of this contrast medium, however,

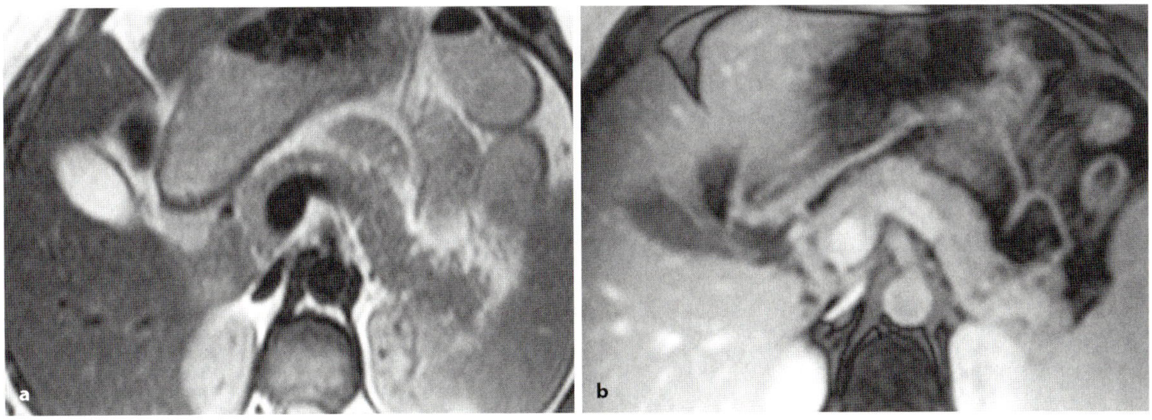

Figure 8.6 a, b

T1-weighted sequence of the pancreas (a: native, b: after intravenous administration of Gd-diethylene triamine pentaacetic acid using fat suppression)

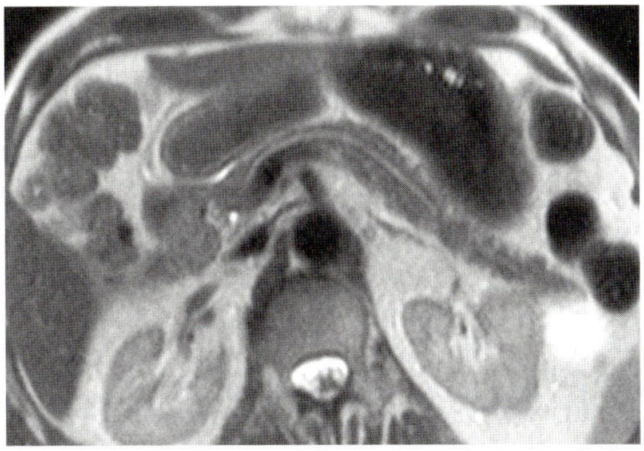

Figure 8.7

T2-weighted imaging of a normal pancreas with delineation of the pancreatic duct

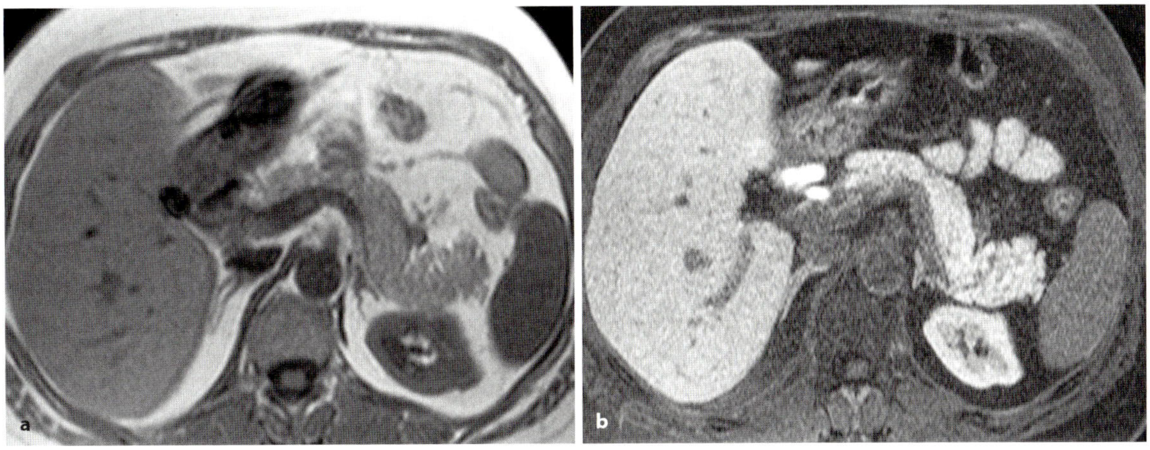

Figure 8.8 a, b

T1-weighted image of the pancreas (a: native, b: after intravenous administration of Mangan)

has not yet found broad acceptance. One reason is that dynamic studies are impossible. In addition, even with this contrast medium, differentiation between pancreatic carcinoma and chronic pancreatitis remains difficult, since both entities present with a reduced concentration [6]. On the other hand, certain tumors such as acinar cell carcinoma show increased uptake of this contrast medium.

Magnetic Resonance Cholangiopancreatography

A comprehensive work-up of pancreatic disorders includes evaluation of the biliary and pancreatic ducts. This can be done rapidly and with adequate quality using MRCP. Many studies have even shown that, for detection of ductal changes within the pancreas and of extrapancreatic changes of the biliary system, MRCP is equivalent to ERCP. In addition, MRCP can be performed without difficulty in patients with stenoses of the stomach and duodenum, large duodenal diverticula, after gastric surgery and after biliodigestive anastomoses – situations in which ERCP is either impossible or associated with very high failure rates.

MRCP is based on very strong T2-weighted sequences in which standing or very slowly flowing fluids are visualized with high signal intensities. Ideally, very rapid sequences are used, although these are associated with the disadvantage of poorer spatial resolution. As a rule, single and multislice techniques are combined, since these are quite complementary.

Single-slice images can be acquired during brief breath-hold phases in thick slices (20–50 mm). Motion artifacts due to peristalsis and respiration are practically negligible. Additional fat suppression increases the contrast between ductal structures and the background and, even without special postprocessing, yields images that are very comparable to ERCP images (Fig. 8.9).

An important advantage of this technique is the short acquisition time, permitting dynamic evaluation. This can be used for work-up of dysfunctions of the sphincter and for evaluating the secretory performance of the pancreas following intravenous administration of secretin. The disadvantage of this technique is that visualization of ductal structures may be compromised by adjacent, fluid-filled structures and by overlying ascites. In order to reduce such artifacts from the stomach or duodenum, patients should either be fasting or can be given contrast medium containing iron oxide shortly before the examination. This latter measure neutralizes gastric and duodenal secretions prior to imaging.

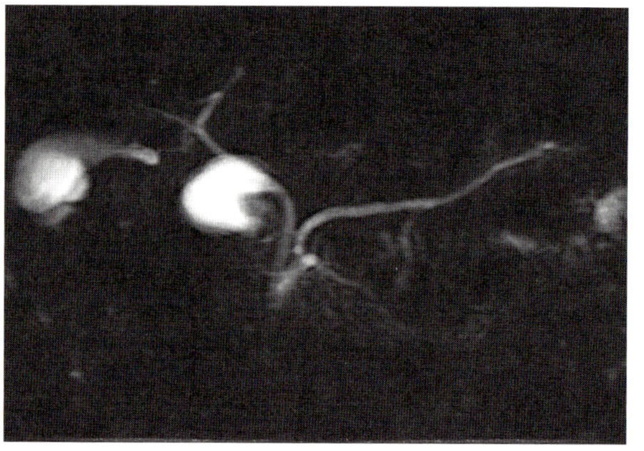

Figure 8.9

Magnetic resonance cholangiopancreatography (MRCP) of a normal ductal system

Multislice techniques generally involve series of slices 3–5 mm in thickness that are acquired with a shorter echo time than with single-slice techniques (100–300 ms). With these settings, both signal-intense fluids and periductal structures are visualized, which is important, especially in cases of malignant obstruction, and can be helpful when artifacts secondary to superposed fluids interfere with diagnosis in single-slice studies. Because the slices are acquired in less than 1 s, motion artifacts do not occur. In addition, image quality is less affected by chemical shift or susceptibility artifacts.

Secretin-Stimulated Dynamic MRCP

The intravenous administration of secretin (1 ml per 10 kg body weight) results in stimulation of water and bicarbonate secretion. This produces better filling of the pancreatic ducts, which is further intensified by a transient contraction of the papilla sphincter that lasts about 5 min. This endogenous "contrast enhancement" permits better evaluation of the main pancreatic duct and often also of the side branches in the head of the pancreas. Here, it is important that with good temporal resolution, both the duodenum and pancreatic duct are visualized over their entire lengths. Good indications include confirmation of pancreas divisum and other ductal variants.

In addition, this method permits dynamic examination of the pancreas (Fig. 8.10), which can be used for semiquantitative estimation of secretory performance and for assessing the exocrine function of the gland [7–9].

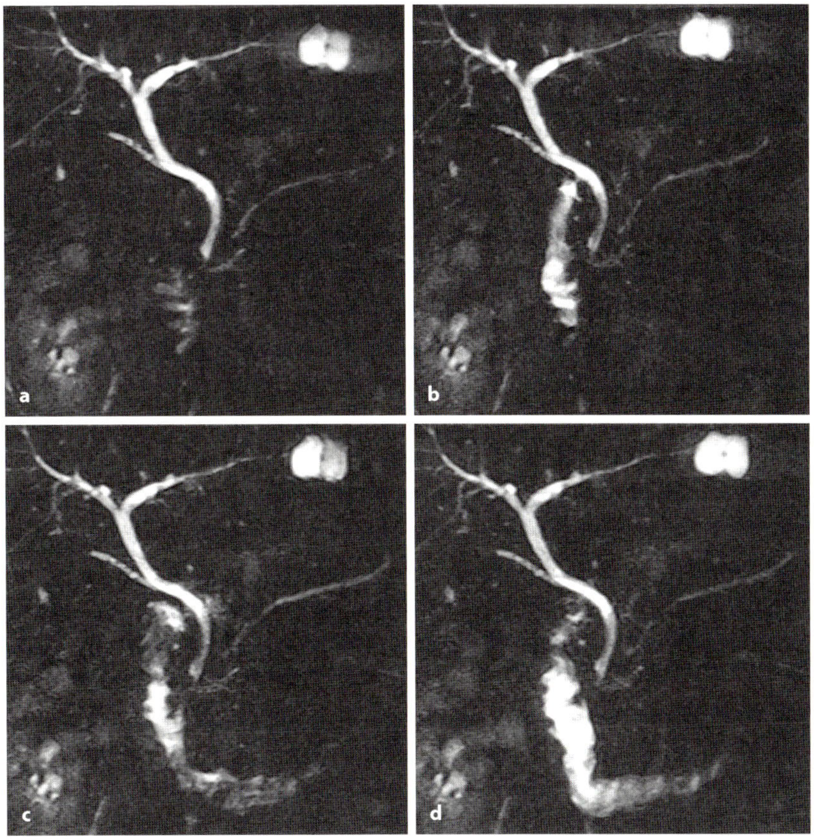

Figure 8.10 a–d

MRCP obtained before and during secretin stimulation slightly improves visualization of the main pancreatic duct and shows an increasing filling of the duodenum due to normal pancreatic secretion

Magnetic Resonance Angiography

Dynamic sequences acquired following intravenous application of gadolinium can be used for assessing arterial and venous vascularization of pancreatic tumors (Fig. 8.11). A three-dimensional gradient echo sequence can also be acquired following gadolinium application for assessing the vascular situation. A novel variation of this technique is the so-called VIBE sequence (volume interpolated breath-hold examination), which provides high resolution and can also be used in hepatobiliary imaging [10].

A Comparison of Methods

Transabdominal ultrasound and EUS have been strongly propagated by internists for the diagnosis of pancreatic disease. Without doubt, transabdominal ultrasound is an outstanding screening method for discovering pancreatic pathology and, in many cases, can be used for follow-up monitoring. If serious therapeutic consequences are expected, EUS is often recommended.

Among radiologists, CT is currently the most frequently recommended method for detecting and characterizing pancreatic diseases. Since the introduction of modern MD-CT scanners, the examination can be performed in a very short time and with very high resolution. A wide range of reconstructions is possible without major time requirements, yielding very useful topographic images. In addition, simultaneous changes involving the lung, liver, adjacent bowel loops, arterial and venous vasculature and lymph nodes can be precisely visualized.

Magnetic Resonance Imaging

As a rule, MRI is not the primary method for diagnosing disorders of the pancreas. This is due in great part to the relatively long examination times, problems of availability, and the relatively high costs of the method. Compared to newer CT technologies, MRI offers less satisfactory resolution, and the previously cited advantages of multiplanar imaging have been met by the at least equivalent performance of MD-CT.

There are, however, a few indications for MRI in the work-up of pancreatic disease:

1. Unsatisfactory or questionable CT results in patients with a high probability of pancreatic disease.

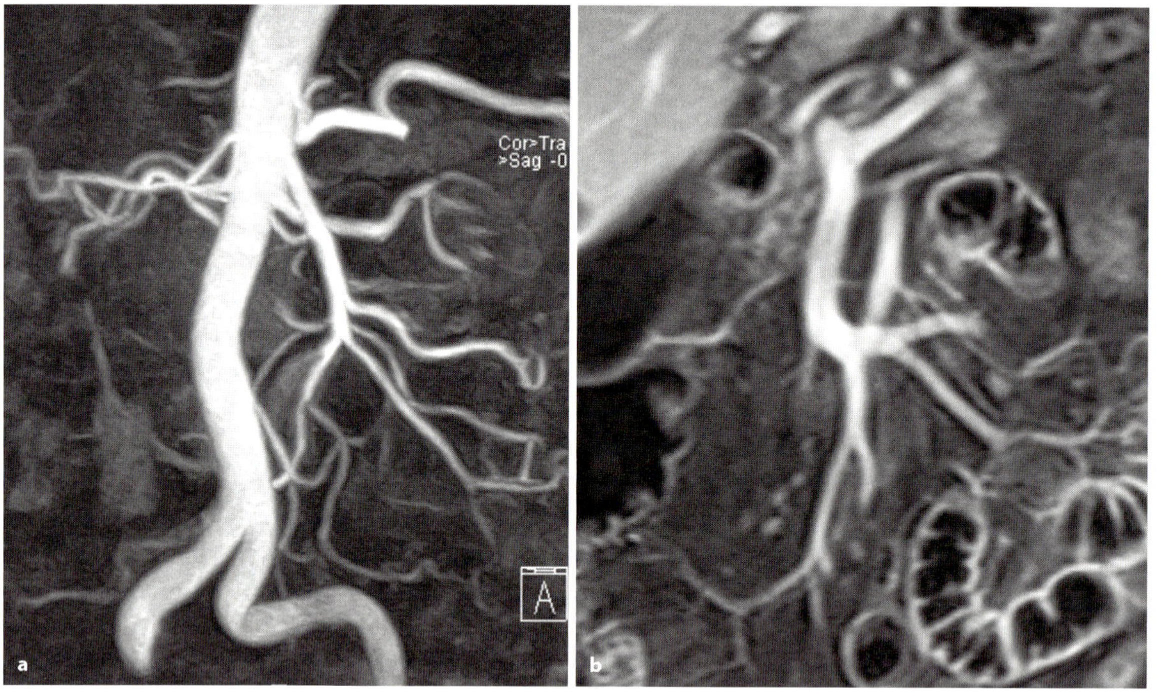

Figure 8.11 a, b

Magnetic resonance angiography of the arterial and venous abdominal vessels

2. Contraindications for iodine-containing contrast media.
3. Patients in whom radiation exposure must be avoided (e.g. pregnancy, children)

The particular strengths of MRI in comparison with other cross-sectional imaging modalities include:

1. Detection of small endocrine tumors.
2. Characterization of questionable parenchymal inhomogeneities at ultrasound or CT (disorders of fat distribution).
3. Cystic tumors of the pancreas.

References

1. Nino-Murcia M, Brooke Jeffrey R, Beaulieu CF, Li KCP, Rubin GD (2001) Multidetector CT of the pancreas and bile duct system. AJR Am J Roentgenol 176:689–693
2. Fenchel S, Fleiter TR, Aschoff AJ, van Gessel R, Brambs HJ, Merkle EM (2004) Effect of iodine concentration of contrast media on contrast enhancement in multislice CT of the pancreas. Br J Radiol 77:821–830
3. Fletcher JG, Wiersema MJ, Farrell MA, Fidler JL, Burgart LJ, Koyama T, Johnson CD, Stephens DH, Ward EM, Harmsen WS (2003) Pancreatic malignancy: value of arterial, pancreatic, and hepatic phase imaging with multi-detector row CT. Radiology 229:81–90
4. McNulty NJ, Francis IR, Platt JF, Cohan RH, Korobkin M, Gebremariam A (2001) Multi-detector row helical CT of the pancreas: effect of contrast-enhanced multiphasic imaging on enhancement of the pancreas, peripancreatic vasculature, and pancreatic adenocarcinoma. Radiology 220:97–102
5. Ly JL, Miller FH (2002) MR imaging of the pancreas. A practical approach. Radiol Clin N Am 40:1289–1306
6. Rieber A, Tomczak R, Nüssle K, Klaus H, Brambs HJ (2000) MRI with mangafodipir trisodium in the detection of pancreatic tumours: comparison with helical CT. Br J Radiol 73:1165–1169
7. Matos C, Metens T, Deviere J, Nicaise N, Braude P, van Yperen G, Cremer M, Struyven J (1997) Pancreatic duct: morphologic and functional evaluation with dynamic MR pancreatography after secretin stimulation. Radiology 203:435–441
8. Fukukura Y, Fujiyoshi F, Sasaki M, Masayuki N (2002) Pancreatic duct: morphologic evaluation with MR cholangiopancreatography after secretin stimulation. Radiology 222:674–680
9. Hellerhoff KJ, Helmberger H, Rösch T, Settles MR, Link TM, Rummeny EJ (2002) Dynamic MR pancreatography after secretin administration: image quality and diagnostic accuracy. AJR Am J Roentgenol 179:121–129
10. Rofsky NM, Lee VS, Laub G, Pollack MA, Krinsky GA, Thomasson D, Ambrosino MM, Weinreb JC (1999) Abdominal MR imaging with a volume interpolated breath-hold examination. Radiology 212:876–884

Chapter 9

H. Saisho

Endoscopic Retrograde Cholangiopancreatography

Pancreatography was first performed by Pillan in 1909 for the study of autopsy specimens [1]. In clinical use, operative pancreatography was established by Doubilet and Mulholland [2], and Leger [3] early in the 1950s. Endoscopic cannulation and pancreatic duct visualization was first reported by McCune in 1968 [4]. In 1970, Oi [5] and Takagi et al. [6] reported retrograde cholangiography as well as pancreatography with the aid of a flexible duodenoscope. Thereafter, endoscopic retrograde cholangiopancreatography (ERCP) was rapidly established as a diagnostic procedure in practice for the pancreas and biliary tract. With the improvement of the instruments and ancillary devices, it has also evolved to become a therapeutic procedure for the management of various pancreatobiliary disorders.

With the development of newer diagnostic imaging procedures over the last quarter of a century, the diagnostic role of ERCP in clinical practice has changed.

Indications

Less invasive imaging techniques than ERCP, that is ultrasound (US), computed tomography (CT), and magnetic resonance imaging (MRI), have proven useful in the diagnosis of pancreatic diseases. In particular, the development of magnetic resonance cholangiopancreatography (MRCP) in the late 1990s has reduced greatly the need for diagnostic ERCP [7]. However, the precise delineation of duct changes is still the diagnostic priority of ERCP for visualizing small or mild abnormalities, thus leading to an early diagnosis [8]. In addition, brush cytology and forceps biopsy as well as pancreatic juice collection for cytology via ERCP are helpful in establishing a tissue diagnosis.

Pancreatic Malignant Tumors

The diagnosis and staging of pancreatic carcinoma is mostly achieved by the combined use of modern US, CT, and MRI. The need for ERCP may remain only in a small group of special cases such as a small carcinoma undefined on conventional imaging and unusual neoplasms including lymphomas and metastatic cancers, the diagnosis of which is apt to be difficult. The latter may present with a smooth narrowing of the pancreatic duct in a compressed fashion (Fig. 9.1). The nature of the tumor, expansive or invasive, will directly reflect upon the radiological features of the stenotic segment, which will be outlined more precisely with ERCP than with MRCP. When an unusual pancreatic mass is suggested by the first-line imaging, ERCP may provide useful information relating to the nature of the tumor pathology.

Besides the highly detailed findings of the distorted pancreatic ducts, the possibility of tissue sampling at the same time is an additional merit of ERCP. Although the sensitivity of pancreatic carcinoma is 30–50% in brush cytology and forceps biopsy via ERCP [9–11], the validity of tissue diagnosis is basically different from that of imaging diagnosis, having the advantage of providing the final diagnosis. ERCP cytology or biopsy sampling should be an integral part of tissue diagnosis including endoscopic-US-guided fine-needle biopsy sampling and percutaneous CT or US-guided biopsy sampling.

Acute Pancreatitis

ERCP is usually unnecessary or contraindicated in the acute stage of pancreatitis except for the treatment of gallstone pancreatitis. In the convalescence stage, ERCP is useful for establishing the critical causes of pancreatitis, including a small cancer of the papilla (Fig. 9.2) or the pancreas, and biliary microcaluculi. Pancreas divisum, which may cause so-called dorsal pancreatitis, is defined almost only by ERCP.

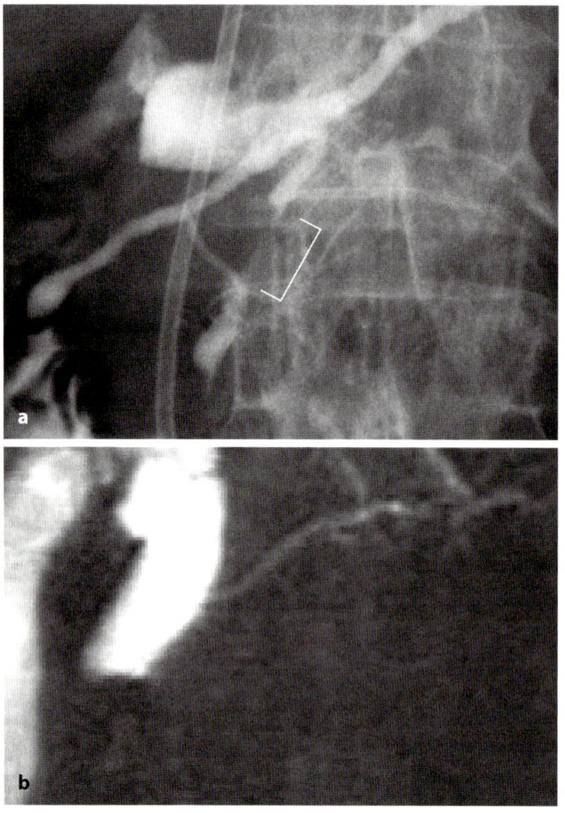

Figure 9.1

a Compressed type of stricture of the main pancreatic duct due to pancreatic malignant lymphoma. Endoscopic retrograde cholangiopancreatography (ERCP) pancreatogram apparently demonstrating a long, smooth, and straightened stenosis (marked with a *white square bracket*) that is a little deviated from the axis of the duct. b Magnetic resonance cholangiopancreatography (MRCP) pancreatogram providing no useful information concerning the strictured segment

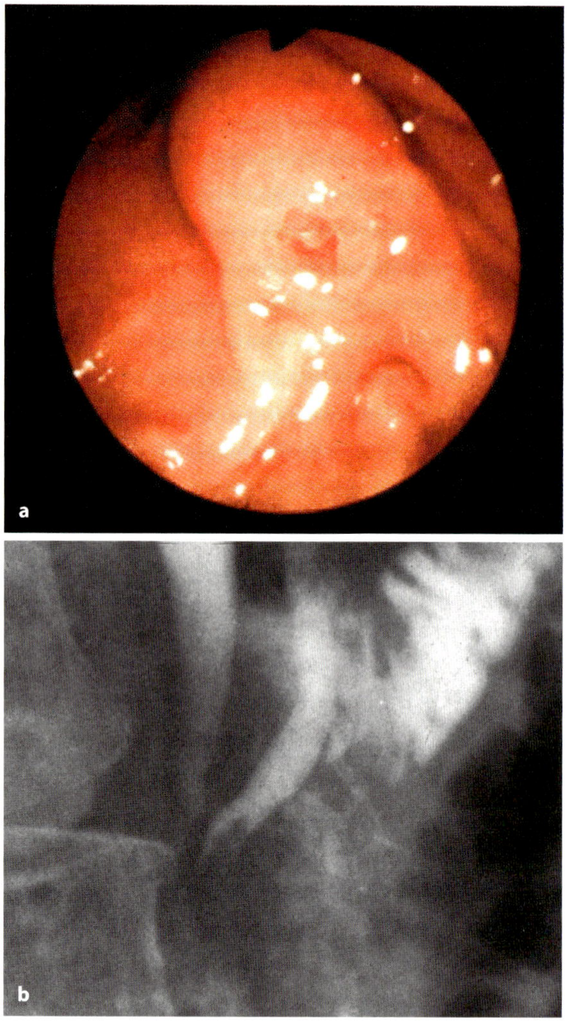

Figure 9.2

A small carcinoma of the papilla of Vater found in a patient with acute pancreatitis. a Duodenoscopic view of the swollen papilla of Vater, and b a small filling defect in the terminal end of the pancreatic duct revealed with ERCP. The diagnosis of carcinoma was finally proven by biopsy sampling in the orifice of the papilla

Chronic Pancreatitis

Calcified concrements in the pancreas, the specific findings for chronic pancreatitis, can be readily demonstrated by US or CT. The role of ERCP has been reduced in diagnosing calcified chronic pancreatitis. MRCP has been also replacing ERCP for the anatomical evaluation of the pancreaticobiliary system prior to planning of therapy in these patients.

In patients with noncalcified chronic pancreatitis, the delineation of the pancreatic ducts is important for the diagnosis. In the absence of pancreatic calcification, duct-caliber irregularity with stenoses and dilatations is the decisive feature of chronic pancreatitis, typically providing the radiological configuration of so-called "chain of lakes" in the main duct as well as in the side branches (Fig. 9.3). The typical changes can also be defined on MRCP. Therefore, ERCP may be saved for difficult cases undefined on MRCP or considered to benefit from qualified duct visualization.

The details of a diffuse or a long irregular narrowing of the pancreatic ducts in autoimmune pancreatitis is mostly defined by ERCP (Fig. 9.4). Brush cytology and forceps biopsy sampling via ERCP may be helpful in diagnosing tumefactive pancreatitis, which is often mistaken for a malignancy.

When the irregularities are presented solely in the side branches, interpretation of the pancreatogram is

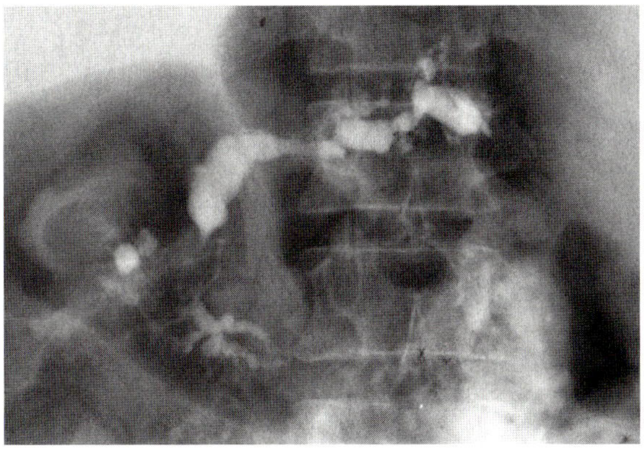

Figure 9.3

ERCP pancreatogram demonstrating multiple stenoses and alternating duct dilatations, a typical configuration of a duct-caliber irregularity in noncalcified chronic pancreatitis

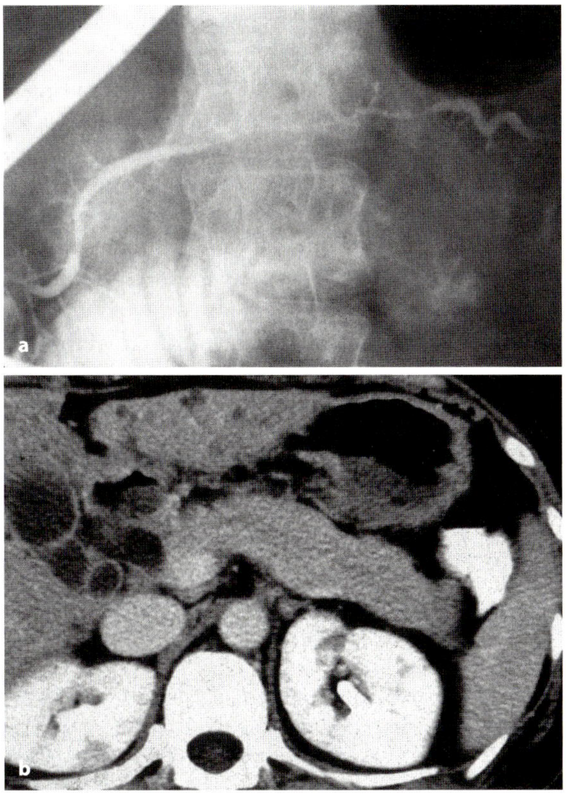

Figure 9.4

Autoimmune pancreatitis. a The characteristic long, irregular narrowing of the main pancreatic duct demonstrated with ERCP. b The enlarged pancreas revealed by computed tomography (CT) images

challenging to the clinician, for these may be found not only in patients with mild pancreatitis, but also in aged people. While up to now the detection of duct branch abnormalities in ERCP are the diagnostic mainstay at an early stage of pancreatitis or mild pancreatitis, these abnormalities are not always pathognomonic in the patients with no pancreatitic symptoms or no history of previous pancreatitis [12].

Few patients had "actual" chronic pancreatitis that could not have been excluded by using other imaging techniques and laboratory work-up. Based on these considerations, diagnostic ERCP is of almost no use for patients with abdominal pain of possible pancreatic or biliary origin, when there are no other objective findings on the biliopancreatic system [13, 14].

Instruments and Accessories for ERCP

Side-viewing video endoscopes with standard 3.2- to large 4.2-mm channels are now the most commonly used. Smaller duodenoscopes are available for examination in neonates and small children. However, the standard endoscope may be used in children over the age of 2 years. A variety of 4-Fr to 6-Fr cannulae are available for intubation and contrast injection into the pancreatic and bile ducts. Brushing catheter and biopsy forceps should be prepared for use as necessary. It is also desirable to have plastic stents or drainage tubes (of 7 or 8 Fr) near at hand for unexpected cases requiring postprocedural duct decompression.

Preoperative Preparation

Disinfection of Instruments

Immediately before the procedure, it is necessary to ensure that the instruments and accessories to be used are clean and sterile. As for the accessories including cannulae, catheters, guide wires, and sampling forceps, disposable devices provided in a sterile state are available and recommended for use for the prevention of cross-infection.

The endoscope should be reprocessed at high standards of disinfection according to accepted protocols and guidelines [15, 16]. In endoscope reprocessing, the cleaning (including brushing and flushing the working and air/water channels) immediately after use is generally the critical step for the removal of blood, secretions, or other debris. Then, after rinsing under running water, disinfection of the endoscope is automatically processed in a disinfection system with a disinfectant solution by following the manufacturer's instructions. In addition to final rinsing, it is necessary to assure correct drying to prevent recontamination of microorganisms during storage.

Patient Preparation

The procedure is performed in the morning after overnight fasting, or when the patient is fasted for at least 6 h prior to the procedure. Lidocaine (Xylocaine) in solution or spray is used for topical pharyngeal anesthesia and any one of the sedatives including diazepam (Valium, Cercine, or Horizone), midazolam (Dormicum), petidine hydrochloride (Opystan), and meperidine hydrochloride (Demerol) is usually given intravenously immediately before the endoscope insertion. Glucagon (0.25–0.5 mg) or Buscopan (20–40 mg) is administered also intravenously to relax the duodenum and to facilitate cannulation.

Prophylactic Use of Antibiotics

Antibiotic prophylaxis is recommended in patients with the high-risk factors described below. Infection of the biliopancreatic system is one of major complications following ERCP. It has been well known that biliary obstruction, a history of previous cholangitis, and pancreatic pseudocyst are the main risk factors for infection. Cholangitis and sepsis are common after ERCP, when the establishment of biliary drainage is incomplete in patients with a biliary obstruction [17, 18]. The pathogens are mainly enteric Gram-negative microorganisms such as *Escherichia coli*, *Klebsiella* spp., and *Enterococcus* spp. [19]. In patients with any one of the risk factors, prophylactic administration of a broad-spectrum antibiotic covering these Gram-negative bacteria is recommended just before the procedure [20]. The addition of antibiotics to the contrast medium may be of no use [21].

Bacterial endocarditis is another potential infection following ERCP, as well as the other upper gastrointestinal endoscopy. Patients at high risk who have heart valve disorders, prosthetic heart valves, and also major vascular disorders including recent (<1 year) synthetic vascular graft placement should be considered for antibiotic prophylaxis. As mentioned elsewhere in authorized guidelines [20, 21], the regimens are important to cover streptcocci and staphylococci, which are the most common pathogens of endocarditis. Otherwise, general use of prophylactic antibiotics is considered unnecessary.

Major Points of the ERCP Technique

The patient is placed prone or in a left lateral decubitus position on a fluoroscopic table. The duodenoscope used in ERCP is a side-viewing instrument, which requires some skill for the operator at several points during the passage through the esophagogastric canal into the descending duodenum. The cannulation of the papilla also requires other delicate techniques critical for ERCP.

Passage of the Esophagogastric Junction into the Stomach

A side-viewing duodenoscope is gently passed through the oropharynx into the esophagus in the angle-free maneuver; sometimes, a brief use of the right-left angle lock may be better to pass the esophageal entrance. While it is slowly advanced into the stomach almost blindly, there may be a resistance on the terminal end of the esophagus. To pass this part smoothly, a bit of a rotating maneuver over the instrument shaft is helpful. When the tip of the instrument comes into the stomach, an adequate amount of air is insufflated to secure the view. Sometimes, the tip of the scope may be trapped in the fundus, curling up in reverse. To avoid this problem, after passing the cardiac entrance, the instrument is rotated counterclockwise to get the view of the longitudinal folds in the greater curvature. Then, it is so advanced as that the tip comes in touch on the folds and rotated clockwise so as to obtain a view of the lesser curvature and the gastric angle downward. Thereafter, with bending the tip slightly upward, it is pushed forwards under visual control until it reaches the pyloric antrum.

Passage of the Pylorus

As the pylorus is approached, it sinks down to the middle of the bottom of view. As the tip of the instrument is further advanced, the view is obstructed in a moment, immediately before it flips into the duodenal bulb. If the view is still obstructed in spite of a pushing maneuver, the instrument is withdrawn to make the second attempt with a corrected adjustment for the direction.

Insertion into the Descending Duodenum

In the duodenal bulb, the tip is bent downward and the instrument is withdrawn a little to detect the superior duodenal angle in the posterior wall, the entrance of the descending duodenum. After the tip is located on this angle, it is intensely bent upward and the entire instrument is rotated clockwise so as to look down the descending duodenum, when necessary, with the help of right angling manipulation. The angling knobs are locked to keep the tip bending as it is, and the "straightening maneuver" is usually performed by pulling the instrument back while applying further clockwise rotation. While any redundant loops of the instrument are straightened in the stomach, paradoxically the tip advances further into the descending part of the duodenum.

When the "straightening maneuver" is not performed well, or afterwards the positioning of the papilla is not appropriate for cannulation, the "pushing maneuver" is an alternative; after the instrument reaches the spot where the descending duodenum is looked down, it is cautiously pushed further into the loop with counterclockwise rotation under visual control. The "pushing maneuver" is often useful for cannulating the minor papilla.

Discovery of the Papilla

When the "straightening maneuver" is completed, the tip has usually advanced distally farther than the papilla of Vater. The bending tip is relaxed, and in withdrawing the instrument slowly, careful observation on the medial wall usually reveals a longitudinal fold and the papilla at the proximal end of this fold.

Cannulation of the Papilla

After the papilla is identified, appropriate repositioning of the instrumental tip is attempted prior to cannulation to get a good face-on view of the papilla in a small look-up position. The positioning is critical to obtain a successful cannulation into the biliary or pancreatic duct.

Contrast Injection

The cannula is brought into view and filled with contrast material. The cannula tip is then carefully advanced and guided into the orifice of the papilla by pressure on the forceps elevator together with attempts to advance the cannula. After the cannula is inserted 5 mm to 2 cm into the papilla, contrast medium is slowly injected under fluoroscopic control. The pancreatic duct is usually outlined first. Sometimes, both the biliary and pancreatic ducts are visualized. To obtain the selective visualization of either one, a deep cannulation into the target duct is required by more careful maneuvering of the cannula tip aligned along the axis of the target duct. In general, cannulation rightwards to the long axis of the duodenum favors the pancreatic duct, whilst upwards angulation favors the bile duct.

Technical Aspects for Radiography

With regard to the gravitational effect, the left lateral position is adequate to facilitate filling of contrast medium in the pancreatic duct system, which runs from right to left across the body. The filling of contrast medium is controlled under television fluoroscopic observation. Overfilling of the pancreatic ducts must be avoided by careful injection of contrast medium.

Although filling of the small branches may not be recognized on the television monitoring screen, they are usually visualized on x-ray films when the whole figure of main pancreatic duct (MPD) is seen clearly on the screen. Excessive contrast medium overfills the duct system, resulting in "acinar filling," which may cause acute pancreatitis.

When the duct systems are filled enough, radiograms are taken after changing the patient's position to the prone or supine, as the lateral radiogram gives a less clear view. If an abnormal finding is noticed, additional films are taken at the proper positions so as to reveal the significant area without superimposing the instrument, the spine, and the contrast medium that has leaked into the intestine.

Then, the cannula and the scope are withdrawn and radiograms are again taken in various projections. At this time, the radiograms can exhibit the natural course and location of the duct systems. The contrast medium in the duct systems is drained through the papilla. The normal pancreatic duct system is completely cleared within a few minutes. Cysts or localized dilatations become more noticeable due to the retained contrast medium.

Interpretation of the Pancreatogram

Normal Pancreatogram

The pancreas is transversely located in the retroperitoneal space between T12 and L2, lying over the spine and aorta. The MPD, which is usually drained by the duct of Wirsung, runs up from the major papilla in the head, and angles to the left so as to run across the spine and slightly cranially in the tail up to the splenic hilum. The duct contour is smooth and gradually tapering toward the tail, diverging into branches to disappear within the tail tip. The maximum diameter, approximately 4 mm on average, is found in the head, while the caliber tends to increase in advancing age [22]. The accessory duct (the duct of Santorini) is found in about 80% of people. This communicates with the MPD in the neck of the pancreas, the transitional zone of the head to the body, and runs to the minor duodenal papilla, situated about 2 cm oroventrally to the major papilla. Many branch ducts join the MPD at right angles to the MPD except in the head, where they are larger and less numerous. The largest one in the head drains the uncinate process. The branch ducts are usually visualized less clearly in the body than in other parts.

Pancreas divisum, in which pancreatic drainage is mainly through the minor papilla, has been reported in 3–9% of autopsy and ERCP series [1, 23, 24]. In our ERCP experience in Japan [22], it was found in only 20 (1.6%) of 1263 patients having no pancreatic diseases, and among them only 8 patients (0.6%) had complete divisum in which the small duct Wirsung was isolated from the main drainage (the duct of Santorini) and terminated into a fine network within the head of the pancreas.

Abnormal Pancreatogram

Ductal Stenosis or Obstruction

Ductal stenosis or obstruction is an essential finding in either neoplasms or inflammatory processes of the pancreas. An isolated stenosis with upstream dilatation is usually indicative of pancreatic carcinoma. Duct obstruction, or contrast stop, is also usually due to tumors. In particular, the "double duct stricture" sign, concurrent obstruction at the same level in the common bile duct and MPD, is almost specific to carcinoma of the pancreas head [25] (Fig. 9.5). However, some inflammatory processes may present with a stenosis or an obstruction that mimics those found in patients with pancreatic carcinoma. Endoscopic brush cytology or forceps biopsy sampling via the papilla may be considered to obtain a definite diagnosis for the selected patients when the pancreatograms are confusing.

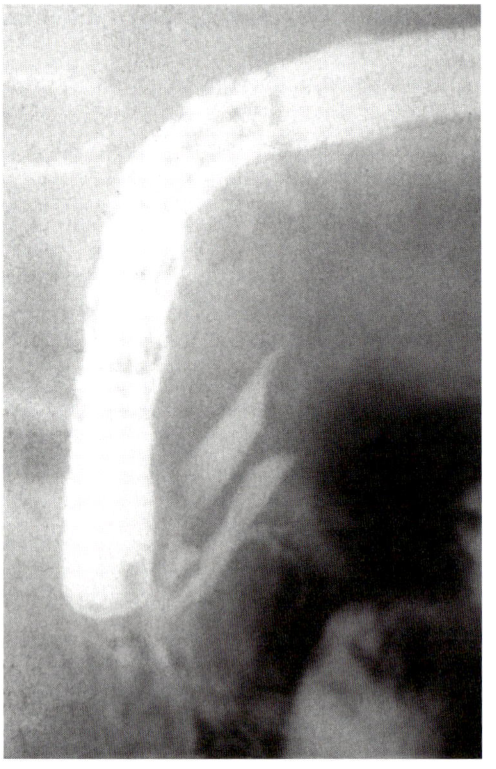

Figure 9.5

ERCP pancreatogram demonstrating the "double- duct stricture" sign due to carcinoma of the pancreas head

Variations of Caliber

The duct configuration of multiple stenoses and alternating segmental dilatations, well noted as irregular dilatations, is characteristic for advanced chronic pancreatitis. It is frequently associated with contrast defects due to pancreatic stones. The variation in caliber may reflect the irregular distribution of inflammatory and fibrotic processes in the pancreas.

Irregular Narrowing of the MPD

Diffuse or elongated irregular narrowing of the MPD with or without a mild dilatation upstream is found in another type of chronic pancreatitis or autoimmune pancreatitis [26, 27]. In this type of pancreatitis, a focal or global enlargement of the pancreas is usually revealed on medical imaging, and this is challenging

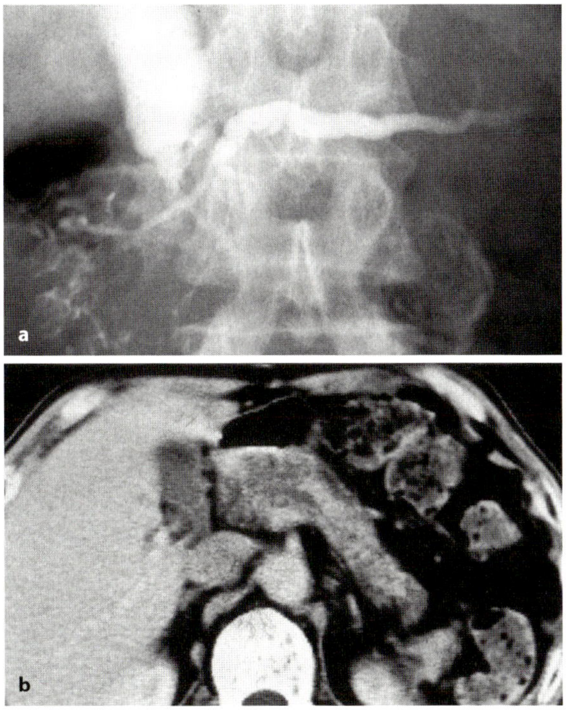

Figure 9.6

Tumefactive pancreatitis (autoimmune pancreatitis). a ERCP pancreatogram demonstrating a long, irregular narrowing of the main duct in the head with a moderate dilatation accompanied in the upstream. b A focal enlargement of the corresponding site of the pancreas seen in CT images may be confusing to exclude a malignancy

for differentiation from a neoplastic tumor [28]. Even though the duct configuration seems a little bit different from the typical stricture in the case of carcinoma, brush cytology is helpful to solve the problem (Fig. 9.6).

Dilatation of the Pancreatic Ducts

Marked dilatation of the pancreatic ducts with an intraductal mucinous substance is indicative of intraductal papillary mucinous neoplasm (IPMN). When the neoplasm originates in the branch ducts, cystic dilatations in the branches may be found. However, the entire visualization of the pancreatic duct system is usually blocked by the massive amounts of mucin that fill the ducts (Fig. 9.7). MRCP is the tool of choice to display the entire pancreatic duct system in patients with IPMN. Observation of mucinous substance and pancreatic juice sampling for cytology during ERCP is helpful in the diagnosis [11].

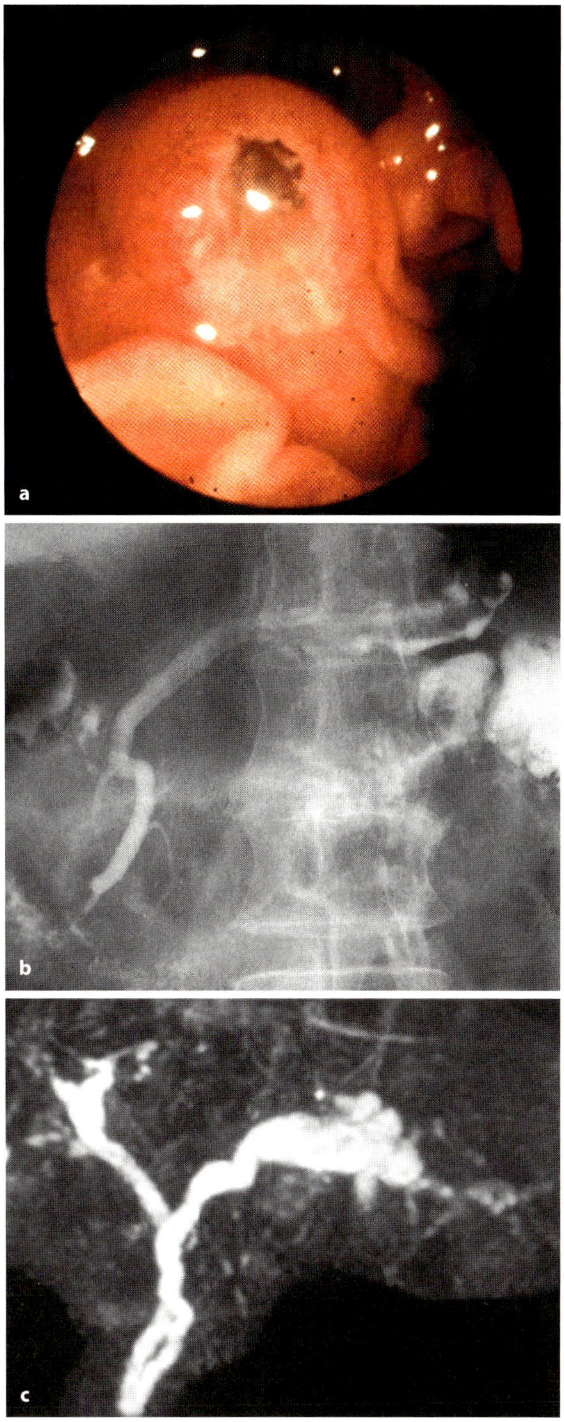

Figure 9.7

Intraductal papillary mucinous neoplasm. a Mucinous substance choked in the loose orifice of the papilla of Vater found on the endoscopic observation is a strong clue for the diagnosis. However, the complete duct delineation is impossible with ERCP due to excessive mucinous substance filled in the ducts (b). c MRCP is better for examining the whole profile of the duct system

Minimal Abnormalities of the Pancreatic Ducts

Minimal abnormalities of the pancreatic ducts such as mild dilatation, low-grade irregularities, and side-branch abnormalities may be found in patients with an early tumor or mild pancreatitis. These mild changes are also seen in aged people at times, and then, the interpretation is an intricate issue in practice. However, the detection of mild duct changes could be the first step for the early diagnosis. In spite of the great progress in modern diagnostic imaging, ERCP remains a mandatory tool because of the high-quality and accurate visualization of the pancreatic ducts.

Complications and Prophylactic Therapy

ERCP is a relatively safe procedure; however, it is always accompanied by the potential risk of complications common to other types of gastrointestinal endoscopy and those peculiar to this procedure. Among the latter complications, pancreatitis and infections are noteworthy and important from the clinical viewpoint.

Post-ERCP Pancreatitis

Pancreatitis is the most frequent complication of ERCP: post-ERCP pancreatitis occurs in 1–7% of cases [17, 18, 29–31] The variation in frequency is thought to be correlated with differences in the definition of post-ERCP pancreatitis, the demography of subjects, and/or ERCP techniques used. The definition of post-ERCP pancreatitis has a consensus as follows: new or worsened abdominal pain with a serum amylase three or more times the upper limits of normal 24 h after the procedure, requiring at least 2 days of hospitalization [32].

The incidence of pancreatitis may be related to the proportion of patients with a high risk for the complication. The patient-related risk factors for pancreatitis have been studied and are now well established [33]. These include young age, female gender, a history of recurrent or post-ERCP pancreatitis, and sphincter of Oddi dysfunction. The frequency of pancreatitis is reported to increase to 40% in patients with multiple risk factors [34].

Technique-related risk factors are also important. The rate of complication probably relates to the endoscopist's level of expertise. In particular, papillary trauma due to repeated attempts at cannulation will cause pancreatitis. Other possible factors include the repeated contrast injection into the pancreatic ducts and the excessive contrast injection at a high pressure. However, pancreatic parenchymal acinarization due to an over-pressured injection of contrast has been recently thought less harmful than considered previously [29, 20, 33].

Prevention of post-ERCP pancreatitis is an important issue in practice. The prophylactic use of pharmacological agents that may prevent pancreatitis is attractive for the selected high-risk patient, because post-ERCP pancreatitis is not predictable for each patient before the procedure. So far, preoperative administration of somatostatin, octreotide, corticosteroids, glycerol trinitrate, heparin, and gabexate mesilate have been attempted with a view to prevention of the complication. Among these agents, somatostatin (a suppressor of pancreatic exocrine secretion) and gabexate (a protease inhibitor) are suggested to be effective in several randomized controlled studies [35–39], but their use has not yet been put into widespread clinical practice. The routine use of these agents is not cost-effective because a considerable number of patients should be treated for one patient's benefit. Randomized controlled trials in the selected subjects with high-risk of post-ERCP pancreatitis are awaited to show a clinical and cost benefit in the prophylactic use of these agents.

Placement of a pancreatic stent is an option with demonstrated efficacy for the prevention of post-ERCP pancreatitis in high-risk patients, particularly for suspected sphincter Oddi dysfunction [40, 41]. However, this method has its own limitation: stent placement following the ERCP procedure would be difficult. In fact, failure rates after biliary intervention ranged from 5% to 10%. Furthermore, failure of stent placement is associated with a high incidence of pancreatitis [42].

Cholangitis and Sepsis

Infectious complication following ERCP is commonly observed in association with incomplete biliary drainage. Two pathways could be attributable to developing the processes: infection of the pancreaticobiliary system by contaminated instrumentation, or invasive spread of already existing intraductal organisms due to ERCP manipulation and contrast injection. The establishment of adequate pancreaticobiliary drainage immediately after ERCP is recognized as the most important way of preventing infective complications. Antibiotics should be used in patients with known cholangitis. In addition, use of postprocedural antibiotics may reduce infectious complications in patients with incomplete biliopancreatic drainage and unexpected filling of pancreatic pseudocysts [19]. But the routine use of prophylactic antibiotics does not appear to reduce this risk and is not recommended [43]. Infection of *Pseudomonas aeruginosa* is rare, but when it is found, incomplete disinfection of the instruments should be considered [44].

Prophylactic antibiotics should be also recommended for patients with heart-valve disorders, prosthetic heart valves, a prior history of endocarditis, systemic-pulmonary shunt, or recent (<1 year) synthetic graft placement [20, 21]. Nonetheless, better skills and experiences of endoscopists and other medical staff can decrease the frequency of complications associated with ERCP. Endoscopists and staff should receive adequate training and ensure that they are exposed to a sufficient case volume to warrant providing this procedure.

References

1. Millbourn E (1950) On the excretory ducts of the pancreas in man, with special reference to their relations to each other, to the common bile duct and to the duodenum: a radiological and anatomical study. Acta Anat 9:1–34
2. Doubilet H, Mulholland JH (1951) Intubation of the pancreatic duct in the human. Proc Soc Exp Biol Med 76:113–114
3. Leger L (1953) Surgical contrast visualization of the pancreatic ducts with a study of pancreatic external secretion. Am J Dig Dis 20:8–12
4. McCune WS, Shorb PE, Moscovitz H (1968) Endoscopic cannulation of the ampulla of Vater. A preliminary report. Ann Surg 167:752–756
5. Oi I (1970) Fiberduodenoscopy and endoscopic pancreatocholangiography. Gastrointest Endosc 17:59–62
6. Takagi K, Ikeda S, Nakagawa Y, et al (1970) Retrograde pancreatography and cholangiography by fiber duodenoscope. Gastroenterology 59:445–452
7. Adamek HE, Albert J, Breer H, et al (2000) Pancreatic cancer detection with magnetic resonance cholangiopancreatography and endoscopic retrograde cholangiopancreatography: a prospective controlled study. Lancet 356:190–193
8. Glasbrenner B, Kahl S, Malfertheiner P (2002) Modern diagnostics of chronic pancreatitis. Eur J Gastroenterol Hepatol 14:935–941
9. Hawes RH (2002) Diagnostic and therapeutic uses of ERCP in pancreatic and biliary tract malignancies. Gastrointest Endosc 56:S201–205
10. Adler DG, Baron TH, Davila RE, et al (2005) ASGE guideline: the role of ERCP in diseases of the biliary tract and the pancreas. Gastrointest Endosc 62:1–8
11. Yamaguchi T, Shirai Y, Ishihara T, et al (2005) Pancreatic juice cytology in the diagnosis of intraductal papillary mucinous neoplasm of the pancreas: significance of sampling by peroral pancreatoscopy. Cancer 104:2630–2636
12. Glasbrenner B, Kahl S, Malfertheiner P (2002) Modern diagnostics of chronic pancreatitis. Eur J Gastroenterol Hepatol 14:935–941
13. Cohen S, Bacon BR, Berlin JA, et al (2002) National Institutes of Health State-of-the-Science Conference Statement: ERCP for diagnosis and therapy, January 14–16, 2002. Gastrointest Endosc 56:803–809
14. Etenad B, Whitcomb DC (2001) Chronic pancreatitis: diagnosis, classification, and new genetic developments. Gastroenterology 120:682–707
15. Nelson DB, Jarvis WR, Rutala WA, et al (2003) Multi-society guideline for reprocessing flexible gastrointestinal endoscopes. Gastrointest Endosc 58:1–8
16. Rey JF, Bjorkman D, Duforest-Rey D, et al (2005) WGO-OMGE practice guideline: endoscope disinfection. http://omge.org/globalguidelines/guide14/g_data14_en.htm 14 Dec
17. Freeman ML (2002) Adverse outcomes of ERCP. Gastrointest Endosc 56:S278–S282
18. Vandervoort J, Soetikno RM, Tham TC, et al (2002) Risk factors for complications after performance of ERCP. Gastrointest Endosc 56:652–656
19. Subhani JM, Kibbler C, Dooley JS (1999) Antibiotic prophylaxis for endoscopic retrograde cholangiopancreatography (ERCP). Aliment Pharmacol Ther 13:103–116
20. Hirota WK, Petersen K, Baron TH, et al (2003) Guidelines for antibiotic prophylaxis for GI endoscopy. Gastrointest Endosc 58:475–482
21. Rey JR, Axon A, Budzynska A, et al (1998) Guidelines of the European Society of Gastrointestinal Endoscopy (ESGE): antibiotic prophylaxis for gastrointestinal endoscopy. Endoscopy 30:318–324
22. Ohto M, Ono T, Tsuchiya Y, Saisho H (1978) Cholangiography and Pancreatography. Igaku-Shoin, Tokyo, New York, pp 81–83
23. Cotton PB (1980) Congenital anomaly of pancreas divisum as cause of obstructive pain and pancreatitis. Gut 21:105–114
24. Delhaye M, Engelholm L, Cremer M (1985) Pancreas divisum: congenital anatomic variant or anomaly? Contribution of endoscopic retrograde dorsal pancreatography. Gastroenterology 89:951–958
25. Kalady MF, Peterson B, Baillie J, et al (2004) Pancreatic duct strictures: identifying risk of malignancy. Ann Surg Oncol 11:581–588
26. Yoshida K, Toki F, Takeuchi T, et al (1995) Chronic Pancreatitis caused by an autoimmune abnormality: proposal of the concept of autoimmune pancreatitis. Dig Dis Sci 40:1561–1568
27. Pearson RK, Longnecker DS, Chari ST, et al (2003) Controversies in clinical pancreatology: Autoimmune pancreatitis: does it exist? Pancreas 27:1–13
28. Levy MJ, Wiesema MJ, Chari ST (2006) Chronic pancreatitis: focal pancreatitis or cancer? Is there a role for FNA/biopsy? Autoimmune pancreatitis. Endoscopy 38:530–535
29. Loperfido S, Angelini G, Benedetti G, et al (1998) Major early complications from diagnostic and therapeutic ERCP: a prospective multicenter study. Gastrointest Endosc 48:1–10
30. Masci E, Toti G, Mariani A, et al (2001) Complications of diagnostic and therapeutic ERCP: a prospective multicenter study. Am J Gastroenterol 96:417–423
31. Mallery JS, Baron TH, Dominitz JA, et al (2003) Complications of ERCP. Gastrointest Endosc 57:633–638

32. Cotton PB, Lehman G, Vennes J, et al (1991) Endoscopic sphincterotomy complications and their management: an attempt at consensus. Gastrointest Endosc 37:383–393
33. Freeman ML, Guda NM (2004) Prevention of post-ERCP pancreatitis: a comprehensive review. Gastrointest Endosc 59:845–864
34. Freeman ML, DiSario JA, Nelson DB, et al (2001) Risk factors for post-ERCP pancreatitis: a prospective, multicenter study. Gastrointest Endosc 54:425–434
35. Cavallini G, Tittobello A, Frulloni L, et al (1996) Gabexate for the prevention of pancreatic damage related to endoscopic retrograde cholangiopancreatography. N Engl J Med 335:919–923
36. Andriulli A, Leandro G, Niro G, et al (2000) Pharmacologic treatment can prevent pancreatic injury after ERCP: a meta-analysis. Gastrointest Endosc 51:100–103
37. Arvanitidis D, Anagnostopoulos GK, Giannopoulos D, et al (2004) Can somatostatin prevent post-ERCP pancreatitis? Results of a randomized controlled trial. J Gastroenterol Hepatol 19:278–282
38. Andriulli A, Solmi L, Loperfido S, et al (2004) Prophylaxis of ERCP-related pancreatitis: a randomized, controlled trial of somatostatin and gabexate mesylate. Clin Gastroenterol Hepatol 2:713–718
39. Andriulli A, Caruso N, Quitadamo M, et al (2003) Antisecretory vs. antiproteasic drugs in the prevention of post-ERCP pancreatitis: the evidence-based medicine derived from a meta-analysis study. JOP 4:41–48
40. Singh P, Das A, Isenberg G, et al (2004) Does prophylactic pancreatic stent placement reduce the risk of post-ERCP acute pancreatitis? A meta-analysis of controlled trials. Gastrointest Endosc 60:544–550
41. Fazel A, Quadri A, Catalono MF, et al (2003) Does a pancreatic duct stent prevent post-ERCP pancreatitis? A prospective randomized study. Gastrointest Endosc 57:291–294
42. Freeman ML, Overby C, Qi D (2004) Pancreatic stent insertion: consequences of failure and results of a modified technique to maximize success. Gastrointest Endosc 59:8–14
43. Harris A, Chan C-H, Torres-Viera C, et al (1999) Meta-analysis of antibiotic prophylaxis in endoscopic retrograde cholangiopancreatography (ERCP) Endoscopy 31:718–724
44. Nelson DB (2003) Infectious disease complications of GI endoscopy: part II, exogenous infections. Gastrointest Endosc 57:695–711

Chapter 10

K. Yamao · H. N. Mizuno · K. Takahashi · Y. Shimizu · T. Koshikawa

Fine-Needle Aspiration Biopsy of the Pancreas

A variety of imaging modalities such as ultrasonography (US), computed tomography (CT), magnetic resonance imaging (MRI), and endoscopic ultrasonography (EUS) have been developed for the demonstration of pancreatic lesions and have remarkably improved the visualization rates of small lesions. Using these imaging modalities, even small lesions less than 2 cm in diameter located in the pancreas can be detected, but differentiating between benign and malignant lesions remains difficult based on their appearance alone. Thus, a tissue sampling method that is definitive, safe, and easy is required.

The tissue sampling methods for pancreatic lesions include a core needle or wedge biopsy [1], fine needle aspiration biopsy [2], and collection of pancreatic juice by direct suction, washing, or brushings during endoscopic retrograde cholangiopancreatography (ERCP) [1,3,4]. Among these sampling methods, fine-needle aspiration biopsy (FNAB) of the pancreas under US, CT, or EUS [5,6] has become established as the most reliable and safe procedure. We describe here endoscopic ultrasound-guided fine-needle aspiration biopsy (EUS-FNAB) with special reference to the pancreas.

Fine-Needle Aspiration Biopsy

FNAB is performed with a 21- to 23-gauze needle. There are three main approaches to FNAB of the pancreas:

1. Intraoperative aspiration biopsy under palpation or direct visualization of the pancreas, or guided by intraoperative ultrasound.
2. Percutaneous transabdominal aspiration biopsy under the guidance of US, CT, ERCP, or angiography.
3. EUS-FNAB.

Intraoperative aspiration biopsy is sometimes performed at the time of palliative surgery. However, diagnostic laparotomies are now rarely performed solely for the purpose of tissue sampling of pancreatic lesions, with the advances in other sampling methods.

US and CT scanning are adequate modalities for localization of the lesion. These cross-sectional imaging modalities allow visualization of the needle path and accurate localization of the depth of the lesion [7]. US-guided FNAB and CT-guided FNAB have been widely evaluated and are now established as useful modalities for sampling of pancreatic lesions. US with a real-time biopsy transducer, which permits simultaneous scanning and observation of the needle path during FNAB, has become the standard method for aspiration biopsy of the pancreas, due to its simplicity and accuracy in obtaining samples [8]. However, clear US images of the entire pancreas cannot always be obtained because of the presence of overlying bowel gas. CT does not have this limitation and generally produces pancreatic images of high quality. If the first attempt under the guidance of US is unsuccessful, CT guidance is valuable. However, CT guidance has several disadvantages, including radiation exposure, longer procedure duration, and greater expense. The diagnostic sensitivity and specificity of US- or CT-guided FNAB for pancreatic carcinoma have been reported to be 74–87% and 78–98%, respectively [9–13]. The complication rate of US- or CT-guided FNAB is comparatively low at 1.6–4.9% compared with core-needle biopsy or wedge biopsy.

ERCP permits visualization of pancreatic ducts and bile ducts. Small pancreatic cancer can be detected as a localized stricture or obstruction of the pancreatic duct. Some cases with pancreatic head cancer presenting with obstructive jaundice may undergo an endoscopic or percutaneous drainage procedure. The opacified pancreatic ducts or biliary ducts may provide a visible landmark for fluoroscopic biopsy [14]. Angiography may visualize an encasement of blood vessels by a tumor growth. However, ERCP and angiography cannot display the pancreatic mass itself. Furthermore, the appropriate depth of the needle may be difficult to ascertain fluoroscopically, unless biplane fluoroscopy is available [15].

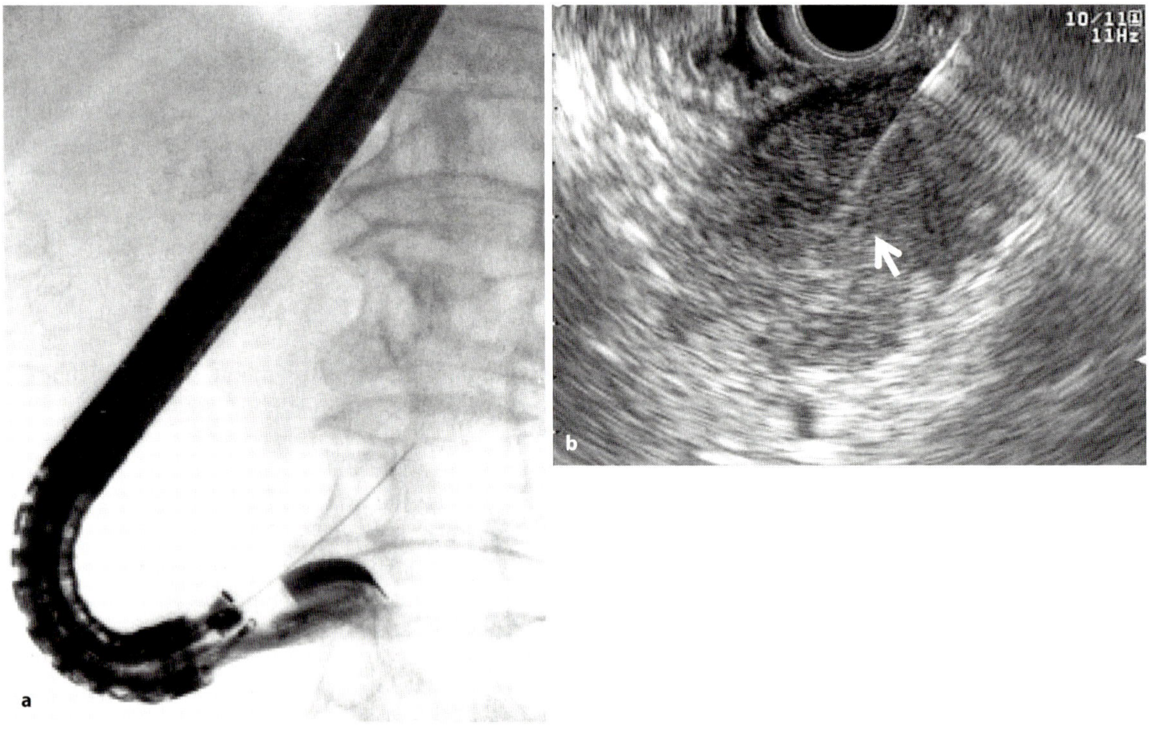

Figure 10.1

a Fluoroscopic image showing endoscopic ultrasound-guided fine-needle aspiration (EUS-FNA) from the second portion of the duodenum for pancreatic head tumor. b Endoscopic ultrasound displaying a fine needle (*white arrow*) puncturing a hypoechoic pancreatic tumor

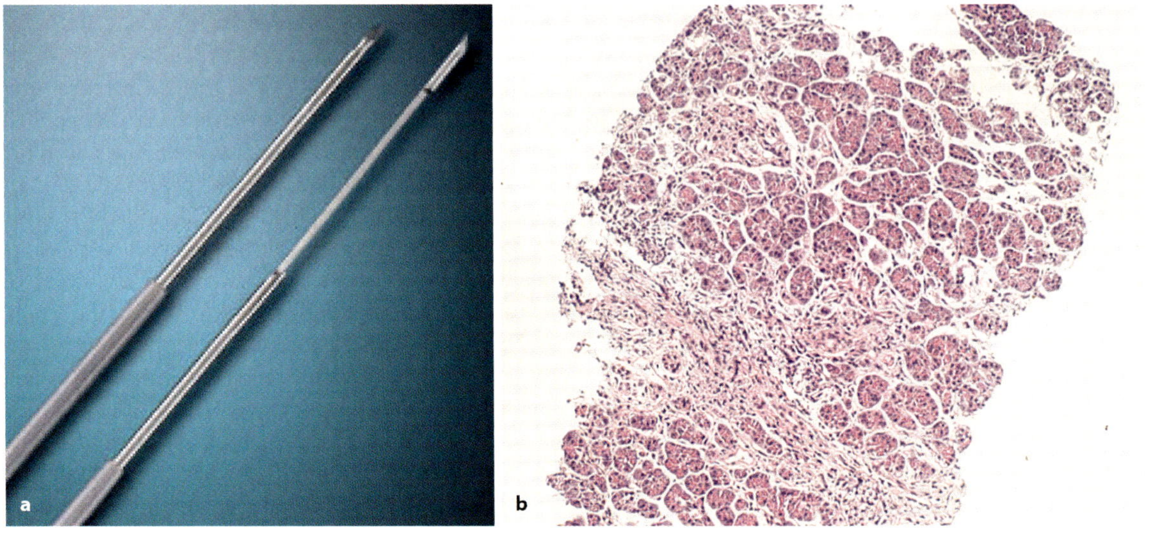

Figure 10.2

a A 19-gauge trucut biopsy needle for EUS-FNA. b A pancreatic tissue specimen large enough for histopathological and immunohistochemical study obtained with the aid of a trucut biopsy needle

EUS is a combination of endoscopy and intraluminal ultrasonography. Because EUS enables ultrasonographic images of high resolution to be obtained, it is now a widely accepted modality for detecting pancreatobiliary diseases, determining the invasion depth of gastrointestinal malignancies, and often visualizing lesions more precisely than other imaging modalities. However, whether the lesion is malignant or benign cannot be discerned solely from the findings of EUS [16]. Thus, EUS-FNAB was developed to enhance the diagnostic capabilities of EUS by providing additional pathological findings (Figs. 10.1 and 10.2). At the beginning of 1992, Vilmann et al. (5) published the first case report of direct EUS-guided FNAB of a lesion in the pancreatic head using a curved linear array echoendoscope. More than 10 years have passed since EUS-FNAB was first performed for pancreatic disease, and this technique is now popular worldwide. EUS-FNAB has several advantages compared to US- or CT-guided biopsy [17]: (1) The ability to sample lesions (including lymph nodes) too small to be identified by other methods ; (2) The ability to biopsy the lesion through a segment of the intestinal wall, which typically becomes part of the resection specimen, thereby minimizing the risk of needle tract seeding; (3) Procurement of additional staging information through the EUS examination. The diagnostic accuracy, sensitivity, and specificity of EUS-FNAB for pancreatic neoplasm in different studies are 76–95%, 64–94% and 93–100%, respectively [18]. The complication rate of EUS-FNAB appears to be around 1–2% [19].

Indications and Contraindications of FNAB

A fundamental principle for establishing the indications of any tissue sampling method is determining whether the information obtained has the potential to affect patient management. The current indications of EUS-FNAB of the pancreas include [20,21]:

1. Differentiating between benign and malignant pancreatic lesions.
2. Staging of pancreatic cancer (e.g., lymphadenopathy, ascites/pleural effusion, liver metastasis).
3. Obtaining histological evidence in cases of unresectable pancreatic cancer before chemotherapy and/or radiation therapy.

In addition to these indications, Wallace et al. [22] have described additional indications for EUS-FNAB of the pancreas: (1) reluctance of patients to undergo major surgery without a definitive diagnosis, and (2) to document the absence of malignancy when the pretest probability of malignancy is low.

Pathological confirmation of malignancy is absolutely necessary in a patient with inoperable pancreatic cancer who is a candidate for chemotherapy and/or radiation therapy. Some doctors claim that histological evidence need not be obtained when imaging modalities show typical findings of pancreatic cancer. However, a few patients with locally advanced pancreatic cancer who undergo chemotherapy and radiation therapy can survive more than 3 years. Taking this into account, in the absence of pretreatment histological evidence of malignancy, the length of treatment cannot be determined if the treatment is very effective and the patient survives longer than expected.

More controversial is the role of FNAB in patients suspected of having pancreatic cancer that appears to be resectable on other imaging studies. One view is that a tissue diagnosis will not alter management, and is therefore unnecessary. This is because FNAB for pancreatic masses has a comparatively low negative predictive value for malignancy. Thus, a negative FNAB for cancer will not exclude the diagnosis and the patient will be explored anyway. In addition, the risk of tumor seeding caused by FNAB is stressed in the dissenting opinions against this indication. On the other hand, the diagnostic accuracy of FNAB, especially EUS-FNAB, has recently been shown to be almost identical to that of endoscopic biopsy in gastrointestinal cancers, leading to a false negative result in around 5% of patients in our hospital.

Establishment of a histological diagnosis may alter the choice of treatment and choice of operative procedure even when surgery is planned. Some patients, especially those at high risk for surgery, as well as surgeons, are eager to see the histological evidence of malignancy when major surgery is scheduled. Further studies are required to determine the role of FNAB in patients suspected of having pancreatic cancer who appear to be resectable on other imaging studies.

To document the absence of malignancy when the pretest probability of malignancy is low is very important in clinical practice. The present authors make it a rule to perform FNAB at least once before following up suspected cases of an inflammatory mass caused by autoimmune pancreatitis or alcoholic intake, and benign cystic pancreatic neoplasm suspected to be serous cystic neoplasm or benign cyst without high risk stigmata for malignancy. The "wait and watch" approach seems to be very risky in cases of pancreatic mass lesions. Recently, immunohistochemical staining of EUS-FNAB specimens is being used increasingly to define the histological type of pancreatic cancer (e.g., duct cell adenocarcinoma, acinar cell carcinoma, endocrine tumor), malignant lymphoma, autoimmune pancreatitis, and so on.

The contraindications to tissue sampling methods include situations in which the result of the procedure will not affect management, inability to clearly visualize the lesion, the cancer or vessel is located between the gut and the target, and the patient is at high risk of bleeding and needle tract seeding [20,23].

Biopsy Procedure

Mild sedation may be desirable if the patient is particularly anxious. Once a pancreatic mass is identified with US or EUS, color Doppler is used to ensure the absence of major vessels in the needle track. The lesion is then punctured under real-time US guidance. When the needle has entered the target of interest, the stylet is removed and negative pressure is applied with a 10- to 20-ml syringe. However, reduced negative (1–2 ml) pressure or no suction may result in less bloody aspirate, particularly with vascular tumors or lymph nodes. In addition to tailoring the degree of suction to the type of lesion, an adequate number of back and forth motions of the needle inside the lesion is very important to improve the chance of obtaining an adequate specimen. Some ten or more motions are commonly used during each needle pass. A simultaneous rotary motion of the needle helps to obtain an adequate specimen. Aspiration should be discontinued before withdrawing the needle from the lesion to avoid contamination of the aspirated specimen with material from outside the lesion.

The cellular aspirate may be aspirated through the needle into the suction syringe, but commonly remains within the long needle lumen. This material should be expressed onto a slide by passing the stylet through the needle lumen, and smeared immediately. The adequacy of the aspirated material for cytological or histological diagnosis can be determined by macroscopic inspection. A "worm-like tissue specimen" in the blood may be judged as adequate material. Tissue fragments, if any, may be placed in formalin for histologic processing. The pancreatic mass is punctured repeatedly, preferably in the presence of a cytopathologist/cytotechnician who, on quick review of the slides, can indicate the presence of cancer cells or an adequate specimen. The aspirated material mixed with blood is usually prepared on slides or placed directly into fixative for hematoxylin and eosin (H-E) staining. When a cytopathologist or cytotechnician is in attendance, the aspirated material is spread onto a plate, and visible tissue fragments are picked up with small tweezers and spread onto glass slides. One slide is air-dried for on-site interpretation and the other slide is fixed in ethanol for Papanicolaou staining. Any remaining material goes into a fixative or cell preservative for later cell block preparation for H-E staining or immunohistochemical staining.

Most clinicians believe that histopathology is a more sensitive technique than cytology for obtaining histological evidence of gastrointestinal cancers. Furthermore, cytology is considered unnecessary when an endoscopic biopsy is available. However, cytology (or FNAB) has been reported to be an equally or more sensitive technique than histopathology in the diagnosis of breast or thyroid cancer, as cytology has been determined to be a safe, accurate, fast, and economic (SAFE) technique [24]. On the other hand, histopathology combined with immunohistochemical analysis may be helpful in determining specific etiology. As to the needle technology for EUS-FNAB, the shapes of the tips and the diameter of the needle have been continuously developed and improved. Needles range from 19 to 22 gauge, with a depth of penetration of up to 10 cm. A large size, 19-gauze trucut needle is now commercially available. Although specimens obtained by EUS-FNAB using 22-gauge needles can be processed for histopathology, in most cases, specimens obtained with the aid of a trucut needle are more suitable for histopathological and immunohistochemical analysis [25,26]. Thus, an aspiration system in which both cytopathology and histopathology are available needs to be established.

Complications of FNAB

While complications of open and wedge biopsies of the pancreas occurred in 2–20% of patients [1], the complication rate of US- or CT-guided FNAB is comparatively low at 1.6–4.9% [9,11,13]. The complication rate of EUS-FNAB appears to be 1–2% [18]. The major complications reported with EUS-FNAB are infection, bleeding, pancreatitis, and duodenal perforation.

The risk of acute pancreatitis after EUS-FNAB of pancreatic masses was estimated in 19 centers, and was found to occur at a frequency of 0.29% of all procedures in a retrospective analysis and 0.64% in a prospective study [27]. Thus, although FNAB for pancreatic lesions is a good modality for guiding further treatment, due to the high technical reliability of pancreatic tissue sampling, the possibility of acute pancreatitis needs to be well considered.

Needle tract seeding by US-guided or CT-guided fine-needle biopsy has been documented. According to available reports, the frequency of needle tract seeding ranges from 0.003% to 0.009% [28,29]. Overall, the frequency of needle tract seeding by transabdominal biopsy was very low, but a higher risk was reported for pancreatic carcinoma (five out of eight reported cases). Whether tumor seeding by EUS-FNAB occurs or not has not been fully determined, but so far there have been quite a few reports of seeding possibly caused by EUS-FNAB [23].

Thus, FNAB of the pancreas should be carefully performed with special concern for complications peculiar to pancreatic biopsy such as acute pancreatitis and tumor seeding.

Interpretation of Pancreatic FNAB

The highlights of various pancreatic lesions sampled by EUS-FNAB and stained using Diff Quick, Papanicolaou, and H-E are detailed below.

Normal Pancreas

The pancreas is composed of exocrine tissue (acinar cells and ductal epithelial cells), endocrine tissue (islet cells of Langerhans), and surrounding connective tissue [15]. Normal pancreatic aspirate obtained by FNAB contains two groups of cell populations including many acinar cells, a few clusters of ductal epithelial cells, and mesothelial cells [1,7]. Islet cells are seldom aspirated due to their sparse distribution.

Ductal cells typically appear as cohesive sheets of uniform tall columnar or cuboidal cells with delicate mosaic cell borders [15]. Nuclei are spherical and even in size, with a fine chromatin pattern and inconspicuous nucleoli.

Acinar cells are typically displayed as a single cell or in small clusters of overlapping uniform cells with indistinct cell borders. Nuclei are small, and round to oval with a finely granular chromatin pattern, and the cytoplasm is granular in appearance due to the presence of zymogen granules [15]. In addition, some fibroblasts and endothelial cells can also be seen in the smear.

Inflammatory Change

The reactive ductal epithelium in inflammatory lesions is sometimes difficult to differentiate cytologically from a well-differentiated tubular adenocarcinoma. The cytological characteristics of pancreatitis include sparse cellularity and frequent presence of both benign and atypical epithelial cell fragments admixed with variable amounts of acute and chronic inflammation (Fig. 10.3a). Cells are loosely aggregated with some pleomorphism, but lack three-dimensional clusters, and have small nuclei with a preserved nuclear/cytoplasmic ratio [15]. A biopsy specimen often shows a decreased number of acinar cell clusters and fibrous tissue with infiltration by inflammatory cells (Fig. 10.3b).

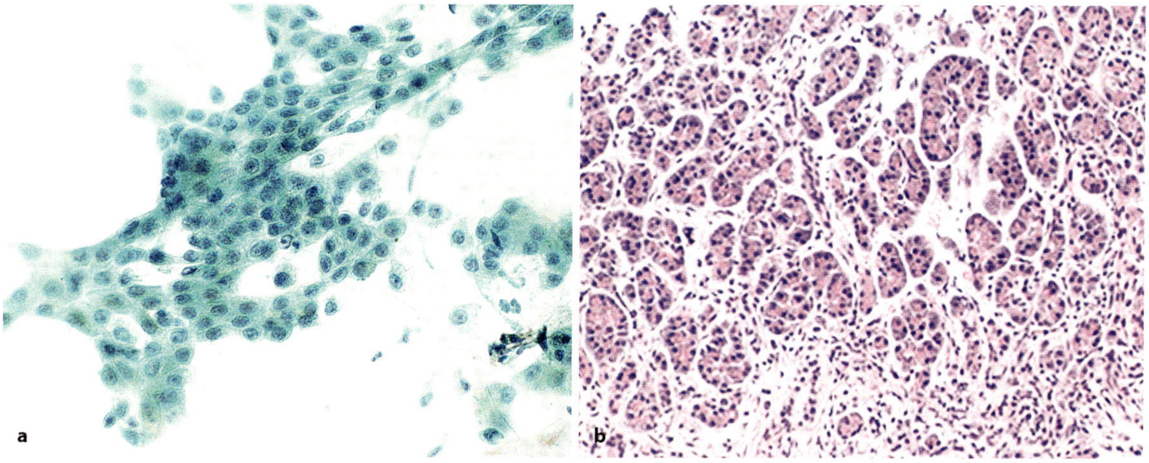

Figure 10.3

Chronic pancreatitis. a Papanicolaou stain (magnification, ×60). b Hematoxylin and eosin (H&E) stain (magnification, ×60)

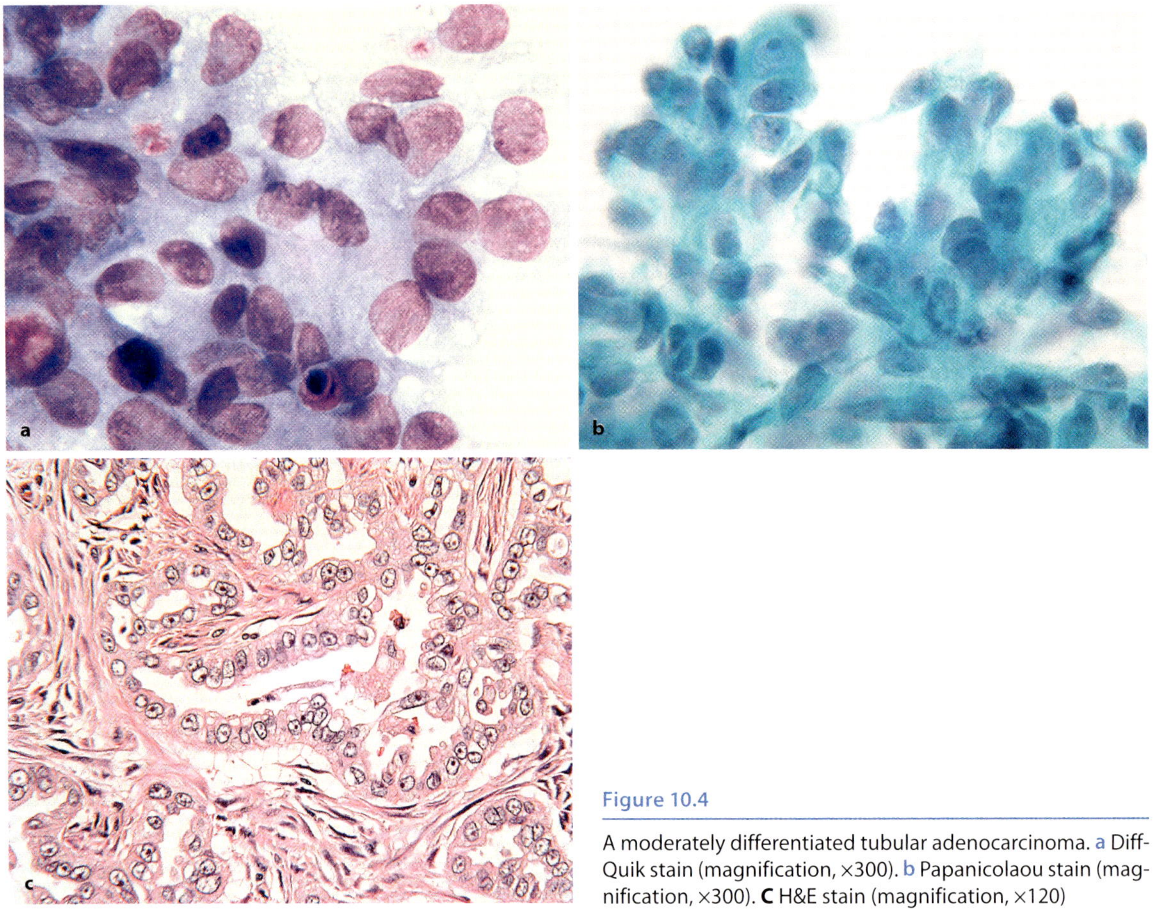

Figure 10.4

A moderately differentiated tubular adenocarcinoma. a Diff-Quik stain (magnification, ×300). b Papanicolaou stain (magnification, ×300). C H&E stain (magnification, ×120)

Solid Neoplasms

Ductal Adenocarcinoma

The cytological features of pancreatic ductal adenocarcinoma include nuclear enlargement with anisonucleosis, nuclear crowding and overlapping, irregular nuclear contour, and irregular chromatin distribution (Fig. 10.4a, b) [1,15]. A three-dimensional and loosely cohesive cluster of cells with nuclear enlargement and anisonucleosis are seen. Additional features, such as the presence of single cells, necrosis, and mitotic figures are also found [15]. Some pancreatic carcinomas show extreme desmoplasia, and FNAB cannot provide sufficient cells to allow a diagnosis. A histopathological specimen shows a structural atypia with small and irregularly distorted tubules in addition to cellular atypia (Fig. 10.4c).

A well-differentiated ductal adenocarcinoma may be difficult to distinguish from reactive epithelium associated with chronic pancreatitis [1]. In particular, a cytological diagnosis of malignancy is sometimes difficult because of a lesser degree of cellular atypia. The cytological features seen in well-differentiated adenocarcinomas include uniform cells with round or oval nuclei and two-dimensional clusters (Fig. 10.5a, b). In contrast, a histopathological diagnosis of malignancy is comparatively easy to make because the tissue specimen shows cellular and structure atypia (Fig. 10.5c).

Adenosquamous Carcinoma

Adenosquamous carcinoma has a coexistent malignant component showing squamous differentiation. Adenocarcinoma cells show secretory activity and squamous carcinoma cells show evidence of keratinization [30].

Undifferentiated (Anaplastic) Carcinoma

Undifferentiated carcinoma aspirates contain epithelial tumor cells that vary greatly in size and shape along with marked nuclear pleomorphism. Cytological features include poorly cohesive, irregularly

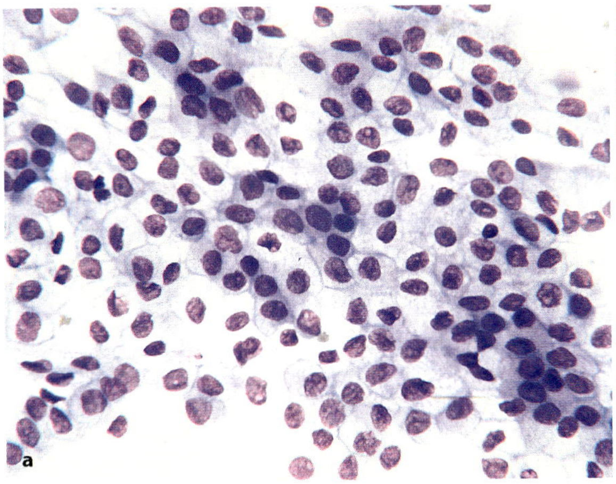

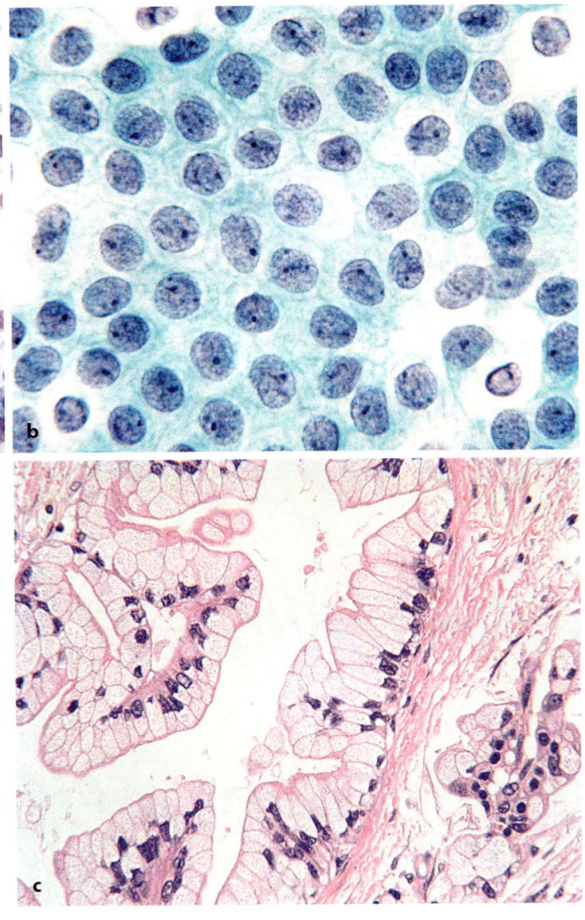

Figure 10.5

A well-differentiated tubular adenocarcinoma. a Diff-Quik stain (magnification, ×120). b Papanicolaou stain (magnification, ×300). C H&E stain. ×120.

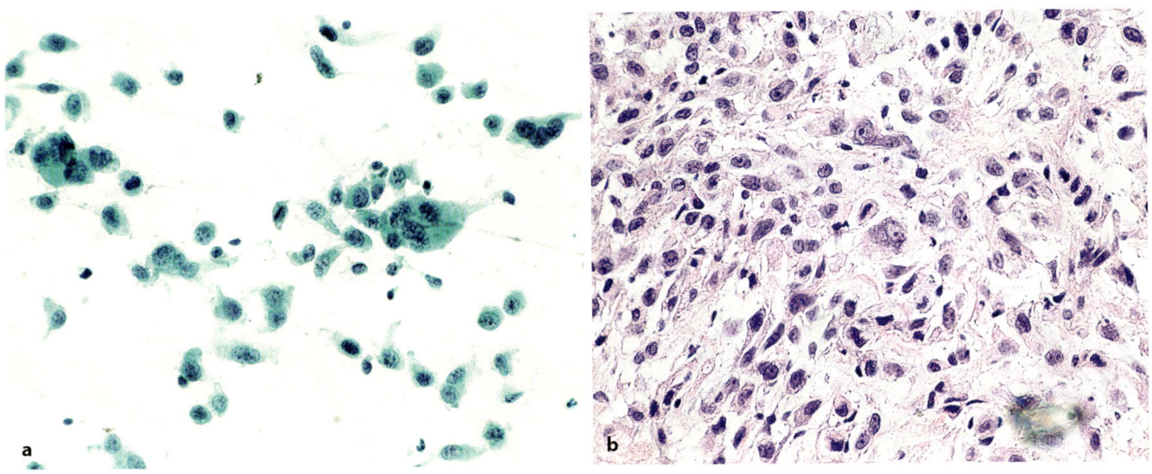

Figure 10.6

An undifferentiated adenocarcinoma. a Papanicolaou stain (magnification, ×60). b H&E stain (magnification, ×60) shaped, and bizarre giant cells with some cells showing multinucleation (Fig. 10.6a). The tumor cells mixed with bizarre giant cells do not form tubular structures in biopsy specimens (Fig. 10.6b). Positive immunostaining for epithelial membrane antigen is present in the tumor cells, thus indicating an epithelial histogenesis.

Small Cell Carcinoma

Undifferentiated small-cell carcinoma is a high-grade carcinoma with neuroendocrine differentiation that is morphologically similar to small cell carcinoma occurring in the lung. The aspirated tumor cells are seen singly or in small loose clusters [31]. They have an ill-defined, very scanty cytoplasm and round, heavily stained nuclei with inconspicuous nucleoli. Immunohistochemical staining both for cytokeratin as an epithelial marker, and for chromogranin and synaptophysin as neuroendocrine markers are positive in tumor cells.

Signet Ring Cell Carcinoma

Signet ring cell carcinoma exhibits noncohesive single cells that display prominent cytoplasmic mucin that displaces the nucleus to the periphery of the cell, and frequently deforms the nucleus into a crescent shape [8]. Although three-dimensional cell clusters with nuclear enlargement and anisonucleosis are occasionally observed, a definite cytological diagnosis of signet ring cell carcinoma is difficult to make (Fig. 10.7a). Histopathology shows characteristic features of this carcinoma including noncohesive and crescent-shaped single cells (Fig. 10.7b).

Acinar Cell Carcinoma

The aspirate from an acinar cell carcinoma is similar to that seen with an islet cell tumor [32,33]. Cells are displayed singly and in small cell groups and can be arranged in loosely cohesive acinar structures. (Fig. 10.8a). The cytoplasm is granular in appearance due to the presence of zymogen granules. Nuclei are relatively small, and round to oval. The biopsy specimen shows an acinar structure composed of eosinophilic cells (Fig. 10.8b). Positive immunostaining for trypsin, chymotrypsin, lipase, and alpha-fetoprotein support the diagnosis of acinar cell carcinoma [8,32,33].

Endocrine Tumors

Aspirates are typically cellular, consisting of a relatively even mixture of single cells and small cohesive cell groups (Fig. 10.9a) [15]. Individual cells are round to cuboidal with dense, homogenous, and well-defined cytoplasm. Nuclei are small, round to oval, contain fine, evenly dispersed chromatin and an inconspicuous nucleolus, and are eccentrically placed within the cytoplasm. A biopsy specimen shows a trabecular, ribbon-like, or cobble-stone-like appearance with various degree of cellular atypia (Fig. 10.9b). Positive immunohistochemical staining for chromogranin and synaptophysin confirms the presence of neuroendocrine cells [32,34]. The immunohistochemical demonstration of neurosecretory granules differentiates a pancreatic endocrine neoplasm from acinar cell carcinoma and solid-pseudopapillary, tumor.

Solid-Pseudopapillary Tumor

Solid-pseudopapillary tumors arise within the tail of the pancreas in adolescent girls and young women [8]. Cytologic smears are cellular, showing slender papillary-like fronds with delicate endothelium lined vascular channels and attached epithelial cells (Fig. 10.10a) [15]. Neoplastic cells radiate out from a central fibrovascular core, and are recognized by the perpendicularly placed spindled endothelial cells (Fig. 10.10c). Immunostaining for α1-antitrypsin, α1-antichymotrypsin, and vimentin may be positive in this tumor.

Metastatic Tumors

Metastatic tumors of the pancreas from other organs have been reported, and include breast, lung, stomach, colonic, ovarian, uterine, esophageal, and renal carcinoma, malignant melanoma, lymphoma, and leukemia. Metastatic tumors are diagnosed more or less easily depending on the type of primary tumor. In general, the site of primary tumors may be difficult to identify by cytology alone, but can be determined by histopathology and immunohistochemical studies.

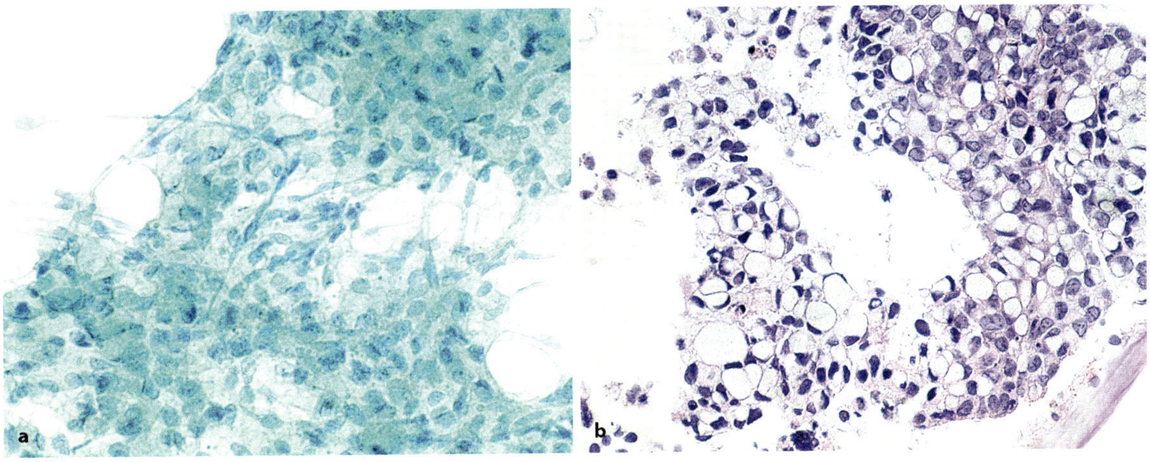

Figure 10.7

Signet ring cell carcinoma. a Papanicolaou stain (magnification, ×60). b H&E stain (magnification, ×60)

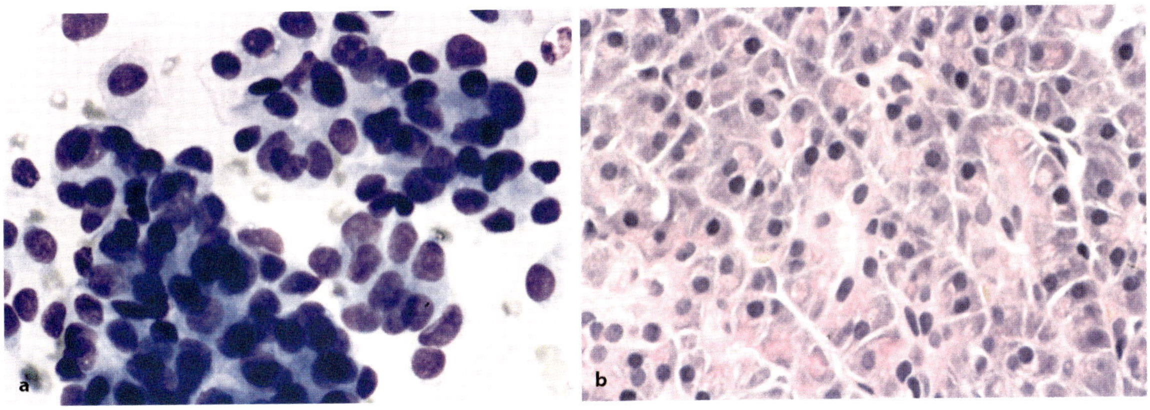

Figure 10.8

Acinar cell carcinoma. a Diff-Quik stain (magnification, ×200). b H&E stain (magnification, ×200)

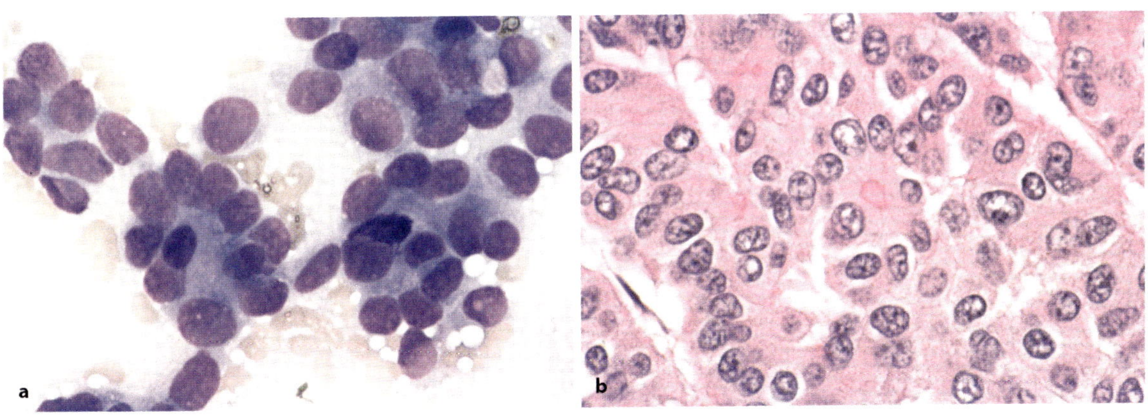

Figure 10.9

Endocrine tumor. a Diff-Quik stain (magnification, ×200). b H&E stain (magnification, ×200)

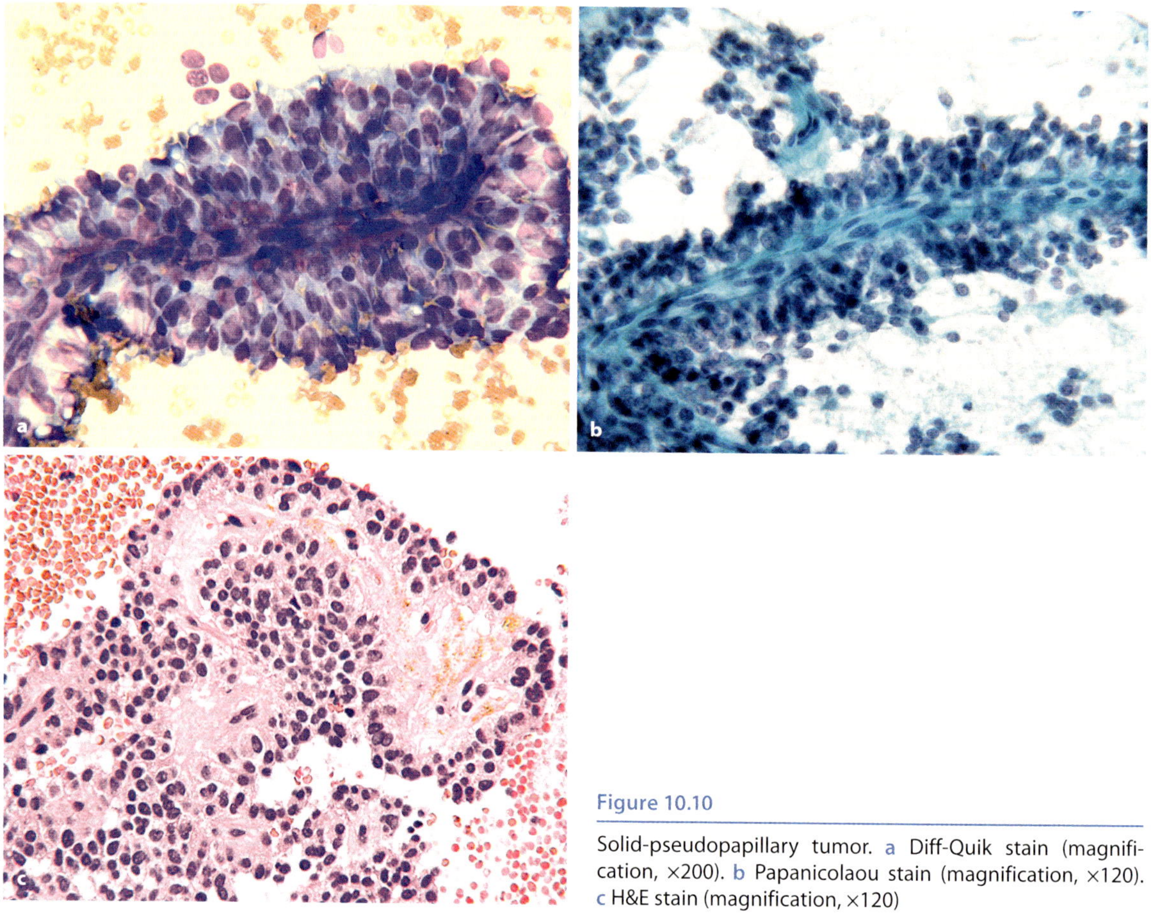

Figure 10.10

Solid-pseudopapillary tumor. a Diff-Quik stain (magnification, ×200). b Papanicolaou stain (magnification, ×120). c H&E stain (magnification, ×120)

References

1. Kloppel G (1984) Pancreatic biopsy. In: Kloppel G, Heitz PU (eds). Pancreatic Pathology. Churchill Livingstone, Edinburgh, pp 114–122
2. Hajdu SI (1989) The value and limitations of aspiration cytology in the diagnosis of primary tumors: a symposium. Acta Cytol 33:741–790
3. Goodale RL, Gail-Peczalska K, Dressel T, Samuelson J (1981) Cytologic studies for the diagnosis of pancreatic cancer. Cancer 47:1652–1655
4. Osnes M, Serck-Hanssen A, Kristensen O, Swensen T, Aune S, Myren J (1979) Endoscopic retrograde brush cytology in patients with primary and secondary malignancies of the pancreas. Gut 20:279–284
5. Vilmann P, Jacobsen GK, Henriksen FW, Hancke S (1992) Endoscopic ultrasonography with guided fine needle aspiration biopsy in pancreatic disease. Gastrointest Endosc 38:172–173
6. Chang KJ, Nguyen P, Erickson RA, Durbin TE, Katz KD (1997) The clinical utility of endoscopic ultrasound-guided fine-needle aspiration in the diagnosis and staging of pancreatic carcinoma. Gastrointest Endosc 45:387–393
7. Grossman M, Burnett K (1985) Diagnostic needle aspiration of the pancreas. In: Berk JE, Haubrich WS, Kaiser MK, Roth JLA, Schaffner F (eds) Gastroenterology, 4th edn. , WB Saunders, Philadelphia, pp 3962–3970
8. Solcia EN, Capella C, Kloppel G (1997) Tumor of the pancreas. In: Atlas of Tumor Pathology, 3rd series. Armed Forces Institute of Pathology, Washington DC, pp 247–257
9. Di Stasi M, Lencioni R, Solmi L, Magnolfi F, Caturelli E, De Sio I, Salmi A, Buscarini L (1998) Ultrasound-guided fine needle biopsy of pancreatic masses: results of a Multicenter Study. Am J Gastroenterol 93:1329–1333
10. Zheng M, Liu LX, Zhu AL, Qi SY, Jiang HC, Xiao ZY (2003) K-ras gene mutation in the diagnosis of ultrasound guided fine-needle biopsy of pancreatic masses. World J Gastroenterol 9:188–191
11. Sperti C, Pasquali C, Di Prima F, Rugge M, Petrin P, Costantino V, Canton A, Pedrazzoli S (1994) Percutaneous CT-guided fine needle aspiration cytology in the differential diagnosis of pancreatic lesions. Ital J Gastroenterol 26:126–131
12. David O, Green L, Reddy V, Kluskens L, Bitterman P, Attal H, Prinz R, Gattuso P (1998) Pancreatic masses: A multi-institutional study of 364 fine-needle aspiration biopsies with histopathologic correlation. Diagn Cytopathol 19:423–427
13. Zech CJ, Helmberger T, Wichmann MW, Holzknecht N, Diebold J, Reiser MF (2002) Large core biopsy of the pancreas under CT fluoroscopy control: results and complications. J Comput Assist Tomogr 26:743–749

14. Ho CS, McLoughlin MJ, Mchattie JD, Tao LC (1977) Percutaneous fine needle aspiration biopsy of the pancreas following endoscopic retrograde cholangiopancreatography. Radiology 125:351–353
15. Staerkel GA (2005) Fine-needle aspiration biopsy of the pancreas: indication and interpretations. In: Von Hoff AA, Evans DB, Hruban RH (eds) Pancreatic Cancer. Jones and Bartlett, Sudbury pp 225–234
16. Rosch T, Classen M (1991) Endosonography – What are the limits in gastroenterological diagnostics? Endoscopy 23:144–146
17. Wiersema MJ, Norton ID (2005) Endoscopic ultrasound guided fine needle aspiration biopsy. Version 13.2
18. Bhutani MS (1999) Endoscopic ultrasound guided fine needle aspiration of pancreas. In: Bhutani M (ed) Interventional Endoscopic Ultrasonography. Harwood Academic, The Netherlands, pp 65–72
19. Wiersema MJ, Vilmann P, Giovannini M, Chang KJ, Wiersema LM (1997) Endosonography-guided fine-needle aspiration biopsy: diagnostic accuracy and complication assessment. Gastroenterology 112:1087–1095
20. Hawes RH (1998) Indications for EUS-directed FNA. Endoscopy 30:155–157
21. Irisawa A, Hikichi T, Yamao K, Bhutani MS, Obara K, Takenoshita S, et al (2003) Interventional endoscopic ultrasonography for pancreatic tumor: EUS-guided fine needle aspiration biopsy and injection. Nippon Shokakibyo Gakkai Zasshi 100:280–291 (in Japanese with English abstract)
22. Wallace MB, Woodwaed T, Raimond M (2004) Endoscopic ultrasound and guided fine-needle aspiration for pancreatic cancer. Dig Endosc 16:S093–096
23. Yamao K (2005) Complications of endoscopic ultrasound-guided fine-needle biopsy (EUS-FNAB) for pancreatic lesions. J Gastroenterol 40:921–923
24. DeMay R (1996) Aspiration Cytology. In: DeMay R (ed) The Art and Science of Cytopathology. ASCP, Chicago, pp 463–1208
25. Levy MJ, Jondal ML, Clain J, Wiersema MJ (2003) Preliminary experience with an EUS-guided trucut biopsy needle compared with EUS-guided FNA. Gastrointest Endosc 57:101–106
26. Itoi T, Itokawa F, Sofuni A, Nakamura K, Tsuchida A, Yamao K, et al (2005) Puncture of solid pancreatic tumors guided by endoscopic ultrasonography: a pilot study series comparing Trucut and 19-gauge and 22-gauge aspiration needles. Endoscopy37:362–366
27. Eloubeidi MA, Gress FG, Savides TJ, Wiersema MJ, Kochman ML, Ahmad NA, et al (2004) Acute pancreatitis after EUS-guided FNA of solid pancreatic masses: a pooled analysis from EUS centers in the United States. Gastrointest Endosc 6:385–389
28. Fornari F, Civardi G, Cavanna L, Di Stasi M, Rossi S, Sbolli G, et al (1989) Complications of ultrasonically guided fine-needle abdominal biopsy. Results of a multicenter Italian study and review of the literature. The Cooperative Italian Study Group. Scand J Gastroenterol 24:949–955
29. Smith EH (1991) Complications of percutaneous abdominal fine-needle biopsy. Radiology 178:253–258
30. Wilcyznski SP, Valente BF, Atkinson BF (1984) Cytodiagnosis of adenosquamous carcinoma of the pancreas. Use of intraoperative fine needle aspiration. Acta Cytol84:733–736
31. Frable WJ (1983) Thin Needle Aspiration Biopsy. WB Saunders, Philadelphia, pp 222–251
32. Labate AM, Klimstra DS, Zakowski MF (1997) Comparative cytologic features of pancreatic acinar cell carcinoma and islet cell tumor. Diagn Cytopathol 16:112–116
33. Samuel LH, Frierson HF (1996) Fine needle aspiration cytology of acinar cell carcinoma of the pancreas: a report of two cases. Acta Cytol 40:585–591
34. Collins BT, Cramer HM (1996) Fine needle aspiration cytology of islet cell tumors Diagn Cytopathol 15:37–45

Chapter 11

S. N. Reske

FDG-PET and PET/CT in Pancreatic Cancer

Pancreatic cancer, the fourth most common cause of cancer deaths, has a very poor prognosis, with a 3% 5-year survival rate [1], accounting for 30,000 deaths yearly in the USA [2]. The majority of patients present with advanced disease, resulting in a low resection rate, especially if the patient is seen outside of regional specialist units [3]. Without resection, the overall median survival is 4–6 months, with an estimated 5-year survival rate of 0.4–5% [4]; chemotherapy has only a modest effect, improving survival by just a few weeks or months [5]. High mortality rates are related to the highly aggressive nature of the tumor, the nonspecific symptoms leading to late presentations, and the diagnostic limitations of current imaging modalities [6]. Patients who undergo pancreatic resection demonstrate a median survival of 10–18 months and a 5-year survival rate of 17–24%. The late presentation is responsible in part for the poor overall survival and poor long-term survival rates. Since pancreatic tumors may have a better prognosis when detected at an early stage, before metastases occur, imaging studies that can detect small isolated lesions could be valuable.

Standards of Care

Currently, the standard of care for patients with suspected pancreatic cancer includes imaging with ultrasonography, endosonography, and computed tomography (CT), and then either needle biopsy sampling or open laparoscopy depending upon whether the mass appears malignant or benign. Masses that appear malignant and resectable may undergo laparoscopy, while masses that appear rather benign or malignant but unresectable undergo biopsy. Biopsy, although safer then laparoscopy, is associated with complications, the most concerning of which is acute pancreatitis. Approximately 5% of individuals will have minor complications and the diagnostic yield of endoscopic ultrasound-guided biopsy is about 68%.

Imaging Techniques

The limitations of CT in detecting pancreatic carcinoma include difficulty in identifying small lesions in the pancreas (false negatives), difficulty in differentiating pancreatic carcinoma from mass-forming pancreatitis (false positives), and indeterminate results. Mass-forming pancreatitis occurs when the inflammation associated with pancreatitis affects only a portion of the pancreas, creating the appearance of a mass on imaging tests. As chronic pancreatitis is a risk factor for pancreatic carcinoma, mass-forming pancreatitis is not uncommon in the patient population being investigated. Adjunct testing with an imaging study that relies upon a different imaging technique has been suggested as a way to address these limitations of CT. The use of [^{18}F]fluorodeoxyglucose (FDG) positron emission tomography (PET; FDG-PET) has several theoretical advantages over conventional imaging. FDG-PET uses a radiotracer-labeled glucose analogue, FDG, to monitor the functional activity of specific regions of interest and to compare it with the baseline background activity of a nearby area. The pancreas typically has a very low uptake of FDG, while pancreatic adenocarcinoma has a high uptake due to the upregulated expression of glucose transporters at the cellular membrane of pancreatic cancer cells (Fig. 11.1) [7]. In addition, pancreatic carcinoma cells lack the enzymes to break down FDG, essentially resulting in storage of FDG within the tumor tissue, further enhancing its signal intensity as compared with the normal surrounding areas (Fig. 11.2). As FDG-PET relies upon detection of functional activity rather than lesion size, it may possess an advantage in the differentiation of benign from malignant pancreatic lesions. For these reasons, it has been suggested that FDG-PET should be added as an adjunct to CT to reduce the overall false-positive, false-negative, and indeterminate rates [8–17]. Reducing the false-positive rate prevents unnecessary laparoscopy and/or biopsy; reducing the false-negative rate may permit earlier detection of small,

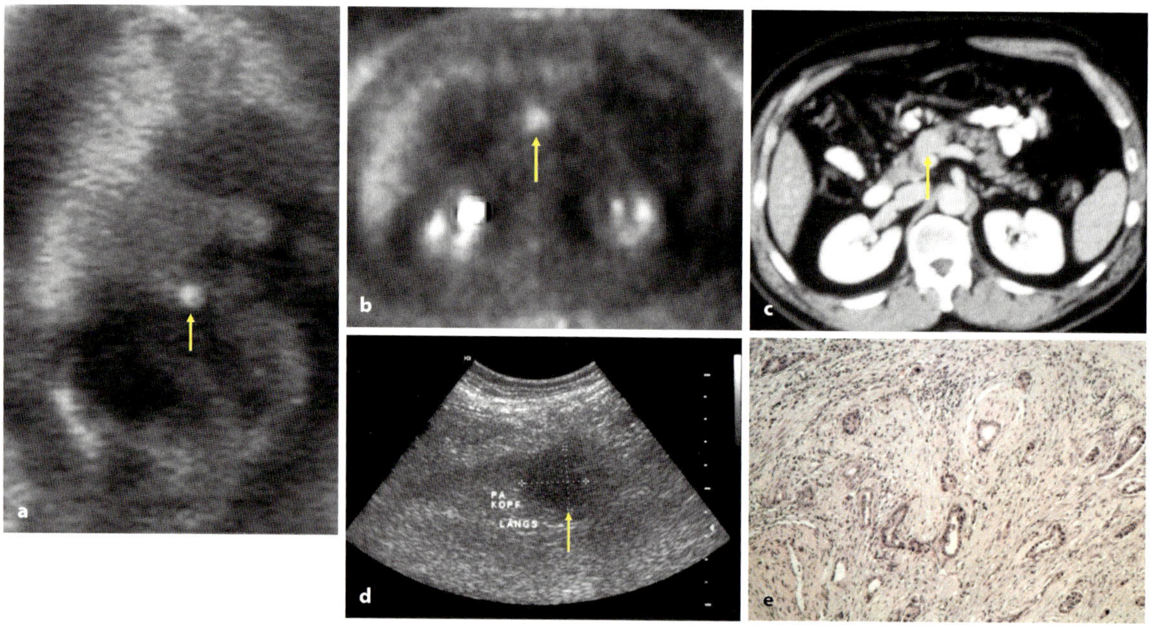

Figure 11.1

Ductal pancreatic adenocarcinoma pT2. [18F]fluorodeoxyglucose (FDG) positron emission tomography (FDG-PET) shows focally increased FDG uptake in the head of the pancreas (*arrows*,a,b) corresponding to CT lesion (*arrow*,c) and ultrasonography (*arrow*, d). Histology (hematoxylin and eosin stain) shows adenocarcinoma of the pancreas (e)

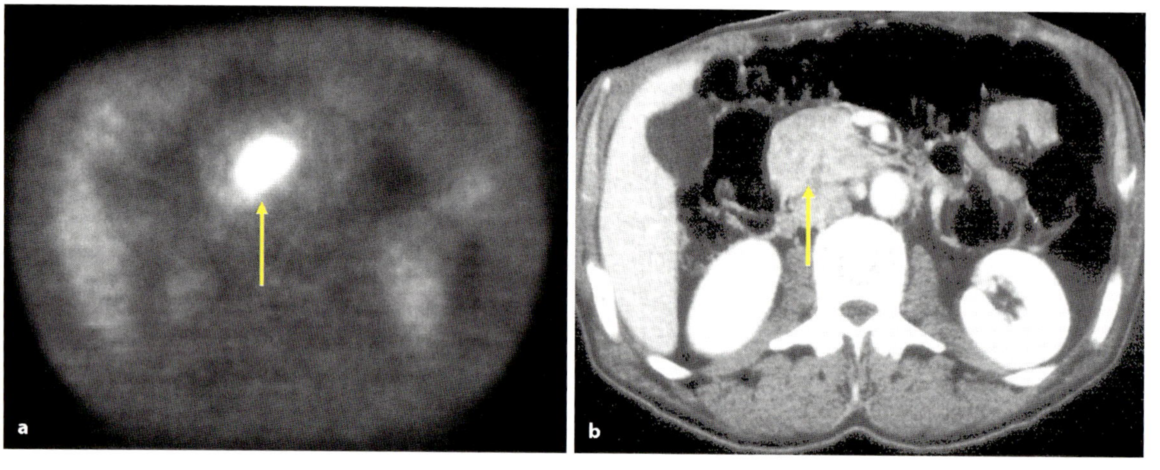

Figure 11.2

FDG-PET (a) and corresponding CT (b), transverse sections. Large mass seen on CT (*arrow*) in the head of the pancreas with intensive FDG uptake within the central part of the lesion (*arrow*)

localized tumors during a period when they may be more amenable to cure; and reducing the indeterminate rate has the benefits of both reducing the false-positive and false-negative rates.

Comparison of CT and FDG-PET

Several studies have been performed comparing FDG-PET to CT for the differentiation of benign from malignant pancreatic lesions (Table 11.1). The most relevant studies up to the publication year of 2001 have been summarized in a recent meta-analysis [18]. The pooled sensitivity and specificity for CT across

Table 11.1. Description of studies included in analysis [18]. *PET* Positron emission tomography, *CT* computed tomography

Author	Year	PET total	CT total	Population	PET sensitivity[a]	PET specificity[a]	CT sensitivity[a]	CT specificity
Delbeke et al. [16]	1999	65	65	Suspected carcinoma	92% (81–96)	58% (34–79)	64% (51–78)	62% (32–85)
Nakamoto et al. [22]	2000	47		Suspected carcinoma	100% (87–100)	80% (56–93)		
Zimny et al. [15]	1997	105		Suspected carcinoma	89% (79–95)	53% (35–70)		
Diederichs et al. [9]	1999	122	101	Referred resection	88% (74–94)	87% (75–94)	95% (84–99)	91% (78–97)
Bares et al. [25]	1994	40	40	Mass or pancreatitis	89% (70–97)	85% (54–97)	100% (87–100)	23% (6–54)
Ho et al. [17]	1996	14	14	Mass or pancreatitis	100% (63–100)	67% (24–94)	25% (5–64)	100% (54–100)
Keogan et al. [26]	1998	37	37	Mass of dilated duct	88% (68–97)	83% (51–97)	75% (53–89)	93% (51–97)
Bares et al. [20]	1993	15	15	Mass	92% (62–100)	100% (16–100)	95% (75–100)	50% (3–97)
Kalady et al. [27]	2002	54	54	Mass	88% (73–95)	92% (62–100)	65% (39–85)	87% (72–95)
Kato et al. [28]	1995	24		Mass	93% (66–100)	78% (40–96)		
Koyoma et al. [29]	2001	86	86	Mass	82% (70–90)	81% (58–94)	91% (80–96)	38% (19–61)
Sendler et al. [21]	2000	42	42	Mass	81% (52–85)	64% (32–87)	74% (55–87)	73% (40–93)
Imdahl et al. [30]	1999	48	48	Known Ca or pancreatitis	96% (79–100)	100% (84–100)	50% (35–65)	44% (15–77)
Inokuma et al. [31]	1995	46	46	Clinical symptoms	94% (80–99)	82% (48–97)	89% (72–96)	73% (40–93)
Papos et al. [32]	2001	22	22	Clinical symptoms	100% (54–100)	88% (61–98)	100% (54–100)	56% (31–79)
Rajput et al. [33]	1998	13	13	Clinical symptoms	82% (48–97)	100% (16–100)	73% (40–93)	0% (0–84)
Kasperk et al. [34]	2001	103	103	Suspected carcinoma	92% (83–96)	58% (34–79)	85% (75–91)	89% (66–98)

[a] Sensitivity and specificity are reported as the calculated value with the 95% confidence interval

Table 11.2. Results of PET and CT for individuals with a false positive (*FP*) or false negative (*FN*) on either imaging test [18]. *NA* Not available

Study	No without cancer	CT false positives (FP) CT FP correctly dx by PET/CT FP	PET false positives (FP) PET FP correctly dx by CT/PET FP	No with cancer	CT false negatives (FN) CT FN correctly dx by PET/CT FN	PET false negatives (FN) PET FV correctly dx by CT/PET FN
Delbeke et al. [16]	13	2/5	0/3	52	18/18	0/0
Keogan et al. [26]	12	0/2	0/2	22	2/2	0/1
Kalady et al. [27]	13	4/5	01	41	1/4	3/5
Koyoma et al. [29]	21	6/8	3/5	65	4/6	5/7
Sendler et al. [21]	11	NA/3	3/4	31	7/8	8/9
Imdahl et al. [30]	21	4/4	0/0	27	5/5	1/1
Inokuma et al. [35]	11	3/3	2/2	35	2/4	0/2
Papos et al. [32]	16	5/7	0/2	6	0/0	0/0
Rajput et al. [33]	2	2/2	0/0	11	3/3	2/2

all studies was 81% (95% confidence interval, CI, 72–88%) and 66% (95% CI 53–77%), respectively. When combining the nine studies from Table 11.2, the pooled sensitivity and specificity for PET in those with a positive CT was 92% (95% CI 87–95%) and 68% (95% CI 51–81%), respectively, and in those with a negative CT those figures were 73% (95% CI 50–88%) and 86% (95% CI 75–93%), respectively. The areas under the ROC curve for PET were higher in both those with a positive CT (0.94) and a negative CT (0.93) than for CT alone (0.82), suggesting that the addition of PET as an adjunct test would improve the ability to discriminate between patients with and without pancreatic cancer. The sensitivity was 92% and the specificity 88% for the abnormal prior imaging group, and 86% and 89%, respectively for the normal prior imaging group. There was a strong trend toward a lower test performance for PET in individuals with a negative CT.

Other Findings

In the five studies [14, 15, 19–21] that evaluated the effect of hyperglycemia on the sensitivity and specificity of PET, all concluded that hyperglycemia increased the number of false-negative results (Fig. 11.3). The average sensitivity for detecting pancreatic cancer decreased by 4%, from 92 to 88% in individuals with hyperglycemia [18].

Several studies on FDG-PET in pancreatic cancer have been published since 2001, covering new imaging technologies such as PET/CT, technical-software-based fusion imaging, technically improved data acquisition and analysis, response to chemotherapy, and diagnosis of relapse.

In general, diagnostic studies comparing CT, magnetic resonance tomography (MRT) or endoscopic ultrasonography (EUS) and PET have found increased sensitivity of CT, MRT, or EUS imaging compared to earlier studies, probably related to improved imaging equipment used in these studies (Table 11.3). Although the specificity of FDG-PET has generally improved compared to standard imaging technology, most authors found little additional value of FDG-PET for the diagnosis of pancreatic cancer, given the lack of information regarding T-staging and resectability through FDG-PET.

It appears, however, that virtually all studies excluding one case report, did not use PET/CT equipment, which is now regarded as a standard PET imaging procedure in oncology. It is therefore believed that the value of FDG-PET/CT in the diagnosis and staging of pancreatic cancer is currently unknown and needs to be prospectively studied.

Beyond use of adequate imaging technology, PET-based imaging of pancreatic cancer may be improved by delayed imaging (i.e., 2 h instead of 1 h post-FDG injection) due to increased detectability of primaries, and liver and lymph node metastases [22, 23], and normalization to tumoral FDG uptake to blood glucose concentration.

In a recent report, the value of FDG-PET (n=31) for the diagnosis of recurrent pancreatic cancer was compared to CT (n=14) or MRI (n=17) [24]. All 31 patients relapsed and 25/31 patients had local relapse; 23 of the 25 relapsing patients relapsed early after surgery. FDG-PET detected 22/23 (96%) patients with "initial" relapse; that number for CT/MRI was 9/23 (39%). FDG-PET detected 5/12 (42%) liver metastases and CT/MRT detected 11/12 (92%). PET detected 7/9 ab-

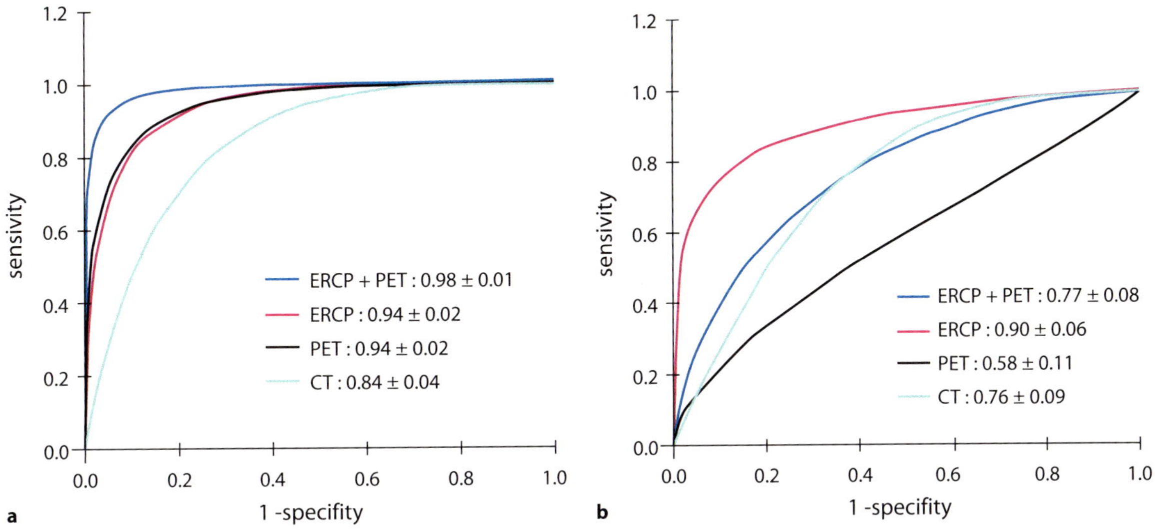

Figure 11.3

ROC analysis of CT, endoscopic retrograde cholangiopancreatography (*ERCP*) and FDG-PET in pancreatic cancer. Comparison of CT, ERCP, and FDG-PET in euglycemic (a) and hyperglycemic (b) patients. Note the markedly reduced performance of FDG-PET in hyperglycemic patients [19]

Table 11.3. FDG-PET in the diagnosis of pancreatic cancer – recent publications. *sens* Sensitivity, *spec* specificity, *SUV* standardized uptake value [41], *EUS* endoscopic ultrasonography, *MRT* magnetic resonance tomography

Author	Publication Year	CT *N*	CT sens (%)	CT spec (%)	PET *N*	PET sens (%)	PET spec (%)	
Koyoma and Okamura [36]	2001	86	94	62	86	82	81	SUV$\geq$2.2
		(MRT 86)	79	70	86	91	76	
Papós and Takacs [32]	2002	22	100	50	22	100	88	
Valinas and Barrier [37]	2002				22	64		Gamma camera, PET
Rasmussen and Sorensen [38]	2004				20	75	80	SUV$\geq$3.5
					20	92	75	
Borbath et al. [39]	2005	59	MRT 97.5		59	87,5		
		59	EUS 98					
Lytras et al. [40]	2005	112	89	65	112	73	60	
		small-volume metastases 112	20	94	112	22	91	
Ruf et al. [24]	2005	focal relapse 31	39		31	96		
		liver metastases 12	92		12	42		

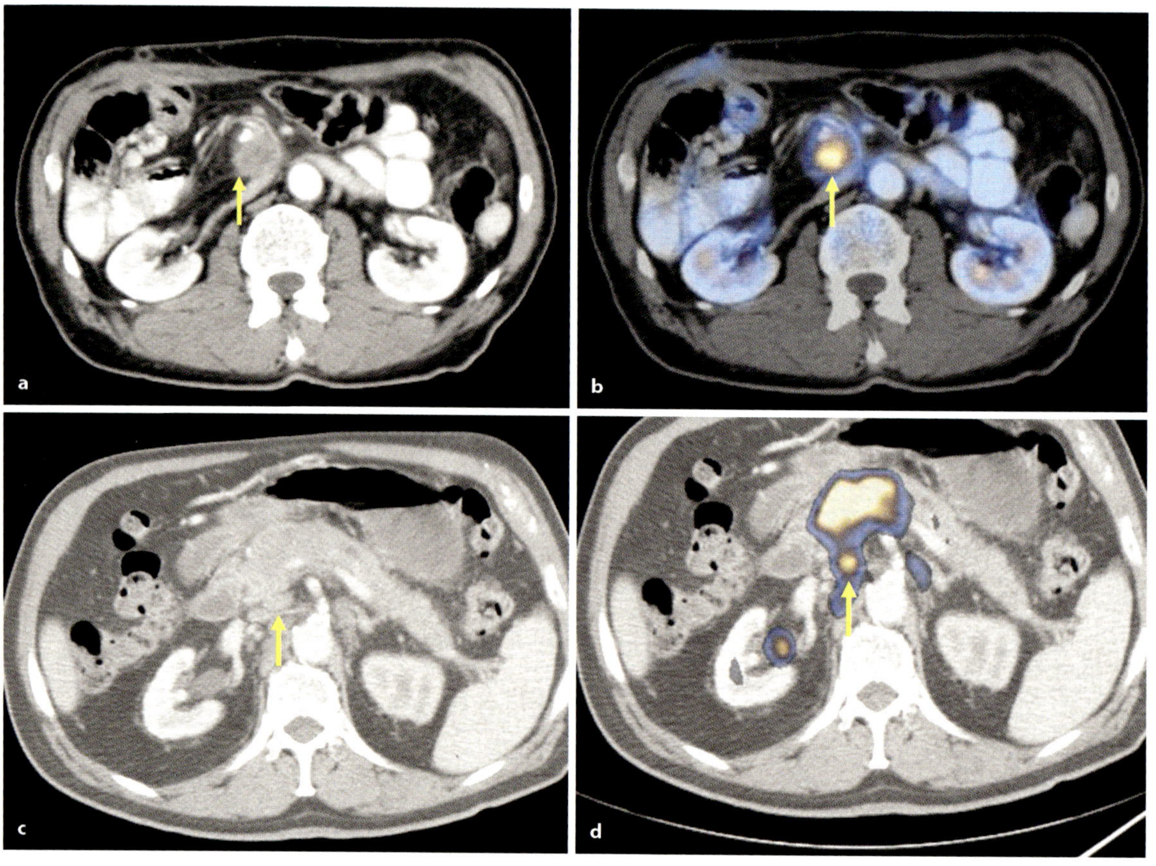

Figure 11.4

FDG-PET/CT in adenocarcinoma of pancreatic head (*arrow*, CT a, PET/CT fusion imaging b) with regional nodal involvement (*arrows*, CT c, PET/CT fusion imaging d)

dominal lesions and CT/MRT detected none [24]. The authors concluded that FDG-PET was much more sensitive for detecting local relapse of pancreatic cancer and was advantageous for showing nonlocoregional abdominal deposits, whereas CT/MRT was more sensitive for detecting liver metastases. The preliminary results of an ongoing study in our institution basically confirmed these data, when FDG-PET/CT is used (Figs. 11.4–11.6).

It must be kept in mind, however, that at present, standard imaging techniques such as EUS, spiral CT and magnetic resonance cholangiopancreatography are not able to reliably detect small cancer lesions (<1 cm). Furthermore, even small pancreatic carcinomas (<1 cm) are frequently incurable. Detection of pancreatic intraepithelial neoplasia (PanIN) is virtually impossible with the standard diagnostic modalities. Thus new diagnostic tools using novel technology for targeting of cancer (or PanIN)-specific genetic changes are urgently needed, in particular for the screening of high-risk populations. Development of novel diagnostic approaches using up-to-date genetic analyses and molecular and diagnostic imaging technology is currently being pursued in a large EU-sponsored consortium of basic and clinical scientists (MolDiag-Paca: Novel molecular diagnostic tools for the prevention and diagnosis of pancreatic cancer. EU Contract no.: PL018771).

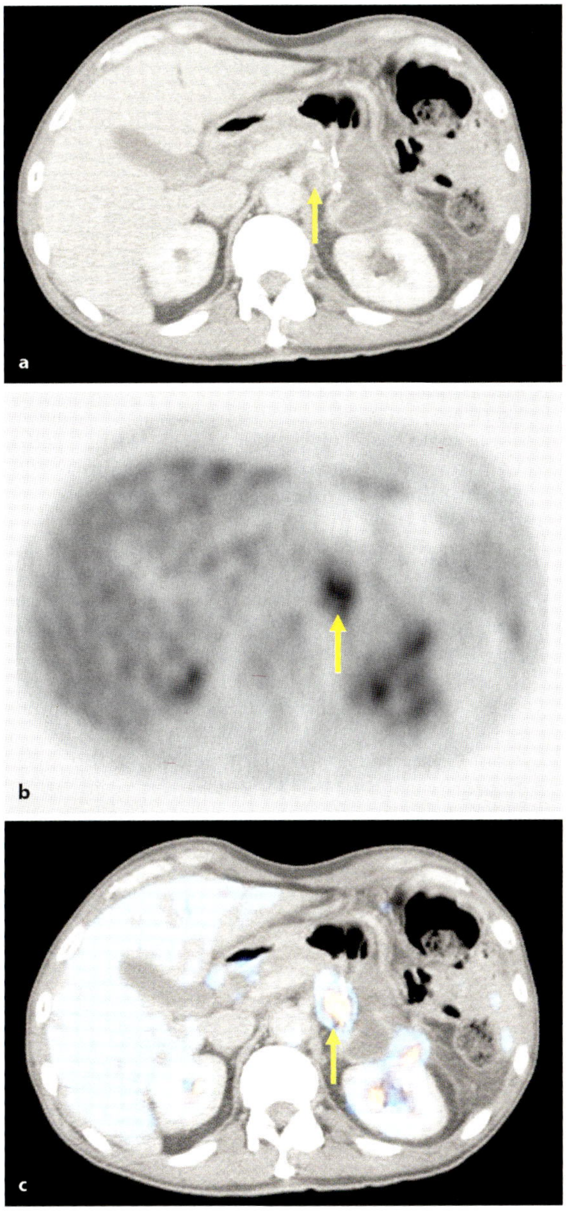

Figure 11.5

Local relapse of pancreatic adenocarcinoma in an indeterminate mass, as judged from CT (*arrow*, a). FDG-PET shows a focal hypermetabolic mass (*arrow*, b). PET/CT fusion imaging localizes the hypermetabolic mass just below the clip material within the mass seen on CT (*arrow*, c) indicative of local relapse, which was confirmed by resection

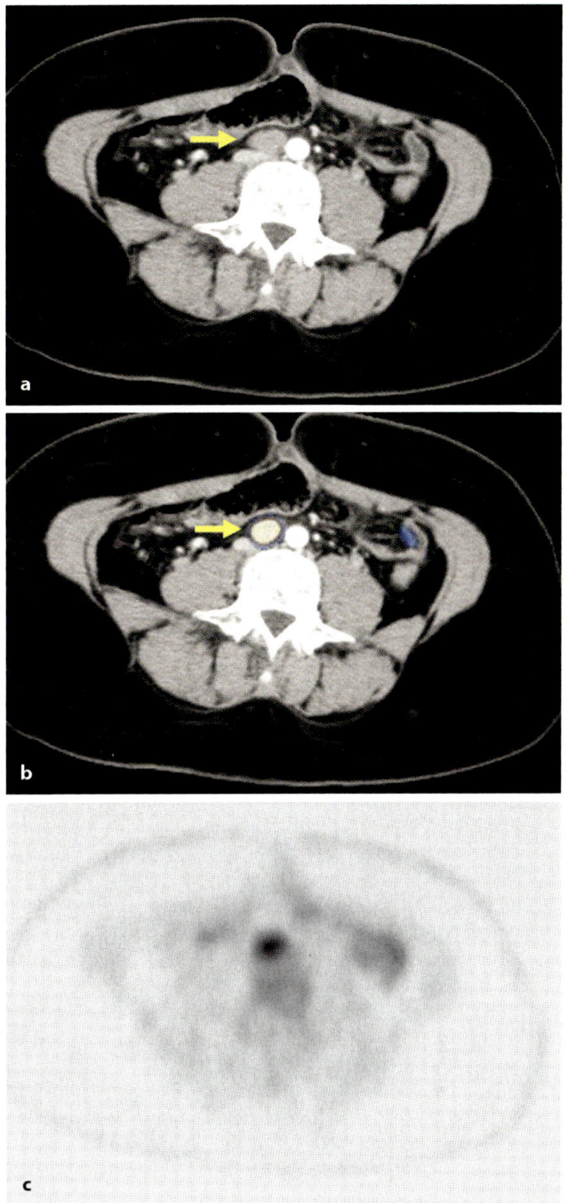

Figure 11.6

Nodal relapse in a para-aortic lymph node after Whipple's resection of pancreatic cancer. Highly increased focal FDG uptake (*arrow*, a) precisely localized in an enlarged aortocaval lymph node seen on CT (*arrow*, b and PET/CT (*arrow*, c)

References

1. Warshaw AL, Castillo CFD (1992) Pancreatic carcinoma. New Engl J Med 326:455–465
2. Jemal A, Murray T, Samuels A, Ghafoor A, Ward E, Thun MJ (2005) Cancer statistics, 2005. CA Cancer J Clin 53:5–26
3. Andren-Sandberg A, Neoptolemos JP (2002) Resection for pancreatic cancer in the new millennium. Pancreatology 2:431–439
4. Bramhall SR, Allum WH, Jones AG, Allwood A, Cummins C, Neoptolemos JP (1995) Treatment and survival in 13,560 patients with pancreatic cancer, and incidence of the disease, in the West Midlands: an epidemiological study. Br J Surg 82:111–115
5. Shore S, Raraty MG, Ghaneh P, Neoptolemos JP (2003) chemotherapy for pancreatic cancer. Aliment Pharmacol Ther 18:1049–1069
6. Maringhini A, Ciambra M, Raimondo M, Baccelliere P, Grasso R, Dardanoni G, et al (1993) Clinical presentation and ultrasonography in the diagnosis of pancreatic cancer. Pancreas 8:146–150
7. Reske SN, Grillenberger KG, Glatting G, Port M, Hildebrandt M, Gansauge F, et al (1997) Overexpression of glucose transporter 1 and increased FDG uptake in pancreatic carcinoma. J Nucl Med 38:1344–1348
8. Zimny M, Fass J (2000) Fluorodeoxyglucose positron emission tomography and the prognosis of pancreatic carcinoma. Scand J Gastroenterol 35:883–888
9. Diederichs CG, Staib L, Vogel J, Glasbrenner B, Glatting G, Brambs HJ, et al (2000) Values and limitations of 18F-fluorodeoxyglucose-positron-emission tomography with preoperative evaluation of patients with pancreatic masses. Pancreas 20:109–116
10. Stollfuss JC, Glatting G, Friess H, Kocher F, Berger HG, Reske SN (1995) 2-(fluorine-18)-fluoro-2-deoxy-D-glucose PET in detection of pancreatic cancer: value of quantitative image interpretation. Radiology 195:339–344
11. Fröhlich A, Diederichs C, Staib L, Beger H, Reske S (1997) FDG-PET in the detection of pancreatic cancer liver metastases. J Nucl Med 38:145P
12. Fröhlich A, Diederichs CG, Staib L, Vogel J, Beger HG, Reske SN (1999) Detection of liver metastases from pancreatic cancer using FDG PET. J Nucl Med 40:250–255
13. Friess H, Langhans J, Ebert M, Beger H, Stollfuß J, Reske S, et al (1995) Diagnosis of pancreatic cancer by 2[18-F]-fluoro-deoxy-D-glucose positron emission tomography. Gut 36:771–777
14. Bares R, Klever P, Hauptmann S, Hellwig D, Fass J, Cremerius U, et al (1994) F-18 fluorodeoxyglucose PET in vivo evaluation of pancreatic glucose metabolism for detection of pancreatic cancer. Radiology 192:79–86
15. Zimny M, Bares R, Fass J, Adam G, Cremerius U, Dohmen B, et al (1997) Fluorine-18 fluorodeoxyglucose positron emission tomography in the differential diagnosis of pancreatic carcinoma: a report of 106 cases. Eur J Nucl Med 24:678–682
16. Delbeke D, Rose M (1999) Optimal interpretation of FDG PET in the diagnosis, staging and management of pancreatic carcinoma. J Nucl Med 40:1784–1791
17. Ho CL, Dehdashti F, Griffeth LK, Buse PE, Balfe DM, Siegel BA (1996) FDG-PET evaluation of indeterminate pancreatic masses. J Comp Assist Tomogr 20:363–369
18. Orlando LA, Kulasingam SL (2004) Meta-analysis: the detection of pancreatic malignancy with positron emission tomography. Aliment Pharmacol Ther 20:1063–1070
19. Diederichs C, Staib L, Glatting G, Beger H, Reske S (1998) FDG-PET: elevated plasma glucose reduces both uptake and detection rate of pancreatic malignancies. J Nucl Med 39:1030–1033
20. Bares R, Klever P, Hellwig D, Hauptmann S, Fass J, Hambuechen U, et al (1993) Pancreatic cancer detected by positron emission tomography with 18-F-labelled deoxyglucose: method and first results. Nucl Med Commun 14:596–601
21. Sendler A, Avril N (2000) Preoperative evaluation of pancreatic masses with positron emission tomography using 18F-fluorodeoxyglucose: diagnostic limitations. World J Surg 24:1121–1129
22. Nakamoto Y, Higashi T, Sakahara H, Tamaki N, Kogire M, Doi R, et al (2000) Delayed 18F-fluoro-2-deoxy-D-glucose positron emission tomography scan for differentiation between malignant and benign lesions in the pancreas. Cancer 89:2547–2554
23. Nishiyama Y, Yamamoto Y, Monden T, Sasakawa Y, Tsutsui K, Wakabayashi H, et al (2005) Evaluation of delayed additional FDG PET imaging in patients with pancreatic tumour. Nucl Med Commun 26:895–901
24. Ruf J, Lopez Hanninen E, Oettle H, Plotkin M, Pelzer U, Stroszczynski C, et al (2005) Detection of recurrent pancreatic cancer: comparison of FDG-PET with CT/MRI. Pancreatology 5:266–272
25. Bares R, Klever P, Hauptmann S, Hellwig D, Fass J, Cremerius U, et al (1994) F-18 fluorodeoxyglucose PET in vivo evaluation of pancreatic glucose metabolism for detection of pancreatic cancer. Radiology 192:79–86
26. Keogan MT, Tyler D, Clark L, Branch MS, McDermott VG, DeLong DM, et al (1998) Diagnosis of pancreatic carcinoma: role of FDG PET. AJR Am J Roentgenol 171:1565–1570
27. Kalady MF, Clary BM (2002) Clinical utility of positron emission tomography in the diagnosis and management of periampullary neoplasms. Ann Surg Oncol 9:799–806
28. Kato T, Fukatsu H, Ito K, Tadokoro M, Ota T, Ikeda M, et al (1995) Fluorodeoxyglucose positron emission tomography in pancreatic cancer: an unsolved problem. Eur J Nucl Med 22:32–39
29. Koyama K, Okamura T, Kawabe J, Nakata B, Chung KH, Ochi H, et al (2001) Diagnostic usefulness of FDG PET for pancreatic mass lesions. Ann Nucl Med 15:217–224
30. Imdahl A, Reinhardt MJ, Nitzsche EU, Mix M, Dingeldey A, Einert A, et al (2000) Impact of 18F-FDG-positron emission tomography for decision making in colorectal cancer recurrences. Langenbecks Arch Surg 385:129–134
31. Inokuma T, Tamaki N, Torizuka T, Fujita T, Magata Y, Yonekura Y, et al (1995) Value of fluorine-18-fluorodeoxyglucose and thallium-201 in the detection of pancreatic cancer. J Nucl Med 36:229–235
32. Papos M, Takacs T (2002) The possible role of F-18 FDG positron emission tomography in the differential diagnosis of focal pancreatic lesions. Clin Nucl Med 27:197–201
33. Rajput A, Stellato TA, Faulhaber PF, Vesselle HJ, Miraldi F (1998) The role of fluorodeoxyglucose and positron emission tomography in the evaluation of pancreatic disease. Surgery 124:793–797, discussion 797–798
34. Kasperk RK, Riesener KP, Wilms K, Schumpelick V (2001) Limited value of positron emission tomography in treatment of pancreatic cancer: surgeon's view. World J Surg 25:1134–1139

35. Inokuma T, Tamaki N, Torizuka T, Magata Y, Fujii M, Yonekura Y, et al (1995) Evaluation of pancreatic tumors with positron emission tomography and F-18 fluorodeoxyglucose: comparison with CT and US. Radiology 195:345–352
36. Koyama K, Okamura T (2001) Diagnostic usefulness of FDG PET for pancreatic mass lesions. Ann Nucl Med 15:217–224
37. Valinas R, Barrier A (2002) 18 F-fluorodeoxyglucose positron emission tomography for characterization and initial staging of pancreatic tumors. Gastroenterol Clin Biol 26:888–892
38. Rasmussen I, Sorensen J (2004) Is positron emission tomography using 18F-fluorodeoxyglucose and 11C-acetate valuable in diagnosing indeterminate pancreatic masses? Scand J Surg 93:191–197
39. Borbath I, Van Beers BE, Lonneux M, Schoonbroodt D, Geubel A, Gigot JF, et al (2005) Preoperative assessment of pancreatic tumors using magnetic resonance imaging, endoscopic ultrasonography, positron emission tomography and laparoscopy. Pancreatology 5:553–561
40. Lytras D, Connor S, Bosonnet L, Jayan R, Evans J, Hughes M, et al (2005) Positron emission tomography does not add to computed tomography for the diagnosis and staging of pancreatic cancer. Dig Surg 22:55–61
41. Zasadny KR, Wahl RL (1993) Standardized uptake values of normal tissues at PET with 2-[fluorine-18]-fluoro-2-deoxy-D-glucose: variations with body weight and a method for correction. Radiology 189:847–850

Chapter 12

K. Schütte · S. Kahl · P. Malfertheiner

Laboratory Diagnosis of Exocrine and Endocrine Dysfunctions in Inflammatory and Neoplastic Lesions

The pancreas has a central function in digestion and the control of glucose homeostasis. Its exocrine function is not exhausted during the prandial phase. In the interdigestive phase pancreatic secretion is tightly coordinated with the migrating motor complex (MMC), and bursts of enzyme and bicarbonate secretion occur in association with MMC phase III every 80–120 min. During the interdigestive phase bicarbonate secretion amounts to approximately 25% of the maximum secretion during the postprandial phase and the maximal pancreatic enzyme secretion is around 10% of the maximal digestive secretion.

The physiological role of the interdigestive pancreatic secretion (complemented by bile secretion) is believed to be that of a housekeeper that allows the small bowel to be cleansed of bacterial overgrowth and other detrimental collections within the luminal site. Obviously both the digestive and interdigestive functions of the exocrine pancreas as well as pancreatic hormone production are heavily affected by inflammatory and neoplastic pancreatic diseases and their treatment.

Maldigestion of carbohydrate, protein, and fat caused by decreased activity of amylase, trypsin, and lipase is the result of exocrine pancreatic insufficiency. The clinical picture of exocrine pancreatic insufficiency is dominated by the consequences of deficient lipase activity, resulting in steatorrhea. Carbohydrate tolerance disorders are the result of endocrine pancreatic insufficiency.

This chapter gives an overview of the most important laboratory function tests for the diagnosis of exocrine and endocrine pancreatic dysfunctions.

Exocrine and Endocrine Dysfunctions in Acute Pancreatitis

Inhibition of pancreatic secretion to put the gland to rest has been one of the key management aspects of the disease for a long time. Studies of different models of acute pancreatitis in rats have shown evidence of an impaired response to exogenous stimulation of the pancreas during acute pancreatitis [1]. The theory of an imbalance between the synthesis of pancreatic enzymes and the release of exocrine pancreatic secretion has been developed. Very few studies though have reported on pancreatic function during acute pancreatitis in humans, showing data that are in contrast to the experimental results as most of the patients examined showed normal exocrine pancreatic secretory activity during the acute state of the disease [2].

The frequency, severity, and duration of exocrine pancreatic dysfunction following acute pancreatitis is defined by several factors such as the severity of the attack (edematous or necrotizing pancreatitis, extend of necrosis) and the etiology of the disease (mainly alcoholic or nonalcoholic pancreatitis) [3]. The study of the functional sequelae following acute pancreatitis is limited by several problems. There is usually no information available on the pancreatic function before the acute disease, resulting in difficulties distinguishing between disorders occurring as a consequence of acute pancreatitis or in the context of chronic pancreatitis (CP). The results of studies done on this topic are also very much influenced by the test used to assess exocrine pancreatic function, as most noninvasive tests are not suited for the detection of mild exocrine pancreatic insufficiency.

Impairment of exocrine pancreatic function after acute pancreatitis has been demonstrated in several studies, but the results concerning the severity and length of the dysfunction are conflicting. There is evidence that episodes of alcoholic etiology and severe attacks resulting in parenchymal necrosis do more often result in exocrine pancreatic insufficiency. Functional recovery is possible months, but also years after acute pancreatitis [4].

The metabolic response during acute pancreatitis may depend on the one hand on acute stress caused by a systemic inflammatory response and on the other hand on damage to the Langerhans' islets as a consequence of pancreatic inflammation and necrosis. During the course of acute pancreatitis, hyperglycemia can often be observed in the early phase. As hyperinsulinemia as a response to hyperglycemia has also been reported, a relative endocrine pancreatic insufficiency during acute pancreatitis has been hypothesized. In spite of hyperglycemia, serum basal levels of glucagon are increased during the early phase of acute pancreatitis caused by several factors such as alteration of pancreatic α cells due to pancreatic inflammation and high levels of circulating catecholamines.

Similar to exocrine pancreatic function, the endocrine function during acute pancreatitis depends on the severity of the disease, mainly on the existence and extent of pancreatic necrosis. After resolution of acute pancreatitis, endocrine pancreatic function usually returns to normal within several months in the case of edematous pancreatitis. Following necrotizing pancreatitis, alterations of endocrine function persist in more than 50% of patients [5].

Exocrine and Endocrine Dysfunctions in CP

The diagnosis of CP is based on the clinical history, morphological abnormalities, and functional impairment of the pancreas. CP is a dynamic disease that is characterized by a progressive loss of pancreatic parenchyma, caused by inflammation, tissue destruction, and following biosynthesis of fibrotic tissue. In clinical routine, histopathology of fibrotic changes does not play any role. In the clinical setting, diagnosis of CP is based on typical symptoms, a suggestive history, and on typical morphological changes, shown by imaging methods. Impairment of exocrine and endocrine pancreatic function may be present in different degrees, depending on the current stage of the disease.

According to Amman et al., the course of the disease is classified into three different stages (Table 12.1) [6]: (1) early stage, characterized by recurrent acute attacks without any or with only mild impairment of pancreatic function; (2) later in the course of the disease complications occur (pseudocysts, cholestasis, segmental portal hypertension), increasing pain (more frequent acute attacks, increasing pain intensity), significantly impaired pancreatic function; (3) end stage of the disease, characterized by less frequent and less intense pain ("burn out of the pancreas") but with marked impairment of pancreatic function (exocrine and/or endocrine). In all stages of the disease, clinical symptoms (pain, weight loss, steatorrhea, diabetes mellitus, local complications) can bee seen in different combinations and degrees.

Table 12.1. Stages of chronic pancreatitis (with typical clinical and morphological pictures, pancreatic function, and recommended diagnostic procedures; adapted from [6]). *EUS* Endoscopic ultrasound, *ERP* endoscopic retrograde pancreatography, *MRP* magnetic resonance pancreatography, *CT* computed tomography, *SCT* spiral computed tomography, *PLT* pancreolauryl test, *FE-1* fecal elastase-1

Stage	Clinical picture		Morphology	Pancreatic function	Diagnostic procedures
	Pain	Complications			
Early	Recurrent acute attacks	No complications	Morphological changes detectable with imaging procedures directed to pancreatic parenchyma and ductal system	Normal pancreatic endocrine and exocrine function	EUS, ERP/MRP, CT, SCT, PLT
Moderate	Increasing pain (number of attacks, intensity, frequency)	Pseudocysts, cholestasis, segmental portal hypertension	Progressive morphological changes, detectable in several imaging procedures	Impairment of pancreatic function in several degrees, but rarely steatorrhea	transabdominal ultrasound, ERP/MRP, EUS, CT, PLT, fasting blood glucose, oral glucose tolerance test
Advanced	Decreasing pain ("burn out of the pancreas")	Pseudocysts, cholestasis, segmental portal hypertension	Calculi	Marked impairment of pancreatic function, more often steatorrhea than in other stages; diabetes mellitus	transabdominal ultrasound, ERP/MRP, CT, FE-1, PLT, fasting blood glucose, (oral glucose tolerance test)

Close correlation between morphological changes and impairment of pancreatic function has been demonstrated in the late stages of the disease, but in the early course of CP there is no correlation between morphology and pancreatic function [7]. In different stages of the disease different morphological examinations and function tests are necessary to establish the diagnosis of CP.

The role of exocrine function tests in the diagnosis of CP remains complementary to imaging methods.

1. Clinical manifestation of exocrine pancreatic insufficiency occurs late in the course of the disease, when approximately 90% of exocrine parenchyma is destroyed [8].
2. The most sensitive test to detect exocrine insufficiency is an invasive test, which requires duodenal intubation and aspiration of duodenal juice after pancreatic stimulation. Only this test is able to detect functional impairment in rather early stages of CP [7].
3. Noninvasive tests of exocrine pancreatic function show high sensitivity only in advanced stages of CP [9].

For clinical decision making (enzyme supplementation), noninvasive pancreatic function tests (pancreolauryl-test, determination of fecal elastase-1) provide adequate information [7]. Invasive tests (with duodenal intubation and aspiration of pancreatic juice) are only available in specialized centers and are used restrictedly to answer scientific questions.

Diabetes mellitus is a frequent complication of chronic pancreatitis that occurs with progressive atrophy of the gland. The incidence of diabetes mellitus in patients with chronic pancreatitis usually goes in parallel with exocrine insufficiency and pancreatic calcifications. The time between diagnosis of chronic pancreatitis and onset of pancreatitis associated diabetes ranges from 7 to 15 years [10]. Due to their low sensitivity and specificity beta-cell functions tests are not helpful in the diagnosis of chronic pancreatitis, but in the course of the disease monitoring of the glucose metabolism is necessary. With regard to the staging of chronic pancreatitis, it seems appropriate to distinguish between normal and abnormal glucose tolerance and overt diabetes.

Exocrine and Endocrine Dysfunctions in Neoplastic Pancreatic Lesions

Malignant pancreatic diseases often become symptomatic by signs of exocrine or endocrine dysfunction resulting in weight loss, steatorrhea, and/or new onset of diabetes mellitus. Longstanding diabetes mellitus type 2 is considered a risk factor for the development of pancreatic carcinoma, but the available data are not conclusive. The overwhelming data from case-control studies suggest that diabetes is a consequence of pancreatic cancer, hypothetically caused by islet-cell abnormalities and altered glucose metabolism as a result of the influence of substances released from the cancer cells [11]. Impaired glucose metabolism can be observed in nearly 80% of patients suffering from pancreatic cancer. Diabetes in patients with pancreatic cancer in most of the cases is of recent onset and therefore presumably caused by the tumor [12].

Tests of exocrine pancreatic function though do not allow a differentiation between inflammatory and neoplastic changes of the organ. Thus, they usually do not play any role in the diagnostic work-up of patients suspected to have malignant pancreatic disease. Assessment of pancreatic function is, however, important during and after the treatment of pancreatic malignancies, as surgical and conservative treatment and possible tumor progression can result in impaired exocrine and endocrine pancreatic function.

Exocrine and Endocrine Function Following Pancreatic Surgery

The digestive and interdigestive functions of the exocrine pancreas as well as pancreatic hormone production are heavily affected by major pancreatic surgery and depend on the type of the surgical procedure as well as on the underlying disease. Only limited data are available on the effect of pancreatic resection on exocrine function (Table 12.2). These data come mostly from series of patients suffering from chronic pancreatitis.

Further deterioration of exocrine pancreatic function is a frequent but not obligatory consequence of pancreatic resection. The degree of pancreatic function impairment is related to the extent of pancreatic parenchyma resection and the functional state of the residual pancreas.

An important additional factor that influences not only exocrine function but also the digestive process in its complexity is gastrectomy. Even partial gastrectomy leads to impaired release of gastrin, pancreatic

Table 12.2. Possible effects of pancreatic surgery on pancreatic physiology (adopted from [52]). *CCK* Cholecystokinin

Procedure	Interdigestive phase		Cephalic		Gastric phase	Intestinal phase				
	Migrating myoelectric complex	Neurotrans-mitters	Vagal nerves	Gastric secretion	Gastric dis-tension	pH of chyme	Passage of chyme	Secretin effect	CCK effects	Islet–acinar axis
Partial duodenopancreatectomy (Whipple's procedure)	+	+	+	+	+	+	+	+	+	+
Pylorus-preserving partial duodenopancreatectomy	+	+	+	–	–	–	–/+	+	+	+
Duodenum preserving partial duodenopancreatectomy (Beger's procedure)	+	+	–/+	–	–	–	–	–	–	+
Pancreatic left resection	?	?	?	–	–	–	–	–	–	+
Lateral side-to-side pancreatico-jejunostomy (Partington-Rochell's procedure)	+	+	+	?	?	?	?	+	+	+
Lateral side-to-side pancreatico-jejunostomy combined with pancreatic left resection (Puestow's procedure)	+	+	+	?	?	?	?	+	+	+
Pylorus-preserving pancreatic head resection combined with lateral pancreaticojejunostomy (Frey's procedure)	+	?	+	–	–	–	–	+	+	+

polypeptide, and cholecystokinin and contributes to further deterioration of exocrine insufficiency [13–15]. Significant adaptation following gastrectomy can be observed, as shown in animal models in which pancreatic weight and enzyme content increased significantly after partial gastrectomy [13]. This observation, which was extended and confirmed in patients undergoing pylorus-preserving pancreatic head resection, is not sufficient to compensate for exocrine insufficiency. After treatment with a proton pump inhibitor (PPI), increased gastrin levels were determined together with an increased volume of the pancreatic remnant [16,17]. Again, this organotrophic effect can not balance the loss of exocrine function.

In a study by Lemaire an even insignificant organotrophic effect was accompanied by a deterioration of exocrine pancreatic insufficiency, while endocrine function was maintained [18].

The influence of different types of surgery on the course of exocrine pancreatic function has been studied in few comparative investigations. In patients who underwent pylorus-preserving pancreatoduodenectomy, different types of pancreatoenterostomy (either pancreaticogastrostomy or pancreaticojejunostomy) were compared. A significant deterioration of pancreatic exocrine function occurred in patients who underwent pancreaticogastrostomy [16]. Early deactivation of pancreatic enzymes by gastric acid is the suggested cause of this phenomenon. However, this is only a minor difference that, as a result of routine administration of a PPI, no clinical important role.

The main determinant of the postoperative course of pancreatic function in chronic pancreatitis is - besides the extent of resection - the inflammatory activity within the remaining portion of the pancreas. Administration of pancreatic enzymes is always required following pancreatic resectional surgery. In pylorus- and duodenum-preserving procedures, additional PPIs are mandatory to avoid early inactivation of orally given pancreatic enzymes by gastric acid. The most important reason for the inadequacy of acid neutralization is insufficient bicarbonate secretion, but increased acid secretion has also been reported. In some patients, PPI treatment leads to increased gastrin levels, which cause an organotrophic effect on the pancreas [16,17]. This could theoretically help to compensate or restore pancreatic function.

The influence of any surgical procedure on endocrine pancreatic function is little studied. However, diabetes mellitus as a sequela of surgical resection is a well recognized and significant clinical problem. The incidence of postoperative diabetes mellitus after Whipple's resection ranges from 20% to 50% [19]. Patients usually suffer from recurrent attacks of hypoglycemia. Insulin sensitivity increases postoperatively. After resection procedures this effect is caused by a simultaneous decrease in glucagon secretion. Therefore, the rate of hypoglycemia due to glucagon deficiency increases significantly and causes a substantial number of deaths and incidences of brain damage. In particular, in patients with alcoholic chronic pancreatitis and insulin-dependent diabetes mellitus, hypoglycemic complications are the main limitations of life expectancy [20].

An improvement of endocrine function can be achieved in certain conditions. In a series of patients with chronic pancreatitis, endocrine pancreatic function was significantly improved after duodenum-preserving pancreatic head resection in a small proportion of patients (11%) [21,22]. This has to be interpreted as a surrogate effect caused by the reduced inflammatory activity after pancreatic resection.

Comparing pylorus-preserving and duodenum-preserving pancreatic head resection, the pylorus-preserving procedure shows a significant impairment of endocrine function compared to the duodenum-preserving procedure [23]. Possible explanations are a lesser amount of resected pancreatic parenchyma and the maintenance of the enteroinsulin axis by preserving the duodenum. Some surgeons who initially recommended an extensive resection, now focus on organ preservation to avoid unnecessary insulin-dependent diabetes and associated complications [24]. The underlying disease is at least as important as any type of surgical resection. If patients with alcoholic chronic pancreatitis continue drinking this is the limiting factor of life expectancy.

Diagnostic Procedures for the Diagnosis of Exocrine Pancreatic Insufficiency

Direct Pancreatic Function Tests

Duodenal intubation tests with humoral stimulation of the pancreas (secretin-cerulein test, SPT; Lundh test) are the only tests able to detect functional impairment at all stages of the disease. They are the gold standard in the evaluation of exocrine pancreatic function and provide the highest sensitivity and specificity. (Table 12.3). Invasive tests, however, are time consuming, expensive, and require manpower and technical equipment and yet provide only minor information for clinical routine. They are therefore only used in specialized centers or to answer scientific questions.

Table 12.3. Sensitivity and specificity of function tests [9, 25–28]. *NBT-PABA N*-benzoyl-L-tyrosyl para-aminobenzoic acid (bentiromide) test

	Sensitivity (%)	Specificity (%)
Tests of exocrine pancreatic function		
Invasive tests		
SCT	≥90–100	>90
Noninvasive tests		
PLT	63–94	85
	63 for mild insufficiency	
	76 for moderate insufficiency	
	94 for severe insufficiency	
NBT-PABA Test	49-72	83
	49 for mild insufficiency	
	64 for moderate insufficiency	
	72 for severe insufficiency	
FE-1	54–95	79–83
	54 for mild insufficiency	
	75 for moderate insufficiency	
	95 for severe insufficiency	
Fecal chymotrypsin	54–89	74
	54 for mild insufficiency	
	53 for moderate insufficiency	
	89 for severe insufficiency	
Mixed triglyceride breath test	63 for mild insufficiency	85
	total 81	

Secretin-Pancreozymin (Cerulein) Test

Due to its high sensitivity and specificity this direct pancreatic function test is still considered to be the gold standard for detection of exocrine pancreatic insufficiency. The idea of aspiration of duodenal content after exogenous stimulation of the pancreas by administration of the hormone secretin as a secretagogue was developed by Lagerloef in 1942 [29]. A variety of modifications in collection time, timing and secretagogue have been made since then, causing difficulties in comparing the test results obtained in different centers. There have been attempts to optimize the test using cholecystokinin or one of its analogues instead of or in addition to secretin.

Following a fasting period of 12 h, a tube with separate gastric and duodenal ports is positioned in the duodenum under fluoroscopic control. Basal pancreatic secretion is measured over a period of 15 min. After intravenous administration of secretin, resulting in an increase in volume and bicarbonate output of the pancreas duodenal content is aspirated in fractions over the period of 1 h and collected on ice for analysis of volume and content of bicarbonate and enzymes. Pancreatic secretion is then stimulated by secretagogues either by rapid injection or by continuous infusion concomitant with aspiration and analysis of duodenal juice. The method of continuous pancreatic stimulation has been shown to be of greater sensitivity [30]. Various centers have standardized their own method as there is no unanimously accepted method of direct pancreatic stimulation testing [31].

Lundh Test

This direct pancreatic function test was first described by Lundh in 1962 [32]. After overnight fasting a tube is positioned in the duodenum under fluoroscopic control. Following a time period of 30 min to allow for a plateau phase to be reached, duodenal content is aspirated over a time period of 30 min to assess the basal pancreatic output. The aspirated juice is kept on ice and analyzed for pH and enzymes. After a standard liquid meal (300 ml of water with a solution of 5% protein, 6% fat, and 15% carbohydrate) the duodenal contents are aspirated in fractions over a period of 2 h. Concentrations of bicarbonate, amylase, trypsin, and lipase are measured.

Table 12.4. Procedure for the modified serum pancreolauryl test. A fluorescein peak at > 4.5 µg/ml is considered a normal result

- Basal blood collection after an overnight fast
- Intravenous administration of secretin (1 U/kg body weight) in bolus
- Consumption of a standard test meal (40 g white bread spread with 20 g butter and 200 ml tea without sugar.
  The content of two capsules of fluorescein dilaurate (1 mmol) is mixed with the butter)
- Intravenous administration of metoclopramid (10 mg) in bolus
- Serum collection at 30, 60, 120, 150, 180, and 240 min for fluorescein measurement

Noninvasive Pancreatic Function Tests

Contrary to the invasive tests, noninvasive tests are applicable in clinical routine. All noninvasive tests, however, have the disadvantage of lower sensitivity in chronic pancreatitis, with only mild to moderate impairment of exocrine pancreatic function.

Oral Function Tests

These include the pancreolauryl test (PLT) and the *N*-benzoyl-L-tyrosyl para-aminobenzoic acid (NBT-PABA or bentiromide) test. The principle of these tests is based on the administration of a complex substrate that, by the effect of a specific pancreatic enzyme, is hydrolyzed with the release of a marker substance. This marker is then absorbed from the gut and detected and quantitated either in urine or serum [33].

In case of the NBT-PAPA test, bentiromide (administered orally) is split by pancreatic chymotrypsin resulting in free p-aminobenzoic acid (PABA), which is then absorbed in the small intestine and excreted in the urine after conjugation in the liver. The oral substrate in the PLT is fluorescein dilaurate, which is hydrolyzed by specific pancreatic arylesterases, releasing in free water-soluble fluorescein that can then be found in serum and urine (Table 12.4). In recent years the diagnostic accuracy of the PLT was further increased in the serum test version [34,35] by the administration of secretin just before and metoclopramide immediately after ingestion of the test breakfast. This promotes a more rapid peak for fluorescein concentration in the serum and enhances the discrimination between unaffected subjects and patients with moderate impairment of pancreatic function.

A continuing limitation of the PLT and PABA test is the fact that their results are influenced by a variety of abnormalities of the anatomical and functional integrity of the upper gastrointestinal tract. In clinical terms, the presence of small bowel diseases, jaundice, abnormal gastric emptying, or status following subtotal or total gastrectomy does not permit a diagnosis of chronic pancreatitis from an abnormal PLT or PABA test result.

Fecal Pancreatic-Enzyme Determination

The low diagnostic value of fecal fat analysis has led to a search for individual enzymes in stool specimens in order to develop a highly sensitive test for exocrine pancreatic insufficiency applicable in the clinical routine setting. Besides the measurement of fecal chymotrypsin, which has been used for many years, an enzyme-linked immunosorbent assay test using monoclonal antibodies against human pancreatic elastase-1 has been established. Elastase-1 is a pancreas-specific enzyme that, in contrast to other pancreatic enzymes, is highly stable through intestinal transit. The commercially available assay detects exclusively human elastase and therefore does not interfere with simultaneous therapeutic pancreatic enzyme supplementation from porcine preparations.

Comparative studies of the diagnostic value of stool tests have shown that measurement of elastase-1 is superior to quantification of fecal chymotrypsin in terms of sensitivity and specificity. The diagnostic accuracy of stool tests for the diagnosis of exocrine pancreatic insufficiency due to chronic pancreatitis, however, should not be overestimated: in early stages of chronic pancreatitis the sensitivity of these tests is low.

Due to the dilutional effects of diarrhea of nonpancreatic origin, artificially low elastase-1 concentrations can be observed.

Breath Tests

Based on the administration of a radioactive ^{14}C- or more recently of a nonradioactive ^{13}C-labeled substrate, noninvasive breath tests have become more widely available. The substrate is administered orally and digested by a specific pancreatic enzyme, and the resulting $^{13}CO_2$ exhalation serves as parameter of exocrine pancreatic function. The ^{13}C-mixed triglyceride [36,37], triolein [38,39], and hiolein [40] breath tests are based on the administration of lipids similar to the triglycerides found in the normal diet. The cholesteryl octanoate breath test utilizes a substrate that is metabolized by pancreatic cholesterol esterase [41,42]. In summary, all of these tests reveal reduced $^{13}CO_2$ exhalation and sometimes even a flat recovery curve in patients with steatorrhea. In patients with normal fat excretion or with mild exocrine insufficiency, the pattern of expired $^{13}CO_2$ is generally normal. Since these tests have a relatively high specificity in the detection of deficient lipolytic activity, they may be used in the diagnostic work-up of patients with chronic diarrhea, in order to rule out the presence of fat malabsorption. A further application is to monitor the efficiency of pancreatic enzyme supplementation [43,44]. None of these tests play a role in the diagnosis of early and moderate chronic pancreatitis. The same holds true for amylase as a specific enzyme tested in the ^{13}C-starch breath test [45,46] The future potential of these tests might be based on the development of ^{13}C-labeled substrates split by specific pancreatic enzymes that are produced in much smaller amounts than amylase and lipase, thus probably allowing the detection of pancreatic damage at an earlier stage. The costs must also be further reduced before ^{13}C-breath tests can be considered for general use in clinical practice [47].

Diagnostic Procedures in Endocrine Pancreatic Disorders

Routine Tests for Beta-Cell Function

The definition of diabetes mellitus, its classification, and the recommendations for diagnosis of the disease have changed a lot during the last decade. Diabetes is defined as an endocrine disorder, the main "symptom" of which is chronic hyperglycemia as a result of disturbed insulin secretion, diminished effect of insulin, or a combination of both. The term "impaired glucose tolerance" (IGT) is still part of the revised classification of diabetes, but is no longer a diagnosis per se, but a term to describe the extent of hyperglycemia. The term "impaired fasting glucose" (IFG) was introduced in the diabetes classification of 1997 by the American Diabetes Association (ADA) [48].

Occasionally Measured Glucose Level

According to the criteria recommended by the ADA, the World Health Organization (WHO), and International Diabetes Federation, diabetes can be diagnosed in cases of classical diabetic symptoms (polyuria, polydipsia, weight loss) or in cases of glucosuria where an occasionally measured plasma glucose level exceeds 11.1 mmol/l, independently of the time of day that the measurement was taken, or the interval since the last meal.

In case of an occasionally measured plasma glucose level being higher than 5.6 mmol/l, further investigation is recommended (measurement of fasting glucose level) [48].

Fasting Glucose Level

The blood glucose level after a fasting period of at least 8 h can be easily used as diagnostic tool for diabetes mellitus. An elevated fasting glucose level (higher than 7.0 mmol/l in venous plasma) measured at two different times is sufficient for the diagnosis of diabetes. In the case of impaired fasting glucose (elevated fasting glucose levels in the range of 5.6–6.9 mmol/l in venous plasma), an oral glucose tolerance test should be carried out. It is important to know that fasting blood glucose levels differ from day to day with a variance of 5%.

Oral Glucose Tolerance Test

The oral glucose tolerance test is the standard endocrine function test to detect IGT (Table 12.5). It was developed to test glucose tolerance after maximal stimulation by measuring the time frame that is needed to lower the elevated blood glucose level after provocation by counter-regulation via insulin release. The test imitates standardized oral food intake and is therefore heavily influenced by enteral function. Motility disorders (delayed gastric emptying, dumping syndrome after Billroth II-resection), duodenal ulcers, or drugs (e.g., oral contraceptives, diuretics, laxatives) can cause false-positive test results. A pro-

Table 12.5. Oral glucose tolerance test (administration of 75 g glucose) according to World Health Organization recommendations

		Capillary whole blood (mmol/l)	Venous plasma (mmol/l)
Diabetes mellitus	Fasting glucose	≥6.1	≥7.0
	2 h	≥11.1	≥11.1
Impaired glucose tolerance	Fasting glucose	<6.1	<7.0
	2 h	7.8–<11.1	7.8–<11.1

longed fasting period before the provocation test is performed can also imitate the picture of IGT. In patients with malabsorption (e.g., due to enteritis, inflammatory bowel diseases, parasite infections, tuberculosis) and in patients treated with biguanides or other blood-glucose-lowering medications, false-negative test results can be observed. In these situations an intravenous glucose-tolerance test would be recommended.

The WHO recommends the oral intake of 75 g glucose in 300 ml of water within 5 min after an overnight fasting period (10–16 h) and after taking a basal blood sample for the determination of fasting glucose levels. During the 3 days preceding the test the patient should have a carbohydrate intake of more than 150 g/day. A second blood sample is taken 2 h after the glucose intake. Smoking is not allowed before or during the test.

A blood glucose level higher than 11.0 mmol/l in venous plasma or capillary whole blood 120 min after the oral intake of 75 g glucose diagnoses diabetes mellitus in combination with elevated fasting glucose levels.

IGT is diagnosed in case of normal fasting glucose levels but elevated glucose levels 2 h after provocation. In capillary whole blood or venous plasma the limit for normal glucose tolerance is 7.8 mmol/l for the 2 h after glucose intake; IGT is diagnosed if this value is in the range of 7.8–11.1 mmol/l.

Determination of C-Peptide and Insulin

Insulin is synthesized in pancreatic beta-cells as inactive proinsulin, which is stored in secretory granules. Proinsulin is split into insulin and c-peptide after activation of the glucose receptors of the beta-cell and then excreted into the circulation. C-peptide can be measured in the plasma as a surrogate of insulin and allows the assessment of insulin secretion in insulin-treated patients, but its long half-life of 30–40 min precludes any study of the kinetics of insulin secretion [49]. The determination of c-peptide does not play any role in diagnosing diabetes mellitus, but it is a tool for the differentiation of the cause of diabetes and for assessment of the secretory capacity of beta cells.

Determination of Glycosylated Hemoglobin

Measurement of blood glucose levels allows judgment on the actual glucose metabolism of the patient. To get an information on the longterm glicemic condition retrospectively, independent of short-term variabilities, other parameters are needed. Dependent on the length and intensity of hyperglycemia, glucose is complexed with various proteins in the body such as hemoglobin and collagens nonenzymatically. In a first reversible step, a Schiff base (aldimine form) is formed between the free aldehyde group of glucose and the free amino group of the protein. This process is a fast one. In a second step, intramolecular conversion leads to the formation of a stable ketoamine molecule (Amadori rearrangement). As erythrocytes are not able to split this molecule the glycosylated hemoglobin can early be eliminated after the death of the erythrocytes, which have a half-life of 60 days. Glycosylated hemoglobin therefore reveals the integrated blood glucose levels of 6–8 weeks.

HbA1c is a fraction of glycosylated hemoglobin consisting of glycosylated hemoglobin A0 with D-glucose at the n-terminal amino acid valine of the beta-chain of hemoglobin. The measurement of glycosylated hemoglobin is not yet a recommended tool for the diagnosis of diabetes mellitus, but it is helpful and recommended for monitoring patients known to suffer from diabetes [50].

Monitored Prolonged Fast

For the diagnosis of hyperinsulinemia the 72-h supervised fast with blood flucose determined is the recommended tool. Inappropriate secretion of insulin in the presence of hypoglycemia is characteristic for insulinoma.

The test requires hospitalization of the patient. During the fasting period consumption of noncaloric caffeine-free beverages and physical activity are not limited. Blood samples for the assessment of glucose, insulin, and c-peptide should be obtained every 4–6 h and in the case of hypoglycemic symptoms. During the entire test the patient should be maintained under observation. If any serious glycopenic symptoms occur, blood samples should be drawn and the test immediately terminated. Glucose should be administered orally or, in case of severe hypoglycemia, intravenously. The test is ended in the case of neuroglycopenic symptoms and a plasma glucose level below 2.5 mmol/l. Some investigators recommend that the patient exercises at the end of the fast if no hypoglycemic symptoms have occurred after 72 h.

Under physiological circumstances during the fasting period the lowering of serum glucose levels is paralleled by low insulin serum levels. In the case of insulinoma serum insulin levels stay high in spite of low glucose levels. The assessment of insulin and c-peptide in the critical blood sample allows the differentiation between endogenously produced insulin and factitious hypoglycemia from exogenous insulin.

Adequate suppression of insulin secretion during prolonged fasting is achieved when serum insulin concentration drops below 5 μU/ml (< 30 pmol/l) with normal blood glucose levels. With adequate suppression of insulin secretion, the concentration of c-peptide serum levels drops below 0.6 ng/ml (< 0.2 nmol/l). If the blood glucose is lower than 2.2 mmol/l, insulin levels should be below 3 μU/ml (< 18 pmol/l). Insulin concentrations above 6 μU/ml (36 pmol/l) are considered as being abnormally elevated if the simultaneous blood glucose concentration is < 2.2 mmol/l. The insulin:glucose ratio in healthy persons is below 0.3, in patients suffering from insulinoma basal values are higher than 0.4 with further increase dury fasting are observed.

Advanced Procedures

As the glucose–insulin system is composed of a complex set of metabolic interactions and regulatory components, highly sophisticated methods to analyze abnormal insulin secretion and sensitivity among diabetic patients – most of them not applicable in clinical routine – have been developed. Various indices such as HOMA (homeostasis model assessment) and QUICKI (quantitative insulin sensitivity check index) to calculate insulin sensitivity and secretion by mathematical handling of the fasting levels of glucose and insulin have been introduced. However, these methods are not able to give any clue as to the dynamic state of the relationship between insulin secretion and sensitivity. The gold standard for measurement of insulin sensitivity is the euglycemic hyperinsulinemic clamp technique. It is performed by infusing insulin at a constant rate to achieve physiological suprabasal levels. Glucose serum levels are monitored frequently and glucose is infused at variable rates to maintain near-constant glycemia, which is equivalent to normal fasting glucose levels. At steady state, when endogenous glucose production is suppressed, the glucose infusion rate is assumed to equal the amount of glucose needed in tissues. To study the dynamic situation after intravenous glucose injection as a tool to study the beta-cell response to a stimulus, the intravenous glucose tolerance test with frequent sampling at the beginning was developed. The magnitude and kinetics of insulin secretion is then determined by using the so-called "minimal model." The test allows direct stimulation of the beta-cell without the confounding effects of incretins or gastrointestinal hormones and possible problems related to gastric emptying [51].

References

1. Andersson E, Andersson R (2001) Exocrine insufficiency in acute pancreatitis. Scand J Gastroenterol 11:1035–1039
2. Dominguez-Munoz JE, Pieramico O, Büchler M, Malfertheiner P (1995) Exocrine pancreatic secretion in the early phase of acute pancreatitis. Scand J Gastroenterol 30:186–191
3. Dominguez-Munoz JE, Malfertheiner P (1997) Exocrine pancreatic function during and following acute pancreatitis. In: Malfertheiner P, Dominguez-Munoz JE, Schulz HU, Lippert H (eds) Diagnostic Procedures in Pancreatic Disease. Springer Verlag, Berlin Heidelberg, pp 81–85
4. Migliori M, Pezzilli R, Tomassetti P, Gullo L (2004) Exocrine pancreatic function after alcoholic or biliary acute pancreatitis. Pancreas 28:359–363
5. Dominguez-Munoz JE, di Sebastiano P, Malfertheiner P(1997) Endocrine pancreatic function during and following acute pancreatitis. In: Malfertheiner P, Dominguez-Munoz JE, Schulz HU, Lippert H (eds) Diagnostic Procedures in Pancreatic Disease. Springer Verlag, Berlin Heidelberg, pp 87–90
6. Ammann RW, Akovbiantz A, Largiader F, Schueler G (1984) Course and outcome of chronic pancreatitis. Longitudinal study of a mixed medical-surgical series of 245 patients. Gastroenterology 86:820–828
7. Malfertheiner P, Buchler MW (1989)Correlation of imaging and function in chronic pancreatitis. Radiol Clin North Am 27:51–64
8. DiMagno EP, Go VL, Summerskill WH (1973) Relations between pancreatic enzyme outputs and malabsorption in severe pancreatic insufficiency. N Engl J Med 288:813–815
9. Lankisch PG (1993) Function tests in the diagnosis of chronic pancreatitis. Critical evaluation. Int J Pancreatol 14:9–20

10. Glasbrenner B, v Tirpitz C, Malfertheiner P, Adler G (1997) Endocrine pancreatic function in the diagnosis and staging of chronic pancreatitis. In: Malfertheiner P, Dominguez-Munoz JE, Schulz HU, Lippert H (eds) Diagnostic Procedures in Pancreatic Disease. Springer Verlag, Berlin Heidelberg, pp 303–309
11. Yalniz M, Pour PM (2005) Diabetes mellitus: a risk factor for pancreatic cancer? Langenbecks Arch Surg 390:66–72
12. Gullo L (1999) Diabetes and the risk of pancreatic cancer. Ann Oncol 10 Suppl 4:79–81
13. Malfertheiner P, Buchler M, Glasbrenner B, Schafmayer A, Ditschuneit H (1987) Adaptive changes of the exocrine pancreas and plasma cholecystokinin release following subtotal gastric resection in rats. Digestion 38:142–151
14. Buchler M, Malfertheiner P, Fischbach W, Beger HG (1987) Adaptive changes in rat exocrine pancreas following subtotal colectomy. Eur Surg Res 19:31–39
15. Friess H, Bohm J, Muller MW, Glasbrenner B, Riepl RL, Malfertheiner P, Buchler MW (1996) Maldigestion after total gastrectomy is associated with pancreatic insufficiency. Am J Gastroenterol 91:341–347
16. Jang JY, Kim SW, Park SJ, Park YH (2002) Comparison of the functional outcome after pylorus-preserving pancreatoduodenectomy: pancreatogastrostomy and pancreatojejunostomy. World J Surg 26:366–371
17. Jang JY, Kim SW, Han JK, Park SJ, Park YC, Joon AY, Park YH (2003) Randomized prospective trial of the effect of induced hypergastrinemia on the prevention of pancreatic atrophy after pancreatoduodenectomy in humans. Ann Surg 237:522–529
18. Lemaire E, O'Toole D, Sauvanet A, Hammel P, Belghiti J, Ruszniewski P (2000) Functional and morphological changes in the pancreatic remnant following pancreaticoduodenectomy with pancreaticogastric anastomosis. Br J Surg 87:434–438
19. Stone WM, Sarr MG, Nagorney DM, McIlrath DC (1988) Chronic pancreatitis. Results of Whipple's resection and total pancreatectomy. Arch Surg 123:815–819
20. Sato T, Noto N, Matsuno S, Miyakawa K (1981) Follow-up results of surgical treatment for chronic pancreatitis. Present status in Japan. Am J Surg 142:317–323
21. Beger HG, Schlosser W, Friess H, Buchler MW (1999) Duodenum-preserving head resection in chronic pancreatitis changes the natural course of the disease: a single-center 26-year experience. Ann Surg 230:512–519
22. Bittner R, Butters M, Buchler M, Nagele S, Roscher R, Beger HG (1994) Glucose homeostasis and endocrine pancreatic function in patients with chronic pancreatitis before and after surgical therapy. Pancreas 9:47–53
23. Buchler MW, Friess H, Muller MW, Wheatley AM, Beger HG (1995) Randomized trial of duodenum-preserving pancreatic head resection versus pylorus-preserving Whipple in chronic pancreatitis. Am J Surg 169:65–69
24. Frey CF, Child CG, Fry W (1976) Pancreatectomy for chronic pancreatitis. Ann Surg 184:403–413
25. Leodolter A, Kahl S, Dominguez-Munoz JE, Gerards C, Glasbrenner B, Malfertheiner P (2000) Comparison of two tubeless function tests in the assessment of mild-to-moderate exocrine pancreatic insufficiency. Eur J Gastroenterol Hepatol 12:1335–1338
26. Lankisch PG. Exocrine pancreatic function tests. Gut 1982;23:777–798
27. Siegmund E, Löhr JM, Schuff-Werner P (2004) Die diagnostische Validität nichtinvasiver Pankreasfunktionstests-eine Metaanalyse. Z Gastroenterol 42:1117–1128
28. Weaver LT, Amarri S, Swart GR (1998) 13C mixed triglyceride breath test. Gut 43 (Suppl 3):S13–S19
29. Lagerloef HO (1942) Pancreatic function and pancreatic disease: studied by means of secretin. Acta Med Scand 128 (Suppl):1–289
30. Gullo L (1997) Direct pancreatic functions tests in the diagnosis and staging of chronic pancreatitis. In: Malfertheiner P, Dominguez-Munoz JE, Schulz HU, Lippert H (eds) Diagnostic Procedures in Pancreatic Disease. Springer Verlag, Berlin Heidelberg, pp 303–309
31. Chowdhury RS, Forsmark CE (2003) Pancreatic function testing. Aliment Pharmacol Ther 17:733–750
32. Lundh G (1962) Pancreatic exocrine function in neoplastic and inflammatory disease: a simple and reliable new test. Gastroenterology 42:275–280
33. Rünzi M, Layer P (1997) Oral pancreatic function tests in the diagnosis and staging of chronic pancreatitis. In: Malfertheiner P, Dominguez-Munoz JE, Schulz HU, Lippert H (eds) Diagnostic Procedures in Pancreatic Disease. Springer Verlag, Berlin Heidelberg, pp 253–260
34. Malfertheiner P, Büchler M, Müller A, Ditschuneit H (1987) Fluorescein dilaurate (FDL) serum test – a rapid tubeless pancreatic function test. Pancreas 2:53–60
35. Dominguez-Munoz JE, Malfertheiner P (1998) Optimized serum pancreolauryl test for differentiating patients with and without chronic pancreatitis. Clin Chem 44:869–875
36. Ghoos YF, Vantrappen GR, Rutgeerts PJ, Schurmans PC (1981) A mixed triglyceride breath test for intraluminal fat digestive capacity. Digestion 22:239–247
37. Vantrappen GR, Rutgeerts PJ, Ghoos YF, Hiele ML (1989) Mixed triglyceride breath test: a noninvasive test of pancreatic lipase activity in the duodenum. Gastroenterology 96:1126–1134
38. Newcomer AD, Hofmann AF, DiMagno EP, Thomas PJ, Carlson GL (1979) Triolein breath test: a sensitive and specific test for fat malabsorption. Gastroenterology 76:6–13
39. Mylvaganam K, Hudson PR, Ross A, Williams CP (1986) 14C triolein breath test: a routine test in the gastroenterology clinic? Gut 27:1347–1349
40. Lembcke B, Braden B, Caspary WF (1996) Exocrine pancreatic insufficiency: accuracy and clinical value of the uniformly labeled 13C-Hiolein breath test. Gut 39:668–674
41. Cole SG, Rossi S, Stern A, Hofmann AF (1987) Cholesteryl octanoate breath test. Preliminary studies on a new noninvasive test of human pancreatic exocrine function. Gastroenterology 93:1372–1380
42. Ventrucci M, Cipolla A, Ubalducci GM, Roda A, Roda E (1998) 13C labelled cholesteryl octanoate breath test for assessing pancreatic exocrine insufficiency. Gut 42:81–87
43. Mundlos S, Kuhnelt P, Adler G (1990) Monitoring enzyme replacement treatment in exocrine pancreatic insufficiency using the cholesteryl octanoate breath test. Gut 31:1324–1328
44. Adler G, Mundlos S, Kuhnelt P, Dreyer E (1993) New methods for assessment of enzyme activity: do they help to optimize enzyme treatment? Digestion 54:3–9
45. Patel VP, Jain NK, Agarwal N, Gee Varghese PJ, Pitchumoni CS (1986) Comparison of bentiromide test and rice flour breath hydrogen test in the detection of exocrine pancreatic insufficiency. Pancreas 1:172–175
46. Loser C, Mollgaard A, Aygen S, Hennemann O, Fölsch UR (1997) 13C-starch breath test-comparative clinical evaluation of an indirect pancreatic function test. Z Gastroenterol 35:187–194

47. Glasbrenner B, Kahl S, Malfertheiner P (2002) Modern diagnostics of chronic pancreatitis. Eur J Gastroenterol Hepatol 14:935–941
48. American Diabetes Association (2004) Diagnosis and classification of diabetes mellitus. Diabetes Care 27 (Suppl 1): S5–S10
49. Vague P, Nguyen L (2001) Rationale and methods for the estimation of insulin secretion in a given patient. From research to clinical practice. Diabetes 51 (Suppl 1) S240–244
50. American Diabetes Association (2004) Tests of glycemia in diabetes. Diabetes care 27 (Suppl 1):S91–S93
51. Ahren B, Pacini G (2004) Importance of quantifying insulin secretion in relation to insulin sensitivity to accurately assess beta cell function in clinical studies. Eur J Endocrinol 150:97–104
52. Kahl S, Malfertheiner P (2004) Exocrine and endocrine pancreatic insufficiency after pancreatic surgery. Best Pract Res Clin Gastroenterol 18:947–955

Chapter 13

J. Mössner

Guidelines, Clinical Evaluation, Short Track

History may reveal known gallbladder stones or alcohol abuse as potential causes of acute pancreatitis. Physical findings are dependent upon the severity of the disease. However, serum laboratory parameters and imaging procedures are mandatory not only for diagnosis, but also for decision making for further therapeutic options. Contrast-enhanced computed tomography (CT) is the most accurate, noninvasive, single method for evaluating the severity of acute pancreatitis. Detection of bacterial infection of necrosis is mandatory to decide between the continuation of conservative treatment or indication for either surgery or endoscopically transgastral or transcutaneous CT-guided drainages. In chronic pancreatitis, leading symptoms are upper relapsing abdominal pain and weight loss. There are numerous imaging procedures that can be used to diagnose chronic pancreatitis and its complications. Due to rapid technical improvements, comparative trials between CT, magnetic resonance (MR) cholangiopancreatography (MRCP), endoscopic retrograde cholangiopancreatography (ERCP), and endosonography are mostly outdated at the time of publishing. Endosonography has probably the highest sensitivity in diagnosing early changes in chronic pancreatitis. Pancreatic function tests are usually not necessary for further therapeutic decisions. Up to now there are no reliable and cost-effective screening methods for detecting early pancreatic cancer. Diagnosis of pancreatic cancer at a stage where the disease can be cured is a rather rare event. Transabdominal sonography may already diagnose metastatic disease. However, most patients with suspicion of pancreatic cancer will have an abdominal CT to detect the tumor. MR imaging (MRI) in combination with MR-angiography and MRCP ("one-stop shopping") is probably the most reliable method for the decision as to whether the patient can still be operated with R0 resection as a main goal. Despite the use of all imaging procedures, in up to 25% irresectability is only seen during operation. Another unresolved problem is the early diagnosis of pancreatic cancer in patients with chronic pancreatitis. Positron emission tomography (PET) does not help very much in the differentiation between chronic inflammation and pancreatic cancer. The following chapter presents some recent comparative trials of various imaging procedures regarding their sensitivity and specificity in the diagnosis of the three leading diseases of the exocrine pancreas (i.e., acute and chronic pancreatitis, and pancreatic cancer). However, due to the lack of comparative trials stratified to the various stages of each disease, the diagnostic recommendations (i.e., "short track") cannot completely avoid the subjective recommendations of the author.

Acute Pancreatitis

History

Gallstones and excessive alcohol abuse are the most important risk factors for acute pancreatitis. Sometimes acute pancreatitis is initiated by large fatty meals and/or acute alcohol excess. Thus, history may reveal known gallbladder stones or alcohol abuse. Amongst numerous rare causes, such as drugs (e.g., angiotensin converting enzyme inhibitors, L-asparaginase, azathioprine, 6-mercaptopurine, estrogens, sulfasalazine, 5-aminosalicylic acid, thiazides, valproic acid), hyperlipidemia, hypercalcemia, trauma, and viral infection (mumps), one has to mention diagnostic and therapeutic ERCP. According to a prospective multicenter study, when endosonography was performed to confirm or exclude a biliary origin of acute pancreatitis, age, gender, and alanine transaminase levels at admission were the only factors predictive of a biliary cause [32].

The typical symptoms of acute pancreatitis are severe, knifelike pain located in the upper and midepigastric abdomen combined with nausea, vomiting, and anorexia [54]. Pain may radiate to the back like a belt. The onset of pain is rather rapid, but not as rapid as in perforated duodenal or gastric ulcer. At the beginning, pain may be colic-like, and later more diffuse and felt deep in the abdomen. Pain may gradually increase; mostly it is steady and very severe. In mild pancreatitis, pain resolves after a few days but may return after the patient starts to eat. In severe attacks, pain progresses.

Physical Findings

The physical findings are dependent upon the severity of the disease. Abdominal tenderness varies from mild to severe. In severe pancreatitis, the patient looks severely ill, lies still, and often has abdominal distention. One will find tenderness in the upper abdomen. In necrotizing pancreatitis, a progression to peritonitis is possible. Due to the inflammation of an organ located retroperitoneally, signs of peritonism are usually absent at the beginning. In metabolic or hereditary cases and in cases associated with alcohol abuse, the onset may be less abrupt [54].

Rarely seen, but typical for a severe course, is a brownish discoloration of the skin (i.e., ecchymosis) due to the spread of the inflammation to flanks (Grey-Turner-sign) and the periumbilical region (Cullen-sign). When these signs are present, the prognosis is usually worse. On auscultation, bowel sounds are reduced or absent as signs of paralytic ileus. Tachycardia and fall in blood pressure are already symptoms of the beginning shock syndrome. Shock and fall in hemoglobin may be caused by gastrointestinal bleeding (peptic ulcer, Mallory-Weiss-syndrome), or intra-abdominal or retroperitoneal bleeding, splenic lesions, or vessel arrosions. Flushing of the face is the consequence of the release of vasoactive substances. Fever may be present initially due to aseptic inflammation, and later as a sign of sepsis due to infected necrosis. Fever over 38.5°C, chills, shock, leukocytosis above 16,000/μl, thrombocytopenia, and metabolic acidosis are signs of a septic course, the most severe complication. Further clinical signs of a severe course are hypotension, shock, oligo-, anuria, dyspnea, bleedings, precoma, and coma. Shallow respiration and tachypnea can be caused by subdiaphragmatic exudates, leading to painful breathing.

Severe vomiting may be due to duodenal compression caused by the inflammatory mass of the head of the pancreas or due to paralytic ileus. Jaundice may be seen when the distal bile duct is compressed. Ascites and ileus lead to an increase in the abdominal circumference. In alcoholic pancreatitis, when liver damage is also present, one may see typical liver skin signs, such as, for example, spider angiomas and thickening of the palmar sheaths.

Necrosis, Abscess, Sepsis

Necrosis of the pancreas is a potentially very harmful complication. Primarily there are no bacteria in the pancreas. Paralytic ileus favors the penetration of bacteria from the gut into the pancreas. Infected necrosis is the source for sepsis causing an increase in mortality. Leukocytosis is seen even in uncomplicated pancreatitis. However, leukocytosis is especially prominent in sepsis. The presence of fever is an indication for contrast-enhanced CT to detect necrosis and perform fine-needle aspiration (FNA) microbiology. Contrast-enhanced CT remains the most accurate noninvasive single method for evaluating the severity of acute pancreatitis [20, 24, 30].

Shock

Due to fluid and blood losses into the retroperitoneum and fluid losses caused by paralytic ileus, blood circulation is endangered. Measurement of blood pressure, pulse rate, and central venous pressure is mandatory for the early detection of shock syndrome. In necrotizing pancreatitis, blood penetrates not only the retroperitoneum, but may also penetrate the intestine. This may cause severe blood loss. Furthermore, bleeding may be caused by stress ulcerations of the stomach and duodenum. Disturbances in serum electrolytes can be marked due to enormous fluid losses. Hypocalcemia may also result from fat necrosis.

Acute Kidney Failure

Severe volume losses and toxic damage of the renal tubuli are responsible for kidney failure. Measurement of 24-h urinary excretion is obligatory. Values below 40 ml/h are critical. Elevation of serum creatinine may be seen after a delay. Serum levels of creatinine and urea have to be determined to detect renal failure.

Acute Respiratory Distress Syndrome, Shock Lung

Analysis of blood oxygen and carbon dioxide and acid–base status are mandatory to detect respiratory insufficiency and determine indications for artificial ventilation (decrease of oxygen partial pressure of <65 mmHg). Auscultation of the lungs and chest x-ray are not very helpful in this regard.

Obstruction of the Common Bile Duct

In obstruction of the bile outlet due to impacted bile stones or an inflammatory mass of the pancreatic head, one will see cholestasis in serum parameters such as elevation of gamma-glutamyl transferase, alkaline phosphatase, and bilirubin. Jaundice is only seen in marked obstruction.

Disseminated Intravascular Coagulation

In disseminated intravascular coagulation one will find hematomas of the skin. It is very important to establish patients at risk of having a severe, potentially lethal course of the disease. Numerous various scoring systems, such as the Atlanta criteria, Ransons's score, CT severity index, Acute Physiology and Chronic Health Evaluation II (APACHE II) score, Glasgow score, Multi Organ System Score, and urinary trypsinogen activation peptide are available (for further literature see [13, 14, 31, 37, 41, 49, 54, 55]). Besides the CT severity index, these all include the combination of clinical parameters and various laboratory values, which will be discussed in another chapter. None of these scoring systems is simple, really easy to perform, or absolutely reliable to early detect those patients at risk.

Systemic inflammatory response syndrome (SIRS) is rather easy to detect and monitor. SIRS is characterized by two or more of the following signs: temperature >38°C or <36°C; heart rate >90 beats/min; respiratory rate >20/min; arterial carbon dioxide partial pressure <32 mmHg; leukocytosis >12,000/µl; leukopenia <4000/µl. The course of SIRS is highly predictive of further prognosis [40].

A differential diagnosis of chronic pancreatitis is described in Table 13.1.

Short Track

Diagnosis and Clarification of Etiology

Pancreatitis is mostly proven when abdominal pain and elevation of serum lipase more than three times above normal are present [27]. In fulminant pancreatitis and delayed diagnostic work up, serum lipase can already be normal due to loss of pancreatic acini [56]. Patient history may already help to discriminate between biliary and alcohol-induced pancreatitis or rare causes such as drugs. MRCP can be used to detect bile duct stones, with high sensitivity [46]. However, endosonography is probably the most sensitive method to detect bile duct stones and has replaced diagnostic ERCP. In contrast to ERCP, endosonography imposes only a minor risk of inducing or aggravating pancreatitis. Endosonography is also the most sensitive method for detecting early pancreatic changes characteristic of chronic pancreatitis [45]. In a recent study using endosonography to confirm or exclude a biliary origin of acute pancreatitis, it was reported that age, gender, and alanine transaminase level at admission were the only factors predictive of a biliary cause [32]. Acute pancreatitis should not be declared as idiopathic as long endosonography has not excluded abnormalities such as bile duct stones [42].

Evaluation of Severity of the Disease

Serum levels of lipase or other pancreatic enzymes do not correlate with the severity of the disease. Other parameters such as trypsinogen activation peptide, polymorphonuclear-elastase, and hematocrit are either not evaluated in larger trials or are not routinely available, such as determination of interleukin-6.

Table 13.1. Differential diagnosis of acute pancreatitis. *CT* Computed tomography, *ECG* electrocardiogram, *CK* cholecystokinin

Diagnosis	Diagnostic procedures
Perforation of gastric or duodenal ulcer	Free air: abdominal plain x-ray: upright or left-sided position
Acute cholecystitis	History of colic possible, pain in right upper abdomen, sonography
Occlusion of mesenteric artery	History of postprandial pain, angiography
Aneurysma dissecans of abdominal aorta	Sonography, CT
Ileus	Abdominal plain x-ray
Acute appendicitis	History, physical examination, laboratory, sonography
Left-sided ureter colic	Sonography, urography
Heart infarction	History, ECG, troponin, CK, CK-MB
Lung embolus with pleuritis	Physical examination, D-dimer, chest x-ray, echocardiography, chest CT, perfusion scintigraphy

Obesity is certainly a risk factor of both the severity and mortality of the disease [36]. Serum C-reactive protein and contrast-enhanced CT are the most reliable methods of detecting pancreatic necrosis [5, 6, 9]. MRI may be as sensitive and has not the risk to deteriorate renal function. However, severely ill patients are more difficult to handle in MRI as compared to CT. To evaluate the development and extension of pancreatic necrosis, CT is better performed not earlier than 2 days after the clinical onset of pancreatitis. However, CT is often indicated in patients with acute abdomen of unknown origin. A normal pancreas in CT excludes pancreatitis as a cause of acute abdomen. Up to now there are no simple screening techniques and laboratory parameters for predicting the further course of the disease. Ranson's score, the Imrie-Glasgow score, APACHE II score, and Atlanta criteria have been offered to characterize the severity of the disease and to predict prognosis [10, 13, 22, 43, 48]. These criteria, however, are not routinely used by all experts treating patients with acute pancreatitis. A recent study reported that the interobserver agreement of the Atlanta classification for categorizing peripancreatic collections in acute pancreatitis on CT was rather poor [8]. The Marshall score is used to monitor organ failure. Rapid resolution of organ failure (i.e., within 48 h) is suggestive of a good prognosis, in contrast to persistent organ failure [23].

Detection of bacterial infection of necrosis is mandatory to decide between continuation of conservative treatment or indication for either surgery or endoscopically transgastral or transcutaneous CT-guided drainages. CT- or ultrasonographically guided FNA are standard [7, 18, 44]. Further signs of infected necrosis or sepsis are provided by measurements of rectal temperature (>38.5°C), hematocrit (<35%), and oxygen partial pressure (<60 mmHg) [9].

Chronic Pancreatitis

History

In the industrialized nations, up to 80% of all cases of chronic pancreatitis are caused by alcohol abuse. Thus, by careful history, consumption of more than 80 g of alcohol per day can be found. Alcohol-induced chronic pancreatitis may evolve from acute pancreatitis [3]. Alcohol consumption is often associated with cigarette smoking. Smoking per se does not seem to be a risk factor for chronic pancreatitis. In less than 5%, a family history of pancreatic diseases, especially chronic pancreatitis, can be found. In hereditary chronic pancreatitis, an autosomal dominant disease with a penetrance rate of about 80%, mutations of the cationic trypsinogen are reported. In alcoholic pancreatitis these mutations are almost absent [50]. In patients with so-called idiopathic chronic pancreatitis, a serum elevation of IgG4 and detection of antibodies against carbonic anhydrase should be suspicious for autoimmune pancreatitis [4].

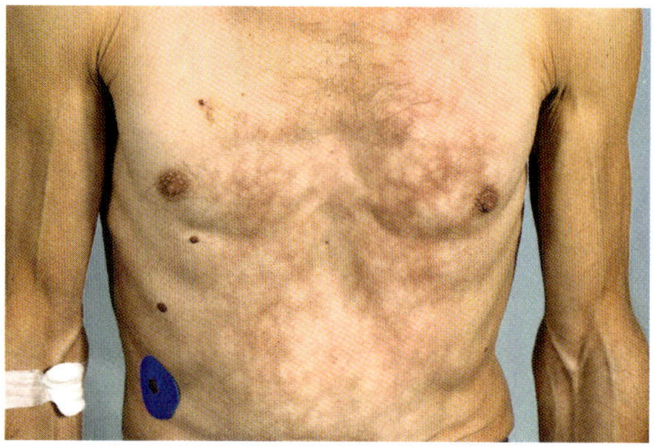

Figure 13.1

Patient with chronic pancreatitis: "erythema ab igne" due to chronic application of heat to alleviate pain

Table 13.2. Causes of pain in chronic pancreatitis

Hypertension of ducts due to obstruction
Stones, scars, pseudocysts
Inflammatory infiltration of sensory nerves
Retroperitoneal effusions
Ischemia
Compression/distension of biliary duct, duodenum, pancreatic "capsule"
Inflammatory mass, pseudocyst
Extrapancreatic causes
Ulcer, meteorism due to steatorrhea
Psychological disorders due to alcoholism

Leading symptoms are upper relapsing abdominal pain and weight loss later during the course of the disease [16, 47]. The disease may be classified according to different stages. In early stage I, patients are either pain free or report noncharacteristic upper abdominal discomfort. Pain may be intermittent and lasts for days and weeks. Pain is felt deep in the abdomen and sometimes like a belt with radiation into the back. Pain may improve by application of local heat (Fig. 13.1) and in a more sitting forward position. Pain is described as piercing and penetrating. In stage II,

Table 13.3. Symptoms caused by pancreatic pseudocysts

Pathophysiology	Symptoms and clinical findings
Dependent on size, localization and speed of enlargement	Pain
Compression of duodenum and/or stomach	Pain, vomiting
Rupture into the abdomen	Pancreatic ascites
Infection of ascites	Peritonitis
Rupture into the gut	Spontaneous "healing"
Connection with pleura	Pleural effusion, dyspnea
Erosion of vessels	Life threatening bleeding
Thrombosis of splenic vein	Fundic varices, bleeding

patients have intermittent, often severe pain attacks or chronic pain. There is a wide variation regarding length of pain (days to weeks), interval between pain attacks, and the severity of pain. There are numerous causes of pain (Table 13.2) and these causes may vary during the course of the disease. At the clinical beginning of the disease the first acute attack can often not be differentiated from acute pancreatitis. Severe courses like necrotizing pancreatitis needing intensive care are possible. In most cases, acute relapses can be treated conservatively. During stage II, complicated courses like the formation of pseudocysts are typical. Some patients experience a decrease in severity of their relapses due to the destruction of pancreatic parenchyma, which is a substrate for inflammation [2]. Pain may "burn out." This observation by the Zürich group, however, has not been uniformly confirmed.

Pseudocysts may lead to a wide variety of symptoms (Table 13.3). Jaundice may be caused by bile outlet obstruction due to the inflammatory mass of the pancreatic head, fibrosis of the distal bile duct, or by a pseudocyst. Biliary obstruction in chronic pancreatitis alone does not seem to cause pain [25].

In stage III, symptoms of exocrine and endocrine insufficiency are dominant. Diabetes is more difficult to control in alcoholics with chronic pancreatitis due to several reasons, such as lack of anti-insulin hormones (i.e., glucagon), noncompliance, and dietary faults (sometimes due to pain attacks caused by eating). Steatorrhea may lead to bacterial overgrowth, causing pain due to meteorism. Treatment with porcine pancreatic extracts may improve abdominal discomfort. However, the assumption that pancreatic enzymes inhibit pancreatic enzyme secretion via a negative-feedback mechanism and thus are beneficial in the treatment of pain is not supported by clinical studies [38].

Due to long-term cigarette smoking, patients may report symptoms of severe arteriosclerosis, such as "claudicatio intermittens," angina pectoris, and pneumonia. Symptoms due to lung cancers, and cancers of the throat and esophagus are also not uncommon.

About 5% of all patients never experienced pain attacks and may present at the first time already with symptoms of severe exocrine insufficiency, such as weight loss and steatorrhea. During the first years of the disease, with often noncharacteristic abdominal symptoms, diagnosis may be difficult.

Autoimmune pancreatitis is receiving increasing attention. Without imaging procedures such as MRI, MRCP, and endosonography, and certain serum parameters, such as the presence of antibodies against carbonic anhydrase and elevation of IgG4, it is not able to make a diagnosis just by clinical means. Sometimes these patients have additional symptoms due to other concomitant autoimmune disorders such as Sjogren's syndrome.

Physical Findings

Pain in the upper abdomen by deep palpation is a rather unspecific sign and can be seen in numerous abdominal diseases. Rarely, one can feel a large pancreatic pseudocyst. One has to pay attention to the typical signs of chronic alcohol and nicotine abuse such as yellow fingertips and liver skin signs when alcoholic liver damage is also present. In rare cases, but highly specific for chronic pancreatitis, a brownish discoloration of the skin located in the upper abdomen can be seen, so called "erythema ab igne" (Fig. 13.1). These skin changes are caused by continuous slight burning injuries due to the application of heat to improve abdominal pain.

The body mass index may be normal in the beginning of the disease. Chronic alcoholics who smoke

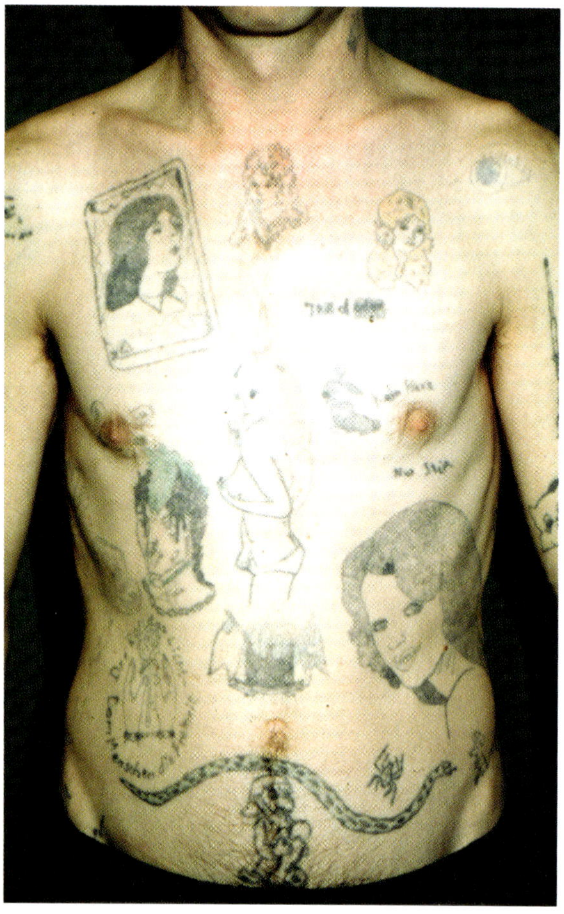

Figure 13.2

Patient with chronic pancreatitis: underweight and many tattoos

heavily are seldom overweight and are often malnourished. Decrease of body weight during the early stages of chronic pancreatitis may be caused by several factors such as fear of eating due to abdominal pain and inadequate intake of calories (i.e., alcoholic beverages instead of food). Weight loss in the later stages of the disease is caused by exocrine insufficiency or due to the development of cancers (i.e., lung, esophagus, pancreas). At least in our region, which is a formerly heavily industrialized city that currently has a high unemployment rate, many patients with chronic alcohol-induced pancreatitis belong to a lower social class. These patients very often have tattoos (Fig. 13.2).

Many patients avoid fatty meals because they cause pain. Thus, visible steatorrhea, even in severe exocrine insufficiency, is not usual. Furthermore, detection of fatty stools just by visual evaluation is not very reliable [29].

Differential and early diagnosis of pancreatic cancer remains a challenge both in patients with suspicion of autoimmune pancreatitis and in patients with known long-lasting chronic pancreatitis. One has to pay attention to symptoms of alcohol withdrawal such as hallucinations, disorientation, and agitations.

Short Track

Diagnosis and Further Therapy

There are various imaging procedures used to diagnose chronic pancreatitis and its complications. Due to rapid technical improvements, comparative trials between CT, MRI, ERCP, and endosonography are mostly outdated at the time of publishing. Figure 13.3 proposes a not-evidence-based algorithm of how to proceed when chronic pancreatitis is suspected. Endosonography probably has the highest sensitivity or diagnosing early changes in chronic pancreatitis [15, 52]. Endosonography is also used by most experts prior to endoscopic drainage of pseudocysts to avoid puncture of vessels within the wall of the pseudocysts and to check for the nearest distance of the pseudocyst to either the stomach or duodenum. To evaluate the cause of pain in chronic pancreatitis and for decision making as to whether to continue with conservative treatment or better recommend surgery, both transabdominal sonography and CT are very often "straight forward" (Fig. 13.4).

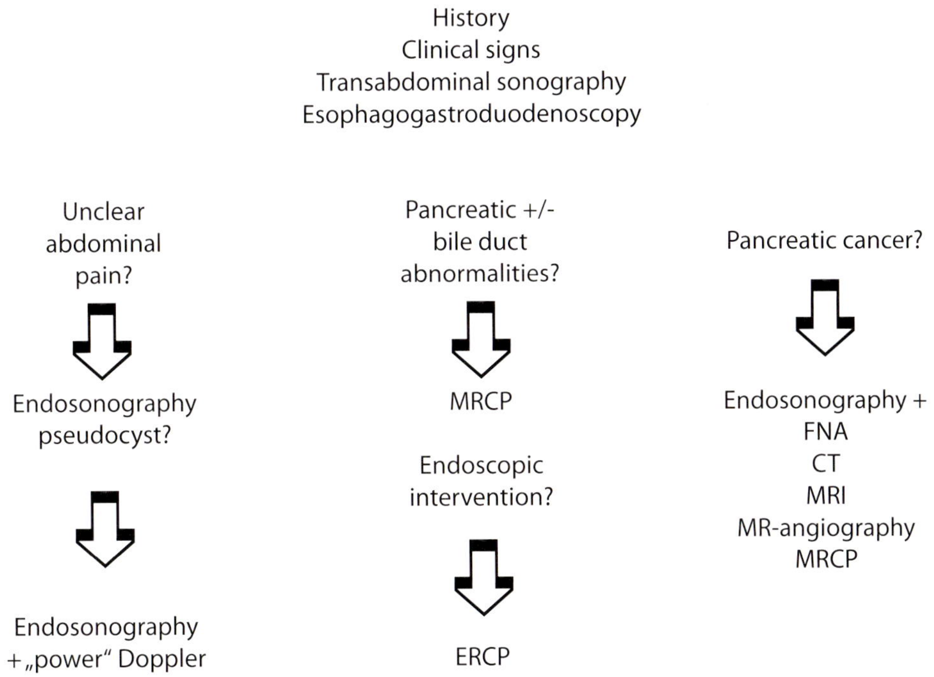

Figure 13.3

Diagnostic algorithm in suspected chronic pancreatitis

Pancreatic Cancer

History

Pancreatic cancer is one of the most devastating diseases; its associated mortality, incidence, and prevalence are almost identical. Patients rarely survive beyond 5 years; indeed most patients die within 6 months after diagnosis. Familial cancer syndromes, smoking, and to a lesser extent being overweight and having type II diabetes are known risk factors for pancreatic cancer [11, 39, 53]. There are speculations that the incidence of pancreatic cancer could be reduced by 30% if people didn't smoke. However, due to the "epidemic" of being overweight in industrialized countries, the high prevalence of smoking and the lack of reliable and cost-effective screening methods to detect early pancreatic cancer, the ability to diagnose pancreatic cancer at a stage where the disease can be really cured is still an unfulfilled dream. Even when cancer can be completely resected, most patients experience early local recurrence or metastasis.

Chronic pancreatitis is an established risk factor for pancreatic cancer [34]. However, most patients with alcoholic pancreatitis die due to their "lifestyle." Death is caused by diseases as a consequence of heavy smoking and alcohol, such as, for example, cancers, accidents, and pneumonia [35]. Patients with hereditary pancreatitis suffer from pancreatitis for decades, usually are very compliant, and do not drink or smoke. These patients have an increased risk of developing pancreatic cancer over the age of 40 or 50 years. Unfortunately, we have no reliable diagnostic procedures that will enable an early diagnosis of pancreatic cancer. There are no larger trials that demonstrate any advantage for endosonography, CT, or positron emission tomography scan when applied annually in these patients.

Usually there are no suspicious symptoms that could lead to an early diagnosis. Most patients present with obstructive jaundice caused by compression of the bile duct in the head of the pancreas. In less than one-quarter of the patients, a nontender gallbladder is palpable (i.e., Courvoisier's sign). Epigastric or back pain, vague abdominal symptoms, and weight loss are also characteristic of pancreatic cancer [17]. Pain, jaundice, or both are seen in more than 90% of all patients [26]. Other symptoms include fatigue, anorexia, and sometimes vomiting. More than one half of cases have distant metastasis at diagnosis. In cases of jaundice due to a tumor close to the papilla of Vater or due

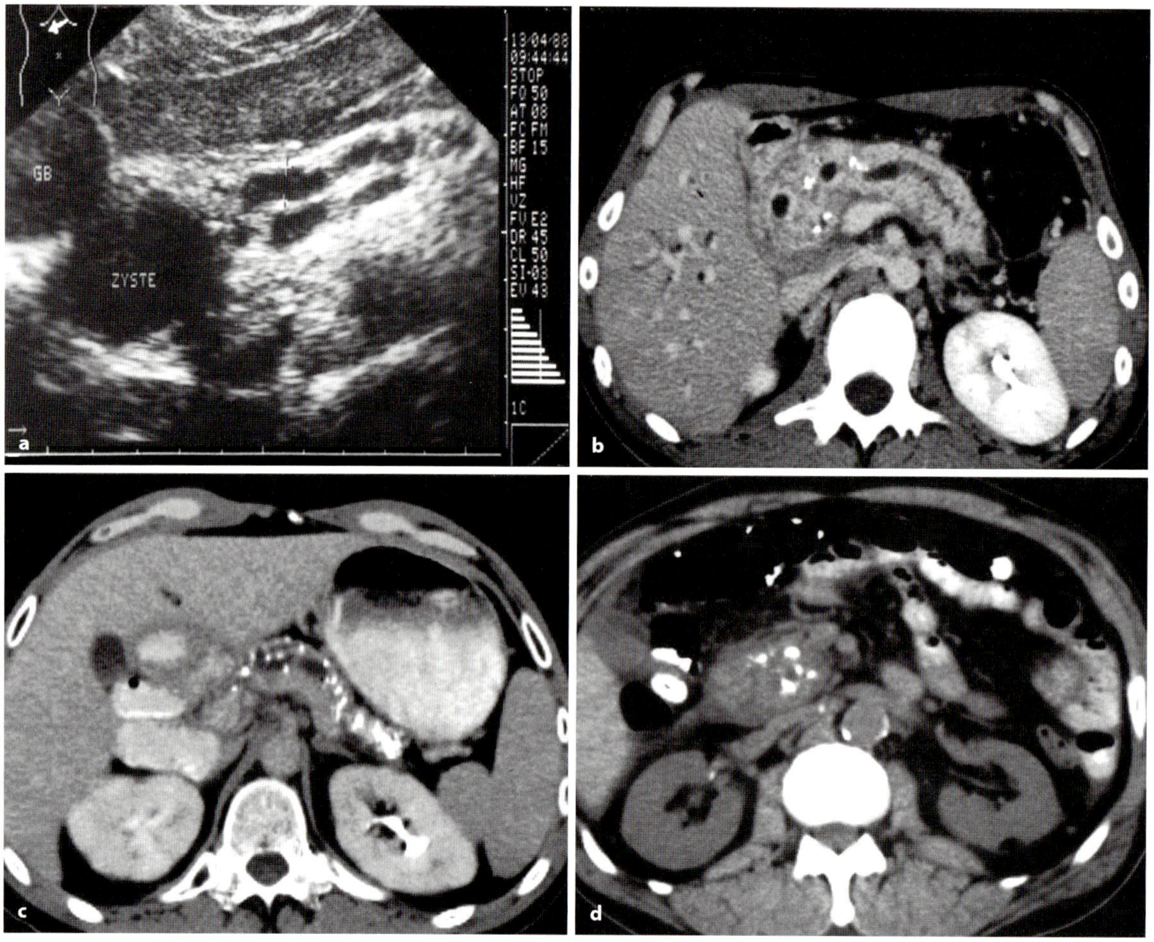

Figure 13.4

Typical complications of chronic pancreatitis. a Transabdominal sonography: pseudocyst leading to pancreatic duct dilatation and bile duct obstruction with gallbladder enlargement. b Computed tomography (CT) scan: inflammatory mass of pancreatic head leading to pancreatic duct obstruction. Numerous calcifications can be seen in the pancreatic head. c CT scan: pancreatic duct enlargement, pancreatic parenchymal atrophy, numerous calcifications. d CT scan: inflammatory mass of pancreatic head

to a tumor of the papilla itself, the tumor may still be rather small and resection with curative intention may be possible. However, very often one will find already a large tumor that can not be resected, or the patient has already liver metastases. Tumors of the distal pancreas without metastases are usually not accompanied by jaundice. They may remain painless until advanced stages [53]. However, according to an Italian study of 305 pancreatic cancer patients, there seem to be some hints with which to make an earlier diagnosis: 49.5% of these patients had some prior disturbances, 35.4% 6 months or less, before pain or jaundice, such as anorexia and/or early satiety and/or asthenia [19]; 4.6% had diabetes 7–24 months before; 1.3% had acute pancreatitis 8–26 months before. Diabetes is usually already a symptom of advanced disease.

Physical Findings

Jaundice and signs of severe weight loss are already very often seen when patients present for the first time. Rarely, the pancreatic tumor can be palpated directly.

Short Track

Diagnosis

Despite the impressive technical improvements in imaging procedures such as MRI in combination with MR-angiography and MRCP ("one stop shopping") or multislice CT and endosonography, most cases of pancreatic cancers are diagnosed at a rather late stage.

In a study from Berlin, MR assessment of pancreatic lesions with regards to differentiation between benign and malignant had an accuracy of about 90%. The positive- and negative-predictive values for cancer nonresectability were 90% and 83%, respectively [33]. MRCP has replaced diagnostic ERCP, since it has a similar sensitivity and specificity [1]. There are no cost-effective screening procedures suitable for mass screening, or at least for screening of patients at risk, such as patients with hereditary chronic pancreatitis, patients with a family history of pancreatic cancer, and patients with Peutz-Jeghers syndrome. One recent study proposed annual endoscopic ultrasound (EUS) and CT in these patients at risk [12]. Furthermore, it is still very difficult to diagnose pancreatic cancer in patients with chronic pancreatitis. Analyses of pancreatic secretions for the existence of ki-ras mutations have been disappointing [51]. EUS-guided FNA may be slightly superior to CT/ultrasound-guided FNA for the diagnosis of pancreatic malignancy [21]. EUS-FNA samples with equivocal cytology can be tested for microsatellite loss and ki-ras point mutations. This additional analysis may improve the diagnostic accuracy and prevent unnecessary surgery [28].

References

1. Adamek HE, Albert J, Breer H, Weitz M, Schilling D, Riemann JF (2000) Pancreatic cancer detection with magnetic resonance cholangiopancreatography and endoscopic retrograde cholangiopancreatography: a prospective controlled study. Lancet 356:190–193
2. Ammann RW, Akovbiantz A, Largiader F, Schueler G (1984) Course and outcome of chronic pancreatitis. Longitudinal study of a mixed medical-surgical series of 245 patients. Gastroenterology 86:820–828
3. Ammann RW, Heitz PU, Klöppel G (1996) Course of alcoholic chronic pancreatitis: a prospective clinicomorphological long-term study. Gastroenterology 111:224–231
4. Aparisi L, Farre A, Gomez-Cambronero L, Martinez J, De Las Heras G, Corts J, Navarro S, Mora J, Lopez-Hoyos M, Sabater L, Ferrandez A, Bautista D, Perez-Mateo M, Mery S, Sastre J (2005) Antibodies to carbonic anhydrase and IgG4 levels in idiopathic chronic pancreatitis: relevance for diagnosis of autoimmune pancreatitis. Gut 54:703–709
5. Arvanitakis M, Delhaye M, De Maertelaere V, Bali M, Winant C, Coppens E, Jeanmart J, Zalcman M, Van Gansbeke D, Devière J, Matos C (2004) Computed tomography and magnetic resonance imaging in the assessment of acute pancreatitis. Gastroenterology 126:715–723
6. Balthazar EJ, Freeny PC, van Sonnenberg E (1994) Imaging and intervention in acute pancreatitis. Radiology 193:297–306
7. Beger HG, Bittner R, Block S, Büchler M (1986) Bacterial contamination of pancreatic necrosis. A prospective clinical study. Gastroenterology 91:433–438
8. Besselink MG, van Santvoort HC, Bollen TL, van Leeuwen MS, Lameris JS, van der Jagt EJ, Strijk SP, Buskens E, Freeny PC, Gooszen HG; Dutch Acute Pancreatitis Study Group (2006) Describing computed tomography findings in acute necrotizing pancreatitis with the Atlanta classification: an interobserver agreement study. Pancreas 33:331–335
9. Block S, Büchler M, Bittner R, Beger HG (1987) sepsis indicators in acute pancreatitis. Pancreas 2:499–505
10. Bradley ELIII (1993) A clinically based classification system for acute pancreatitis. Summary of the International Symposium on Acute Pancreatitis, Atlanta, Ga, September 11 through 13, 1992. Arch Surg 128:586–590
11. Calle EE, Rodriguez C, Walker-Thurmond K, Thun MJ (2003) Overweight, obesity, and mortality from cancer in a prospectively studied cohort of U.S. adults. N Engl J Med 348:1625–1638
12. Canto MI, Goggins M, Hruban RH, Petersen GM, Giardiello FM, Yeo C, Fishman EK, Brune K, Axilbund J, Griffin C, Ali S, Richman J, Jagannath S, Kantsevoy SV, Kalloo AN (2006) Screening for early pancreatic neoplasia in high-risk individuals: a prospective controlled study. Clin Gastroenterol Hepatol 4:766–781
13. Chatzicostas C, Roussomoustakaki M, Vlachonikolis IG, Notas G, Mouzas I, Samonakis D, Kouroumalis EA (2002) Comparison of Ranson, APACHE II and APACHE III scoring systems in acute pancreatitis. Pancreas 25:331–335
14. Chen YT, Chen CC, Wang SS, Chang FY, Lee SD (2005) Rapid urinary trypsinogen-2 test strip in the diagnosis of acute pancreatitis. Pancreas 30:243–247
15. Conwell DL, Zuccaro G, Purich E, Fein S, Vargo JJ, Dumot JA, Vanlente F, Lopez R, Trolli P (2007) Comparison of endoscopic ultrasound chronic pancreatitis criteria to the endoscopic secretin-stimulated pancreatic function test. Dig Dis Sci 52:1206–1210
16. Etemad B, Whitcomb DC (2001) Chronic pancreatitis: diagnosis, classification, and new genetic developments. Gastroenterology 120:682–707
17. Freelove R, Walling AD (2006) Pancreatic cancer: diagnosis and management. Am Fam Physician 73:485–492
18. Gerzof SG, Banks PA, Robbins AH, Johnson WC, Spechler SJ, Wetzner SM, Snider JM, Langevin RE, Jay ME (1987) Early diagnosis of pancreatic infection by computed tomography-guided aspiration. Gastroenterology 93:1315–1320
19. Gullo L, Tomassetti P, Migliori M, Casadei R, Marrano D (2001) Do early symptoms of pancreatic cancer exist that can allow an earlier diagnosis? Pancreas 22:210–213
20. Gurleyik G, Emir S, Kilicoglu G, Arman A, Saglam A (2005) Computed tomography severity index, APACHE II score, and serum CRP concentration for predicting the severity of acute pancreatitis. JOP 6:562–567
21. Horwhat JD, Paulson EK, McGrath K, Branch MS, Baillie J, Tyler D, Pappas T, Enns R, Robuck G, Stiffler H, Jowell P (2006) A randomized comparison of EUS-guided FNA versus CT or US-guided FNA for the evaluation of pancreatic mass lesions. Gastrointest Endosc 63:966–975
22. Imrie CW (1994) Acute pancreatitis. Curr Opin Gastroenterol 10:496–501
23. Johnson CD, Abu-Hilal M (2004) Persistent organ failure during the first week as a marker of fatal outcome in acute pancreatitis. Gut 53:1340–1344
24. Ju S, Chen F, Liu S, Zheng K, Teng G (2006) Value of CT and clinical criteria in assessment of patients with acute pancreatitis. Eur J Radiol 57:102–107

25. Kahl S, Zimmermann S, Genz I, Schmidt U, Pross M, Schulz HU, Malfertheiner P (2004) Biliary strictures are not the cause of pain in patients with chronic pancreatitis. Pancreas 28:387–390
26. Kalser MH, Barkin J, MacIntyre JM (1985) Pancreatic cancer. Assessment of prognosis by clinical presentation. Cancer 56:397–402
27. Keim V, Teich N, Fiedler F, Hartig W, Thiele G, Mössner J (1998) A comparison of lipase and amylase in the diagnosis of acute pancreatitis in patients with abdominal pain. Pancreas 16:45–49
28. Khalid A, Nodit L, Zahid M, Bauer K, Brody D, Finkelstein SD, McGrath KM (2006) Endoscopic ultrasound fine needle aspirate DNA analysis to differentiate malignant and benign pancreatic masses. Am J Gastroenterol 101:2493–2500
29. Lankisch PG, Droge M, Hofses S, Konig H, Lembcke B (1996) Steatorrhoea: you cannot trust your eyes when it comes to diagnosis. Lancet 347:1620–1621
30. Lempinen M, Puolakkainen P, Kemppainen E (2005) Clinical value of severity markers in acute pancreatitis. Scand J Surg 94:118–123
31. Leung TK, Lee CM, Lin SY, Chen HC, Wang HJ, Shen LK, Chen YY (2005) Balthazar computed tomography severity index is superior to Ranson criteria and APACHE II scoring system in predicting acute pancreatitis outcome. World J Gastroenterol 11:6049–6052
32. Levy P, Boruchowicz A, Hastier P, Pariente A, Thevenot T, Frossard JL, Buscail L, Mauvais F, Duchmann JC, Courrier A, Bulois P, Gineston JL, Barthet M, Licht H, O'Toole D, Ruszniewski P (2005) Diagnostic criteria in predicting a biliary origin of acute pancreatitis in the era of endoscopic ultrasound: multicentre prospective evaluation of 213 patients. Pancreatology 5:450–456
33. Lopez Hanninen E, Amthauer H, Hosten N, Ricke J, Böhmig M, Langrehr J, Hintze R, Neuhaus P, Wiedenmann B, Rosewicz S, Felix R (2002) Prospective evaluation of pancreatic tumors: accuracy of MR imaging with MR cholangiopancreatography and MR angiography. Radiology 224:34–41
34. Lowenfels AB, Maisonneuve P, Cavallini G, Ammann RW, Lankisch PG, Andersen JR, DiMagno EP, Andren-Sandberg A, Domellof L (1993) Pancreatitis and the risk of pancreatic cancer. International Pancreatitis Study Group. N Engl J Med 328:1433–1437
35. Lowenfels AB, Maisonncuve P, Cavallini G, Ammann RW, Lankisch PG, Andersen JR, DiMagno EP, Andren-Sandberg A, Domell`f L, Di Francesco V, Pederzoli P, Löhr-Happe A, Krag F, Boyle P, Pitchumoni CS, Wynn PS, Melton LJ (1994) Prognosis of chronic pancreatitis; an international multicenter study. Am J Gastroenterol 89:1467–1471
36. Martinez J, Johnson CD, Sanchez-Paya J, de Madaria E, Robles-Diaz G, Perez-Mateo M (2006) Obesity is a definitive risk factor of severity and mortality in acute pancreatitis: an updated meta-analysis. Pancreatology 6:206–209
37. McKay CJ, Imrie CW (1999) Staging of acute pancreatitis. Is it important? Surg Clin North Am 79:733–743
38. Mössner J (1999) palliation of pain in chronic pancreatitis: use of enzymes. Surg Clin N Am 79:861–872
39. Mössner J (2005) What is the epidemiological impact of pancreatic cancer? In: Dominguez-Munoz JE (ed) Clinical Pancreatology for Practising Gastroenterologists and Surgeons. Blackwell, Oxford, pp 331–350
40. Mofidi R, Duff MD, Wigmore SJ, Madhavan KK, Garden OJ, Parks RW (2006) Association between early systemic inflammatory response, severity of multiorgan dysfunction and death in acute pancreatitis. Br J Surg 93:738–744
41. Neoptolemos JP, Kemppainen EA, Mayer JM, Fitzpatrick JM, Raraty MG, Slavin J, Beger HG, Hietaranta AJ, Puolakkainen PA (2000) Early prediction of severity in acute pancreatitis by urinary trypsinogen activation peptide: a multicentre study. Lancet 355:1955–1960
42. Norton SA, Alderson D (2000) Endoscopic ultrasonography in the evaluation of idiopathic acute pancreatitis. Br J Surg 87:1650–1655
43. Ranson IHC, Rifkind RM, Roses DF (1975) Prognostic signs and the role of operative management in acute pancreatitis. Surg Gynecol Obstet 139:69–80
44. Rau B, Pralle U, Mayer JM, Beger HG (1998) Role of ultrasonographically guided fine-needle aspiration cytology in the diagnosis of infected pancreatic necrosis. Br J Surg 85:179–184
45. Scheiman JM, Carlos RC, Barnett JL, Elta GH, Nostrant TT, Chey WD, Francis IR, Nandi PS (2001) Can endoscopic ultrasound or magnetic resonance cholangiopancreatography replace ERCP in patients with suspected biliary disease? A prospective trial and cost analysis. Am J Gastroenterol 96:2900–2904
46. Shanmugam V, Beattie GC, Yule SR, Reid W, Loudon MA (2005) Is magnetic resonance cholangiopancreatography the new gold standard in biliary imaging? Br J Radiol 78:888–893
47. Steer ML, Waxman I, Freedman S (1995) Chronic pancreatitis. N Engl J Med 332:1482–1490
48. Talamini G, Bassi C, Falconi M, Sartori N, Frulloni L, Di Francesco V, Vesentini S, Pederzoli P, Cavallini G (1996) Risk of death from acute pancreatitis. Role of early, simple "routine" data. Int J Pancreatol 19:15–24
49. Taylor SL, Morgan DL, Denson KD, Lane MM, Pennington LR (2005) A comparison of the Ranson, Glasgow, and APACHE II scoring systems to a multiple organ system score in predicting patient outcome in pancreatitis. Am J Surg 189:219–222
50. Teich N, Mössner J, Keim V (1999) Screening for mutations of the cationic trypsinogen gene: are they of relevance in chronic alcoholic pancreatitis? Gut 44:413–416
51. Trümper L, Menges M, Daus H, Kohler D, Reinhard JO, Sackmann M, Moser C, Sek A, Jacobs G, Zeitz M, Pfreundschuh M (2002) Low sensitivity of the ki-ras polymerase chain reaction for diagnosing pancreatic cancer from pancreatic juice and bile: a multicenter prospective trial. J Clin Oncol 20:4331–4337
52. Wallace MB, Hawes RH, Durkalski V, Chak A, Mallery S, Catalano MF, Wiersema MJ, Bhutani MS, Ciaccia D, Kochman ML, Gress FG, Van Velse A, Hoffman BJ (2001) The reliability of EUS for the diagnosis of chronic pancreatitis: interobserver agreement among experienced endosonographers. Gastrointest Endosc 53:294–299
53. Warshaw AL, Fernandez-del Castillo C (1992) Pancreatic carcinoma. N Engl J Med 326:455–465
54. Whitcomb DC (2006) Clinical practice. Acute pancreatitis. N Engl J Med 354:2142–2150
55. Williams M, Simms HH (1999) Prognostic usefulness of scoring systems in critically ill patients with severe acute pancreatitis. Crit Care Med 27:901–907
56. Yadav D, Agarwal N, Pitchumoni CS (2002) A critical evaluation of laboratory tests in acute pancreatitis. Am J Gastroenterol 97:1309–1318

Acute Pancreatitis

Chapter 14 Etiology and Epidemiology of Acute Pancreatitis *131*
P. G. Lankisch, P. Maisonneuve, A. B. Lowenfels

Chapter 15 Epidemiology and Intervention During the Clinical Course of Biliary Acute Pancreatitis *143*
R. C. Carter, C. W. Imrie

Chapter 16 Pathogenesis and Pathophysiology of Acute Pancreatitis *153*
M. L. Steer, G. Perides

Chapter 17 Natural Course of Acute Pancreatitis *163*
H. G. Beger, B. M. Rau

Chapter 18 Classification of Severe Acute Pancreatitis *173*
R. Isenmann

Chapter 19.1 Biochemical Diagnosis, Staging, and Prediction *181*
B. M. Rau

Chapter 19.2 Imaging Diagnosis of Acute Pancreatitis *193*
E. J. Balthazar

Chapter 20 Nonsurgical Management of Acute Pancreatitis *203*
P. A. Banks, K. J. Mortele

Chapter 21.1 Indications for the Surgical Management of Necrotizing Pancreatitis *211*
H. G. Beger, B. M. Rau

Chapter 21.2 Debridement and Closed Packing for the Treatment of Necrotizing Pancreatitis *219*
M. Reinblatt, C. Fernandez-del-Castillo, A. L. Warshaw

Chapter 21.3 Necrosectomy and Redressing *225*
P. Götzinger

Chapter 21.4 Necrosectomy and Closed Lavage *231*
B. M. Rau, H. G. Beger

Chapter 21.5 Infected Necrosis – Minimally Invasive Necrosectomy *241*
R. Carter, A. P. Wysocki

Chapter 21.6 Benefits and Limitations of Necrosectomy *249*
O. Mann, T. Strate, E. Yekebas, J. Izbicki

Chapter 22 Surgical Management of Pancreatic Abscess *253*
R. Bittner, B. M. Rau, H. G. Beger

Chapter 23 Surgical Management of Pseudocysts after Acute Pancreatitis *259*
B. M. Rau, H. G. Beger

Chapter 24 Interventional Management of Pancreatic Fluid Collections and Abscesses *271*
T. H. Baron

Chapter 25 Pancreatic and Intestinal Fistulas *281*
G. Tsiotos, J. Tsiaoussis

Chapter 26 Late Outcome after Necrosectomy *289*
I. H. Nordback, J. Sand

Chapter 14

P. G. Lankisch · P. Maisonneuve · A. B. Lowenfels

Etiology and Epidemiology of Acute Pancreatitis

Acute pancreatitis is a potentially fatal disease. To ameliorate the course of the disease and to prevent a fatal outcome it would be of importance to know more about its etiology and epidemiology. At present, several factors are thought to play an etiological role in the development of acute pancreatitis; however, not all of them have thus far been established as significant and some may only cause pancreatitis when acting with others. Indeed, in many cases of acute pancreatitis, combinations of factors are assumed to be interacting. To know more about the epidemiology of the disease in different countries and races would perhaps give an insight into the development of acute pancreatitis under special conditions. More information about both the etiology and epidemiology of acute pancreatitis could help us to either prevent the disease or, once it has been established, to use therapeutic measures more selectively.

Etiology

General Remarks

The list of etiological factors of acute pancreatitis is long (Table 14.1). The most frequent etiologies of acute pancreatitis are biliary tract disease and alcoholism, which account for about 60–80% of patients. In about 10%, rare etiologies are responsible, but in 10–30% of patients, the etiology remains unknown. A discussion of all of the details of possible etiological factors would be beyond the limit of a book on current surgical therapy of diseases of the pancreas. In the following, therefore, the most important aspects of etiology will be explored.

Obstructive Causes

The most common obstructive cause of acute pancreatitis is gallstones. The peak incidence occurs between 50 and 60 years of age, and more women than men are affected. However, acute pancreatitis seems to occur more frequently in male patients with gallstones than in women with gallstone disease [1]. In the majority of patients with so-called biliary pancreatitis, stones are found in the gallbladder but not in the common bile duct, and stones impacted in the distal common bile duct are reported in only 3–5% of patients with acute pancreatitis [2]. The frequency of acute pancreatitis is inversely proportional to the size of stones [3]. Both stone-related factors (small and multiple stones) and anatomical factors (e.g., a large cystic duct) may contribute to the development of biliary pancreatitis [4].

In a study from Lüneburg county (Germany), the crude incidence rates for biliary pancreatitis in the general population were 5.7 for men and 9.7 for women. However, the rate of biliary pancreatitis in male patients with gallstones was distinctly higher than that for female patients: 75.0 versus 58.1 per 100,000 inhabitants per year. These gender-related differences were especially apparent in the older individuals (Fig. 14.1). Over a 20- or 30-year period, the risk of developing biliary pancreatitis in patients with asymptomatic gallstones is unlikely to be greater than 2% [5]. Therefore, the low frequency of pancreatitis among patients with gallstones implies that other, as yet undetected, environmental or genetic factors are important.

Annular pancreas, obstructing periampullary polyps, or intraluminal duodenal diverticulae may lead to acute pancreatitis probably by obstructing the duodenum and thus inducing an inflow of chymus into the pancreatic duct under high pressure. More recently, acute pancreatitis has been described as a result of herniation of the afferent loop of the Billroth-II gastrectomy or obstruction of the duodenum in ventral hernias [6, 7].

Pancreatic carcinoma, either obstructing the duct system or involving the gland itself, or both, may induce acute pancreatitis. Two studies, one on patients with all types of pancreatic carcinoma [8] and the other on ampullary carcinoma only [9], reported an incidence of acute pancreatitis in 13.8% and 14.6%,

Table 14.1. Etiological factors for acute pancreatitis, modified according to Trivedi and Pitchumoni [98]

- Obstructive
  - Biliary tract disease (cholelithiasis, choledocholithiasis)
  - Duodenal disorders (annular pancreas, obstructing periampullary polyps, or intraluminal duodenal diverticulae, or obstructing afferent loop after gastrectomy, or obstruction of the duodenum in ventral hernias)
  - Tumors (ampullary or pancreatic)
  - Congenital anomalies (pancreas divisum)
  - Worms (ascariasis, clonorchiasis)
  - Foreign bodies obstructing the papilla
  - Sphincter of Oddi dysfunction
- Toxic
  - Alcoholism
  - Scorpion venom
  - Organophosphates
  - Drugs[a]
- Metabolic
  - Hypertriglyceridemia (types I, IV, and V)
  - Hypercalcemia (primary or secondary)
  - Uremia
- Traumatic
  - Accidental, blunt trauma to the abdomen
  - Iatrogenic, postendoscopic retrograde cholangiopancreatography, postendoscopic sphincterotomy, postoperative
- Genetic/hereditary
  - Hereditary pancreatitis
- Infections
  - Parasitic: ascariasis, clonorchiasis
  - Viral: mumps, rubella, hepatitis A, B, C, Coxsackie virus B, echo virus, adenovirus, cytomegaly virus, Epstein-Barr virus, human immunodeficiency virus
  - Bacterial: mycoplasma, *Campylobacter jejuni*, leptospirosis, legionella, *Mycobacterium tuberculosis*, *Myobacterium avium complex*
- Vascular
  - Ischemic: hypoperfusion, embolism
  - Vasculitis: systemic lupus erythematosus, nodular periarteritis, malignant hypertension
- Idiopathic

[a] see tables 14.2 und 14.3

respectively, and of hyperamylasemia in an additional 9.8% and 7.3%, respectively.

A recent survey on acute pancreatitis secondary to pancreatic carcinoma [10] showed that the diagnosis of pancreatic carcinoma as the underlying cause of acute pancreatitis is not that easy. The patients described in this study had a mean of two (range 1–15) episodes of acute pancreatitis before the diagnosis of pancreatic carcinoma, and this was associated with a delay of 34 weeks from acute pancreatitis to diagnosis of pancreatic cancer.

Pancreas divisum results from incomplete fusion of the dorsal and ventral ductal systems. When associated with accessory duct obstruction, its role as an

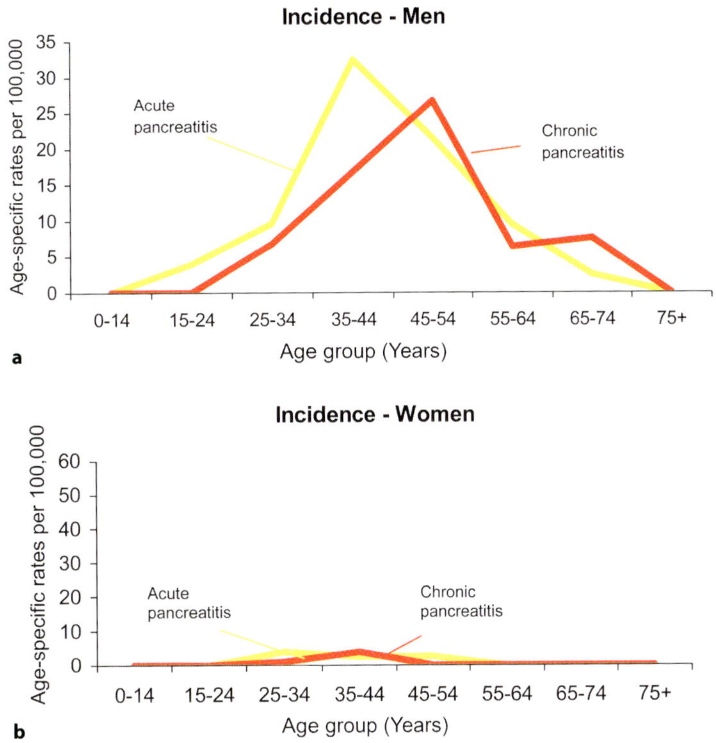

Figure 14.1

Estimated frequency of biliary acute pancreatitis in Lüneburg county among men (a) and women (b) during 1988–1995 [5]

etiological factor for acute pancreatitis is still not definitely clarified. Authors in favor of an association have hypothesized that an accessory papillary and Santorini's duct are too small to accept total pancreatic secretion, resulting in eventually obstructive pain in pancreatitis.

Other causes of obstructive acute pancreatitis may be worms and foreign bodies. Among the latter, dental filaments, cornhusk bristles, and vegetables have been described.

Sphincter of Oddi Dysfunction

Clinical studies have suggested that sphincter of Oddi dysfunction may be an etiological factor in recurrent pancreatitis, hence strengthening die hypothesis that sphincter of Oddi motility is involved in its pathogenesis [11–13].

Toxins

Whereas alcohol abuse is generally considered to be a major etiological factor of acute pancreatitis, it is not clear whether an episode of acute alcohol-induced pancreatitis represents an attack of acute or chronic pancreatitis. The diagnosis of acute pancreatitis implies that prior to the attack the pancreas was perfectly normal in all structural and functional aspects. With few exceptions, however, the antecedent state of the gland is unknown. Nevertheless, in the absence of signs of chronic pancreatitis (e.g., calcifications), the initial attacks of pancreatitis in an alcoholic are assumed to be "acute pancreatitis." Furthermore, it is unknown how much alcohol is needed to induce alcoholic pancreatitis, and studies designed to assess the etiology of the disease vary considerably in this regard. Some believe that > 80 g alcohol/day for more than 5 years or social or weekend abuse [14] is likely to induce acute pancreatitis. We consider alcohol abuse to be the cause of acute pancreatitis when the patient or his relatives report regular alcohol consumption of at least 60 g per day of pure alcohol in any form, or when an excessive amount of alcohol has been consumed immediately before the attack. However, there are many other definitions.

In another study from Lüneburg county (Germany), the crude incidence rates for alcoholic pancreatitis for men and women in the general population, between 1988 and 1995, were 10.1 and 1.3 per 100,000 inhabitants per year, respectively. However, the risk of developing acute pancreatitis, in heavy drinkers (≥ 60 g alcohol/day) was almost the same for men and women: 91.5 versus 81.9 patients per 100,000 heavy drinkers per year. Over a 20- or 30-year period, the

Table 14.2. Proposed classification for medications associated with drug-induced pancreatitis [98]

Class I drug

- At least 20 reported cases of acute pancreatitis
- At least 1 case with positive rechallenge

Class II drug

- >10 but <20 reported cases of acute pancreatitis with or without positive rechallenge

Class III drug

- All medications implicated in pancreatitis (i.e., class I, class II) and those with ≤10 reported cases or unpublished reports in pharmaceutical or Food and Drug Association files

Table 14.3. Medications associated with pancreatitis (modified according to Trivedi and Pitchumoni [98])

Medication (Class I)	Medication (Class II)
Didanosine	Rifampicin
Asparaginase	Lamivudine
Azathioprine	Octreotide
Valproic acid	Carbamazepine
Pentavalent antimonials	Acetaminophen
Pentamidine	Phenformin
Mercaptopurine	Interferon $\alpha_{2\text{-b}}$
Mesalamine	Enalapril
Various estrogens	Hydrochlorothiazide
Opiates	Cisplatin
Tetracycline	Erythromycin
Cytarabine	Cyclopenthiazide
Steroids	
Sulfamethoxazole/ trimethoprim	
Sulfasalazine	
Furosemide	
Sulindac	

risk of developing alcoholic pancreatitis in this group is unlikely to be more than 2–3% [15]. Similar to biliary disease, the low frequency of pancreatitis among heavy drinkers indicates that there are as yet other undetected environmental or genetic factors.

At one time, poisoning by the sting of *Tityus trinitatis* was the most common cause of acute pancreatitis in Trinidad [16]. Subsequent intensive studies have led to the scorpion's extinction on the island, but have clarified the underlying mechanism of acute scorpion venom pancreatitis. The venom acted directly on the canine pancreas, on the one hand stimulating exocrine pancreatic enzyme secretion, and on the other hand contracting the sphincter of Oddi [17]. Thus, obstruction plays a pathogenetic role in this form of acute pancreatitis.

Both painful and almost painless acute pancreatitis have been reported after cutaneous exposure to an organophosphate insecticide [18] and as a complication of organophosphate poisoning [19].

Among adverse drug reactions, pancreatitis is often ignored because of the difficulty implicating a drug as its cause. The surgeon should have a high index of suspicion for drug-induced pancreatitis, especially in specific subpopulations such as geriatric patients, who may be on multiple medications, AIDS patients, cancer patients, and patients receiving immunomodulating agents. A new classification for medications associated with drug-induced pancreatitis has been formulated (Table 14.2). Based on this classification, medications associated with pancreatitis are summarized in Table 14.3.

Metabolic Causes

Hyperlipemia may occur during acute pancreatitis. When it persists, it may have been the cause of the disease. All types of acute and chronic pancreatitis have been described in patients with primary hyperparathyroidism. Hypercalcemia that stimulates pancreatic enzyme secretion in humans and animals may play a role.

Acute renal failure is a well-known severe complication of acute pancreatitis. The vice versa situation, acute pancreatitis complicating chronic renal failure, has been reported less frequently [20]. In one study, half of patients who died of uremia had a histological evidence of acute pancreatitis [21]. Three recent studies have shown that acute pancreatitis occurs more frequently and also more heavily in peritoneal dialysis patients as compared to hemodialysis patients and also in the general population [22, 23, and Lankisch et al. unpublished data].

Traumatic Causes

Pancreatic injury occurs more frequently after a penetrating than after a blunt abdominal trauma. The degree of injury may range from mild contusion to fracture. Acute pancreatitis is the consequence of disruption of the ductular, vascular, and parenchymatous continuity, and subsequent extravasation of enzymes.

The incidence of acute pancreatitis following endoscopic retrograde cholangiopancreatography (ERCP) has been reported to be 5.1%, and following endoscopic sphincterotomy (ES) it is found to be 7.1% [24]. Compared to acute pancreatitis of other origins, ERCP-induced acute pancreatitis tends to be a more severe disease [25].

Risk factors for post-ERCP pancreatitis are young age, female gender, suspected sphincter of Oddi dysfunction, prior post-ERCP pancreatitis, recurrent pancreatitis, absence of chronic pancreatitis, pancreatic duct injection, pancreatic sphincterotomy, balloon dilatation of intact biliary sphincter, difficult or failed cannulation, precut (access) sphincterotomy and, of course, inexperience of the investigator [26].

Acute pancreatitis may occur after sphincter of Oddi manometry with an overall risk of between 4.2% and 14.5% [27–29]. Acute pancreatitis seems to be mild in most patients; it occurs more frequently after catheterization of the pancreatic duct and of the bile duct, and more frequently in patients with than without signs of chronic pancreatitis [27]. The frequency of acute pancreatitis caused by sphincter of Oddi manometry may be reduced by using modern techniques [28, 29].

Postoperative acute pancreatitis may occur after a variety of interabdominal procedures including biliary tract operation, gastric resections, colectomies, and splenectomies. How such surgical procedures lead to acute pancreatitis is unknown. Postoperative pancreatitis can also occur after surgery in areas distant from the pancreas (e.g., after parathyroidectomy). Finally, acute pancreatitis has been reported following different transplantation procedures, including cardiopulmonary transplantation [30, 31], liver transplantation [32, 33], and renal transplantation [34, 35].

Hereditary Pancreatitis

Hereditary pancreatitis is an uncommon variety of pancreatitis. It generally follows an autosomal dominant inheritance and is associated with germline mutations in the cationic trypsinogen [36]. When an idiopathic pancreatitis occurs in a young patient, surgeons should suspect hereditary pancreatitis even in the absence of a family history [37] and genetic testing is recommended [38].

Infections

Acute pancreatitis, usually mild, often subclinical, and healing with disappearance of the infection, has been described in association with mumps [39, 40], infectious mononucleosis [41, 42], Coxsackie B virus [43], ECHO viruses, *Mycoplasma pneumoniae* infections [44–46], varicella, and measles [43, 47, 48]. Acute pancreatitis may also complicate fulminant viral hepatitis [49–51]. Furthermore, acute pancreatitis may occur in cases of salmonellosis and campylobacter infection [52–54], as well in tuberculosis and sarcoidosis [55–57].

More recently, hyperamylasemia in acute pancreatitis has been described in human immunodeficiency virus (HIV)-infected patients. Acute pancreatitis was found in 40% of HIV patients and was of mild to moderate severity. The inflammation is commonly associated with gallstones, intravenous drug abuse, pentamidine intake, and *Pneumocystis carinii*, and *Mycobacterium avium* intracellular infections. The usefulness of predictors commonly used to identify the severity of pancreatitis remains a matter of controversy [58, 59].

Vascular Disease

Because of the very efficient collateral blood supply of the pancreas, primary vascular disease is rarely the sole causative factor for pancreatitis. In most cases, local ischemia of the pancreas must be accompanied by other noxious factors in order to induce acute pancreatitis. So-called idiopathic pancreatitis has been attributed to a combination of stenosing atheromatosis in pancreatic vessels and shock. Diffuse vascular injury to the pancreas, as resulting from necrotizing angiitis caused by amphetamines, malignant hypertension, nodular periarteritis, and systemic lupus erythematosus, may result in pancreatitis. The exact etiological links are unknown [1]. More recently, cases of nonocclusive visceral ischemia associated with severe acute pancreatitis have also been described [60].

Idiopathic Acute Pancreatitis

Although numerous actual and potential etiological factors have been identified, the cause of acute pancreatitis is obscure in several cases. After gallstones and alcoholism, idiopathic etiology is the third main cause in most reported series. Two studies have indicated that the majority of cases of idiopathic pancreatitis are caused by biliary sludge and microlithiasis. No recurrence of acute pancreatitis occurred among patients following endoscopic sphincterotomy, gallbladder removal, or treatment with ursodeoxycholic acid [61, 62]. It is important to perform imaging procedures, either ultrasound, contrast-enhanced computed tomography, or magnetic resonance cholangiopancreatography, in patients with idiopathic acute pancreatitis about 2 or 3 months after the acute attack so that a pancreatic carcinoma is not overlooked [10]. In contrast to previous beliefs, patients with acute pancreatitis secondary to pancreatic carcinoma may survive a first attack, and pancreatic carcinoma as the underlying etiology may not be recovered even after further episodes of acute pancreatitis [10].

Etiological Factors and National Differences

Gullo et al. [14] performed a multicenter study of 1,068 patients from 5 European countries who were admitted to hospital because of acute pancreatitis between January 1990 and December 1994. The etiological factors varied considerably (Table 14.4) [14]. Gallstone disease occurred much more frequently in Greece and Italy compared to Germany, Hungary, and France [14]. The percentage of dominance of one particular etiological factor for acute pancreatitis may vary over the years.

A national or center change in the major etiology of acute pancreatitis is possible and has been demonstrated at least twice. Mero [63] found a change of etiology from gallstone disease (1967–1968) to alcohol abuse (1977–1978), during which time there was a 2.5-fold rise in the consumption of alcohol in Finland.

In a recent study, Lindkvist et al. [64] reported on 929 first attacks of acute pancreatitis in Malmö, the third largest city in Sweden. It is the only hospital serving the city, and there are no referrals of patients to or from this hospital. Thus, the risk of selection bias is low. During the period between 1985 and 1999, the total incidence of acute pancreatitis increased by 3.9% per year, probably due to an increase in biliary pancreatitis of 6.6% per year. This correlated with an increase in the incidence of other gallstone-related conditions and obesity. In contrast, alcohol-induced pancreatitis decreased during this period by 5.1% per year, and this correlated with a decrease in the incidence of delirium tremens, mortality from liver cirrhosis, and incidence of lung cancer. Between 1980 and 1996, the amount of legally sold alcohol in Malmö decreased by about 36%. This decrease was due to a marked reduction in the sales of hard liquor, whereas the sale of wine and beer was stable [64]. Interestingly, a specific correlation of acute pancreatitis with hard liquor, but not wine and beer, had been reported earlier in Sweden [65].

Etiological Factors and Prognosis of the Disease

It has frequently been questioned whether the etiology of acute pancreatitis has any effect on the severity of the prognosis of the disease. Two large studies, one comprising of 190 patients with a first attack of acute

Table 14.4. Acute pancreatitis in five European countries: Etiology in 1,068 patients [14]

Country	Patients (n)	Gallstones (n)	(%)	Alcohol (n)	(%)
Germany	232	81	34.9	88	37.9
Hungary	483	116	24.0	293	60.7
France	65	16	24.6	25	38.5
Greece	84	60	71.4*	5	6.0*
Italy	204	123	60.3*	27	13.2*
Total	**1068**	**396**	**37.1**	**438**	**41.0**

*$P < 0.01$ versus the corresponding values of Germany, Hungary, and France

pancreatitis [66], the other comprising 602 such patients [67], showed that the etiology had no influence on the mortality of the disease. However, the etiology may have an impact on the cause of the disease.

Patients with alcohol-induced acute pancreatitis more frequently have pancreatic necrosis than patients with other etiologies and the need for artificial ventilation in alcoholics is high [68]. Whether this is due to a higher incidence of smokers in this group, who presumably have some lung damage prior to acute pancreatitis, is unknown, but it should be a subject for future prospective studies. Some investigations have shown that alcohol abuse per se has a negative effect on the lung [69, 70].

Several groups have investigated the development of pancreatic pseudocysts in acute pancreatitis of different etiologies. In two of these studies, the incidence of pancreatic pseudocysts was the same in all etiological subgroups [71, 72]. In contrast, Thomson et al. [73] found that patients with alcohol-induced pancreatitis were more likely to develop pancreatic pseudocysts than those patients with biliary acute pancreatitis. In these studies, a differentiation between fluid collections and pancreatic pseudocysts was not clarified. Whether a higher incidence of fluid collections/pseudocysts in patients with alcohol-induced acute pancreatitis indicates a later progression from acute to chronic pancreatitis, remains an open question [74].

Finally, as indicated earlier, the etiology of acute pancreatitis and the absence or presence of initial organ failure has an impact on the later course of the disease. Patients with alcohol abuse and initial organ failure (arterial partial pressure of oxygen ≤ 60 mmHg and/or serum creatinine > 2 mg/dl after rehydration) deteriorated more significantly than other subgroups, requiring artificial ventilation and/or dialysis treatment. If, on admission, there was no initial organ failure, there were no differences within the etiological subgroups. Thus, patients with alcohol-induced acute pancreatitis plus initial organ failure represent a major risk group, requiring special attention and intensive care. If necessary, they should be transferred to a specialized center. In addition, patients with no initial organ failure are at lower risk of organ failure and usually do not need intensive care [75].

Recommended Search for the Cause of Acute Pancreatitis

Several investigations, which are summarized in Table 14.5, may be helpful for surgeons to determine the cause of acute pancreatitis.

Table 14.5. Investigations helpful to determine the cause of acute pancreatitis (modified according to [99])

History	Previous gall stones Alcohol intake Family history[a] Drug intake Exposure to known viral causes or prodromal syndromes
Initial investigation on admission	Ultrasound of the gallbladder
Follow-up investigations (recovery phase)	Fasting plasma lipids Fasting plasma calcium Viral antibody titers Repeat biliary ultrasound, perform magnetic resonance cholangio-pancreaticography or contrast-enhanced computed tomography, if necessary
Further investigations (usually appropriate for recurrent idiopathic acute pancreatitis)	Further ultrasound, endoscopic ultrasound (if necessary) Autoimmune markers Sphincter of Oddi manometry Pancreatic function tests to exclude chronic pancreatitis

[a] Genetic analysis is only indicated in the presence of a family history of one or more of the following: acute pancreatitis, recurrent undiagnosed abdominal pain, pancreatic carcinoma, or type 1 diabetes mellitus

Table 14.6. Undetected fatal acute pancreatitis in different countries

Author(s)	Time period	Deceased patients (*n*)	Percentage of deceased patients for whom the diagnosis was made post mortem
Corfield et al. [77]	1968–1979	125	35 %
Wilson and Imrie [91]	1974–1984	126	42 %
Lankisch et al. [92]	1980–1985	43	30 %
Mann et al. [93]	1988–1992	50	12 %
Appelros and Borgstöm [84]	1985–1994	31	52 %

Epidemiology

General Remarks

Data on the epidemiology of acute pancreatitis vary considerably. This may be explained by several factors.

1. Data concerning the epidemiology of acute pancreatitis are limited and only available from eight countries, which are mainly European [73, 76–90], therefore, little is known about the epidemiology of the disease in most of the world.
2. The time periods vary considerably among the reports, as well as the availability and/or the use of imaging procedures such as ultrasound or computed tomography. This may lead to an underestimation of the disease.
3. The reports come from different types of centers. This may have an influence not only on the incidence rate, but also on the etiology. An urban hospital is more likely to report on alcohol-induced pancreatitis, whereas a rural hospital is more likely to report on biliary pancreatitis.
4. Death certificates, as a basis for epidemiological studies, are unreliable.
5. The post mortem ratios differ considerably. A substantial number of diagnoses are made at the post mortem and not during the patient's lifetime (Table 14.6) [77, 84, 91–93]. This may also lead to an underestimation of the disease.
6. The referral rates differ from country to country. This is attributable to the criteria laid down by the general practitioners and/or health insurance companies. A study from the Netherlands [94] showed that only 2% of patients who definitely had acute pancreatitis were not referred to hospital and thus, in hospital-based studies, the incidence of acute pancreatitis will not be underestimated. However, the diagnosis of acute pancreatitis made by general practitioners was, when checked, not substantiated in 24%, probable in 24%, and definite only in 53%.
7. Different centers use different diagnostic criteria. The "usual suspects" for the diagnosis of acute pancreatitis are abdominal pain and increased serum enzyme levels. However, it is unclear what the enzyme levels should be in order to diagnose or evaluate the severity of the disease. The current use of > 3 times the upper limit of normal as a cut-off point for pancreatic enzymes in the diagnosis of acute pancreatitis, can be misleading. We found that patients with only mildly increased amylase/lipase levels can also have or develop acute pancreatitis [95]. When patients were divided into two groups according to the serum enzyme levels (group 1, ≤ 3n, group 2, > 3n), 31% (amylase) and 18% (lipase) were in the first group. However, there were no significant differences between either group with regard to organ failure, fluid collections/pseudocysts, and an indication for a necrosectomy and mortality.
8. Finally, prognostic scores and/or classification systems for imaging procedures are not widely used, and thus information on the severity of the disease is often lacking.

Incidence Rate

The incidence rate of acute pancreatitis per 100,000 inhabitants per year differs considerably. This may be in part due to the fact that some studies included not only first attacks of acute pancreatitis, but also relapses, and some did not clarify this point (Table 14.7). Remarkably, the incidence is high in all Scandinavian countries. In the United Kingdom, it is higher in Scotland than in England (Table 14.4) [73, 76–90].

The increased incidence of acute pancreatitis was significantly correlated with alcohol consumption in The Netherlands [78] and in Finland [87]. It was also associated with an increase in male, but not in female patients in Finland [87], Scotland [96], and Denmark [82]. In contrast, a recent study from Denmark has shown that between 1981 and 2000, there was an in-

Table 14.7. Overall incidence of acute pancreatitis in various countries, ranked according to the 1st year of assessment. Reports are grouped according to the declaration of first attacks only (*), the summing up of first attacks and relapses (**), or if there was no specification as to whether the report contained first attacks and relapses (***)

Authors	Location	Period	Incidence (10^5) population/year
Trapnell and Duncan [76]*	Bristol, UK	1961–1967	5.4
Thomson [79]*	North and Northeast Scotland	1968–1980	9.4
Floyd et al. [89]*	North Jutland, Denmark	1981	17.1–18.0
	North Jutland, Denmark	1999	27.1–37.8
Thomson et al. [73]*	Northeast Scotland	1983–1985	24.2
Appelros and Börgstrom [84]*	Malmö, Sweden	1985–1994	23.4
Lindkvist et al. [64]*	Malmö, Sweden	1985-1999	24.7
Gislason et al. [100]*	Western Norway	1986–1995	20.0
Lankisch et al. [81]*	Lüneburg, Germany	1988–1995	19.7
Corfield et al. [77]**	Bristol, UK	1968–1979	7.3
Andersson et al. [101]**	Lund, Sweden	1975–1996	30.0
Goldacre and Roberts [90]**	Southern England	1973–1974	4.9
	Southern England	1975–1986	7.7
	Southern England	1987–1998	9.8
Jaakkola and Nordback [87]***	Finland	1970	46.6
		1989	73.4
Tran and Schilfgaarde [78]***	The Netherlands	1971	6.5
	the Netherlands	1990	10.2
Giggs et al. [80]***	Nottingham, UK	1977–1983	11.7
Worning [82]***	Denmark	1981	26.8
		1990	35.4
McKay et al. [83]***	Scotland	1984–1995	31.8
Eland et al. [85]***	The Netherlands	1985	12.4
		1995	15.9
Go [86]***	United States of America	1987	49.5
			79.8
Halvorsen and Ritland [88]***	Buskerud, Norway	1992	41.5
Toh et al. [102]***	Southern England	1994–1995	14.2

creased incidence of acute pancreatitis, during which time the incidence in women surpassed that in men. This was between 1999 and 2000 (incidence in male patients 1981, 18.0; in 2000, 17.1; in female patients 27.1 and 37.1, respectively, per 100,000 persons per year) [89]. The reasons for this change are unknown.

In Lüneburg county (Germany), where we performed the first epidemiological study in a well-defined German population, the incidence rate of acute pancreatitis was 19.7 per 100,000 inhabitants per year during the period from 1988 to 1995. This was more than three times higher than the same incidence for chronic pancreatitis (6.4 per 100,000 inhabitants per year) [81]. When incidence rates were plotted against age groups, it was shown that acute pancreatitis noticeably peaked in men aged 35–44 years, followed by a similar peak for chronic pancreatitis in those aged 45–54 years. Although distinctly lower, there was an incidence peak for acute pancreatitis in women aged between 25 and 34 years, which was followed by a small peak for chronic pancreatitis in those who were 10 years older (Fig. 14.2) [81]. This time interval suggests either that chronic pancreatitis is the consequence of a necrosis-fibrosis sequence [97], or the development of pancreatic fibrosis without intermittent pancreatic necrosis. In each case it will probably take some time and several attacks of acute pancreatitis before chronic pancreatitis develops [74].

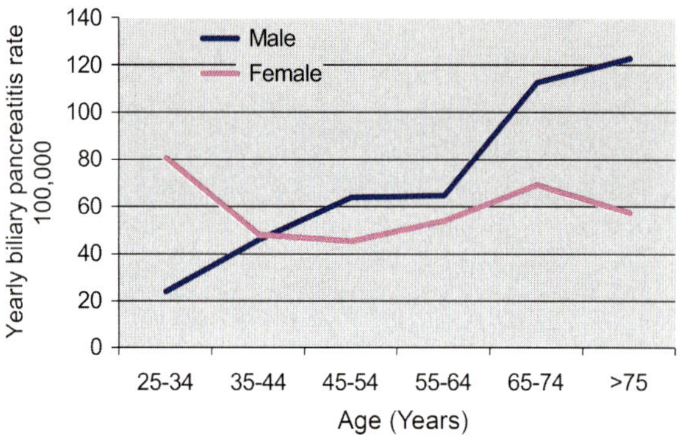

Figure 14.2

Age-specific incidence rates for acute and chronic pancreatitis by etiology in Lüneburg county among men (*blue line*) and women (*pink line*) during 1988–1995 [81]

Outlook

To conclude, we need multicenter studies from different countries in a defined population taken from comparable settings to evaluate the true incidence of acute pancreatitis, the severity, and the outcome. These data could meet the new restrictions of the various health insurance schemes throughout the world and could generate diagnosis-related groups and payment. We need clearer, internationally accepted definitions for alcohol abuse and biliary disease as the etiological factors of acute pancreatitis in order to evaluate and compare the data from different centers. We should pay special attention to patients with a first attack of alcohol-induced acute pancreatitis, because they tend to have a higher incidence of necrotizing pancreatitis and respiratory organ failure and represent an "at risk" group. The higher incidence of fluid collections and/or pseudocysts in this group is probably indicative of a later progression to chronic pancreatitis. These and other open questions concerning the diagnosis, prognosis, and outcome of acute pancreatitis could be answered by groups of pancreatologists or clubs and associations such as the International Association of Pancreatology, the European Pancreatic Club, the American Pancreatic Association, and the Japan Pancreas Society.

Acknowledgments

Patrick Maisonneuve was supported by the Italian Association for Cancer Research (Associazione Italiana per la Ricerca sul Cancro, AIRC). Albert B. Lowenfels was supported in part by the C.D. Smithers Foundation.

References

1. Lankisch PG, Banks PA (1998) Acute pancreatitis: etiology. In: Lankisch PG, Banks PA (eds) Pancreatitis. Springer Verlag, Berlin Heidelberg New York, pp 38–38
2. Wilson C, Imrie CW, Carter DC (1988) Fatal acute pancreatitis. Gut 29:782–788
3. Houssin D, Castaing D, Lemoine J, Bismuth H (1983) Microlithiasis of the gallbladder. Surg Gynecol Obstet 157:20–24
4. Sugiyama M, Atomi Y (2004) Risk factors for acute biliary pancreatitis. Gastrointest Endosc 60:210–212
5. Lowenfels AB, Lankisch PG, Maisonneuve P (2000) What is the risk of biliary pancreatitis in patients with gallstones? Gastroenterology 119:879–880
6. Kaya E, Senyürek G, Dervisoglu A, Danaci M, Kesim M (2004) Acute pancreatitis caused by afferent loop herniation after Billroth II gastrectomy: report of a case and review of the literature. Hepatogastroenterology 51:606–608
7. Lankisch PG, Petersen F, Brinkmann G (2003) An enormous ventral (epigastric) hernia as a cause of acute pancreatitis: Pfeffer's closed duodenal loop model in the animal, first seen in a human. Gastroenterology 124:865–866
8. Köhler H, Lankisch PG (1987) Acute pancreatitis and hyperamylasaemia in pancreatic carcinoma. Pancreas 2:117–119
9. Robertson JFR, Imrie CW (1987) Acute pancreatitis associated with carcinoma of the ampulla of Vater. Br J Surg 74:395–397
10. Mujica VR, Barkin JS, Go VLW, Study Group Participants (2000) Acute pancreatitis secondary to pancreatic carcinoma. Pancreas 21:329–332
11. Toouli J, Roberts-Thomson IC, Dent J, Lee J (1985) Sphincter of Oddi motility disorders in patients with idiopathic recurrent pancreatitis. Br J Surg 72:859–863
12. Toouli J, Di Francesco V, Saccone G, Kollias J, Schloithe A, Shanks N (1996) Division of the sphincter of Oddi for treatment of dysfunction associated with recurrent pancreatitis. Br J Surg 83:1205–1210
13. Chen JWC, Saccone GTP, Toouli J (1998) Sphincter of Oddi dysfunction and acute pancreatitis. Gut 43:305–308
14. Gullo L, Migliori M, Oláh A, Farkas G, Levy P, Arvanitakis C, Lankisch P, Beger H (2002) Acute pancreatitis in five European countries: etiology and mortality. Pancreas 24:223–227
15. Lankisch PG, Lowenfels AB, Maisonneuve P (2002) What is the risk of alcoholic pancreatitis in heavy drinkers? Pancreas 25:411–412
16. Bartholomew C (1970) Acute scorpion pancreatitis in Trinidad. Br Med J 1:666–668
17. Sankaran H, McGeeney FK, Bartholomew C, Raghupathy E (1987) Mechanism of scorpion toxin-induced pancreatitis in dogs. Biochem Arch 3:41–46
18. Marsh WH, Vukov GA, Conradi EC (1988) Acute pancreatitis after cutaneous exposure to an organophosphate insecticide. Am J Gastroenterol 83:1158–1160
19. Lankisch PG, Müller C-H, Niederstadt H, Brand A (1990) Painless acute pancreatitis subsequent to anticholinesterase insecticide (parathion) intoxication. Am J Gastroenterol 85:872–875
20. Pitchumoni CS, Arguello P, Agarwal N, Yoo J (1996) Acute pancreatitis in chronic renal failure. Am J Gastroenterol 91:2477–2482
21. Baggenstoss AH (1948) The pancreas in uremia: a histopathologic study. Am J Pathol 24:1003–1011

22. Bruno MJ, van Westerloo DJ, van Dorp WT, Dekker W, Ferwerda J, Tytgat GNJ, Schut NH (2000) Acute pancreatitis in peritoneal dialysis and haemodialysis: risk, clinical course, outcome, and possible aetiology. Gut 46:385–389
23. Quraishi ER, Goel S, Gupta M, Catanzaro A, Zasuwa G, Divine G (2005) Acute pancreatitis in patients on chronic peritoneal dialysis: an increased risk? Am J Gastroenterol 100:2288–2293
24. Sherman S, Lehman GA (1991) ERCP- and endoscopic-sphincterotomy-induced pancreatitis. Pancreas 6:350–367
25. Fung ASY, Tsiotos GG, Sarr MG (1997) ERCP-induced acute necrotizing pancreatitis: is it a more severe disease? Pancreas 15:217–221
26. Freeman ML, Guda NM (2004) Prevention of post-ERCP pancreatitis: a comprehensive review. Gastrointest Endosc 59:845–864
27. Rolny P, Anderberg B, Ihse I, Lindström E, Olaison G, Arvill A (1990) Pancreatitis after sphincter of Oddi manometry. Gut 31:821–824
28. Sherman S, Troiano FP, Hawes RH, Lehman GA (1990) Sphincter of Oddi manometry: decreased risk of clinical pancreatitis with use of a modified aspirating catheter. Gastrointest Endosc 36:462–466
29. Wehrmann T, Stergiou N, Schmitt T, Dietrich CF, Seifert H (2003) Reduced risk for pancreatitis after endoscopic microtransducer manometry of the sphincter of Oddi: a randomized comparison with the perfusion manometry technique. Endoscopy 35:472–477
30. Adiseshiah M, Wells FC, Cory-Pearce R, Wallwork J, English TAH (1983) Acute pancreatitis after cardiac transplantation. World J Surg 7:519–521
31. Aziz S, Bergdahl L, Baldwin JC, Weiss LM, Jamieson SW, Oyer PE, Stinson EB, Shumway NE (1985) Pancreatitis after cardiac and cardiopulmonary transplantation. Surgery 97:653–661
32. Eghtesad B, Reyes JD, Ashrafi M, Arzate J, Osorio G, Fung JJ, Mazariegos GV (2003) Pancreatitis after liver transplantation in children: a single-center experience. Transplantation 75:190–193
33. Alexander JA, Demetrius AJ, Gavaler JS, Makowka L, Starzl TE, Van Thiel DH (1988) Pancreatitis following liver transplantation. Transplantation 45:1062–1065
34. Viale P, Montanaro D, Bresadola F, Risaliti A (2005) Acute pancreatitis after kidney transplantation. Am J Gastroenterol 100:1620–1620
35. Slakey DP, Johnson CP, Cziperle DJ, Roza AM, Wittmann DH, Gray DWR, Roake JA, Britton J, Morris PJ, Adams MB (1997) Management of severe pancreatitis in renal transplant recipients. Ann Surg 225:217–222
36. Whitcomb DC, Gorry MC, Preston RA, Furey W, Sossenheimer MJ, Ulrich CD, Martin SP, Gates LK, Jr., Amann ST, Toskes PP, Liddle R, McGrath K, Uomo G, Post JC, Ehrlich GD (1996) Hereditary pancreatitis is caused by a mutation in the cationic trypsinogen gene. Nat Genet 14:141–145
37. Simon P, Weiss FU, Zimmer KP, Rand S, Brinkmann B, Domschke W, Lerch MW (2002) Spontaneous and sporadic trypsinogen mutations in idiopathic pancreatitis. J Am Med Assoc 288:2122–2122
38. Ellis I, Lerch MM, Whitcomb DC (2001) Genetic testing for hereditary pancreatitis: guidelines for indications, counselling, consent and privacy issues. Pancreatology 1:405–415
39. Feldstein JD, Johnson FR, Kallick CA, Doolas A (1974) Acute hemorrhagic pancreatitis and pseudocyst due to mumps. Ann Surg 180:85–88
40. Witte CL, Schanzer B (1968) Pancreatitis due to mumps. J Am Med Assoc 203:1068–1069
41. Wislocki LC (1966) Acute pancreatitis in infectious mononucleosis. N Engl J Med 275:322–323
42. Hedström SÅ, Belfrage I (1976) Acute pancreatitis in two cases of infectious mononucleosis. Scand J Infect Dis 8:124–126
43. Imrie CW, Ferguson JC, Sommerville RG (1977) Coxsackie and mumps virus infection in a prospective study of acute pancreatitis. Gut 18:53–56
44. Mårdh P-A, Ursing B (1973) Acute pancreatitis in mycoplasma pneumoniae infections. Br Med J 2:240–241
45. Mårdh P-A, Ursing B (1974) The occurrence of acute pancreatitis in mycoplasma pneumoniae infection. Scand J Infect Dis 6:167–171
46. Freeman R, McMahon MJ (1978) Acute pancreatitis and serological evidence of infection with *mycoplasma pneumoniae*. Gut 19:367–370
47. Kirschner S, Raufman J-P (1988) Varicella pancreatitis complicated by pancreatic pseudocyst and duodenal obstruction. Dig Dis Sci 33:1192–1195
48. Adler JB, Mazzotta SA, Barkin JS (1991) Pancreatitis caused by measles, mumps, and rubella vaccine. Pancreas 6:489–490
49. Achord JL (1968) Acute pancreatitis with infectious hepatitis. J Am Med Assoc 205:129–132
50. Geokas MC, Olsen H, Swanson V, Rinderknecht H (1972) The association of viral hepatitis and acute pancreatitis. Calif Med 117:1–7
51. Lankisch PG, Rahlf G, Schmidt H, Creutzfeldt W (1975) Pankreatitis bei Virushepatitis und Coma hepaticum. Z Gastroenterol 13:407–412
52. Gallagher P, Chadwick P, Jones DM, Turner L (1981) Acute pancreatitis associated with campylobacter infection. Br J Surg 68:383–383
53. Pönkä A, Kosunen TU (1981) Pancreas affection in association with enteritis due to campylobacter fetus ssp. jejuni. Acta Med Scand 209:239–240
54. De Bois MHW, Schoemaker MC, Van der Werf SDJ, Puylaert JBCM (1989) Pancreatitis associated with *Campylobacter jejuni* infection: diagnosis by ultrasonography. Br Med J 298:1004–1004
55. Rushing JL, Hanna CJ, Selecky PA (1978) Pancreatitis as the presenting manifestation of miliary tuberculosis. West J Med 129:432–436
56. McCormick PA, Malone D, Fitzgerald MX, FitzGerald O (1985) Pancreatitis in sarcoidosis. Br Med J 290:1472–1473
57. Peters MJ, Jones MG, Moulton J, Breslin ABX (1990) Sarcoidosis presenting as recurrent alcohol-induced pancreatitis. Med J Aust 153:104–107
58. Parithivel VS, Yousuf AM, Albu E, Kaul A, Aydinalp N (1999) Predictors of the severity of acute pancreatitis in patients with HIV infection or AIDS. Pancreas 19:133–136
59. Gan I, May G, Raboud J, Tilley J, Enns R (2003) Pancreatitis in HIV infection: predictors of severity. Am J Gastroenterol 98:1278–1283
60. Yasuda T, Takeyama Y, Ueda T, Hori Y, Nishikawa J, Kuroda Y (2003) Nonocclusive visceral ischemia associated with severe acute pancreatitis. Pancreas 26:95–97
61. Ros E, Navarro S, Bru C, García Pugés A, Valderrama R (1991) Occult microlithiasis in "idiopathic" acute pancreatitis: prevention of relapses by cholecystectomy or ursodeoxycholic acid therapy. Gastroenterology 101:1701–1709
62. Lee SP, Nicholls JF, Park HZ (1992) Biliary sludge as a cause of acute pancreatitis. N Engl J Med 326:589–593

63. Mero M (1982) Changing aetiology of acute pancreatitis. Ann Chir Gynaecol 71:126–129
64. Lindkvist B, Appelros S, Manjer J, Borgström A (2004) Trends in incidence of acute pancreatitis in a Swedish population: is there really an increase? Clin Gastroenterol Hepatol 2:831–837
65. Schmidt DN (1991) Apparent risk factors for chronic and acute pancreatitis in Stockholm county. Int J Pancreatol 8:45–50
66. Uhl W, Isenmann R, Curti G, Vogel R, Beger HG, Büchler MW (1996) Influence of etiology on the course and outcome of acute pancreatitis. Pancreas 13:335–343
67. Lankisch PG, Burchard-Reckert S, Petersen M, Lehnick D, Schirren CA, Stöckmann F, Köhler H (1996) Etiology and age have only a limited influence on the course of acute pancreatitis. Pancreas 13:344–349
68. Lankisch PG, Assmus C, Pflichthofer D, Struckmann K, Lehnick D (1999) Which etiology causes the most severe acute pancreatitis? Int J Pancreatol 26:55–57
69. Lange P, Groth S, Mortensen J, Appleyard M, Nyboe J, Jensen G, Schnohr P (1988) Pulmonary function is influenced by heavy alcohol consumption. Am Rev Respir Dis 137:1119–1123
70. Garshick E, Segal MR, Worobec TG, Salekin CMS, Miller MJ (1989) Alcohol consumption and chronic obstructive pulmonary disease. Am Rev Respir Dis 140:373–378
71. Schulze S, Baden H, Brandenhoff P, Larsen T, Burcharth F (1986) Pancreatic pseudocysts during first attack of acute pancreatitis. Scand J Gastroenterol 21:1221–1223
72. Nguyen B-LT, Thompson JS, Edney JA, Bragg LE, Rikkers LF (1991) Influence of the etiology of pancreatitis on the natural history of pancreatic pseudocysts. Am J Surg 162:527–531
73. Thomson SR, Hendry WS, McFarlane GA, Davidson AI (1987) Epidemiology and outcome of acute pancreatitis. Br J Surg 74:398–401
74. Lankisch PG (1999) Progression from acute to chronic pancreatitis. A physician's view. Surg Clin North Am 79:815–827
75. Lankisch PG, Pflichthofer D, Lehnick D (1999) Acute pancreatitis: which patient is most at risk? Pancreas 19:321–324
76. Trapnell JE, Duncan EHL (1975) Patterns of incidence in acute pancreatitis. Br Med J 2:179–183
77. Corfield AP, Cooper MJ, Williamson RCN (1985) Acute pancreatitis: a lethal disease of increasing incidence. Gut 26:724–729
78. Tran DD, Van Schilfgaarde R (1994) Prevalence and mortality from acute pancreatitis in the Netherlands during 1971–1990. Digestion 55:342–343
79. Thomson HJ (1985) Acute pancreatitis in North and North-East Scotland. J R Coll Surg Edinb 30:104–110
80. Giggs JA, Bourke JB, Katschinski B (1988) The epidemiology of primary acute pancreatitis in Greater Nottingham: 1969–1983. Soc Sci Med 26:79–89
81. Lankisch PG, Assmus C, Maisonneuve P, Lowenfels AB (2002) Epidemiology of pancreatic diseases in Lüneburg County – a study in a defined German population. Pancreatology 2:469–477
82. Worning H (1994) Acute interstitial (edematous) pancreatitis in Denmark. In: Bradley EL III (ed) Acute Pancreatitis: Diagnosis and Therapy. Raven, New York, pp 269–269
83. McKay CJ, Evans S, Sinclair M, Carter CR, Imrie CW (1999) High early mortality rate from acute pancreatitis in Scotland, 1984–1995. Br J Surg 86:1302–1305
84. Appelros S, Borgström A (1999) Incidence, aetiology and mortality rate of acute pancreatitis over 10 years in a defined urban population in Sweden. Br J Surg 86:465–470
85. Eland IA, Sturkenboom MJCM, Wilson JHP, Stricker BHC (2000) Incidence and mortality of acute pancreatitis between 1985 and 1995. Scand J Gastroenterol 35:1110–1116
86. Go VLW (1994) Etiology and epidemiology of pancreatitis in the United States. In: Bradley EL III (ed) Acute Pancreatitis: Diagnosis and Therapy. Raven, New York, pp 239–239
87. Jaakkola M, Nordback I (1993) Pancreatitis in Finland between 1970 and 1989. Gut 34:1255–1260
88. Halvorsen F-A, Ritland S (1996) Acute pancreatitis in Buskerud County, Norway. Incidence and etiology. Scand J Gastroenterol 31:411–414
89. Floyd A, Pedersen L, Lauge Nielsen G, Thorlacius-Ussing O, Sorensen HT (2002) Secular trends in incidence and 30-day case fatality of acute pancreatitis in North Jutland County, Denmark. A register-based study from 1981–2000. Scand J Gastroenterol 37:1461–1465
90. Goldacre MJ, Roberts SE (2004) Hospital admission for acute pancreatitis in an English population, 1963–98: database study of incidence and mortality. Br Med J 328:1466–1469
91. Wilson C, Imrie CW (1988) Deaths from acute pancreatitis: why do we miss the diagnosis so frequently? Int J Pancreatol 3:273–282
92. Lankisch PG, Schirren CA, Kunze E (1991) Undetected fatal acute pancreatitis: why is the disease so frequently overlooked? Am J Gastroenterol 86:322–326
93. Mann DV, Hershman MJ, Hittinger R, Glazer G (1994) Multicentre audit of death from acute pancreatitis. Br J Surg 81:890–893
94. Eland IA, Sturkenboom MJCM, van der Lei J, Wilson JHP, Stricker BHC (2002) Incidence of acute pancreatitis. Scand J Gastroenterol 37:124–124
95. Lankisch PG, Burchard-Reckert S, Lehnick D (1999) Underestimation of acute pancreatitis: patients with only a small increase in amylase/lipase levels can also have or develop severe acute pancreatitis. Gut 44:542–544
96. Wilson C, Imrie CW (1990) Changing patterns of incidence and mortality from acute pancreatitis in Scotland, 1961–1985. Br J Surg 77:731–734
97. Klöppel G, Maillet B (1991) Chronic pancreatitis: evolution of the disease. Hepatogastroenterology 38:408–412
98. Trivedi CD, Pitchumoni CS (2005) Drug-induced pancreatitis. An update. J Clin Gastroenterol 39:709–716
99. Working Party of the British Society of Gastroenterology; Association of Surgeons of Great Britain and Ireland; Pancreatic Society of Great Britain and Ireland; Association of Upper GI Surgeons of Great Britain and Ireland. (2005) UK guidelines for the management of acute pancreatitis. Gut 54 (Suppl 3):iii1–iii9
100. Gislason H, Horn A, Hoem D, Andrén-Sandberg Å, Imsland AK, Søreide O, Viste A (2004) Acute pancreatitis in Bergen, Norway. Scand J Surg 93:29–33
101. Andersson R, Andersson B, Haraldsen P, Drewsen G, Eckerwall G (2004) Incidence, management and recurrence rate of acute pancreatitis. Scand J Gastroenterol 39:891–894
102. Toh SKC, Phillips S, Johnson CD (2000) A prospective audit against national standards of the presentation and management of acute pancreatitis in the South of England. Gut 46:239–243

Chapter 15

R. C. Carter · C. W. Imrie

Epidemiology and Intervention During the Clinical Course of Biliary Acute Pancreatitis

Friedrich first described the association between alcohol and abdominal pain, vomiting, and pancreatic inflammation in 1878, and Reginald Fitz, a Harvard pathologist, described the hemorrhagic and suppurative complications that can arise as a result of this process. It was not until 1901 that Eugene Opie proposed the common channel theory of how gallstones caused acute pancreatic inflammation. This resulted from his post mortem study of a patient in whom fatal acute pancreatitis (AP) was associated with the impaction of a single small gallstone in the ampulla of Vater.

Gallstone disease is an important cause of morbidity in the Western world. Operations on the biliary tree are more frequent than any other major surgical intervention in the abdomen. Gallstones are usually classified as being either ivory/yellow cholesterol or black pigment types. Cholesterol stones are smooth or faceted, single or multiple, and on cross-section show a laminated and/or crystalline appearance. The cholesterol in gallstones is mainly in the form of cholesterol monohydrate crystals and anhydrous cholesterol, with lesser amounts of an alternative crystalline form of anhydrous cholesterol.

Pigment stones are usually smaller, more numerous, irregular in shape and amorphous or crystalline on cross-section. They are formed mainly of the calcium salts of unconjugated bilirubin deposited in a glycoprotein matrix. As with cholesterol stones, pigment stones demonstrate layering of calcium bilirubinate salts and a glycoprotein matrix. In the Western world, 70% of stones are at least in part formed from cholesterol. Predominantly brown-colored stones are a mixture of cholesterol and pigment, often laid down in concentric alternating layers.

It is estimated that between 10 and 20% of the adult population in the Western world have gallstones. Age, country of origin, race, gender, drug therapy, obesity, diabetes, diet, liver disease, blood dyscrasias, and inflammatory bowel disease have all been associated with increased prevalence. The majority of patients with gallstones are asymptomatic and remain so, although 10–15% of asymptomatic patients will develop symptoms within 10 years. It is apparent that people do not die because of the presence of gallstones and the risk of major complications is low. Uncomplicated biliary colic is the first manifestation of gallstones for most patients. However, AP can be the first indication that stones are present. Indeed, the majority of patients with this etiology are unaware of their gallstones until the attack of AP takes place.

The predominant cause of AP in most societies is biliary in origin. The association with alcohol is often overstated and many patients with a possible alcohol history may have coexistent cholelithiasis. In addition, probably two-thirds of the idiopathic group consist of patients with bile crystals, cholesterolosis, or biliary sludge.

AP is more likely to occur in the presence of a wide cystic duct and small, multiple stones (<3 mm). A common pancreatobiliary channel of > 5mm is more frequently found in gallstone patients with AP than in those with standard biliary disease presentations. It is unclear whether pancreatic duct obstruction by transient impaction of a stone within this common channel is sufficient to initiate an attack, or whether biliopancreatic reflux of bile is also required.

Transient hold up of stone(s) is customary, as fecal recovery of stones in most gallstone-associated AP was demonstrated first in Rosario (Argentina) [1], then in Akron (Ohio, USA), and also in Leeds (UK). This repeated proof in several countries of the accuracy of the initial thoughts of Juan Acosta is very important with respect to the comprehension of the likely pathogenesis of gallstone-related AP.

Not all patients with a biliary etiology will have evidence of residual gallstones within the gallbladder. A patient with a wide cystic duct may pass a single stone once formed, such that subsequent imaging, including endoscopic ultrasound (EUS) may prove negative. New stones may form in 18–36 months and trigger a further attack of AP. Surgeons with an extended experience in the management of AP have found that cholecystectomy in recurrent AP proves therapeutic. This observation underlines the truth of the previous data and was noted more than 30 years ago [2].

Diagnosis of Gallstones as the Cause of AP

Whilst the most accurate means of diagnosis of gallstones is fecal sieving this is impractical in clinical practice. Abdominal X-ray is of little value as only 15% of gallstones are radio-opaque. Abdominal ultrasound is the initial mode of diagnosis and should be performed within 24 h of admission. Bowel gas can be troublesome in obtaining good visualization of the bile ducts and gall bladder. The investigation needs to be repeated if this problem is noted. Stones of 4 mm in diameter may be at the limit of small size detectability for standard ultrasonic techniques.

Contrast-enhanced computed tomography (CT) is commonly performed within the first few days following admission to identify angiographic and morphological changes to the pancreas, but the sensitivity for the detection of small gallstones is poor. Magnetic resonance imaging (MRI) is rarely feasible during the acute phase of an attack, but it is very good for delineation of the anatomy and contents of the extrahepatic biliary tree. Magnetic resonance cholangiopancreatography is often under-utilized.

Most patients with AP initially labeled as idiopathic have a biliary cause for their pancreatitis. EUS has been shown to be highly accurate for the identification of gallbladder sludge, microlithiasis, and common bile duct (CBD) stones. It is claimed in expert hands to be able to delineate 1- to 2-mm diameter stones and is an appropriate second-line investigation within the idiopathic group. Careful investigation usually lowers the percentage of patients with an unidentified etiology to less than 5%. This subject has been well reviewed recently [3].

Circumstantial evidence pointing toward a biliary etiology may be obtained from routine liver function tests, with a raised bilirubin, and in particular elevations of transaminases (transferases) in the first 48 h in hospital, being suggestive of gallstones. Occasionally, cholangitis and AP coexist, with the biliary sepsis being a very important element in these patients such that organ dysfunction may originate in the biliary sepsis. Intravenous antibiotic therapy with urgent endoscopic retrograde cholangiopancreatography (ERCP) and sphincterotomy and CBD stone clearance are required. This is the major indication for urgent ERCP in this phase of the illness.

Initial Management

Aggressive fluid resuscitation and attention to fluid balance represents the single key element of initial management, optimizing organ perfusion and oxygenation, and are essential regardless of the etiology of pancreatic inflammation. In the most severely ill patients, fluid needs may exceed 5 l in the initial 12–18 h. the provision of high-flow oxygen is very important and checks of the adequacy of this move to achieve satisfactory oxygenation are crucial. Full mechanical ventilation may be required. Control of analgesic needs is usually with morphine. Some prefer to use spinal nerve blocks. A detailed description of supportive measures is beyond the scope of this chapter, and have been described elsewhere.

Sustained organ failure is the most important indicator of disease severity. Transient easily correctable organ failure within 48 h of hospital admission is not associated with a high mortality and morbidity [4]. Patients who have a modified Marshall score of 2 or more beyond 48 h invariably feature respiratory failure. Renal, cardiac, and hematological failures are the most frequent of the other systems to be compromised.

The Role of Antibiotics

The place of prophylactic antibiotic single-dose intravenous therapy in covering ERCP procedures is not under debate. For the few with severe accompanying biliary sepsis manifested by rigors and obstructive jaundice, longer antibiotic therapy is necessary. However, the use of prophylactic intravenous antibiotics in the initial stages of severe AP of any cause is not proved. The only two truly randomized controlled studies have failed to show any benefit from such drugs being routinely prescribed [5,6]. In the German study, ciprofloxacin and metronidazole were given versus placebo, while in the multinational study, meropenem was tested against a placebo. Neither study found the main end point of infected pancreatic necrosis less frequently in the treatment group of patients. Mortality was also not lowered by antibiotic therapy. Prior to the publication of these two important papers, a series of less-well-controlled studies were reported suggesting that prophylactic antibiotic therapy was beneficial. The numbers of patients were less and the study designs suboptimal, so less weight is to be given to this evidence. Assessment of the current situation remains equivocal, and prompts the recommendation that antibiotics should be prescribed only with specific clinical and microbiological culture/Gram stain indications.

Early Nasoenteral Feeding

This is a therapeutic development of the last 11 years and is to be encouraged. Randomized clinical trials have shown the benefit of early nasojejunal feeding compared to intravenous total parenteral nutrition [7,8]. Early nasogastric feeding has also been shown to be practical in many patients [9].Furthermore, in a randomized trial it was found to be as effective as nasojejunal feeding [10]. As a practical matter, it can be started earlier without the inconvenience and risk of endoscopy, which is utilized in the placement of most nasojejunal feeding tubes.

Intervention in Biliary Pancreatitis

Preventive Measures

The majority of patients with biliary pancreatitis will settle after a short period of conservative management, subsequent intervention being aimed at the prevention of a second episode.

Cholecystectomy

Cholecystectomy (with operative cholangiography) is the treatment of choice and the rate of recurrence of AP in patients with gallstones has been reported in 29–63% of cases if the patient is discharged from the hospital without additional treatment [11]. The timing of cholecystectomy depends on the clinical situation. In mild gallstone-associated AP, cholecystectomy should be performed as soon as the patient has recovered from the attack and preferably during the same hospital stay. In severe gallstone-associated AP, the timing of cholecystectomy varies, taking into account the requirement for additional interventions for complications of that severe attack. Cholecystectomy (with cholangiogram) should be combined with any open/laparoscopic intervention for late complications, as described below.

When younger men are excluded, any cohort of AP patients will have a very high probability of stone etiology. Indeed, the single stone required to cause an attack can have passed already into the gut. For this reason, the threshold to perform cholecystectomy as a prophylactic action is low. During the operation it is wise to remember that the diameter of the cystic duct is likely to be larger than at an average cholecystectomy. Careful and accurate dissection to display the main structures on the lateral border of the CBD and common hepatic duct is therefore warranted. Intraoperative cholangiography via the cystic duct may indicate the need for opening of the CBD and stone retrieval. If intraoperative imaging and inspection by choledochoscopy reveals a clear duct after exploration and stone removal, primary CBD closure is sensible. Should doubt exist regarding CBD clearance of stones, then a latex T-tube external duct drainage should be performed. Check cholangiography via the T-tube is usual at 6–7 days, with ERCP stone removal prior to removal of the T-tube after 12–24 h of side-arm clamping without symptoms/signs of CBD obstruction.

Endoscopic Sphincterotomy to Prevent Further Attacks

Following an attack of either mild or severe gallstone-associated AP, comorbidity may prevent the patient proceeding to cholecystectomy. In these circumstances, elective prophylactic endoscopic sphincterotomy (whether there are or are not any stones in the main bile ducts) may be considered as an alternative. In medium-term follow-up studies, the risk of developing a further attack of AP is less than 1%, although more may develop other biliary symptoms [12,13]. In patients with severe pancreatitis and a postinflammatory fluid collection, particularly those containing significant necrosis, there is a significant risk of introducing infection during the ERCP procedure and it is advisable to delay this action until clinical and laboratory markers of inflammatory response resolve.

Operations and Other Procedures Used During the Acute Phase of Biliary Pancreatitis

The following section will describe the basic steps involved in undertaking these procedures. The variability of the presentation and pathology demands flexibility and real-time modification of the techniques, and consequently these are aimed at providing a generic outline rather than a dogmatic protocol. The choice of procedure is influenced by the clinical condition of the patient, the presence of infection, the timing of intervention, and whether the peripancreatic collection is "solid predominant" or "fluid predominant" on CT or MRI (Fig. 15.1).

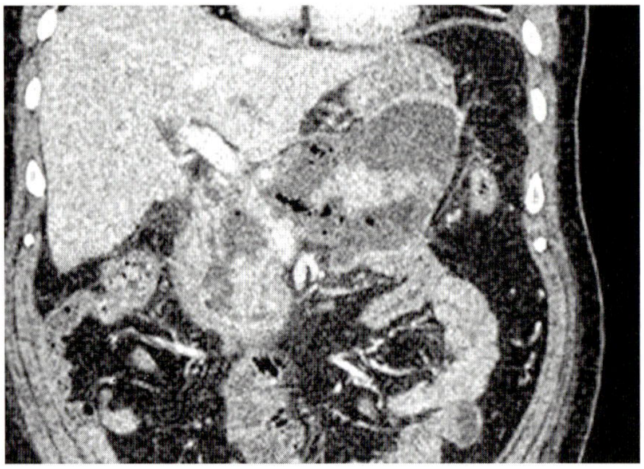

Figure 15.1

Coronal computed tomography (CT) scan showing a postinflammatory fluid collection with central necrosis and gas within the collection, indicating probable infection

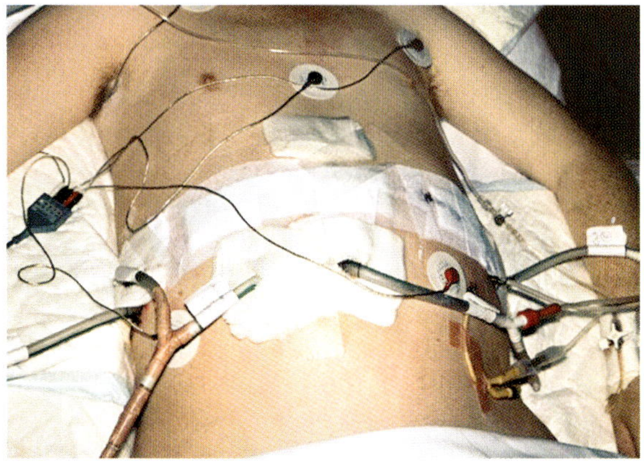

Figure 15.2

Patient postnecrosectomy with multiple intra-abdominal inflow and outflow drains for closed lavage of the Beger type. Average lavage duration 23 days

Pancreatic Necrosectomy

Surgery is usually required for the management of complications rather than for the necrosis itself and there is no role for early laparotomy and resective procedures. The most common procedure for infected pancreatic necrosis in a patient failing to respond to conservative treatment is an open necrosectomy. This may be performed by an open anterior, left lateral retroperitoneal, anterior laparoscopic, or a percutaneous approach.

Open Anterior Approach

1. A laparotomy is performed through a transverse, gently superior curving incision. The exact length of the surgical incision and its location will be guided to some degree by imaging information, especially CT scan.
2. Access to drain the peripancreatic and pancreatic infected necrotic tissue is through the lesser sac or by dividing the gastrocolic omentum. Both hepatic and splenic flexures of the colon may need to be mobilized inferiorly to expose the anterior aspect of a pancreatic collection. Once entry to the abscess cavity is obtained (often aided by aspiration identification), suction aspiration of the pus and digital removal of necrotic tissue is performed. Sharp dissection is avoided, as this can to lead to significant hemorrhage.
3. Cholecystectomy +/– operative cholangiogram should be performed if it is probable or proved that gallstones are the etiology of the AP.

Closed Lavage Approach

Having cleared the cavity of all necrotic tissue, the abdomen is closed after the careful location of paired large-diameter (28–32 French gauge, FG) drains [14]. We usually employ 4–6 plastic drains and check adequate flow communication during surgery (Fig. 15.2). Postoperative lavage with body temperature saline or dialysis fluid at a rate of 250 ml/h follows. This may be necessary for 2–6 weeks (median of 23 days in the Ulm experience).

Open Packing Approach

In the event of a significant coagulopathy resulting in oozing of blood, such that placement of drains is thought unwise, the necrosectomy cavity may be packed with large cotton packs enclosed in petroleum jelly (Vaseline)-impregnated mesh (Jelonet, Smith and Nephew), as described in the next section (Fig. 15.3). After 48–72 h, and having restored normal or "near normal" coagulation, a re-laparotomy should permit pack removal and creation of a closed lavage system (section "Preventive Measures," above) as recommended by the Ulm team of Professor Beger in the 1980s.

In addition to having a role in the temporary control of hemorrhage, the open packing technique has been used as the primary technique to maintain control of sepsis [15]. This laparostomy technique requires repeated pack changes every 48–72 h. While these pack changes are initially performed under general anesthesia, later in the process this may be

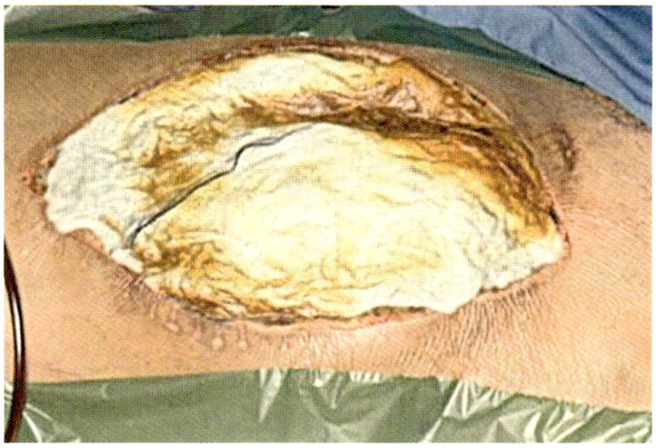

Figure 15.3

Open packed laparostomy wound using large cotton packs. Betadine antiseptic coloration and plastic Steridrape applied over the site

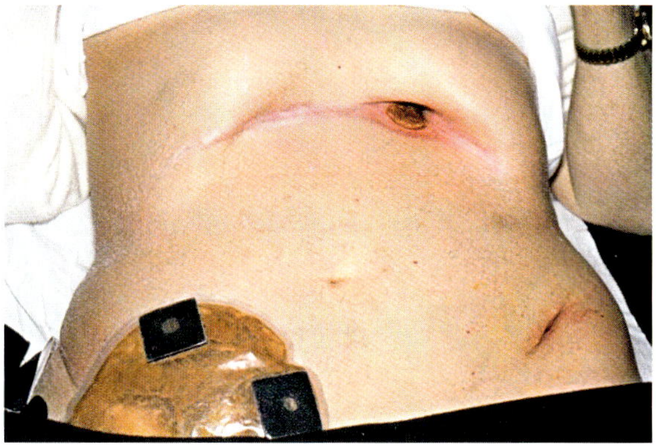

Figure 15.4

Healed transverse laparostomy wound in a patient who had needed ascending and transverse colectomy with end ileostomy in addition to open packing of the necrotic cavity. No wound suture of any layer was employed

achieved under sedation. A higher enteric fistula rate tends to occur, and procedures are more labor intensive. Consequently, laparostomy has not been adopted as widely as the closed lavage technique described in section "Preventive Measures," above. The French have an alternative system of packing such large cavities utilizing the minimally adherent Mickulicz packs, which are available in their hospitals. Where the whole thickness of the abdominal wall is left to heal by granulation, the process takes approximately 10–14 weeks. Somewhat surprisingly, only one-third of the patients have a wound hernia once this healing has taken place (Fig. 15.4).

Closed Packing Approach

A variation of this technique is that of closed packing [16], whereby multiple soft Penrose drains containing cotton gauze to pack the cavity are utilized following completion of the necrosectomy. These are subsequently removed at intervals, allowing the cavity to collapse around the drains.

Lateral Retroperitoneal Approach

1. A left-flank incision is performed and the colon mobilized medially, allowing retroperitoneal access to the lesser sac.
2. The pus is aspirated and necrotic material is then removed by blunt finger dissection.
3. The cavity is managed by either lavage with drainage or packing as described above. This approach was mainly reported from France [17]. Problems were encountered that limited enthusiasm for this technique such that few have followed this path. Visibility tends to be suboptimal and this probably is a factor in complications. Enteric fistulas and hemorrhage occurred in over 35% of patients, while colonic necrosis was noted in 15%.

Video-Assisted Retroperitoneal Debridement

This is a form of halfway house procedure between the open lateral retroperitoneal approach and percutaneous necrosectomy described below). It originated in The Netherlands and was subsequently reported from the USA [18].

1. Using a 5- to 6-cm oblique left lateral skin incision, a laparoscope is introduced along the line of a percutaneously CT-guided plastic drain.
2. Copious suction and lavage removes much of the liquid component within the cavity.
3. The retroperitoneal tunnel alongside the laparoscope is developed to allow the parallel insertion of large grasping forceps, such as sponge holding forceps.
4. Solid necrotic material within the cavity can then be visualized and removed piecemeal.
5. Maintenance of access and continued control of sepsis may be obtained by postoperative closed lavage, or closed or open packing, as described above.

Anterior Laparoscopic Approach

This mimics the open necrosectomy approach described above, with the exception that standard laparoscopic ports are utilized for access instead of a bilateral subcostal incision.

1. Using a cut-down technique, a blunt port is inserted subumbilically.

2. Further 10-mm and 5-mm ports are inserted to provide both operative access and upward retraction of the colon to expose the transverse mesocolon.
3. The lesser sac is entered by opening the transverse mesocolon or gastrocolic omentum, and the pus and necrotic material are removed through this opening. Postoperatively, tube drainage is used to enable both lavage and drainage of the necrosectomy cavity. The technical challenges presented by this approach have limited its general application.

Percutaneous Necrosectomy

This procedure was developed in Glasgow [19] and involves the dilatation of a percutaneous CT-guided drain tract to promote adequate drainage and lavage of the area of infected pancreatic and peripancreatic infected necrosis/abscess cavity. This has the advantage of being technically simple to perform.

1. Under CT guidance, a percutaneous catheter is inserted into the abscess cavity. This is usually a left-flank approach (approximately 85% of patients) inferior and anterior to the lower pole of the spleen, posterior to the proximal descending colon, and anterior to the left kidney. Less frequently, the right anterior oblique approach (occasionally combined with the left-flank approach) is employed (Fig. 15.5). In some patients, this immediately precedes the next stages of therapy. For others, a delay to await the potential clinical benefits of the percutaneous drainage (with a van Sonnenberg or similar drain) alone is wise. This is particularly the case in the most severely compromised patients in terms of respiratory and additional organ failures, as drainage of pus can be associated with clinical improvement.
2. Usually under general anesthetic (local anesthesia has been used by some), a guide wire is inserted into the drain, and the tract dilated to 34 FG using either a balloon dilatation system or a series of graduated dilators. The balloon dilator we have used is that of Cook Medical (UNBS 10-15), with a balloon length of 55 cm. The alternative, which we used in our early experience, is the standard urological Amplatz Dilator System (260100 BOSRW).
3. At the initial procedure, an Amplatz Plastic sheath 32FG is then inserted to maintain tract integrity. Pus of varying density may spontaneously extrude at this point. Using an operating nephroscope, the cavity can then be explored and any easily movable solid necrotic material taken out under visual aid (Fig. 15.6). Tissue that appears dead but is still adherent to adjacent structures should be left to a subsequent exploration. The initial procedure is best regarded as one of optimum drainage of pus combined with the establishment of a valuable lavage system.
4. At the end of the procedure, a simple plastic 32 FG tube drain (Portex/similar) with a parallel 8 FG umbilical inflow lavage catheter (secured together by nonabsorbable sutures) is sutured to skin for continuous postoperative lavage, usually at a rate of 250 ml/h with body temperature fluid (Fig. 15.7). A larger-diameter modified nephroscope has been designed by one of us (CRC) to make the operation easier and safer. This was in collaboration with Olympus in Hamburg and has prototype identifiers of S841/1for the scope and S1447/1 for the stainless steel sleeve. This tool allows utilization of many

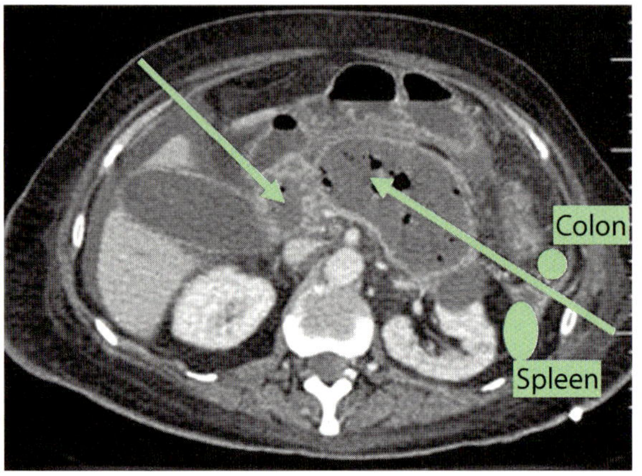

Figure 15.5

The preferred routes for CT-guided access drainage

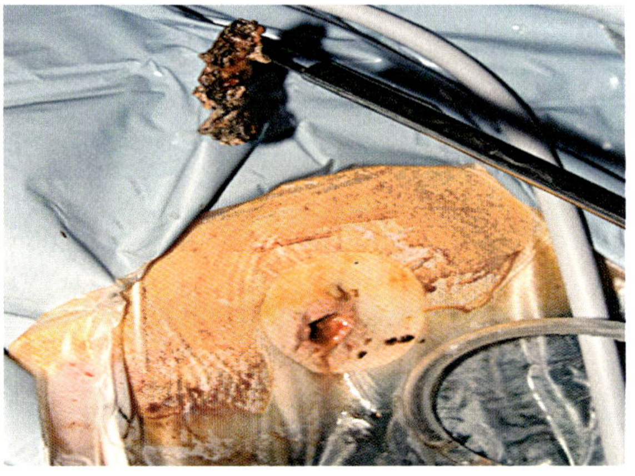

Figure 15.6

Piecemeal removal of retroperitoneal necrosis during percutaneous necrosectomy via the customary left flank approach

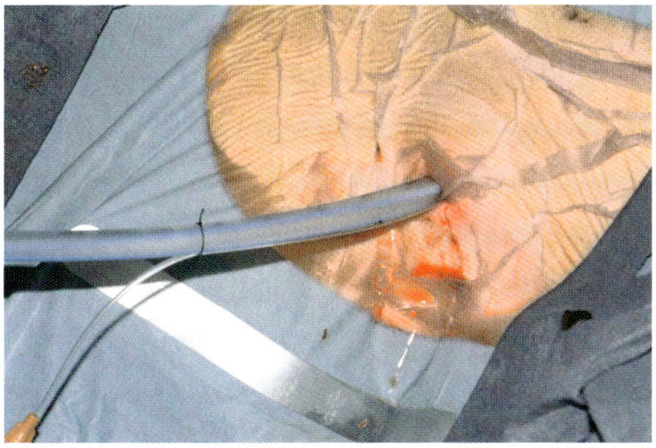

Figure 15.7

A 32 FG Portex outflow drain placed along the drain tract, with a 8FG inflow umbilical catheter sutured alongside to allow "closed" postoperative lavage

standard (5 mm) laparoscopic instruments that will not pass through the operating channel of a standard nephroscope.

5. When clinically and/or radiologically indicated, further percutaneous necrosectomy procedures will be required in most patients at varying time intervals after the initial operation. The indication for reintervention is usually clinical or biochemical signs of sepsis or a planned procedure following 10–12 days of continuous lavage, when a significant degree of separation of necrotic tissue may be expected. The average patient undergoes three procedures, each of which is less traumatic than open operations, as measured by the requirement for intensive care and postoperative elevation of C-reactive Protein.

Management of Pseudocyst

The use of the term pseudocyst in this context is often misleading as by definition a pseudocyst should contain minimal or no solid material. Endoscopic cystogastrostomy (with or without EUS control) is becoming increasingly common and is the approach of choice where necrosis is minimal. In the postacute biliary patient, with an organized peripancreatic fluid collection arising within 1–3 months of an attack, the majority of collections will have a significant amount of solid material within them. This is often underestimated by CT scanning. In this circumstance, therefore, we prefer to describe a fluid collection as either "solid predominant" (as in infected or sterile necrosis) or "fluid predominant" (as would be described as a pseudocyst on CT). Even in the "fluid predominant" collections, there may be a significant amount of debris, and drainage through small-aperture endoscopic stents may be suboptimal.

Surgical drainage of postacute collections is particularly useful for postinflammatory cysts containing significant necrotic debris. This procedure is performed for drainage of a pseudocyst either into a Roux loop of jejunum or, more commonly, into the posterior wall of the stomach. Definitive management of cholelithiasis by cholecystectomy is usually performed simultaneously.

Open Cystogastrostomy

1. Transverse/longitudinal skin and body wall incision.
2. The anterior aspect of the stomach is identified and a longitudinal gastrotomy is performed of approximately 10–15 cm length. Imaging evidence as to the location of the pancreatic pseudocyst and palpation at surgery will determine the optimum placement of this gastrotomy incision.
3. The exact site of the retrogastric pseudocyst from within the stomach is then confirmed using palpation with or without intraoperative ultrasound. Needle puncture and aspiration is the final confirmation prior to incision.
4. The anterior wall of the pseudocyst is opened using a diathermy scalpel and the edge is oversewn with interrupted heavy 1:0 absorbable suture as there is a tendency to bleed significantly. The length of the cystogastrostomy is usually 5–10 cm. Biopsy sampling of the anterior wall of the pseudocyst is advised.
5. Fluid is aspirated and any necrotic material within the cyst is removed.
6. The anterior wall of the stomach is then closed using a continuous 3:0 polydioxone or similar suture, and the abdominal wound closed without drainage.

Laparoscopic Cystogastrostomy

A subumbilical open cut down technique allows insertion of a blunt port and creation of a pneumoperitoneum. The laparoscope is introduced through this port site.

There are two techniques for laparoscopic cystogastrostomy: (1) intraluminal, where the ports are placed inside the stomach and the operation is performed from within an inflated stomach (Fig. 15.8), and (2) transgastric, where a standard anterior gastrotomy is performed laparoscopically to allow access to the posterior gastric wall.

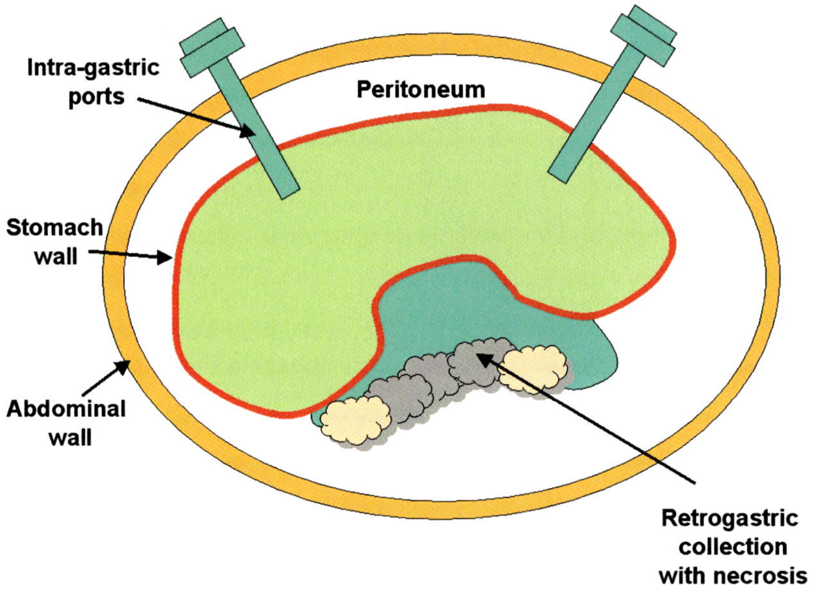

Figure 15.8

Line diagram illustrating the insertion of the laparoscopic ports through both the abdominal wall and the stomach wall, allowing intraluminal surgery

Intraluminal Approach

1. Accessing the intragastric lumen. This is assisted by passing a standard flexible endoscope into the stomach, tilting the patients into a reverse Trendelenburg position with a right-side-down tilt and then instilling 100 ml of H_20 into the duodenum to act as a water seal sump, allowing insufflation of the gastric lumen without distending the small bowel with CO_2.
2. Retention of the ports and obtaining an adequate intragastric gas seal is facilitated by the use of dilating laparoscopic "Step" ports (2×12 mm plus sometimes 1×5 mm ports; VersaStep Plus: Tyco Auto Suture VS 101012P) rather than using standard ports or balloon-tipped ports. The "Step" ports, having been introduced into the peritoneal cavity, are then advanced before dilatation through the anterior gastric wall into the gastric lumen, thereby allowing access to the posterior gastric wall. These are placed in the upper abdomen, with the exact positions being determined by the position of the stomach, the aim being to insert a 12-mm port into the most dependent portion of the greater curve, an antral 12-mm port and sometimes a higher greater curve 5-mm port, depending on access. The 12-mm antral port provides access for the intraoperative ultrasound and the linear stapling device.
3. An ultrasound probe, aided by a Doppler facility, can be used to identify the site of cyst puncture, usually by diathermy puncture using laparoscopic scissors. The puncture orifice is dilated and the fluid content of the cyst aspirated. Biopsy of the pseudocyst wall is also advised.
4. The puncture site is then extended along the posterior gastric wall using a laparoscopic stapling device, over a distance of 10–15 cm (Endo GIA :Tyc 030445 or similar device).
5. Solid material can be withdrawn into the gastric lumen and the cavity lavaged.
6. Having ensured hemostasis, which will occasionally require suture legation of the staple line, the ports are removed from the anterior aspect of the stomach wall and the defects repaired by suture.

Transgastric Laparoscopic Approach

Although the stomach wall is usually easily seen draped over the anterior aspect of the pseudocyst, the ability to insert the trocars in a position to allow adequate intraluminal access is often compromised. In this situation a transgastric laparoscopic approach may be used, which is technically easier in such circumstances.

1. The blunt port is inserted as described above and if a transgastric approach thought suitable, two standard 12-mm ports are inserted to optimize triangulation and avoid the rib margin.
2. An anterior gastrotomy is performed over a length of 10–15 cm.

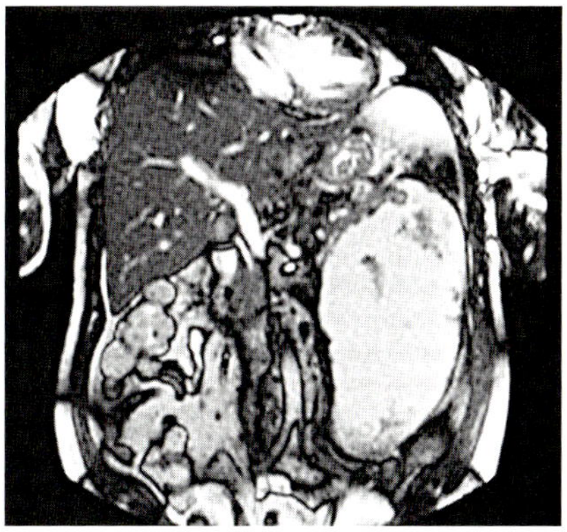

Figure 15.9

A coronal magnetic resonance view of a large pancreatic pseudocyst with no apposition to the gastric wall, which was treated by open cystojejunostomy

3. An anterior retraction suture is inserted through the abdominal wall utilizing a straight needle (Biosyn 3:0 Tyco SN643 or similar). This is passed through the anterior–superior leaf of the gastrotomy to retract this edge up to the anterior abdominal wall, allowing access to the lumen of the stomach.
4. Steps 3–5 of the intraluminal approach are then performed, draining the pseudocyst and creating a cystgastrotomy over 10–15 cm.
5. The anterior gastrotomy is then repaired using a running suture.

Cystojejunostomy

Where the site of the pseudocyst precludes drainage into the posterior aspect of the stomach, a Roux loop can be used as an alternative. The location of the abdominal wall incision will be determined by the imaging evidence of the location of the pseudocyst (Fig. 15.9).

1. The anterior wall of the pseudocyst is dissected and a safe anastomotic site chosen.
2. The Roux loop of jejunum is first prepared using standard staple and cut division of the proximal jejunum approximately 20–25 cm beyond the duodenojejunal flexure.
3. The distal limb of jejunum is then brought up to lie adjacent to the anterior wall of the pseudocyst, and its position can once again be confirmed by intraoperative ultrasound or needle aspiration.
4. Prior to this, bowel continuity can be restored by end-to-side hand-sewn jejunojejunostomy using a continuous 3:0 absorbable suture (Maxon ,Vicryl or similar) so that the distal free limb of jejunum is 50 cm in length. Alternatively, this anastomosis can be made by a side-to-side staple and cut technique with hand suture closure of the areas needed to access the entry of the stapling instrument.
5. The pseudocyst is opened and drained with removal of friable necrotic material (as already described). A biopsy of the wall is taken for pathological examination. Pseudocyst fluid is sent for culture and biochemical analysis of amylase/lipase and albumin.
6. The posterior surface of the Roux loop is opened and a side-to-side anastomosis to the pseudocyst wall is performed using a continuous suture technique (abdominal wall closure without a drain).

Laparoscopic Cystoenterostomy

The same procedure may be performed laparoscopically if the cyst is not in apposition with the stomach wall.

1. Standard subumbilical 10- to 12-mm blunt port placement using a cut-down technique.
2. Three further 12-mm standard laparoscopic ports are placed in an arc around the collection to optimize triangulation, depending on the site of the collection.
3. Measurement of the distance of the small bowel is facilitated by wrapping a SteriStrip around one of the laparoscopic graspers 5 and 10 cm from the tip. The site for the jejunal division is approximately 20–25 cm from the duodenojejunal flexure. The mesentery is divided using an ultrasonic dissector and the bowel divided with the aid of a laparoscopic linear stapler (Endo GIA: Tyc 030445 or similar device).
4. A 50-cm length of distal jejunum is then measured, and jejunal continuity restored by a functional side-to-side anastomosis. This is performed by creating two small enterotomies, and two firings (proximal and distal) of a laparoscopic linear stapler. The defect on the anterior aspect of the anastomosis is closed using a continuous running suture.
5. The distal limb of jejunum is approximated to the prepared anterior wall of the pseudocyst.
6. The pseudocyst is opened using laparoscopic diathermy scissors. Fluid is aspirated and sent for analysis. Tissue is taken from the pseudocyst wall for histology. Friable necrotic tissue from within the pseudocyst is removed.
7. The anastomosis is either hand sutured or the linear stapler again employed, with suture closure of the entry site of the linear stapler.
8. The ports are removed with closure of the entry points.

References

1. Acosta JM, Ledesma CL (1974) Gallstone migration as a cause of acute pancreatitis. N Engl J Med 290:484–487
2. Imrie CW (1974) Observations on acute pancreatitis. Br J Surg 61:539–544
3. Wilcox CM, Varadarajulu S, Eloubeidi M (2006) Role of endoscopic evaluation in idiopathic pancreatitis: a systematic review. Gastrointest Endosc 63:1037–1045
4. Buter A, Imrie CW, Carter CR, Evans S, McKay CJ (2002) Dynamic nature of early organ dysfunction determines outcome in acute pancreatitis. Br J Surg 89:298–302
5. Dellinger EP, Tellado JM, Soto NE, Ashley SW, Barie PS, Duernier T, Imrie CW, Johnson CD, Knaebel HP, Laterre PF, Maravi-Poma E, Kissler JJO, Sanchez-Garcia M, Utzolino S (2007) Early antibiotic treatment for severe acute necrotizing pancreatitis: a randomized, double-blind, placebo-controlled study. Ann Surg 245:674–683
6. Isenmann R, Runzi M, Kron M, Kahl S, Kraus D, Jung N, Maier L, Malfertheiner P, Goebell H, Beger HG (2004) Prophylactic antibiotic treatment in patients with predicted severe acute pancreatitis: a placebo-controlled, double-blind trial. Gastroenterology 126:997–1004
7. Kalfarentzos F, Kehagias J, Mead N, Kokkinis K, Gogos CA (1997) Enteral nutrition is superior to parenteral nutrition in severe acute pancreatitis: results of a randomized prospective trial. Br J Surg 84:1665–1669
8. Olah A, Pardavi G, Belagyi T, Nagy A, Issekutz A, Mohamed GE (2002) Early nasojejunal feeding in acute pancreatitis is associated with a lower complication rate. Nutrition 18:259–262
9. Eatock FC, Brombacher GD, Steven A, Imrie CW, McKay CJ, Carter R (2000) Nasogastric feeding in severe acute pancreatitis may be practical and safe. Int J Pancreatol 28:25–31
10. Eatock FC, Chong P, Menezes N, Murray L, McKay CJ, Carter CR, Imrie CW (2005) A randomized study of early nasogastric versus nasojejunal feeding in severe acute pancreatitis. Am J Gastroenterol 100:432–439
11. Kelly TR, Wagner DS (1988) Gallstone pancreatitis: a prospective randomised trial of the timing of surgery. Surgery 104:600–605
12. Davidson BR, Neoptolemos JP, Carr-Locke DL (1988) Endoscopic sphincterotomy for common bile duct calculi in patients with gall bladder in situ considered unfit for surgery. Gut 29:114–120
13. Welbourn CR, Beckly DE, Eyre-Brook IA (1995) Endoscopic sphincterotomy without cholecystectomy for gall stone pancreatitis. Gut 37:119–120
14. Beger HG, Buchler M, Bittner R, Block S, Nevalainen T, Roscher R (1988) Necrosectomy and postoperative local lavage in necrotizing pancreatitis. B J Surg 75:207–212
15. Bradley EL III (1987) Management of infected pancreatitis necrosis by open drainage. Ann Surg 206:542–550
16. Fernandez-Del Castillo C, Rattner DW, Makary MA, Mostafavi A, McGrath D, Warshaw AL (1998) Debridement and closed packing for the treatment of necrotizing pancreatitis. Ann Surg 228:676–684
17. Fagniez PL, Rotman N, Kracht M (1989) Direct retroperitoneal approach to necrosis in severe acute pancreatitis. Br J Surg 76:264–267
18. Horvath KD, Kao LS, Wherry KL, Pellegrini CA, Sinanan MN (2001) A technique for laparoscopic-assisted percutaneous drainage of infected pancreatic necrosis and pancreatic abscess. Surg Endosc 15:1221–1225
19. Carter CR, McKay CJ, Imrie CW (2000) Percutaneous necrosectomy and sinus tract endoscopy in the management of infected pancreatic necrosis: an initial experience. Ann Surg 232:175–180

Chapter 16

M. L. Steer · G. Perides

Pathogenesis and Pathophysiology of Acute Pancreatitis

Conventionally, the distinction between acute and chronic pancreatitis is based on the issue of reversibility, in other words, can the functional and morphological pancreatic changes associated with the disease be completely reversed if the inciting cause(s) are removed and if no further attacks occur? This characteristic of so-called "acute pancreatitis" appears to be critical to its natural history and, at the extremes of its spectrum, it appears to distinguish acute pancreatitis from chronic pancreatitis, both in terms of its various inciting causes (i.e., its pathogenesis) and in terms of the cellular events that mediate its evolution (i.e., its pathophysiology). At the center of the spectrum, however, that distinction may break down and it must be recognized that there may exist considerable overlap, in terms of both pathogenesis and pathophysiology, between acute and chronic pancreatitis. This chapter will summarize current concepts regarding both the pathogenesis and the pathophysiology of acute pancreatitis. Our knowledge regarding the former is based primarily on clinical observations, while that regarding the latter is almost entirely based on observations made using models of acute pancreatitis induced in experimental animals.

Pathogenesis of Acute Pancreatitis

Biliary tract stones and prolonged ethanol abuse account for most attacks of pancreatitis, but the relative contributions of these so called "etiologies" depends upon the type of pancreatitis involved. Ethanol abuse is an unusual cause of clinical acute pancreatitis, but it is the most common cause of chronic pancreatitis; in contrast, the vast majority of patients with acute pancreatitis develop their disease as a consequence of biliary tract stone disease, but stone disease is only a rare cause of chronic pancreatitis. Viewed in this context, some 70–80% of patients with acute pancreatitis develop their pancreatitis attack as a complication of biliary tract stone disease (Table 16.1) and the inciting event leading to pancreatitis usually involves passage of a stone (or stones) into (or through) the terminal biliary-pancreatic ductal system. Of the remaining 20–30% of patients with acute pancreatitis, most (roughly 15% of all patients with acute pancreatitis) develop their disease in association with no recognized cause. They are said to have "idiopathic acute pancreatitis" although, as further insights into the pathogenesis of pancreatitis are gained, the cause of pancreatitis in most of this group may eventually be identified. Regardless, by combining these observations we can conclude that roughly 80–90% of patients with acute pancreatitis have either biliary acute pancreatitis or idiopathic acute pancreatitis.

Table 16.1. Etiologies of acute pancreatitis. *ERPC* Endoscopic retrograde cholangiopancreatography

Biliary tract stones	Pancreatic duct obstruction
Ethanol abuse	Hereditary
Medications	Trauma
ERCP	Hyperlipidemia
Hypercalcemia	Infections
Ischemia	Trauma
Parasites	Postoperative

Over the past century, many other causes of acute pancreatitis have been identified (Table 16.1), but clearly, together they account for relatively few attacks of the disease. With its emergence as a commonly employed clinical procedure, either alone or combined with other forms of instrumentation such as sphincterotomy or biliary manometry, endoscopic retrograde cholangiopancreatography currently accounts for a significant fraction of these patients. Another significant fraction of the patients develop their pancreatitis as a result of exposure to certain potentially disease-inducing drugs such as thiazide diuretics, furosemide, 6-mercaptopurine, dideoxyinosine, pentamidine, tetracycline, valproic acid, and sulfonamides. Finally, a small fraction of the remaining patients can be identified who develop their disease as a result of pancreatic trauma, metabolic disorders such as hyperlipidemia, infectious processes such as mumps or Coxsackie virus infection, genetic abnormalities such as those underlying the development of hereditary pancreatitis, or mechanical events, including tumors and pancreas divisum, which can cause relative pancreatic duct obstruction. The other identified causes of acute pancreatitis, even taken together, probably account for less than 1% of patients with the disease.

Mechanisms Responsible for Biliary Pancreatitis

Reports by Acosta and Ledesma [1] and by Acosta et al. [2] have shown that the onset of biliary pancreatitis is associated with the passage of biliary tract stones either into or through the terminal biliopancreatic ductal system, and studies performed by many investigators over the past two centuries have examined the potential mechanisms by which such stones might trigger pancreatic inflammation. In a general sense, three theories have been advanced: the common channel theory, the pancreatic duct obstruction theory and the duodenal reflux theory. The common channel theory, originally proposed by Opie in 1901 [3], suggests that the offending stone, or perhaps edema triggered by passage of that stone, causes obstruction of the most distal, common biliopancreatic drainage channel (i.e., duct) and, in the process, this event creates a more proximal common channel that permits bile to reflux into the pancreatic ductal system from the bile duct. According to the common channel theory of Opie, that reflux of bile into the pancreatic ductal system is injurious and it triggers pancreatitis, although the mechanisms by which such bile reflux might cause injury to the pancreas have not been clearly identified. Although not so well known, the second theory by which the onset of biliary pancreatitis might be explained was actually also developed by Opie in 1901 [4]. This so called duct obstruction theory suggests that impaction of the offending stone in the distal bile duct, or edema triggered by that stone, causes pancreatic duct obstruction, and that this obstruction causes pancreatic ductal hypertension leading to ductal disruption and pancreatic injury. Finally, for reasons of completeness, mention should also be made of the third, or duodenal reflux theory, by which the onset of biliary pancreatitis might be explained. According to this theory [5], during passage of the offending stone into the duodenum, the sphincter of Oddi is rendered incompetent and, as a result, duodenal juices containing activated digestive enzymes can reflux into the pancreatic ductal system and cause pancreatic injury. Given the low incidence of recurrent, acute pancreatitis after biliopancreatic sphincterotomy, the duodenal reflux theory would seem a very unlikely explanation for acute pancreatitis, but establishing the validity of one or the other of the competing theories has proven both difficult and highly controversial.

We attempted to resolve this controversy in a series of studies that employed an animal model of acute pancreatitis developed in the American opossum by Senninger et al. [6]. They had shown that obstruction of the biliopancreatic ductal system in this primitive species triggered time-dependent severe necrotizing pancreatitis. In our studies (7), we ligated the opossum common bile duct, main pancreatic duct, and common biliopancreatic duct in ways that elicited either isolated pancreatic duct obstruction, isolated bile duct obstruction, or combined pancreatic and bile duct obstruction. In the latter case, we created two subgroups of animals, those with bile and pancreatic duct obstruction that permitted bile reflux into the pancreatic duct and those in which the ductal obstructions were noncommunicating and reflux was not possible. We then compared the time-dependence and severity of the resulting pancreatitis in each of our experimental groups and found that both the time-dependent evolution and the severity of the resulting pancreatitis were identical for all groups of animals with pancreatic duct obstruction, regardless of whether or not bile reflux was possible. In addition, we found that bile duct obstruction, either with or without reflux, did not worsen the severity of pancreatitis induced by pancreatic duct obstruction. Based on these observations, we concluded that biliary pancreatitis is triggered by pancreatic duct obstruction and that the common channel theory and bile reflux into the pancreatic duct are not valid explanations for the evolution of that disease.

Where Pancreatitis Begins

Considerable controversy has surrounded the question of where, within the pancreas, acute pancreatitis might begin. Some have argued that pancreatitis begins in periductal areas as a result of pancreatic duct disruption triggered by ductal hypertension (or even bile reflux into the pancreatic ductal system) [8]. They suggest that this might trigger pancreatitis by allowing digestive enzymes in pancreatic juice to gain access to the gland parenchyma. Others have suggested that pancreatitis begins in perilobular areas as a result of alterations in parenchymal perfusion during the early stages of the disease [9]. They suggest that this might trigger pancreatitis by making watershed structures, including peripancreatic fat and the periphery of lobules, ischemic. Finally, some investigators have argued that pancreatitis begins within pancreatic acinar cells as a result of as yet to be defined alterations in acinar cell biology.

We have employed the opossum model of pancreatitis to examine these three competing theories [10]. We induced pancreatitis by ligating the terminal biliopancreatic duct and sacrificed the opossums at short, timed intervals. We found that the earliest changes we could identify were localized to acinar cells. Within 6 h of duct ligation, foci of acinar cells appeared necrotic and, by 12 h after duct ligation, those foci had enlarged and coalesced. Evidence of perilobular or periductal injury was not observed until 24 h had elapsed following duct ligation. These observations, made with the opossum model, suggested to us that pancreatitis begins within pancreatic acinar cells. The remainder of this review will be devoted to the mechanisms responsible for the early intra-acinar cell changes of pancreatitis and to the relationship between those changes and the eventual severity of a pancreatitis attack.

Pathophysiology of Acute Pancreatitis

Digestive Injury and Inflammation

Injury to the pancreas caused by digestive enzymes that are normally synthesized and released by the gland is generally believed to be the immediate cause of pancreatitis. This belief is based on three frequently made observations: (1) the pancreas normally synthesizes a wide variety of digestive enzymes which might, theoretically, injure the gland; (2) the morphologic changes of pancreatitis resemble those that might be seen during digestive injury; (3) activated pancreatic digestive enzymes can be detected within the pancreas during the early stages of both experimental and clinical pancreatitis. On the other hand, for the most part the potentially harmful enzymes that are synthesized and secreted by pancreatic acinar cells are, under physiological conditions, synthesized and secreted as inactive proenzymes or zymogens, and activation occurs only when these enzymes reach the duodenum where enterokinase activates trypsinogen and the resulting trypsin activates the other zymogens. Furthermore, potent trypsin inhibitors are synthesized and cotransported with trypsinogen and the other zymogens through the cell so that small amounts of prematurely activated trypsin might be inhibited before further zymogen activation has occurred. How, then, might trypsin and the other digestive enzymes become prematurely activated within acinar cells, and how might this lead to pancreatitis? Because of the central importance of this question to the pathogenesis of pancreatitis, it is not surprising that considerable experimental effort has been devoted toward defining the mechanisms by which premature, intrapancreatic (and even intra-acinar cell) activation of those zymogens, to a degree sufficient to cause pancreatitis, might occur.

In addition to pancreatic injury, acute pancreatitis is characterized by an acute intrapancreatic inflammatorv process. In severe cases, that inflammatory process is not confined to the pancreas but, rather, it becomes systemic and it is manifested by the systemic immune response syndrome as well as distant organ injury including an acute lung injury that may clinically present as the adult respiratory response syndrome. It is generally believed that these inflammatory processes play a critical role in determining the severity of a pancreatitis attack and, as has been extensively documented, the severity of pancreatitis is closely related to both its morbidity and its mortality. It is not surprising, therefore, that considerable experimental effort has also been devoted toward defining the mechanisms that regulate these inflammatory events and toward developing potentially therapeutic or prophylactic methods of aborting them.

To a great extent, the remainder of this review will focus on both of these issues, the intra-acinar cell activation of digestive enzymes and the regulation of inflammatory events during the early stages of pancreatitis. Unfortunately, studies dealing with both of these issues using clinical material have not been possible because most patients with pancreatitis are not identified during this early stage of their disease and because access to pancreatic tissue during the early stages of pancreatitis is usually not possible. As a consequence, most of the studies dealing with these issues have been conducted using models of the disease in experimental animals. Not surprisingly, therefore, the relevance of those studies to the clinical situation has been frequently challenged and this issue remains the subject of considerable emotion and controversy, which can only be eventually resolved when and if such studies lead to the identification of clinically useful pancreatitis treatments. To date, unfortunately, that has not been the case, but efforts at achieving that goal continue.

Table 16.2. Experimental models of acute pancreatitis

Model	Animal	Time	Severity
Retrograde duct injection	Rat, Mouse	Hours–Days	Severe
Diet-induced	Mouse	Days	Severe and Lethal
Secretagogue-induced	Rat, Mouse	Hours	Mild to Moderate
Duct Obstruction	Opossum	Days	Severe
Closed duodenal loop	Rat	Days	Severe
Arginine-induced	Rat, Mouse	Days	Severe
Secretagogue + injection	Rat	Hours	Variable

Experimental Models of Acute Pancreatitis

The various experimental models of pancreatitis are listed in Table 16.2. The oldest and the classical model of acute pancreatitis involves retrograde injection of bile (or bile acids with or without trypsin) into the pancreatic duct of rats [11] or larger animals including dogs and cats. Unfortunately, this model of severe pancreatitis has proven to be difficult to control and, in many cases, the extensive mechanical injury elicited with this model may prelude mechanistic studies focused on cell biological events. In the mid-1970s, this field of research was suddenly stimulated by the description of two newer, more controllable, experimental models. One involved feeding young female mice an ethionine-supplemented, choline-deficient diet which, within 5 days of its start, elicited lethal hemorrhagic pancreatic necrosis (i.e., diet-induced pancreatitis) [12]. The other model involved exposing rats to doses of the cholecystokinin analog cerulein that were in excess of those that elicited a maximal rate of digestive enzyme secretion from the exocrine pancreas [13]. Within hours of the start of this supramaximal stimulation, extensive edematous pancreatitis was observed and, subsequently, this so-called secretagogue-induced model has been employed extensively in efforts to characterize early acinar cell events in pancreatitis. Similar treatment of mice leads to a more severe, hemorrhagic and necrotizing pancreatitis but, in both species, the secretagogue-induced disease is self-limited and reversible. Because of its simplicity, high reproducibility, and relatively low cost, the secretagogue-induced models of pancreatitis elicited in either rats or mice have been employed extensively and they are, by far, the best characterized of the pancreatitis models. As noted previously, pancreatitis can also be elicited by ligating the biliopancreatic duct of the American opossum [6]. Although this model would appear to be justified by clinical observations linking biliopancreatic duct obstruction to pancreatitis, it is an infrequently used model because of its relatively high cost and because of difficulties encountered when working with these wild, parasite-infected, animals. Several other models of pancreatitis have also been described, including one elicited by the creation of a closed duodenal loop in rats [14], one elicited by giving rats toxic doses of L-arginine [15], and another, in rats, which combines bile salt injection into the pancreatic duct with supramaximal secretagogue stimulation [16]. These latter models are only used infrequently and it is not clear whether they offer any particular advantages over the more frequently described and better-characterized models mentioned previously.

Digestive Enzyme Activation and the "Colocalization Theory"

Along with other proteins, digestive enzymes are assembled within the cisternae of the rough endoplasmic reticulum of acinar cells. They are transported vectorially to the Golgi stacks where newly synthesized proteins are sorted prior to being intracellularly transported to their ultimate destinations. Most of the digestive enzymes, destined for secretion from the cell, are synthesized as inactive proenzymes or zymogens. They pass through the Golgi apparatus and are packaged within condensing vacuoles, which migrate toward the luminal surface of the cell. During this migration, the contents of those vacuoles become increasingly more electron-dense, as condensing vacuoles mature into zymogen granules. Eventually, the zymogen granules undergo regulated fusion/fission at the luminal surface and their contents are extruded into the acinar lumen – a space that is continuous with the ductal space [17]. In contrast to the simple passage of digestive enzyme zymogens through the Golgi stacks and their packaging into condensing vacuoles, the nonsecretory enzymes destined to undergo transport to lysosomes are posttranslationally glycosylated and then phosphorylated as they pass through the Golgi. The resulting 6-mannose phosphorylated lysosomal hydrolases are bound by 6-mannose-specific receptors, which facilitate their transport to the prelysosomal compartment and away from the secretory pathway [18]. This process, however, is incomplete and some lysosomal hydrolases escape segregation as they are trapped within the secretory pathway [19]. In addition, a fraction of newly synthesized lysosomal hydrolases is transported to a subspecies of lysosomes that are themselves capable of being secreted (i.e., secretory lysosomes) [20]. Together, these two phenomena account for the observation that a small fraction of newly synthesized lysosomal hydrolases appear in exocrine pancreatic secretions.

The vast majority of digestive enzyme zymogens remain unactivated as they pass through the acinar cell and, after their exocytosis from acinar cells, through the ductal space. Activation normally occurs when they reach the duodenum, where the brush border enzyme enterokinase activates trypsinogen and trypsin activates the other zymogens. Trypsinogen can also be activated by the lysosomal hydrolase cathepsin B [21] (and, perhaps, by other lysosomal hydrolases), but that activation is minimized under physiological conditions because the two types of enzyme (lysosomal and zymogen) are mostly segregated from each other.

More than two decades ago, we hypothesized that a breakdown in this segregation might occur during the early stages of acute pancreatitis and that the colocalization of digestive enzyme zymogens with lysosomal hydrolases could lead to intra-acinar cell activation of trypsinogen catalyzed by the lysosomal hydrolase cathepsin B [22]. Furthermore, we suggested that if that were to occur, activation of the other zymogens by the newly generated trypsin might also occur and that might lead to the cell injury that underlies pancreatitis.

In the subsequent two decades, many studies have been performed by our group as well as others, which have used the various models of experimental pancreatitis to test this so-called colocalization theory and, for the most part, the predictions of that theory have been borne out. Lysosomal hydrolases including cathepsin B have been shown to be capable of activating trypsinogen [21], and colocalization of digestive zymogens and lysosomal hydrolases, documented by subcellular fraction and/or immunolocalization techniques, has been found in virtually all of the experimental models of acute pancreatitis [23–26]. The mechanisms responsible for the colocalization phenomenon appear to differ between the different models. In the diet-induced model, it appears to reflect fusion of zymogen granules with lysosomes (crinophagy) [23], while in the secretagogue model, it appears to reflect crinophagy as well as missorting of lysosomal hydrolases as they traverse the Golgi stacks [24]. In the duct-obstruction opossum model, colocalization reflects the fact that some of the secreted digestive zymogens are taken up by acinar cells and incorporated within the endocytic/lysosomal compartment following their endocytosis [24]. In all cases, however, colocalization has been found to occur prior to the appearance of cell injury and to be coincident with the onset of digestive enzyme activation [27]. Both the colocalization of digestive enzyme zymogens with lysosomal hydrolases and the intra-acinar cell activation of trypsinogen have been observed to occur at the same site [28]. Interventions that prevent colocalization have been shown to prevent zymogen activation and to reduce the severity of pancreatitis [29]. In addition, either genetic or pharmacological interventions that interfere with cathepsin-B-induced activation of trypsinogen by either deleting or inhibiting cathepsin B have also been shown to reduce the severity of pancreatitis [30]. Finally, in vitro systems have been developed with which supramaximal secretagogue stimulation can be shown to promote the colocalization phenomenon and cause both intra-acinar cell digestive enzyme activation and acinar cell injury/necrosis [31, 32]. Very recently, these in-vitro systems have been exploited to examine, in molecular terms, potential mechanisms that are involved in the colocalization phenomenon. De Lisle has shown that it may involve a change in zymogen or lysosomal hydrolase processing within the Golgi, while Lu et al. [33] and Perides et al. [34] have shown that in addition to the rise in calcium and activation of protein kinase C that follow physiological stimulation of acinar cells with cholecystokinin, the colocalization phenomenon and intra-acinar cell activation of zymogens is further increased by cyclic AMP and activation of protein kinase A. Very recently, Gorelick's group [35] has reported studies that suggest that release of the ryanodine-sensitive, rather than the inisitol-trisphosphate-sensitive, pool of calcium is responsible for intracellular activation of zymogens during supramaximal secretagogue stimulation. It is likely that future studies using these in vitro systems will further expand our understanding of the molecular events that couple supramaximal secretagogue stimulation with intracellular zymogen activation and acinar cell injury. Whether or not these same events play critical roles in the early stages of clinical pancreatitis is obviously open to question, but it is hoped that this further understanding of the effects of supramaximal stimulation will permit the development of clinically useful interventions that suppress those events and, furthermore, that suppression of those events will beneficially effect the course of clinical pancreatitis.

Inflammation and Pancreatitis

Acute intrapancreatic inflammation is one of the hallmarks of acute pancreatitis, and systemic inflammatory syndromes are typically observed in cases of severe acute pancreatitis. Considerable experimental effort has been devoted toward achieving an understanding of the events that underlie and regulate the extent of these inflammatory processes, and a complex picture has emerged. Central to that picture is the concept that intracellular zymogen activation and the onset of the inflammatory process are parallel but, to a considerable extent, independent phenomena. The events responsible for the former have been summarized above and, to a great extent, they are not dependent upon the early events that mediate inflammation. It is likely that zymogen activation and the acinar cell injury that is triggered by zymogen activation eventually leads to acinar cell necrosis, which itself further promotes inflammation. Regardless of these later events, however, the early events responsible for inflammation have already been triggered before zymogen activation and cell injury/necrosis have occurred.

The vast majority of the studies exploring the inflammation-related issues of pancreatitis have been performed using either the secretagogue-induced models of experimental pancreatitis or in vitro systems that involve exposing rodent pancreatic acini to supramaximally stimulating concentrations of cerulein. In the absence of complimentary studies using other models and other in vitro systems, the ability to generalize the observations reported to date must be considered tentative at best and, as noted previously, their relevance to the issue of clinical acute pancreatitis remains uncertain. In spite of these caveats, however, they are noteworthy and they may lead to important insights that allow for the development of clinically useful therapies for pancreatitis.

To date, the reported studies examining inflammatory events in rodents exposed to supramaximal secretagogue stimulation or rodent pancreatic acini exposed to supramaximally stimulating concentrations of cerulein have shown that these interventions result in a rather broad-spectrum triggering of responses. At very early stages, there is upregulation of stress kinase activating cascades [36–39] involving p-38 mitogen activated protein kinase (p38-MAPK), extracellular signal-regulated kinases 1 and 2 (ERK1/2), and N-terminal jun kinase (JNK). In addition, the inflammation-related transcription factors AP-1 and NF-κB are activated [40–43] and the expression of a large number of inflammatory mediators is altered [44–50]. To a great extent, these inflammatory mediators are known to have overlapping effects, and defining those effects has proven difficult. Perhaps the most successful strategy has involved the use of genetically modified mouse strains that either do not express the gene responsible for a mediator or, less frequently, overexpress that gene. Those studies have indicated that some of the relevant mediators trigger proinflammatory events such as increased vascular permeability (i.e., edema) or the activation and recruitment to the pancreas of inflammatory cells while other mediators exert anti-inflammatory effects [51–54]. Ultimately, the extent of the inflammatory response in pancreatitis reflects the balance between these two opposing phenomena.

Other Acinar Cell Events that may Play Roles in the Pathogenesis of Acute Pancreatitis

In addition to intracellular zymogen activation and the triggering of an inflammatory reaction, several other events have been observed during the early stages of some models of experimental pancreatitis and shortly after supramaximal stimulation of acini under in vitro conditions. While it is likely that many, if not all, of these events play important roles in the pathogenesis of pancreatitis, a detailed description of these events is beyond the scope of this review. For the sake of completeness, however, they will be briefly mentioned.

Cytoskeletal Changes

Profound cytoskeletal changes within acinar cells are observed shortly after either in vivo or in vitro supramaximal stimulation [55]. The subapical f-actin web becomes disorganized and f-actin is redistributed from its subapical location to the basolateral region of the cell. Most of the evidence suggests that the subapical f-actin web plays an important role in regulating secretion from acinar cells [56], and this redistribution phenomenon has been thought to be the basis for the inhibition of secretion that accompanies supra-maximal secretagogue stimulation. Recent studies, however, challenge this conclusion since, under appropriate conditions, the redistribution phenomenon can be observed in the absence of inhibited secretion [34]. Its role in pancreatitis, however, remains to be established.

Reactive Oxygen Species and Glutathione

Several experimental studies have indicated that pancreatic levels of reactive oxygen species are increased during the early stages of pancreatitis [57–60] and that acinar cell levels of reduced glutathione are diminished [61]. It is likely that both of these changes contribute to acinar cell injury during pancreatitis, but they appear to occur subsequent to intraacinar cell zymogen activation and the early inflammatory events described above. Taken together, these findings suggest that reactive oxygen species and reduced glutathione play important secondary, but not primary, roles in the pathogenesis of pancreatitis.

Proteinase-Activated Receptor-2

Pancreatic acinar cells express functional proteinase-activated receptors belonging to the PAR2 class [62, 63]. In other systems, PAR2 has generally been considered as a proinflammatory receptor, activation of which worsens inflammatory processes [64]. In the case of pancreatic PAR2, however, this interesting tethered ligand receptor appears to promote anti-inflammatory events and deletion of PAR2 markedly worsens acute pancreatitis [65, 66]. Since trypsin is the primary activator of PAR2, these findings suggest the provocative teleologically based hypothesis that pancreatic PAR2 has evolved because it mediates a protective response to prematurely activated trypsinogen within the pancreas. The mechanisms responsible for this protection are as yet undefined but preliminary observations suggest that they involve the downregulation of proinflammatory signals during the early phases of pancreatitis [67].

Heat Shock Proteins

Heat shock proteins (HSPs) are generated by pancreatic cells during the early stages of pancreatitis and there is considerable evidence that at least two types of HSP (HSP27 and HSP70) exert a protective effect on pancreatitis severity [68, 69]. The mechanisms responsible for this protection have not been fully established, but there is the suggestion that prior activation of the HSP system might be of prophylactic benefit in the management of pancreatitis.

Apoptosis/Necrosis

While the earliest events in pancreatitis appear to promote acinar cell injury, the cellular response to that injury and the mode of cell death after injury may have profound effects on the subsequent course and severity of pancreatitis. In a general sense, cells die by either apoptosis or necrosis. In the former, sometimes referred to as programmed cell death, the dead cells are eliminated by being phagocytosed by neighboring cells and little or no inflammatory reaction is triggered. Necrosis, on the other hand, involves cell disruption and the triggering of an intense inflammatory response. Considerable evidence has now accumulated that suggests that the induction of apoptosis lessens the severity of pancreatitis, while the induction of necrosis makes pancreatitis more severe [70]. Commitment to one or the other form of cell death appears to occur relatively early during the course of an attack and many of the mediators that appear to regulate the severity of pancreatitis have been shown to act by altering the balance between apoptosis and necrosis.

Inflammatory and Neural Cells

Most of this review has focused on events involving pancreatic acinar cells during pancreatitis, but there is also evidence that events involving other cell types may play equally important roles in mediating acute pancreatitis. The inflammatory response to pancreatitis described above results in pancreatic generation of many pro- and anti-inflammatory mediators. Some of those mediators function to activate and recruit a variety of inflammatory cells to the pancreas. Among these responsive cells, neutrophils and macrophages may be of primary importance because they can generate additional proinflammatory signals and because, by releasing reactive factors, they may worsen the severity of pancreatic injury. Nerve cells may also play important roles in mediating the early events in pancreatitis via their ability to trigger neurogenic inflammation in response to release of agents such as substance P [71] or in response to PAR2 stimulation [72].

Summary

Acute pancreatitis is a complex but poorly understood disease that can be triggered by several associated processes. Biliary tract stone disease is the most frequent cause of acute pancreatitis, and most of the evidence suggests that the offending stone triggers pancreatitis by obstructing the pancreatic duct. By as yet unidentified mechanisms, that obstruction triggers changes in pancreatic acinar cells, which lead to digestive zymogen/lysosomal hydrolase colocalization, cathepsin-B-catalyzed trypsinogen activation, and acinar cell injury/necrosis. By parallel pathways, it also triggers a series of acinar cell inflammatory events that culminate in the elaboration of several pro- and anti-inflammatory mediators that regulate the severity of pancreatitis. The pathophysiology of acute pancreatitis is also dependent upon several other events including acinar cell cytoskeletal changes, the generation or reactive oxygen species, depletion of reduced glutathione, activation of PAR2, generation of HSPs, the balance between apoptosis and necrosis, the activation and/or recruitment of inflammatory cells to the pancreas, and the triggering of neurogenic inflammation Our understanding of each of these phenomena is still in its infancy but, with further elucidation, it is hoped that methods of treating and/or preventing acute pancreatitis will be identified.

References

1. Acosta JM, Ledesma CL (1974) Gallstone migration as a cause of acute pancreatitis. N Engl J Med 290:484–487
2. Acosta MJ, Rossi R, Ledesma CL (1977) The usefulness of stool screening for diagnosing cholelithiasis in acute pancreatitis. A description of the technique. Am J Dig Dis 22:168–172
3. Opie EL (1901) The etiology of acute hemorrhagic pancreatitis. Bull Johns Hopkins Hosp 12:182–192
4. Opie EL (1901) The relationship of cholelithiasis to disease of the pancreas and fat necrosis. Am J Med Surg 12:27–40
5. McCutcheon AD (1964) Reflux of duodenal contents in the pathogenesis of pancreatitis. Gut 25:260–265
6. Senninger N, Moody FG, Coelho JC, Van Buren DH (1986) The role of biliary obstruction in the pathogenesis of acute pancreatitis in the opossum. Surgery 99:688–693
7. Lerch MM, Saluja AK, Runzi M, Dawra R, Saluja M, Steer ML (1993) Pancreatic duct obstruction triggers acute necrotizing pancreatitis in the opossum. Gastroenterology 104:853–861
8. Foulis AK (1980) Histological evidence of initiating factors in acute necrotising pancreatitis in man. J Clin Pathol 33:1125–1131
9. Kloppel G, Dreyer T, Willemer S, Kern HF, Adler G (1986) Human acute pancreatitis: its pathogenesis in the light of immunocytochemical and ultrastructural findings in acinar cells. Virchows Arch A Pathol Anat Histopathol 409:791–803
10. Lerch MM, Saluja AK, Dawra R, Ramarao P, Saluja M, Steer ML (1992) Acute necrotizing pancreatitis in the opossum: earliest morphological changes involve acinar cells. Gastroenterology 103:205–213
11. Aho HJ, Koskensalo SM, Nevalainen TJ (1980) Experimental pancreatitis in the rat. Sodium taurocholate-induced acute haemorrhagic pancreatitis. Scand J Gastroenterol 15:411–416
12. Lombardi B, Estes LW, Longnecker DS (1975) Acute hemorrhagic pancreatitis (massive necrosis) with fat necrosis induced in mice by DL-ethionine fed with a choline-deficient diet. Am J Pathol 79:465–480
13. Lampel M, Kern HF (1977) Acute interstitial pancreatitis in the rat induced by excessive doses of a pancreatic secretagogue. Virchows Arch A Pathol Anat Histol 373:97–117
14. Pfeffer RB, Stasior O, Hinton JW (1957) The clinical picture of the sequential development of acute hemorrhagic pancreatitis in the dog. Surg Forum 8:248–251
15. Tani S, Itoh H, Okabayashi Y, Nakamura T, Fujii M, Fujisawa T, Koide M, Otsuki M (1990) New model of acute necrotizing pancreatitis induced by excessive doses of arginine in rats. Dig Dis Sci 35:367–374
16. Schmidt J, Rattner DW, Lewandrowski K, Compton CC, Mandavilli U, Knoefel WT, Warshaw AL (1992) A better model of acute pancreatitis for evaluating therapy. Ann Surg 215:44–56
17. Palade G (1975) Intracellular aspects of the process of protein synthesis. Science 189:347–358
18. Kornfeld S (1986) Trafficking of lysosomal enzymes in normal and disease states. J Clin Invest 77:1–6
19. Hirano T, Saluja A, Ramarao P, Lerch MM, Saluja M, Steer ML (1991) Apical secretion of lysosomal enzymes in rabbit pancreas occurs via a secretagogue regulated pathway and is increased after pancreatic duct obstruction. J Clin Invest 87:865–869
20. Bossi G, Griffiths GM (2005) CTL secretory lysosomes: biogenesis and secretion of a harmful organelle. Semin Immunol 17:87–94
21. Figarella C, Miszczuk-Jamska B, Barrett AJ (1988) Possible lysosomal activation of pancreatic zymogens. Activation of both human trypsinogens by cathepsin B and spontaneous acid. Activation of human trypsinogen 1. Biol Chem Hoppe Seyler 369 Suppl:293–298
22. Steer ML, Meldolesi J, Figarella C (1984) Pancreatitis. The role of lysosomes. Dig Dis Sci 29:934–938
23. Koike H, Steer ML, Meldolesi J (1982) Pancreatic effects of ethionine: blockade of exocytosis and appearance of crinophagy and autophagy precede cellular necrosis. Am J Physiol 242:G297–307
24. Lerch MM, Saluja AK, Runzi M, Dawra R, Steer ML (1995) Luminal endocytosis and intracellular targeting by acinar cells during early biliary pancreatitis in the opossum. J Clin Invest 95:2222–2231
25. Saluja A, Hashimoto S, Saluja M, Powers RE, Meldolesi J, Steer ML (1987) Subcellular redistribution of lysosomal enzymes during caerulein-induced pancreatitis. Am J Physiol 253: G508–516
26. Saluja A, Saluja M, Villa A, Leli U, Rutledge P, Meldolesi J, Steer M (1989) Pancreatic duct obstruction in rabbits causes digestive zymogen and lysosomal enzyme colocalization. J Clin Invest 84:1260–1266
27. Grady T, Saluja A, Kaiser A, Steer M (1996) Edema and intrapancreatic trypsinogen activation precede glutathione depletion during caerulein pancreatitis. Am J Physiol 271: G20–26

28. Hofbauer B, Saluja AK, Lerch MM, Bhagat L, Bhatia M, Lee HS, Frossard JL, Adler G, Steer ML (1998) Intra-acinar cell activation of trypsinogen during caerulein-induced pancreatitis in rats. Am J Physiol 275:G352–362
29. Singh VP, Saluja AK, Bhagat L, van Acker GJ, Song AM, Soltoff SP, Cantley LC, Steer ML (2001) Phosphatidylinositol 3-kinase-dependent activation of trypsinogen modulates the severity of acute pancreatitis. J Clin Invest 108:1387–1395
30. van Acker GJ, Saluja AK, Bhagat L, Singh VP, Song AM, Steer ML (2002) Cathepsin B inhibition prevents trypsinogen activation and reduces pancreatitis severity. Am J Physiol Gastrointest Liver Physiol 283:G794–800
31. Leach SD, Modlin IM, Scheele GA, Gorelick FS (1991) Intracellular activation of digestive zymogens in rat pancreatic acini. Stimulation by high doses of cholecystokinin. J Clin Invest 87:362–366
32. Saluja AK, Donovan EA, Yamanaka K, Yamaguchi Y, Hofbauer B, Steer ML (1997) Cerulein-induced in vitro activation of trypsinogen in rat pancreatic acini is mediated by cathepsin B. Gastroenterology 113:304–310
33. Lu Z, Kolodecik TR, Karne S, Nyce M, Gorelick F (2003) Effect of ligands that increase cAMP on caerulein-induced zymogen activation in pancreatic acini. Am J Physiol Gastrointest Liver Physiol 285:G822–828
34. Perides G, Sharma A, Gopal A, Tao X, Dwyer K, Ligon B, Steer ML (2005) Secretin differentially sensitizes rat pancreatic acini to the effects of supramaximal stimulation with caerulein. Am J Physiol Gastrointest Liver Physiol 289: G713–721
35. Husain SZ, Prasad P, Grant WM, Kolodecik TR, Nathanson MH, Gorelick FS (2005) The ryanodine receptor mediates early zymogen activation in pancreatitis. Proc Natl Acad Sci U S A 102:14386–14391
36. Clemons AP, Holstein DM, Galli A, Saunders C (2002) Cerulein-induced acute pancreatitis in the rat is significantly ameliorated by treatment with MEK1/2 inhibitors U0126 and PD98059. Pancreas 25:251–259
37. Dabrowski A, Grady T, Logsdon CD, Williams JA (1996) Jun kinases are rapidly activated by cholecystokinin in rat pancreas both in vitro and in vivo. J Biol Chem 271:5686–5690
38. Dabrowski A (2003) Exocrine pancreas; molecular basis for intracellular signaling, damage and protection – Polish experience. J Physiol Pharmacol 54 Suppl 3:167–181
39. Wagner AC, Metzler W, Hofken T, Weber H, Goke B (1999) p38 map kinase is expressed in the pancreas and is immediately activated following cerulein hyperstimulation. Digestion 60:41–47
40. Blinman TA, Gukovsky I, Mouria M, Zaninovic V, Livingston E, Pandol SJ, Gukovskaya AS (2000) Activation of pancreatic acinar cells on isolation from tissue: cytokine upregulation via p38 MAP kinase. Am J Physiol Cell Physiol 279: C1993–2003
41. Gukovsky I, Gukovskaya AS, Blinman TA, Zaninovic V, Pandol SJ (1998) Early NF-kappaB activation is associated with hormone-induced pancreatitis. Am J Physiol 275:G1402–1414
42. Han B, Logsdon CD (1999) Cholecystokinin induction of mob-1 chemokine expression in pancreatic acinar cells requires NF-kappaB activation. Am J Physiol 277:C74–82
43. Steinle AU, Weidenbach H, Wagner M, Adler G, Schmid RM (1999) NF-kappaB/Rel activation in cerulein pancreatitis. Gastroenterology 116:420–430
44. Fink GW, Norman JG (1997) Specific changes in the pancreatic expression of the interleukin 1 family of genes during experimental acute pancreatitis. Cytokine, 9:1023–1027
45. Denham W, Fink G, Yang J, Ulrich P, Tracey K, Norman J (1997) Small molecule inhibition of tumor necrosis factor gene processing during acute pancreatitis prevents cytokine cascade progression and attenuates pancreatitis severity. Am Surg 63:1045–1049; discussion 1049–50
46. Frossard JL, Past CM (2002) Experimental acute pancreatitis: new insights into the pathophysiology. Front Biosci 7: d275–287
47. Frossard JL, Saluja AK, Mach N, Lee HS, Bhagat L, Hadenque A, Rubbia-Brandt L, Dranoff G, Steer ML (2002) In vivo evidence for the role of GM-CSF as a mediator in acute pancreatitis-associated lung injury. Am J Physiol Lung Cell Mol Physiol 283:L541–548
48. Osman MO, Gesser B, Mortensen JT, Matsushima K, Jensen SL, Larsen CG (2002) Profiles of pro-inflammatory cytokines in the serum of rabbits after experimentally induced acute pancreatitis. Cytokine 17:53–59
49. Vaccaro MI, Ropolo A, Grasso D, Calvo EL, Ferreria M, Iovanna JL, Lanosa G (2000) Pancreatic acinar cells submitted to stress activate TNF-alpha gene expression. Brioche Biopsy's Rees Common 268:485–490
50. Gerard C, Frossard JL, Bhatia M, Saluja A, Gerard NP, Lu B, Steer M (1997) Targeted disruption of the beta-chemokine receptor CCR1 protects against pancreatitis-associated lung injury. J Clin Invest 100:2022–2027
51. Bhatia M, Saluja AK, Singh VP, Frossard JL, Lee HS, Bhagat L, Gerard C, Steer ML (2001) Complement factor C5a exerts an anti-inflammatory effect in acute pancreatitis and associated lung injury. Am J Physiol Gastrointest Liver Physiol 280: G974–978
52. Cuzzocrea S, Mizzen E, Dug L, Centurion T, Piccolo A, McDonald MC, de Sara A, Capote AP, Thiemermann C (2002) Absence of endogenous interleukin-6 enhances the inflammatory response during acute pancreatitis induced by cerulein in mice. Cytokine 18:274–285
53. Norman JG, Fink GW, Sexton C, Carter G (1996) Transgenic animals demonstrate a role for the IL-1 receptor in regulating IL-1beta gene expression at steady-state and during the systemic stress induced by acute pancreatitis. J Surg Rees 63:231–236
54. Tietz AB, Wagner AC, Gastec M, Goke B, Schafer C (2004) Gene deletion of MAPKAPK-1 inhibits TNF-a and protects against cerulein-induced pancreatitis. Gastroenterology 126 (Suppl 2):A105
55. O'Konski MS, Pandol SJ (1990) Effects of caerulein on the apical cytoskeleton of the pancreatic acinar cell. J Clin Invest 86:1649–1657
56. Muallem S, Kwiatkowska K, Xu X, Yin HL (1995) Actin filament disassembly is a sufficient final trigger for exocytosis in nonexcitable cells. J Cell Biol 128:589–598
57. Sanfey H, Bulkley GB, Cameron JL (1984) The role of oxygen-derived free radicals in the pathogenesis of acute pancreatitis. Ann Surg 200:405–413
58. Schoenberg MH, Buchler M, Gaspar M, Stinner A, Younes M, Melzner I, Bultmann B, Beger HG (1990) Oxygen free radicals in acute pancreatitis of the rat. Gut 31:1138–1143
59. Rutledge PL, Saluja AK, Powers RE, Steer ML (1987) Role of oxygen-derived free radicals in diet-induced hemorrhagic pancreatitis in mice. Gastroenterology 93:41–47

60. Guice KS, Miller DE, Oldham KT, Townsend CM Jr, Thompson JC (1986) Superoxide dismutase and catalase: a possible role in established pancreatitis. Am J Surg 151:163–169
61. Neuschwander-Tetri BA, Ferrell LD, Sukhabote RJ, Grendell JH (1992) Glutathione monoethyl ester ameliorates caerulein-induced pancreatitis in the mouse. J Clin Invest 89:109–116
62. Kawabata A, Nishikawa H, Kuroda R, Kawai K, Hollenberg MD (2000) Proteinase-activated receptor-2 (PAR-2): regulation of salivary and pancreatic exocrine secretion in vivo in rats and mice. Br J Pharmacol 129:1808–1814
63. Sharma A, Tao X, Gopal A, Ligon B, Steer ML, Perides G (2005) Calcium dependence of proteinase-activated receptor 2 and cholecystokinin-mediated amylase secretion from pancreatic acini. Am J Physiol Gastrointest Liver Physiol 289: G686–695
64. Coughlin SR, Camerer E (2003) PARticipation in inflammation. J Clin Invest 111:25–27
65. Namkung W, Han W, Luo X, Muallem S, Cho KH, Kim KH, Lee MG (2004) Protease-activated receptor 2 exerts local protection and mediates some systemic complications in acute pancreatitis. Gastroenterology 126:1844–1859
66. Sharma A, Tao X, Gopal A, Ligon B, Andrade-Gordon P, Steer ML, Perides G (2005) Protection against acute pancreatitis by activation of protease-activated receptor-2. Am J Physiol Gastrointest Liver Physiol 288:G388–395
67. Tao X, Sharma A, Dwyer K, DeLuca N, Steer ML, Perides G (2004) Par-2 activation protects against pancreatitis by inhibiting nuclear translocation of p38 MAPK and ERK 1/2. Pancreas 29:356
68. Kubisch C, Dimagno MJ, Tietz AB, Welsh MJ, Ernst SA, Brandt-Nedelev B, Diebold J, Wagner AC, Goke B, Williams JA, Schafer C (2004) Overexpression of heat shock protein Hsp27 protects against cerulein-induced pancreatitis. Gastroenterology 127:275–286
69. Bhagat L, Singh VP, Song AM, van Acker GJ, Agrawal S, Steer ML, Saluja AK (2002) Thermal stress-induced HSP70 mediates protection against intrapancreatic trypsinogen activation and acute pancreatitis in rats. Gastroenterology 122:156–165
70. Kaiser AM, Saluja AK, Sengupta A, Saluja M, Steer ML (1995) Relationship between severity, necrosis, apoptosis in five models of experimental acute pancreatitis. Am J Physiol 269:C1295–1304
71. Bhatia M, Saluja AK, Hofbauer B, Frossard JL, Lee HS, Castagliuolo I, Wang CC, Gerard N, Pothoulakis C, Steer ML (1998) Role of substance P and the neurokinin 1 receptor in acute pancreatitis and pancreatitis-associated lung injury. Proc Natl Acad Sci U S A 95:4760–4765
72. Hoogerwerf WA, Shenoy M, Winston JH, Xiao SY, He Z, Pasricha PJ (2004) Trypsin mediates nociception via the proteinase-activated receptor 2: a potentially novel role in pancreatic pain. Gastroenterology 127:883–891

Chapter 17

Natural Course of Acute Pancreatitis

H. G. Beger · B. M. Rau

Acute pancreatitis comprises a mild, self-limiting disease, and in about one-third of patients an inflammatory process that causes local and systemic complications, frequently resulting in a systemic organ dysfunction. With regard to pathomorphological, radiological, biochemical, and bacteriological data, several clinical subgroups have been defined that require different management approaches (Table 17.1). Pathomorphologically, acute pancreatitis ranges from edematous-interstitial pancreatitis, which is restricted to the pancreas, to a necrotizing process that includes pancreatic, retroperitoneal, and peripancreatic tissues. Since the initial description by Fitz in 1889 [1] the variability of the clinical manifestations in terms of local and systemic complications has stimulated investigators to study experimental acute pancreatitis, but clinical management approaches remain challenging.

Experimental and clinical data have produced considerable progress in the understanding of the pathophysiological events during the early stage of acute pancreatitis. However, the underlying pathogenetic processes responsible for the inflammatory cascade and the alteration in the acinus and duct cell compartments of the pancreas, the first hit to acinus and duct cells, are still unknown to a large extent in humans. Therefore, management of human acute pancreatitis has been empiric, and there are still conflicting opinions regarding therapeutic approaches. With the development of clinical-based multiparameter scores, such as the RANSON and the APACHE II systems [2–5], an important step toward the clinical stratification of severity was made.

At the beginning of the 1980s, the morphological features of pancreatic necrosis was established by the definition of infected necrosis, sterile necrosis, pancreatic abscess, and postacute pseudocysts as the principal determinants of clinical severity and overall survival [6–8]. The introduction of contrast-enhanced computed tomography (CECT) as a standard diagnostic measure for the early detection of necrosis has allowed the development of a basic staging system and resulted in an understanding of the correlation between the degree of pathomorphological changes in the pancreas and the pattern and frequency of local and systemic complications [8–13].

Table 17.1. Classification of acute pancreatitis based on pathomorphological and bacteriological criteria

1.	Interstitial-edematous pancreatitis
2.	Necrotizing pancreatitis with sterile necrosis
3.	Necrotizing pancreatitis with infected necrosis
4.	Necrotizing pancreatitis with pancreatic and retroperitoneal fatty tissue necrosis
5.	Pancreatic abscess
6.	Postacute pseudocysts

Classification of Acute Pancreatitis

Based on the Ulm data of the late 1980s, a new classification of acute pancreatitis has been proposed (Table 17.1). Pathomorphological and bacteriological criteria are corner stones for the differentiation of subgroups of acute pancreatitis [14]. There are five different pathomorphological entities of acute pancreatitis: (1) acute interstitial-edematous pancreatitis, (2) acute necrotizing pancreatitis with sterile or infected necrosis, (3) necrotizing pancreatitis with retroperitoneal fatty tissue necrosis, (4) postacute pancreatic pseudocysts, and (5) pancreatic abscess. During the following years this fundamental classification was supplemented by clinical and pathomorphological data put together at the international symposium in Atlanta 1993 [14]. The Atlanta classification has now been accepted worldwide as a clinical classification system, with the exception of the definition of systemic organ complications (Table 17.2).

The macroscopic and histological features of edematous-interstitial pancreatitis are interstitial edema, intrapancreatic tissue necrosis, intra- and

Table 17.2. Severe acute pancreatitis Atlanta classification [14]. *MOFS* Multiple organ failure syndrome

Local complications	Systemic complications
Pancreatic tissue necrosis	MOFS
Infected necrosis	Organ failure
Abscess	lung
Extended sterile necrosis	kidney
Pseudocyst	liver
Fluid collections	cardiocirculatory
Ascites	G7 bleeding
Pleural effusions	

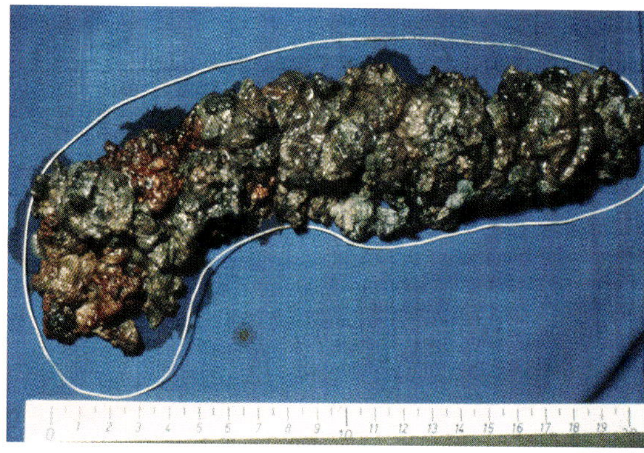

Figure 17.1

Operative specimen of hemorrhagic necrotizing pancreatitis

peripancreatic fatty tissue necrosis, and peripancreatic fluid collections [15]. Peripancreatic and remote retroperitoneal intra-abdominal fatty tissue necrosis may be present or absent [16]. Large retroperitoneal fatty tissue necrosis occurs as a separate entity in a minority of patients, but is mostly connected to extended intrapancreatic parenchymal necrosis. Most patients with acute pancreatitis – according to our own experience about two-thirds of the patients – suffer from edematous-interstitial pancreatitis, which is a self-limiting disease that responds well to vigorous fluid replacement and pain management.

Necrotizing pancreatitis is characterized macroscopically by focal or diffuse areas of devitalized pancreatic parenchyma and peripancreatic fatty tissue necrosis extending to different retroperitoneal spaces up to the pelvis. Intrapancreatic hemorrhage is variably present (Fig. 17.1). Microscopically, necrotizing pancreatitis includes extensive interstitial fatty tissue necrosis with vessel wall injury and necrosis affecting the acinus and ductal cells as well as the islet cell compartment. Infection of necrosis occurs in about 20–35% of all patients with necrotizing pancreatitis [11, 15–17].

In the clinical setting of acute pancreatitis, postacute pseudocysts and pancreatic abscess are late consequences of the disease. In both subgroups of acute pancreatitis, an inflammatory wall has developed that separates the process from the surrounding tissue and may be located within or around the pancreas [7, 12]. In half of patients with necrotizing pancreatitis, pancreatic pseudocysts have a connection with the pancreatic duct system, which has a major impact on treatment modalities. Postacute pseudocysts and pancreatic abscess develop after the necrotizing inflammatory process. In most instances postacute pseudocysts exhibit a combination of necrotic debridement and fluid accumulation in the pseudocystic cavity. Pancreatic abscesses are different from infected necrosis, they appears after the 3rd and 6th week of necrotizing pancreatitis. Both features are different with respect to clinical symptomatology and associated mortality [12, 18, 19]. The peripancreatic fluid collection that arises early during the course of acute pancreatitis is frequently a sign of severity; it does not have a wall surrounding it and has to be discriminated from postacute pseudocysts (Table 17.2).

Clinical Course

Acute pancreatitis is not a stable disease. The frequency and severity of local and systemic complications increase with increasing amounts of intrapancreatic and retroperitoneal necroses (Table 17.3). The beginning of the disease is marked by a sudden onset of abdominal pain located in the epigastrium, in the left upper quadrant in association with gallstone disease, or after large food and alcohol consumption. The pain frequently radiates into the middle of the back. In about 80% of patients there is an association between the clinical symptoms and elevations in the serum concentration of pancreatic enzymes (pancreatic amylase, pancreatic lipase, and elastase). Nausea and vomiting present are in most cases. In about two-thirds of patients with acute pancreatitis the disease takes a mild course and is associated only with minimal organ dysfunction. Clinical improvement can easily be achieved by fluid replacement, pain treatment, and continuation of enteral nutrition combined with a short period of parenteral food supplementation (if necessary). However, a small group of patients with interstitial-edematous pancreatitis may develop systemic complications (e.g., pulmonary and renal

Table 17.3. Clinical course of acute pancreatitis and severe acute pancreatitis. *D* Day, *HA* hospital admission, *ESAP* early severe acute pancreatitis, *IN* infected necrosis, *SPN* sterile pancreatic necrosis, *CARS* compensatory anti-inflammatory syndrome

	Clinical	Pathophysiologic process
Early D1–D2 after HA	Hypovolemia	Fluid sequestration
	Abdominal pain	Liberation of pro- and anti-inflammatory cytokines
ESAP in about 20%	Organ-Dysfunction	
	Pulmonary	Endotoxemia
	Renal	Hypovolemia
	Cardiocirculatory	Liberation of vasoactive substances
	Liver	Disturbance of blood coagulation
	Intestine	Translocation of endotoxin and bacteria
Late >2 weeks after HA	Local and systemic	CARS
	septic complications	
	IN, SPN	Immunosuppression
		Anti-inflammatory reaction

dysfunctions). Intensive care treatment results in resolution of the complications and cure of the attack [18–21]. The initial 24–72 h after the onset of symptoms are the crossroads where about 20–30% of all patients with acute pancreatitis take a severe clinical course of the disease. On the basis of clinical and experimental observations this period is characterized by an initial hypovolemic state. In severe acute pancreatitis hypotension or even shock is frequently observed, and is the leading feature as a result of fluid sequestration into the pancreas, the peripancreatic areas, and the abdominal cavity [20, 21]. Simultaneously, the first evidence of the subsequent systemic hyperinflammation leads to organ dysfunction involving the lungs, the kidney, the cardiocirculatory systems and the splanchnicus respective intestinal compartments (Table 17.3) [22, 23]. Based on computed tomography data, these patients with extended pancreatic necrosis demonstrate a strong morphological correlation between clinical severity and extent of intra- and extrapancreatic necrosis [8].

Early Severe Acute Pancreatitis

Patients who develop local complications, necrosis, infected necrosis, and retroperitoneal tissue necrosis frequently suffer systemic complications. Pulmonary, renal, cardiocirculatory, hepatic, and intestinal organ dysfunctions are considered systemic signs of severity. As evidenced by contrast-enhanced computed tomography observations and of C-reactive protein measurements, necrotizing pancreatitis develops early in the course, mostly in the 1st week of the disease. A subgroup of patients suffers an early severe form of acute pancreatitis (ESAP). In these cases, organ failure or even multiorgan failure occurs within 72 h after the onset of acute pancreatitis and is observed at hospital admission. By that time, most of the patients have developed necrotizing pancreatitis with extended necrosis. Despite application of maximum intensive care treatment measures, 30–50% of patients with ESAP do not respond and develop a complicated course involving multisystems organ failure. They have a high risk of mortality. The early mortality associated with severe acute pancreatitis is caused by systemic inflammatory response syndrome associated with early multiorgan insufficiency syndrome (Table 17.4) [23–27].

If the patient with severe acute pancreatitis has survived the critical early period of the disease, a septic complication caused by translocated bacteria, mostly Gram-negative microbes from the intestine, leads to infected necrosis. Infected necrosis leading to sepsis determines the patient's morbidity and late outcome. Pathomorphologically and bacteriologically, the septic phase of necrotizing pancreatitis peaks in the 3rd week of the disease. Infected necrosis is observed in up to 70% of the patients with extended necrosis, but occurs in a about 17% of all patients with severe acute pancreatitis. A pancreatic abscess develops in about 5% of patients with necrotizing pancreatitis [12, 24]. However, patients with extended necrosis, inside and outside of the pancreas, combined with retroperitoneal fatty tissue necrosis frequently suffer a sepsis-like syndrome without bacterial infection

Table 17.4. Acute pancreatitis – pattern of inflammation [57, 65]. *IAP* Interstitial-edematous pancreatitis, *SAP* severe acute pancreatitis, *NP* necrotizing pancreatitis, *OF* organ failure, *SIRS* systemic inflammatory response syndrome

MAP →	15–28% →	SAP
IAP/NP<50%		IN/SPN>50%
Proinflammatory cytokines		Pro-/anti-inflammatory cytokines
SIRS →	OF/MOF →	SEPSIS → MOFS
	ESAP<72 h	Immunosuppression (2nd–3rd week)
	Early mortality	Late mortality
	42–60%	22–33%

Table 17.5. Acute pancreatitis: evidence of compartmentalization of the inflammatory response. *TNF-α* Tumor necrosis factor α, *IL* interleukin, *IFγ* interferon gamma-8, *PGF-β* prostaglandin F-β, *MIF* macrophage migration inhibitory factor, *ICAM-1* intercellular adhesion molecule 1, *HLA-DR* major histocompatibility complex, class II, DR, *E/L/P* endothelial/leukocyte/platelet

Local		Systemic
Proinflammatory		Pro-/anti-inflammatory (CARS)
TNF-α		IL-6
IL-1β		IL-10
IL-2		PGF-β
IL-6		IL-1Ra
IL-8		sTNF-aRI/II
IFγ-8		PGE_2
MIF		Catecholamines
Endothelial response*:	First 3 days of	↓
	ICAM-1	
	E-/L-/P-selectine	
		Immunosuppression
		Deactivation of monocytes
		Reduction of HLA-DR expression**
		Loss of antigen-presenting activity

*Chooklin et al. 2005 [68]
**Mentula et al. 2004 [69].
Granger et al. 2005 [65]
Reijnen et al. 2001 [67]

and without a septic focus. Patients with extended sterile necrosis (>50% pancreatic necrosis on CECT) frequently develop local complications and systemic organ failure syndrome that affects the lungs, kidneys, liver, cardiovascular compartments, and the intestine [27–30]. These patients suffer increasing and persistent upper abdominal complaints: upper abdominal pain, prolonged and severe adynamic ileus, and frequently a palpable mass in the upper abdomen [19, 31, 32].

Pattern of Inflammation

The tissue response of the pancreas to an injury like necrotizing pancreatitis leads to liberation of proinflammatory cytokines, chemokines and other biological active compounds. Anti-inflammatory or modulatory molecules are also produced by the local inflammatory processes (Table 17.4) [33–40]. At the beginning of the disease, the blood contains a complex mixture of mediators including proinflammatory and anti-inflammatory cytokines and other biologically active compounds like prostaglandin F-α, catecholamines, and corticosteroids, which result after the initial inflammatory period in an immunosuppressed status. Measurements in humans have strong about compartmentalization of the inflammatory reaction within the body. High concentrations of local inflammatory cytokines exist simultaneously with predominantly anti-inflammatory compounds in the blood compartments of the systemic circulation (Table 17.5). A large body of data accumulated from animal experiments and humans have demonstrated convincingly a strong correlation between the circulating levels of cytokines and biologically active compounds, and the development of organ insufficiency, and eventually multiorgan failure syndrome [37–40].

Presence of Necrosis

Experimental and clinical observations have shown that development of pancreatic necrosis results in a dramatic increase in local and associated systemic organ complications and an increased risk of mortality compared to patients with interstitial-edematous pancreatitis. Most patients who develop early or late organ failure in association with acute pancreatitis suffer a necrotizing course [6, 25, 26]. Data derived from autopsy and surgical studies reveal that more than 80% of deaths as a result of acute pancreatitis are correlated with the presence of necrosis [25–27]. Edematous-interstitial pancreatitis parenchymal pancreatic necroses are present but not dominant. In 205 patients evaluated prospectively by preoperative CECT and intraoperative measurement of the extent of necrosis, 39% displayed focal necrosis (i.e., involving <30% of the pancreatic parenchyma), 37% displayed extended necrosis, (i.e., involving 30–50% of the pancreatic parenchyma), and 25% displayed necrosis involving >50% of the pancreatic parenchyma. The corresponding mortality rates were 8%, 18%, and 26%, respectively (Table 17.6) [49].

Extrapancreatic, Retroperitoneal Tissue Necrosis

Fatty tissue necrosis is also a pathomorphological feature of edematous-interstitial and necrotizing acute pancreatitis. However, in addition to the presence of pancreatic parenchymal necrosis, the occurrence and extent of a necrotizing process into the extrapancreatic retroperitoneal fatty tissue spaces – including the tissue compartments of the mesentery of the small and large bowel, the perirenal fat, and the retroperitoneal para- and retrocolic compartments – are important factors determining the course of the disease and strongly effect the clinical severity and mortality [6, 27, 30, 32]. Involvement of the large bowel, particularly the mesentery of the colon transversum and the large bowel wall, in necrotizing pancreatitis has been shown to be a deleterious complication [32]. The presence of extrapancreatic fatty tissue necrosis increases significantly the morbidity and mortality. In addition, patients who suffer intrapancreatic parenchymal necrosis and retroperitoneal fatty tissue necrosis have a significantly higher risk of bacterial contamination of the necrotic tissue.

Table 17.6. Pathomorphological factors related to mortality from necrotizing pancreatitis (n=205 patients) [49]

Factor	Patients *(n)*	Mortality *(n)*	*p*
Intrapancreatic necrosis			
30%	79 (39%)	6	
50%	75 (37%)	18	<0.0001
Subtotal/total	51 (25%)	26	
Extrapancreatic necrosis			
Positive	96 (47%)	33	
Negative	109 (53%)	17	<0.02
Pancreatogenic ascites			
Positive	115 (56%)	42	
Negative	90 (44%)	8	<0.01
Bacterial infection			
Positive	56 (41%)	18	
Negative	82 (59%)	8	<0.01

Table 17.7. Spectrum and frequency of bacteria in patients with pancreatic abscess and in infected pancreatic necrosis [11, 12, 41, 42]. *S. Staphylococcus*, *E. Escherichia*

Pancreatic abscess		Infected pancreatic necrosis		Infected necrosis after prior antibiotic treatment	
Polymicrobial abscess	62%	Polymicrobial infection	62%		
S. aureus	15%	*Enterococci*	21%		
Enterococci	15%	*S. aureus*	11%		
		S. epidermidis	9%		
		Gram positive	41%	Gram positive	84%
E. Coli	14%	*E. coli*	28%		
Klebsiella	9%	*Klebsiella*	13%		
Pseudomonas	9%	*Pseudomonas*	3%		
Proteus	6%	*Proteus*	2%	Gram negative	40%
		Gram negative	46%		
Others	13%			Fungi	36%
Fungi	7%	Candida	6%	Anaerobes	4%
Anaerobes	12%	Anaerobes	7%		

Bacterial and Fungal Infection of Pancreatic Necrosis

Pathophysiologically infection of pancreatic necrosis develops as a consequence of an increase in the permeability of the intestinal membranes. Endotoxins and bacterial translocation of Gram-negative and positive germs from the intestinal compartments are the pathophysiologic processes that determine morbidity. In patients suffering necrotizing pancreatitis, the overall infection rate of pancreatic tissue in acute pancreatitis is 17% (median) and may increase in the 3rd week of the disease to 70% [6, 11, 17, 18]. The definition of pancreatic infection includes several different pathomorphological entities, infected necrosis, pancreatic abscess, and infected pancreatic pseudocysts. The bacteriological analysis of intraoperative smears or aspirates from percutaneous fine-needle puncture of the necrosis reveals predominantly Gram-negative microbes derived from the intestine [17, 41]. *Escherichia coli* is the most frequent pathogen, followed by *Enterococcus* and *Klebsiella*; a monomicrobial infection will be identified in half of patients with infected necrosis, and a polymicrobial infection in one-third (Table 17.7). Enterobacteria, *Staphylococcus*, anaerobes or fungi are found in fewer than 20% of cases (Table 17.8) [11, 12, 41, 42]. Experimental evidence and clinical observations suggest that there are several pathophysiological roots for bacterial translocation into the pancreas. The most important root of bacterial infection occurs via translocation from the large and small bowels into the lymph compartments of the intestine. Other modes of infection are microperforation of the transverse colon, hematogenous infection, migration by macrophages and polymorphonuclear leukocytes that have incorporated living bacteria. It has been demonstrated by prospective clinical trials that infection is an increasing and time-dependent process during necrotizing pancreatitis. Contamination rates were 25% in the 1st week, 44% in the 2nd week, and peaks above 60% in the 3rd week of necrotizing pancreatitis (Fig. 17.3) [6, 11, 17, 18]. Despite the high standards of therapeutic measures including application of antibiotics, early enteral nutrition, and vigorous fluid replacement, the mortality for infected necrosis is considerably higher than for noninfected patients with sterile pancreatic necrosis) (Tabelle 17.6). However, it has been demonstrated that even with infected necrosis nonsurgical management is effective, depending on the amount and types of bacteria growing in the necrotic tissue. Conversely, patients with extended sterile necrosis have a high risk of systemic complications and of developing multisystem organ failure syndrome without a septic focus. The mortality in this subgroup of patients with extended sterile necrosis lies between 35 and 68% [41, 43–53].

Table 17.8. Severe acute pancreatitis – high-risk group pancreatic fungal infection. *AB* Antibiotic, *LOH* length of hospital stay, *EBM* evidence-based medicine

- Definition of primary and secondary infection and contamination are missing
- Late occurrence of fungal infection in NP
- Increasing incidence of Candida in necrosis:
  - before AB prophylaxis ~7% [11]
  - after routine AB prophylaxis 12–41% [59–63, 66, 67]
- Hospital mortality ~50% [64]
- LOH significantly extended
- Antifungal prophylaxis presently not established by EBM

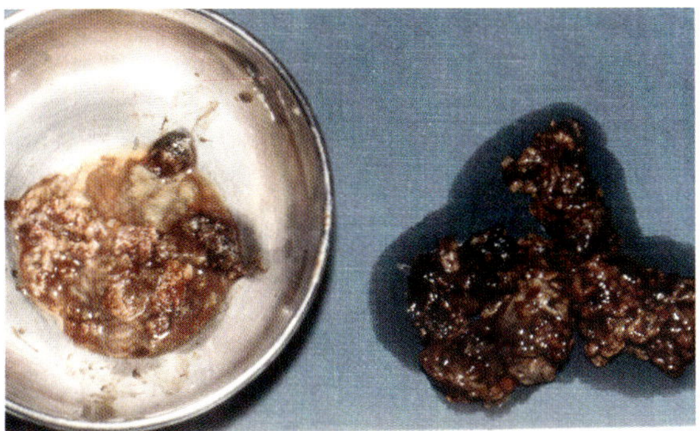

Figure 17.2

Operative specimen of infected necrosis

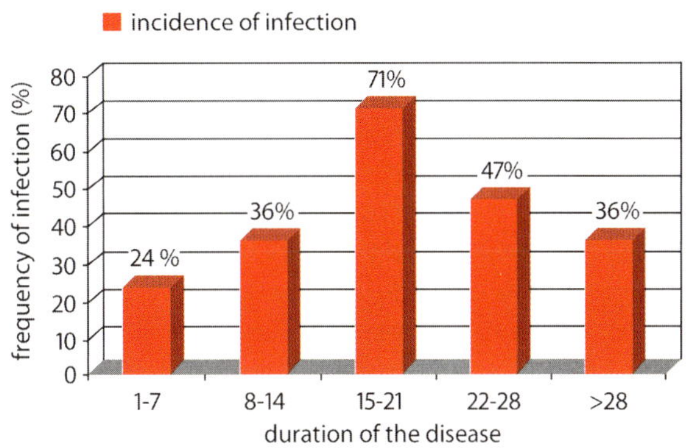

Figure 17.3

Incidence of infected necrosis in relation to the disease ratio. (With permission from Beger et al. 1986 [11])

Determinants of the Natural Course

At the beginning of the 1980s necrotizing pancreatitis was associated with high mortality rate. Knowledge about the natural history of the disease was restricted to either autopsy cases and surgical specimens or clinical observations. Later, based on improved multidisciplinary experience in terms of histopathology, biochemistry, radiology, and bacteriology, hospital mortality decreased. The introduction of the ATLANTA classification, clinicopathological correlation became possible, thus opening the door to new therapeutic, and in particular, surgical concepts. As a result, the overall hospital mortality rate for patients afflicted with necrotizing pancreatitis decreased to a level below 35% in high-volume centers (Table 17.9) [54–56]. Based on large, prospectively accumulated data, several authors have been able to define independent factors determining the outcome of patients with severe acute pancreatitis. These are early multisystems organ failure syndrome associated with early severe acute pancreatitis [57, 58], infected necrosis, pancreatic abscess, extended necrosis (involving >50% of the pancreatic parenchyma, as defined using CECT), necrosis with *Candida* infection, and age >70 years [59–64, 66].

Table 17.9. Mortality in severe acute pancreatitis

First week – ESAP – MOFS	
60% of all deaths	Renner [25]
54% of all deaths	McKay [51]
42% of all deaths	Isenmann [52]
Third/fourth week – infected necrosis – bacterial sepsis - MOFS	
27.5% of all deaths	Takeda [53]
33% of all deaths	LeMee [54]
22% of all deaths	Garg [55]
27.1% of all deaths	Rau [56]

Long-Term Outcome

Surgical treatment of acute pancreatitis is not the first choice of treatment. In biliary acute pancreatitis, laparoscopic cholecystectomy is recommended, or in the case of common bile duct stones, endoscopic sphincterotomy and stone extraction are recommended after the disappearance of the acute inflammatory process during the same hospital period. In necrotizing pancreatitis, surgical necrosectomy (whether using open surgical access or a minimally invasive technique of debridement) is indicated in patients with sepsis caused by infected necrosis and in patients with extended sterile necrosis causing severe systemic organ dysfunction and sepsis without a septic focus. In patients with pancreatic abscess, the first choice is interventional surgical management. In most cases, necrotizing pancreatitis includes only parts of the tissue; from this knowledge, the classical surgical resection technique has declined as a therapeutic option in the setting of necrotizing pancreatitis to avoid a resection of vital pancreatic tissue. Careful necrosectomy is the basic principal of any surgical technique in necrotizing pancreatitis. Surgical treatment regimes combine tissue-preserving digital necrosectomy, in most instances with a postoperative continuous evacuation of retroperitoneal debrides and exudates.

Following necrotizing pancreatitis, long-term morbidity remains high. Endocrine and exocrine insufficiency will develop in about half of patients and is proportional to the extent of pancreatic necrosis.

In terms of the maintenance of the exocrine function, patients with necrotizing pancreatitis develop an exocrine insufficiency of more than 70%. Every second patient who survives necrotizing pancreatitis requires continuous treatment with pancreatic enzyme supplementation. The largest published series concerned with long-term survival and quality of life after severe acute pancreatitis has been published by Halonen et al. [50]. The study, which included hospital records of 283 consecutive patients with severe acute pancreatitis, indicated that patients surviving severe acute pancreatitis have a good quality of life that was comparable to that of a normal population. After a median follow-up period of surviving patients of 66 months, 87% of patients who were working a year before the attack of severe acute pancreatitis returned to work. However, 10% of the patients died in the late follow-up years after having survived their last attack of severe acute pancreatitis. They died mostly from alcoholism and pancreas-related disease and were mainly diabetics. In this follow-up series the mortality rate was 25%. A hospital mortality rate of 25% and a late mortality rate of 10% give a realistic risk figure of about one-third of all patients with an episode of severe acute pancreatitis who will finally die from the disease. In European industrialized countries, alcohol-induced acute pancreatitis is a major feature of patients with acute pancreatitis; these patients have a high rate of continuous drinking after hospitalization. Late morbidity is therefore connected to continuous alcohol consumption rather than the late consequences of acute pancreatitis.

References

1. Fitz RH (1989) Acute pancreatitis: a consideration of pancreatic hemorrhage, hemorrhagic, suppurative and gangrenous pancreatitis, and of disseminated fat necrosis. Boston Med Surg J 70:181–187
2. Ranson JHC, Rifkind KM, Roses DF, Fink SD, Eng K, Localio SA (1974) Objective early identification of severe acute pancreatitis. Am J Gastroenterol. 61:443–451
3. Imrie CW (1974) Observations on acute pancreatitis. Br J Surg 61:539–544
4. Knaus WA, Draper EA, Wagner DP, Zimmermann JE (1985) APACHE II: a severity of disease classification system. Crit Care Med 13:818–829
5. Wilson C, Heath DI, Imrie CW (1990) Prediction of outcome in acute pancreatitis: a comparative study of APACHE II, clinical assessment and multiple factor scoring systems. Br J Surg 77:1260–1264
6. Beger HG, Krautzberger W, Bittner R, Block S, Büchler M (1985) Results of surgical treatment of necrotizing pancreatitis. World J Surg 9:972–979
7. Beger HG, Kunz R, Bittner R (1987) Prognostic criteria in necrotizing pancreatitis. In: Beger HG, Büchler M (eds) Acute Pancreatitis. Springer, Berlin, pp 198–200
8. Block S, Maier W, Bittner R, Büchler M. Malfertheiner P, Beger HG (1986) Identification of pancreatic necrosis in severe acute pancreatitis: imaging procedures versus clinical staging. Gut 27:1035–1042
9. Kivisaari L, Schröder T, Sainio V, Somer K, Standertskjöld-Nordenstam C-G (1987) CT evaluation of acute pancreatitis: 8 years clinical experience and experimental evidence. Acta Radiol 377:20–24

10. Freeny PC (1993) Incremental dynamic bolus computed tomography of acute pancreatitis. Int J Pancreatol 13:147–158
11. Beger HG, Bittner R, Block S, Büchler M (1986) Bacterial contamination of pancreatic necrosis. Gastroenterology 49:433–438
12. Bittner R, Block S, Büchler M, Berger HG (1987) Pancreatic abscess and infected necrosis: different local septic complications in acute pancreatitis. Dig Dis Sci 32:1082–1087
13. Beger HG (1991) Surgery in acute pancreatitis. Hepatogastroenterology 38:92–96
14. Bradley EL III (1993) A clinically based classification system for acute pancreatitis. Summary of the International Symposium on Acute Pancreatitis, Atlanta, Ga, September 11 through 13, 1992. Arch Surg 128:586–590
15. Bockman DE (1994) Pathology of edematous (interstitial) pancreatitis. In: Bradley EL III (ed) Acute Pancreatitis: Diagnosis and Therapy. Raven, New York, pp 241–247
16. Klöppel G, Maillet B (1993) Pathology of acute and chronic pancreatitis. Pancreas 8:659–670
17. Gerzof SG, Banks PA, Robbins AH, Johnson WC, Spechler SJ, Wetzner SM, Snider JM, Langevin RE, Jay ME (1987) Early diagnosis of pancreatic infection by computed tomography-guided aspiration. Gastroenterology 93:1315–1320
18. Bradley EL III, Allen K (1991) A prospective longitudinal study of observation versus surgical intervention in the management of necrotizing pancreatitis. Am J Surg 161:19–24
19. Grace PA, Williamson RCN (1993) Modern management of pancreatic pseudocysts. Br J Surg 80:573–581
20. Banks PA (1986) Acute pancreatitis: clinical presentation. In: Go VLW, Brooks FP, DiMagno EP, Gardner JD, Lebenthal E, Scheel GA (eds) The Exocrine Pancreas. Raven, New York, pp 475–479
21. Beger HG, Bittner R, Büchler M, Hess W, Schmitz JE (1986) Hemodynamic data pattern in patients with acute pancreatitis. Gastroenterology 90:74–79
22. Carey LC (1979) Extra-abdominal manifestations of acute pancreatitis. Surgery 86:337–342
23. McFadden DW (1991) Organ failure and multiple organ system failure in pancreatitis. Pancreas 6:37–43
24. Widdison AL, Karanjia ND (1993) Pancreatic infection complicating acute pancreatitis. Br J Surg 80:148–154
25. Renner IG, Savage WT, Pantoia JL, Renner VJ (1985) Death due to acute pancreatitis: a retrospective analysis of 405 autopsy cases. Dig Dis Sci 30:1005–1018
26. Teerenhovi O (1988) Fatal fulminant pancreatitis. Surg Res Commun 3:207
27. Jimenez G, Aldrete JS (1983) Clinical implications derived from the morphological classification of 89 patients with acute pancreatitis. J Clin Gastroenterol 5:137–142
28. Uhl W, Büchler M, Malfertheiner P, Isenmann R, Martini M, Beger HG (1991) Pancreatic necrosis develops within four days after the acute attack. Gastroenterology 100:A123
29. Rau B, Seifert T, Schoenberg MH, Brambs HJ, Beger HG (1995) Contrast enhanced CT: does it accentuate severity of necrotizing pancreatitis in humans? Pancreas 11:445 (Abstract)
30. Balthazar EJ, Robinson DL, Megibow AJ (1990) Acute pancreatitis: value of CT in establishing prognosis. Radiology 174:331–336
31. Foitzik T, Bassi DG, Schmidt J, Lewandrowski KB, Fernandez del Castillo C, Rattner DW, Warshaw AL (1994) Intravenous contrast medium accentuates the severity of acute necrotizing pancreatitis in the rat. Gastroenterology 106:207–214
32. Aldridge MC, Francis ND, Glazer G, Dudley HAF (1989) Colonic complications of severe acute pancreatitis. Br J Surg 76:362–367
33. McMahon MJ, Lankisch PG (1987) Peritoneal lavage and dialysis for the treatment of acute pancreatitis. In: Beger HG, Büchler M (eds) Acute Pancreatitis. Springer, Berlin. pp 278–284
34. Büchler M, Malfertheiner P, Schädlich H, Nevalainen TJ, Friess H, Beger HG (1989) Role of phospholipase A2 in human acute pancreatitis. Gastroenterology 97:1521–1526
35. Heath DI, Wilson C, Gudgeon AM, Jehanli A, Shenkin A, Imrie CW (1994) Trypsinogen activation peptides (TAP) concentrations in the peritoneal fluid of patients with acute pancreatitis and their relation to the presence of histologically confirmed pancreatic necrosis. Gut 35:1311–1315
36. Puolakkainen P, Valtonen V, Paananen A, Schröder T (1987) C-reactive protein (CRP) and serum phospholipase A2 in the assessment of the severity of acute pancreatitis. Gut 28:764–771
37. Uhl W, Büchler M, Malfertheiner P, Martini M, Beger HG (1991) PNM-elastase in comparison with CRP, antiproteases and LDH as indicators of necrosis in human acute pancreatitis. Pancreas 6:253–259
38. Buttenschön K, Berger D, Hiki N, Buttenschön DC, Vasilescu C, Chick-Torab FG, Seidelmann M, Beger HG (2000) Endotoxin and antiendotoxin antibodies in patients with acute pancreatitis. Eur J Surg 166:459–466
39. Wilson C, Heads A, Shenkin A, Imrie CW (1989) C-reactive protein, antiproteases and complement factors as objective markers of severity in acute pancreatitis. Br J Surg 76:177–181
40. Gross V, Leser H-G, Heinisch A, Schölmerich J (1993) Inflammatory mediators and cytokines – new aspects of the pathophysiology and assessment of severity of acute pancreatitis. Hepatogastroenterology 40:522–530
41. Bassi C, Falconi M, Girelli R, Nifosi F, Elio A, Martini N, Pederzoli P (1989) Microbiological findings in severe pancreatitis. Surg Res Commun 5:1–4
42. Medich DS, Lee TK, Melhem MF, Rowe MI, Schraut WH, Lee KK (1993) Pathogenesis of pancreatic sepsis. Am J Surg 165:46–50
43. Rau B, Pralle U, Uhl W, Schoenberg MH, Beger HG (1995) Management of sterile necrosis in instances of severe acute pancreatitis. J Am Coll Surg 181:279–288
44. Yeo CT, Bastidas JA, Lynch-Nyhan A, Fishman EK, Zinner MJ, Cameron JL (1990) The natural history of pancreatic pseudocysts documented by computed tomography. Surg Gynecol Obstet 170: 411–417
45. Schoenberg MH, Rau B, Beger HG (1995) Diagnose und Therapie des primären Pankreasabszesses. Chirurg 66:588–596
46. Mitchell CJ, Playforth MJ, Kellenher J, McMahon MJ (1983) Functional recovery of the exocrine pancreas after acute pancreatitis. Scand J Gastroenterol 18:5–8
47. Büchler M, Malfertheiner P, Block S, Beger HG (1985) Morphologische und funktionelle Veränderungen des Pankreas nach akuter nekrotisierende Pankreatitis. Z. Gastroenterol 23:79–83
48. Angelini G, Cavallini G, Pederzoli P, Bovo P, DiFrancesco V, Frulloni L, Sgabri L, Talamini G, Castagnini A (1993) Long-term outcome of acute pancreatitis: a prospective study with 118 patients. Digestion 54:143–147

49. Beger HG, Büchler M (1986) Decision-making in surgical treatment of acute pancreatitis: operative or conservative management of necrotizing pancreatitis. Theor Surg 1:61–68
50. Halonen KI, Pettila V, Leppaniemi AK, Kemppainen EA, Puolakkainen PA, Haapiainen RK (2003) Long-term health-related quality of life in survivors of severe acute pancreatitis. Intensive Care Med 29:782–786
51. McKay CJ, Evans S, Sinclair M, Carter CR, Imrie CW (1999) High early mortality rate from acute pancreatitis in Scotland, 1984–1995. Br J Surg 86:1302–1305
52. Isenmann R, Rau B, Beger HG (2001) Early severe acute pancreatitis: characteristics of a new subgroup. Pancreas 22:274–278
53. Takeda K, Matsuno S, Sunamura M, Kobari M (1998) Surgical aspects and management of acute necrotizing pancreatitis: recent results of a cooperative national survey in Japan. Pancreas 16:316–322
54. Le Mee J, Paye F, Sauvanet A, O'Toole D, Hammel P, Marty J, Ruszniewski P, Belghiti J (2001) Incidence and reversibility of organ failure in the course of sterile or infected necrotizing pancreatitis. Arch Surg 136:1386–1390
55. Garg PK, Madan K, Pande GK, Khanna S, Sathyanarayan G, Bohidar NP, Tandon RK (2005) Association of extent and infection of pancreatic necrosis with organ failure and death in acute necrotizing pancreatitis. Clin Gastroenterol Hepatol 3:159–166
56. Rau B, Bothe A, Beger HG (2005) Surgical treatment of necrotizing pancreatitis by necrosectomy and closed lavage: changing patient characteristics and outcome in a 19-year, single center series. Surgery 138:28–39
57. Mentula P, Kyläanpäa, Kemppainen E, Jansson SE, Sarna S, Poulakkainen P, Haapiainen R, Repo H (2004) Plasma anti-inflammatory cytokines and monocyte human leukocyte antigen-DR expression in patients with acute pancreatitis. Scand J Gastroenterol 39:178–187
58. Isenmann R, Rau B, Beger HG (2001) Early severe acute pancreatitis: characteristics of a new subgroup. Pancreas 22:274–278
59. Edwards JE, Bodey GP, Bowden RA, Buchner T, de Pauw BE, Filler SG, Ghannoum MA, Glauser M, Herbrecht R, Kauffmann CA, Kohno S, Martino P, Meunier F, Mori T, Pfaller MA, Rex JH, Rogers TR, Rubin RH, Solomkin J, Viscoli C, Walsh TJ, White M (1997) International Conference for the development of a consensus on the management and prevention of severe candidal infections. Clin Infect Dis 25:43–59
60. Grewe M, Tsiotos GG, Luque de-Leon E, Sarr MG (1999) Fungal infection in acute necrotizing pancreatitis. J Am J Surg 188:408–414
61. Aloia T, Solomkin J, Fink AS (1994) *Candida* in pancreatic infection: a clinical experience. Am Surg 60:793–796
62. Hoerauf H, Hammer S, Mueller-Myhsok B, Rupprecht H (1998) Intra-abdominal *Candida* infection during acute necrotizing pancreatitis has a high prevalence and is associated with increased mortality. Crit Care Med 26:2010–2015
63. Isenmann R, Schwarz M, Rau B, Trautmann M,Schober W, Beger HG (2002) Characteristics of infection with *Candida* species in patients with necrotizing pancreatitis. World J Surg 26:372–376
64. Shanmugam N, Isenmann R, Barkin JS, Beger HG (2003) Pancreatic fungal infection. Pancreas 27:133–138
65. Granger J, Ramich D (2005) Acute pancreatitis: models, markers and mediators. Shock 24:45–51
66. Ho HS, Frey CF (1997) The role of antibiotic prophylaxis in severe acute pancreatitis. Arch Surg 132:487–492
67. Reijnen MM, van Goor H, Falk P, Hedgren M, Holmdahl L (2001) Sodium hyaluronate increases the fibrinolytic response of human peritoneal mesothelial cells exposed to tumor necrosis factor alpha. Arch Surg 136:291–296
68. Chooklin S, Perejaslov A (2005) Interlukin 18 and adhesion molecules in acute pancreatitis. Pancreas 29:367–368
69. Mentula P, Kylanpaa ML, Kemppainen E, Jansson SE, Sarna S, Puolakkainen P, Haapiainen R, Repo H (2005) Early prediction of organ failure by combined markers in patients with acute pancreatitis. Br J Surg 92:68–75

Chapter 18

R. Isenmann

Classification of Severe Acute Pancreatitis

The first classification system for acute pancreatitis was reported by Fitz, who, in 1889, separated patients dying from the disease into hemorrhagic, suppurative, and gangrenous forms. As this was a postmortem classification, the clinical usefulness of this system was limited [1]. The introduction of serum amylase in 1929 as reliable diagnostic parameter of the disease can be regarded as a first major breakthrough for the classification of acute pancreatitis. With the increasing knowledge about the pathogenesis of the disease, its natural course and its different pathological features, various idiosyncratic definitions and descriptions were used for different entities of acute pancreatitis, but most of them were poorly defined. Terms such as "pancreatic abscess," "pancreatic phlegmon," or "pancreatic collections" were used synonymously and a confusion was created, which Bradley called "the Pancreatic Tower of Babel" [2]. The lack of a precise definition of the different forms of acute pancreatitis made it difficult to analyze and to compare different clinical studies and, even more important, to allocate patients to the treatment that the different subgroups deserved.

In the late 1980s and early 1990s, it became evident that a uniformly accepted, comprehensive definition of acute pancreatitis and its complications was urgently needed. By that time, sophisticated diagnostic imaging tools (such as contrast-enhanced computed tomography, CECT, scanning) had become available that enabled the differentiation of pathomorphologic entities of acute pancreatitis and facilitated their classification.

The Atlanta Classification

In the majority of cases, acute pancreatitis is a self-limiting disease and complete functional restitution of the gland is the rule. Nevertheless, 10–15% of the patients develop severe courses characterized by life-threatening complications such as multiple organ failure and/or severe sepsis. These cases are associated with mortality rates of 15–25%, even if the patients are transferred to specialized centers with expertise in the treatment of this disease [3–5].

The current classification of severe acute pancreatitis (SAP) is based on a consensus found on the International Symposium on Acute Pancreatitis held in Atlanta in 1992 [6]. The consensus group comprised anatomists, gastroenterologists, internists, surgeons, pathologists, and radiologists, providing a broad basis for acceptance of the new classification.

The Atlanta classification has introduced the term "severe acute pancreatitis" in differentiation to "mild acute pancreatitis." Patients suffering from SAP bear a high risk of developing life-threatening complications and complicated courses of the disease.

SAP is today defined by occurrence of one or more systemic (organ failure) or local complication during the course of the disease. The Atlanta classification defines six systemic complications that characterize the severe form of acute pancreatitis:

1. Pulmonary insufficiency (arterial oxygen tension of 60 mmHg or less)
2. Renal insufficiency (serum creatinine >2.0 mg/dl after rehydration)
3. Shock (systolic blood pressure of 90 mmHg or less over at least 15 min)
4. Gastrointestinal bleeding (>500 ml/24 h)
5. Coagulopathy (platelets 100,000/mm^3 or less, fibrinogen less than 1.0 g/l and fibrin split products more than 80 μg/ml)
6. Metabolic disturbances (serum calcium <7.5 mg/dl)

In addition, two of the most widely used scoring systems were accepted for discrimination between mild acute pancreatitis and SAP: the Ranson criteria (three or more criteria) and the Acute Physiology And Chronic Health Evaluation (APACHE) II score (eight or more points)

From the pathomorphological point of view, four entities were defined that characterize SAP:

1. Pancreatic necrosis, defined by diffuse or focal area(s) of nonviable pancreatic parenchyma, typically associated with peripancreatic fat necrosis.
2. Acute fluid collections, defined as peripancreatic collections of fluid, located in or near the pancreas, lacking a wall of surrounding granulation or fibrous tissue.
3. Acute pseudocyst, defined as a collection of pancreatic juice enclosed by a wall of fibrous or granulation tissue.
4. Pancreatic abscess, defined as a circumscribed intra-abdominal collection of pus, usually in proximity to the pancreas, containing little or no pancreatic necrosis.

Shortcomings of the Atlanta Classification

In a potential lethal disease such as SAP, severity has to be defined by the patients' individual risk of death. For almost 10 years, the Atlanta classification has been the standard classification of SAP and its complications. One of the major advantages of the Atlanta classification is that it allows comparison of data gathered from different institutions and that it provides a reliable base for the definition of the complications of the disease. SAP is based on a combination of morphologic, clinical, and diagnostic criteria. In particular, the clear definition of systemic complications of acute pancreatitis has been a pivotal progress.

Nevertheless, during the past years, it became clear that the Atlanta classification has some shortcomings with regard to the definition of severity. The reasons for this are manyfold. Improvements in the intensive care management of acute pancreatitis have led to a decrease in the mortality of some systemic complications, such as pulmonary failure. In addition, patients are nowadays receiving stage-adopted forms of treatment. For example, it is accepted that the indication for surgical necrosectomy should be limited to patients with infected pancreatic necrosis, whereas the overwhelming majority of sterile necrosis can be managed by conservative treatment [7–9]. In the following, we will discuss some facts and findings that we think should be taken into consideration when our current definition of SAP is undergoing revision.

Pancreatic Necrosis and Pancreatic Abscess

Beyond any doubt, the development of pancreatic necrosis is one of the major complications of acute pancreatitis. The overwhelming majority of deaths can be attributed to this morphologic entity. Necrotizing pancreatitis can easily be diagnosed by CECT, and with a mortality of 15–30%, there is no doubt that patients with necrotizing pancreatitis should be treated in units having expertise with this disease [10–13]. Necrotizing pancreatitis is the underlying condition in most patients developing organ failure during pancreatitis [14,15]. Nevertheless, the past years have shown that the entity of pancreatic necrosis can be divided into several subgroups with different prognoses.

The most severe form of acute pancreatitis is characterized by bacterial infection of necrotizing pancreatitis. The term "infected pancreatic necrosis" is usually used in this situation [10,16]. The patients develop septic multiple organ failure and have a long and complicated course. Surgical treatment is mandatory and the mortality even in specialized centers is reported to be up to 25–30% [12,13,16,17]. In contrast, patients with necrotizing pancreatitis but without signs of sepsis are characterized as having "sterile pancreatic necrosis." This subgroup has a significantly better prognosis, with a mortality of 5–10%, and today it is accepted that the overwhelming majority of these patients can be managed without surgery [3,8,9,18]. The incidence of both systemic organ failure and infected pancreatic necrosis are correlated with the extent of necrotic pancreatic parenchyma, and it has been shown that a considerable percentage of patients with limited pancreatic necrosis do not even develop systemic complications [14,19].

These facts show that today, the mere presence of pancreatic necrosis should no longer be accepted as a criterion for SAP. For defining severity, additional complications have to be present, such as systemic organ failure or bacterial infection.

The Atlanta classification discriminates between "pancreatic necrosis" and "pancreatic abscess." Both are regarded as criteria of severity, but both are different clinical entities. This is based on observations that both entities have different clinical courses and that the prognosis of encapsulated infected collections in the pancreatic and peripancreatic region is significantly better than that of diffuse infected areas, as it is the common finding in infected pancreatic necrosis [3,5,20,21]. Nevertheless, there obviously exists a link between pancreatic necrosis and pancreatic abscess, and the question is: when does necrotizing pancreatitis end and when does pancreatic abscess start? [22]. We have learned from well-designed studies that the optimal time for surgery in patients with necrotizing pancreatitis is around the 4th–5th week after onset of the disease [9,13], which is the time when necrotic areas usually become encapsulated and abscess formation is about to start. This apparently shows that both entities are closely linked. Given a mortality of 5–10% for pancreatic abscess in larger studies [20,21], the prognostic relevance of abscess formation is arguable. This discrepancy in mortality is the reason why the authors doubt that pancreatic abscess should be classified as "severe" pancreatitis.

Organ Failure as an Indicator of Severity

Another major disadvantage of the Atlanta classification is that several criteria for severity are common in patients with acute pancreatitis, regardless of their individual risk of death. Patients classified as having a severe attack of acute pancreatitis should have a high risk for a complicated or even fatal course, and it should be the purpose of any classification of acute pancreatitis to identify this cohort of patients. The systemic complications that define severity in the Atlanta classification were chosen according to the information available at the time of the consensus. It is important to note that the Atlanta criteria base the diagnosis of SAP on both local morphologic and/or systemic features. It must be emphasized that according to this definition, SAP is not necessarily associated with the morphologic presence of local complications, such as pancreatic necrosis. But this reveals one of the shortcomings of this classification: a patient with pulmonary failure, not even requiring artificial ventilation, might be classified as suffering from SAP as well as a patient suffering from transient renal dysfunction. It is a well-known finding among pancreatologists that these systemic complications are frequent in acute pancreatitis; they are commonly transient and most patients recover with an uneventful course [23].

Meanwhile, it has become apparent that some complications do not necessarily correlate with poor outcome [15,19]. Some of the criteria of severity appear to be redundant; their value with regard to mortality appears to be limited.

The limitations of the Atlanta criteria have been demonstrated using data from 260 patients with necrotizing pancreatitis who were treated at the Department of Abdominal Surgery of the University Hospital of Ulm. The eight clinical Atlanta criteria of severity were analyzed by a multiple logistic regression analysis for their prognostic value in predicting death. Surprisingly, only three of the eight criteria could be identified as important risk factors of death. Multiple logistic regression revealed that only an APACHE II score of eight or more points, renal insufficiency, and shock were the best parameters to identify patients with a high risk for a lethal course (Table 18.1).

Table 18.1 Results of the multiple logistic regression of the eight Atlanta criteria for their prognostic value in predicting fatal outcome. Data were gather from 260 patients with necrotizing pancreatitis treated at the University Hospital of Ulm. *APACHE II* Acute Physiology And Chronic Health Evaluation II

	Odds ratio	95% Confidence limits	*p*-value
APACHE II score (8 or more points vs. less than 8 points)	7.8	[1.8 : 34.9]	0.0007
Renal Insufficiency (yes vs. no)	3.0	[1.3 : 6.6]	0.0078
Shock (yes vs. no)	4.4	[2.0 : 9.5]	< 0.0001

Table 18.2. Modified classification system: crude odds ratios and confidence limits. *MOF* Multiple organ failure

	Crude odds ratio	95% Confidence limits
APACHE II score 8 or more points	13.3	[3.1 : 56.5]
Renal insufficiency	7.0	[3.6 : 13.6]
Shock	9.4	[4.86 : 18.21]
Catecholamines	11.3	[5.7 : 22.2]
Dialysis/hemofiltration	5.1	[2.1 : 12.6]
MOF at admission	5.0	[2.7 : 9.3]
Age > 70 years	3.0	[1.3 : 7.0]
Bacterial infection of pancreatic necrosis	2.0	[1.1 : 3.7]
Mechanical ventilation	4.2	[2.1 : 8.6]

Table 18.3. Results of the multiple logistic regression analysis of fatal outcome: independent risk factors identified from the modified classification system

	Odds ratio	95% confidence limits	*p*-value
APACHE II score 8 or more points	5.3	[1.1 : 25.5]	0.0163
Application of catecholamines	3.5	[1.5 : 8.1]	< 0.0001
Renal insufficiency	2.6	[1.1 : 6.2]	0.0293

Today there is ongoing discussion about which clinical criteria correlate with clinical outcome. For example, Halonen and colleagues identified several clinical features, such as transferal admission from other hospitals or advanced age, which were associated with an increased risk of death [24]. Other groups reported that [15,16,25] advanced age [5,24,26], mechanical ventilator support [27], pressure support, dialysis [24], transfer from other hospitals to referral centers [28], or obesity [29,30] were relevant factors associated with high mortality rates. Nevertheless, they are not recognized as risk factors by our current definition of SAP. Therefore, in a second step, a modified classification of severity was constructed from the data of the 260 Ulm patients. This classification was based on the results of the logistic regression analysis of the Atlanta criteria, and included the three criteria identified as risk factors of death. In addition, six other variables, regarded as promising candidates to define poor prognosis, were added to this modified classification system. These variables were: age more than 70 years, bacterial infection of pancreatic necrosis (proven by positive fine-needle aspiration or positive intraoperative smears), the necessity of mechanical ventilation, application of catecholamines, dialysis/hemofiltration, and whether the patients presented with organ failure at admission. The crude odds ratios that were calculated for these variables were different, which means that all of these parameters were associated with an increased risk of death (Table 18.2). The most pronounced effect with regard to the odds ratios was found for an APACHE II score of eight or more points, application of catecholamines, and development of shock. In contrast to that, the effect of dialysis/hemofiltration, renal insufficiency, organ failure at admission, an age of more than 70 years, bacterial infection of pancreatic necrosis, and need of mechanical ventilation on mortality was less pronounced, with minor relevance for the prognosis of the patient.

In order to assess simultaneously the effects of the nine modified classification criteria, the variables again were analyzed by a multiple logistic regression with variable selection. This analysis identified the APACHE II score, renal insufficiency and application of catecholamines as important risk factors for a lethal outcome (Table 18.3). The conclusion from these results is that it appears to be reasonable to restrict the number of criteria of any future classification system to a limited number of variables. Some of the current Atlanta criteria are redundant and it appears to make little sense to provide a classification system with numerous criteria of severity as long as three or four of them are enough to identify patients with poor prognosis.

Dynamics of Organ Failure

Thirty years ago, Imrie and Blumgart demonstrated the significance of pulmonary insufficiency in patients with severe acute pancreatitis [31]. Forty-five percent of their patients with acute pancreatitis developed arterial oxygen tension levels of less than 60 mmHg breathing air. This is one of the first reports about the impact of organ failure on the course of patients with SAP. Today, organ failure is a typical complication in patients with acute pancreatitis. The intention of the Atlanta classification was to clearly define the different characteristic types of organ failure as criteria for SAP. On the basis of this definition, it has become clear during recent years, that if organ failure occurs, the persistence and progression of these complications, rather than the mere occurrence, are determining the course. Varying percentages of patients with pancreatic necrosis on CECT do not develop organ dysfunction. As far as we know from the literature, 20–50% of the patients recover from necrotizing pancreatitis without having organ failure [14,15,19].

If organ failure develops, this is a dynamic process and not necessarily a criterion of severity. In a British series, early organ failure resolved without further complications in 62% of the patients [32]. Other studies show that pulmonary failure according to the Atlanta definition is present in 50–60% of patients with SAP [14,15,33]. These patients are classified as suffering from a severe attack of the disease regardless of the fact that pulmonary insufficiency might resolve spontaneously without further intervention [23]. The risk of death increases considerably only if pulmonary failure progresses and the patient requires mechanical ventilation, justifying this episode of pancreatitis being defined as severe [24]. This is the reason why today, it is evident that a valid definition of SAP should take into account the dynamics of organ failure. Persistent or progressive organ failure is more likely to be a good indicator of severity than a laboratory or clinical parameter exceeding a specific cut-off level for a limited period of time.

Early Severe Acute Pancreatitis

Systemic complications that occur during the 1st week after onset of pancreatitis can be transient without further clinical relevance. Nevertheless, there has been increasing evidence that this early organ dysfunction is of considerable clinical impact [34–37]. As a consequence, the relevance of early organ failure has been addressed by several studies during recent years. Today, it is clear that a group of patients with SAP will have early organ failure within the first 7–10 days after on set of symptoms. This clinical entity has been defined as early severe acute pancreatitis (ESAP) [34,35,37]. Depending on patient selection in the different studies, organ failure resolves within a limited period of time and is associated with low mortality. However, organ function that is unresolved or progresses carries a considerable mortality of up to 50% [37]. The percentage of patients that recover from early organ failure is a matter of controversy. In our personal series of patients, we found a progression of early organ failure in 79%. ESAP was associated with an extremely high mortality of 42% (Table 18.4).

Extended Pancreatic Necrosis

There has been some controversy during the past years over whether the amount of necrotic parenchyma present constitutes a prognostic factor in patients with necrotizing pancreatitis. In some series, no correlation between the extent of pancreatic necrosis and the incidence of systemic complications was found [15,19]. Today, the amount of necrosis in and around the pancreas can easily be defined by CECT and there is clinical evidence to suggest that patients with an extent of necrosis of more than 50% of the gland can be regarded as a special clinical entity. In our experience, the extent of necrosis is directly correlated with the incidence of organ failure in patients with sterile pancreatic necrosis [14]. Not surprisingly, the subgroup of patients with subtotal to total necrosis of the pancreas could be defined as a special clinical entity covering a mortality risk of up to 26% [38]. It therefore seems reasonable to regard patients with extended pancreatic necrosis as candidates for a severe course. This is underlined by the fact that extended pancreatic necrosis is a risk factor for developing infected pancreatic necrosis, as the incidence of bacterial infection is closely correlated with the amount of necrotic parenchyma.

Future Classifications of Acute Pancreatitis

It seems to be important to stress that a revised classification system of acute pancreatitis should not only consist of clinical criteria, but also, as it has been during the past 10 years, of morphologic and diagnostic features. With regard to this, the Atlanta classification remains of undoubted value. If the classification is undergoing revision, this should take into account the findings that have been made during the past years

Table 18.4. Clinical course and outcome of early severe acute pancreatitis (*ESAP*) and severe acute pancreatitis (*SAP*) without organ failure at admission. *ICU* Intensive care unit

	ESAP (47 patients)	SAP (111 patients)	*p*
Mean ICU treatment (days ± SD)	44.7 ± 43.3	21.1 ± 22.5	<0.0001
Mean hospitalization (days ± SD)	66.4 ± 54.1	44.9 ± 36.5	0.01
Infected necrosis	11 patients (23%)	23 patients (21%)	n.s.
Surgical treatment	42 patients (89%)	66 patients (60%)	0.0002
Days between onset and operation (mean ± SD)	5.6 ± 5.5	16.6 ± 8.2	0.01
Mortality	20 patients (42%)	16 patients (14%)	0.0003

Table 18.5. Proposal for a modification of the Atlanta classification, introducing "complicated acute pancreatitis" for clinical entities with mortality rates of 5–10%. *CECT* Contrast-enhanced computed tomography

Complicated acute pancreatitis
Acute pancreatitis with organ failure, irrespective of pancreatic necrosis
Necrotizing pancreatitis on CECT
Pancreatic abscess
Pancreatic pseudocyst
Peripancreatic collections
Severe acute pancreatitis
Infected necrosis
Necrotizing pancreatitis with organ failure of three or more organ systems and/or organ failure persisting at least 72 h or longer
Early severe acute pancreatitis

From the author's view, it seems to be reasonable that the term "mild acute pancreatitis" remains a part of the classification of acute pancreatitis. This should be attributed to entities with a low risk of death, not exceeding 3–5%. According to our current knowledge, this applies mainly to patients with edematous pancreatitis without systemic complications or patients with postacute pancreatic pseudocysts or peripancreatic fluid collections.

For clinical entities that are associated with local or systemic complications that bear a mortality of 5–10%, the term "complicated acute pancreatitis" would be more appropriate than "severe acute pancreatitis." According to our personal experience, this applies to patients presenting with solitary or transient organ failure, irrespective of the presence of pancreatic necrosis, necrotizing pancreatitis on CECT (but not with total to subtotal necrosis), or with pancreatic abscess.

The term "severe acute pancreatitis" should be applied to courses with organ failure of three or more organ systems and/or organ failure persisting at least 72 h or longer. As ESAP defines a subgroup of patients with very poor prognosis and complicated courses, this apparently justifies this entity to be classified as severe. Nevertheless, pancreatic infection is the most severe complication of necrotizing pancreatitis and, as a matter of fact, patients with signs of local pancreatic infection (but not with pancreatic abscess) should be classified as suffering from SAP (Table 18.5).

Conclusion

Our current classification of SAP has proven to be valuable for more than 15 years. Nevertheless, our knowledge about acute pancreatitis has increased during this period of time, and I believe that a revision is necessary within the near future. This revision should take into consideration new subgroups and entities of acute pancreatitis that have been defined during recent years [37].

References

1. Fitz RH (1889) Acute pancreatitis. A consideration of pancreatic hemorrhage, hemorrhagic suppurative and gangrenous pancreatitis and dissemination necrosis. Boston Med Surg J 120:181–186
2. Bradley ELI (1999) A natural history-based clinical classification system for acute pancreatitis. In: Büchler MW, Uhl W, Friess H, Malfertheiner P (eds) Acute Pancreatitis – Novel Concepts in Biology and Therapy. Blackwell Science, Berlin – Vienna, pp 181–192
3. Nathens AB, et al (2004) Management of the critically ill patient with severe acute pancreatitis. Crit Care Med 32:2524–2536
4. Mitchell RMS, Byrne MF, Baillie J (2003) Pancreatitis. Lancet 361:1447–1455
5. Pitchumoni CS, Patel NM, Shah P (2005) Factors influencing mortality in acute pancreatitis: can we alter them? J Clin Gastroenterol 39:798–814
6. Bradley ELI (1993) A clinically based classification system for acute pancreatitis. Arch Surg 128:586–590
7. Bradley ELI, Allen K (1991) A prospective longitudinal study of observation versus surgical intervention in the management of necrotizing pancreatitis. Am J Surg 161:19–25
8. Rau B, Pralle U, Uhl W, Schoenberg MH, Beger HG (1995) Management of sterile necrosis in instances of severe acute pancreatitis. J Am Coll Surg 181:279–288
9. Büchler MW, Gloor B, Müller CA, Friess H, Seiler CA, Uhl W (2000) Acute necrotizing pancreatitis: treatment strategy according to the status of infection. Ann Surg 232:619–626
10. Beger HG, Isenmann R (1999) Surgical management of necrotizing pancreatitis. Surg Clin North Am 79:783–800
11. Isenmann R, Wittau M, Henne-Bruns D (2003) Candidainfektionen in der Abdominalchirurgie. Chemother J 12 (Suppl 22):3–6
12. Tsiotos GG, et al (1998) Management of necrotizing pancreatitis by repeated operative necrosectomy using a zipper technique. Am J Surg 175:91–98
13. Fernandez Del-Castillo C, et al (1998) Debridement and closed packing for the treatment of necrotizing pancreatitis. Ann Surg 228:676–684
14. Isenmann R, Rau B, Beger HG (1999) Bacterial infection and extent of necrosis are determinants of organ failure in patients with acute necrotizing pancreatitis. Br J Surg 86:1020–1024
15. Tenner S, et al (1997) Relationship of necrosis to organ failure in severe acute pancreatitis. Gastroenterology 113:899–903
16. Bradley ELI (1993) A fifteen year experience with open drainage for infected pancreatic necrosis. Surg Gynecol Obstet 177:215–222
17. Beger HG, Bittner R, Block S, Büchler M (1986) Bacterial contamination of pancreatic necrosis – a prospective clinical study. Gastroenterology 91:433–438
18. Malangoni MA, Martin AS (2005) Outcome of severe acute pancreatitis. Am J Surg 189:273–277
19. Lankisch PG, Pflichthofer D, Lehnick D (2000) No strict correlation between necrosis and organ failure in acute pancreatitis. Pancreas 20:319–322
20. Bassi C, et al (1990) Pancreatic abscess and other pus-harbouring collections related to pancreatitis: a review of 108 cases. World J Surg 14:505–512
21. Bittner R, Block S, Büchler M, Beger HG (1987) Pancreatic abscess and infected pancreatic necrosis. Different local septic complications in acute pancreatitis. Dig Dis Sci 32:1082–1087
22. Warshaw AL (2000) Pancreatic necrosis: to debride or not to debride, that is the question. Ann Surg 232:627–629
23. McKay CJ, Imrie CW (1999) Staging of acute pancreatitis: is it important? Surg Clin North Am 79:733–743
24. Halonen KI, et al (2000) Severe acute pancreatitis: prognostic factors in 270 consecutive patients. Pancreas 21:266–271
25. Widdison AL, Karanjia ND (1993) Pancreatic infection complicating acute pancreatitis. Br J Surg 80:148–154
26. Pezelli R, Billi P, Morselli-Labate AM. Severity of acute pancreatitis: relationship with etiology, sex and age. HepatoGastroenterology 45:1859–1864
27. Dervenis C, et al (1999) Diagnosis, objective assessment of severity, and the management of acute pancreatitis. Int J Pancreatol 25:195–210
28. de Beaux AC, Palmer KR, Carter DC (1995) Factors influencing morbidity and mortality in acute pancreatitis; an analysis of 279 cases. Gut 37:121–126
29. Martinez J, et al (1999) Obesity: a prognostic factor of severity in acute pancreatitis. Pancreas 19:15–20
30. Lankisch PG, Schirren CA (1990) Increased body weight as a prognostic parameter for complications in the course of acute pancreatitis. Pancreas 5:625–629
31. Imrie CW, Blumgart LH (1975) Acute pancreatitis: a prospective study on some factors in mortality. Bull Soc Int Chir 6:601–603
32. Kourtesis G, Wilson SE, Williams RA (1990) The clinical significance of fluid collections in acute pancreatitis. Am Surg 12:796–799
33. Appelros S, Lindgren S, Borgström A (2001) Short and long term outcome in severe acute pancreatitis. Eur J Surg 167:281–286
34. Isenmann R, Rau B, Beger HG (2001) Early severe acute pancreatitis – characteristics of a new subgroup. Pancreas 22:274–278
35. Tao H-Q, Zhang J-X, Zou S-C (2004) Clinical characteristics and management of patients with early acute severe pancreatitis: experience from a medical center in China. World J Gastroenterol 10:919–921
36. Johnson CD, Abu-Hilal M, Members of the British Acute Pancreatitis Study Group (2004) Persistent organ failure during the first week as a marker of fatal outcome in acute pancreatitis. Gut 53:1340–1344
37. Vege SS, Chari ST (2005) Organ failure as an indicator of severity of acute pancreatitis: time to revisit the Atlanta Classification. Gastroenterology 128:1134–1135
38. Isenmann R, Rau B, Zöllner U, Beger HG (2001) Management of patients with extended pancreatic necrosis. Pancreatology 1:63–68

B. M. Rau

Biochemical Diagnosis, Staging, and Prediction

A broad spectrum of parameters have been suggested for the diagnosis and severity stratification of acute pancreatitis and can be classified into activated pancreas- and leukocyte-derived proteases, cytokines, chemokines, and acute-phase reactants. An ideal biochemical parameter for acute pancreatitis should be disease-specific, reliably predict the development of necrosis and/or organ failure during the early stage, and accurately indicate pancreatic infections within the later course of the disease. Currently, there is no single biochemical variable that meets all of these demands; however, there are several useful markers for diagnostic and prognostic purposes.

The diagnosis of acute pancreatitis still relies on the measurement of systemic amylase or lipase concentrations, which remain the "gold standard" despite the recent discovery of several more pancreas-specific enzymes. For an early severity stratification of acute pancreatitis into mild and severe forms within 48 h of symptom onset trypsinogen activation peptide (TAP), carboxypeptidase B activation peptide (CAPAP), polymorphonuclear (PMN)-elastase, serum amyloid A protein (SAA), interleukin (IL)-6, and IL-8 have proven to be good candidates. Because fully automated assays have become available IL-6, IL-8, SAA, and PMN-elastase are interesting parameters in this respect.

Severity stratification beyond 48 h after the onset of symptoms as well as monitoring the course of acute pancreatitis is still the major domain of the acute-phase proteins. C-reactive protein (CRP) is the parameter of choice for the differentiation of mild from severe acute pancreatitis as well as for monitoring purposes due to its fast and widespread availability at low cost. Whereas the development of pancreatic infections or prognosis in terms of nonsurvival can not be reliably predicted by any of the acute-phase proteins or cytokines, procalcitonin (PCT) has emerged as the most promising variable in this setting, followed by IL-8, which is a good candidate to monitor evolving septic multiorgan failure. PCT and IL-8 determinations are available as fully automated tests, thus problems with the assay practicability are no longer a point of issue.

Background

During the past decade, major advances in our understanding of the natural history of acute pancreatitis with identification of relevant prognostic factors [1–3] have driven its management toward conservative intensive care, with a marked reduction of aggressive surgical approaches. Hence, it has been well recognized that immediate and goal-directed treatment considerably influences the course and outcome of this disease [4]. Therefore, early and reliable diagnosis of the disease itself and subsequent complications requiring specific intervention are central issues for clinicians. Since their introduction in the 1980s, contrast-enhanced computed tomography (CE-CT) and guided fine-needle-aspiration (FNA) have become indispensable for diagnosing local complications such as pancreatic necrosis and infection, and still represent cornerstones for morphology-based severity stratification and management alike. However, despite beeing highly accurate, neither CE-CT nor FNA are universally available, they carry the risk of potential complications, and they constitute considerable cost factors.

The era of laboratory markers in acute pancreatitis found its beginnings after the introduction of serum amylase measurements by Elman et al. in 1929, which for the first time enabled a noninvasive diagnosis of acute pancreatitis [5]. This laboratory test profoundly improved the knowledge about the natural course of the disease since it became evident that a mild course with uneventful recovery was the rule rather than the exception, yet severity stratification or assessment of specific complications was not possible. In his hallmark paper published almost four decades later Trapnell et al. provided the first evidence that acute pancreatitis is reflected by abnormalities of many serum/plasma variables [6]. During the subsequent years, much effort has been made in the search for biochemical parameters that allow an early stratification of patients at risk to develop complications such as necrosis, septic complications, or organ failure. Although a still increasing array of potentially useful parameters is currently available, their large-scale clinical use is often limited by time-consuming and expensive assay procedures. In this chapter, the most important biochemical markers for the diagnosis and severity stratification of acute pancreatitis are discussed.

Biochemical Diagnosis of Acute Pancreatitis

The diagnosis of acute pancreatitis relies on the determination of increased pancreatic enzymes in patients with acute abdominal pain along with specific changes in imaging procedures. However, some patients with acute pancreatitis do not present with the typical clinical picture of sudden-onset upper abdominal pain and the disease is not considered in the differential diagnosis [7, 8]. Clinically suspected acute pancreatitis is usually first diagnosed by the determination of increased pancreatic enzymes in the systemic circulation, whereas urinary enzymes have shown no advantage in this respect [9–13]. A host of serum enzymes such as serum amylase and lipase, amylase isoenzymes, trypsinogen-2, pancreatic elastase-1 (P-elastase-1), phospholipase A2 (PLA2), or procarboxypeptidase B are available to diagnose acute pancreatitis. However, elevated amylase and lipase levels continue to be the "gold standard" among these serum markers.

Amylase and Lipase

The sensitivity of serum amylase and lipase in the diagnosis of acute pancreatitis is difficult to evaluate since the definition of the disease relies on the presence of increased serum enzymes [14]. Although this definition suggests a sensitivity of 100% irrespective of the enzyme measured, imaging or autopsy-based findings have shown that pancreatic enzymes may be below the diagnostic cutoff in a variable proportion of patients [7, 8, 15–17]. There are three major factors that interfere with the diagnostic sensitivity of these tests:

1. The time interval since symptom onset and first blood analysis: Within the first 24 h of symptom onset nearly all enzymes are elevated and no differences in sensitivity are observed. Amylase is the first enzyme to return back to normal concentrations, and as such, after the first in-hospital day it is the least sensitive among the enzymatic tests for pancreatitis. Amylase is cleared faster than lipase or trypsin, lipase and trypsin faster than pancreatic elastase, PLA2, or procarboxypeptidase B [18–21]. Rapid normalization usually indicates early resolution of the disease, or less frequently, extensive destruction of the pancreatic parenchyma with cessation of enzyme production [16, 20].
2. Alcoholic etiology: Patients with alcoholic acute pancreatitis frequently present with normal or only slightly elevated pancreatic enzyme concentrations, and serum amylase levels are reported to be normal in one-third of these patients [17]. In addition, normoamylasemia closely correlated with the number of previous attacks (0.7 versus 0.4, $p<0.01$) [16], suggesting considerable loss of viable parenchyma that is no longer able to produce sufficient amounts of enzymes [16, 20]. Since the pancreas contains about 4.5 times more lipase than amylase [22] lipase is less affected in this setting. Thus, elevated lipase levels are found in more than two-thirds of patients with normal amylase [16, 19].
3. Hypertriglyceridemia: Hyperlipidemia specifically interferes with the amylase assay, which leads to normal results in both serum and urine in up to 50% of hypertriglyceridemic patients with clinical symptoms and computed-tomography-proven pancreatic inflammation indicating acute pancreatitis [23]. A circulatory inhibitor rather than the triglyceride itself has been found to cause this problem [24]. Additional enzymes such as lipase should be determined in all situations with normal amylase levels and clinically suspected acute pancreatitis.

The greatest limitation of both serum amylase and lipase is their lack of specificity, albeit lipase performs somewhat better than amylase [25]. In addition to acute pancreatitis there are several conditions that increase serum amylase levels including diseases and derangements of the biliary tract, liver, intestine, genitourinary tract, lungs, breast, prostate, central nervous system, and the salivary glands [12]. Abnormal serum amylase levels also occur in the presence of metabolic disturbances such as renal failure, liver dysfunction, diabetic ketoacidosis, shock, eating disorders, abdominal and nonabdominal trauma, as well as with the use of various drugs [12, 26]. Persistent hyperamylasemia may be a normal variant [27] and has been described as a benign abnormality in many members of certain families [28]. Extrapancreatic injuries causing elevated lipase levels include mumps, types I and IV hyperlipoproteinemias, peptic ulcer, acute cholecystitis, posthepatic obstructive jaundice, liver diseases, small-bowel obstruction, intestinal infarction, perforated bowel, acute renal failure, trauma, fat embolism, or diabetic ketoacidosis [12]. Recently, inflammatory bowel disease and, as observed for amylase, familial pancreatic hyperenzymemia have been included among the causes of lipase elevation [12, 29].

Finally, the technique to determine amylase and lipase concentrations and the cutoff level indicating "abnormal" levels significantly influences the specificity of either enzyme in diagnosing acute pancreatitis. More than 100 techniques of amylase determinations have been reported in the literature creating a wide range of "normal" values that differ quantitatively and in methods of expression as either Somogyi units (SU) or international units (IU) [30, 31]. As far as lipase is concerned, the reference point determined as "abnormal" may differ even for identical methods [22, 30]. As with amylase, different authors have arbitrarily used different cutoff values for lipase ranging from the upper reference range itself [32] to more than two [15] or even three times above the upper normal limit [33]. Unfortunately, no international reference method or cutoff value has yet been adopted toward establishing a standardized tool.

The advantage of serum amylase and lipase lies in its technical simplicity, ready availability in all hospitals and low cost. Considering the low sensitivity of amylase in specific subsets of patients, lipase should be used whenever the diagnosis remains unclear, and imaging studies should be accomplished, if the clinical suspicion for acute pancreatitis is still high. Depending on the etiology of acute pancreatitis, amylase appears to be the better test for biliary-induced acute pancreatitis, whereas lipase performs better for alcoholic or other causes. Simultaneous evaluations of amylase and lipase do not improve accuracy [13, 15]. Both enzymes are of no value in predicting severity or complications. Table 19.1.1 summarizes the sensitivity and specificity rates of both tests in the diagnosis of acute pancreatitis.

Other Tests to Diagnose Acute Pancreatitis

Dissatisfaction with the limited diagnostic accuracy of amylase and lipase determinations has driven the development of new assays for more specific enzymes (Table 19.1.1).

Pancreatic Isoamylase

Pancreatic isoamylase, which accounts for about 40% of total amylase, allows the differentiation of pancreatic from extrapancreatic hyperamylasemeia with a higher specificity than total amylase in diagnosing acute pancreatitis. However, the most important differential diagnoses such as penetrating peptic ulcers, small-bowel obstruction, cholecystitis, or intestinal ischemia are frequently associated with elevated serum pancreatic isoamylase, because a secondary pancreatic involvement occurs under these circumstances [34]. In general, no convincing benefit of isoamylase

Table 19.1.1. Clinical value of laboratory tests for the diagnosis of acute pancreatitis based on the results of multicenter trials or at least two adequately powered ($n \geq 50$ patients) clinical studies. *tr-FIA* Time-resolved fluorometric immunoassay, *ELISA* enzyme-linked immunosorbent assay, *RIA* radioimmunoassay, *PLA2* phospholipase A2

Parameter	Sensitivity[a]	Specificity[a]	Assay	References
Amylase[b]	68–100%	70–100%	Various routine methods	[15, 18, 19, 25, 31–33, 36–38, 40, 41, 44]
Lipase	85–100%	73–100%	Various routine methods	[15, 18, 19, 25, 32, 33, 35, 37, 38, 41]
P-isoamylase	78–97%	85–92%	Various routine methods	[18, 32, 35, 39]
Trypsinogen-2	85–95%	83–97%	tr-FIA, dipstick	[36–38]
Pancreatic elastase-1	66–100%	85–96%	ELISA	[18, 39–41]
Type I PLA2	90–100%	≈75%	tr-FIA, RIA	[20, 35]
Procarboxypeptidase B	95–100%	82–95%	RIA, ELISA	[21, 43, 44]

[a] Sensitivity and specificity with large variations depending on the cutoff value and time of assessment after disease onset

[b] Limitations: delayed estimation, alcoholic etiology, hyperlipidemia, macroamylasemia, extrapancreatic inflammatory disorders

or isoenzymes for a more reliable diagnosis of acute pancreatitis could be shown in large prospective studies [35], and their measurement therefore has been largely abandoned [12].

Trypsinogen-2

Trypsinogen-2 is another pancreas-specific enzyme that has been found to be of diagnostic and prognostic value in acute pancreatitis. In the largest prospective study by Kemppainen et al. comprising 500 patients with acute abdominal pain, a urinary trypsinogen-2 dipstick test was compared with a quantitative urinary trypsinogen-2 assay, a urinary dipstick test for amylase, and serum and urinary amylase assays [36]. The urinary trypsinogen-2 dipstick test (cutoff 50 ng/ml) achieved a sensitivity of 94%, including all patients with severe pancreatitis, and a specificity of 95%. The serum amylase assay had a sensitivity of 85% (cutoff value of 300 IU/l) and a specificity of 91%. More pronounced differences were found by comparing the urinary trypsinogen-2 dipstick with serum lipase or amylase in a subsequent study of the same group [37]. Quantitative testing of trypsinogen-2 plasma concentrations showed similar results with almost no differences of admission values compared with serum amylase and lipase for diagnostic purposes. However, in contrast to serum amylase and lipase, trypsinogen-2 concentrations remain clearly elevated for at least 1 week after symptom onset [38]. Besides acute pancreatitis, elevated trypsinogen-2 concentrations are also found in nonacute pancreatic disorders such as chronic pancreatitis and pancreatic cancer, in other abdominal malignancies, and in cholangitis. Despite the high specificity of trypsinogen-2 and the availability of a fast and easy test system, the diagnostic advantages are still limited so that a large-scale use beyond academic purposes cannot be recommended.

Pancreatic Elastase-1

P-elastase-1 determinations suffer from similar shortcomings to those of trypsinogen-2. P-elastase-1 has been found to be of equal or lower diagnostic accuracy than serum amylase and lipase during the early stages of acute pancreatitis [18, 39–41]. A large prospective evaluation of this enzyme in 567 patients with clinically suspected acute pancreatitis found a diagnostic accuracy of 80% for P-elastase-1 and 97% for serum amylase [40]. As with other pancreas-specific enzymes, pancreatic disorders other than acute pancreatitis interfere with the specificity of the test, which is available as enzyme-linked assay or radioimmunoassay only. A clear advantage of p-elastase-1 is the extremely long persistence beyond the 1st week after onset of acute pancreatitis, which may be of value in cases with late presentation and where the diagnosisis in doubt. However, the disadvantages of elastase-1 determinations clearly prohibit a role of this test for the routine management of patients with acute pancreatitis.

Further pancreatic enzymes such as PLA2 [42] and procarboxypeptidase B [43, 44] have been shown to be of diagnostic value in acute pancreatitis. However, since these enzymes are outperformed by amylase and lipase in terms of their diagnostic accuracy, adequate assay techniques, and cost, they are no useful screening tests for diagnosing acute pancreatitis.

Biochemical Stratification of the Severity of Acute Pancreatitis

Ever since the first classification system of acute pancreatitis was established in Marseille in 1965 [45], the definition of "severe" disease has been linked to the development of specific complications with an increased risk of mortality [14]. The fact that acute pancreatitis is characterized by an extreme variability of clinical presentation with rapidly or insidiously evolving complications underpins a fascination with predictive or prognostic systems that have a long tradition for more than five decades.

Severity assessment means objective quantification of the actual overall severity of illness. Early and reliable stratification of severity is required for targeting individual patients for interventions against evolving complications or for referral to specialist centers and for comparing patients for scientific purposes or recruitment into clinical trials. Per definition, clinical severity is the sum of the clinical course and ultimate outcome. Outcome itself, usually reflected by nonsurvival, forms the "gold standard" for evaluation of systems to assess severity and prognosis. There are various approaches to assess severity and prognosis that can be inferred from the patient's medical history, clinical signs and symptoms, diagnostic imaging procedures, and laboratory variables. An ideal laboratory test for biochemical severity stratification of acute pancreatitis should be simple in test performance, readily available under routine and emergency conditions, accurate, and inexpensive. Given these attributes, a still growing panel of laboratory variables has been considered as an attractive alternative to imaging procedures or multiple parameter scoring systems in terms of availability, accuracy, and cost (Table 19.1.2).

Table 19.1.2. Clinical value of relevant biochemical parameters for the prediction of severity, infected necrosis/septic shock, and death in patients with acute pancreatitis based on results of meta-analyses, multicenter trials or at least two adequately powered (n ≥ 50 patients) clinical studies. *<48h* Within 48 h of disease onset, *>48h* beyond 48 h of disease onset, *IA* immunoassay, *TAP* trypsinogen activation peptide, *CAPAP* carboxypeptidase B activation peptide, *PMN* polymorphonuclear, *IL* Interleukin, *CRP* C-reactive protein, *SAA* serum amyloid A protein, *PCT* procalcitonin, *MODS* multiorgan dysfunction syndrome, *n.a.* data not available

Parameter	Severity	Infection	Death	Assay	References
Pancreatic proteases					
TAP	yes (<48h)	no	n.a.	ELISA	[52, 70–73]
CAPAP	yes (<48h)	no	n.a.	RIA	[43, 75, 76]
Leukocyte-derived proteases					
PMN-elastase	yes (<48h)	no	yes (>48h)	ELISA, fully automated IA	[92–96]
Type II PLA2	yes (<48h)	yes (>48h)	n.a.	tr-FIA	[78, 99, 100]
Cytokines/chemokines					
IL-6	yes (<48h)	no	no	automated IA	[85–89]
IL-8	yes (<48h)	septic MODS	yes (>48h)	automated IA	[86–89]
Acute-phase proteins					
CRP	yes (>48h)	no	no	automated IA	[16, 52, 55, 57, 67, 68, 71, 72, 77–79, 82, 86]
SAA	yes (<48h)	no	no	automated IA	[79, 82]
Others					
PCT	no	yes (>48h)	yes (>48h)	Semi- and fully automated IA, dipstick	[81, 105–109]

Routine Laboratory Parameters

Since the introduction of the Ranson [46] and Imrie [47] scores, single laboratory components such as hematocrit, creatinine or blood urea nitrogen, and blood glucose continue to be extensively investigated, either alone or in combination, to predict complications and thus "severe" disease.

Hematocrit

Admission hematocrit and its changes during fluid resuscitation have been paid specific attention as a prognostic variable. An admission hematocrit of >44% was found to be closely associated with complications in terms of necrosis and organ failure [48] or pancreatic infections [49]. Other authors reported that a hematocrit of >50% predicts "severe" acute pancreatitis as defined by the Atlanta system [50]. However, admission hematocrit values of >41% to >44% failed to predict severity, organ failure, or death in several other large studies, and even subsequent changes in terms of an increase or decrease within 24 h after treatment did not yield better results [51–55]. Yet, an overall high negative predictive value (NPV) of around 90% excluding "severe" acute pancreatitis at an admission hematocrit of <44% [48, 54] and <40% [51] was reported by some authors. In addition, hematocrit is not able to predict fatal attacks of acute pancreatitis [51, 56, 57]. Taken together, hematocrit may serve as a rough estimate to exclude severe attacks, but is no reliable means to predict severity or any other specific complication accurately.

Creatinine/Blood Urea Nitrogen

Creatinine and blood urea nitrogen (BUN) are laboratory surrogate parameters that indicate and define renal failure alike. Renal failure, defined as creatinine >2 mg/dl (177 μmol/l) by the Atlanta classification belongs to the most serious organ complications in acute pancreatitis and has been shown to be an independent risk factor for fatal outcome [51, 56–61]. However, the widely used cutoff level of >2.0 mg/dl is frequently not reached at the day of hospital admission and limits the use of this variable for "early" risk estimation. In addition, few studies have provided sensitivity and specificity rates for either creatinine or

BUN alone for predicting nonsurvival. As far as disease severity in terms of local or systemic complications is concerned, admission BUN achieved no satisfactory test performance [55, 62, 63] by reaching a maximum sensitivity of 79% and a specificity of 67% (positive predictive value, PPV 43%, NPV 91%) only [62].

Blood Glucose

Blood glucose levels at admission have been shown to correlate with pancreatic necrosis, organ failure, and fatal outcome in acute pancreatitis. In some studies, elevated admission blood glucose at various cutoff levels ranging from 150 mg/dl to 250 mg/dl was even found to be an independent risk factor for local or systemic complications [62], organ failure [55], and death [51, 57]. Normal admission glucose levels in nondiabetic patients can exclude local and systemic complications as well as fatal attacks with a high NPV. However, the overall test performance is not better than observed for hematocrit and laboratory parameters of renal function.

Pancreatic Proteases and Antiproteases

The protease–antiprotease imbalance has been attributed a key role in the pathophysiology of acute pancreatitis since the mid 1980s. Ever since the "autodigestion" theory of Chiari in 1989 [64], trypsinogen activation is believed to be one of the earliest intracellular events that triggers a cascade of other pancreatic proenzymes in acute pancreatitis. In addition, high concentrations of trypsinogen and other proteases have been measured in peripancreatic exudates and in the systemic circulation and correlate well with the extent of pancreatic damage and overall disease severity [65].

Antiproteases

The role of antiproteases as biochemical markers of severity has been addressed by several clinical studies. Hedstrom et al. could show that the trypsin-2-α1-antitrypsin complex in serum is superior to trypsinogen-2, CRP, and amylase in diagnosing acute pancreatitis and is able to differentiate between severe and mild attacks within 12 h after hospital admission [66]. The α2-macrogobulin is another antiprotease, which binds to pancreatic proteases such as trypsin or elastase. In severe attacks, the protease–antiprotease complex is rapidly degraded from the systemic circulation by macrophages and causes an early and pronounced decrease of α2-macroglobulin levels [1, 67, 68]. Although early disease prediction and severity stratification may be possible by means of antiproteases, neither the diagnostic accuracy nor the assay procedures are appropriate for use under routine conditions.

Activation Peptides

Trypsinogen activation peptide (TAP) and carboxypeptidase B activation peptide (CAPAP) account for the most important activation peptides in acute pancreatitis. The results of several studies clearly indicate that measuring activation peptides is superior to that of leaking proenzymes such as trypsinogen-2 to predict severity, which is attributable to the high stability of the cleaved propeptide in the systemic circulation [69].

TAP is by far the most extensively investigated activation peptide in acute pancreatitis. TAP is known to be disease specific, not influenced by the underlying etiology of acute pancreatitis and is detectable in the systemic circulation and in urine alike. Since its first description in 1990 by Gudgeon et al. [52] the clinical usefulness of this parameter has been investigated extensively, three multicenter trials have been published with the common endpoint "severe disease" according to the Atlanta classification. A United States trial showed that urinary TAP achieved a sensitivity of 100% and a specificity of 85% (PPV not recorded, NPV 100%) in predicting a severe attack of acute pancreatitis within 48 h of disease onset [70]. Two subsequent European multicenter trials showed somewhat less favorable results, with a sensitivity and specificity of 58% and 73%, respectively (PPV 39%, NPV 86%) [71] as well as 46% and 80%, respectively (PPV 28%, NPV 90%) [72], for urinary TAP within 24 h using the same cutoff levels. The test performed better at 48 h after disease onset, with a sensitivity of 83% and a specificity of 72% (PPV 44%, NPV 94%) [71]. Corresponding results were found in a multicenter study for admission plasma TAP concentrations [73]. On the other hand, overall accuracy rates of urinary TAP in predicting a severe attack did not exceed 75%, even 48 h after the onset of acute pancreatitis, which was also achieved by clinical scoring systems. Moreover, it is still not known whether early prediction of specific complications such as organ failure or death is possible. Unfortunately, the very early burst-like secretion of TAP with a rapid decline makes discrimination between severe and mild cases no longer possible after 72 h. Therefore, monitoring the progression of the disease to severe organ failure or septic complications, which usually develops beyond 48 h after symptom onset, is hardly possible.

The current enzyme-linked immunosorbent assay (ELISA) technique prohibits the analysis of this parameter in the daily laboratory routine.

The activation peptide CAPAP possesses diagnostic and prognostic properties in acute pancreatitis and has been found to correlate well with disease severity as defined by Atlanta [43, 74–76]. CAPAP can be measured in the plasma and urine and is more stable than TAP due to its larger size. As observed for TAP, the highest diagnostic accuracy in predicting pancreatic necrosis is obtained by measuring this activation peptide in urine, with excellent accuracy rates of about 90% throughout several studies [43, 75, 76]. Unfortunately, CAPAP levels also rapidly decline and are thus not useful in depicting severe cases in the later course of the disease. Moreover, the CAPAP assay is currently available as a radioimmunoassay only, which prohibits an introduction of this parameter to clinical routine analysis at present.

According to the published literature, assessment of pancreatic protease activation peptides is one of the very few approaches to an early severity stratification of acute pancreatitis within 48 h of disease onset. Measurement of these variables may be of specific interest for specialized centers whenever early severity stratification for clinical trials or improved interinstitutional comparison of patients is an issue. However, from an economical and practical standpoint, a large-scale clinical application of TAP or CAPAP will be unlikely. Because many patients with acute pancreatitis are admitted or referred beyond the 48-h diagnostic window after disease onset the general need for very early markers of severity has to be questioned. Even if the development of an "immunostick" for a single or combined assessment of activation peptides is developed in the future, the clinical use of these parameters will probably remain a scientific one due to the limited indication and therefore persisting high cost.

Acute-Phase Proteins

Acute-phase proteins constitute a family of inflammatory proteins that are predominantly synthesized in the liver in response to various infectious and non-infectious stimuli. The most famous member is CRP, and more recently SAA accomplished the spectrum of acute-phase reactants for biochemical severity stratification of acute pancreatitis. Both parameters share an essential feature for a large-scale routine application: they have become available as fully automated immunoassays.

C-Reactive Protein

Severity stratification of acute pancreatitis by CRP has a long tradition and still represents the "gold standard" new biochemical parameters have to compete with [1, 16, 52, 55, 57, 67, 68, 71, 72, 77–79]. The practicability of the assay procedure, the cost, and the availability have rendered CRP as a widely established means for both severity stratification and monitoring the course of the disease. CRP is the parameter of choice to differentiate necrotizing from interstitial edematous acute pancreatitis [80]. However, the majority of the studies focused on the discrimination between mild and severe acute pancreatitis and obtained a diagnostic accuracy of between 70 and 80% at a cutoff level of >150 mg/l within the first 48 h after disease onset [68, 71, 72]. Higher cutoff levels up to 200 mg/l and more have been reported beyond this interval, yielding even better results [67]. As well documented for all acute-phase proteins, CRP is not useful for the prediction of infected necrosis, organ failure, or death within the 1st week after disease onset [55, 81]. Another shortcoming of CRP is the relatively long delay of its induction with systemic peak values at 72–96 h after disease onset, thus making very early severity assessment impossible.

Serum Amyloid A

SAA is another acute-phase reactant for the severity stratification of acute pancreatitis, and has been evaluated by two adequately powered studies so far [79, 82]. A common finding of both studies was an earlier release with a wider dynamic range of SAA than observed for CRP. However, these studies are not quite comparable, because they differ in endpoint analysis and assay techniques applied. The multicenter study found that SAA was a better early predictor of severe acute pancreatitis than CRP by using a conventional ELISA technique [82]. The study of our group could not demonstrate any advantage of SAA over CRP in stratifying severity at any time point during the course of acute pancreatitis by using a fully automated assay technique [79]. Further studies will be needed to define a convincing clinical benefit of SAA over CRP determinations to justify the still higher cost of this alternative acute-phase reactant.

Among the acute-phase proteins, CRP still remains the gold standard in predicting severity beyond 48 h after the onset of acute pancreatitis. This readily available, fast, and inexpensive test is still the reference parameter among the indicators of necrosis and severe disease according to the Atlanta classification.

Cytokines and Chemokines

A wealth of experimental and clinical studies have convincingly outlined that cytokines and chemokines play a key role in the pathophysiology of acute pancreatitis by promoting local tissue destruction and mediating distant organ complications [83]. Since the early 1990s, the first clinical reports about the role of cytokine measurements in acute pancreatitis appeared in the literature and still continue to address this topic. The development of fast and fully automated assay techniques have overcome the problem of the conventional ELISA measurements; however, the vast majority of the cytokine and chemokine family members play no role as biochemical markers for the severity assessment of acute pancreatitis in the clinical setting. So far, only the cytokine IL-6 and the chemokine IL-8 have crossed the threshold from pathophysiological importance to clinical application [80].

Interleukin-6

Systemic concentrations of IL-6 have been found to be early and excellent predictors of severity. A large number of clinical studies have shown uniformly that IL-6 is dramatically increased in complicated attacks [55, 84–89]. The rise of IL-6 concentrations generally occurs 24–36 h earlier than that of CRP, with significantly elevated levels as long as complications persist. One of the first series in 24 patients by Heath et al. from Glasgow found a sensitivity of 100% and a specificity of 71% (PPV 71%, NPV 100%) at a cutoff level of >130 IU/ml for IL-6 in predicting a severe attack within 36 h of disease onset [84], and even better results have been reported [86]. Beyond discriminating mild from severe attacks, IL-6 closely correlates with evolving organ failure [55, 87, 88], while early prediction of death has rarely been the subject of investigation, but does not seem to be possible [85]. IL-6 has been introduced as a routine parameter in some laboratories and represents an easy and rapid means to select patients at risk to develop severe disease.

Interleukin-8

IL-8 was initially described as an early marker of disease severity within the 1st day after onset of symptoms, with a rapid decease after 3–5 days [86, 90, 91] and reveals obvious parallels with IL-6. However, our group described an even more interesting aspect of IL-8 assessment beyond simple discrimination between mild and severe attacks. In patients with necrotizing pancreatitis who developed septic multiorgan failure or died in the later stages of the disease, IL-8 has proven to be an excellent marker for monitoring this life-threatening complication [81]. As for IL-6, a fully automated assay is available for IL-8, and the use of this chemokine for disease monitoring has become possible on a daily routine basis. However, the relatively high cost still prohibits a large-scale application of both IL-6 and IL-8 in clinical practice.

Leukocyte-Derived Enzymes/Proteases

The activation of different leukocyte subsets has been well recognized as an important pathophysiological step for the development of diseases severity and pancreatitis-associated organ failure. Beyond their pathophysiological importance, several PMN-derived proteolytic enzymes have been described as good biochemical markers for the severity stratification of acute pancreatitis.

PMN-Elastase

Enhanced systemic release of PMN elastase is an early feature in severe attacks with peak values even before CRP and other parameters begin to rise [90, 92–95]. In a Spanish multicenter trial by Dominguez-Munoz et al. in 182 patients, PMN-elastase reached sensitivity and specificity rates of more than 90% (PPV >80%, NPV >90%) in predicting severe acute pancreatitis within 24–48 h of disease onset [93]. Concentrations rapidly decline in patients with an uneventful recovery, while a persistent elevation of this enzyme was observed in nonsurvivors [92]. The PMN-elastase test has not been adopted into routine laboratories because of problems with the assay and the reproducibility of the test results. Very recently, the same Spanish group has evaluated a new, routinely applicable assay, which has overcome the previous disadvantages, in a multicenter study and confirmed the excellent results of their previous studies [96]. However, as already several excellent parameters are available for a fast and accurate early severity stratification of acute pancreatitis, the fate of PMN-elastase measurement has yet to be established.

Phospholipase A2

In addition to type I PLA2, which is of pancreatic origin, type II, or synovial type PLA2 is secreted by activated neutrophils [97]. Whereas type I PLA2 is of no prognostic value, synovial type PLA2 provides a good discrimination between severe and mild attacks of acute pancreatitis throughout the course of the disease [78, 98, 99]. Interestingly, a more recent study of our group has outlined a new diagnostic aspect of type II PLA2 in acute pancreatitis: the course of type II PLA2 concentrations is closely correlated with the development of pancreatic infections in patients with necrotizing pancreatitis [100]. Unfortunately, no assay for clinical routine analysis has yet been developed for measuring type II PLA2. Therefore, this interesting and potentially useful parameter continues to play a role in a scientific respect only.

Procalcitonin

Ever since its first description in 1993 [101], an extensive number of reports have largely confirmed that PCT is the first biochemical variable that closely correlates with the presence of bacterial or fungal infections and severe sepsis [102]. Since infection of necrosis is a major complication with significant impact on management and outcome [1, 103, 104], biochemical stratification of patients at risk would be an attractive approach. In a cohort study comprising 50 patients with acute pancreatitis, our group first described a highly significant correlation of elevated PCT levels and the subsequent development of infected necrosis. At a cutoff level of 1.8 ng/ml, PCT was able to predict this complication with a sensitivity and specificity of more than 90% within the first days after disease onset [81]. This observation was confirmed by several subsequent studies [105]. In addition, a large Finnish study by Kylanpaa-Back et al. showed that PCT at a cut-off level of >0.4 ng/ml was able to predict subsequent organ failure with a sensitivity of 94% and a specificity of 73% (PPV 58%, NPV 97%) already 24 h after hospital admission [106]. Even by using a semiquantitative PCT strip test in another study by the same authors in 162 acute attacks all patients who developed subsequent organ failure were correctly identified within 24 h of admission [107]. An international multicenter trial conducted by our group in 104 patients with severe acute pancreatitis has shown that PCT is able to predict major complications such as clinically relevant pancreatic infections or death, with a sensitivity of 79% and a specificity of 93% (PPV 65%, NPV 97%) at a cut-off level of >3.8 ng/ml within 48–96 h after onset of symptoms [108]. Notably, PCT is of limited value for simple stratification of patients as "mild" or "severe" according to the Atlanta classification [109]. PCT determinations have become available as fully automated assay for routine use; a semiquantitative strip test is an alternative for a fast and easy quantification.

On the basis of the data available at present, PCT is one of the most promising parameters for an early stratification of patients at risk of developing most serious complications as well as for monitoring the course of acute pancreatitis. In terms of the assay technique, PCT meets all demands to be run under clinical routine and emergency conditions.

References

1. Buchler M, Malfertheiner P, Schoetensack C, Uhl W, Beger HG (1986) Sensitivity of antiproteases, complement factors and C-reactive protein in detecting pancreatic necrosis. Results of a prospective clinical study. Int J Pancreatol 1:227–235
2. Isenmann R, Rau B, Beger HG (2001) Early severe acute pancreatitis: characteristics of a new subgroup. Pancreas 22:274–278
3. Johnson CD, Abu-Hilal M (2004) Persistent organ failure during the first week as a marker of fatal outcome in acute pancreatitis. Gut 53:1340–1344
4. Heinrich S, Schafer M, Rousson V, Clavien PA (2006) Evidence-based treatment of acute pancreatitis: a look at established paradigms. Ann Surg 243:154–168
5. Elman R, Arneson N, Graham EA (1929) Value of blood amylase estimations in the diagnosis of pancreatic disease: a clinical study. Arch Surg 19:943–967
6. Trapnell JE (1966) The natural history and prognosis of acute pancreatitis. Ann R Coll Surg Engl 38:265–287
7. Wilson C, Imrie CW (1988) Deaths from acute pancreatitis: why do we miss the diagnosis so frequently? Int J Pancreatol 3:273–281
8. Lankisch PG, Schirren CA, Kunze E (1991) Undetected fatal acute pancreatitis: why is the disease so frequently overlooked? Am J Gastroenterol 86:322–326
9. Saxon EI, Hinkley WC, Vogel WC, Zieve L (1957) Comparative value of serum and urinary amylase in the diagnosis of acute pancreatitis. AMA Arch Intern Med 99:607–621
10. Thomson HJ, Obekpa PO, Smith AN, Brydon WG (1987) Diagnosis of acute pancreatitis: a proposed sequence of biochemical investigations. Scand J Gastroenterol 22:719–724
11. Fabris C, Basso D, Naccarato R (1992) Urinary enzymes excretion in pancreatic diseases. Clinical role and pathophysiological considerations. J Clin Gastroenterol 14:281–284
12. Yadav D, Agarwal N, Pitchumoni CS (2002) A critical evaluation of laboratory tests in acute pancreatitis. Am J Gastroenterol 97:1309–1318
13. Werner M, Steinberg WM, Pauley C (1989) Strategic use of individual and combined enzyme indicators for acute pancreatitis analyzed by receiver-operator characteristics. Clin Chem 35:967–971
14. Bradley EL III (1993) A clinically based classification system for acute pancreatitis. Summary of the International Symposium on Acute Pancreatitis, Atlanta, Ga, September 11–13, 1992. Arch Surg 128:586–590

15. Keim V, Teich N, Fiedler F, Hartig W, Thiele G, Mossner J (1998) A comparison of lipase and amylase in the diagnosis of acute pancreatitis in patients with abdominal pain. Pancreas 16:45–49
16. Clavien PA, Robert J, Meyer P, Borst F, Hauser H, Herrmann F, Dunand V, Rohner A (1989) Acute pancreatitis and normoamylasemia. Not an uncommon combination. Ann Surg 210:614–620
17. Spechler SJ, Dalton JW, Robbins AH, Gerzof SG, Stern JS, Johnson WC, Nabseth DC, Schimmel EM (1983) Prevalence of normal serum amylase levels in patients with acute alcoholic pancreatitis. Dig Dis Sci 28:865–869
18. Ventrucci M, Pezzilli R, Gullo L, Plate L, Sprovieri G, Barbara L (1989) Role of serum pancreatic enzyme assays in diagnosis of pancreatic disease. Dig Dis Sci 34:39–45
19. Gwozdz GP, Steinberg WM, Werner M, Henry JP, Pauley C (1990) Comparative evaluation of the diagnosis of acute pancreatitis based on serum and urine enzyme assays. Clin Chim Acta 187:243–254
20. Kitagawa M, Hayakawa T, Kondo T, Shibata T, Sakai Y, Sobajima H, Ishiguro H, Nakae Y (1991) The diagnostic value of serum pancreatic phospholipase A2 (PLA2) in pancreatic diseases. Gastroenterol Jpn 26:62–68
21. Rau B, Cebulla M, Uhl W, Schoenberg MH, Beger HG (1998) The clinical value of human pancreas-specific protein procarboxypeptidase B as an indicator of necrosis in acute pancreatitis: comparison to CRP and LDH. Pancreas 17:134–139
22. Tietz NW, Shuey DF (1993) Lipase in serum – the elusive enzyme: an overview. Clin Chem 39:746–756
23. Toskes PP (1990) Hyperlipidemic pancreatitis. Gastroenterol Clin North Am 19:783–791
24. Mishkin S, Bates J, O'Hashi J, Schneider P, Sniderman AD, Wolf RO (1976) Possible mechanisms of normal amylase activity in hyperlipemic pancreatitis. Can Med Assoc J 115:1016–1019
25. Kazmierczak SC, Catrou PG, Van Lente F (1993) Diagnostic accuracy of pancreatic enzymes evaluated by use of multivariate data analysis. Clin Chem 39:1960–1965
26. Lott JA (1991) The value of clinical laboratory studies in acute pancreatitis. Arch Pathol Lab Med 115:325–326
27. Warshaw AL, Hawboldt MM (1988) Puzzling persistent hyperamylasemia, probably neither pancreatic nor pathologic. Am J Surg 155:453–456
28. Gullo L (2000) Familial pancreatic hyperenzymemia. Pancreas 20:158–160
29. Heikius B, Niemela S, Lehtola J, Karttunen TJ (1999) Elevated pancreatic enzymes in inflammatory bowel disease are associated with extensive disease. Am J Gastroenterol 94:1062–1069
30. Tietz NW (1997) Support of the diagnosis of pancreatitis by enzyme tests – old problems, new techniques. Clin Chim Acta 257:85–98
31. Butler J, Bates D (2003) Serum amylase and acute pancreatitis. Emerg Med J 20:550–551
32. Steinberg WM, Goldstein SS, Davis ND, Shamma'a J, Anderson K (1985) Diagnostic assays in acute pancreatitis. A study of sensitivity and specificity. Ann Intern Med 102:576–580
33. Gumaste VV, Roditis N, Mehta D, Dave PB (1993) Serum lipase levels in nonpancreatic abdominal pain versus acute pancreatitis. Am J Gastroenterol 88:2051–2055
34. Pieper–Bigelow C, Strocchi A, Levitt MD (1990) Where does serum amylase come from and where does it go? Gastroenterol Clin North Am 19:793–810
35. Sternby B, O'Brien JF, Zinsmeister AR, DiMagno EP (1996) What is the best biochemical test to diagnose acute pancreatitis? A prospective clinical study. Mayo Clin Proc 71:1138–1144
36. Kemppainen EA, Hedstrom JI, Puolakkainen PA, Sainio VS, Haapiainen RK, Perhoniemi V, Osman S, Kivilaakso EO, Stenman UH (1997) Rapid measurement of urinary trypsinogen-2 as a screening test for acute pancreatitis. N Engl J Med 336:1788–1793
37. Kylanpaa-Back ML, Kemppainen E, Puolakkainen P, Hedstrom J, Haapiainen R, Korvuo A, Stenman UH (2002) Comparison of urine trypsinogen-2 test strip with serum lipase in the diagnosis of acute pancreatitis. Hepatogastroenterology;49:1130–1134
38. Hedstrom J, Kemppainen E, Andersen J, Jokela H, Puolakkainen P, Stenman UH (2001) A comparison of serum trypsinogen-2 and trypsin-2-alpha1-antitrypsin complex with lipase and amylase in the diagnosis and assessment of severity in the early phase of acute pancreatitis. Am J Gastroenterol 96:424–430
39. Malfertheiner P, Buchler M, Stanescu A, Uhl W, Ditschuneit H (1987) Serum elastase 1 in inflammatory pancreatic and gastrointestinal diseases and in renal insufficiency. A comparison with other serum pancreatic enzymes. Int J Pancreatol 2:159–170
40. Millson CE, Charles K, Poon P, Macfie J, Mitchell CJ (1998) A prospective study of serum pancreatic elastase-1 in the diagnosis and assessment of acute pancreatitis. Scand J Gastroenterol 33:664–668
41. Wilson RB, Warusavitarne J, Crameri DM, Alvaro F, Davies DJ, Merrett N (2005) Serum elastase in the diagnosis of acute pancreatitis: a prospective study. ANZ J Surg 75:152–156
42. Kaiser E (1999) Phospholipase A2: its usefulness in laboratory diagnostics. Crit Rev Clin Lab Sci 36:65–163
43. Muller CA, Appelros S, Uhl W, Buchler MW, Borgstrom A (2002) Serum levels of procarboxypeptidase B and its activation peptide in patients with acute pancreatitis and non-pancreatic diseases. Gut 51:229–235
44. Chen CC, Wang SS, Chao Y, Chen SJ, Lee SD, Wu SL, Jeng FS, Lo KJ (1994) Serum pancreas-specific protein in acute pancreatitis. Its clinical utility in comparison with serum amylase. Scand J Gastroenterol 29:87–90
45. Sarles H (1965) Proposal adopted unanimously by the participants of the symposium on pancreatitis at Marseille, 1963. Bibl Gastroenterol 7:VII–VIII
46. Ranson JH, Lackner H, Berman IR, Schinella R (1977) The relationship of coagulation factors to clinical complications of acute pancreatitis. Surgery 81:502–511
47. Imrie CW, Benjamin IS, Ferguson JC, McKay AJ, Mackenzie I, O'Neill J, Blumgart LH (1978) A single-centre double-blind trial of Trasylol therapy in primary acute pancreatitis. Br J Surg 65:337–341
48. Brown A, Orav J, Banks PA (2000) Hemoconcentration is an early marker for organ failure and necrotizing pancreatitis. Pancreas 20:367–372
49. Sun B, Li HL, Gao Y, Xu J, Jiang HC (2003) Factors predisposing to severe acute pancreatitis: evaluation and prevention. World J Gastroenterol 9:1102–1105
50. Gan SI, Romagnuolo J (2004) Admission hematocrit: a simple, useful and early predictor of severe pancreatitis. Dig Dis Sci 49:1946–1952
51. Lankisch PG, Mahlke R, Blum T, Bruns A, Bruns D, Maisonneuve P, Lowenfels AB (2001) Hemoconcentration: an early marker of severe and/or necrotizing pancreatitis? A critical appraisal. Am J Gastroenterol 96:2081–2085

52. Gudgeon AM, Heath DI, Hurley P, Jehanli A, Patel G, Wilson C, Shenkin A, Austen BM, Imrie CW, Hermon-Taylor J (1990) Trypsinogen activation peptides assay in the early prediction of severity of acute pancreatitis. Lancet 335:4–8
53. Pezzilli R, Morselli-Labate AM (2001) Hematocrit determination (HCT) as an early marker associated with necrotizing pancreatitis and organ failure. Pancreas 22:433–435
54. Khan Z, Vlodov J, Horovitz J, Jose RM, Iswara K, Smotkin J, Brown A, Tenner S (2002) Urinary trypsinogen activation peptide is more accurate than hematocrit in determining severity in patients with acute pancreatitis: a prospective study. Am J Gastroenterol 97:1973–1977
55. Mentula P, Kylanpaa ML, Kemppainen E, Jansson SE, Sarna S, Puolakkainen P, Haapiainen R, Repo H (2005) Early prediction of organ failure by combined markers in patients with acute pancreatitis. Br J Surg 92:68–75
56. Eachempati SR, Hydo LJ, Barie PS (2002) Severity scoring for prognostication in patients with severe acute pancreatitis: comparative analysis of the Ranson score and the APACHE III score. Arch Surg 137:730–736
57. Talamini G, Bassi C, Falconi M, Sartori N, Frulloni L, Di Francesco V, Vesentini S, Pederzoli P, Cavallini G (1996) Risk of death from acute pancreatitis. Role of early, simple "routine" data. Int J Pancreatol 19:15–24
58. Halonen KI, Leppaniemi AK, Puolakkainen PA, Lundin JE, Kemppainen EA, Hietaranta AJ, Haapiainen RK (2000) Severe acute pancreatitis: prognostic factors in 270 consecutive patients. Pancreas 21:266–271
59. Company L, Saez J, Martinez J, Aparicio JR, Laveda R, Grino P, Perez-Mateo M (2003) Factors predicting mortality in severe acute pancreatitis. Pancreatology 3:144–148
60. Kong L, Santiago N, Han TQ, Zhang SD (2004) Clinical characteristics and prognostic factors of severe acute pancreatitis. World J Gastroenterol 10:3336–3338
61. Halonen KI, Pettila V, Leppaniemi AK, Kemppainen EA, Puolakkainen PA, Haapiainen RK (2002) Multiple organ dysfunction associated with severe acute pancreatitis. Crit Care Med 30:1274–1479
62. Radenkovic D, Bajec D, Karamarkovic A, Stefanovic B, Milic N, Ignjatovic S, Gregoric P, Milicevic M (2004) Disorders of hemostasis during the surgical management of severe necrotizing pancreatitis. Pancreas 29:152–156
63. Heath DI, Meng WC, Anderson JH, Leung KL, Lau WY, Li AK (1997) Failure of the Hong Kong criteria to predict the severity of acute pancreatitis. Int J Pancreatol 22:201–206
64. Chiari H (1896) Über die Selbstverdauung des menschlichen Pankreas. Zeitschrift für Heilkunde 17:69–96
65. Frossard JL (2001) Trypsin activation peptide (TAP) in acute pancreatitis: from pathophysiology to clinical usefulness. JOP 2:69–77
66. Hedstrom J, Sainio V, Kemppainen E, Haapiainen R, Kivilaakso E, Schroder T, Leinonen J, Stenman UH (1996) Serum complex of trypsin 2 and alpha 1 antitrypsin as diagnostic and prognostic marker of acute pancreatitis: clinical study in consecutive patients. BMJ 313:333–337
67. Wilson C, Heads A, Shenkin A, Imrie CW (1989) C-reactive protein, antiproteases and complement factors as objective markers of severity in acute pancreatitis. Br J Surg 76:177–181
68. Dominguez-Munoz JE, Carballo F, Garcia MJ, Miguel de Diego J, Gea F, Yanguela J, de la Morena J (1993) Monitoring of serum proteinase–antiproteinase balance and systemic inflammatory response in prognostic evaluation of acute pancreatitis. Results of a prospective multicenter study. Dig Dis Sci 38:507–513
69. Borgstrom A, Appelros S, Muller CA, Uhl W, Buchler MW (2002) Role of activation peptides from pancreatic proenzymes in the diagnosis and prognosis of acute pancreatitis. Surgery 131:125–128
70. Tenner S, Fernandez-del Castillo C, Warshaw A, Steinberg W, Hermon-Taylor J, Valenzuela JE, Hariri M, Hughes M, Banks PA (1997) Urinary trypsinogen activation peptide (TAP) predicts severity in patients with acute pancreatitis. Int J Pancreatol 21:105–110
71. Neoptolemos JP, Kemppainen EA, Mayer JM, Fitzpatrick JM, Raraty MG, Slavin J, Beger HG, Hietaranta AJ, Puolakkainen PA (2000) Early prediction of severity in acute pancreatitis by urinary trypsinogen activation peptide: a multicentre study. Lancet 355:1955–1960
72. Johnson CD, Lempinen M, Imrie CW, Puolakkainen P, Kemppainen E, Carter R, McKay C (2004) Urinary trypsinogen activation peptide as a marker of severe acute pancreatitis. Br J Surg 91:1027–1033
73. Kemppainen E, Mayer J, Puolakkainen P, Raraty M, Slavin J, Neoptolemos JP (2001) Plasma trypsinogen activation peptide in patients with acute pancreatitis. Br J Surg 88:679–680
74. Pezzilli R, Morselli-Labate AM, Barbieri AR, Plate L (2000) Clinical usefulness of the serum carboxypeptidase B activation peptide in acute pancreatitis. JOP 1:58–68
75. Appelros S, Petersson U, Toh S, Johnson C, Borgstrom A (2001) Activation peptide of carboxypeptidase B and anionic trypsinogen as early predictors of the severity of acute pancreatitis. Br J Surg 88:216–221
76. Saez J, Martinez J, Trigo C, Sanchez-Paya J, Grino P, Company L, Laveda R, Penalva JC, Garcia C, Perez-Mateo M (2004) A comparative study of the activation peptide of carboxypeptidase B and trypsinogen as early predictors of the severity of acute pancreatitis. Pancreas 29:e9–14
77. Gurleyik G, Cirpici OZ, Aktekin A, Saglam A (2004) [The value of Ranson and APACHE II scoring systems, and serum levels of interleukin-6 and C-reactive protein in the early diagnosis of the severity of acute pancreatitis]. Ulus Travma Derg 10:83–88
78. Puolakkainen P, Valtonen V, Paananen A, Schroder T (1987) C-reactive protein (CRP) and serum phospholipase A2 in the assessment of the severity of acute pancreatitis. Gut 28:764–771
79. Rau B, Steinbach G, Baumgart K, Gansauge F, Grunert A, Beger HG (2000) Serum amyloid A versus C-reactive protein in acute pancreatitis: clinical value of an alternative acute-phase reactant. Crit Care Med 28:736–742
80. Rau B, Schilling MK, Beger HG (2004) Laboratory markers of severe acute pancreatitis. Dig Dis 22:247–257
81. Rau B, Steinbach G, Gansauge F, Mayer JM, Grunert A, Beger HG (1997) The potential role of procalcitonin and interleukin 8 in the prediction of infected necrosis in acute pancreatitis. Gut 41:832–840
82. Mayer JM, Raraty M, Slavin J, Kemppainen E, Fitzpatrick J, Hietaranta A, Puolakkainen P, Beger HG, Neoptolemos JP (2002) Serum amyloid A is a better early predictor of severity than C-reactive protein in acute pancreatitis. Br J Surg 89:163–171
83. Rau BM, Kruger CM, Schilling MK (2005) Anti-cytokine strategies in acute pancreatitis: pathophysiological insights and clinical implications. Rocz Akad Med Bialymst 50:106–115

84. Heath DI, Cruickshank A, Gudgeon M, Jehanli A, Shenkin A, Imrie CW (1993) Role of interleukin-6 in mediating the acute phase protein response and potential as an early means of severity assessment in acute pancreatitis. Gut 34:41–45
85. Brivet FG, Emilie D, Galanaud P (1999) Pro- and anti-inflammatory cytokines during acute severe pancreatitis: an early and sustained response, although unpredictable of death. Parisian Study Group on Acute Pancreatitis. Crit Care Med 27:749–755
86. Chen CC, Wang SS, Lee FY, Chang FY, Lee SD (1999) Proinflammatory cytokines in early assessment of the prognosis of acute pancreatitis. Am J Gastroenterol 94:213–218
87. Mayer J, Rau B, Gansauge F, Beger HG (2000) Inflammatory mediators in human acute pancreatitis: clinical and pathophysiological implications. Gut 47:546–552
88. Dugernier TL, Laterre PF, Wittebole X, Roeseler J, Latinne D, Reynaert MS, Pugin J (2003) Compartmentalization of the inflammatory response during acute pancreatitis: correlation with local and systemic complications. Am J Respir Crit Care Med 168:148–157
89. Stimac D, Fisic E, Milic S, Bilic-Zulle L, Peric R (2006) Prognostic values of IL-6, IL-8, and IL-10 in acute pancreatitis. J Clin Gastroenterol 40:209–212
90. Gross V, Andreesen R, Leser HG, Ceska M, Liehl E, Lausen M, Farthmann EH, Scholmerich J (1992) Interleukin-8 and neutrophil activation in acute pancreatitis. Eur J Clin Invest 22:200–203
91. Pezzilli R, Billi P, Miniero R, Fiocchi M, Cappelletti O, Morselli-Labate AM, Barakat B, Sprovieri G, Miglioli M (1995) Serum interleukin-6, interleukin-8, and beta 2-microglobulin in early assessment of severity of acute pancreatitis. Comparison with serum C-reactive protein. Dig Dis Sci 40:2341–2348
92. Gross V, Scholmerich J, Leser HG, Salm R, Lausen M, Ruckauer K, Schoffel U, Lay L, Heinisch A, Farthmann EH, Gerok W (1990) Granulocyte elastase in assessment of severity of acute pancreatitis. Comparison with acute-phase proteins C-reactive protein, alpha 1-antitrypsin, and protease inhibitor alpha 2-macroglobulin. Dig Dis Sci 35:97–105
93. Dominguez-Munoz JE, Carballo F, Garcia MJ, de Diego JM, Rabago L, Simon MA, de la Morena J (1991) Clinical usefulness of polymorphonuclear elastase in predicting the severity of acute pancreatitis: results of a multicentre study. Br J Surg 78:1230–1234
94. Uhl W, Buchler M, Malfertheiner P, Martini M, Beger HG (1991) PMN-elastase in comparison with CRP, antiproteases, and LDH as indicators of necrosis in human acute pancreatitis. Pancreas 6:253–259
95. Viedma JA, Perez-Mateo M, Agullo J, Dominguez JE, Carballo F (1994) Inflammatory response in the early prediction of severity in human acute pancreatitis. Gut 35:822–827
96. Dominguez-Munoz JE, Villanueva A, Larino J, Mora T, Barreiro M, Iglesias-Canle J, Iglesias-Garcia J (2006) Accuracy of plasma levels of polymorphonuclear elastase as early prognostic marker of acute pancreatitis in routine clinical conditions. Eur J Gastroenterol Hepatol 18:79–83
97. Nevalainen TJ, Hietaranta AJ, Gronroos JM (1999) Phospholipase A2 in acute pancreatitis: new biochemical and pathological aspects. Hepatogastroenterology 46:2731–2735
98. Nevalainen TJ, Gronroos JM, Kortesuo PT (1993) Pancreatic and synovial type phospholipases A2 in serum samples from patients with severe acute pancreatitis. Gut 34:1133–1136
99. Bird NC, Goodman AJ, Johnson AG (1989) Serum phospholipase A2 activity in acute pancreatitis: an early guide to severity. Br J Surg 76:731–732
100. Mayer J, Rau B, Grewe M, Schoenberg MH, Nevalainen TJ, Beger HG (1998) Secretory phospholipase A2 in patients with infected pancreatic necroses in acute pancreatitis. Pancreas 17:272–277
101. Assicot M, Gendrel D, Carsin H, Raymond J, Guilbaud J, Bohuon C (1993) High serum procalcitonin concentrations in patients with sepsis and infection. Lancet 341:515–518
102. Simon L, Gauvin F, Amre DK, Saint-Louis P, Lacroix J (2004) Serum procalcitonin and C-reactive protein levels as markers of bacterial infection: a systematic review and meta-analysis. Clin Infect Dis 39:206–217
103. Uhl W, Warshaw A, Imrie C, Bassi C, McKay CJ, Lankisch PG, Carter R, Di Magno E, Banks PA, Whitcomb DC, Dervenis C, Ulrich CD, Satake K, Ghaneh P, Hartwig W, Werner J, McEntee G, Neoptolemos JP, Buchler MW (2002) IAP Guidelines for the Surgical Management of Acute Pancreatitis. Pancreatology 2:565–573
104. Working Party of the British Society of Gastroenterology; Association of Surgeons of Great Britain and Ireland; Pancreatic Society of Great Britain and Ireland; Association of Upper GI Surgeons of Great Britain and Ireland (2005) UK guidelines for the management of acute pancreatitis. Gut 54 Suppl 3:iii1–9
105. Rau B, Kruger CM, Schilling MK (2004) Procalcitonin: improved biochemical severity stratification and postoperative monitoring in severe abdominal inflammation and sepsis. Langenbecks Arch Surg 389:134–144
106. Kylanpaa-Back ML, Takala A, Kemppainen EA, Puolakkainen PA, Leppaniemi AK, Karonen SL, Orpana A, Haapiainen RK, Repo H (2001) Procalcitonin, soluble interleukin-2 receptor, and soluble E-selectin in predicting the severity of acute pancreatitis. Crit Care Med 29:63–69
107. Kylanpaa-Back ML, Takala A, Kemppainen E, Puolakkainen P, Haapiainen R, Repo H (2001) Procalcitonin strip test in the early detection of severe acute pancreatitis. Br J Surg 88:222–227
108. Rau B, Kemppainen E, Gumb A, Büchler MW, Wegscheider K, Bassi C, Puolakkainen P, Beger HG (2007) Early assessment of pancreatic infections and overall prognosis in severe acute pancreatitis by procalcitonin (PCT): a prospective international multicenter study. Ann Surg 245:745–754
109. Purkayastha S, Chow A, Athanasiou T, Cambaroudis A, Panesar S, Kinross J, Tekkis P, Darzi A (2006) Does serum procalcitonin have a role in evaluating the severity of acute pancreatitis? A question revisited. World J Surg 30:1713–1721

E. J. Balthazar

Imaging Diagnosis of Acute Pancreatitis

The beneficial use of noninvasive imaging methods for the diagnosis and evaluation of patients suspected of acute pancreatitis has been widely acknowledged in the literature. For the first time in history, developed only in the last 25 years and with ever increasing accuracy, new imaging modalities such as sonography, computerized tomography (CT), and magnetic resonance imaging (MRI) have allowed the direct visualization of the pancreatic gland, as well as of morphologic abnormalities of the pancreatic gland and retroperitoneum associated with acute pancreatitis.

Background

Acute pancreatitis is mainly a diffuse, nonspecific inflammatory condition related to a great number of diverse etiologic factors, most frequently cholelithiasis and chronic alcohol abuse. The triggering events at the cellular level are still poorly understood, but in most patients, the common precipitating factor is the extravasation of activated pancreatic secretions, which is responsible for many of the pathophysiologic consequences that follow [1–3]. The beginning of the pathologic process is similar to a chemical burn precipitated by autodigestive injuries, which vary greatly in extent and severity depending upon the degree of trypsinogen activation and amount of extravasation of pancreatic enzymatic secretions. Interstitial edema, acinar cell damage, microvascular injuries with thrombosis and obliteration of the capillary network, and zones of ischemia and necrosis are seen frequently in the pancreatic gland. Inflammatory reaction, retroperitoneal fat necrosis, patchy retroperitoneal hemorrhage, and peripancreatic fluid collections often develop in the adjacent retroperitoneum [4].

For practical clinical use, acute pancreatitis was classified by the International Symposium on Acute Pancreatitis in 1992 in Atlanta (USA) into mild and severe acute pancreatitis [5]. This classification is based on the detection and severity of distal organ dysfunction induced by the release of pro- and anti-inflammatory mediators (clinical and laboratory parameters) as well as on the presence and extent of pancreatic necrosis.

Mild pancreatitis, previously referred to as edematous or interstitial pancreatitis, is a self-limiting disease with no mortality and absent or minimal systemic manifestations that resolve rapidly without morbidity. It occurs in about 70–80% of patients. Conversely, severe acute pancreatitis, previously called necrotizing or hemorrhagic pancreatitis, is a potentially lethal disease that exhibits severe systemic manifestations and distal organ failure, has a protracted clinical course that is plagued by abdominal complications, and a significant mortality rate [2, 3]. These patients exhibit different degrees of pancreatic necrosis and a mortality rate of 10–23% that is further increased when secondary contamination (infected necrosis) occurs [2, 3, 6]. Individuals with severe pancreatitis are monitored in intensive care units, metabolic abnormalities are corrected, organ functions supported, and follow up imaging studies, mainly CT examinations, performed.

Noninvasive modern imaging studies play a triple role in the evaluation of patients with acute pancreatitis:

1. To confirm the clinical diagnosis and elicit the etiology of an acute attack, mainly with CT and sonographic examinations. Conversely, to detect other intraperitoneal acute conditions that may mimic pancreatitis clinically.
2. In combination with clinical and laboratory parameters (Ranson, Acute Physiology and Chronic Health Evaluation II numerical systems) to stage the severity of an acute attack of pancreatitis.
3. Finally, to detect abdominal complications on follow up imaging examinations, frequently developing in patients with severe pancreatitis.

The use of imaging studies in the cohort of patients with acute pancreatitis is justified by the obvious limitations of clinical examination (physical and laboratory findings) in detecting intra-abdominal disease. Diagnosis is hampered by the lack of specificity of subjective complaints and physical findings as well as by some deficiencies in the sensitivity and specificity of serum amylase and lipase levels. Hyperamylasemia, the essential diagnostic test, has an uncertain sensitivity of about 80–95% [7]. Serum amylase levels tend to rise at the beginning of an acute attack of pancreatitis, but show a propensity of rapid decline to normal levels within 24–72 h. Serum lipase levels decrease more slowly and thus are more reliable when there is delay in the initial blood sampling. Furthermore, several relatively common acute intra-abdominal disorders such as acute biliary disease, perforated peptic ulcer, closed loop small bowel obstruction, and acute ischemic bowel disease may present with hyperamylasemia, decreasing the specificity of this test. In one large series, of the 20% of patients with acute abdominal conditions who presented with hyperamylasemia, only 75% had acute pancreatitis. With the use of imaging modalities, particularly CT imaging, most of these shortcomings can be obviated.

Imaging Modalities

Initial radiologic examinations, conventional chest films, abdominal films, and barium upper gastrointestinal examinations, although sometimes useful, are mostly disappointing in the evaluation of patients with acute pancreatitis. These modalities are unable to visualize the pancreatic gland, rely mainly on secondary findings involving adjacent intestinal segments, and lack clinically acceptable sensitivity and specificity levels. The development of more reliable noninvasive imaging modalities in the last 25 years has resulted in dramatic improvements, which become indispensable for making clinical decisions regarding the management of patients with acute pancreatitis.

Ultrasonography

Despite steady technical developments, abdominal sonography plays a limited role in the evaluation of patients with acute pancreatitis [8]. In many patients, obesity and/or overlying gas in the transverse colon hinders adequate visualization of the pancreatic gland, rendering the examination suboptimal. Ultrasonography, however, has a prominent role in establishing the etiology of an acute attack of pancreatitis by detecting biliary stones. Sonographic examinations are operator dependent, but in experienced hands have a >95% sensitivity in the diagnosis of gallstones and 50–60% sensitivity in the detection of common duct stones. This information is highly beneficial since it influences the management of these patients. In addition, sonography is used to detect large fluid collections and to follow up pancreatic pseudocysts. Because of variable specific individual anatomic factors, inconstant results, and dependence on a skillful and experienced operator, abdominal ultrasound abnormalities have been reported in anywhere from 33–90% of patients with acute pancreatitis [8].

Computerized Tomography

Abdominal imaging study performed on a multidetector CT (MDCT) unit during a bolus of intravenous (IV) iodinated contrast material has become the examination of choice for acute pancreatitis. The examination is highly reliable, being able to visualize the pancreatic gland in almost all individuals, it can be performed fast on sick patients, and it is available in most medical centers in the developed world [9, 10].

CT Technique

The objectives of the examination are to obtain high-resolution images, increase conspicuity of the pancreatic gland, and virtually eliminate respiratory and streak artifacts. The technical protocols used vary slightly in different institutions based on available equipment, local factors, and individual preferences. In our experience, excellent results are obtained with a two-phase acquisition technique. We administer a rapid bolus of 150 ml of 60% nonionic contrast material at 3–4 ml/s after the digital scout film of the abdomen is taken. The first phase of the image acquisition, which is the arterial dominant phase, starts at 35 s after the beginning of the IV contrast administration. Processing data is acquired over the pancreatic gland and adjacent structures, usually from the top of the vertebral body (T12) to the superior edge of the vertebral body (L4). The second, portal dominant phase starts at about 80 s and acquires data over the entire abdomen from the top of the diaphragm to the symphysis pubis. Once computer data are generated, images can be viewed as planar two-dimensional axial images or they can be reconstructed into coronal, oblique, or sagittal planes at a commercially available work station. Images can be stored and examined on printed films, workstations, or picture archiving and communication systems (PACS). In our institution, examinations are reviewed on a PACS with axial images of 2.5 mm collimation for the first, arterial dominant phase and 5 mm collimation for the second, portal dominant phase. Since the multidetector acquisition data contain hundreds of images, the use of films has become wasteful and impractical.

Normal Pancreas

On CT the pancreatic gland is seen in the upper abdomen as a sharply contoured and homogeneously enhanced structure with a smooth outer surface or a corrugated acinar configuration. There are slight variations in the size of the gland, with smaller atrophic glands seen in the older population. The head of the pancreas is larger, measuring about 3–4 cm in the anteroposterior diameter, with a gradual transition into the pancreatic body and a smaller tapering tail situated in the splenic hilum. A common normal variant is a slightly enlarged bulbous tail exhibiting similar gland texture and enhancing values as the rest of the gland. The splenic artery and vein are located posterior to the body of the pancreas, which is a useful morphologic hallmark that helps in the identification of the gland in cachectic individuals. In the majority of patients a normal pancreatic duct measuring no more than 1–2 mm in thickness, traversing the entire gland, can be detected.

Basic attenuation values of a normal pancreas obtained without IV contrast administration are about 50 HU, similar to the liver and spleen. Lower attenuation values should be expected with fatty infiltration of the pancreas. Homogeneous gland enhancement occurs after the IV contrast administration, with values as high as 150 HU in the arterial dominant phase and about 100 HU in the portal dominant phase of acquisition. Slight density variations between different segments of pancreatic gland, usually no more than 10–20 HU, are sometimes seen in normal individuals.

Diagnosis of Acute Pancreatitis

A wide spectrum of radiologic findings from a relatively normal gland, to subtle changes or profound morphologic alterations affecting the pancreatic gland and retroperitoneal structures can be seen in acute pancreatitis [9, 10]. In about 14–28% of patients with hyperamylasemia and abdominal pain presumed to have pancreatitis, the gland appears relatively normal on CT imaging. Based on vast accumulated experience, a normal CT examination may be seen only with very mild, self-limiting forms of pancreatitis, while characteristic CT abnormalities are detected in all patients with moderate or severe forms of acute pancreatitis.

In the great majority of patients, acute pancreatitis is a diffuse inflammatory process affecting the entire gland. In the milder clinical forms the gland may be enlarged, show subtle interstitial heterogeneous densi-

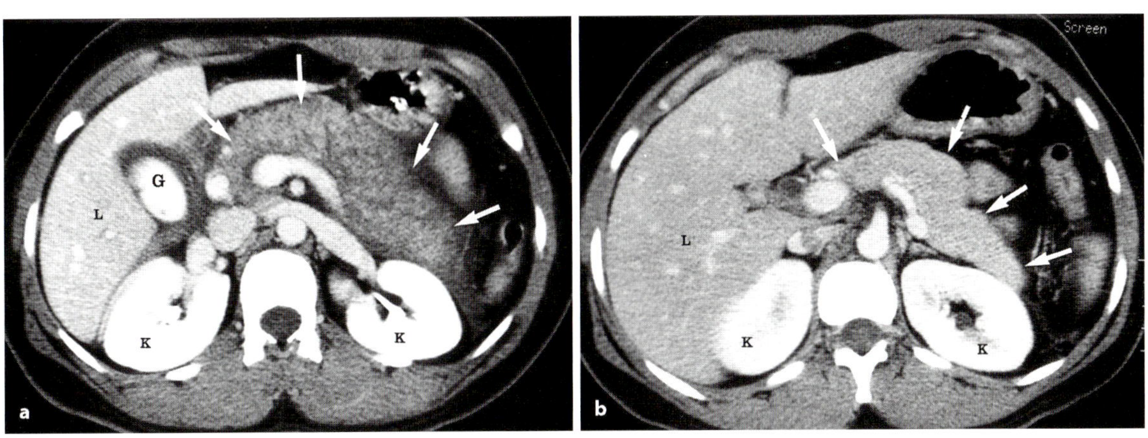

Figure 19.2.1

Acute pancreatitis in a 27-year-old woman following endoscopic retrograde cholangiopancreatography examination. a The pancreas (*arrows*) is markedly enlarged, slightly heterogeneous, but enhanced throughout. Grade B pancreatitis, no necrosis, computed tomography (CT) severity index 2. b Follow up CT examination 1 week later reveals a normal pancreas (*arrows*). *K* Kidneys, *L* liver, *G* contrast-enhanced gallbladder

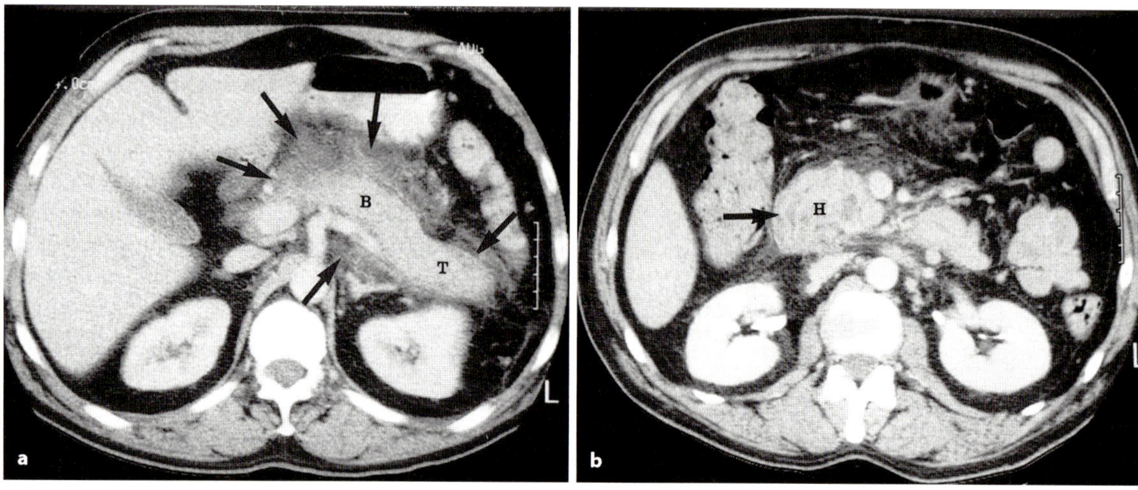

Figure 19.2.2

Acute pancreatitis in 45-year-old alcoholic man. a The body (*B*) and tail (*T*) of pancreas are enhanced homogeneously. There is extensive peripancreatic inflammatory stranding (*arrows*) indicative of acute pancreatitis. b The head of the pancreas (*H*) is enlarged and mildly heterogeneous (*arrow*). Grade C pancreatitis, no necrosis, CT severity index 3

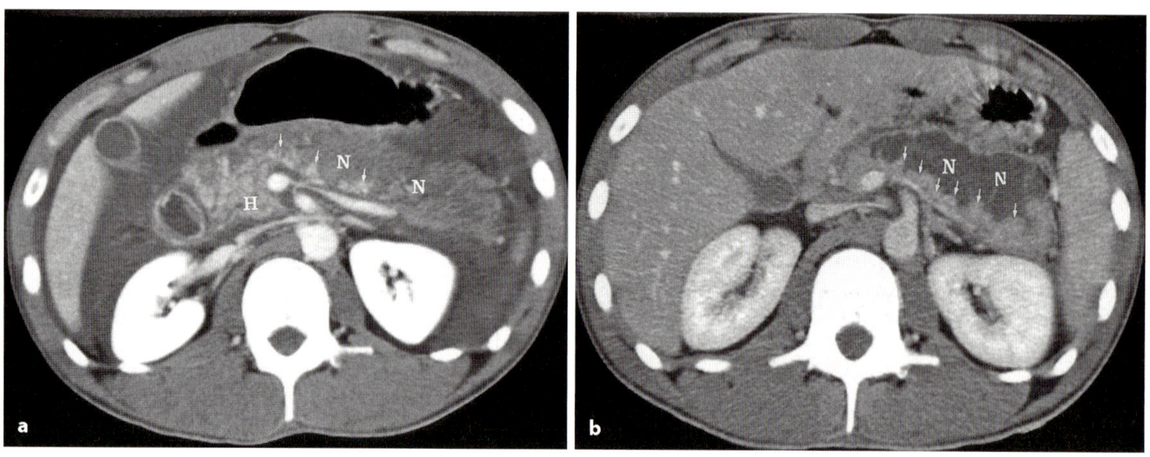

Figure 19.2.3

Acute pancreatitis in a 44-year-old alcoholic man. a Initial CT examination reveals massive peripancreatic fluid collections and lack of enhancement of most of the body and tail of pancreas, consistent with necrosis (*N*). The head (*H*) of the pancreas is enhanced. Grade E pancreatitis with approximately 50% necrosis, CT severity index 8. b Follow up CT examination 3 weeks later better defines the extent of liquefied necrosis and the residual viable pancreatic tissue (*arrows*) on the posterior aspect of the gland. Fluid collections have resolved

ties, may exhibit variable degrees of homogeneous parenchymal enhancement depending on the extent of hyperemia and/or edema induced by the acute attack of pancreatitis (Fig. 19.2.1). Subtle peripancreatic densities called stranding having a dirty, lace-like appearance begin to appear and may coalesce into small, ill-defined heterogeneous fluid collections (Fig. 19.2.2). These collections, usually of 20–40 HU detected in the retroperitoneum adjacent to the pancreatic gland, are very characteristic indicators of acute pancreatitis. They may be developing in the presence of a relatively normal-looking pancreatic gland, are induced by the extravasation of activated pancreatic enzymes, and represent a combination of fat necrosis, extravasated exudates, inflammatory reaction, and patchy areas of hemorrhage.

In the moderate and more severe forms of disease there are larger heterogeneous fluid collections located in the left and right anterior pararenal spaces and lesser peritoneal sac. Fluid collections tend to involve predominantly the left pararenal space, but when massive they can dissect fascial planes and extend into the lower abdomen and pelvis. Enzymatic exudates may involve the mesocolon, small bowel mesentery, duodenum, splenic flexure of the colon, and can enter the peritoneal cavity presenting as ascites (Fig. 19.2.3). Free peritoneal fluid has been observed in 7% of cases of acute pancreatitis, incidence, which probably relates to the severity of an acute attack [11].

The fate of the developing retroperitoneal fluid collections, seen in about 50% of patients with acute pancreatitis, is unpredictable. In the majority of patients they tend to resolve over a 1- to 2-week period. In other patients, however, they increase in volume, become partially encapsulated, and eventually develop into pseudocysts or linger on and become infected pancreatic abscesses. The natural history of the fluid collections detected at the beginning of an acute attack appears to be related to the amounts of extravasated peripancreatic fluid and the presence of associated conspicuous parenchymal changes indicative of gland necrosis.

Failure of the pancreatic gland to enhance for at least 30 HU over basic measurement values, during the IV contrast administration is consistent with ischemia and leads to pancreatic necrosis in most instances (Fig. 19.2.3). The process may be diffuse, affecting the entire gland, or it may be patchy, affecting only parts of the gland. The depiction of this phenomenon at the onset of an acute attack heralds the presence of a severe attack, of a protracted clinical course, and of a high incidence of local complications. Ischemic tissue tends to liquefy within the first 2 or 3 days and it may disrupt the pancreatic ductal system, allowing larger amounts of pancreatic secretions to extravasate in the retroperitoneum. With CT imaging, the extent of pancreatic necrosis can be quantified by dividing necrosis into severe, involving >50% of the gland, moderate, involving 30–50% of the gland, and mild or focal when necrotic tissue involves <30% of the pancreas (Fig. 19.2.3).

The diagnostic sensitivity of CT imaging in acute pancreatitis varies from 77 to 92%, being heavily dependent on the severity of an acute attack. However, when present, the CT findings are characteristic and reliable with very few exceptions, leading to a reported specificity approaching 100%.

Segmental Pancreatitis

In up to 15% of patients the acute attack of pancreatitis involves exclusively or predominantly either the tail or more often the head of the pancreas [11]. This presentation occurs mostly in patients with repeated episodes of pancreatitis. It manifests as a focal enlargement of the pancreatic gland and discrete peripancreatic stranding, and it is associated with milder clinical forms of acute pancreatitis. When unfamiliar with this appearance, the CT may be misinterpreted as pancreatic carcinoma (Fig. 19.2.4).

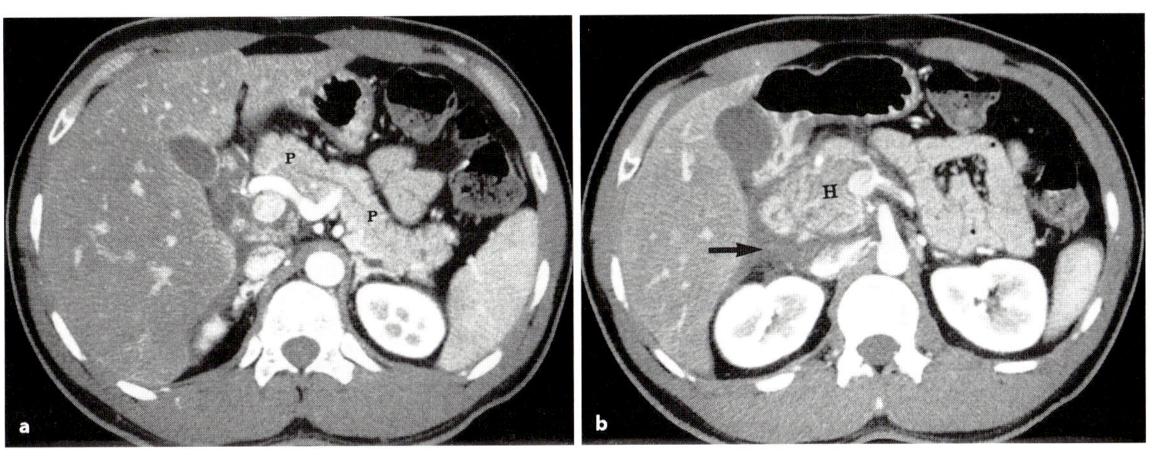

Figure 19.2.4

Segmental pancreatitis affecting mainly the head of pancreas in a 28-year-old alcoholic man with a previous history of pancreatitis. **a** The body and tail of the pancreas are unremarkable (*P*). **b** The head of the pancreas (*H*) is enlarged and there is extravasated fluid in the right anterior pararenal space (*arrow*), indicative of focal pancreatitis

Groove Pancreatitis

A more chronic and severe form of segmental pancreatitis involving the head of the pancreas, associated with intrinsic duodenal inflammatory changes and biliary obstruction, has been described as groove pancreatitis. In addition to an enlarged, heterogeneous head of the pancreas, pancreatic secretions collect in the groove between the head of the pancreas and duodenal sweep. About 50% of these patients exhibit clinical signs of jaundice, duodenal stricture, and/or gastric outlet obstruction. The syndrome is apparently caused by excessive alcohol intake following repeated episodes of pancreatitis [12].

Associated Carcinoma of the Pancreas with Pancreatitis

About 1–2% of patients with solitary or multiple clinical attacks of acute pancreatitis have unsuspected carcinoma of the pancreas. MDCT examination is able to detect carcinoma of the pancreas in the majority of these patients. Most of these patients are older, present with milder segmental forms of pancreatitis, and display dilatation of the pancreatic duct with an abrupt cut-off produced by a small, low-attenuated pancreatic neoplasm. When these findings are observed, endoscopic sonography and fine-needle aspiration of the soft tissue mass can confirm the CT diagnosis [13].

Autoimmune Pancreatitis

This is a more unusual form of segmental or diffuse pancreatitis that is caused by an autoimmune mechanism and sometimes associated with other autoimmune disorders. Focal or diffuse homogeneous enlargement of the pancreas with a sharp contour and occasionally with a peripheral rim of hypoattenuation may be seen on CT. Compression and/or strictures of the common duct manifesting clinically as jaundice may occur. Radiographically, the entity may be mistaken as pancreatic carcinoma or lymphoma. Endoscopic ultrasound-guided biopsy shows a lymphocytic infiltrate, fibrosis, plasma cells, and absent malignant cells. Serum markers of autoimmune disorders (elevated IgG and antinuclear antibody levels) contribute to confirm the diagnosis. Resolution of symptoms and a return to a normal size of the pancreas is the rule with good response to steroid therapy [14].

Acute Exacerbation of Chronic Pancreatitis

Reactivation of the inflammatory process in patients with a history of chronic pancreatitis can induce acute attacks characterized by a sudden onset of abdominal pain and elevated serum amylase levels. Depending on the degree of parenchymal damage (fibrosis, atrophy), the acute episodes vary in severity but are mostly mild, self-limiting exacerbations of a chronic disease. CT imaging detects stigmata of chronic pancreatitis such as parenchymal atrophy, pancreatic duct dilatation, and intraductal calcifications as well as the peripancreatic stranding and small fluid collections seen in acute pancreatitis. The recent peripancreatic inflammatory changes that occur as well as the acute clinical symptoms usually resolve with conservative therapy, while the chronic morphologic changes of chronic pancreatitis are stable and permanent.

CT Staging of Acute Pancreatitis

An early accurate assessment of the severity of an acute attack of pancreatitis is essential for the improved management of these patients. In great measure, the previously described CT abnormalities, and particularly the ability of MDCT to detect pancreatic necrosis, contribute to this evaluation.

For over 20 years, radiologic observations and clinical investigations have attempted to correlate the presence, extent, and severity of CT abnormalities with morbidity and mortality in acute pancreatitis. In our original 1985 report [11], performed on the older and slower CT scanners without a bolus IV contrast administration, we classified the severity of this disease into five separate grades: grade A, normal pancreas, grade B pancreatic enlargement, grade C pancreatic abnormalities and peripancreatic stranding, grade D small single peripancreatic fluid collection, and grade E multiple large heterogeneous fluid collections and/or retroperitoneal extraluminal air (Figs. 19.2.1–19.2.3). In our group of patients, clinical and CT follow up examinations have shown that most complications and all lethal attacks had occurred in patients with grades D and E, those who had developed fluid collections. Combined mortality for grade D and E patients was 14% and morbidity was 54% as compared with no mortality and a morbidity rate of only 4% in patients with initial grades A, B, or C. The advantages of this grading system are that it can be performed without intravenous contrast administration or with slower injection rates, on older CT scanners, and using 5-mm collimation.

Further advances in CT staging have been achieved when a causal relationship between lack of pancreatic

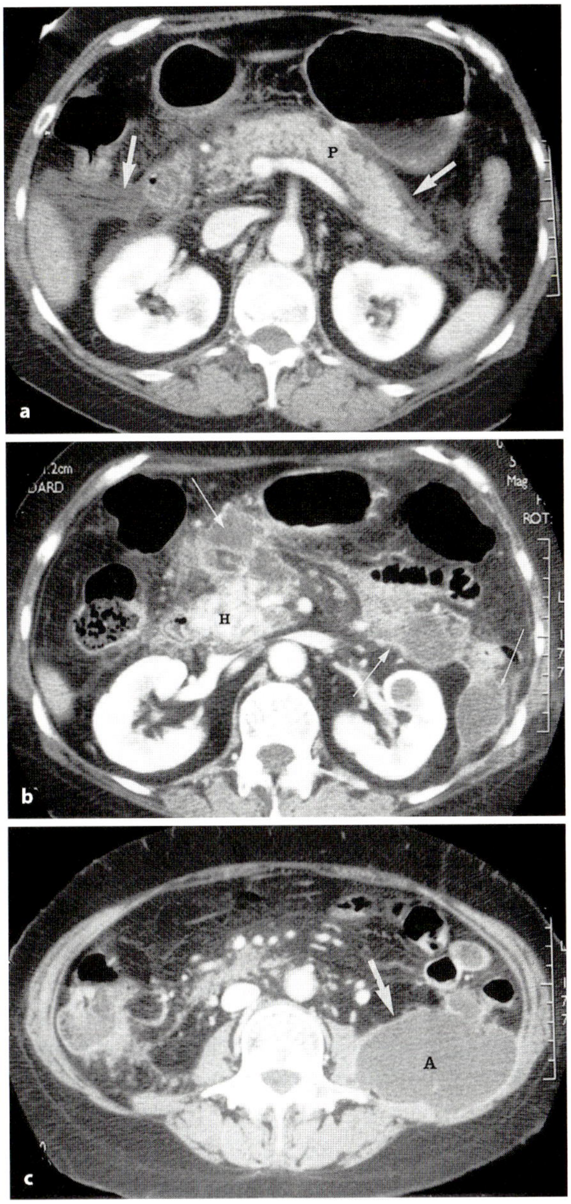

Figure 19.2.5

Acute gallstone pancreatitis in a 66-year-old woman. **a** The pancreas is normally enhanced with peripancreatic extravasated fluid (*arrows*). Grade D pancreatitis without necrosis. **b, c** Follow up CT examination 4 weeks later reveals multiple partially loculated fluid collections (*arrows*). Patient developed fever, and percutaneous aspiration of the large fluid collection in the left flank (*A*) revealed a pyogenic abscess

enhancement and the development of pancreatic necrosis has been recognized. With few exceptions, necrosis appears at the beginning of an acute attack and remains relatively stable in size and location. The necrotic tissue undergoes liquefaction in the following few days and becomes better defined when compared with the adjacent viable enhancing pancreatic tissue (Fig. 19.2.3). In our 1990 paper [15] we documented an excellent correlation between the presence of pancreatic necrosis (areas of lacking enhancement) and severity of the disease. Patients with normal parenchymal enhancement had no mortality and only a 6% morbidity rate, whereas patients with necrosis exhibited a 23% mortality and 82% morbidity rate. Furthermore, the extent of pancreatic necrosis has prognostic significance since the mortality and morbidity in patients with extensive (>30%) necrosis far exceeded those observed in patients with smaller, patchy areas of necrosis. Thus, the early detection of pancreatic necrosis by CT imaging has acquired great clinical significance, being used as a prognostic indicator of the severity of disease.

While the early detection of necrosis by CT imaging should be considered the most important imaging prognostic indicator of severity of disease, a smaller incidence of local complications do occur (22% in our experience) in grade E patients with large fluid collections but with normally enhanced pancreatic glands (Fig. 19.2.5) [15, 16]. For this reason I have combined the described CT prognostic indicators into a single CT grading system called the "CT severity index". Patients graded A–E are assigned 0–4 points, to which 2, 4, and 6 points are added for up to 30%, 50%, and >50% necrosis, respectively. The resulting severity score between 0 and 10 points correlates well with severity of disease at the beginning of an acute attack of pancreatitis. Patients with low numbers have mild forms of pancreatitis, while patients with high numbers of 7–10, have a 17% mortality and >90% complication rate [15].

Complications of Acute Pancreatitis

A variety of systemic and local complications that occur in patients with severe pancreatitis are responsible for the reported overall 2–10% mortality rates [1–3]. Most life-threatening complications should be expected to develop in patients with necrotizing pancreatitis. The early complications, which account for 20–50% of the mortality, seen at the onset within the first 2–3 days of an acute attack, are organ failures and systemic toxic manifestations with various clinical expressions, detected and monitored by clinical means [1, 17]. Ominous abdominal complications usually occur between the 2nd and 5th week following an acute attack, after the initial violent systemic manifestations subside. Other complication, mostly vascular in nature, may be detected later or after several episodes of pancreatitis.

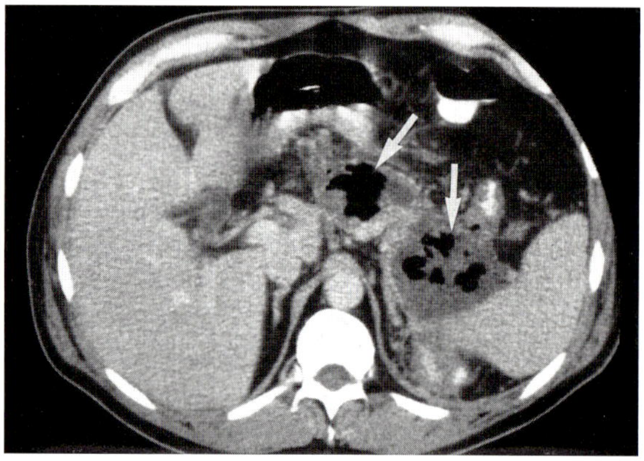

Figure 19.2.6

Infected pancreatic necrosis in a 65-year-old man following an attack of acute pancreatitis. CT axial image at the level of the pancreas shows liquefaction of the necrosed gland replaced by fluid and collections of air (*arrows*). The patient expired

Infected Pancreatic Necrosis and Pancreatic Abscess

Over 50% of the mortality associated with acute pancreatitis is related to the development of local abdominal complications, mostly secondary infections of devitalized pancreatic tissue, fat necrosis, and lingering fluid collections. Infected necrosis is defined as a secondary bacterial contamination of nonviable pancreatic tissue that occurs in about 40–70% of patients with devitalized pancreatic parenchyma (Fig. 19.2.6) [2]. Pancreatic abscess is a similar contamination of peripancreatic fluid collection of low viscosity and of water density that occurs in about 3% of patients with acute pancreatitis, mostly within 3–4 weeks of the onset of an acute attack (Fig. 19.2.5C) [5]. Pancreatic abscess usually resolves with antibiotic therapy and percutaneous drainage procedures, while thicker, infected necrotic pancreatic tissue is more amenable to surgical necrostomy, debridement, sump drainage, and lavage. The mortality rate of infected necrosis is about twice that of pancreatic abscess and is as high as 40–80% in some reports [2, 3, 18].

The source of contamination is subject to controversy; probably translocation of bacteria through the intestinal wall, via the lymphatic system, hematogenously born, or due to microperforations. The most common organisms are *Escherichia coli*, enterobacter, klebsiella, anaerobes, and fungus.

On CT imaging there are no specific signs of infection unless bubbles of air are detected in the infected tissues (Fig. 19.2.6). This occurs, however, in only about 12–18% of cases [19]. In the other majority of patients, CT images will detect solitary or multiple poorly encapsulated collections of heterogeneous or homogeneous low-attenuated fluid that fail to resolve 3–4 weeks after the onset of an acute attack of pancreatitis (Fig. 19.2.5). In these patients, infection should be suspected when sepsis (fever, chills, elevated white count) develops. The diagnosis can be confirmed by percutaneous aspiration under CT or sonography guidance and bacteriologic examination.

Pancreatic Pseudocyst

Pancreatic pseudocyst is defined as a fully encapsulated enzymatic fluid collection located either in the pancreas or, often, in the vicinity of the gland, that requires more than 4 weeks to evolve [5, 19]. This complication occurs when the initial peripancreatic fluid collections fail to resolve or they are increasing in size because of an injury and communication with the pancreatic ductal system. Pseudocysts occur in 3–10% of cases of acute pancreatitis, most often at the site of a focal area of pancreatic necrosis [20].

On CT imaging pseudocysts appear as round or oval fully encapsulated collections with low attenuated (< 15 HU) fluid content that vary greatly in size from 1 cm to > 15 cm in diameter (Fig. 19.2.7). They can dissect fascial planes and travel into the lower abdomen and pelvis, or superiorly into the mediastinum. Pseudocysts have no septations, no peripheral nodules, and show no intraluminal enhancement. Highly attenuated cystic fluid or fluid-fluid levels denote the presence of intracystic hemorrhage. In most instances these morphologic characteristics enable us to distinguish pseudocysts from other pancreatic cystic tumors [20].

The fate of acute pancreatic pseudocysts that communicate with the pancreatic ductal system is unpredictable. These pseudocysts are unstable and prone to fluctuations in size, spontaneous resolution, or recurrences following draining procedures. As expected, young pseudocysts (<6 weeks) have a high rate of resolution, whereas older pseudocysts (>12 weeks) tend to persist. Conversely, chronic pseudocysts that show a thicker calcified capsule and have lost the connection to the pancreatic duct are stable and constant but respond well to surgical or draining procedures.

Complications of pseudocysts such as rupture, hemorrhage, or infection can occur at any time but are relatively rare (Fig. 19.2.7). These complications are more common in larger and symptomatic pseudocysts. Pain, obstructive symptoms, jaundice, secondary infection with sepsis, and intra-abdominal hem-

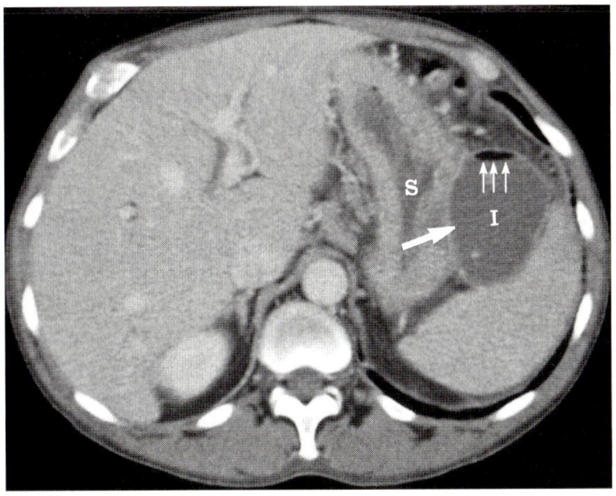

Figure 19.2.7

Infected pseudocyst in a 45-year-old man following acute pancreatitis. Encapsulated round fluid collection in the left upper quadrant between the stomach (*S*) and spleen, which contains a small amounts of air (*small arrows*). Aspiration revealed infected pseudocyst (*I*)

orrhage are all indications for an aggressive surgical approach guided by the CT findings. In patients with smaller, acute, or stable pseudocysts seen in asymptomatic individuals, a more conservative approach with routine follow up CT examinations may be justified.

Other Complications

Extravasated and activated pancreatic secretions may lead to a wide range of other complications affecting hollow viscous and solid organs in proximity to the pancreas [20]. The location and extent of injuries lead to different clinical manifestations that can be diagnosed and assessed by CT imaging. Among the late complications, sudden abdominal hemorrhage, venous occlusions, and pseudoaneurysms are the most important [20]. Massive intra-abdominal hemorrhage can occur at any time, usually after 1 year following an acute attack, and are often attributed to ruptured pseudoaneurysms of the splenic, gastroduodenal, or pancreaticoduodenal arteries. Pseudoaneurysms are apparently common complications of acute pancreatitis detected by CT in asymptomatic individuals. Early detection with IV-contrast CT imaging followed by angiographic embolization is the recommended treatment of choice.

Splenic vein thrombosis is a common vascular complication that develops in 1–3% of patients following pancreatitis. The developing syndrome, called left-sided portal hypertension is produced by obstruction of the splenic vein and massive enlargement of collateral pathways leading to enlarged gastric varices on the posterior wall of the gastric fundus. Patients are asymptomatic until hematemesis intervenes.

The massive and chronic accumulation of intraperitoneal fluid, rich in amylase, caused by a disruption of the pancreatic duct with a fistulous communication to the peritoneal cavity, defines a more unusual syndrome called "pancreatic ascites." Chronic pancreatic ascites is a debilitating syndrome that is difficult to properly manage and control. Endoscopic retrograde cholangiopancreatography followed by dilatation of strictures or pancreatic duct stent placement is advocated [20].

Magnetic Resonance Imaging

While CT is the gold standard for the diagnosis and staging of acute pancreatitis, MRI has become a reliable secondary imaging modality used as a complimentary examination, or more often in patients in whom IV-contrast CT studies are contraindicated [21]. Contraindications include allergic reactions, renal insufficiency with nephrotoxic reactions, and ionizing radiation in pregnant women. MRI can visualize the inflamed pancreatic gland, can detect complex fluid collections and pseudocysts, and it is more sensitive than CT for the diagnosis of choledocholithiasis. However, MRI is more expensive, takes longer to perform, is difficult to perform in critically ill patients, and is less available.

MRI examination includes several sequences, T1-weighted images, fat-suppressed images, single-shot, fast spin-echo, T2-weighted images, and IV (gadolinium chelate)-enhanced three-dimensional images to maximize the contrast between normal parenchyma and nonenhanced pancreatic necrosis. Reconstruction can be performed in any plane without loss of spatial resolution. Peripancreatic stranding or fluid is shown on T2-weighted, fat-suppressed images or post-gadolinium-chelate gradient echo images. Pseudocysts are depicted as homogeneous high signal lesions on T2-weighted images without internal debris. Hemorrhagic fluid can be easily detected; however, infection may be difficult to diagnose as MRI is insensitive to small bubbles of air [21].

Summary

State-of-the-art imaging modalities are essential in the evaluation of patients with acute pancreatitis. The gold standard of imaging study is IV-contrast-enhanced MDCT or, when this is either not available or contraindicated, MRI. The role of these modalities is threefold:

1. To confirm the clinical diagnosis, detect pancreatitis not suspected clinically, or detect other intra-abdominal catastrophes misdiagnosed clinically as acute pancreatitis.
2. Assist in the initial staging of the severity of an acute attack.
3. Depict a variety of local complications that occur following episodes of severe acute pancreatitis.

Imaging modalities, and particularly MDCT, have become an indispensable investigative tool in the evaluation and management of patients with acute pancreatitis.

References

1. Steinberg W, Tenner S (1994) Acute pancreatitis. N Engl J Med 330:1198–1210
2. Beger HG, Rau B, Mayer J, et al (1997) Natural course of acute pancreatic. World J Surg 21:130–135
3. Banks PA (1994) Acute pancreatitis: medical and surgical management. Am J Gastroenterol 89:S78–85
4. Kloppel G (1994) Pathology of severe acute pancreatitis. In: Bradley EL III (ed) Acute Pancreatitis: Diagnosis and Therapy. Raven, New York, pp 35–46
5. Bradley EL III (1993) A clinically based classification system for acute pancreatitis. Arch Surg 128:586–590
6. Dervenis C, Johnson CD, Bassi C, et al (1999) Diagnosis, objective assessment of severity, and management of acute pancreatitis. Int J Pancreatol 25:195–210
7. Clavien PA, Robert J, Meyer P, et al (1989) Acute pancreatitis and normoamylasemia: not an uncommon combination. Ann Surg 210:614–620
8. Jeffrey RB (1989) Sonography in acute pancreatitis. Radiol Clin North Am 27:5–17
9. Balthazar EJ (1989) CT diagnosis and staging of acute pancreatitis. Radiol Clin Am 27:19–37
10. Clavien PA, Hauser, Meyer P, et al (1988) Value of contrast-enhanced computerized tomography in the early diagnosis of acute pancreatitis. A prospective study of 202 patients. Am J Surg 155:457–466
11. Balthazar EJ, Ranson JHC, Naidich, et al (1985) Acute pancreatitis: prognostic value of CT. Radiology 156:767–772
12. Becker V, Mischke U (1991) Groove pancreatitis. Int J Pancreatol 10:173–182
13. Balthazar EJ (2005) Pancreatitis associated with pancreatic carcinoma preoperative diagnosis: role of CT imaging in detection and evaluation. Pancreatology 330–344
14. Sahani DV, Kalva SP, Farrell J, et al (2004) Autoimmune pancreatitis: imaging features. Radiology 233:345–352
15. Balthazar EJ, Robinson DL, Megibow AJ, et al (1990) Acute pancreatitis: value of CT in establishing prognosis. Radiology 174:331–336
16. Balthazar EJ (2002) Acute pancreatitis: assessment of severity with clinical and CT evaluation. Radiology 223:603–613
17. Lowham A, Lavelle J, Leese T (1999) Mortality from acute pancreatitis. Int J Pancreatol 25:103–106
18. Bassi C (1994) Infected pancreatic necrosis. Int J Pancreatol 16:1–10
19. Balthazar EJ, Freeny PC, VanSonnenberg E (1994) Imaging and intervention in acute pancreatitis. Radiology 193:297–306
20. Balthazar EJ (2002) Complications of acute pancreatitis: clinical and CT evaluation. Radiol Clin North Am 40:1211–1227
21. Semelka RC, Ascher SM (1993) MR imaging of the pancreas. Radiology 188:593–602

Chapter 20

P. A. Banks · K. J. Mortele

Nonsurgical Management of Acute Pancreatitis

Almost all patients with interstitial pancreatitis and the majority with necrotizing pancreatitis are managed nonsurgically. In one recent report, 64% of patients with necrotizing pancreatitis were managed nonsurgically [1]. Those who required surgery either had infected necrosis or late complications of sterile necrosis (primarily persistent pain with inability to tolerate oral feeding). As innovative nonsurgical options become increasingly available for infected necrosis and for the late complications of sterile necrosis (such as radiologic and endoscopic techniques), the need for surgical treatment may decrease even further. This chapter will review nonsurgical management of acute pancreatitis.

Assessment of the Severity of Acute Pancreatitis at Admission

It is important to establish risk factors of severity as early as possible after admission. This information will help determine which patients should be transferred to an intensive care unit in a hospital that specializes in the care of acute pancreatitis. Accurate risk factors of severity will also facilitate the randomization of appropriate patients in prospective trials of new therapy for severe acute pancreatitis.

Risk factors at admission that have been identified include advanced age (possibly >55 years of age and certainly >70 years of age), obesity (with a body mass index of >30), and organ failure [2]. Mortality is particularly high among patients who develop multisystem organ failure [1] and those who have persistent organ failure during the 1st week of illness (that is, organ failure that persists for >48 h) [3]. In addition, the majority of all deaths as a result of acute pancreatitis occur during the first two episodes, and comparably fewer for each succeeding episode. Finally, in terms of imaging abnormalities that can be identified at admission, a pleural effusion and/or pulmonary infiltrates on X-ray is associated with increased morbidity, and a computed tomography (CT) grade of E according to the Balthazar-Ranson scoring system (that is, two or more well-defined fluid collections) is associated with increased morbidity and mortality (Table 20.1 and Fig. 20.1) [2].

In some reports, hemoconcentration at admission (hematocrit ≥44 at admission) has correlated with the development of necrotizing pancreatitis [4]. In the absence of hemoconcentration at admission, few patients develop necrotizing pancreatitis.

Table 20.1. Balthazar-Ranson computed tomography (CT) severity index

CT Grade	Score	Necrosis	Score
A	0	None	0
B	1	< 33%	2
C	2	33–50%	4
D	3	> 50%	6
E	4		

A – Normal pancreas

B – focal or diffuse enlargement of the pancreas

C – Intrinsic pancreatic abnormalities with inflammatory changes in peripancreatic fat

D – Single, ill-defined fluid collection

E – Two or more poorly defined collections or presence of gas in or adjacent to the pancreas

CT grade (0–4) + necrosis (0–6) = total score (maximum score, 10)

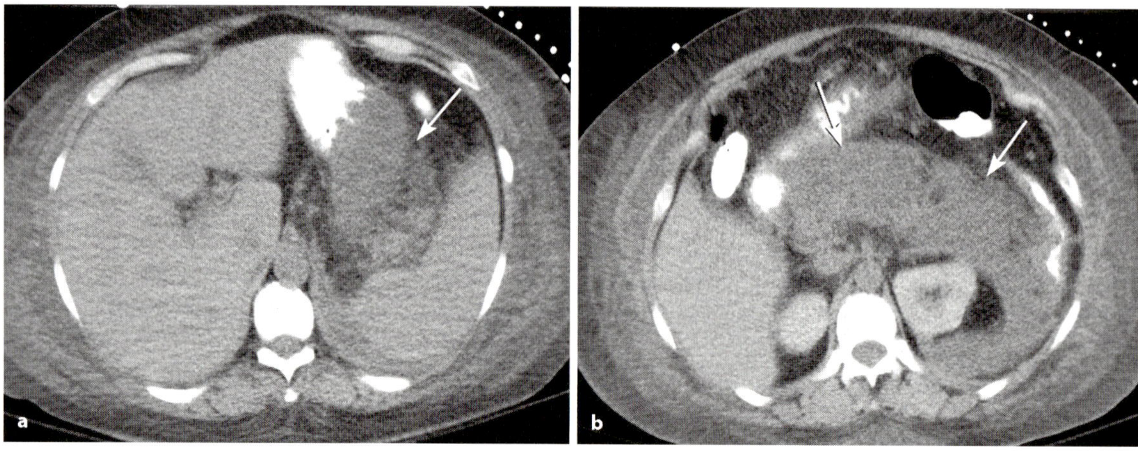

Figure 20.1

Axial unenhanced computed tomography (CT) images through the upper abdomen (a) and pancreatic bed (b) showing localized fluid collection (*arrow* in a) next to the stomach and extensive inflammation and fluid accumulation in the anterior and posterior pararenal spaces. Note the hypodense and swollen pancreatic gland (*arrows* in b). The presence of two fluid collections is compatible with a grade E pancreatitis (Balthazar Score)

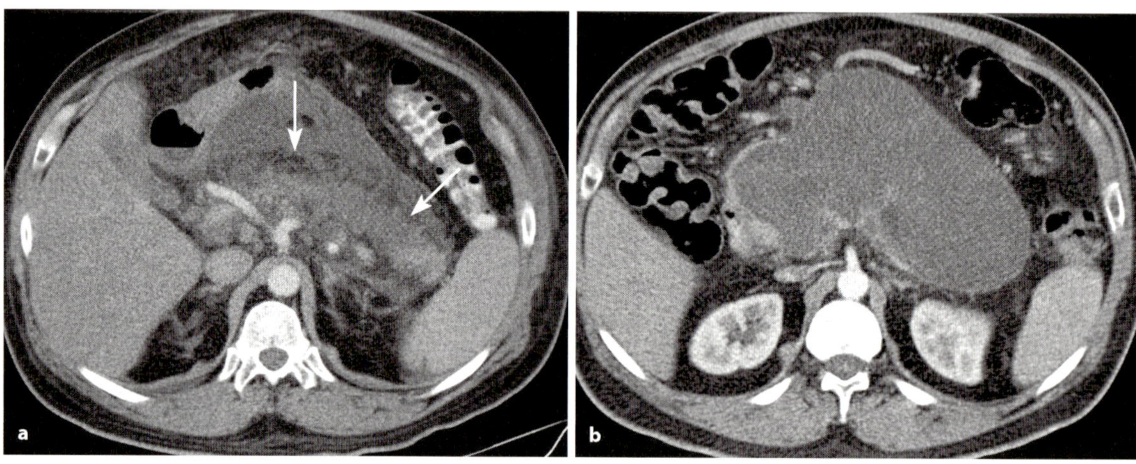

Figure 20.2

Axial contrast-enhanced CT images through the pancreatic bed obtained 8 weeks apart show (a) subtotal necrosis of the pancreas (*arrows*) with peripancreatic inflammation and (b) organized necrosis in the pancreatic bed (CT severity index = 10). The patient remains asymptomatic. For this reason, there is no indication for either surgical or nonsurgical management. His treatment consists of medications for diabetes mellitus and steatorrhea

At admission, Acute Physiology and Chronic Health Evaluation (APACHE)-II score combined with an obesity score to derive an APACHE-O score appears also to be a useful marker for severity in acute pancreatitis [5]. Ranson score developed at 48 h in recent studies has been shown to be a relatively poor predictor of severity. Plasma levels of C-reactive protein > 150 mg/l within the first 72 h of disease correlates very well with the development of necrosis but may not peak until 36–72 h after admission.

Determination of the Severity of Acute Pancreatitis During Hospitalization

According to the Atlanta symposium, the two most important markers of severity of acute pancreatitis are pancreatic necrosis and organ failure. Contrast-enhanced CT scan (particularly contrast-enhanced, thin-section, multidetector row CT scan) is very reliable for distinguishing interstitial from necrotizing

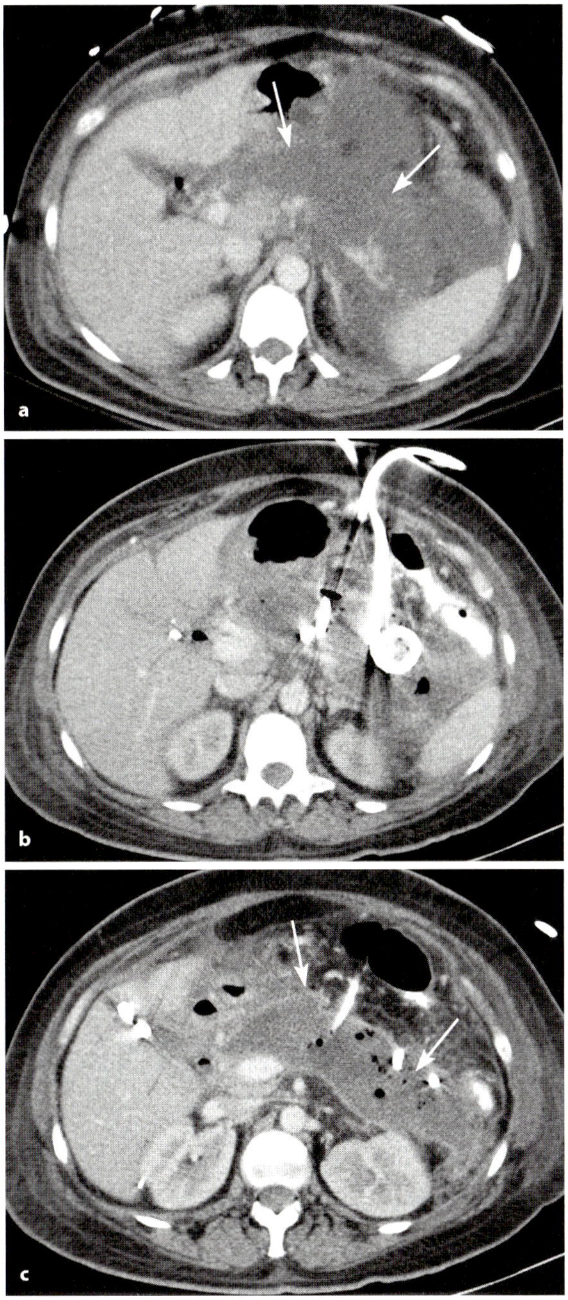

Figure 20.3

a Axial contrast-enhanced CT image showing severe pancreatitis with subtotal necrosis of the pancreas (*arrows*) with peripancreatic inflammation and fluid accumulation (CT severity index = 10). b Infected necrosis was documented in the same patient by percutaneous CT-guided aspiration, and initially the patient was managed conservatively with aggressive CT-guided catheter drainage (12–18 Fr catheters). **c** Persistence of undrained infected material (*arrows*) resulted in the need for surgical debridement

pancreatitis after 2–3 days of hospitalization. The Balthazar-Ranson CT index can be utilized to provide a formal assessment of the severity of acute pancreatitis (Table 20.1; Figs. 20.2 and 20.3).

The criteria for organ failure as established by the Atlanta symposium have not been utilized in uniform fashion. There is reasonable agreement that the three major components of organ failure are shock (systolic blood pressure ≤ 90 mmHg), hypoxemia (oxygen tension < 60 mmHg), and renal impairment (creatinine > 2.0 mg/dl after rehydration). However, in some reports, different thresholds for organ failure are utilized, while in other reports additional criteria for organ failure are utilized, including gastrointestinal bleeding (> 500 cc/24 h), leukocytosis, thrombocytopenia, and hypocalcemia [2].

It has become increasingly clear that organ failure (and particularly multisystem organ failure) is a more powerful determinant of survival than extent of pancreatic necrosis [1]. For example, in one study of patients with organ failure, the mortality associated with interstitial pancreatitis was that of necrotizing pancreatitis (approximately 15%), and the mortality associated with necrotizing pancreatitis was not correlated with the Balthazar-Ranson score [6]. Also, the mortality associated with necrotizing pancreatitis in the absence of organ failure is very low (usually < 10%), whereas that in the presence of multisystem organ failure is 36–48% [2]. In one report, the mortality of sterile necrosis and infected necrosis was the same when associated with multisystem organ failure (47 vs. 50%) [1]. Hence, sustained organ failure at admission and the development of multisystem organ failure during the hospitalization are powerful prognostic indicators in necrotizing pancreatitis. These relationships in interstitial pancreatitis have not been fully characterized.

Nonsurgical Management

Supportive Care

All patients with acute pancreatitis require aggressive fluid replacement to overcome hypovolemia caused by vomiting, diaphoresis, third-space losses, and increased vascular permeability [7]. Early aggressive fluid resuscitation, especially in patients who exhibit hemoconcentration at admission, may help prevent pancreatic necrosis [8]. It is also recommended that supplemental oxygen be administered and that measurements of oxygen saturations be determined at frequent intervals during the first 24–48 h, especially if narcotic agents are administered to control pain. Careful bedside management includes frequent measurement of vital signs and intake and output of fluids, and careful monitoring of intravenous fluid resuscitation. It is recommended that hematocrit be measured at 12 and 24 h to be sure that hemoconcentration is corrected in a timely fashion.

The choice of narcotic agent as well as the amount and frequency administered should be determined by experienced physicians and, if need be, by a dedicated pain service. Patient-controlled anesthesia can be utilized for refractory severe pain.

During the first several days of hospitalization, bowel rest and supportive care, with particular attention to recognition of early organ failure is the hallmark of treatment. A contrast-enhanced CT scan performed before the 3rd day has not been shown to add substantially to the quality of patient care. If intravenous contrast is utilized, fluid resuscitation should have already taken place to avoid the deleterious effects of intravenous contrast on renal function. It should also be kept in mind that the recognition of pancreatic necrosis is made more easily after 3–4 days than at admission.

Transfer to an Intensive Care Unit

Transfer to an intensive care unit is required for patients with sustained hypoxemia, hypotension that does not respond to a bolus of intravenous fluid, and possibly evidence of renal insufficiency that does not respond to a fluid bolus. Transfer to an intensive care unit should also be considered when there is a need for aggressive fluid resuscitation in older patients with underlying cardiovascular disease and when there is evidence of respiratory fatigue even in the absence of hypoxemia, persistent oliguria, and tachycardia. An intensive care unit provides maximal coordinated care that can optimize fluid resuscitation and provide proper minute-by-minute supervision and treatment for organ dysfunction. This supervision and treatment may include pressor agents for persistent hypotension, intubation with assisted ventilation and renal dialysis when required. These measures are supportive. There is currently no specific treatment that will prevent the deterioration of organ failure.

Transfer to an intensive care unit for these indications should take place for both interstitial pancreatitis complicated by organ failure and necrotizing pancreatitis similarly complicated by organ failure.

Nutritional Support

When oral intake cannot be restored within 1 week of hospitalization, nutritional support is required. There are many reasons to consider enteral feeding rather than total parenteral nutrition (TPN) under these circumstances. First, enteral feeding avoids complications such as blood stream infection and hyperglycemia that may occur with TPN. Second, in severe acute pancreatitis, enteral feeding may prevent the increases in intestinal permeability to bacteria and endotoxins that contribute to infected necrosis and organ failure. Thus far, there have been numerous prospective trials that have compared enteral feeding with TPN. Most studies have been underpowered and have included patients with varying degrees of illness. There is good evidence that enteral feeding is safer and less expensive than TPN, but less convincing evidence that enteral feeding improves morbidity and mortality.

There has been concern that enteral feeding delivered within the duodenum may exacerbate pancreatitis by increasing pancreatic enzyme synthesis and secretion [9]. As a result, several investigators have recommended that enteral feeding be delivered to at least the mid-jejunum rather than to the distal duodenum or even the proximal jejunum. The need for enteral feeding delivered to the jejunum has been recently challenged in one study, which concluded that nasogastric feeding was comparable to nasojejunal feeding in terms of safety and patient outcome [10]. Additional larger studies will be required to determine whether nasogastric feeding is an acceptable alternative and whether nasojejunal (or nasogastric) enteral feeding improves morbidity and mortality in acute pancreatitis.

Use of Prophylactic Antibiotics

In interstitial pancreatitis, whether associated with organ failure or not, prophylactic antibiotics do not play a role in therapy. In necrotizing pancreatitis, there have been six randomized prospective but not double-blind studies that have evaluated whether the use of antibiotics results in a decrease in infected necrosis and an improvement in mortality. These studies have generally concluded that there is a decrease in morbidity, but none has shown a decrease in mortality. A more recent multicenter, double-blind, placebo-controlled trial was conducted in Germany on the effectiveness of ciprofloxacin and metronidazole in reducing morbidity and mortality. The conclusion of the study was that there was no difference in the prevalence of infected necrosis, organ failure, or mortality in the two groups [11].

Additional studies will be required to determine whether prophylactic antibiotics decrease the prevalence of infected necrosis and improve mortality [12]. It is of interest that in recent studies of patients with necrotizing pancreatitis there appears to be a decrease in the prevalence of infected necrosis compared to previous studies [11]. The explanation is unclear, but could be related to more vigorous fluid resuscitation resulting in improved perfusion of the gut, stabilization of gut integrity, and reduction in the translocation of bacteria.

There is increasing concern that the prolonged use of potent antibiotics such as carbipenems may result in an increased prevalence of fungal infections and possibly also an increased mortality [13]. Additional studies will be required to determine the significance of superimposed fungal infections on the natural history of acute pancreatitis. The role of prophylactic antifungal agents has not been fully defined. At the present time, prophylactic antibiotic therapy is not recommended in necrotizing pancreatitis. Antibiotic therapy should be reserved for treatment of specific infections, such as those originating in the blood stream, lung, or urinary tract [2].

Treatment of Infected Necrosis

For many years, the prevailing concept has been that early recognition of infected necrosis may improve morbidity and mortality of infected necrosis. The key component of this strategy is the use of CT- or ultrasound-guided percutaneous aspiration for Gram stain and culture when pancreatic infection is suspected. During the first 7–10 days, leukocytosis and fever are common, but usually resolve slowly. After 10–14 days, pancreatic infection should be suspected if there is a significant increase in white blood count or temperature, or if organ failure develops. Pancreatic infection should also be suspected if leukocytosis and fever and/or organ failure persist for >7–10 days after admission.

The role of guided percutaneous aspiration in the care of patients has recently been questioned [14]. First, while the safety of guided percutaneous aspiration has generally been upheld in all studies, some investigators now question the accuracy of this technique. For example, whereas most infections are identified the first time percutaneous aspiration is utilized, some infections are identified after several negative aspirations performed at weekly intervals. In this circumstance, the question has been raised as to whether the initial negative aspirates were truly negative or did not detect a pancreatic infection that had already taken place. It is not possible to reconcile these two interpretations.

Secondly, in some medical centers, imaging-guided percutaneous aspiration is thought to be unnecessary because the standard of care in these institutions is to place all patients with necrotizing pancreatitis on prophylactic antibiotic therapy without making an attempt to ascertain if the patient has sterile or infected necrosis [14]. In these institutions, surgery is not performed unless the patient fails to improve or shows evidence of clinical deterioration. It has therefore been reasoned that there is no value of knowing at an earlier time interval whether a patient has sterile or infected necrosis.

There are several reasons to recommend imaging-guided percutaneous aspiration when pancreatic infection is strongly suspected and to withhold potent antibiotics unless infected necrosis is documented. First, even if surgery is not offered among patients with infected necrosis unless there is clinical deterioration, a case can be made for imaging-guided percutaneous aspiration to determine the sensitivity of organisms that are recovered and to utilize the most appropriate antibiotic coverage. Secondly, because the prevalence of fungal infections has increased among patients who have received antibiotics in necrotizing pancreatitis, the use of prophylactic antibiotics should be discouraged. At the present time, imaging-guided percutaneous aspiration is recommended when pancreatic infection is suspected, and antibiotics should be reserved for patients who are determined to have infected necrosis based on Gram stain and culture [15].

If imaging-guided percutaneous aspiration reveals the presence of infected necrosis, the standard of care for many years has been prompt surgical debridement unless patients are unacceptable surgical candidates [16, 17]. More recently, this strategy has been called into question. In particular, there has been strong consideration for the continuation of antibiotic therapy until the acute inflammatory response has subsided, with the view that surgery that is deferred for several weeks is more easily accomplished with one intervention [18]. There has also been one report that infected necrosis in many instances can be treated with prolonged use of antibiotics without the eventual need for surgery [19]. The role of delayed surgery versus urgent surgery and the role of prolonged medical therapy without surgery will require additional study.

Surgical alternatives including minimally invasive retroperitoneal necrosectomy will be described in another chapter. A nonsurgical alternative for the treatment of infected necrosis is percutaneous catheter drainage [20]. While the experience with this technique has been limited, there may be a role for percutaneous catheter drainage as a temporary measure to allow stabilization of the patient such that a safer surgical necrosectomy can be done at a later time (Fig. 20.3). On occasion, prolonged percutaneous catheter drainage with the use of multiple radiologically placed catheters that are upsized as needed has resulted in complete eradication of infected necrosis after several weeks or months. This radiologic approach requires a team of dedicated radiologists who are prepared to make daily bedside rounds to supervise the catheter care and also to obtain a CT scan whenever needed, with further radiologic interventions in timely fashion as indicated. Percutaneous radiologic techniques have not been directly compared with surgical techniques or prolonged antibiotic therapy. Endoscopic drainage of infected necrosis within the first several weeks of illness has not been widely utilized and has not been compared with other forms of intervention.

A pancreatic abscess (representing eventual liquefaction and secondary infection of a residual area of pancreatic necrosis or an infected peripancreatic pseudocyst) does not usually develop until 4–6 weeks after the onset of severe acute pancreatitis. Percutaneous catheter drainage and occasionally endoscopic drainage are suitable alternatives to surgical drainage.

Treatment of Sterile Necrosis

During the first several weeks of sterile necrosis, some patients exhibit severe systemic toxicity with pronounced leukocytosis, fever, and organ failure. Early intervention (whether surgical, radiologic, or endoscopic) within the first 2–3 weeks for sterile necrosis has been considered as a possible method of improving organ failure, preventing the development of infected necrosis, reducing systemic toxicity, and treating abdominal pain that may be associated with expanding fluid collections. Reports thus far (which are mostly anecdotal) would indicate that surgical debridement and attempted percutaneous debridement using multiple catheters are ineffective in improving morbidity and mortality. Similarly, early stenting of the pancreatic duct to prevent the extravasation of pancreatic fluid with the view that this technique might improve organ failure, reduce systemic toxicity, or treat abdominal pain have not been subjected to prospective trials. There is concern that the introduction of a stent into the pancreatic duct would lead to infection of the surrounding necrotic tissue. Hence, early intervention by these various modalities is not recommended. However, after 3 weeks, the diffuse inflammatory process usually resolves considerably, and the necrotic pancreas and inflamed peripancreatic area become encapsulated in a structure that has frequently been called a pseudocyst, but more recently has been termed organized necrosis. By this time, organ failure has usually also improved. In the absence of symptoms, there is no need for surgical or nonsurgical intervention (Fig. 20.2). However, on occasion, organized necrosis is associated with intractable abdominal pain, preventing oral intake of food, intractable nausea, and vomiting because of obstruction of the stomach or duodenum, or general lingering symptoms including malaise, anorexia, and low-grade fever suggestive of the presence of infected necrosis. Under these circumstances, there is a role for nonsurgical rather than surgical intervention. Radiologic percutaneous debridement has been attempted in this setting, but unless large percutaneously placed catheters fully evacuate the semisolid necrotic material, retained necrotic material becomes secondarily infected. In general, percutaneous debridement should be reserved for centers with considerable experience in therapeutic radiologic techniques.

Endoscopic cyst-gastrostomy is an alternative to surgical cyst-gastrostomy or Roux-en-y cyst-jejunostomy. This technique has been utilized when the organized necrosis is firmly attached to the posterior wall of the stomach (or duodenum). Once endoscopic ultrasound targets a safe route to open the posterior wall of the stomach (or duodenum) without risk of damaging a nearby vessel, the opening can then be expanded with balloon dilatation and the instrument itself advanced into the cavity of organized necrosis to remove all necrotic debris. Double pigtail catheters are then placed between the stomach (or duodenum) and the cavity. However, the opening itself may close down around the catheters, thereby creating a closed space and the possibility for secondary infection. Should this take place, the patient may become severely toxic and require either surgical or radiologic treatment, or possibly another attempt at endoscopic drainage. In one study of patients treated by endoscopic debridement, there were numerous complications including infections as well as recurrences [21]. This technique should be reserved for centers with particular interest in therapeutic endoscopic maneuvers. Thus far, endoscopic debridement has not been compared with surgical debridement in a randomized prospective trial.

Treatment of Pancreatic Ductal Disruption

Occasionally in interstitial pancreatitis, and more commonly in necrotizing pancreatitis, the main pancreatic duct becomes disrupted either partially (most commonly in the genu) or completely ("disconnected duct syndrome"). A disruption is suggested when a series of CT scans show a progressive increase in size of fluid collections or persistence of a loculated fluid collection. In the absence of symptoms, no treatment is required. When there is evidence of persisting or increasing pain, endoscopic retrograde cholangiopancreatography (ERCP) should be performed to document the presence of a ductal disruption. Medical treatment of a symptomatic disruption is rarely successful. Occasionally, therapy including nasojejunal feeding (or TPN) coupled with subcutaneous injections of octreotide may reduce pancreatic flow and facilitate closure of a ductal disruption.

Recent reports have shown that endoscopic therapy is the treatment of choice, especially if the disruption is partial and if the pancreatic stent inserted into the pancreatic duct bridges the disruption [22]. The stent is generally left in place for 4–6 weeks and is then removed if pancreatic imaging by ERCP indicates that the disruption has healed. Endoscopic stent therapy is generally unsuccessful if the pancreatic stent is inserted only to the area of the disruption without actually bridging it. When pancreatic necrosis is extensive, the placement of a pancreatic stent to overcome a focal disruption may result in secondary infection of the nearby necrosis.

At times, the entire mid-portion of the pancreas becomes necrotic, with persistence of residual viable parenchyma in both the head and remnant tail of the pancreas. If there is a large gap in the integrity of the main pancreatic duct due to extensive necrosis of the middle portion of the pancreas, endoscopic stent therapy should not be attempted. First, it is virtually impossible to make a connection to the duct in the tail of the pancreas with a wire inserted via the ampulla across the zone of necrosis. Secondly, even if a connection could be made and a stent introduced over the wire to bridge the gap, there is a high likelihood of infection of the surrounding necrosis. Accordingly, endoscopic stent therapy is not recommended in the presence of extensive pancreatic necrosis either during the first several weeks or later after organized necrosis has developed.

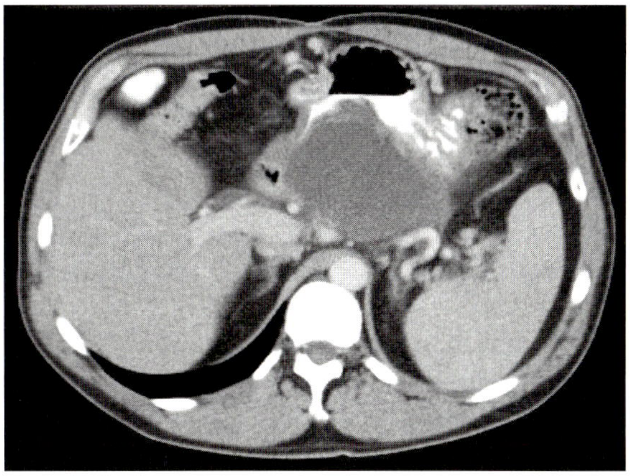

Figure 20.4

Axial contrast-enhanced CT image of a patient suffering from severe abdominal pain several months following surgical debridement for infected necrosis shows a well-defined fluid collection in the lesser sac. Persistent secretion of pancreatic juice from a viable remnant tail presumably caused this collection. It was possible to drain the collection endoscopically because of its proximity to the stomach

Treatment of a Remnant Tail of the Pancreas

Following treatment of organized necrosis in the mid-portion of the pancreas (whether by surgical, endoscopic, or radiologic techniques), there is frequently a small area in the tail of the pancreas that remains viable and continues to secrete pancreatic fluid. This fluid may accumulate in the pancreatic bed in the area where the necrosis had been eliminated. Accumulation of this fluid implies that the enteric communication has not remained open (whether created surgically or endoscopically). In the absence of symptoms, there is no need for further therapy. However, if the pancreatic fluid becomes secondarily infected or causes abdominal pain, additional attempts can be made to drain this collection nonsurgically, such as with endoscopic cyst-gastrostomy or prolonged percutaneous drainage (Fig. 20.4). If these efforts fail, a surgical procedure will then be indicated, such as a surgical cyst-gastrostomy or resection of the tail of the pancreas.

Biliary Sphincterotomy in Gallstone Pancreatitis

There have been three published randomized controlled studies of urgent ERCP and biliary sphincterotomy in gallstone pancreatitis. While many have interpreted the overall results of these studies to favor endoscopic sphincterotomy in severe gallstone pancreatitis, other have interpreted the data to conclude that urgent endoscopic sphincterotomy may improve the morbidity but not the mortality associated with necrotizing pancreatitis [23].

There is general agreement that for endoscopic sphincterotomy to be helpful, it must be performed very early in the course of acute pancreatitis, preferably within 24–48 h of the onset of symptoms. Patients who might benefit from early endoscopic sphincterotomy are those who show early evidence of organ failure. One explanation for organ failure would be a retained common bile duct stone causing ascending cholangitis. Endoscopic sphincterotomy in this circumstance can be life saving. It remains unproven whether organ failure in severe acute pancreatitis can be improved by endoscopic sphincterotomy with removal of an obstructing common bile duct stone [2]. In mild biliary pancreatitis, endoscopic sphincterotomy is indicated for patients who are not likely to undergo a laparoscopic cholecystectomy for several weeks because of comorbid disease and for those whose comorbid disease preludes laparoscopic cholecystectomy.

References

1. Perez A, Whang EE, Brooks DC, Moore FD Jr, Hughes MD, Sica GT, Zinner MJ, Ashley SW, Banks PA (2002) Is severity of necrotizing pancreatitis increased in extended necrosis and infected necrosis? Pancreas 25:229–233
2. Banks PA, Freeman ML (2006) Practice guidelines in acute pancreatitis. Am J Gastroenterol 101:2379–2400
3. Johnson CD, Abu-Hilal M (2004) Persistent organ failure during the first week as a marker of fatal outcome in acute pancreatitis. Gut 53:1340–1344
4. Brown A, Orav J, Banks PA (2000) Hemoconcentration is an early marker for organ failure and necrotizing pancreatitis. Pancreas 20:367–372
5. Johnson CD, Toh SK, Campbell MJ (2004) Combination of APACHE-II score and an obesity score (APACHE-O) for the prediction of severe acute pancreatitis. Pancreatology 4:1–6
6. Malangoni MA, Martin AS (2005) Outcome of severe acute pancreatitis. Am J Surg 189:273–277
7. Tenner S (2004) Initial management of acute pancreatitis: critical issues during the first 72 hours. Am J Gastroenterol 99:2489–2494
8. Brown A, Baillargeon JD, Hughes MD, Banks PA (2002) Can fluid resuscitation prevent pancreatic necrosis in severe acute pancreatitis? Pancreatology 2:104–107
9. Kaushik N, Pietraszewski M, Holst JJ, O'Keefe SJD (2005) Enteral feeding without pancreatic stimulation. Pancreas 31:353–359
10. Eatock FC, Chong P, Menezes N, Murray L, McKay CJ, Carter CR, Imrie CW (2005) A randomized study of early nasogastric versus nasojejunal feeding in severe acute pancreatitis. Am J Gastroenterol 100:432–439
11. Isenmann R, Runzi M, Kron M, Kahl S, Kraus D, Jung N, Maier L, Malfertheiner P, Goebell H, Beger HG (2004) Prophylactic antibiotic treatment in patients with predicted severe acute pancreatitis: a placebo-controlled, double-blind trial. Gastroenterology 126:997–1004
12. Brown A (2004) Prophylactic antibiotic use in severe acute pancreatitis: hemlock, help, or hype? Gastroenterology 126:1195–1198
13. Beger HG, Rau B, Isenmann R, Schwarz M, Gansauge F, Poch B (2005) Antibiotic prophylaxis in severe acute pancreatitis. Pancreatology 5:10–19
14. Pappas TN (2005) Con: computerized tomographic aspiration of infected pancreatic necrosis: the opinion against its routine use. Am J Gastroenterol 100:2373–2374
15. Banks PA (2005) Pro: computerized tomographic fine needle aspiration (CT-FNA) is valuable in the management of infected pancreatic necrosis. Am J Gastroenterol 100:2371–2372
16. Nathens AB, Curtis JR, Beale RJ, Cook DJ, Moreno RP, Romand JA, Skerrett SJ, Stapleton RD, Ware LB, Waldmann CS (2004) Management of the critically ill patient with severe acute pancreatitis. Crit Care Med 32:2524–2536
17. Werner J, Feuerbach S, Uhl W, Buchler MW(2005) Management of acute pancreatitis: from surgery to interventional intensive care. Gut 54:426–436
18. Vege SS, Baron TH (2005) Management of pancreatic necrosis in severe acute pancreatitis. Clin Gastroenterol Hepatol 3:192–196
19. Runzi M, Niebel W, Goebell H, Gerken G, Layer P. 2005. Severe acute pancreatitis: nonsurgical treatment of infected necroses. Pancreas 30:195–9
20. Shankar S, vanSonnenberg E, Silverman SG, Tuncali K, Banks PA (2004) Imaging and percutaneous management of acute complicated pancreatitis. Cardiovasc Intervent Radiol 27:567–580
21. Baron TH, Harewood GC, Morgan DE, Yates MR (2002) Outcome differences after endoscopic drainage of pancreatic necrosis, acute pancreatic pseudocysts, and chronic pancreatic pseudocysts. Gastrointest Endosc 56:7–17
22. Varadarajulu S, Noone TC, Tutuian R, Hawes RH, Cotton PB (2005) Predictors of outcome in pancreatic duct disruption managed by endoscopic transpapillary stent placement. Gastrointest Endosc 61:568–575
23. Ayub K, Imada R, Slavin J (2004) Endoscopic retrograde cholangiopancreatography in gallstone-associated acute pancreatitis. Cochrane Database Syst Rev 18:CD003630

H. G. Beger · B. M. Rau

Indications for the Surgical Management of Necrotizing Pancreatitis

Unlike edematous acute pancreatitis, necrotizing pancreatitis is associated with morphologic changes causing functional impairment that may not recover to normal even years after the acute attack. About one-third of patients suffering from acute pancreatitis develop severe pathomorphological local complications (Table 21.1.1).

The etiology of acute pancreatitis plays an important role in the decision making for surgical and non-surgical management. Biliary pancreatitis is almost uniformly associated with a complete recovery of the gland [1]. In patients with biliary acute pancreatitis of different severity, pancreatic function has been assessed by the secretin-cerulein test 1 year after the acute attack and showed normal exocrine function in all subjects. To prevent the recurrence of acute biliary pancreatitis, the gallbladder should be removed in mild edematous disease within 2 weeks of acute pancreatitis after resolution of symptoms or during the same hospital stay [2]. It has been demonstrated that early (emergency) endoscopic retrograde cholangiopancreatography and endoscopic sphincterotomy reduces significantly [3, 4] morbidity and mortality in biliary seosis [3–5]. There is some evidence, that irrespective of the severity, significantly more patients suffer from exocrine dysfunction after alcoholic pancreatitis as compared with biliary pancreatitis.

Evidence regarding the persistence of endocrine and exocrine insufficiency after an acute attack of severe acute pancreatitis has been published with insufficiency rates of 30–60% in the long-term follow-up [6, 7].

Table 21.1.1. Acute pancreatitis – incidence of local complications. The Ulm experience: data collected from 1568 patients between February 1982 and May 2001 (Department of General Surgery, University of Ulm). *pts* Patients, *NP* necrotizing pancreatitis

Complication	*n*	Incidence
Interstitial-edematous pancreatitis	1071 pts	68.3%
Necrotizing pancreatitis	497 pts	31.7%
NP-sterile necrosis	227 pts	63.2%
NP – primary infected necrosis	132 pts	36.8%
Pancreatic abscess	42 pts	2.7%
Postacute pseudocyst	96 pts	6.1%

The Role of Antibiotic Prophylaxis in Infected Necrosis to Avoid Surgery

Late morbidity and mortality in patients with severe acute pancreatitis is caused by infection of necrosis. Infected necrosis is observed in about 25–70% of all patients with necrotizing pancreatitis and in 7% of all patients with acute pancreatitis. Pancreatic abscess, which is a different infective entity of acute pancreatitis, has been observed in 10% of patients with necrotizing pancreatitis and in 3% of all patients with acute pancreatitis (Table 21.1.2).

It was believed that antibiotic therapy would result in a reduction of infectious complications, hospital mortality, and the number of required surgical interventions. Based on the data regarding the penetration of different antibiotics into pancreatic tissue and the highest penetration rate of imipenem into the necrotic parenchyma, randomized prospective clinical trials have been performed to evaluate the effects of prophylactic antibiotic treatment [8]. Several prospective randomized clinical trials have shown that prophylactic antibiotic treatment in cases with contrast-enhanced computed tomography (CECT)-proven necrotizing pancreatitis reduces the incidence of infection of necroses and leads to a decrease in the need for surgical necrosectomy [9, 10]. A significant reduction in hospital mortality has been objectified in two trials [11, 12]; however, with regard to reduction of infected necrosis and reduction of hospital mortality the results of randomized, controlled trials are conflicting [13]. A selective decontamination of the intestine was evaluated in a Dutch trial including more than 100

Table 21.1.2. Incidence of pancreatic infection in 427 patients with necrotizing pancreatitis (i.e., pancreatic necrosis/extrapancreatic fatty tissue necrosis, pancreatic abscess, or postacute pseudocyst). Data collected between May 1982 and December 1996 at the Department of General Surgery, University of Ulm, Germany. *AP* Acute pancreatitis

	n	% of NP	% of AP
Infected necrosis	99 pts	23.2%	6.9%
Pancreatic abscess	40 pts	9.4%	2.8%
Infected pseudocyst after AP	7 pts	1.6%	10.1%
TOTAL	146 pts	34.2%	10.1%

Table 21.1.3. Antibiotic prophylaxis in severe acute pancreatitis – results of two double-blind randomized controlled trials: Isenmann et al. 2004 [15] (ciprofloxacin, metronidazole) and Dellinger et al. 2006 [16] (meropenem). *NS* Not significant

	Isenmann [15]	p-value	Dellinger [16]	p-value
Patients	114		100	
Treatment (n)	58		50	
Placebo (n)	41		50	
Infection				
Treatment	12%	NS	18%	NS
Placebo	14%		12%	
Need for surgery				
Treatment	17%	NS	26%	NS
Placebo	11%		20%	
Hospital mortality				
Treatment	12%	NS	20%	NS
Placebo	9%		18%	

Table 21.1.4. Infected necrosis response to nonsurgical management. *IN* Infected necrosis, *OF* organ failure, *Ø Compl.* No complications

Study	Patients with IN *n*	Patients with OF *n*	Ø Compl.	Nonsurgical management	Hospital mortality
Le Mée 2001 [17]	27	14 (52%)	–	4 (15%)	0%
Rünzi 2005 [18]	28	10 (36%)	6 (21%)	16 (57%)	12.5%
Rau 2005 [19]	11	10 (91%)	–	11 (100%)	9.1%

patients with severe acute pancreatitis [14]. By selective decontamination of the gut in combination with intravenous antibiotics, the authors observed a significantly decreased morbidity and mortality from Gram-negative sepsis. However, the selective decontamination group received additionally intravenous cefotaxim; whereas the control group did not. The clinical relevance of the Dutch data with regard to the role of prophylactic intravenous antibiotics in preventing pancreatic infections, therefore, remains conflicting and unconvincing. Contrary results were recently published from two randomized, multicenter, double-blind, controlled clinical trials, using ciprofloxaxin/metronidazole in the one and meropenem in the other study (Table 21.1.3). Both trials included more than 100 patients and, on basis of the double-blind, randomized, multicentric study protocol, were unable to confirm a reduction of infected necrosis or overall pancreatic infections. Hospital mortality and frequency of surgical intervention were similar in the treatment and control groups of either study. Meta-analysis including the double-blind randomized, controlled trials conclude that prophylactic antibiotic treatment is ineffective in terms of lowering the rate of infected necrosis and the clinical consequences [15, 16].

Patients who suffer from infected necrosis, as evidenced by CECT and bacterial/fungal positive fine-needle aspiration without having clinical signs of sepsis or other systemic complications do not need surgical necrosectomy. Several groups reported convincing results following nonsurgical management in small groups of patients who had infected necrosis and prophylactic antibiotic treatment but showed no clinical signs of sepsis [17–19]. The hospital mortality in this group of patients was about 10% (Table 21.1.4).

Sterile Pancreatic Necrosis and Surgical Intervention

About 20% of patients with acute pancreatitis develop a severe course with pathomorphological signs of pancreatic tissue necrosis and fatty tissue necroses in the retroperitoneal spaces. Most patients with sterile necrotizing pancreatitis respond to intensive care unit (ICU) treatment and are not candidates for surgical intervention. However about 5% of patients with necrotizing pancreatitis develop a severe type with extended necrosis involving more than 50% of the pancreas (Table 21.1.5). The contention that conservative management is usually blessed with a successful outcome in patients with sterile pancreatic necrosis has been revised after the demonstration that patients with extended sterile pancreatic necrosis have a very high risk of mortality [20]. Banks reported a mortality of 38% in a group of 26 patients with sterile pancreatic necrosis and at least one systemic complication [21]. Evidence suggests that early surgical intervention is not helpful in patients with necrosis. All patients with higher Acute Physiology and Chronic Health Evaluation II (APACHE II) scores – those with a recorded systolic blood pressure of <80 mmHg and with renal or pulmonary complications as well as a high body mass index – had a high risk of death. However, up to now there are no prospective data supporting the hypothesis concept that early surgical intervention within the 1st week after symptom onset may improve organ failure and thus lower mortality.

Surgical intervention of patients suffering from extended, sterile pancreatic necrosis should be based, on the criteria of nonresponse to prolonged maximum intensive care treatment beyond the 2nd week after symptom onset (Table 21.1.6). Fifty percent of patients with extended sterile necrosis will develop infected necrosis in the later course of disease. Patients suffering from early severe acute pancreatitis show systemic complications on the basis of early extended (>50%), sterile pancreatic necrosis. Patients with extended sterile, pancreatic necrosis (>50f) show clinical signs of sepsis as in infected necrosis, but have negative FNP. The authors consider an indication for surgery in patients with extended sterile necrosis if they do not respond to maximum intensive care treatment after a period of at least 1 week despite maximum ICU support [20, 22]. However, it has to be emphasized that this issue remains controversial throughout the current literature.

Table 21.1.5. Morbidity associated with sterile pancreatic necrosis. Unpublished data. Department of General Surgery, University of Ulm

Pancreatic necrosis	Pain every day	Leukocytosis[a]	Palpable abdominal mass	Pulmonary insuff.[b]	Renal insuff.[c]	Hepatic insuff.[d]	Shock[e]	Sepsis[f]
Focal (43 pts)	86%	65.1%	30.2%	23.3%	16.3%	25.6%	4.7%	2.3%
Extended (31 pts)	93.5%	74.2%	45.2%	25.8%	12.9%	32.5%	6.5%	12.9%
Subtotal/Total (21 pts)	95%	85.7%	33.3%	47.6%	52.4%	47.6%	14.3%	19.0%

[a] >12,000 leukocytes/mm^3

[b] Arterial oxygen tension <60 mmHg or mechanical ventilation

[c] Creatinine 1.4 mg/dl

[d] Serum glutamic oxaloacetic transaminase >50 μ/l

[e] Systolic blood pressure <80 mmHg for more than 15 min

[f] Temperature >38.5°C+leukocyte count <4000/mm^3 or >12,000/mm^3, thrombocytopenia (platelet count <150,000/mm^3)+base excess >4 mMol for more than 48 h

Table 21.1.6. Severe acute pancreatitis high-risk groups: extended sterile necrosis (i.e., involving >50% of the pancreas). *CECT* contrast-enhanced computed tomography, *MOF* multiorgan failure, *ESAP* early severe acute pancreatitis

Extended sterile necrosis (>50%, CECT, Balthazar grade D+E)

- >75% develop early OF/MOF
  - pulmonary insufficiency
  - cardiocirculatory dysfunction
  - renal insufficiency
- 27% develop infected necrosis (by the 3rd week) [40]
- 34% of patients suffering from ESAP have extented (>50%) necroses [28]
- Hospital mortality in patients with necrosis >50% is significantly higher than in those with to focal necrosis [41]

The Role of Surgery in the Management of Necrotizing Pancreatitis

The severity of necrotizing pancreatitis is determined by the amount of necrosis of pancreatic parenchyma and the extent of retroperitoneal fatty tissue necrosis. Necrotizing pancreatitis including up to 30% of the pancreas (CECT data) is not strongly related to severity of acute pancreatitis. However, almost every patient with >50% pancreatic parenchymal necrosis suffers from clinically severe acute pancreatitis. CECT investigation of necrotizing pancreatitis reveals frequently superficial pancreatic parenchymal necrosis encoating vital pancreatic core tissue. For this reason the application of extended pancreatic resection techniques (e.g., hemipancreatectomy or subtotal pancreatosplenectomy), as advocated in the 1960s and 1970s, have uniformly been abandoned as a therapeutic option in acute necrotizing pancreatitis. These techniques are associated with high early morbidity and mortality rates of 50–80%. Endocrine insufficiency was found in up to 90% of the resected cases in long-term follow-up studies [23, 24]. Surgical treatment regimens combining a tissue-preserving digital debridement of devitalized tissue with a postoperative additional technique to provide further evacuation of retroperitoneal debris and exudates using either open or closed approaches are associated with lower mortality rates and preserve the endocrine and exocrine function. A carefully performed retrospective analysis of patients with necrotizing pancreatitis comparing classic pancreatic resection and digital necrosectomy has revealed the development of diabetes mellitus in 100% of patients after resection and in 52% after necrosectomy [25]. The following techniques are currently in use for the debridement of pancreatic/extrapancreatic necrosis (Table 21.1.7):

1. Open necrosectomy with postoperative closed continuous lavage of the lesser sac and the abdominal cavity.
2. Open necrosectomy with open packing and planned relaparotomy
3. Retroperitoneal or ventral laparoscopic necrosectomy with staged lavage
4. Endoscopic transgastric necrosectomy and lavage and drainage
5. Percutaneous interventional drainage and lavage

Timing of Surgery for Necrotizing Pancreatitis

Nowadays there is clearly no more doubt that surgery is not the first choice of treatment for patients suffering from severe acute pancreatitis. To predict local and systemic complications, several approaches have been developed and evaluated (Table 21.1.8). The daily APACHE II, the sequential organ failure (SOFA) assessment and the multiorgan failure score have a moderate-to-reliable positive predictive value to predict organ failure/multiorgan dysfunction syndrome (MODS) early in the course of acute pancreatitis [26]. As an established biochemical routine parameter, C-reactive protein offers reasonable sensitivity and specificity to predict the development of local or systemic complications within 72–96 h after disease onset. Recently, the use of procalcitonin (PCT) has been found to have a high sensitivity and specifity to predict early organ failure [27]. Moreover, a prospective international multicenter trial could show that PCT allows accurate early assessment of clinically relevant complications such as severe pancreatic infections or nonsurvival [28].

About 5–8% of the patients suffer from early severe acute pancreatitis with single or multiple systemic complications, mostly pulmonary insufficiency and

Table 21.1.7. Surgical management: algorithm for acute pancreatitis. *SIRS* systemic inflammatory response syndrome, *ICU* intensive care unit

	Treatment principle
Interstitial-edematous pancreatitis	Nonsurgical[a]
Peripancreatic fluid collections	Nonsurgical
	Interventional to interrupt SIRS
Necrotizing pancreatitis	
Sterile necrosis	Nonsurgical
Sterile >50%	Surgical necrosectomy if nonresponse to maximum ICU management
Infected necrosis	Surgery + continuous lavage
	Laparoscopic/endoscopic/interventional management/lavage
Pancreatic abscess	Interventional drainage + lavage
	Surgical drainage if sepsis persists after interventional drainage
Postacute pseudocyst	Interventional drainage
	Extrapancreatic localization
	Surgical drainage
	Intrapancreatic localization

[a] Except biliary tract surgery for biliary pancreatitis

Table 21.1.8. Approaches to predict OF and MOF or infected necrosis in acute pancreatitis [26]. *MODS* Multiorgan dysfunction syndrome, *PPV* positive predictive value, *NPV* negative predictive value, *APACHE II* Acute Physiology and Chronic Health Evaluation II score, *PCT* procalcitonin, *CRP* C-reactive protein

	Cut-off	Sensitivity	Specificity	PPV	NPV
Prediction of OF/MODS [26]					
APACHE II (48 h[a])	>13	59%	88%	59%	88%
SOFA (48 h[a])	> 4	73%	90%	73%	90%
MOF (48 h[a])	> 2	80%	69%	47%	91%
Prediction of MODS and infected necrosis [28]					
PCT (72–96h[b])	≥3.8 ng/ml	80%	90%4	7%	98%
CRP (72–96h[b])	≥440 mg/l	40%	96%	50%	94%
Ranson 1974 [42]	1–2	3–4	5–6	7–8	
Mortality		0.9%	16.4%	40%	100%

[a] Within 48 h of disease onset
[b] Within 72–96 h of disease onset

cardiocirculatory dysfunction [29]. The first choice of treatment is intensive care management. Patients suffering from early severe acute pancreatitis with two or more organ failures require maximum intensive care treatment with vigorous fluid replacement and, in the case of severe organ failure, mechanical ventilation, dialysis/hemofiltration, and vasopressors. Most patients with clinical MODS demonstrate on CECT extended sterile necrosis (Fig. 21.1.1). Several groups recommended persistence of intensive care treatment until disappearance of the organ dysfunction for these patients. However, hospital mortality in patients with early severe acute pancreatitis ranges between 42 and 60% [29–32]. In the author's opinion, patients with early severe acute pancreatitis and CECT-proven extended necrosis (>50%) of the pancreas should have

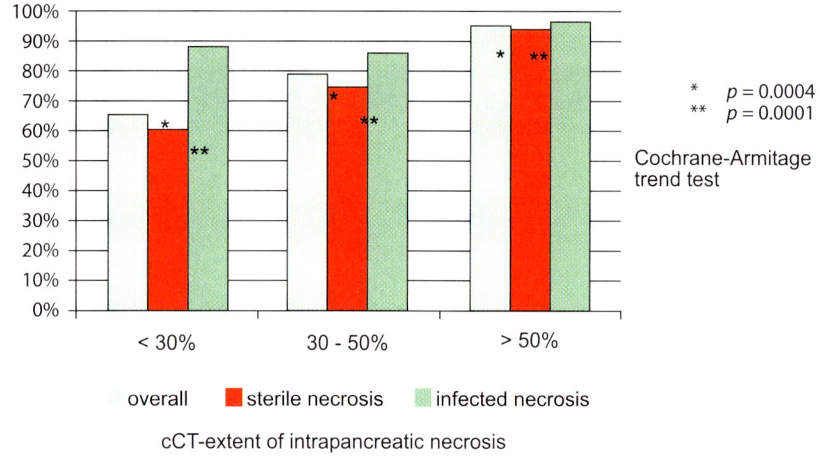

Figure 21.1.1

Organ failure and extent of necrosis. The incidence of organ failure is related to the extent of pancreatic necrosis in patients with sterile necrosis, but not in those with infected necrosis (taken, with permission, from Isenmann et al. 1999 [43]). *cCT* Contrast-enhanced computed tomography

surgical debridement if organ failure is nonresponsive to maximum intensive care treatment for more than 1 week (Table 21.1.7). However, neither the persistence of intensive care treatment until successful management of systemic organ complications nor the definition of nonresponders with subsequent necrosectomy has been evaluated by controlled clinical trials. However, empirical data from several studies completed since the 1990s strongly recommend postponement of surgery for as long as possible, usually beyond the 2nd week of the disease or later, when necrotic tissue can be well distinguished from viable pancreatic parenchyma and dissection of necrotic tissue is technically applicable without major blood loss [33–35]. The degree of functional insufficiency after necrotizing pancreatitis depends on the severity of the necrotizing attack, but is generally not related to the surgical technique of debridement [36]. Studies evaluating pancreatic function in patients after an acute attack have revealed that the development of functional pancreatic impairment strongly correlated with the extent of pancreatic necrosis [36–38]. In patients with severe acute pancreatitis and infected necrosis, surgical management is mandatory because of aedequate focus control in order to present further local and systemic complications [36–40]. The goal of surgical treatment is the interruption of the ongoing autodestruction and local/systemic sepsis by necrosectomy and evacuation of infected and biological active material in and around the pancreas, using additional ccontinuous closed lavage or planned reoperations. The disappearance of the clinical signs of sepsis occurs within 2–4 days after the successful operative intervention.

References

1. Pareja E, Artigues E, Aparisi L, Fabra R, Martinez V, Trullenque R (1906) Exocrine pancreatic changes following acute attack of biliary pancreatitis. Pancreatology 2:478–483
2. Uhl W, Warshaw A, Imrie C, Bassi C, McKay CJ, Lankisch PG, et al (2002) IAP guidelines for the surgical management of acute pancreatitis. Pancreatology 2:565–573
3. Fan ST, La SC, Mok FPT, LoCH, Rheng SS, Wong J (1993) Early treatment of acute biliary pancreatitis by endoscopic papillotomy. N Engl J Med 328:228–232
4. Neoptolemos JP, London NJ, James D, Carr-Locke DL, Bailey IA, Fossard DP (1988) Controlled trial of urgent endoscopic retrograde cholangiopancreatography and endoscopic sphincterotomy versus conventional treatment for acute pancreatitis due to gallstones. Lancet 11:979–983
5. Fölsch UR, Nitsche R, Lüdtke R, Hilgers RA, Creutzfeldt W (1997) Early ERCP and papillotomy compared with conservative treatment for acute biliary pancreatitis. The German Study Group on Acute Biliary Biliary Pancreatitis. N Engl J Med 336:237–242
6. Büchler M, Hauke A, Malfertheiner P (1987) Follow-up after acute pancreatitis – morphology and function. In: Beger HG, Büchler M (eds) Acute Pancreatitis – Research and Clinical Management. Springer-Verlag, Berlin, Heidelberg, pp 367–374
7. Tsiotos GG, Luque-de LE, Sarr MG (1998) Long-term outcome of necrotizing pancreatitis treated by necrosectomy. Br J Surg 85:1650–1653
8. Büchler M, Malfertheiner P, Friess H, Isenmann R, Vanek E, Grimm H, et al (1992) Human pancreatic tissue concentration of bactericidal antibiotic. Gastroenterology 103:1902–1908

9. Pederzoli P, Bassi C, Vesentini S, Campedelli A (1993) A randomized clinical trial of antibiotics prophylaxis of septic complications in acute necrotising pancreatitis with imipenem. Surg Gynaecol Obstet 176:480–483
10. Spicak J, Hubaczovai M, Antos F, Bairtovai J, Cech P, Kasalickyi M, et al (2002) Antibiotics in the treatment of acute pancreatitis – findings from a randomized multi-centre prospective study. Cesk Gastroenterol Hepatol 56:183–189
11. Sainio V, Kemppainen E, Puolakkainen P, Taavitsainen M, Kivisaari L, Valtonen V (1995) Early antibiotic treatment in acute necrotizing pancreatitis. Lancet 346:663–667
12. Delcenserie R, Yzet T, Ducroix JP (1996) Prophylactic antibiotics in treatment of severe acute alcoholic pancreatitis. Pancreas 13:198–201
13. Schwarz M, Isenmann R, Meyer H, Beger HG (1997) Antibiotic use in necrotizing pancreatitis. Results of a controlled study. Dtsch Med Wochenschr 122:356–361
14. Luiten EJT, Hop WCJ, Lange JF, Bruining HA (1995) Controlled clinical trial of selective decontamination of the treatment of severe acute pancreatitis. Ann Surg 222:57–65
15. Isenmann R, Rünzi M, Kron M, Kahl S, Kraus D, Jung N, et al (2004) Prophylactic antibiotic treatment in patients with predicted severe acute pancreatitis: a placebo-controlled, double-blind trial. Gastroenterology 126:997–1004
16. Dellinger EP, Telado JM, Soto N (2007) Prophylactic antibiotic treatment in patients with severe acute pancreatitis: a double-blind placebo-controlled study. Ann Surg 245:674–683
17. Le Mée, Paye F, Sauvanet A, O'Toole D, Hammel P, Marty J, et al (2001) Incidence and reversibility of organ failure in the course of sterile and infected necrotizing pancreatitis. Arch Surg 136:1386–1390
18. Rünzi M, Niebel W, Goebell H, Gerken G, Layer P (2005) Non-surgical treatment of infected necrosis in severe acute pancreatitis. Pancreas 30:195–199
19. Rau BM, Bothe A, Beger HG (2005) Surgical treatment of necrotizing pancreatitis by necrosectomy and closed lavage: changing patient characteristics and outcome in a 19-year, single-center series. Surgery 138:28–39
20. Rau B, Pralle U, Uhl W, Schoenberg MH, Beger HG (1995) Management of sterile necrosis in instances of severe necrotizing pancreatitis. J Am Coll Surg 181:279–288
21. Tenner S, Sica G, Hughes M, Noordhoek E, Feng S, Zinner M, et al (1997) Relationship of necrosis to organ failure in severe acute pancreatitis. Gastroenterology 113:899–903
22. Isenmann R, Beger HG (2001) Bacterial infection of pancreatic necrosis: role of bacterial translocation; impact of antibiotic treatment. Pancreatology 1:79–89
23. Nordback IH, Auvinen OA (1985) Long-term results after pancreas resection for acute necrotizing pancreatitis. Br J Surg 72:687–689
24. Eriksson J, Doepel M, Widen E, Halme L, Ekstrand A, Groop L, et al (1992) Pancreatic surgery, not pancreatitis, is the primary cause of diabetes after acute fulminant pancreatitis. Gut 33:843–847
25. Halonen KI, Pettila V, Leppaniemi AK, Kemppainen EA, Puolakkainen PA, Haapiainen RK (2003) Long-term health-related quality of life in survivors of severe acute pancreatitis. Intensive Care Med 29:782–786
26. Rau BM, Kemppainen E, Bassi C, Uhl W, Büchler MW, Puolakkainen P, et al (2005) Assessment of major complications and overall prognosis by the SOFA-, APACHE II- and MOF-score in severe acute pancreatitis: Results of an international multicenter study. Pancreatology 5:76 (abstract)
27. Kylanpaa-Back ML, Takala A, Kemppainen E, Puolakkainen P, Haapiainen R, Repo H (2001) Procalcitonin strip test in the early detection of severe acute pancreatitis. Br J Surg 88:222–227
28. Rau BM, Kemppainen EA, Gumbs AA, Büchler MW, Wegscheider K, Bassi C, et al (2007) Early assessment of pancreatic infections and overall prognosis in severe acute pancreatitis by procalcitonin (PCT): a prospective international multicenter study. Ann Surg 245:745–754
29. Mier J, Leon EL, Castillo A, Robledo F, Blanco R (1997) Early versus late necrosectomy in severe necrotising pancreatitis. Am J Surg 173:71–75
30. Isenmann R, Rau B, Beger HG (2001) Early severe acute pancreatitis: characteristics of a new subgroup. Pancreas 22:274–278
31. Renner IG, Savage WT, Pantoza JL, Renner VJ (1985) Death due to acute pancreatitis. A retrospective analysis of 405 autopsy cases. Dig Dis Sci 30:1005–1018
32. McKay CJ, Evans S, Sinclair M, Carter CR, Imrie CW (1999) High early mortality rate from acute pancreatitis in Scotland, 1984–1995. Br J Surg 86:1302–1305
33. Rattner DW, Legermate DA, Lee MJ, Mueller PR, Warshaw AL (1992) Early surgical debridement of symptomatic pancreatic necrosis is beneficial irrespective of infection. Am J Surg 163:105–109
34. Tsiotos GG, Luque-de LE, Soreide JA, Bannon MP, Zietlow SP, Baerga-Varela Y, et al (1998) Management of necrotizing pancreatitis by repeated operative necrosectomy using a zipper technique. Am J Surg 175:91–98
35. Bradley EL (1987) Management of infected pancreatic necrosis by open drainage. Ann Surg 206:542–550
36. Angelini G, Cavallini G, Pederzoli P, Bovo P, Bassi C, Di Francesco V, et al (1993) Long-term outcome of acute pancreatitis: a prospective study with 118 patients. Digestion 54:143–147
37. Mitchell CJ, Playforth MJ, Kelleher J, McMahon MJ (1983) Functional recovery of the exocrine pancreas after acute pancreatitis. Scand J Gastroenterol 18:5–8
38. Boreham B, Ammori BJ (2003) A prospective evaluation of pancreatic exocrine function in patients with acute pancreatitis: correlation with extent of necrosis and pancreatic endocrine insufficiency. Pancreatology 3:303–308
39. Sarr MG, Nagorney DM, Mucha PJ, Farnell MB, Johnson CD (1991) Acute necrotizing pancreatitis: management by planned, staged pancreatic necrosectomy/debridement and delayed primary wound closure over drains. Br J Surg 78:576–581
40. Rau BM, Bothe A, Kron M, Beger HG (2006) Role of early multisystem organ failure as major risk for pancreatic infections and death in severe acute pancreatitis. Clin Gastroenterol Hepatol 4:1053–1061
41. Takeda K, Matsuno S, Sunamura M, Kobari M (1998) Surgical aspects and management of acute pancreatitis: recent results of a cooperative national survey in Japan. Pancreas 16:316–322
42. Ranson JH, Rifkind KM, Roses DF, Fink SD, Eng K, Spencer FC (1974) Prognostic signs and the role of operative management in acute pancreatitis. Surg Gynecol Obstet 139:69–81
43. Isenmann R, Rau B, Beger HG (1999) Bacterial infection and extent of necrosis are determinants of organ failure in patients with acute necrotizing pancreatitis. Br J Surg 86:1020–1024

M. Reinblatt · C. Fernandez-del-Castillo · A. L. Warshaw

Debridement and Closed Packing for the Treatment of Necrotizing Pancreatitis

Over the past two decades, considerable progress has been made regarding the pathogenesis, diagnosis, and management of necrotizing pancreatitis (NP). The widespread availability of contrast-enhanced computed tomography (CT) and the use of percutaneous needle aspiration to assess for infection in pancreatic necrosis have led to a greater understanding of the natural history of NP and to significant improvements in patient care. Nevertheless, challenges remain regarding the indications, timing, and methods of debridement for tissue necrosis in severe pancreatitis.

Necrotizing Pancreatitis

Pancreatic and peripancreatic necrosis are the hallmarks of severe acute pancreatitis. The management of these patients requires a multidisciplinary team comprising surgeons, endoscopists, intensivists, and interventional radiologists. Pancreatic necrosis occurs in approximately 10–20% of patients with acute pancreatitis and is most commonly attributable to long-term ethanol abuse or biliary tract stone disease [1].

Experimental pancreatitis models have significantly improved our understanding of the etiology, progression, and severity of pancreatitis. Biliary pancreatitis is caused by pancreatic ductal outflow obstruction and disease severity is associated with the duration of the obstruction. The earliest morphologic change in pancreatitis occurs in acinar cells. The secretion of digestive enzymes from acinar cells is blocked, resulting in colocalization of these enzymes with lysosomal hydrolases, and premature activation within the acinar cells. The acinar cell response to injury may be an important determinant of the severity of pancreatitis. Acinar cells may undergo either apoptosis or necrosis, with reports suggesting an inverse relationship between the severity of pancreatitis and the extent of apoptosis associated with that attack. Further elucidation of these cellular pathways will broaden our understanding of the disease and may ultimately help reduce disease severity [2, 3].

The natural course of severe acute pancreatitis progresses through three phases. The 1st week after the onset of symptoms is characterized by the systemic inflammatory response syndrome (SIRS) resulting from the release of inflammatory mediators, which lead to the development of pulmonary, cardiovascular, and renal insufficiency. At this point, SIRS may proceed and contribute to the development of pancreatic necrosis, in part through impairment of microcirculatory perfusion of the pancreas. The second phase is characterized by that necrosis, with or without symptoms. If the necrotic tissues become infected, there is a third phase in which sepsis and its complications are the dominant issue [4, 5].

The risk of developing pancreatic necrosis with subsequent infection is determined by the severity of the initial attack and is most often heralded by multiple organ failure [6, 7]. Secondary infection of pancreatic and peripancreatic necrosis develops in 40–70% of patients with severe pancreatitis and is found in 80% of patients dying from acute pancreatitis [8–10]. Patients with necrosis involving greater than 30% of the gland have a 12-fold increased risk of sepsis compared to patients with less extensive necrosis [11]. The pathogens isolated from infected pancreatic necrosis are most commonly enteric Gram-negative organisms (65–70%), with Escherichia coli predominating (25–35%), followed by Gram-positive organisms (20%), and anaerobes (10–15%). Fungal organisms are found more frequently later in the disease course, which may be promoted by the prolonged use of antibiotics in these patients [12]. Prophylactic, broad-spectrum antibiotics have been shown to reduce infection in NP but not to improve survival. Many questions remain unanswered regarding the best drug, timing, and duration of antimicrobial therapy [8, 10].

Rationale for Operative Debridement of Necrotizing Pancreatitis

There is general agreement that surgical management of NP is required in patients who have infected pancreatic necrosis, usually proven by a positive culture or Gram stain obtained by fine needle aspiration (FNA) of the necrosum. If treated by antibiotics alone, the vast majority of these patients will die. Despite the consensus that patients with infected pancreatic necrosis require intervention for debridement and drainage, controversy remains regarding the need for similar treatment for sterile pancreatic necrosis. Most patients with significant pancreatic necrosis, in the absence of infection, can be treated successfully with supportive management even in the face of organ failure [8]. However, some will die from SIRS and organ failure, which can be produced by sterile necrosis or from unrecognized infection; others will remain symptomatic until the sterile necrosis has been evacuated [13, 14].

The current indications for operative intervention are:

1. Infected pancreatic necrosis as evidenced by bacteriologically positive FNA.
2. Nonresponders to maximal supportive therapy.

Except in the circumstances of uncertain diagnosis, peritonitis with concern for visceral infarction, perforation, or evidence of infection, there are advantages to delaying surgical intervention as long as patients continue to respond to conservative management. Necrosis occurs within days of onset of pancreatitis but evolves and extends; effective demarcation of the devitalized tissues is generally incomplete for a few weeks. Experience has led to a consensus that the optimal time for debridement may be in the 3rd or 4th week. Earlier surgical intervention is undertaken for proven bacterial infection with signs of sepsis, or for a deteriorating clinical course despite maximal supportive therapy [10].

Diagnostic Work-up

When NP is suspected because of clinical severity [15] or serum markers such as C-reactive protein [16] or polymorphonuclear leukocyte elastase [17], contrast-enhanced CT [18], or magnetic resonance imaging (MRI) are the investigations of choice [19]. Widespread CT availability and advances in CT imaging, such as spiral scanning, provide improved delineation of necrotic and viable pancreatic tissues. CT can be used to predict NP, as evidenced by poor pancreatic perfusion, with an 85–100% sensitivity, but only a 50–57% specificity. CT imaging may overestimate the degree of necrosis, but provides critical mapping for surgical debridement. MRI avoids the use of irradiation and large doses of toxic contrast media; however, it takes longer to complete the study and may not be readily available [19].

Percutaneous FNA of pancreatic necrosis is reserved for those patients who are neither clinically stable nor so critically ill as to unequivocally require operative intervention. FNA is particularly useful for the critically ill patient in the 1st weeks of illness, since sterile necrosis might justify continued supportive care, while infected necrosis would mandate debridement. Although radiologically guided FNA has been reported to have a sensitivity of 98% and specificity of 99.5% in the diagnosis of infected necrosis [20], recent studies suggest either that the sensitivity of a single aspirate may be as low as 60% or that infection may occur subsequent to the first FNA [21]. In either case, repetition of the aspiration as much as five times may be required before the infection is proven [21]. Although the clinical signs of infection generally appear later, infection of pancreatic necrosis occurs early, with 25% of positive aspirates occurring in the 1st week of symptoms, and 50% within the first 2 weeks [20].

Procedure-Relevant Preparation

Patients with severe NP require close monitoring and aggressive fluid replacement, which may require the use of an intensive care unit. The consensus of clinical and experimental data is for the use of prophylactic antibiotics in patients with NP. Imipenem or the combination of a quinolone with metronidazole are favored because of their documented bioavailability in pancreatic tissue, and their efficacy against those organisms most frequently recovered from infected necrosis [22–24].

Patients with organ failure or those who fail to improve within the first 72 h are unlikely to resume oral intake within an acceptable time. These patients may therefore benefit from the early institution of total parenteral nutrition [24] or enteral tube feedings [25] while awaiting the resumption of gastrointestinal activity. Disruption of pancreatic duct integrity by the necrotizing process may be the basis of relapsing pain and inflammation upon attempts at oral feeding.

Surgical Technique

Our technique for operative debridement of pancreatic necrosis comprises three major principles:

1. As complete evacuation of necrotic material and fluid collections as possible, while preserving all viable tissues.
2. Packing to tamponade ooze from granulations on the walls of the cavity.
3. Placement of drains to allow egress of residual retroperitoneal debris and to channel pancreatic secretions as a contained fistula.

A recent contrast-enhanced CT is invaluable to guide the operative exploration and to ensure that all areas of necrosis and fluid collections are evacuated. We prefer an upper-midline incision above the umbilicus. This approach allows excellent access to the area of interest, preserves the rectus abdominis muscles, and does not interfere with peripancreatic drain placement.

The lesser sac may be approached through the gastrohepatic omentum, gastrocolic omentum, or transverse mesocolon. Entering the lesser sac through the transverse mesocolon is often the simplest, fastest, and safest route [26]. Severe inflammatory reaction in the gastrocolic omentum may obliterate the visualization of these organs and make the access between the stomach and transverse colon (widely advocated by others) difficult and dangerous. In contrast, the transverse mesocolon to the left and right of the ligament of Treitz is thin and avascular, and the necrotic tissues and fluid almost necessitate through in this region, resulting in rapid, easy, and safe access (Fig. 21.2.1). The middle colic vessels are often thrombosed; however, if additional access is needed, they may be ligated without negative effects, should they remain patent. After the retrogastric space is developed by blunt dissection, a hand placed through the opening in the mesocolon into the lesser sac can safely guide subsequent division of the gastrocolic omentum while avoiding inadvertent injury to the stomach or colon. Furthermore, entry through the mesocolon permits drains to be placed in a more dependent position once the debridement is completed.

The necrotic tissues are separated gently by finger and instrument dissection and removed bluntly through the mesocolon (Fig. 21.2.2). Extensions of the cavity are explored digitally to insure against leaving the irregular material that can serve as a culture medium for postoperative abscesses. The body and tail of the pancreas, if necrotic, may form a coherent sequestrum that comes out as a single unit. This pancreatic dissection is also performed bluntly, ligating and tying any firm attachments. Minor bleeding from the cavity walls is usually from granulation tissue, but is easily controlled with packing (see below and Fig. 21.2.3). Even the major vessels in the region may be thrombosed, but major hemorrhage may ensue from false aneurysms, stumps of eroded arteries, or from major veins. Hemostasis by suture ligature can be challenging but vital since packing is unlikely to assure control of hemorrhage. Occasionally, postop-

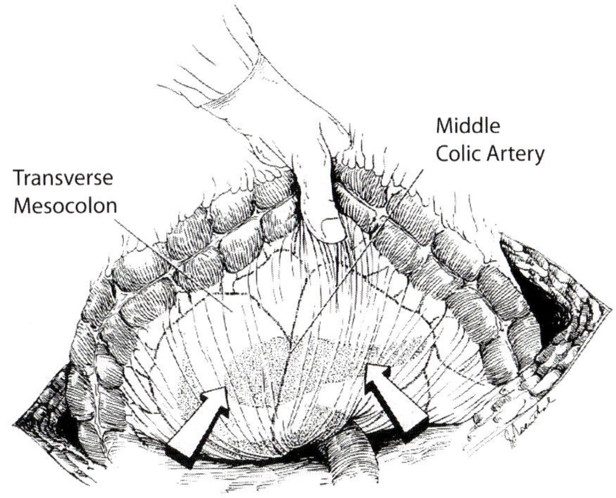

Figure 21.2.1

Access via the transverse mesocolon simplifies entry into the lesser sac [24]

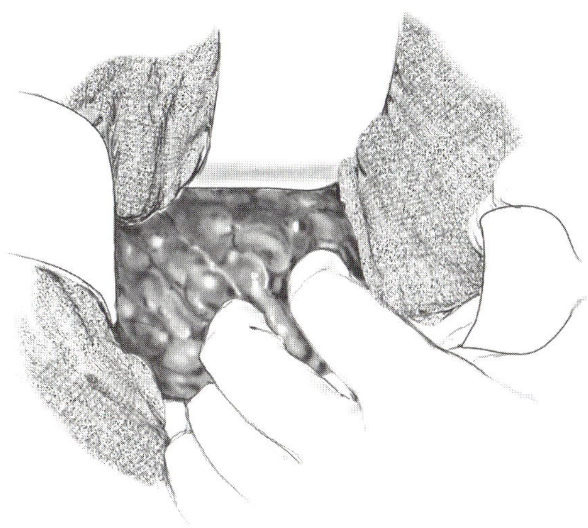

Figure 21.2.2

Blunt debridement of the lesser sac through the transverse mesocolon [24]

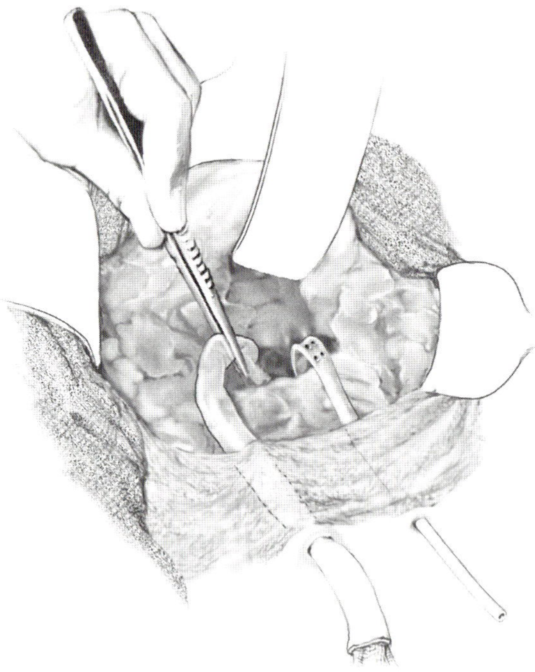

Figure 21.2.3

Packing of the cavity with stuffed Penrose and Jackson-Pratt drains [26]

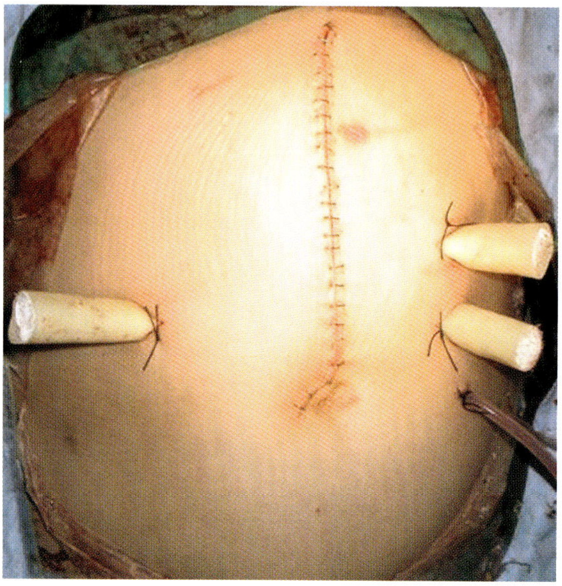

Figure 21.2.4

Jackson-Pratt and stuffed Penrose drains are brought out through separate stab wounds [26]

erative angiographic embolization may be necessary. The spleen is generally viable despite splenic vessel thrombosis and should be preserved if possible. Necrotic visceral segments, most commonly the splenic flexure of the colon, should be resected; proximal diversion with a stoma, rather than attempted reanastomosis, is mandatory in this setting. Closure of gastric or duodenal perforations, while unavoidable, are likely to break down and fistulize.

The head of the pancreas may not be adequately accessed by approach through the left side of the transverse mesocolon, but can be reached through the right side of the transverse mesocolon (Fig. 21.2.1) or via a plane posterior to the second and third portions of the duodenum after a Kocher maneuver. If there are fluid collections or necrotic tissues in the pararenal and retrocolic spaces, these regions must be opened and drained as well. These areas are often accessible through the same transmesocolic approach used to drain the pancreatic bed, but sufficient exposure of the retroperitoneum may sometimes also require mobilization of the hepatic and/or splenic flexures of the colon.

Every effort should be taken to drain all fluid and remove as much necrotic tissue as possible. Aerobic and anaerobic cultures of the material should be planted. The thoroughness of the initial debridement is the most critical factor in determining the need for reexploration for recurrent sepsis and for survival. After blunt dissection, further debridement can be achieved with copious irrigation and gentle abrasion with the fingertips covered by a sponge. However, overenthusiastic debridement is liable to injure the viscera, particularly the stomach and duodenum, which may be part of the confines of the cavity.

Following debridement, the resulting cavities are relatively stiff. These regions can be filled with 1-inch (2.5-cm) soft latex (Penrose) drains "stuffed" with gauze (as many as necessary to fill the space in order to inhibit capillary bleeding from granulations). Closed suction drains are placed in each major extension of the cavity (Fig. 21.2.4). The drains are brought out through the omentum and then through separate exits in the abdominal wall. The midline abdominal wound is sutured primarily [24–26].

Early Postoperative Course

The stuffed Penrose drains that were placed in the operating room are removed beginning 1 week after the operation to allow compartmentalization of the drain tracts. One drain is removed every day or two to allow the residual cavity to close sequentially around the drains. The closed suction drains are the last to be removed and are withdrawn only when their output is minimal. Should a pancreatic fistula develop, as determined by drain output and fluid amylase level, the drain tract is left to mature and the drain is gradually advanced to encourage the fistula to close. More than 90% of pancreatic fistulas will not require later surgical internal diversion or resection of the pancreatic source of the leak. Enteric fistulas will require treatment somewhat more commonly (10–20%).

The surgical debridement of pancreatic necrosis may result in several complications, which are the direct result of operative technique. In an effort to diminish blood loss, necrosectomy should be limited to easily debrided tissue and gentle, blunt dissection. Severe bleeding encountered intraoperatively may require mass ligation and temporary packing, as significant retroperitoneal inflammation may prevent direct vascular control. The preservation of vessels in the mesocolon and retroperitoneum helps to reduce the development of colonic ischemia. Delaying debridement until the 3rd week reduces the resection of viable pancreatic tissue, which may prevent the development of pancreatic insufficiency and fistula formation. Thorough operative debridement with methodical exploration of the lesser sac and retroperitoneum will minimize the need for reexploration and the development of residual abscesses [26].

Long-Term Postoperative Outcome

Surgical treatment of NP in appropriately selected patients has led to significantly decreased mortality from the disease. In an early report of debridement and drainage followed by closed packing of the resulting cavity, the postoperative mortality was only 6% [26]. Contrary to many other experiences, there was no significant difference in outcomes between sterile or infected necrosis. Although further percutaneous drainage of residual or recurrent collections is required in 20% of patients, the need for reoperation was acceptably low at 12%. A single surgical procedure without further intervention was effective in 69% of patients [26]. Our expanded experience continues to bear out these findings [14], although the current mortality rate is a bit higher (11%), in part due to differences in patient mix and selection.

Pancreas-related morbidity is common following these procedures. Pancreatic fistula, although managed conservatively in over 90%, occurred in 41% of patients, and an enteric fistula in 15%. Pancreatic insufficiency, especially diabetes mellitus, is proportional to the degree of pancreatic necrosis [14]. The median postoperative hospital stay following debridement and closed packing was 19 days, with the mean period of time before patients returned to their regular activities of 5 months [14, 26]. Patients who recover from NP can be expected to have good functional outcome and quality of life [26, 27].

References

1. Beger HG, Uhl W (1990) Severe acute pancreatitis. II: the surgical approach. Clin Intensive Care 1:223–227
2. Steer ML (1997) Pathogenesis of necrotizing pancreatitis. Probl Gen Surg 13:1–9
3. Bhatia M (2004) Apoptosis versus necrosis in acute pancreatitis. Am J Physiol Gastrointest Liver Physiol 286:189–196
4. Tenner S, SicaG, Hughes M, et al (1997) Relationship of necrosis to organ failure in severe acute pancreatitis. Gastroenterology 113:899–903
5. Beger HG, Bittner R, Block S, et al (1986) Bacterial contamination of pancreatic necrosis. A prospective clinical study. Gastroenterology 91:433–438
6. Ranson JHC, Spencer FC (1997) Prevention, diagnosis and treatment of pancreatic abscesses. Surgery 82:96–105
7. Isenmann R, Rau B, Beger HG (1999) Bacterial infection and extent of necrosis are determinants of organ failure in patients with acute necrotizing pancreatitis. Br J Surg 86:1020–1024
8. Buchler MW, Gloor B, Muller C, et al (2000) Acute necrotizing pancreatitis: Treatment strategy according to the status of infection. Ann Surg 232:619–626
v9. Renner IG, Savage WT, Pantoja JL, et al (1985) Death due to acute pancreatitis. Dig Dis Sci 30:1005–1018
10. Uhl W, Warshaw L, Imrie C, et al (2002) IAP guidelines for the surgical management of acute pancreatitis. Pancreatology 2:565–573
11. Vesentini C, Bassi C, Talamini G, et al (1993) Prospective comparison of C-reactive protein level, Ranson score and contrast-enhanced computed tomography in the prediction of septic complications of acute pancreatitis. Br J Surg 80:755–757
12. Deziel DJ, Doolas A (1990) Pancreatic abscess and pancreatic necrosis: current concepts and controversies. Probl Gen Surg 7:415–427
13. Rattner DW, Legermate DA, Lee MJ, et al (1992) Early surgical debridement of symptomatic pancreatic necrosis is beneficial irrespective of infection. Am J Surg 163:105–109
14. Rodriguez JR, Razo AO, Targarona J (2008) Debridement and closed packing for sterile or infected necrotizing pancreatitis – Insights into indications and outcomes in 167 patients. Ann Surg (in press)

15. Larvin M, MacMahon MJ (1989) APACHE II score for assessment and monitoring of acute pancreatitis. Lancet 2:201–205
16. Riche FC, Cholley BP, Laisne MJ, et al (2003) Inflammatory cytokines, C reactive protein, and procalcitonin as early predictors of necrosis infection in acute necrotizing pancreatitis. Surgery 133:257–262
17. Ikei S, Ogawa M, Yamaguchi Y (1988) Blood concentrations of polymorphonuclear leukocyte elastase and interleukin-6 are indicators for the occurrence of multiple organ failures at the early stage of acute pancreatitis. J Gastroenterol Hepatol 13:1274–1283
18. Balthazar EJ, Freeny PC, van Sonnenberg E (1994) Imaging and intervention in acute pancreatitis. Radiology 193:297–306
19. Simms MD, Johnson CD (1997) Diagnosis of necrotizing pancreatitis using contrast-enhanced CT. Probl Gen Surg 13:10–21
20. Tenner SM, Banks PA (1997) Radiologic-guided percutaneous fine needle aspiration in the evaluation of suspected pancreatic infection. Probl Gen Surg 13:61–66
21. Ashley SW, Perez A, Pierce E, et al (2001) Necrotizing pancreatitis: Contemporary analysis of 99 consecutive cases. Ann Surg 234:572–580
22. Mithofer K, Fernandez-del Castillo C, Ferraro MJ, et al (1996) Antibiotic treatment improves survival in experimental acute necrotizing pancreatitis. Gastroenterology 110:232–240
23. Luiten EJ, Hop WCJ, Lange JF, et al (1995) Controlled clinical trial of selective decontamination for the treatment of severe acute pancreatitis. Ann Surg 222:57–65
24. Fernandez-del Castillo C, Warshaw AL, Rattner DW (1997) Closed packing and drainage following debridement for necrotizing pancreatitis. Probl Gen Surg 13:126–130
25. Avgerinos C, Delis S, Rizos S, et al (2003) Nutritional support in acute pancreatitis. Dig Dis 21:214–219
26. Fernandez-del Castillo C, Rattner DW, Makary MA, et al (1998) Debridement and closed packing for the treatment of necrotizing pancreatitis. Ann Surg 228:676–684
27. Doepel M, Eriksson J, Halme L, et al (1993) Good long-term results in patients surviving acute pancreatitis. Br J Surg 80:1583–1586

P. Götzinger

Necrosectomy and Redressing

Acute pancreatitis has a variable clinical presentation ranging from mild to severe. Pancreatic necrosis remains the most severe form and accounts for the majority of morbidity and mortality related to acute pancreatitis. Death occurs usually only in patients with necrotizing pancreatitis and is commonly associated with failure of at least one organ system [1].

Contrast-enhanced abdominal computed tomography (CT) is the current gold standard in the clinical diagnosis of pancreatic necrosis. The lack of contrast enhancement of the pancreatic gland, indicating disruption of normal pancreatic microcirculation, correlates well with the findings of necrosis at surgery and clinical outcomes [2].

Clinical studies have demonstrated that pancreatic necrosis develops over a couple of days, and with few exceptions remains stable during a given episode of acute pancreatitis. Demarcation of pancreatic necrosis evolves 2–3 weeks after onset of the disease, even if the exact demarcation process still has not been clearly and objectively evaluated [3].

The natural course of acute pancreatitis proceeds in two phases. During the first 24 h after onset of initial symptoms about 20–30% of all patients with acute pancreatitis take a severe clinical course of their disease. This period is characterized as the initial hypovolemic stage where arterial hypotension or even shock is the leading symptom. Simultaneously the systemic toxic phase caused by the release of inflammatory mediators or cytokines induces organ dysfunction involving the lungs, liver, kidney, and cardiorespiratory system. In patients with severe acute pancreatitis (SAP), organ failure is common and often occurs in the absence of infection. The second phase at the end of the 2nd week after the onset is dominated by septic complications caused by infection of pancreatic necrosis, which furthermore increases the incidence of organ failure [4]. Approximately 40–70% of patients with necrotizing pancreatitis suffer from infection of pancreatic necrosis, which has become the most important risk factor of death from SAP. The extent of pancreatic necrosis and the duration of the disease increase the risk of local pancreatic infection. It's incidence tends to peak in the 3rd week of the disease, although infection might occur at any moment during the course of the disease [5].

Most conditions requiring operative intervention in acute pancreatitis are due to necrosis of the pancreas or peripancreatic tissue.

Indication for Surgical Treatment

There are several incontrovertible indications for operative intervention in patients with SAP: Infection of pancreatic necrosis can be proven by fine-needle aspiration, or evidence of gas in the contrast-enhanced CT scan, suspected or confirmed intra-abdominal catastrophe including intestinal infarction or perforation, exsanguinating hemorrhage, or abdominal compartment syndrome [5–8]. The indication for surgical intervention in patients with sterile necrosis is less clear. There is evidence that patients with extensive pancreatic necrosis and persisting multiple organ failure despite maximal intensive care benefit from surgical intervention [9].

The patient must be assessed daily for deterioration with these possibilities in mind, since timely surgical intervention is essential. Medical intensive care is appropriate unless indication for operation arises, and then surgery is required [10].

Rationale and Goals of Surgical Treatment

The rationale for surgical debridement of pancreatic necrosis is based on two principles. The first is to remove the necrotic pancreatic tissue as well as pancreatogenic ascites out of the peritoneal cavity and the lesser sac. During the course of SAP, fluid exudes into the peripancreatic area and the abdominal cavity. This exudate contains biologically active enzymes that lead, via absorption through the thoracic duct, to an increased incidence of systemic complications such as the development of single or multiple organ failure [11]. A possibility to approach this problem is to debride the necrotic tissue and to evacuate fluid and remove the septic foci to prevent further local and systemic inflammatory active metabolites and bacteria. Secondly, as much as possible viable pancreatic tissue should be preserved. The amount of remaining pancreatic parenchyma strongly influences the quality of long-term results concerning endo- and exocrine pancreatic function [12].

Timing of Surgery

To date, the timing of necrosectomy in SAP remains a matter of discussion. Proponents of early surgery state that patients would benefit from the early removal of pancreatic necrosis, leading to a reduction in the multisystemic complications related to enzymes and toxic substances [13,14]. So in the past early surgical intervention was favored, especially in the presence of deteriorating systemic organ function, but led to inordinately high mortality rates [15,16].

At present, there is general agreement that surgical intervention should be delayed as long as the patient benefits from intensive care medicine. By deferring surgery, a proper demarcation of pancreatic and peripancreatic necrosis can take place. The demarcation of necrotic masses from viable tissue enables an easier and safer debridement with a greater likelihood of sparing pancreatic tissue, and leads to successful surgical control of pancreatic necrosis. Thus, the risk of bleeding and the surgery-related loss of vital tissue that predisposes to surgery-induced endocrine and exocrine pancreatic insufficiency can be minimized by this approach. The literature reveals only one prospective randomized trial that compared early (within 72 h of symptoms) with late (at least 12 days after onset) pancreatic resection/debridement in patients with severe pancreatitis, the mortality rates were 56% and 27%, respectively [17]. Although this was not a statistically significant difference, the study was stopped because of a very high mortality rate in the early group. This high mortality rate in patients who were operated early in this study was independent of the bacteriologic status of pancreatic necrosis. Although there were some caveats in this study because of small numbers and limited power of comparison, the concept of delaying surgery being beneficial to the patients complies with the current opinion of recent published studies [18,19].

In a recent study we showed that the benefit of delaying surgery is due to a ceased demarcation process of nonviable tissue. This demarcation is a precondition for sufficient debridement, leading to successful surgical control of pancreatic necrosis in one or few surgical steps. By analyzing the time of operative treatment it could be shown that necrosectomy performed later than 3 weeks after onset of the disease, was associated with a higher rate of successful debridement of pancreatic necrosis, leading to less reoperations and lower mortality. The very early debridement (within the first 3 weeks) may be associated with an inordinately high mortality rate, stressing the importance of a conservative approach towards SAP [20,21].

Operative Treatment of Pancreatic Necrosis - Necrosectomy

The accepted surgical management of necrotizing pancreatitis is the removal of necrotic pancreatic tissue and pancreatogenic ascites from the peritoneal cavity and the lesser sac. We use the open approach for the surgical treatment of SAP. Blunt debridement is combined with laparotomy for drainage and access for revisions to further remove local debris.

Operative access is gained either by way of a midline or bilateral subcostal incision. Careful exploration is performed to assess the extent of pancreatic and extrapancreatic necrosis, including a Kocher's mobilization of the second part of the duodenum. Furthermore, the right and left colon are mobilized. It is possible to approach the lesser sac through the gastrohepatic omentum or the gastrocolic omentum. If opening of the lesser sac is not possible because of a bounded inflammatory process, direct access from the infracolic compartment via the left transverse mesocolon (space of Riolan) is an alternative. The access through the mesocolon also allows drains to be placed in a more exact position once the debridement is completed.

It is important to send fluid collection from the necrotic region for aerobic and anaerobic culture. Good demarcated pancreatic and peripancreatic necrotic tissues are then removed bluntly. Granulation or significant vascular structures may cause significant bleeding. Hemostasis can be difficult and may require packing of the cavity. Removal of the spleen should be avoided unless the splenic tissue is necrotic.

From the left-sided approach, the head of the pancreas cannot always be completely reached. If there is significant necrosis in this area, as established by CT scan, this region can be reached through the right side of the transverse mesocolon or via a plane poste-

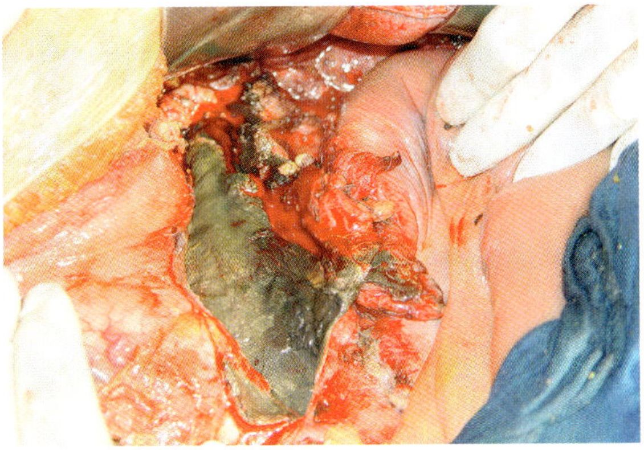

Figure 21.3.1

Necrotic cavity after sufficient debridement of pancreatic necrosis

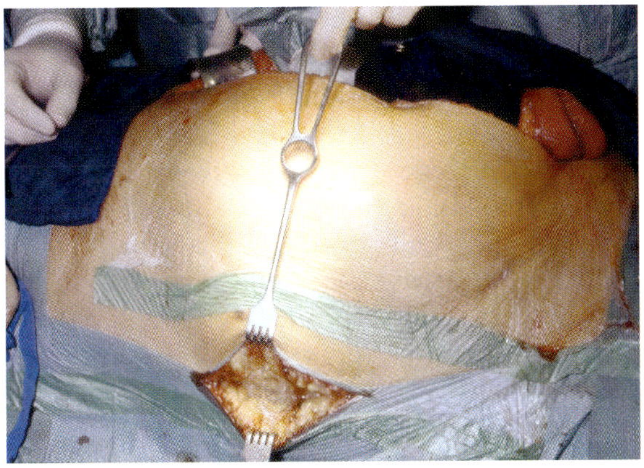

Figure 21.3.2

Creating a laparostoma with the aid of a right-sided dorso-lumbar incision

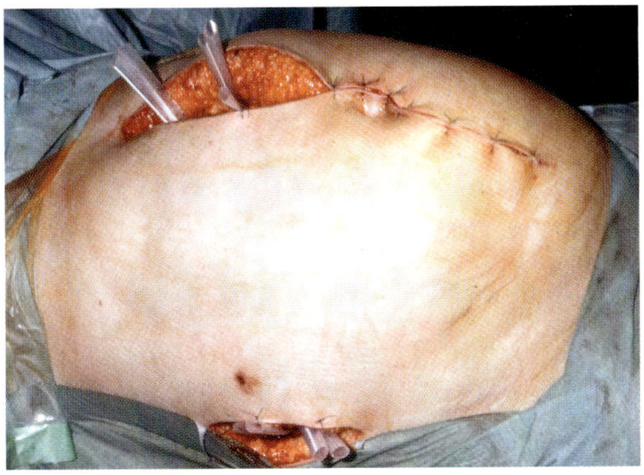

Figure 21.3.3

Placing multiple easy-flow drains through the median and lateral laparostoma

rior to the second and third part of the duodenum. Furthermore, it is important to drain all fluid collections from the pararenal and retrocolic spaces. If it is not possible to reach these collections through the same transmesocolic approach, access via the gastrocolic omentum is an alternative.

The sufficient surgical control of pancreatic and peripancreatic necrosis, and the continuous evacuation of fluid have impacted on the need for further re-explorations, thus affecting patients survival. Every effort should therefore be made to remove most of the necrotic tissue and to drain all fluid collections at the first surgical procedure. By means of blunt dissection and generous irrigation with warm isotonic saline, it should be possible to remove most of the necrotic tissue (Fig. 21.3.1). After sufficient debridement there remain cavities, which are often stiff and may bleed from the granulated surface. In these spaces we place 4-10 easy-flow drains, that are brought out through laparostoma placed on either the left or right side (Figs. 21.3.2 and 21.3.3). These drains are not removed unless the daily quantum of fluid loss is less than 20 ml. Another possibility is to remove these drains in a stepwise fashion, resulting in a fistula due to a mature fistula tract. This fistula will close over a given period.

Reoperation: "On Demand" and Preplanned

For treatment of intra-abdominal infection, source control has been identified as the most important determinant affecting patient outcome. The same is true for the operative treatment of SAP [21]. Regarding operative therapy, most surgical concepts, such as aggressive local debridement, continuous postoperative lavage, and relaparotomy, attempt to control local necrosis, even if SAP is an intermittent disease.

Surgical source control means the complete removal of pancreatic or peripancreatic necroses by blunt debridement or nonanatomical resection. Surgical control of pancreatic necrosis can be achieved either by first operation or subsequent reoperation. Subsequent reoperations are based upon two concepts according to either a preplanned schedule or the individual need of the patient (referred to as "on demand"). In contrast to the planned repeated laparotomy concept of fixed reoperations every 48–72 h, patients are reoperated on demand if organ dysfunction persists despite 48 h of maximal intensive supporting therapy (Table 21.3.1). Postoperative drainage is provided either by open packing and/or lateral laparostomy.

Table 21.3.1. Criteria for organ system failure. paO_2 Arterial oxygen tension

Organ system	Criteria
Cardiovascular dysfunction:	Mean arterial pressure ≤ 50 mmHg, need for treatment with catecholamines (except low-dose dopamine) or fluid resuscitation, or both, to achieve adequate cardiac output and perfusion rate
Pulmonary dysfunction:	Tachypnea (>20 beats/min), decrease in arterial oxygen saturation (<90%), paO_2<60 mmHg, need for mechanical ventilation
Renal dysfunction:	Deterioration of creatinine clearance (<30 ml/min) and/or creatinine concentration greater than 2 mg/dl, or both, after rehydration, need for continuous hemofiltration/dialysis
Hepatic dysfunction:	Isolated increase of serum bilirubin above 3 mg/dl, deterioration of liver synthesis (prothrombin time <50%).

The literature reveals that the strategy of operative revisions (preplanned vs. on demand) has no influence on mortality. Patients with planned reoperations, however, may have a higher reoperation rate than patients who are reoperated on demand, resulting in a higher rate of intestinal fistulas [21].

In conclusion, surgical control of pancreatic or peripancreatic necrosis is a precondition for survival. If reoperations are part of the surgical concept it does not affect the outcome if these operative revisions are done on demand or preplanned.

Complications and Long-Term Outcome

Pancreatic necrosis requiring operative treatment continues to be an extraordinary and complex disease that demands a large investment of medical resources if a good clinical outcome is expected. Nevertheless, SAP causes high mortality rates that most often result from multiorgan dysfunction syndrome, occurring either early (within the first 14 days) or 2 weeks or more after the onset of symptoms due to septic or other complications. Table 21.3.2 shows the results and main complications of patients with SAP who were treated by open debridement and reoperation either on demand or preplanned.

Long-term outcome data concerning recovery and pancreatic function are scarce. Most available data refer to function after resection, which is accompanied by a high incidence of diabetes. It has to be expected that about two-thirds of debrided patients will develop exocrine and endocrine insufficiency [22].

Immunologic Implications on Reoperation for SAP

Inflammatory events are thought to play an important role in the pathogenesis of acute pancreatitis, but the exact mechanisms that trigger the inflammatory and necrotizing processes are not completely understood. Several studies have reported a possible role for proinflammatory cytokines in mediating steps in the pathogenesis of acute pancreatitis and its systemic complications. In this specific disease monocytes and macrophages are not only of interest for their cytokine secretion, but also to their cell surface markers, such as human leukocyte antigen DR (HLA-DR) and CD14. Changes in HLA-DR expression have been reported in patients who develop infections after surgery. CD14 functions as a receptor for the complex between lipopolysaccharide (LPS) and LPS-binding protein, thereby playing a key role in LPS-induced cell activation and inflammatory responses to Gram-negative bacterial infection.

The epitopes of peripheral blood monocytes, reflecting the immunological functions of these cells, are altered profoundly during the course of SAP. These alterations correlate with the severity of the disease, whereas operative treatment does not alter the expression of these cell surface markers [23].

Table 21.3.2. Surgical treatment of severe acute pancreatitis. Descriptive data and complications. *APACHE* Acute Physiology and Chronic Health Evaluation, *ICU* intensive care unit

	Patients *n*	APACHE II Score	Reoperation (%)	ICU - Duratiuon (days)	Hospital stay days	Bleeding complication (%)	Pancreatic fistula (%)	Intestinal fistula (%)	Incisional hernia (%)	Mortality (%)
Büchler [5]	86	12.6 (5–28)	22	–	44 (11–209)	7	29	0	–	10
Fernandez-del Castillo [9]	64	9 (9–23)	17	–	41 (7–82)	3	53	16	–	6,2
Connor [25]	88	9 (1–21)	–	1 (0–66)	93 (8–300)	11	13	5	2	28
Götzinger [21]	240	16 (8–35)	74	26 (3–185)	39 (11–215)	16.5	45	22	24	39
Branum [24]	50	–	48	23 (0–119)	54 (9-186)	–	17	16	–	12
Tzovaras [26]	44	11 (5–21)	32	23 (1–95)	55 (11–126)	–	10	14	23	18

References

1. Baron T, Morgan D (1999) Acute necrotizing pancreatitis. N Engl J Med 340:1412–1417
2. Balthazar EJ (2002) Acute pancreatitis: assessment of severity with clinical and CT evaluation. Radiology 223:603–613
3. Isenmann R, Büchler M, Uhl W, Malfertheiner P, Martini M, Beger HG (1993) Pancreatic necrosis: an early finding in severe acute pancreatitis. Pancreas 8:358–361
4. Beger HG, Rau B, Mayer J, Pralle U (1997) Natural course of acute pancreatitis. World J Surg 21:130–135
5. Büchler MW, Gloor B, Müller CA, Friess H, Seiler CA, Uhl W (2000) Acute necrotizing pancreatitis: treatment strategy according to the status of infection. Ann Surg 232:619–626
6. Gecelter G, Fahoum B, Gardezi S, Schein M (2002) Abdominal compartment syndrome in severe acute pancreatitis: an indication for a decompressing laparotomy? Dig Surg 19:402–404
7. Bradley EL (2000) Indications for surgery in necrotizing pancreatitis–a millennial review. 1:1–3
8. Baron TH, Morgan DE (1999) Acute necrotizing pancreatitis. N Engl J Med 340:1412–1417
9. Fernandez-del Castillo C, Rattner DW, Makary MA, Mostafavi A, McGrath D, Warshaw AL (1998) Debridement and closed packing for the treatment of necrotizing pancreatitis. Ann Surg 228:676–684
10. Nathens A, Curtis J, Beale R, Cook D, Moreno R, Romand J, Skerrett S, Stapleton R, Ware L, Waldmann C (2004) Management of the critically ill patient with severe acute pancreatitis. Crit Care Med 32:2524–2536
11. Mayer AD, Airey M, Hodgson J, McMahon MJ (1985) Enzyme transfer from pancreas to plasma during acute pancreatitis. The contribution of ascitic fluid and lymphatic drainage of the pancreas. Gut 26:876–881
12. Broome AH, Eisen GM, Harland RC, Collins BH, Meyers WC, Pappas TN (1996) Quality of life after treatment for pancreatitis. Ann Surg 223:665–670
13. Orlando R, Welch JP, Akbari CM (1993) Techniques and complications of open packing of infected pancreatic necrosis. Surg Gynecol Obstet 177:65–71
14. Rau B, Pralle U, Uhl W, et al (1995) Management of sterile necrosis in instances of severe acute pancreatitis. J Am Coll Surg 181:279–288
15. Fernandez-Cruz L, Navarro S, Valderrama R, Saenz A, Guarner L, Aparisi L, Espi A, Jaurietta E, Marruecos L, Gener J (1994) Acute necrotizing pancreatitis: a multicenter study. Hepatogastroenterology 41:185–189
16. Smadja C, Bismuth H (1986) Pancreatic debridement in acute necrotizing pancreatitis: an obsolete procedure? Br J Surg 73:408–410
17. Mier J, Leon EL, Castillo A, Robledo F, Blanco R (1997) Early versus late necrosectomy in severe necrotizing pancreatitis. Am J Surg 173:71–75
18. Hungness ES, Robb BW, Seeskin C, Hasselgren PO, Luchette FA (2002) Early debridement for necrotizing pancreatitis: is it worthwhile? J Am Coll Surg 194:740–744
19. Hartwig W, Maksan SM, Foitzik T, Schmidt J, Herfarth C, Klar E (2002) Reduction in mortality with delayed surgical therapy of severe pancreatitis. J Gastrointest Surg 6:481–487
20. Götzinger P, Wamser P, Exner R, Schwanzer E, Jakesz R, Függer R, Sautner (2003) Surgical treatment of severe acute pancreatitis: timing of operation is crucial for survival. Surg Infect 4:205–211

21. Götzinger P, Sautner T, Kriwanek S, Beckerhinn P, Barlan M, Armbruster C, Wamser P, Függer R (2003) Surgical treatment for severe acute pancreatitis: extent and surgical control of necrosis determine outcome. World J Surg 26:474–478
22. Büchler M, Hauka A, Malfertheiner P (1987) Follow-up after acute pancreatitis: morphology and function. In: Beger HG, Büchler M (eds) Acute pancreatitis: research and clinical management. Springr Verlag, Berlin, pp 367–374
23. Götzinger P, Sautner T, Spittler A, Barlan M, Wamser P, Roth E, Jakesz R, Függer R (2000) Severe acute pancreatitis causes alterations in HLA-DR and CD14 expression on peripheral blood monocytes independently of surgical treatment. Eur J Surg 166:628–632
24. Branum G, Galloway J, Hirchowitz W, Fendley M, Hunter J (1998) Pancreatic necrosis: results of necrosectomy, packing, and ultimate closure over drains Ann Surg 227:870–877
25. Connor S, Alexakis N, Raraty MG, Ghaneh P, Evans J, Hughes M, Garvey CJ, Sutton R, Neoptolemos JP (2005) Early and late complications after pancreatic necrosectomy. Surgery 137:499–505
26. Tzovaras G, Parks R, Diamond T, Rowlands B (2004) Early and long-term results of surgery for severe necrotising pancreatitis. Dig Surg 21:41–46

B.M. Rau · H.G. Beger

Necrosectomy and Closed Lavage

Acute pancreatitis is characterized by an extreme variability in clinical presentation and outcome that has plagued the study and management of this disease ever since its first description by Reginald Fitz in 1889 [1]. At that time the diagnosis of acute pancreatitis was restricted to the most severe cases by means of clinical symptoms – surgery was a desperate attempt to lower the excessively high mortality rates. Sir Berkeley Moynihan summed up the prevailing opinion at the turn of the century: "recovery from this disease, apart from operation, is so rare that no case should be left untreated" [2]. The development of serum amylase assays in 1925 as a reliable means to diagnose acute pancreatitis substantially changed the general understanding of the natural course of this disease [3]. It became evident that in the majority of patients a mild course with spontaneous recovery was the rule rather than the exception. As a consequence, the therapeutic approach was directed toward conservative management [4,5].

However, mortality rates among patients with severe disease continued to be high and physicians felt the need to reassess the role of surgery in this specific setting [6,7]. These efforts culminated in a variety of surgical approaches ranging from conservative simple peripancreatic drainage [8–10] to aggressive operative techniques such as total pancreatectomy [11–16]. In the subsequent years, clinical observations flanked by novel diagnostic imaging procedures helped us to gain further insights into the pathophysiological background of acute pancreatitis. It became evident that complications develop in about 20% of all patients, and these are closely related to the morphological features of intra- and extrapancreatic necrosis [17–20]. Several factors have been identified as the main determinants of outcome in this severely ill group of patients: (1) the extent of intra- and extrapancreatic necrosis [10,18–20], (2) infection of pancreatic necrosis [21,22], and, most recently (30) early onset [23–26] and persisting [27,28] multiorgan dysfunction syndrome.

Considering the individuality and dynamics of the natural course of acute pancreatitis, physicians became aware that any single therapeutic concept would be unlikely to be successful for each of these patients during the different stages of the disease. Therefore, a multidisciplinary approach of improved intensive care management and the combination of widespread necrosectomy with some form of drainage of the peripancreatic space markedly decreased the mortality of necrotizing pancreatitis to about 20% in the past 20 years [29]. Besides simple drainage, two major additional concepts were introduced in the 1980s and have gained widespread acceptance because they provide further evacuation of necrotic or infected pancreatic and peripancreatic tissue: the open approach by either controlled packing or repeated, planned reoperative debridement [30–35], and the closed approach with continuous lavage [36–42] or simple drainage [43–48].

Despite the benefits of these new surgical concepts, postoperative morbidity and procedure-related complications still remained a major point of concern. Bearing in mind the prognostic importance of infection, a completely conservative approach was attempted during the early 1990s in the subset of patients with sterile necrosis, for which the mortality rates were surprisingly favorable as long as infection was absent [49–51]. In this context, several new diagnostic and therapeutic protocols, such as guided fine-needle aspiration (FNA) of necrosis [52,53], early endoscopic retrograde cholangiopancreatography (ERCP) in patients with acute biliary pancreatitis [54], prophylactic antibiotics [55], and early enteral feeding [56] helped to correctly diagnose or even to decrease the occurrence of subsequent complications, most importantly infections. Thus, the therapeutic pendulum once again swung away from operative toward conservative approaches [38,57–60]. Currently, the overall percentage of patients with necrotizing pancreatitis ultimately subjected to operative treatment has decreased to less than 20%.

Rationale for Necrosectomy and Debridement

The general rationale for necrosectomy of devitalized pancreatic tissue is based on two major aspects. First, local focus control by removal of necrotic intra- and extrapancreatic tissue as well as pancreatogenic ascites from the lesser sac and the peritoneal cavity in order to interrupt the ongoing inflammatory process and the systemic release of the various inflammatory mediators that account for remote organ failure [61–63], and second the preservation of still vital intact pancreatic tissue.

Local Focus Control

Contrary to what was previously accepted, early pancreatic resection or necrosectomy within the 1st week after disease onset neither prevents necrosis from becoming infected nor improves organ failure [26,64,65], and should therefore be avoided whenever possible. Experimental and clinical observations have shown that exudation of fluid into the peripancreatic area and the abdominal cavity is one of the main characteristics of severe acute pancreatitis within the early course. Analysis of these exudates revealed a high concentration of activated enzymes and vasoactive and inflammatory mediators [62,63,66]. Despite this important pathophysiological background, the ultimate benefit of removing pancreatogenic ascites by early peritoneal lavage alone on morbidity and mortality remains controversial [67,68]. However, a thorough analysis of randomized controlled trials with detailed stratification of local and systemic severity still showed some beneficial effects if lavage was carried out for at least 4 days or longer. Significant reductions in pancreatic sepsis, organ failure, early deaths, and length of hospital stay were observed [15,69], thus supporting the lavage concept, especially as an adjunct of necrosectomy [69–72].

In the later course of necrotizing pancreatitis septic multiorgan failure as a consequence of infected pancreatic necrosis or pancreatic abscess is a well-established determinant of outcome. The only way to approach this problem is a thorough evacuation of the septic focus to prevent further local and systemic bacterial spread [22,35,73].

Preservation of Vital, Intact Pancreatic Tissue

Experience over the past years has shown that the necrotizing process is often represented by fatty tissue necrosis in and around the gland [74]. Pancreatectomy is difficult to justify, even in patients with macroscopically total pancreatic necrosis, as in many cases only the superficial areas of the gland are necrotic and can easily be mistaken intraoperatively as total pancreatic necrosis [12,18]. The amount of remaining pancreatic parenchyma strongly influences the quality of long-term results concerning endo- and exocrine pancreatic function [75–81].

Indications for Necrosectomy

Operative debridement should generally be restricted to those patients with necrotizing pancreatitis in whom conservative or interventional treatment fails. The initial treatment for all patients with necrotizing pancreatitis should include maximum intensive care management with aggressive fluid resuscitation and should be continued for at least 2 weeks after the onset of symptoms. Although organ failure is a frequent and early finding in necrotizing pancreatitis, it responds well to in intensive care treatment and is reversible in at least 50% of patients [38,49,50,82,83]. Therefore, prolonged intensive care unit (ICU) treatment allows selection of patients who do not require surgery. Another important reason for the need for a conservative basic treatment concept is the clinical observation that effective necrosectomy of devitalized tissue is not possible unless demarcation of the necrotic areas occurs at the end of the 2nd week after disease onset (Fig. 21.4.1).

Operative debridement is indicated in patients with sterile necrosis who are suffering from persisting abdominal discomfort, weight loss, inability to return to a regular oral diet, or persisting organ failure despite conservative treatment for more than 2–3 weeks. In our own series of patients with sterile necrosis, the percentage of operatively treated patients significantly ($p<0.0005$) decreased from 61% in the time period May 1982 to April 1993, to 35% in the time period May 1993 to May 2001 [41]. Although there is continuing controversy about an indication for necrosectomy or intervention in patients with sterile necrosis, a group of patients with persisting abdominal or systemic complications over several weeks represent a small entity that still requires operative treatment [35,41,46].

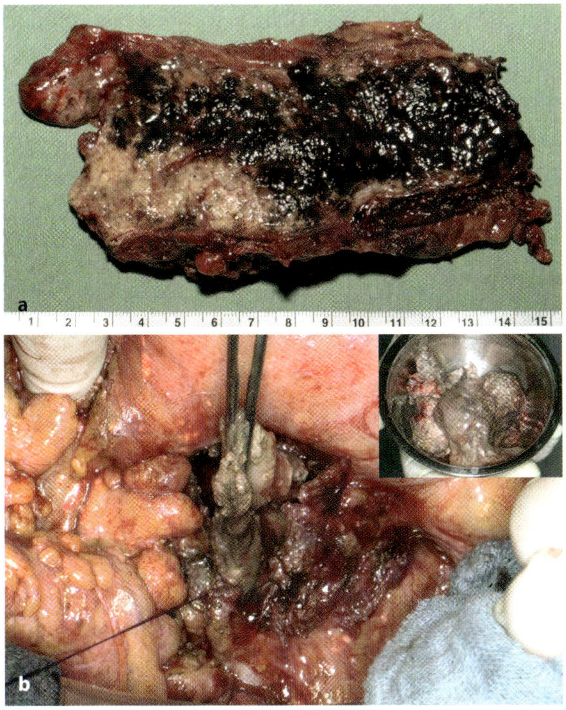

Figure 21.4.1

Demarcation of intrapancreatic necrosis in necrotizing pancreatitis. Pancreatic parenchymal necrosis in a patient on day 4 (a) and on week 14 (b) after onset of symptoms

The presence of documented infection of pancreatic necrosis is a uniformly accepted indication for open or interventional drainage. Very recently, the dogma of infected necrosis as an absolute indication for immediate surgery has also been challenged. Rünzi et al. reported a series of 88 consecutive patients with clinically severe acute necrotizing pancreatitis of whom 28 (32%) developed FNA-proven infected necrosis 19 days after disease onset. An entirely conservative approach resulted in an extremely favorable mortality rate of 12% (16 of 28); delayed surgical intervention was performed on the remaining 12 patients after 36 days following disease onset with a mortality rate of 17% [60]. Although these results require further evaluation, increasing empirical evidence suggests that even in the presence of proven pancreatic infections, extended conservative treatment protocols seem to carry a favorable outcome. On the other hand, a clear relationship between infected necrosis and associated septic multiorgan failure, the ultimate determinant of death, has been well established [22,73]. It therefore remains to be proven how much conservative treatment a critically ill patient with infected necrosis can bear before systemic sepsis becomes uncontrolled and a point of no return is reached.

Finally, operative intervention is indicated in any patient with clinical signs of acute abdomen in whom other complications such as intestinal perforations cannot be ruled out.

Timing of Necrosectomy

As mentioned above, the timing of operative intervention is generally recommended to be delayed as long as possible, at least 2 weeks after symptom onset [84]. However, the only study ever conducted on this issue by Mier et al. was discontinued before its completion because the odds ratio clearly favored delaying operative therapy for at least 12 days after disease onset irrespective of the status of infection [85]. In contrast, patients undergoing "early" debridement did so within the first 72 h after symptom onset, a time interval during which necrosectomy is not performed in most centers, and hasn't been since the 1990s. On the other hand, Fernandez-Castillo et al. from the Boston group has shown that delaying debridement beyond the 4th week after the onset of symptoms does not confer an additional advantage in terms of overall outcome and cost [46]. Taking an average cut-off of <2 weeks for "early" and >2 weeks after symptom onset for "late" debridement, there are still studies that did not find a difference in outcome [37,39,86,87]. In a multiple logistic regression analysis of our own patient series with sterile necrosis who underwent operative treatment, the timing of operative intervention was a not risk factor for either subsequent pancreatic infections or for nonsurvival [26]. A general problem in comparing these studies is the lack of uniform definitions of "early" versus "delayed" and a precise stratification of type and severity of organ failure, thus making interinstitutional comparisons difficult. Therefore, the recommendation that operative treatment should be delayed at least until the 2nd week after onset of necrotizing pancreatitis is supported largely by empirical data [48,88–92] and is reasonable, although convincing prospective randomized data are lacking.

Diagnostic Work-Up

In general, all patients with clinical severe acute pancreatitis should undergo close clinical and laboratory evaluation on a daily basis. The imaging procedure of choice is contrast-enhanced helical computed tomography (CECT), which is a widely available and well-established tool for estimating the extent of intra- and extrapancreatic necrosis [17]. Percutaneous FNA, either guided by ultrasound or CT, with Gram-stain and culture of the aspirate is still the "gold-standard" for the diagnosis of the presence of infection [52,53]. In cases of biliary severe acute pancreatitis, early ERCP should be performed to exclude or treat impacted prepapillary gallstones [54].

Most of the aforementioned diagnostic tests are indispensable for an accurate severity stratification and are of high prognostic relevance, as discussed in detail elsewhere in this section. However, if the indication for operative debridement has been established, the ultimately essential diagnostic procedure providing all necessary information for the surgeon is CECT.

Surgical Techniques

A variety of different approaches have been advocated for the surgical management of this disease during the past few decades. They include a wide spectrum of techniques ranging from conservative, nonresecting methods to aggressive, extensively resecting procedures. From a historical perspective, neither nonresecting, conservative strategies such as peritoneal and lesser-sac lavage [10,14,15,67] or triple-tube drainage [8,9] alone nor aggressive resection modalities such as partial or total pancreatectomy [11–16] have brought about a significant reduction in the overall mortality of severe acute pancreatitis. The underlying reason for this is the fact that none of the protocols sufficiently addressed the pathophysiological background of the disease. Peritoneal dialysis as an intra-abdominal treatment modality neither approaches the retroperitoneum nor provides evacuation of necrotic or infected foci. Although triple-tube drainage is aimed at two important factors, the retroperitoneal drainage of toxic exudate and the inhibition of exocrine pancreatic secretion, necrosectomy is not performed. In contrast, pancreatic resection modalities are aimed at the radical removal of the gland. The removal of still viable pancreatic parenchyma, healthy duodenum, stomach, and biliary tract exposes the severely ill patient to additional stress. Thus, these aggressive approaches, which clearly represent overtreatment, are linked to high postoperative morbidity and increased risk of late morbidity, and have been abandoned.

The most appropriate procedure in the surgical management of necrotizing pancreatitis is the careful removal of necrosis and preservation of vital pancreatic tissue. This simple change in the intraoperative management has reduced the mortality rate from >50% to about 20% [29,43]. Despite the initial necrosectomy and simple drainage of the peripancreatic bed, recurrent intra-abdominal sepsis continues to be a major problem [30]. The cause of recurrent sepsis is probably multifactorial, but most commonly due to either inadequate peripancreatic drainage or incomplete necrosectomy as a result of the ongoing necrotizing process.

Necrosectomy and Continuous Closed Lavage of the Lesser Sac

In an attempt to provide further evacuation of peripancreatic exudates as well as to promote further debridement, in the early 1980s we introduced and established the concept of postoperative closed local lavage of the lesser sac and necrotic cavities for the treatment of necrotizing pancreatitis [20,70]. Between May 1982 and May 2001 a total of 285 patients were treated according to this protocol [41]. Table 21.4.1 shows the clinical severity in the operatively treated patient group with sterile and infected necrosis, which was significantly higher than in patients managed by conservative means. The preoperative extent of intrapancreatic necrosis was assessed by CECT in 92 patients with sterile necrosis and in 103 patients with infected necrosis. Limited necrosis involving less than 30% of the pancreatic parenchyma was more frequent ($p<0.003$) in the sterile (46%) than in the infected group (24%). In contrast, extended necrosis involving more than 30% of the pancreatic parenchyma was observed more frequently in the infected than in the sterile group ($p<0.003$). Necrosectomy was performed 5.5 days (median) after disease onset (range 0.5–143 days) in patients with sterile necrosis and 20.1 days (median) after disease onset (range 1.2–207 days) in patients with infected necrosis ($p<0.0001$).

The concept of necrosectomy includes surgical removal of devitalized peri- and intrapancreatic tissue and emptying of fluid collections. Depending on the surgeon's preference, access to the abdomen is achieved by a midline or a bilateral subcostal incision. However, the midline incision enables a better exploration of the whole abdomen, especially in the case of

Table 21.4.1. Clinical severity in operatively treated patients with sterile and infected necrosis, and in conservatively treated patients. Clinical severity was assessed within the preoperative course, during surgery, and during the overall course in conservatively treated patients. *OP sterile* Operated with sterile necrosis, *OP Infected* operated with infected necrosis, *Conservative* conservatively treated patients, *APACHE II* Acute Physiology and Chronic Health Evaluation II

Variable	OP Sterile (*n*=145)	OP Infected (*n*=140)	Conservative (*n*=107)
Ranson	5 (0–0)	5 (0–9)	3.5 (0–11)[a]
APACHE II (24 h)	12 (0–28)	11 (0–27)	8 (1–29)[a]
Pulmonary failure	*n*=100 (64%)	*n*=102 (72%)	*n*=55 (51%)[b]
Mechanical ventilation	*n*=74 (42%)	*n*=49 (31%)	*n*=15 (14%)[a]
Renal failure	*n*=46 (23%)	*n*=31 (25%)	*n*=14 (13%)[b]
Dialysis/hemofiltration	*n*=19 (10%)	*n*=12 (9%)	*n*= 5 (5%)
Cardiocirculatory failure	*n*=51 (25%)	*n*=46 (28%)	*n*=16 (15%)[a]
Vasopressors	*n*=46 (21%)	*n*=45 (26%)	*n*=15 (14%)*

[a] Conservative versus operative treatment: p<0.001
[b] Conservative versus operative treatment: p<0.005

extended extrapancreatic necrosis affecting the paracolic spaces. After division of the gastrocolic ligament, the lesser sac is exposed and necrosectomy is performed either digitally or by the careful use of instruments that permit the preservation of still vital pancreatic parenchyma (Fig. 21.4.2A). After surgical debridement, an extensive intraoperative lavage is performed using 6–12 l of isotonic saline in order to clear the surface of the pancreatic bed and the extrapancreatic spaces affected by fatty-tissue necrosis (Fig. 21.4.2B). For postoperative continuous local lavage, large-bore, single- (Charr. 24–28) and double-lumen (Charr. 16–18) catheters are placed into the lesser sac and extravulnarily brought out through either side of the lateral abdominal wall at the level of the retroperitoneal spaces. At the end of the procedure, the gastrocolic and duodenocolic ligaments are sutured to create a closed compartment for a regionally restricted lavage (Fig. 21.4.2C, E). The abdomen is then closed by running or interrupted slowly absorbable sutures (Fig. 21.4.2D).

In cases of paralytic ileus, we prefer a loop ileostomy for intestinal decompression (in 26% of our operatively treated patients) because it can be easily taken down during a minor surgical procedure, usually 6 months after hospital discharge and complete recovery. Initial postoperative continuous lavage is done with fluid amounts of 24 l/day using a commercial, hyperosmolar, potassium-free dialysis fluid (CAPD, Fresenius, Germany). If the peritoneal cavity is also affected, local lavage is combined with a short-term peritoneal lavage.

This mechanical "flow-through" technique allows atraumatic and continuous removal of further devitalized tissue, elimination of microorganisms, and biologically active compounds during the postoperative course. In general, there is no need for routine reoperations unless specific indications such as persistent pancreatic sepsis, intra-abdominal abscesses, or bleeding occur. Lavage therapy is stopped when the effluent is clear without signs of active pancreatic enzymes (amylase and lipase levels) or a positive bacteriology. ICU monitoring is not necessary during lavage therapy and thus helps to limit further escalating costs in the treatment of these patients. Table 21.4.2 shows the incidence of postoperative complications in our own series of 285 operatively treated patients with necrotizing pancreatitis [41]. Intraoperative bacteriology revealed primary infected necrosis in 140 out of 392 patients (36%) with necrotizing pancreatitis; the overall complication rate was significantly higher in this group. Table 21.4.3 shows the results in terms of hospital stay, duration of ICU treatment, reoperations, and mortality. Main indications for relaparotomy were recurrent systemic sepsis with or without organ failure due to local sequestration of infected fluid or abscesses, and bleeding from the pancreatic or retroperitoneal areas. Intestinal fistulae were rare indications for reoperation; pancreatic fistulae could be successfully managed by conservative means with only few exceptions. Relaparotomy was necessary in less than 50% of patients, and the in-hospital stay was significantly longer in the infected group; ICU treatment was required for up to 4 weeks. We achieved a

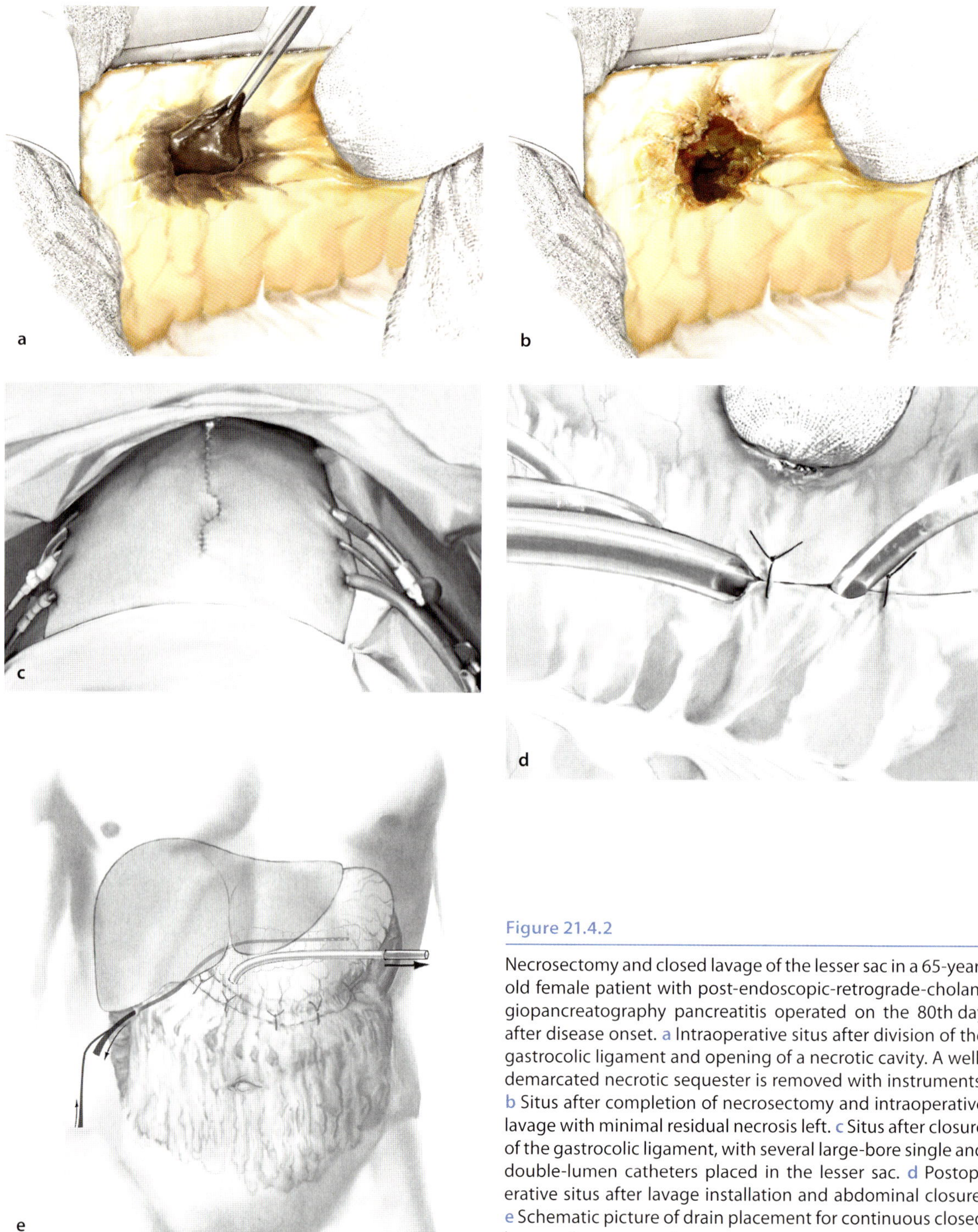

Figure 21.4.2

Necrosectomy and closed lavage of the lesser sac in a 65-year-old female patient with post-endoscopic-retrograde-cholangiopancreatography pancreatitis operated on the 80th day after disease onset. a Intraoperative situs after division of the gastrocolic ligament and opening of a necrotic cavity. A well-demarcated necrotic sequester is removed with instruments. b Situs after completion of necrosectomy and intraoperative lavage with minimal residual necrosis left. c Situs after closure of the gastrocolic ligament, with several large-bore single and double-lumen catheters placed in the lesser sac. d Postoperative situs after lavage installation and abdominal closure. e Schematic picture of drain placement for continuous closed lavage after necrosectomy

postoperative mortality rate of 25% with no difference between patients with sterile and infected necrosis. In a reviewed series, the cumulative mortality, incidence of postoperative pancreatic fistulae, and bleeding of open necrosectomy with postoperative continuous closed lavage was 21%, 18%, and 11%, respectively (Table 21.4.4).

Table 21.4.2. Postoperative complications after necrosectomy and closed lavage in patients with sterile and infected necrosis. *n.s.* Not significant

Complication	OP sterile (n=142)[b]	OP infected (n=135)[b]	p
No complications	n=55 (39%)	n=30 (22%)	0.006
Complications[a]	n=87 (61%)	n=105 (78%)	0.004
Abscess	n=38 (27%)	n=45 (33%)	n.s.
Fistula:			
Pancreatic	n=33 (23%)	n=40 (30%)	n.s.
Biliary	n=1 (1%)	n=7 (5%)	n.s.
Small bowel	n=10 (7%)	n=18 (13%)	n.s.
Large bowel	n=6 (4%)	n=17 (13%)	0.01
Wound infection	n=19 (13%)	n=18 (13%)	n.s.
Sepsis	n=56 (39%)	n=81 (60%)	0.001
Bleeding	n=26 (18%)	n=18 (13%)	n.s.

[a] Figures represent the total number of complications per group. Most patients had more than one complication

[b] Previous operation at referring hospital without further operative intervention at our department: sterile group n=3 patients, infected group n=5 patients (excluded from analysis)

Table 21.4.3. Overall results of necrosectomy and closed lavage in patients with sterile and infected necrosis. *ICU* Intensive care unit, *reop* reoperated

	OR sterile (n=145)	OR infected (n=140)	p
Hospitalization[a] (days)	45 (2–209)	64 (1–238)	<0.007
ICU treatment[a] (days)	22 (2–189)	27 (1–238)	n.s.
Lavage duration[a] (days)	23 (1–163)	29 (1–132)	n.s.
Frequency of reop	n=63 (43%)	n=71 (51%)	n.s.
Reop patient[b]	2 (1–41)	1 (1–26)	n.s.
Conversion to scheduled relaparotomies	n=13 (9%)	n=9 (6%)	n.s.
Mortality	n=33 (23%)	n=38 (27%)	n.s.

[a] Data are presented as median, range

[b] Including patients switched to programmed reoperations

Table 21.4.4. Review: results of necrosectomy and closed lavage since 1989. *n.r.* Not recorded

Authors	Patients (n)	Deaths (n)	%	Fistulae n (%)	Bleeding n (%)
Larvin et al. 1989 [36]	14	3	21%	0	1 (7%)
Pederzoli et al. 1990 [37]	191	40	18%	15 (8%)	17 (9%)
Büchler et al. 2000 [38]	28	6	21%	8 (29%)	2 (7%)
De Waele et al. 2000 [39]	17	9	53%	3 (18%)	0
Wig et al. 2004 [40]	58	17	29%	9 (16%)	8 (14%)
Besselink et al. 2006	53	13	25%	n.r.	17 (32%)
Farkas et al. 2006 [42]	220	17	8%	24 (11%)	6 (3%)
Rau et al. 2005 [41]	285	72	25%	77 (27%)	44 (15%)
Total	866	177	20%	136 (17%)	95 (11%)

References

1. Fitz RH (1889) Acute pancreatitis: a consideration of pancreatic hemorrhage, hemorrhagic, suppurative and gangrenous pancreatitis. Boston Med Surg J 70:181–235
2. Moynihan B (1925) Acute pancreatitis. Ann Surg 81:132–142
3. Elman R, Arneson N, Graham EA (1929) Value of blood amylase estimations in the diagnosis of pancreatic disease: a clinical study. Arch Surg 19:943–967
4. Paxton JR, Payne JH (1948) Acute pancreatitis: a statistical review of 307 established cases of acute pancreatitis. Surg Gynecol Obstet 86:69–75
5. Lewison EF (1940) Acute pancreatitis. Arch Surg 41:1008–1037
6. Pollock AV (1959) Acute pancreatitis: analysis of 100 patients. Br Med J 1:6–14
7. Trapnell JE (1966) The natural history and prognosis of acute pancreatitis. Ann R Coll Surg 38:265–287
8. McCarthy MC, Dickerman RM (1982) Surgical management of severe acute pancreatitis. Arch Surg 117:476–480
9. Hesselink EJ, Sloof MJH, Bleichrodt RP, Van Schilfgaarde R (1987) Conservative surgical treatment for acute pancreatitis: the Lawson procedure. Neth J Surg 39:79–82
10. Teerenhovi O, Nordback I, Eskola J (1989) High volume lesser sac lavage in acute necrotizing pancreatitis. Br J Surg 76:370–373
11. Watts GT (1963) Total pancreatectomy for fulminant pancreatitis. Lancet 13:384
12. Alexandre JH, Guerrieri MT (1981) Role of total pancreatectomy in the treatment of necrotizing pancreatitis. World J Surg 5:369–377
13. Aldridge MC, Ornstein M, Glazer G, Dudley HAF (1985) Pancreatic resection for severe acute pancreatitis. Br J Surg 72:796–800
14. Kivilaakso E, Lempinen M, Mäkelaäinen A, Nikki P, Schröder T (1984) Pancreatic resection versus peritoneal lavation for acute fulminant pancreatitis. Ann Surg 199:426–431
15. Schröder T, Sainio V, Kivisaari L, Puolakkainen P, Kivilaakso E, Lempinen M (1991) Pancreatic resection versus peritoneal lavage in acute necrotizing pancreatitis. A prospective randomized trial. Ann Surg 214:663–666
16. Nordback I, Auvinen O, Pessi T, Autio V (1986) Complications after pancreatic resection for acute necrotizing pancreatitis. Acta Chir Scand 152:49–54
17. Block S, Maier W, Bittner R, Buchler M, Malfertheiner P, Beger HG (1986) Identification of pancreas necrosis in severe acute pancreatitis: imaging procedures versus clinical staging. Gut 27:1035–1042
18. Leger L, Chiche B, Louvel A (1981) Pancreatic necrosis and acute pancreatitis. World J Surg 5:315–317
19. Hollender LF, Meyer C, Marrie A, Costa Jda S, Castellanos JG (1981) Role of surgery in the management of acute pancreatitis. World J Surg 5:361–368
20. Beger HG, Krautzberger W, Bittner R, Block S, Büchler M (1985) Results of surgical treatment of necrotizing pancreatitis. World J Surg 9:972–979
21. Beger HG, Bittner R, Block S, Büchler M (1986) Bacterial contamination of pancreatic necrosis. A prospective clinical study. Gastroenterology 49:433–438
22. Widdison AL, Karanjia ND (1993) Pancreatic infection complicating acute pancreatitis. Br J Surg 80:148–154
23. Isenmann R, Rau B, Beger HG (2001) Early severe acute pancreatitis: characteristics of a new subgroup. Pancreas 22:274–278
24. Tao HQ, Zhang JX, Zou SC (2004) Clinical characteristics and management of patients with early acute severe pancreatitis: experience from a medical center in China. World J Gastroenterol 10:919–921
25. Poves Prim I, Fabregat Prous J, Garcia Borobia FJ, Jorba Marti R, Figueras Felip J, Jaurrieta Mas E (2004) Early onset of organ failure is the best predictor of mortality in acute pancreatitis. Rev Esp Enferm Dig 96:705–713
26. Rau BM, Bothe A, Kron M, Beger HG (2006) The role of early multisystem organ failure as major risk factor for pancreatic infections and death in severe acute pancreatitis. Clin Gastroenterol Hepatol 4:1053–1061
27. Buter A, Imrie CW, Carter CR, Evans S, McKay CJ (2002) Dynamic nature of early organ dysfunction determines outcome in acute pancreatitis. Br J Surg 89:298–302
28. Johnson CD, Abu-Hilal M (2004) Persistent organ failure during the first week as a marker of fatal outcome in acute pancreatitis. Gut 53:1340–1344
29. Beger HG, Rau B, Isenmann R (2000) Necrosectomy or anatomically guided resection in acute pancreatitis. Chirurg 71:274–280
30. Bradley EL III (1993) A fifteen year experience with open drainage for infected pancreatic necrosis. Surg Gynecol Obstet 177:215–222
31. Orlando R III, Welch JP, Akbari CM, Bloom GP, Macaulay WP (1993) Techniques and complications of open packing of infected pancreatic necrosis. Surg Gynecol Obstet 177:65–71
32. Tsiotos GG, Luque-de-Leon E, Soreide JA, Bannon MP, Zietlow SP, Baerga-Varela Y, Sarr MG (1998) Management of necrotizing pancreatitis by repeated operative necrosectomy using a zipper technique. Am J Surg 175:91–98
33. Bosscha K, Hulstaert PF, Hennipman A, Visser MR, Gooszen HG, van Vroonhoven TKMV, van der Werken C (1998) Fulminant acute pancreatitis and infected necrosis: results of open management of the abdomen and "planned" reoperations. J Am Coll Surg 187:255–262
34. Branum G, Galloway J, Hirchowitz W, Fendley M, Hunter J (1998) Pancreatic necrosis: results of necrosectomy, packing, and ultimate closure over drains. Ann Surg 227:870–877
35. Gotzinger P, Sautner T, Kriwanek S, Beckerhinn P, Barlan M, Armbruster C, Wamser P, Fugger R (2002) Surgical treatment for severe acute pancreatitis: extent and surgical control of necrosis determine outcome. World J Surg 26:474–478
36. Larvin M, Chalmers AG, Robinson PJ, McMahon MJ (1989) Debridement and closed cavity irrigation for the treatment of pancreatic necrosis. Br J Surg 76:465–471
37. Pederzoli P, Bassi C, Vesentini S, Iacono C, Nicoli N, Mangiante G, Corra S, Falconi M, Nifosi F, Girelli R (1990) Necrosectomy by lavage in the surgical treatment of severe necrotizing pancreatitis. Acta Chir Scand 156:775–780
38. Büchler MW, Gloor B, Müller CA, Friess H, Seiler C, Uhl W (2000) Acute necrotizing pancreatitis: treatment strategy according to the status of infection. Ann Surg 232:619–626
39. De Waele JJ, Hesse UJ, Pattyn P, Decruyenaere J, de Hemptinne B (2000) Postoperative lavage and on demand surgical intervention in the treatment of acute necrotizing pancreatitis. Arch Chir Belg 100:16–20
40. Wig JD, Mettu SR, Jindal R, Gupta R, Yadav TD (2004) Closed lesser sac lavage in the management of pancreatic necrosis. J Gastroenterol Hepatol 19:1010–1015
41. Rau B, Bothe A, Beger HG (2005) Surgical treatment of necrotizing pancreatitis by necrosectomy and closed lavage: changing patient characteristics and outcome in a 19-year single center series. Surgery 138:28–39

42. Farkas G, Marton J, Mandi Y, Leindler L (2006) Surgical management and complex treatment of infected pancreatic necrosis:18 year experience at a single center. J Gastrointest Surg 10:278–285
43. Wilson C, McArdle CS, Carter DC, Imrie CW (1988) Surgical treatment of acute necrotizing pancreatitis. Br J Surg 75:119–123
44. Howard JM (1989) Delayed debridement and external drainage of massive pancreatic or peripancreatic necrosis. Surg Gynecol Obstet 168:25–29
45. Villazon A, Villazon O, Terrazas F, Rana R (1991) Retroperitoneal drainage in the management of the septic phase of severe acute pancreatitis. World J Surg 15:103–108
46. Fernandez-del Castillo C, Rattner DW, Makary MA, Mostafavi A, McGrath D, Warshaw AL (1998) Debridement and closed packing for the treatment of necrotizing pancreatitis. Ann Surg 228:676–684
47. Oleynikov D, Cook C, Sellers B, Mone MC, Barton R (1998) Decreased mortality from necrotizing pancreatitis. Am J Surg 176:648–653
48. Bhansali S, Shah S, Desai SB, Sunawala JD (2003) Infected necrosis complicating acute pancreatitis: experience with 131 cases. Indian J Gastroenterol 22:7–10
49. Bradley EL III, Allen K (1991) A prospective longitudinal study of observation versus surgical intervention in the management of necrotizing pancreatitis. Am J Surg 161:19–25
50. Rau B, Pralle U; Uhl W, Schoenberg MH, Beger HG (1995) Management of sterile necrosis in instances of severe acute pancreatitis. J Am Coll Surg 181:279–288
51. Uomo G, Visconti M, Manes G, Calise F, Laccetti M, Rabitti PG (1996) Nonsurgical treatment of acute pancreatitis. Pancreas 12:142–148
52. Gerzof SG, Banks PA, Robbins AH, Johnson WC, Spechler SJ, Wetzner SM, Snider JM, Langevin RE, Jay ME (1987) Early diagnosis of pancreatic infection by computed tomography-guided aspiration. Gastroenterology 93:1315–1320
53. Rau B, Pralle U, Mayer JM, Beger HG (1998) The role of ultrasonographically guided fine-needle aspiration cytology in the diagnosis of infected pancreatic necrosis. Br J Surg 85:179–184
54. Ayub K, Imada R, Slavin J (2004) Endoscopic retrograde cholangiopancreatography in gallstone-associated acute pancreatitis. Cochrane Database Syst Rev 4:CD003630
55. Mazaki T, Ishii Y, Takayama T (2006) Meta-analysis of prophylactic antibiotic use in acute necrotizing pancreatitis. Br J Surg 93:674–684
56. McClave SA, Chang WK, Dhaliwal R, Heyland DK (2006) Nutrition support in acute pancreatitis: a systematic review of the literature. J Parenter Enteral Nutr 30:143–156
57. Aultman DF, Bilton BD, Zibari GB, McMillan RW, McDonald JC (1997) Nonoperative therapy for acute necrotizing pancreatitis. Am Surg 63:1114–1118
58. Ashley SW, Perez A, Pierce EA, Brooks DC, Moore FD Jr, Whang EE, Banks PA, Zinner MJ (2001) Necrotizing pancreatitis: contemporary analysis of 99 consecutive cases. Ann Surg 234:572–580
59. Fotzik T, Klar E, Buhr HJ, Herfarth C (1995) Improved survival in acute necrotizing pancreatitis despite limiting the indications for surgical debridement. Eur J Surg 161:187–192
60. Rünzi M, Niebel W, Goebell H, Gerken G, Layer P (2005) Non-surgical treatment of infected necrosis in severe acute pancreatitis. Pancreas 30:195–199
61. de Beaux AC, Goldie AS, Ross JA, Carter DC, Fearon KC (1996) Serum concentrations of inflammatory mediators related to organ failure in patients with acute pancreatitis. Br J Surg 83:349–353
62. Mayer J, Rau B, Gansauge F, Beger HG (2000) Inflammatory mediators in human acute pancreatitis: clinical and pathophysiological implications. Gut 47:546–552
63. Dugernier TL, Laterre PF, Wittebole X, Roeseler J, Latinne D, Reynaert MS, Pugin J (2003) Compartmentalization of the inflammatory response during acute pancreatitis. Correlation with local and systemic complications. Am J Respir Crit Care Med 168:148–157
64. Teerenhovi O, Nordback I, Isolauri J (1988) Influence of pancreatic resection on systemic complications in acute necrotizing pancreatitis. Br J Surg 75:793–795
65. Smadja C, Bismuth H (1986) Pancreatic debridement in acute necrotizing pancreatitis: an obsolete procedure? Br J Surg 73:408–410
66. Denham W, Yang J, Norman J (1997) Evidence for an unknown component of pancreatic ascites that induces adult respiratory distress syndrome through an interleukin-1 and tumor necrosis factor-dependent mechanism. Surgery 122:295–301
67. Platell C, Cooper D, Hall JC (2001) acute pancreatitis: effect of somatostatin analogs and peritoneal lavage. J Gastroenterol Hepatol 16:689–693
68. Zhang WZ (2003) Early definitive surgery in the management of severe acute pancreatitis. Hepatobiliary Pancreat Dis Int 2:496–499
69. Ranson JHC, Berman RS (1990) Long peritoneal lavage decreases pancreatic sepsis in acute pancreatitis. Ann Surg 211:708–716
70. Büchler M, Block S, Krautzberger W, Bittner R, Beger HG (1985) Necrotizing pancreatitis: peritoneal lavage or bursa lavage? Results of a prospective consecutive controlled study. Chirurg 56:247–250
71. Gebhardt C, Gall FP (1981) Importance of peritoneal irrigation after surgical treatment of hemorrhagic, necrotizing pancreatitis. World J Surg 5:379–385
72. Nieuwenhuijs VB, Besselink MG, van Minnen LP, Gooszen HG (2003) Surgical management of acute necrotizing pancreatitis: a 13-year experience and a systematic review. Scand J Gastroenterol Suppl 239:111–116
73. Rau B, Uhl W, Büchler MW, Beger HG (1997) Surgical treatment of infected necrosis. World J Surg 21:155–161
74. Becker V (1981) Pathology anatomy and pathogenesis of acute pancreatitis. World J Surg 45:303–313
75. Angelini G, Pederzoli P, Caliari S, Fratton S, Brocco G, Marzoli G, Bovo P, Cavallini G, Scuro LA (1984) Long-term outcome of acute necrohemorrhagic pancreatitis: a 4-year follow-up. Digestion 30:131–137
76. Büchler M, Malfertheiner P, Block S, Beger HG (1985) Morphologische und funktionelle Veränderungen des Pankreas nach akuter nekrotisierende Pankreatitis Z Gastroenterol 23:79–83
77. Nordback IH, Auvinen OA (1985) Long-term results after pancreas resection for acute necrotizing pancreatitis. Br J Surg 72:687–689
78. Doepel M, Eriksson J, Halme L, Kumpulainen T, Höckerstedt K (1993) Good long-term results in patients surviving severe acute pancreatitis. Br J Surg 80:1583–1586
79. Kriwanek S, Armbruster C, Dittrich K, Beckerhinn P, Redl E, Balogh B (1996) Langzeitergebnisse nach chirurgischer Therapie der akut nekroitisierenden Pankreatitis. Chirurg 67:244–248

80. Tsiotos GG, Luque-de Leon E, Sarr MG (1998) Long-term outcome of necrotizing pancreatitis treated by necrosectomy. Br J Surg 85:1650–1653
81. Boreham B, Ammori BJ (2003) A prospective evaluation of pancreatic exocrine function in patients with acute pancreatitis: correlation with extent of necrosis and pancreatic endocrine insufficiency. Pancreatology 3:303–308
82. Le Mee J, Paye F, Sauvanet A, O'Toole D, Hammel P, Marty J, Ruszniewski P, Belghiti J (2001) Incidence and reversibility of organ failure in the course of sterile or infected necrotizing pancreatitis. Arch Surg 136:1386–1389
83. Flint R, Windsor JA (2004) Early physiological response to intensive care as a clinically relevant approach to predicting the outcome in severe acute pancreatitis. Arch Surg 139:438–443
84. Uhl W, Warshaw A, Imrie C, Bassi C, McKay CJ, Lankisch PG, Carter R, Di Magno E, Banks PA, Whitcomb DC, Dervenis C, Ulrich CD, Satake K, Ghaneh P, Hartwig W, Werner J, McEntee G, Neoptolemos JP, Büchler MW (2002) IAP Guidelines for the Surgical Management of Acute Pancreatitis. Pancreatology 2:565–573
85. Mier J, Luque-de Leon E, Castillo A, Robledo F, Blanco M (1997) Early versus late necrosectomy in severe necrotizing pancreatitis. Am J Surg 173:71–75
86. Takeda K, Matsuno S, Sunamura M, Kobari M (1998) Surgical aspects and management of acute necrotizing pancreatitis: recent results of a cooperative national survey in Japan. Pancreas 16:316–322
87. De Waele JJ, Hoste E, Blot SI, Hesse U, Pattyn P, de Hemptinne B, Decruyenaere J, Vogelaers D, Colardyn F (2004) Perioperative factors determine outcome after surgery for severe acute pancreatitis. Crit Care 8:504–511
88. Hungness ES, Robb BW, Seeskin C, Hasselgren PO, Luchette FA (2002) Early debridement for necrotizing pancreatitis: is it worthwhile? J Am Coll Surg 194:740–745
89. De Beaux AC, Palmer KR, Carter DC (1995) Factors influencing morbidity and mortality in acute pancreatitis; an analysis of 279 cases. Gut 37:121–126
90. Hartwig W, Maksan SM, Fotzik T, Schmidt J, Herfarth C, Klar E (2002) Reduction in mortality with delayed surgical therapy of severe pancreatitis. J Gastrointest Surg 6:481–487
91. Yang XW, Luo FW, Zhao SD, Yang CM (2002) the relation of laparotomy timing to prognosis in patients with acute necrotizing pancreatitis. Hepatobiliary Pancreat Dis Int 1:604–607
92. Götzinger P, Wamser P, Exner R, Schwanzer E, Jakesz R, Függer R, Sautner T (2003) Surgical treatment of severe acute pancreatitis: timing of operation is crucial for survival. Surg Infect 4:205–211

R. Carter · A. P. Wysocki

Infected Necrosis – Minimally Invasive Necrosectomy

The evolution of the local manifestations of severe acute pancreatitis has been described previously, whereby extension of pancreatic and peripancreatic necrosis occurs within the first 4–5 days in association with peripancreatic edema [1, 2]. The edema within this initially essentially solid inflammatory mass subsequently coalesces into acute fluid collections containing a variable amount of devitalized tissue [3]. With maturity, the demarcation between viable and necrotic tissue becomes established, the collection becoming lined with granulation tissue [4]. In patients with minimal necrosis and an intact pancreatic duct, the process may subsequently resolve or may require intervention for pressure symptoms *(*pseudocyst [3]*)* or late infection *(*pancreatic abscess [3]*)*. Many patients end up with a significant solid component (organized pancreatic necrosis, OPN [4]*)*, which may also require intervention often using modified techniques to address the solid component within the collection. The management of pseudocyst, abscess, and organized pancreatic necrosis is discussed within the relevant chapters.

The early multisystem organ failure with gradual recovery that characterizes the severe end of the clinical spectrum in acute pancreatitis, is thought to result from an initial systemic inflammatory cascade [5]. A late deterioration may occur as a result of a second hit, usually infection [5]. Opinion regarding the role of intervention in those patients who fail to thrive with significant necrosis but without evidence of infection is divided [6]. Intervention in patients with sterile necrosis is, however, becoming the exception rather than the rule [7]. The identification of infection within pancreatic necrosis has generally mandated radical surgical intervention, and the potential role of open debridement with various management strategies of the post-debridement retroperitoneum are discussed in the relevant chapters. A summary is presented in Table 21.5.1.

Approximately one out of ten patients with acute pancreatitis will develop infected pancreatic necrosis, which represents the most severe local complication of the illness [5]. The extent of pancreatic necrosis is correlated with the development of organ failure [8] and infection [8], but the type of infection (Gram negative, Gram positive, or fungal) probably does not affect outcome [9]. It is now recognized that the leading independent predictor of death in patients with severe acute pancreatitis is organ failure persisting longer than 48 h during the 1st week of illness [5].

Rationale for a Minimally Invasive Approach

Most patients demonstrate a deterioration in organ function following any major surgical intervention and, if not self-limiting, this results in the majority of late deaths from acute pancreatitis [5]. The explosion of interventional radiology and minimal access surgery has resulted in the development of new techniques proposed for the management of necrosis-associated pancreatic infection [4, 10]. Further encouragement has been gained from the realization that these techniques minimize the physiological insult to the patient [9]. Whether any reduction in surgical trauma will be reflected in improved overall mortality remains debatable [1].

The comparative rarity and diversity of presentation of these patients has resulted in series describing surgical outcome combining patients with true evolving necrosis along with those who have organized pancreatic necrosis or pancreatic abscess. Pancreatic necrosectomy in the context of this chapter relates to the management of patients developing complications during the first 5 or 6 weeks following the onset of symptoms, with patients often in organ failure. In this setting, collections have a significant solid component with incomplete demarcation of the necrosum.

Table 21.5.1. Summary of key open necrosectomy papers focusing on infected pancreatic necrosis. *AII* APACHE II score, *RS* Ranson score, *CT-SI* computed tomography severity index, *ITU* intensive therapy unit

Unit, year	Method	*n*	Infected necrosis	Mean AII/RS/CT-SI	Mean days from onset to intervention	Mean post-operative length of stay (days)	Mortality	ITU pre-operatively	Morbidity	Reoperations	ITU post-operatively
Warshaw, 1998 [13]	Necrosectomy with closed packing	64	56%	9/-/-	31	41	6%	–	–	17%	45% (median 6 days)
Bradley, 1999 [7]	Necrosectomy with scheduled re-explorations	46	100%	14/-/-	23	–	13%	–	–	–	–
Buchler, 2000 [14]	Necrosectomy with closed lavage	29	100%	13/4/-	22	85	24%	–	44%	26%	–
Beger, 2005 [6]	Necrosectomy with closed lavage	140	100%	11/5/-	20	64	27%	mean 3 days	78%	51% (median 1)	mean 27 days

Table 21.5.2. Percutaneous drainage

Author, year	*n*	Infected necrosis	Mean AII/RS/CT-SI	Timing of intervention (days)	Successful percutaneous drainage alone	Mortality	Duration of drainage (days)	Average catheter exchanges per patient (mean)	Acute surgical management (%)
Freeny, 1998 [10]	34	100%	-/-/8	9 (range 1–48)	47%	12%	25–152 (mean 85)	3.3	24%
Gambiez, 1998 [18]	10	30%	-/3/E	–	30% (0% infected necrosis)	20% (66% infected necrosis)	4–22 (mean 16)	–	70% (100% infected necrosis)
Baril, 2000 [19]	25	76%	-/-/	–	76%	8%	14–56	?0.4	24%

Simple Percutaneous Drainage

The place of image-guided percutaneous management of infected pancreatic necrosis is very difficult to determine from the literature in that many series are small and include patients with pancreatic abscess (Table 21.5.2). Freeny et al. [10] published the first series of patients with infected pancreatic necrosis to be managed by percutaneous drainage alone. A 10- to 28-Fr catheter is placed into the necrosis under computed tomography (CT) guidance. Vigorous catheter irrigation is performed in the radiology department every several days together with a contrast study. Irrigation is performed on the ward three times daily. Catheters are exchanged an average of four times per patient. Less than half of patients recovered without surgery, and mortality in patients with organ failure was 38% [10]. Narrow-bore catheters fail not because the necrotic tissue is not evacuated, but because these become blocked by the putty or cheese-like necrosis resulting in persistently undrained pus and systemic sepsis. The results of that paper [10] illustrate that without the commitment on the part of the radiologist and the use of large-bore drains for aggressive irrigation, radiologically guided percutaneous therapy often results only in temporary sepsis control and should be considered as part of an overall management strategy rather than sufficient treatment on its own.

Minimally Invasive Percutaneous Necrosectomy

Indications for Intervention

Intervention for sterile necrosis is rarely required during the early phase (<6 weeks after disease onset); the management of organized pancreatic necrosis and pseudocyst are discussed elsewhere. Whereas it was traditionally taught that infection mandated urgent intervention, some patients with infected necrosis (proven bacteriology or retroperitoneal gas bubbles on CT scan) manifest little systemic upset, and will either settle without intervention or may be observed until the collection has matured, separation is complete (OPN), and the patient managed at a later stage when the operative risks are minimized. The chief indication for percutaneous necrosectomy is infected pancreatic necrosis associated with systemic signs of sepsis, the aim being to control sepsis whilst minimizing further compromise of organ function.

Procedure-Relevant Preparation

A systemic inflammatory response syndrome [manifested by two or more of the following signs: temperature >38°C or <36°C, heart rate >90 beats/min, respiratory rate >20/min or arterial carbon dioxide tension <32 mmHg (<4.3 kPa), white blood cell count >12,000 cells/mm^3 or <4,000 cells/mm^3, or >10% immature (band) forms] is a consistent feature of acute pancreatitis associated with significant necrosis in the absence of infection. Secondary infection of necrosis is suspected where there is deterioration in organ function or biochemical markers of the inflammatory response (e.g., C-reactive protein) and where alternative sources (e.g., line sepsis, pneumonia) have been excluded. An abdominal CT scan is performed enabling a percutaneous CT-guided fine needle aspiration for Gram stain, and the fluid component of infected necrosis is drained percutaneously using an 8- to 10-Fr pigtail catheter with a side port for lavage. The interventional radiologist chooses the most dependent aspect of the fat plane between the spleen (posteriorly) and colon (anteriorly). Right-sided collections are accessed through the gastrocolic omentum anterior to the duodenum between the liver and colon. The procedure is impossible to perform in the absence of safe percutaneous radiological access. Figure 21.5.1 demonstrates the pre-and postoperative CT scan images. Multiple or bilateral drains may be inserted where there is a complex or additional noncommunicating retroperitoneal collection. Prior to undergoing necrosectomy, the patient is cross-matched for 2 units of packed cells. Informed consent is obtained.

Procedure

Given that fine-bore tube drainage is likely to result in only a transient improvement in the patient's septic state (as indicated above), the patient undergoes operative tract dilatation and debridement within 24–36 h of initial puncture. Under general anesthesia, the patient is placed in a supine position, with sandbags used to optimize access to the drain site. The layout of the operating room is shown in Fig. 21.5.2. The patient is prepped and draped using a Barrier nephroscopy sheet with a drainage bag (1221; Mölnlycke Health Care, Dunstable, UK) to control spilt irrigation fluid; this is connected to the main suction unit. A skin incision (10 mm) is required prior to performing balloon dilatation (UNBS-10-15; Ultraxx Nephrostomy Balloon Set COOK, Hertfordshire, UK) via

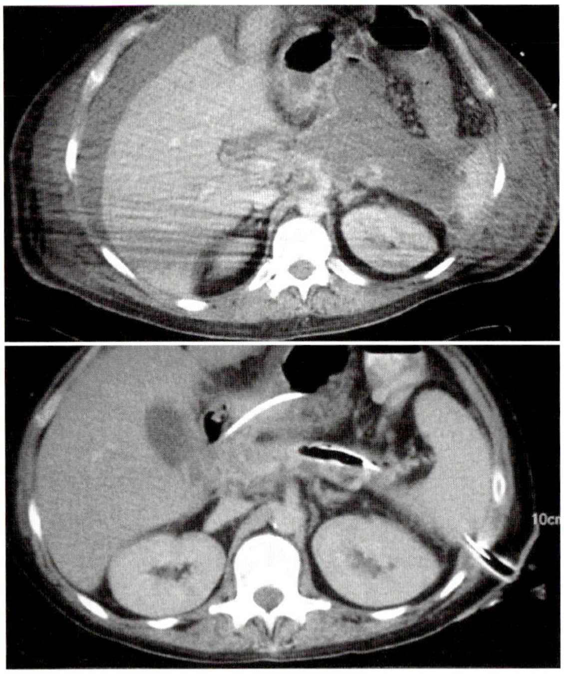

Figure 21.5.1

Computed tomography images taken before (upper) and after (lower) minimally invasive pancreatic necrosectomy for infected necrosis

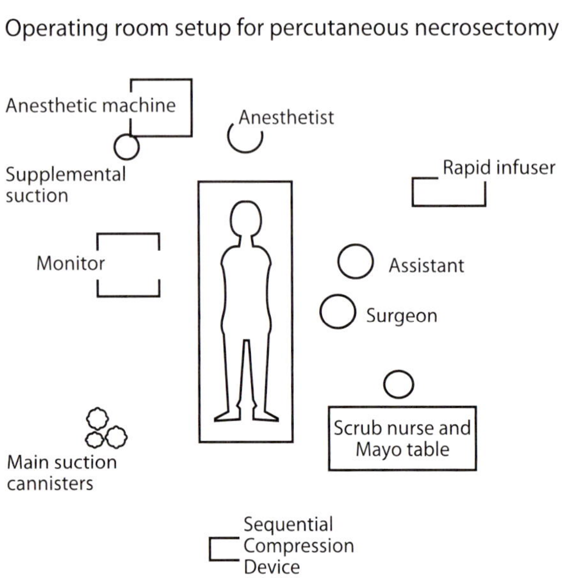

Figure 21.5.2

Operating room setup for percutaneous necrosectomy

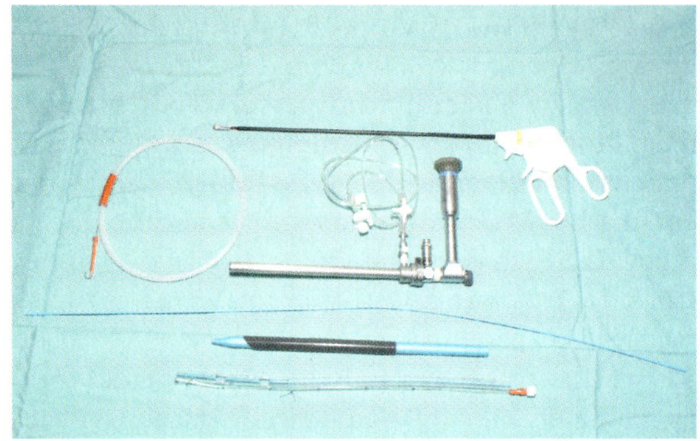

Figure 21.5.3

Rigid scope, Amplatz sheath, and lavage catheter required for percutaneous necrosectomy

the drain tract (alternatively, sequential graduated dilators may be used) to allow insertion of a 34-Fr Amplatz dilator and sheath. Using a nephroscope with a 5-mm working channel (27093BN; Karl Storz Endoscopy, Slough, UK,) copious lavage (normal saline at body temperature via a rapid infuser) and suction is performed until the cavity can be inspected visually (this is connected to the supplemental suction device on the anesthetic machine). Some 10 l of normal saline is used for lavage during each procedure. Gentle traction with the use of a 5-mm laparoscopic grasper (EndoGrasp Tyco Healthcare, Hampshire, UK) enables piecemeal removal of any loose necrotic material. The equipment used is illustrated in Fig. 21.5.3. Under normal circumstances, three types of tissue are encountered: fluffy cloud-like pus which escapes capture by the grasper, typical pale yellow fat necrosis, and silvery-grey necrotic pancreatic parenchyma. Trauma to the viable granulating cavity wall is kept to a minimum in order to minimize venous ooze.

During the primary procedure, debridement is conservative and stopped once a reasonably sized cave has been established; attempts at achieving complete clearance may lead to significant hemorrhage. Secondly, prolonged attempts at debridement during the initial procedure may result is worsening sepsis. An 8-Fr umbilical catheter is sutured to a 32-Fr Portex chest drain (SIMS Portex, Kent, UK) in two positions and this is advanced into the cavity over an 8-Fr stylet (260-120; Microvasive, Boston Scientific, Hertfordshire, UK). The drains are sutured to the skin, brought out via a stoma appliance (to catch any spill), and the umbilical catheter connected to lavage fluid through a blood warmer. Washout is commenced in theater to confirm any bloodstained efflux of fluid is clearing. The chest drain is cut short to minimize outflow resistance. At the second necrosectomy the aim is to develop a path across the entire cavity to ensure that drainage is adequate. Knowledge of the most up-to-date CT scan allows a suitable trajectory of debridement to be chosen. With each subsequent procedure and the passage of time, further tissue separation will take place enabling a thorough debridement in due course.

Intraoperative Issues

The rationale underscoring the procedure is the achievement of sepsis control rather than the completeness of necrotic clearance. Avoiding hemorrhage is the key; therefore, overzealous attempts to achieve complete debridement should be avoided, particularly at the first session. The Amplatz sheath is not usually required at secondary procedures; however, care should be taken to avoid trauma along the track as the nephroscope is passed in and out. Secondly, any tissue that is grasped and does not come away readily should be released. Minor ooze settles spontaneously by the end of the procedure. Venous ooze due to drain-track trauma is managed through tamponade by reinserting the Amplatz sheath. More significant localized bleeding may be locally controlled with a laparoscopic clip applicator (Endo clip 5 mm; Tyco Healthcare, Hampshire, UK), the local application of Floseal (Baxter, Berkshire, UK), or by inflating a balloon catheter within the cavity. Arterial bleeding is best managed by angiographic embolization. In such a setting we would caution against hurried conversion to laparotomy, as this is almost uniformly fatal. Retroperitoneal hemorrhage in this setting carries a 70% mortality [9].

Postoperative Management

Most patients are able to return to the high-dependency unit where deep venous thrombosis prophylaxis with low molecular weight heparin is resumed. Antibiotics are discontinued the next morning unless the patient is in septic shock when tissue culture results indicate choice of antibiotic(s), which are prescribed for 5 days. Oral intake is encouraged, but most patients undergo supplemental peptide-based enteral feeding (Peptisorb; Nutricia Clinical Care, Trowbridge, UK). Continuous lavage at 250 ml/h (Dianil PD1; Baxter Healthcare, Norfolk, UK) is commenced. A careful fluid balance is maintained to ensure that irrigation fluid is not accumulating, although some absorption is often observed. Once the patient's clinical course is satisfactory, they are transferred to the surgical ward where the same treatment is continued.

Indications for repeat abdominal imaging depend on the preoperative CT scan, the likely completeness of necrosectomy, the likelihood of persistent/undrained satellite collections, and the patient's postoperative course (e.g., rigors, persistent tachycardia, or deteriorating biochemical parameters). It is reasonable to reimage after an interval of 7–10 days. Ongoing sepsis may be due to an incompletely drained cavity, the presence of a noncommunicating satellite collection, or another intra-abdominal event.

Planned interval percutaneous necrosectomies are performed approximately 7–10 days apart, depending on the patient's progress, to continue the clearance of the separating necrotic tissue. Little is gained by repeating the procedure within 48 h as no additional tissue separation will have taken place. Once a cavity lined by clean granulation tissue is achieved, necrosectomies are ceased. The Portex drain is replaced by a softer urinary catheter for patient comfort, and irrigation is discontinued.

Outcomes

Confirmed benefits of this approach include [9, 11, 12]: reduced need for intensive care management, not contaminating the peritoneal cavity, ease of access for repeat procedures, and avoidance of the wound complications associated with laparotomy. Connor et al. [9] have for the first time demonstrated that Acute Physiology and Chronic Health Evaluation (APACHE) II score falls after percutaneous retroperitoneoscopic necrosectomy (by average of 1 point), but rises by an average of 1.5 points with open necrosectomy; as such, there is a reduction in the surgical insult on an already unwell patient [9]. This benefit becomes increasingly important when reoperation is required.

When compared to open necrosectomy, the same paper [9] suggests a halving of the mortality rate (19% vs. 39% respectively), this difference only just escaped statistical significance (p=0.06). This benefit was at the expense of an increase in the median length of stay due to the routine need for repeat percutaneous necrosectomies (from 50 to 64 days) [9].

Postoperative Complications

In the three articles describing this procedure (see Table 21.5.3), the following have been noted [9, 11, 12]: conversion to laparotomy, hemorrhage, prolonged gastroparesis, gastric outlet obstruction, fistula in up to 17% (cutaneous, colonic, pleural), communicating pancreatic pseudocyst in up to 20%, occasionally biliary stricture or portal–splenic vein thrombosis. We currently manage colonic fistulae using a diverting loop ileostomy. Almost 90% of pancreaticocutaneous fistulae will heal spontaneously and pancreatic duct stenting or distal pancreatectomy is rarely required. Steatorrhea develops in 25%, and new onset diabetes mellitus is diagnosed in 33% of patients. The incidence of these probably does not differ greatly compared to open necrosectomy. In the patient with gallstones, cholecystectomy with intraoperative cholangiography is performed laparoscopically once the patient has recovered.

Other Minimally Invasive Approaches

When compared to open necrosectomy [6, 7, 13, 14], the potential advantage of minimally invasive approaches may not be limited to the percutaneous necrosectomy technique alone. The following techniques have been described in varying degrees of completeness: percutaneous drainage alone [10], laparoscopic necrosectomy [15], endoscopic transgastric transmural drainage with debridement and irrigation [16], and lumbotomy [17]. It is probably true to suggest that achieving adequate control of sepsis is more relevant than the technique employed. A detailed description of each alternative is beyond the scope of this chapter; however a summary is presented below.

Laparoscopy

Laparoscopic transgastric and transmesocolic necrosectomies have been described [15]. These techniques risk contaminating the peritoneal cavity, are lengthy, and require advanced laparoscopic skill. The advantage of laparoscopy over other minimally invasive techniques is the opportunity of dealing with other intra-abdominal pathology (e.g., colon or gallbladder as well as debriding material) under direct vision. The procedure is not readily repeatable and subsequent radiological intervention may be required. The transgastric approach avoids the middle colic vessels as well as the splenic vein, which are at risk with the

Table 21.5.3. Percutaneous necrosectomy

Author, year	*n*	Infected necrosis	Mean AII/RS/CT-SI	Median days from onset to intervention	Retroperitoneal necrosectomy without laparotomy	Mortality	Median postoperative length of stay (days)	ITU preoperatively (n)	Early morbidity	Median number of operations per patient (range)	ITU postoperatively (n)
Carter, 2000 [11]	10	90%	-/-/-	24	90%	20%	42	3	10%	3 (1–4)	4
Connor, 2003 [12]	24	75%	8/-/-	–	66%	25%	51	9	88%	4 (1–8)	–
Connor, 2005 [9]	47	81%	9/-/6	28	74%	19%	64	16	92%	3 (1–9)	Mean of 0 days

transmesocolic and retroperitoneal approaches, respectively. Published series are difficult to interpret due to unclear definitions of the pathology in question and timing of the intervention, but the advantages are currently unclear. In the largest series dealing with infective complications of necrosis (11 patients) the reader is not advised of the timing of intervention following symptom onset; however, the mortality was 18% with an encouraging median postoperative stay of 21 days [17].

Endoscopy

Baron et al. have evolved the technique of dealing with organized pancreatic necrosis (6 or more weeks from disease onset) [4]. The procedure requires significant expertise: using endoscopic ultrasound guidance, needle-knife fenestration is performed. This is balloon dilated (16–20 mm) and secured with two transmural double pigtail stents (3 cm, 10 Fr) together with a 7-Fr nasocystic lavage catheter. The procedure may be combined with transpapillary pancreatic duct stenting or endoscopic debridement with a stone-retrieval basket. Given that patients typically undergo daily necrosectomy, access to the endoscopy suite may be an issue.

Lumbotomy

The use of a retroperitoneal laparostomy centered on the left 12th rib suffers from difficult postoperative wound management, a high rate of colonic fistulae, and the not infrequent requirement for laparotomy [7]. The procedure may be combined with sinus-track endoscopy. In a recent paper [17], one-third of patients required laparotomy, the mortality was 27% with a median hospital stay of 84 days.

Summary

Percutaneous necrosectomy reduces surgical trauma and immediate postoperative organ compromise. Whether this can be extrapolated into improved ultimate outcome has never been addressed within a clinical trial environment and remains debatable. Adequate and continued control of sepsis remains central to the management of these patients and is more important than the specific method utilized. Percutaneous necrosectomy is probably most appropriate in the critically ill patient with multiple organ failure in whom open surgery carries a prohibitive mortality. Whether the young, premorbidly fit patient without organ failure is more efficiently managed by a one-stage open or laparoscopic necrosectomy remains to be demonstrated.

References

1. Carter R (2003) Management of infected necrosis secondary to acute pancreatitis: a balanced role for minimal access techniques. Pancreatology 3:133–138
2. Werner J, Feuerbach S, Uhl W, Buchler MW (2005) Management of acute pancreatitis: from surgery to interventional intensive care. Gut 54:426–436
3. Bradley EL III (1993) A clinically based classification system for acute pancreatitis. Summary of the International Symposium on Acute Pancreatitis, Atlanta, Ga, September 11 through 13, 1992. Arch Surg 128:586–590
4. Baron TH, Morgan DE, Vickers SM, Lazenby AJ (1999) Organized pancreatic necrosis: endoscopic, radiologic, and pathologic features of a distinct clinical entity. Pancreas 19:105–108
5. Buter A, Imrie CW, Carter CR, et al (2002) Dynamic nature of early organ dysfunction determines outcome in acute pancreatitis. Br J Surg 89:298–302
6. Rau B, Bothe A, Beger HG (2005) Surgical treatment of necrotizing pancreatitis by necrosectomy and closed lavage: changing patient characteristics and outcome in a 19-year, single-center series. Surgery 138:28–39
7. Bradley E III (1999) Operative vs. nonoperative therapy in necrotizing pancreatitis. Digestion 60:19–21
8. Garg PK, Madan K, Pande GK, et al (2005) Association of extent and infection of pancreatic necrosis with organ failure and death in acute necrotizing pancreatitis. Clin Gastroenterol Hepatol 3:159–166
9. Connor S, Alexakis N, Raraty MG, et al (2005) Early and late complications after pancreatic necrosectomy. Surgery 137:499–505
10. Fernandez-del Castillo C, Rattner DW, Makary MA, et al (1998) Debridement and closed packing for the treatment of necrotizing pancreatitis. Ann Surg 228:676–684
11. Buchler MW, Gloor B, Muller CA, et al (2000) Acute necrotizing pancreatitis: treatment strategy according to the status of infection. Ann Surg 232:619–626
12. Freeny PC, Hauptmann E, Althaus SJ, et al (1998) Percutaneous CT-guided catheter drainage of infected acute necrotizing pancreatitis: techniques and results. AJR Am J Roentgenol 170:969–975
13. Gambiez LP, Denimal FA, Porte HL, et al (1998) Retroperitoneal approach and endoscopic management of peripancreatic necrosis collections. Arch Surg 133:66–72
14. Baril NB, Ralls PW, Wren SM, et al (2000) Does an infected peripancreatic fluid collection or abscess mandate operation? Ann Surg 231:361–367
15. Carter CR, McKay CJ, Imrie CW (2000) Percutaneous necrosectomy and sinus tract endoscopy in the management of infected pancreatic necrosis: an initial experience. Ann Surg 232:175–180
16. Connor S, Ghaneh P, Raraty M, et al (2003) Minimally invasive retroperitoneal pancreatic necrosectomy. Dig Surg 20:270–277

17. Cuschieri A (2002) Pancreatic necrosis: pathogenesis and endoscopic management. Semin Laparosc Surg 9:54–63
18. Baron TH, Harewood GC, Morgan DE, Yates MR (2002) Outcome differences after endoscopic drainage of pancreatic necrosis, acute pancreatic pseudocysts, and chronic pancreatic pseudocysts. Gastrointest Endosc 56:7–17
19. Castellanos G, Pinero A, Serrano A, Parrilla P (2002) Infected pancreatic necrosis: translumbar approach and management with retroperitoneoscopy. Arch Surg 137:1060–1063

O. Mann · T. Strate · E. Yekebas · J. Izbicki

Benefits and Limitations of Necrosectomy

Although a lot has been learned about pathophysiology of severe acute pancreatitis Over the last 3 decades, however, treatment has often been detrimental, with a mortality rate of up to 25% [1]. The debate, when and how to operate, is still ongoing. At the beginning of the last century this disease was thought to be incurable if not operated upon [2]. Nowadays a paradigm shift has occurred throughout the medical community. Primary therapy of severe necrotizing pancreatitis consists of conservative treatment, with fluid replacement as the primary goal, sufficient analgesia, and prevention of organ failure as a multidisciplinary intensive care treatment.

Still under debate is early enteral feeding as well as antibiotic treatment [3–6], but both options seem to be viable in the treatment cascade. Furthermore, almost all patients with sterile necrosis can be handled conservatively [7–11]. The exception might be presented by patients with extensive necrosis involving more than 50% of pancreatic parenchyma, since this seems to correlate with a higher incidence of organ failure [12] or patients with multiorgan failure. However, there is no proof that necrosectomy might help those patients either.

Up to now, only patients with fine needle aspiration (FNA)-proven infected necrosis are generally considered to be candidates for surgical therapy, if they present with organ failure [1,12–15]. The timing of surgical intervention seems to be crucial. Early intervention is associated with a high mortality, which decreases significantly if intervention is delayed for 14–21 days [16,17]. The reason behind this might be the fact that the initial phase of up to 14 days is dominated by systemic inflammatory response syndrome (SIRS) due to the release of pro- and anti-inflammatory cytokines, and treatment focuses on excessive fluid reconstitution, whereas the second phase is dominated by sepsis-related morbidity due to septic complications and sepsis-related morbidity due to infected pancreatic necrosis [18–21]. Furthermore, operative treatment should be delayed by at least 2–3 weeks whenever possible to allow demarcation of the necrotic pancreas in order to avoid severe bleeding complications [22].

Since the beginning of this century, not only are new techniques (minimally invasive necrosectomy and endoscopic necrosectomy) being evaluated [23–25], but also the whole concept of operative strategy in cases of infected necrosis are been challenged. In 2002 the International Association of Pancreatology guidelines suggested that the mortality rate of patients with infected necrosis and organ failure is 100% when managed conservatively [14], whereas surgical treatment of patients with infected necrosis could lead to decreased mortality rates of 10–30% [8,9,17,26]. Recently, some reports have shed doubt on whether all patients with infected pancreatic necrosis should undergo surgery [27–29]. Runzi et al. reported on their institutional experience of 28 patients with infected necrosis, of whom 16 (57%) were successfully treated conservatively. Of these, the majority suffered from organ failure [29]. These remarks before the following critical (technical) appraisal should enlighten the reader about the changing treatment strategies in severely sick patients with acute necrotizing pancreatitis. Since it is extremely difficult (and ethically challenging) to design a randomized trial on when and how to operate (or to operate at all), we will most certainly end up with grade B evidence.

Up to now, it is generally agreed that necrotizing pancreatitis with proven infected necrosis as well as septic complications directly caused by pancreatic infection are strong indications for surgical intervention (level B) [14,30,31]. Presently, patients with infected necrosis are rarely managed conservatively without surgical intervention [29]. A recent consensus conference updated the current evidence-based knowledge into 23 recommendations [22]. The jury recommended against pancreatic debridement or drainage for sterile necrosis. Therefore, patients with sterile necrosis should be managed conservatively and undergo surgical intervention only in selected cases, such as persistent organ complications or severe clinical deterioration despite maximum intensive care [17,32].

Table 21.6.1. Different operative strategies

First author	Procedure	Year	Patients (*n*)	Postoperative pancreatic fistula (%)	Mortality (%)
Villazon [46]	Necrosectomy and drainage	1991	18	5.6	22.2
Wilson [47]	Necrosectomy and drainage	1988	14	21.4	28.6
Fernandez-del Castillo [26]	Necrosectomy and closed packing	2000	64	53	6.2
Beger [1]	Necrosectomy and closed lavage	1997	241	20.3	22.4
Pederzoli [48]	Necrosectomy and closed lavage	1990	191	8.3	17.9
Nordback [37]	Necrosectomy + open packing and continuous lavage	1997	33	-	6
Bradley [49]	Necrosectomy + open packing and continuous lavage	1993	71	46.5	14.1
Tsiotos [38]	Necrosectomy + planned relaparotomies with repeated lavage	1998	72	19.4	25.0

The surgical approaches toward pancreatic necrosis are wide-ranging and the optimal procedure is still under debate. The aim of surgical intervention in patients with necrotizing pancreatitis is to eliminate areas of necrotic and infected tissue. Surgical procedures employed to treat severe acute pancreatitis in the past included mobilization, drainage of the pancreatic bed, and extended pancreatic resection. These extended pancreatic resections, which were the major procedure used mainly in Europe from the 1970s throughout the 1980s, have been increasingly avoided in view of the high incidence of postoperative complications, the failure to improve the overall life-saving rate (level 1b–3b) [33,34], and the lowered quality of life in surviving patients because of the impairment of endocrine and exocrine function [33] as a result of removal of vital pancreatic tissue. Preferred surgical techniques currently performed to evacuate necrotic or infected pancreatic and peripancreatic tissue are: (1) necrosectomy combined with open or closed packing, (2) planned staged relaparotomies with repeated lavage, (3) necrosectomy and closed continuous lavage of the retroperitoneum, or (4) simple drainage. Modern agreed principles of surgical intervention include an organ-sparing approach, including the debridement of all infected/necrotic tissue, avoiding intraoperative hemorrhage. It is reported that these approaches are associated with a postoperative mortality of less than 15% in specialized centers, but there has never been a trial that has ever prospectively compared these techniques (Table 21.6.1).

Only one randomized trial has compared pancreatic resection versus continuous peritoneal lavage [34]. Pancreatic resection was associated with increased perioperative morbidity and regular pancreatic parenchyma was removed without need. Since long-term outcome is closely related to the amount of preserved viable pancreatic tissue, the management of patients with infected necrosis has widely changed to limited necrosectomy [35]. There are two main techniques aimed at maximal tissue preservation that are currently used: (1) the "open packing technique," in which repeated necrosectomies are performed in 48-h intervals until all necrosis has resolved and granulation tissue has developed; continuous lavage is often performed thereafter [9], and (2) a single necrosectomy with continuous postoperative lavage (8–10 l/day) through surgically placed drainages has been proposed by Beger [36]. As outlined above, less invasive procedures have been tested but not yet prospectively evaluated. Five prospective trials (level III) used "open packing," [9,16,37–39], whereas two studies investigated the technique described by Beger et al. (level III) [36,40]. Complication rates after surgical treatment were high in all trials, and in the absence of randomized trials, a meta-analysis of the two techniques is impossible. Of note, 25% of patients treated by the procedure reported by Beger et al. required one or more reoperations during the course of their disease for fistulae, intra-abdominal abscesses, or bleeding. "Open packing" is accompanied by a higher morbidity rate mainly due to higher incidences of fistulae, bleeding, and incisional hernias. In addition, mortality rates were slightly higher in the reports on "open packing" [3].

Pancreatic Abscess

Percutaneous or surgical drainage should be performed for pancreatic abscess (recommendation B). If the clinical management of the pancreatic abscess can not be controlled by percutaneous drainage, surgical drainage should be performed (recommendation A). Pancreatic abscess is an indication for surgical intervention, just as for infected pancreatic necrosis. Pus collection is the main lesion in most pancreatic abscess patients, and it has been recently reported that 78–86% of patients can be managed by percutaneous drainage alone (level 3b) [41,42]. If a safe puncture route is assured by ultrasound or CT guidance, this procedure may be the first choice as treatment for pancreatic abscess. However, it should be noted that the favorable results reported for this treatment have all been based on retrospective studies. For example, when severe cases with a Ranson score of 5 or more (level 2b) [43] and cases having multiple abscesses (level 4) [44] were included in the study, the one-stage healing rates of percutaneous drainage declined to 30–47%. When no improvement in clinical findings is observed after percutaneous drainage, surgical drainage should be performed without delay instead of monitoring the clinical course [45].

Summary

There are several indications for surgical intervention in patients with acute necrotizing pancreatitis, such as suspected or confirmed intestinal infarction or perforation, exsanguinating hemorrhage, or abdominal compartment syndrome. The ideal surgical technique for the treatment of pancreatic necrosis remains a matter of debate. In case of infected necrosis, surgical management should favor an organ-preserving approach that involves debridement or necrosectomy combined with a postoperative management concept that maximizes postoperative evacuation of retroperitoneal debris and exudate. Patients with sterile necrosis should be managed conservatively. Only in the case of persistent organ complications or severe clinical deterioration despite maximum intensive therapy should they undergo surgical intervention.

We conclude from these low-ranked studies that careful single necrosectomy and postoperative lavage without planned relaparotomies are less harmful and should be preferred instead of surgical treatment of necrotizing acute pancreatitis, when applicable (level C). Only a few prospective trials on the surgical treatment of acute pancreatitis have been published, and none of them was randomized. Therefore, the level of evidence is generally very low regarding recommendations on surgical treatment. Further studies are mandatory to define the optimal indications, procedures, and timing for surgery. Newer approaches such as laparoscopic, endoscopic, or retroperitoneal procedures might decrease morbidity and mortality in these patients.

References

1. Beger HG, Rau B, Isenmann R (2000) Nekrosektomie oder anatomiegerechte Resektion bei akuter Pankreatitis. Chirurg 71:274–280
2. Moynihan B (1925) Acute pancreatitis. Ann Surg 9:943
3. Heinrich S, Schafer M, Rousson V, Clavien PA (2006) Evidence-based treatment of acute pancreatitis: a look at established paradigms. Ann Surg 243:154–168
4. Mayumi T, Takada T, Kawarada Y, Hirata K, Yoshida M, Sekimoto M, Hirota M, Kimura Y, Takeda K, Isaji S, Koizumi M, Otsuki M, Matsuno S (2006) Management strategy for acute pancreatitis in the JPN Guidelines. J Hepatobiliary Pancreat Surg 13:61–67
5. Pederzoli P, Bassi C, Vesentini S, Campedelli A (1993) A randomized multicenter clinical trial of antibiotic prophylaxis of septic complications in acute necrotizing pancreatitis with imipenem. Surg Gynecol Obstet 176:480–483
6. Whitcomb DC (2006) Clinical practice. Acute pancreatitis. N Engl J Med 354:2142–2150
7. Bassi C, Larvin M, Villatoro E (2003) Antibiotic therapy for prophylaxis against infection of pancreatic necrosis in acute pancreatitis. Cochrane Database Syst Rev 4:CD002941
8. Buchler MW, Gloor B, Muller CA, Friess H, Seiler CA, Uhl W (2000) Acute necrotizing pancreatitis: treatment strategy according to the status of infection. Ann Surg 232:619–626
9. Bradley EL III, Allen K (1991) A prospective longitudinal study of observation versus surgical intervention in the management of necrotizing pancreatitis. Am J Surg 161:19–24
10. Bradley EL III (1996) Indications for debridement of necrotizing pancreatitis. Pancreas 13:219–223
11. Rau B, Pralle U, Uhl W, Schoenberg MH, Beger HG (1995) Management of sterile necrosis in instances of severe acute pancreatitis. J Am Coll Surg 181:279–288
12. Isenmann R, Rau B, Beger HG (1999) Bacterial infection and extent of necrosis are determinants of organ failure in patients with acute necrotizing pancreatitis. Br J Surg 86:1020–1024
13. Rau B, Bothe A, Beger HG (2005) Surgical treatment of necrotizing pancreatitis by necrosectomy and closed lavage: changing patient characteristics and outcome in a 19-year, single-center series. Surgery 138:28–39

14. Uhl W, Warshaw A, Imrie C, Bassi C, McKay CJ, Lankisch PG, Carter R, Di ME, Banks PA, Whitcomb DC, Dervenis C, Ulrich CD, Satake K, Ghaneh P, Hartwig W, Werner J, McEntee G, Neoptolemos JP, Buchler MW (2002) IAP Guidelines for the surgical management of acute pancreatitis. Pancreatology 2:565–573
15. Bassi C, Butturini G, Falconi M, Salvia R, Frigerio I, Pederzoli P (2003) Outcome of open necrosectomy in acute pancreatitis. Pancreatology 3:128–132
16. Mier J, Leon EL, Castillo A, Robledo F, Blanco R (1997) Early versus late necrosectomy in severe necrotizing pancreatitis. Am J Surg 173:71–75
17. Fernandez-del CC, Rattner DW, Makary MA, Mostafavi A, McGrath D, Warshaw AL (1998) Debridement and closed packing for the treatment of necrotizing pancreatitis. Ann Surg 228:676–684
18. Beger HG, Rau B, Isenmann R (2003) Natural history of necrotizing pancreatitis. Pancreatology 3:93–101
19. Isenmann R, Rau B, Beger HG (2001) Early severe acute pancreatitis: characteristics of a new subgroup. Pancreas 22:274–278
20. Buter A, Imrie CW, Carter CR, Evans S, McKay CJ (2002) Dynamic nature of early organ dysfunction determines outcome in acute pancreatitis. Br J Surg 89:298–302
21. Renzulli P, Jakob SM, Tauber M, Candinas D, Gloor B (2005) Severe acute pancreatitis: case-oriented discussion of interdisciplinary management. Pancreatology 5:145–156
22. Nathens AB, Curtis JR, Beale RJ, Cook DJ, Moreno RP, Romand JA, Skerrett SJ, Stapleton RD, Ware LB, Waldmann CS (2004) Management of the critically ill patient with severe acute pancreatitis. Crit Care Med 32:2524–2536
23. Connor S, Ghaneh P, Raraty M, Sutton R, Rosso E, Garvey CJ, Hughes ML, Evans JC, Rowlands P, Neoptolemos JP (2003) Minimally invasive retroperitoneal pancreatic necrosectomy. Dig Surg 20:270–277
24. Cushieri SA (1998) Preface. Semin Laparosc Surg 5:145–146
25. Seewald S, Groth S, Omar S, Imazu H, Seitz U, de WA, Soetikno R, Zhong Y, Sriram PV, Ponnudurai R, Sikka S, Thonke F, Soehendra N (2005) Aggressive endoscopic therapy for pancreatic necrosis and pancreatic abscess: a new safe and effective treatment algorithm (videos) Gastrointest Endosc 62:92–100
26. Fernandez-del CC, Warshaw AL (2000) Parenchymal necrosis: infection and other indications for debridement and drainage. Chirurg 71:269–273
27. Ashley SW, Perez A, Pierce EA, Brooks DC, Moore FD, Jr, Whang EE, Banks PA, Zinner MJ (2001) Necrotizing pancreatitis: contemporary analysis of 99 consecutive cases. Ann Surg 234:572–579
28. Ramesh H, Prakash K, Lekha V, Jacob G, Venugopal A (2003) Are some cases of infected pancreatic necrosis treatable without intervention? Dig Surg 20:296–299
29. Runzi M, Niebel W, Goebell H, Gerken G, Layer P (2005) Severe acute pancreatitis: nonsurgical treatment of infected necroses. Pancreas 30:195–199
30. McFadden DW, Reber HA (1994) Indications for surgery in severe acute pancreatitis. Int J Pancreatol 15:83–90
31. Ranson JH (1995) The current management of acute pancreatitis. Adv Surg 28:93–112
32. McKay CJ, Evans S, Sinclair M, Carter CR, Imrie CW (1999) High early mortality rate from acute pancreatitis in Scotland, 1984–1995. Br J Surg 86:1302–1305
33. Kivilaakso E, Lempinen M, Makelainen A, Nikki P, Schroder T (1984) Pancreatic resection versus peritoneal lavation for acute fulminant pancreatitis. A randomized prospective study. Ann Surg 199:426–431
34. Schroder T, Sainio V, Kivisaari L, Puolakkainen P, Kivilaakso E, Lempinen M (1999) Pancreatic resection versus peritoneal lavage in acute necrotizing pancreatitis. A prospective randomized trial. Ann Surg 214:663–666
35. Tsiotos GG, Luque-de LE, Sarr MG (1998) Long-term outcome of necrotizing pancreatitis treated by necrosectomy. Br J Surg 85:1650–1653
36. Beger HG (1991) Operative management of necrotizing pancreatitis – necrosectomy and continuous closed postoperative lavage of the lesser sac. Hepatogastroenterology 38:129–133
37. Nordback I, Paajanen H, Sand J (1997) Prospective evaluation of a treatment protocol in patients with severe acute necrotising pancreatitis. Eur J Surg 163:357–364
38. Tsiotos GG, Luque-de LE, Soreide JA, Bannon MP, Zietlow SP, Baerga-Varela Y, Sarr MG (1998) Management of necrotizing pancreatitis by repeated operative necrosectomy using a zipper technique. Am J Surg 175:91–98
39. Kalfarentzos FE, Kehagias J, Kakkos SK, Petsas T, Kokkinis K, Gogos CA, Androulakis JA (1999) Treatment of patients with severe acute necrotizing pancreatitis based on prospective evaluation. Hepatogastroenterology 46:3249–3256
40. Beger HG, Buchler M, Bittner R, Block S, Nevalainen T, Roscher R (1988) Necrosectomy and postoperative local lavage in necrotizing pancreatitis. Br J Surg 75:207–212
41. vanSonnenberg E, Wittich GR, Chon KS, D'Agostino HB, Casola G, Easter D, Morgan RG, Walser EM, Nealon WH, Goodacre B, Stabile BE (1997) Percutaneous radiologic drainage of pancreatic abscesses. AJR Am J Roentgenol 168:979–984
42. Baril NB, Ralls PW, Wren SM, Selby RR, Radin R, Parekh D, Jabbour N, Stain SC (2000) Does an infected peripancreatic fluid collection or abscess mandate operation? Ann Surg 231:361–367
43. Lang EK, Paolini RM, Pottmeyer A (1991) The efficacy of palliative and definitive percutaneous versus surgical drainage of pancreatic abscesses and pseudocysts: a prospective study of 85 patients. South Med J 84:55–64
44. Lee MJ, Rattner DW, Legemate DA, Saini S, Dawson SL, Hahn PF, Warshaw AL, Mueller PR (1992) Acute complicated pancreatitis: redefining the role of interventional radiology. Radiol 183:171–174
45. Srikanth G, Sikora SS, Baijal SS, Ayyagiri A, Kumar A, Saxena R, Kapoor VK (2002) Pancreatic abscess: 10 years experience. ANZ J Surg 72:881–886
46. Villazon A, Villazon O, Terrazas F, Rana R (1991) Retroperitoneal drainage in the management of the septic phase of severe acute pancreatitis. World J Surg 15:103–107
47. Wilson C, McArdle CS, Carter DC, Imrie CW (1988) Surgical treatment of acute necrotizing pancreatitis. Br J Surg 75:1119–1123
48. Pederzoli P, Bassi C, Vesentini S, Girelli R, Cavallini G, Falconi M, Nifosi F, Riela A, Dagradi A (1990) Retroperitoneal and peritoneal drainage and lavage in the treatment of severe necrotizing pancreatitis. Surg Gynecol Obstet 170:197–203
49. Bradley EL III (1993) A fifteen year experience with open drainage for infected pancreatic necrosis. Surg Gynecol Obstet 177:215–222

Chapter 22

R. Bittner · B.M. Rau · H.G. Beger

Surgical Management of Pancreatic Abscess

Pancreatic infection is one of the major complication of acute pancreatitis. Due to improvements in surgical and intensive care management, most patients survive the initial phase of severe acute pancreatitis, but their lives are still at risk as soon as septic complications occur. Today, pancreatic infection is regarded as the leading cause of late death in severe acute pancreatitis [1–3] (Table 22.1). Bacterial infection of necrosis occurs in 40–70% of all patients with necrotizing pancreatitis [1,4,5]. Pancreatic abscess develops in about 10% of all patients suffering from a necrotizing pancreatitis and in about 3% of all patients with acute pancreatitis (Table 22.2) [6–8]. The definition of a pancreatic abscess as a distinct clinical entity in the late course of acute pancreatitis, different from infected necrosis, was provided by Bittner et al. [1,9]. The terms pancreatic abscess, pancreatic sepsis, pancreatic phlegmon, and infected necrosis have often been used as a synonym in the past, which has contributed to a considerable confusion about adequate therapeutic approaches and their results [10].

Table 22.1. Pancreatic abscess – high-risk group of severe acute pancreatitis

–	Localized collection of pus, surrounded by pseudocapsule [9]
–	Late after AP/NP (4th–6th week)
–	Necroses present in about 30–50%
–	Polymicrobial bacteria
	< Gram positive
	< aerobic germs
–	Candida infection 7–14%
–	Interventional/laparoscopic drainage + lavage first-choice
–	treatment to interrupt sepsis [25,33,34]

Definition

The term "pancreatic abscess" has been used to describe a heterogeneous group of different kinds of pancreatic infections. Peripancreatic abscess has been considered as an infected pancreatic pseudocyst, often as a sequela of chronic pancreatitis. These various definitions make a valid interpretation of studies and clinical data difficult [10].

Our current definition of pancreatic abscess has emerged from the results of clinical studies [1,9,11] and was accepted by the Atlanta Classification group as a late complication [12]. Pancreatic abscess is defined as a collection of purulent material encapsulated by a wall of fibrotic tissue, located either in the pancreas or in the retroperipancreatic region [3,9,11–13]. It is regarded as a sequel of severe pancreatitis developing in the 3rd–6th week after acute pancreatitis;

Table 22.2. Frequency of pancreatic infection in 427 patients (treated between May 1982 to December 1996 at the Department of Surgery, University of Ulm, Germany) with necrotizing pancreatitis (pancreatic necrosis/extrapancreatic fatty tissue necrosis, pancreatic abscess, or postacute pseudocyst). *NP* Necrotizing pancreatitis, *AP* acute pancreatitis

	Patients (*n*)	% of NP	% of AP
Infected necrosis	99	23.2%	6.9%
Pancreatic abscess	40	9.4%	2.8%
Infected pseudocyst after AP	7	1.6%	10.1%
TOTAL	146	34.2%	10.1%

Table 22.3. Clinical characteristics of infected necrosis and pancreatic abscess

	Infected pancreatic necrosis	Pancreatic abscess
Morphology	Diffuse spread of necrotic tissue	Encapsulated collections of purulent material
Bacteria	Monomicrobial infection in 70–80%	Polymicrobial infection in 40–60%
Clinical appearance	Severely ill, septic patient	Indolent presentation possible, severe septic courses are rare
Hospital admission	During the early phase of acute pancreatitis (2nd to 3rd week)	Usually 1 month after the acute phase of severe pancreatitis
Systemic complications	Frequently present	Frequently absent
Mortality	20–50%	5–10%

the content of the abscess may be either necrotic or purulent. Bacteria identified by fine-needle puncture (FNP) of a pancreatic abscess are polymicrobial, Gram-negative, and Gram-positive, resembling intestinal bacterial patterns. Pancreatic abscess and infected pancreatic necrosis are two different clinical entities of acute pancreatitis. Infected necrosis is characterized by diffuse spread in the retroperitoneum without any signs of encapsulation [1,3] and develops in the first 3 weeks of acute pancreatitis [14]. Pancreatic abscess is regarded as a late sequel of the disease developing after disappearance of acute pancreatitis, mostly in the 4th–6th week after acute pancreatitis (Table 22.3).

In a large series, between 2 and 9% of all patients with necrotizing pancreatitis were reported to develop a pancreatic abscess [3,11,13,15]. In our own series of patients, the frequency of pancreatic abscess was comparable to the rates published in the literature (Table 22.2). Infection of postacute pseudocysts is rare; however, clinically, it resembles pancreatic abscess.

Pathogenesis

The underlying causes of pancreatic abscess are those of acute pancreatitis (Table 22.1). Patients with alcoholic acute pancreatitis have a relatively low risk of abscess formation, where as those who develop postoperative or posttraumatic pancreatitis are frequently complicated by late abscesses [3].

As far as pathogenesis is concerned, pancreatic or peripancreatic necrosis becomes infected by bacterial translocation from the intestine. Pancreatic abscess develops from postacute or peripancreatic exudates or necroses. Bacterial superinfection leads to abscess formation. There are, however, differences between infected necrosis and abscess.

Infected pancreatic necrosis is characterized by a diffuse retroperitoneal spread of pancreatic necrosis or peripancreatic fatty tissue. Its formation is associated with the liberation of biologically active mediators, leading to a systemic response. In contrast to the diffuse inflammation of pancreatic necrosis, pancreatic abscess is a collection of pus surrounded by a fibrotic capsule. This does not necessarily imply that a pancreatic abscess develops solitarily, because a considerable number of patients present with multifocal abscesses. A literature review revealed solitary abscess in only 38% of the patients, whereas multiple abscess formation was found in 62% [3]. Moreover, they are not necessarily located in the pancreas. In our own series, in one-third of cases, abscesses were detected in the pancreas or the lesser sac, while another one-third of patients showed a left-sided location near the pancreatic tail.

Bacterial Spectrum

The bacterial spectrum of pancreatic abscess is similar to the pattern of infected pancreatic necrosis (Table 22.4). Interestingly, the majority of pancreatic abscesses harbor a polymicrobial bacterial or fungal spectrum, whereas monomicrobial infection predominates in infected pancreatic necrosis [3,9,11,16]. As mentioned above, the intestine is most likely source for pancreatic infection, but the ultimate pathway into the lesser sac and into the pancreas remains obscure. There are various routes of bacterial spread under discussion, which include direct transmural penetration from the colon, spread along the lymphatic ducts from the gut, hematogenetic dissemination, and ascending invasion from infected bile [3,16,17].

Table 22.4. Bacteriological findings in pancreatic abscess and infected necrosis [1,9,11,32]

Pancreatic abscess [9,11]		Infected pancreatic necrosis [1]		Infected necrosis after prior antibiotic treatment [5]	
Polymicrobial abscess	62%	Polymicrobial infection	36%		
Staphylococcus aureus	15%	Enterococci	21%		
Enterococci	15%	S. aureus	11%	Gram positive	84%
		S. epidermidis	9%		
		Gram positive	41%		
Escherichia coli	14%	E. coli	28%		
Klebsiella	9%	Klebsiella	13%		
Pseudomonas	9%	Pseudomonas	3%	Gram negative	40%
Proteus	6%	Proteus	2%		
		Gram negative	46%	Fungi	36%
Others	13%			Anaerobes	4%
Fungi	7%	Candida	6%		
Anaerobes	12%	Anaerobes	7%		

Table 22.5. Pancreatic abscess and infected necrosis – two different clinical entities of severe acute pancreatitis [16]. *CRP* C-reactive protein

	Infected pancreatic necrosis (77 patients)	Pancreatic abscess (31 patients)
Time between onset of symptoms and admission	9.2 (0–83) days	29.1 (2–127) days
Hyperamylasemia at admission	65 patients (84.4%)	9 patients (29.0%)
Serum CRP >120 mg/l at admission	77 patients (100%)	0 patients
Duration of hospital stay	62.5 (1–238) days	37.0 (12–140) days
Pulmonary failure	55 patients (71.5%)	7 patients (22.6%)
Renal failure	34 patients (44.2%)	1 patient (9.7%)
Shock	24 patients (31.2%)	3 patients (9.7%)
Mortality	16 patients (20.8%)	2 patients (6.5%)

Clinical Presentation

The typical clinical picture of patients with infected pancreatic necrosis is that of severe sepsis with multi-organ failure and persistence of signs of acute pancreatitis [1,3,15]. In contrast, pancreatic abscess is a local complication in the late course after acute pancreatitis with moderate abdominal symptoms, but only infrequently associated with systemic complications in terms of organ failure. In most cases signs of acute pancreatitis have disappeared.

Fever, leukocytosis, and uncharacteristic upper abdominal pain are frequent symptoms in both groups of patients. Undulating fever has been reported to be one of the characteristics of the abscess patients, arising from intermittent and transient bacteremia [3]. Several studies have shown that none of these three clinical signs can be used for discrimination between pancreatic abscess and infected necrosis. An impotant difference between the two entities is the time to clinical manifestation after onset of acute pancreatitis. Infected necrosis is usually diagnosed early in the course of acute pancreatitis; pancreatic abscess develops several weeks after acute pancreatitis (Table 22.5).

With regard to severity scores pancreatic abscess patients are reported to have a low Acute Physiology and Chronic Health Evaluation II (APACHE II) score and Ranson signs below two points compared with infected pancreatic necrosis. Pulmonary insufficien-

Table 22.6. Laboratory findings and clinical symptoms in pancreatic abscess (data collection, publication 2000–2006) [16]

Finding/Symptom	Frequency (percentage of patients)
Abdominal pain and tenderness	60–90
Fever	75–80
Leukocytosis	60–80
Hyperamylasemia	10–30
Palpable mass	20–50
Pulmonary failure	15–20
Renal failure	5–10

cy, renal failure, and shock are rarely seen in this type of pancreatic infections but are common features in infected pancreatic necrosis [9,11,16]. At the time of hospital admission, leukocytosis is reported to be present in 60–80% of patients [9,11,16,18] regardless of the underlying type of pancreatic infection (Table 22.6). Hyperamylasemia is found only in 10–30% of the abscess patients (Table 22.6), and serum measurements show a statistically significant lower level of C-reactive protein concentrations than those observed in patients with infected necrosis.

Diagnostic Imaging Procedures

Contrast-enhanced computed tomography (CECT) scan is the gold standard for the diagnosis of necrotizing pancreatitis as well as pancreatic abscess. The lack of contrast enhancement in necrotic tissue areas provides information about the extent and location of pancreatic necroses. For pancreatic abscess, the clinical relevance of CECT scanning has been examined in several studies [8–11,13,16]. In our own series pancreatic abscess was correctly diagnosed by CECT scan in 56% of patients. This low sensitivity was due to the inability of this imaging method to discriminate between abscesses and pseudocysts. In the computed tomography (CT) scan, both entities appear as morphological well-defined collections of fluid. The presence of gas in fluid collections is a pathognomonic feature of abscess formation, but only a minority of abscesses contain gas bubbles [11]. Thus, the clinical signs and symptoms of sepsis must be used in combination with CECT scans for the diagnosis of abscesses. Imaging-guided aspiration of potentially infected fluid collections (FNP) provide information about the bacterial content. Using CECT scan and fine-needle aspiration for diagnosis, detection rates of pancreatic abscess are 90–95% [9,13]. The use of ultrasonography in severe acute pancreatitis is limited. Abdominal meteorism is a frequent finding in severe acute pancreatitis and thus precludes the use of ultrasound as a reliable imaging technique of the pancreas. Like CT, ultrasound can be used as guidance for diagnostic aspiration. If CT yields encapsulated fluid collections in the pancreas or the peripancreatic region and the patients suffer from abdominal infection or abdominal sepsis, ultrasound investigations should be used to perform a fine-needle aspiration. The aspirates should be Gram-stained and cultured for further identification of the bacterial/fungal species, and examined for pancreatic enzyme contents.

Clinical Management

Pancreatic abscess is a late consequence after necrotizing pancreatitis that develops after the 1st month of the disease. Antibiotic treatment can only be considered as a supplementary treatment for surgical or interventional drainage of pancreatic abscess. Its purpose is to provide prophylaxis against systemic bacterial dissemination and systemic septic complications. It cannot be expected that systemic antibiotic treatment will lead to a significant reduction of the rate of bacterial infection, because the wall of the pancreatic abscesses is poorly supplied with blood vessels, thus preventing penetration of antibiotic substances into the abscess [32]. Pharmacodynamic investigations suggest that imipenem, quinolones, or third-generation cephalosporins are the most effective antibiotic drugs that will achieve sufficient pancreatic tissue concentrations for the treatment of septic complications of acute pancreatitis [19]. Clinical data have confirmed these results for necrotizing pancreatitis with infected necrosis [20–23].

Interventional Treatment

Progress in the field of ultrasound and CECT has led to various attempts for nonsurgical management of pancreatic abscesses. Interventionally, one or more percutaneous catheters are placed in the region of interest under CT or ultrasound guidance. The first reports documented success rates of 70–100% [24,25]. The interventional approach has limitations set by the amount of necrotic tissue that cannot be evacuated by the catheters and the fact that a considerable percentage of pancreatic abscesses are multifocal or septated

[26]. More recent approaches to drain collections like pancreatic abscess have employed the use of multiple catheters or large-bore catheters up to 30 Fr as a rule. Recently published prospective studies have reported success rates of 40–60% when interventional percutaneous drainage is applied as first-choice treatment for pancreatic abscess [26–29, 33–34].

Surgical Treatment

The standard surgical approach is drainage of the abscess by laparoscopic or open techniques. A variety of surgical procedures have been proposed for pancreatic abscesses: Extensive debridement in combination with either tube drainage [13,18] or open packing [13] debridement with tube drainage and postoperative continuous lavage [9,11,16,30,31], or even open packing with repeated debridement as currently in use [7]. None of these procedures has proven to be superior to the others on the basis of prospective controlled trials. In the authors' institution, a first-choice approach is interventional treatment of pancreatic abscess by percutaneous or retroperitoneal placement of drainage tubes, evacuation of necrotic material, and the institution of a continuous local lavage of the abscess cavity [9,16]. The success rate of minimally invasive surgical approaches, whether they are performed in a transabdominal or retroperitoneal way, is high. The resolution of clinical sepsis signs occurs after successful evacuation of pancreatic abscess in between 2 and 5 days after percutaneous drainage [33–34].

Morbidity and Mortality of Pancreatic Abscess

In comparison with infected pancreatic necrosis, which carries a mortality rate of between 15 and 30%, pancreatic abscess is accompanied by a much lower rate of lethal outcome. Mortality rates of 5–10% are reported by different surgical series [9,11,13,16], regardless of the operative technique applied. Similar observations have been made in terms of specific intensive care support such as mechanical ventilation, dialysis/hemofiltration, and vasopressors, which are rarely necessary in patients with pancreatic abscess.

References

1. Beger HG, Bittner R, Büchler M (1986) Bacterial contamination of pancreatic necrosis. Gastroenterology 91:433–438
2. Isenmann R, Büchler MW (1994) Infection and acute pancreatitis. Br J Surg 81:1707–1708
3. Widdison AL, Karanjia ND (1993) Pancreatic infection complicating acute pancreatitis. Br J Surg 80:148–154
4. Bassi C, Falconi M, Girelli R, Nifosi F, Elio A, Martini N, Pederzoli P (1989) Microbiological findings in severe pancreatitis. Surg Res Commun 5:1–4
5. Gerzof SG, Banks PA, Robbins AH, Johnson WC, Spechler SJ, Wetzner SM, Snider JM, Langevin RE, Jay ME (1987) Early diagnosis of pancreatic infection by computed tomography-guided aspiration. Gastroenterology 93:1315–1320
6. Hurley JE, Vargish T (1987) Early diagnosis and outcome of pancreatic abscesses in pancreatitis. Am Surg 53:29–33
7. Pemberton JH, Becker JM, Dozois RR, Nagorney DM, Ilstrup D, Remine WH (1986) Controlled open lesser sac drainage for pancreatic abscess. Ann Surg 203:600–604
8. Malangoni MA, Richardson JD, Shallcross JC, Seiler JG, Polk HC (1986) Factors contributing to fatal outcome after treatment of pancreatic abscess. Ann Surg 203:605–613
9. Bittner R, Block S, Büchler M, Beger HG (1987) Pancreatic abscess and infected necrosis: different local septic complications in acute pancreatitis. Dig Dis Sci 32:1082–1087
10. Lumsden A, Bradley EL III (1990) Secondary pancreatic infections. Surg Gynecol Obstet 170:459–467
11. Bassi C, Vesentini S, Nifosi F, Girelli R, Falconi M, Elio A, Pederzoli P (1990) Pancreatic abscess and other pus-harboring collections related to pancreatitis: a review of 108 cases. World J Surg 14:505–512
12. Frey C, Reber HA (1993) Clinically based classification system for acute pancreatitis. Pancreas 8:738–743
13. Howard TJ, Wiebke EA, Mogavero G, Kopecky K, Baer JC, Sherman S, Hawes RH, Lehman GA, Goulet RJ, Madura JA (1995) Classification and treatment of local septic complications in acute pancreatitis. Am J Surg 170:44–50
14. Isenmann R, Büchler M, Uhl W, Malfertheiner P, Martini M, Beger HG (1993) Pancreatic necrosis: an early finding in severe acute pancreatitis. Pancreas 8:358–361
15. Beger HG, Büchler M, Bittner R, Block S, Nevalainen T, Roscher R (1988) Necrosectomy and postoperative local lavage in necrotizing pancreatitis. Br J Surg 75:207–212
16. Schoenberg MH, Rau B, Beger HG (1995) Diagnosis and therapy of primary pancreatic abscess. Chirurg 66:588–596
17. Bradley EL (1989) antibiotics in acute pancreatitis. Am J Surg 158:472–478
18. Fink AS, Hiatt JR, Pitt HA, Bennion RS, DeSouza LR, McCoy RD, Meyer JH, Thompson JE Jr, Webster JL, Wilson SE (1988) Indolent presentation of pancreatic abscess. Arch Surg 123:1067–1072
19. Büchler M, Malfertheiner P, Frieß H (1992) Human pancreatic tissue concentration of bacterial antibiotics. Gastroenterology 103:1902–1908
20. Pederzoli P, Bassi C, Vesentini S, Campedelli A (1993) A randomized multicenter clinical trial of antibiotic prophylaxis of septic complications in acute necrotizing pancreatitis with imipenem. Surg Gynecol Obstet 176:480–483
21. Sainio V, Kemppainen E, Puolakkainen P, Taavitsainen M, Kivisaari L, Valtonen V, Haapiainen R, Schroder T, Kivilaakso E (1995) Early antibiotic treatment in acute necrotizing pancreatitis. Lancet 346:663–667

22. Isenmann R, Rünzi M, Kron M, Kahl S, Kraus D, Jung N, Maier L, Malfertheiner P, Goebell H, Beger HG; German Antibiotics in Severe Acute Pancreatitis Study Group (2004) Prophylactic antibiotic treatment in patients with predicted severe acute pancreatitis: a placebo-controlled, double-blind trial. Gastroenterology126:997–1004
23. Dellinger EP, Telado JM, Soto N (2007) Prophylactic antibiotic treatment in patients with severe acute pancreatitis: a double-blind placebo-controlled study. Ann Surg 245:674–683
24. Karlson KB, Martin EC, Fankuchen EI, Mattern RF, Schultz RW, Casarella WJ (1982) Percutaneous drainage of pancreatic pseudocysts and abscesses. Radiology 142:619–624
25. Freeny PC, Lewis GP, Traverso LW, Ryan JA (1988) Infected pancreatic fluid collections: percutaneous catheter drainage. Radiology 167:435–441
26. Mithofer K, Mueller PR, Warshaw AL (1997) Interventional and surgical treatment of pancreatic abscess. World J Surg 21:162–168
27. Lang EK, Paolini RM, Pottmeyer A (1991) The efficacy of palliative and definitive percutaneous versus surgical drainage of pancreatic abscesses and pseudocysts: a prospective study of 85 patients. South Med J 84:55–63
28. Rotman N, Mathieu D, Anglade MC, Fagniez PL (1992) Failure of percutaneous drainage of pancreatic abscess complicating severe acute pancreatitis. Surg Gynecol Obstet 174:141–145
29. van Sonnenberg E, Wittich GR, Chon KS, D'Agostino HB, Casola G, Easter D, Morgan RG, Walzer EM, Nealon WH, Gooacre B, Stabile BE (1997) Percutaneous radiologic drainage of pancreatic abscesses. Am J Roentgenol 168:979–984
30. Nicholson ML, Mortensen NJ, Esoiner HJ (1988) Pancreatic abscess: results of prolonged irrigation of the pancreatic bed after surgery. Br J Surg 75:88–91
31. Stanten R, Frey CF (1990) Comprehensive management of acute necrotizing pancreatitis and pancreatic abscess. Arch Surg 125:1269–1275
32. Gloor B, Muller CA, Wormi M, Stabel PF, Redaelli C, Uhl W, Büchler MW (2001) Pancreatic infection in severe acute pancreatitis. The role of fungus and multiresistant organisms. Arch Surg 136:592–596
33. Carter CR, McKay CJ, Imrie CW (2000) Percutaneous necrosectomy and sinus tract endoscopy in the management of infected pancreatic necrosis: an initial experience. Ann Surg 232:175–180
34. Echenique AM, Sleeman D, Yrizarry J, Scagnelli T, Guerra JJ Jr, Casillas VJ, Huson H, Russell E (1998) Percutaneous catheter-directed debridement of infected pancreatic necrosis: results in 20 patients. J Vasc Interv Radiol 9:565–571

Chapter 23

B. M. Rau · H. G. Beger

Surgical Management of Pseudocysts after Acute Pancreatitis

Pancreatic pseudocysts are a frequent complication of acute pancreatitis and remain a challenging problem. The advent of advanced imaging techniques has improved considerably our knowledge about the natural course of pancreatic pseudocysts and driven the management away from surgery toward conservative approaches. More than 50% of postacute pseudocysts are asymptomatic and resolve spontaneously over time, whereas some form of drainage is required if symptoms or complications arise. To choose the most appropriate approach to drainage, a precise classification into acute- and acute-on-chronic-type pseudocysts with the assessment of pancreatic duct morphology is of central importance. A variety of operative, interventional, radiologic, and endoscopic techniques for cyst drainage are currently available, with a clear shift from open surgery to interventional approaches over the past decades. However, as a result of incorrect or vague terminology, interinstitutional comparison of data is often difficult and controversies in management and outcome are the consequence. A review of well-defined patient series since the 1990s reveals that open surgery of pancreatic pseudocysts carries a long-term recurrence rate of 8% and a hospital mortality of only 3%. The results of recent laparoscopic techniques to pseudocyst drainage in limited patient numbers compares well with the short- and long-term outcome of the open procedures. This chapter provides an overview of the current evidence regarding the natural course, diagnostic aspects, and operative management strategies of postacute pancreatic pseudocysts.

Definition

Pancreatic pseudocysts are the most frequent complication of acute and chronic pancreatitis or pancreatic trauma, and constitute the vast majority of cystic lesions of the pancreas. Morphologically, pancreatic pseudocysts are defined as a collection of pancreatic juice delineated by a nonepithelialized wall of fibrotic tissue [1, 2]. In contrast, true cysts of the pancreas, which are either congenital or neoplastic, possess an epithelium and occur in about 20% of all cystic lesions of the pancreas [3]. Postacute pseudocysts are a late complication after an acute attack requiring 4–6 weeks until complete maturation. The pseudocyst content is usually sterile and rich in pancreatic enzymes. The Atlanta classification has provided a widely used system to define pancreatitis-related local complications since 1993 [1]. However, inconsistent use of terminologies or definitions continues to be a major problem, still causing considerable confusion in comparing treatment algorithms and outcome. There are several local complications that should not be confused with pancreatic pseudocysts as such. The presence of bacteria without clinical signs of sepsis represents contamination only; however, if clinical signs of sepsis are associated, the pseudocyst should rather be termed as pancreatic abscess. Unlike mature postacute pseudocysts, acute fluid collections lack a defined wall because they are only confined by the anatomic space in which they arise, and represent a distinct entity [1]. More recently, the term "organized necrosis" refers to the evolution of necrosis to an encapsulated, circumscribed intra- or extrapancreatic collection of devitalized tissue that develops several weeks after an acute attack of necrotizing pancreatitis [4].

Incidence

The widespread application of imaging techniques such as ultrasonography and computed tomography (CT) has advanced considerably the knowledge of the natural history of postacute pseudocysts, and follow-up studies reveal an incidence of 2–15% [5–8]. Among 1619 patients with acute pancreatitis treated at the Department of General Surgery, University Hospital of Ulm from 1982 to 1999, we observed 120 (7.4%) postacute pseudocysts after a median of 28 days following an acute attack of pancreatitis, of whom 97 were symptomatic and required further treatment [9]. The underlying etiology of postacute pseudocysts varies depending on the geographical area and the age of the patients. Postacute pseudocysts in children and young adults are more commonly secondary to trauma or hereditary pancreatitis [10], whereas pseudocysts related to alcoholic pancreatitis tend to be more frequent in male adults [11, 12]. However, the assessment of a possible relationship between etiology and incidence of postacute pseudocysts is often hampered by the lack of further stratification into true postacute pseudocysts after an acute attack versus pseudocysts in patients with underlying chronic pancreatitis that arise secondary to recurrent episodes of pancreatitis or even without a recognizable preceding episode of acute pancreatitis [11, 13]. In well-defined patients series with postacute pseudocysts following an acute attack, etiology does not seem to play a major role as far as incidence and outcome is concerned [8, 12, 14, 15]. The severity of the preceding acute attack has been shown to be a major determinant of subsequent postacute pseudocyst formation [16, 17].

Pathophysiology

Postacute pseudocysts are the result of trauma, inflammation or necrosis. After an attack of acute pancreatitis, inflammatory cells and granulation tissue form a membrane that consecutively encapsulates the damaged or devitalized tissue. Another possible mechanism of cyst formation is ductular disruption with continuous leakage of pancreatic secretions into the interstitium, which also evokes an inflammatory response [2]. Pseudocysts after acute pancreatitis usually require 4–6 weeks to develop the characteristic membrane, which is stable enough to allow surgical anastomosis and internal drainage [11, 18].

Macroscopically, postacute pseudocysts are round or ovoid and may attain a considerable size of up to 30 cm in diameter, in contrast to the often small, type III pseudocysts in chronic pancreatitis [14]. The location can be extra- or intrapancreatic without any preference concerning the head, body, or tail of the gland. However, large cysts most frequently impose as a separate mass lying beside the pancreas, frequently in the lesser sac, but also extend retroperitoneally between the stomach and the transverse colon or the liver, and occasionally may be located in the mediastinum or the spleen [19–22]. A communication between the cyst cavity and the ductal system may be present in postacute pseudocysts and is frequently associated with underlying chronic pancreatitis [11, 23].

The cyst content is usually watery fluid and often brown in color due to old blood or necrotic tissue. In general, pancreatic enzyme concentrations of amylase, lipase, and trypsin are higher, and protein and albumin levels are lower than systemic concentrations [24–26]. The histological hallmark of pancreatic pseudocysts is the lack of an epithelial lining within the wall of the cavity. Depending on the age, the capsule increases in thickness, but maintains the microscopic architecture of four different zones. However, the pseudocyst wall remains a dynamic structure and even in "old " cysts is subject to continuous biological changes. The possibility of spontaneous resolution as well as recurrence highlights the activity present within the wall of these structures [20].

Natural Course

The first studies on the natural course of pancreatic pseudocysts date back to the mid 1970s, when diagnosis was restricted to clinical symptoms or indirect radiologic imaging techniques. At that time, a spontaneous resolution rate was reported in 10–30% of postacute pseudocysts [27, 28]. In another series, postacute pseudocysts after acute alcoholic pancreatitis were inferred from barium meal studies or angiography and were found to resolve in over 70% within 3–12 weeks. However, the authors were not able to ascertain whether the masses they had studied were pseudocysts rather than inflammatory enlargement of the pancreas [29]. Some years later, Bradley and coworkers conducted the first follow-up study in 54 patients with pancreatic pseudocysts by performing ultrasound, and observed a resolution rate of 40% by 6 weeks after the acute attack; thereafter, resolution was unlikely and the incidence of related complications rose [30]. Similar findings were made by Martin et al. [31] and by Warshaw and Rattner [32] in their surgical series, who observed at best persisting symptoms and at worst an increased risk of complications, if pseudocysts failed to resolve after 6–7 weeks of observation. Follow-up series from Johns Hopkins [33] and the Mayo Clinic [34] using CT scans subsequently confirmed a high spontaneous resolution rate of 50% and more in postacute pseudocysts. On the other hand, both studies challenged the previous conclusions that follow-up for more than 6 weeks after the acute episode is at best useless and at worst hazardous, because resolution in their patients took place up to 1 year of follow-up without increasing complication rates. More recent series continue to report a high resolution rate even after prolonged observation of several months [8, 35].

The size of the pseudocyst has been considered as another important factor in the natural course. Cysts of less than 6–7 cm in diameter are more likely to resolve spontaneously [6, 8, 33–40]. In our series we observed a cyst diameter of less than 6 cm in 83% of 23 patients with asymptomatic postacute pseudocysts and expectant management, whereas in the symptomatic group undergoing surgical or interventional therapy, the cyst diameter was 6 cm or more in 76% [9].

Classification of Postacute Pseudocysts

For an improved, management-driven stratification of pancreatic pseudocysts, D'Egidio and Schein proposed a classification identifying three distinct types in 1991 [11]. Type I, or acute "postnecrotic," pseudocysts occur after an episode of acute pancreatitis without abnormality of the pancreatic duct or the presence of a cyst–duct communication. Type II cysts are also postacute or "postnecrotic" cysts, which develop after an episode of acute-on-chronic pancreatitis. Duct alterations without strictures are the rule, and a pseudocyst–duct communication is frequently found. Type III cysts, defined as "retention" cysts, develop as a consequence of chronic pancreatitis and are uniformly associated with duct strictures and a pseudocyst–duct communication. This was the first attempt at rendering a therapeutic concept to the underlying pathophysiology (Table 23.1). The high effectiveness of this approach was confirmed by a Chinese study comprising 73 patients with pancreatic pseudocysts [23].

Nealon and Walser described recently a corresponding, but more detailed classification system directing the therapeutic approach according to the findings of endoscopic retrograde cholangiopancreatography (ERCP) [41]. Their classification includes seven subsets based on pancreatic ductal anatomy and presence/absence of a cyst–duct communication determining subsequent management (Table 23.2). Both studies allow the clinician to choose the most appropriate approach to patients with pancreatic pseudocysts by avoiding a high failure rate of simple aspiration or percutaneous drainage alone, if pancreatic duct disease is present.

Clinical Presentation

The typical clinical signs and symptoms of postacute pseudocysts become apparent when the characteristic pseudocyst membrane has been formed. Because the acute phase of the preceding acute attack already has subsided at that time, specific organ and systemic

Table 23.1. Classification of pancreatic pseudocysts by D'Egidio and Schein [11]

Characteristics	Type I cyst	Type II cyst	Type III cyst
Synonymous	"postacute"	"postacute-on-chronic"	"retention"
Preceding attack of acute pancreatitis	Yes	Yes	No
Pancreatic duct morphology	Normal	Abnormal	Strictured
Duct–cyst communication	Rarely	Frequently	Always
Chronic pancreatitis	No	Yes	Yes

Table 23.2. Nealon and Walser classification based on ductal anatomy, as assessed by endoscopic retrograde cholangiopancreatography [41]

	Ductal anatomy	Duct–cyst communication
Type I	Normal	No
Type II	Normal	Yes
Type III	Normal with stricture	No
Type IV	Normal with stricture	Yes
Type V	Normal	Complete obstruction
Type VI	Chronic pancreatitis	No
Type VII	Chronic pancreatitis	Yes

Table 23.3. Symptomatic postacute pancreatic pseudocysts: clinical symptoms and systemic disease severity on admission of 97 patients (Department of General Surgery, University of Ulm, 05/1982–12/1999, unpublished data)

Clinical symptoms:	*n*	(%)
Pain	74	(76%)
Nausea/vomiting	26	(27%)
Palpable mass	25	(26%)
Abdominal rebound	12	(12%)
Jaundice	6	(6%)
Sepsis	5	(5%)
Subileus/Ileus	5	(5%)
Disease severity/organ failure:	***n***	**(%)**
Apache II (median, range)	4	(0-14)
Pulmonary insufficiency	3	(3%)
Renal insufficiency	1	(1%)
Shock	1	(1%)

complications are rare, and non-specific clinical symptoms are dominating. On clinical examination, upper abdominal pain, nausea and vomiting, weight loss, ileus, jaundice, or a palpable abdominal mass are frequent findings [29, 37, 40, 42–44]. These symptoms are the consequence of obstruction or compression of adjacent organs or vessels and depend on the location and the size of the cyst [45]. In the occasional catastrophic bleeding from a pancreatic pseudocyst, hematemesis or melaena accompanied by hypotension and shock may occur [34, 43, 46].

The clinical presentation in our own series of 97 symptomatic patients with postacute pseudocysts is shown in Table 23.3. The leading symptom was abdominal pain in 74%, followed by nausea/vomiting and a palpable abdominal mass in about 25% each. Organ failure was observed in less than 5% of all patients, the moderate clinical severity is reflected by low Apache II scores.

Complications

There are five major complications associated with postacute pancreatic pseudocysts: infection, obstruction, hemorrhage, rupture, and internal fistulae. In general, these complications are rare and affect only about 10% of patients, usually after necrotizing attacks of acute pancreatitis.

Infection

Infection occurs variably in initially sterile pseudocysts. If bacteria are isolated from a postacute pancreatic pseudocyst, they often represent contamination only and are most likely of little clinical significance. Bacteriologically positive cyst content is found in 8–55% of pancreatic pseudocysts [15, 47–49]. However, little is known about the incidence of infected pseudocysts, correctly defined as pseudocysts with a non-purulent bacterial positive content in the presence of clinical signs of sepsis such as fever and elevated white blood count [50]. Moreover, it is still unclear as to what extent a transformation of contaminated into infected pseudocysts or even pancreatic abscesses does occur. Upon strict definition, few studies report an infection rate of around 15% [30, 33, 50]; in our series, infected pseudocysts were found in 11% (10 of 89 patients undergoing open surgery).

Obstruction

Obstruction of the alimentary tract most commonly occurs at the esophagogastric junction, the gastric outlet, or the duodenum; the latter is often associated with jaundice. Occasionally, a small or large bowel obstruction may be caused by a postacute pseudocyst. The frequency of obstructive symptoms depends on the size and location of the cyst. In our series, all patients who suffered from obstructive symptoms had either a cyst size of more than 6 cm in diameter or a cyst location close to the duodenum. In terms of obstructive jaundice, fibrotic stricture of the intrapancreatic portion of the common bile duct rather than pressure on the duct by the pseudocyst may be present, thus demanding additional intervention beyond pseudocyst drainage [51].

Rupture

Spontaneous rupture of pancreatic pseudocysts is possible in different ways. The cyst may rupture into the free peritoneal cavity causing signs of acute peritonitis in severe cases, or manifests as pancreatic ascites in a more indolent fashion. The intestinal rupture of a pseudocyst, especially into the stomach, the duodenum, or the colon carries an increased mortality and may be accompanied by significant hemorrhage [52, 53]. In some patients, however, transenteric rupture is the mechanism for sudden resolution of their symptoms without significant complications [52].

Hemorrhage

Hemorrhage is an uncommon, but the most feared and life-threatening complication of postacute pseudocysts, and carries a mortality rate of 20% and higher [22, 54]. Hemorrhage associated with a pancreatic pseudocyst may be due to several pathophysiological conditions. Bleeding can be caused by either the splenic vessels, which are incorporated into the wall of the pseudocyst, or by pseudoaneurysm formation following angiogenesis in the cyst membrane, with leakage into the cyst cavity. Another mechanism is the rupture of a vessel stretched across the internal diameter of an enlarging pseudocyst. Gastrointestinal bleeding from gastric or esophageal varices may occur if left-sided portal hypertension or splenic vein occlusion is caused by the pseudocyst. A rarity is the so called "hemosuccus pancreaticus", if blood passes via the pancreatic duct into the duodenum as a consequence of a ruptured pseudoaneurysm [55].

Internal Fistulae

Internal fistulae result from disruption of a pseudocyst involving the pancreatic duct with subsequent drainage into the peritoneal (pancreatic ascites) or the pleural cavity (pancreatic pleural effusion). In more than half of all patients with internal pancreatic fistulae, an underlying leak from a pseudocyst is found and a history of a preceding episode of alcoholic pancreatitis can be elicited in at least 86% of these patients [56].

Diagnostic Work-Up

Once history, clinical symptoms, and physical examination are suspicious of a pancreatic pseudocyst a patients requires further laboratory tests and imaging procedures for further therapeutic decision making.

Laboratory Evaluation

In instances of postacute pancreatic pseudocysts, biochemical parameters are of limited value. At the time of diagnosis, less than 50% of the patients present with serum amylase or lipase values above normal limits, and an even smaller percentage have leukocytosis, increased C-reactive protein concentrations, or abnormal liver chemistry. On the other hand, abnormal laboratory parameters are suggestive of complications such as obstructive jaundice or infection, and further directs diagnostic work-up toward specific imaging or diagnostic fine-needle aspiration. Therefore, a full laboratory evaluation is strongly recommended in any patient.

In the absence of preceding inflammatory pancreatic disease or trauma, the differential diagnosis of a cystic pancreatic malignancy has to be taken in account. This is of specific importance, because imaging-based differentiation between benign pancreatic pseudocysts and cystadenomas or cystadenocarcinomas is sometimes impossible and may lead to inappropriate treatment with serious consequences [57]. Besides cytologic analysis, biochemical analysis of the cyst fluid for elevated tumor markers such as carinoembryonic antigen (CEA), CA-19-9, CA 72-4, and CA-125 can be helpful in this context. Whereas intracystic fluid of pseudocysts usually contains low levels of CEA, CA-19-9, and CA 125, amylase and lipase content is high [3, 58–60]. Although the sensitivity and positive-predictive value of tumor marker determinations from cyst fluid are less than 50%, specificity and negative-predictive values have been found at 80–98% with CEA yielding the best results [3, 58]. However, in postacute and chronic pseudocysts, one must remember that pancreatic enzymes may degrade over time within the cyst, and in longstanding and/or chronic pseudocysts, amylase or lipase concentrations are low.

Imaging Procedures

Contrast-Enhanced CT and Magnetic Resonance Imaging

Since the early 1980s, radiologic imaging procedures have gained increasing importance for diagnosing pancreatic pseudocysts and have become indispensable for the diagnostic work-up [61]. Thin-section CT with intravenous and oral contrast (contrast-enhanced CT, CE-CT) represents the imaging procedure of choice to evaluate known or suspected cystic lesions of the pancreas. A mature postinflammatory pancreatic pseudocyst appears as a round, low-attenuation, fluid-filled, and mostly unilocular structure surrounded by a contrast-enhancing wall within or adjacent to the pancreas. Although transabdominal ultrasound is an extremely valuable screening method with similar diagnostic accuracy, CE-CT is still superior, because it is less operator-dependent and provides better information about anatomic relationships to surrounding tissue as well as related intra-abdominal pathologies. Due to technical improvements in recent years, magnetic resonance imaging (MRI) is being used with increasing frequency. Contrast-enhanced MRI offers distinct advantages such as lack of radiation exposure, better characterization of morphologic features for sequelae of acute pancreatitis, and differentiating benign from potentially malignant cystic lesions. Limitations are still a lower availability and significantly higher cost compared with CE-CT.

Endoscopic Retrograde Cholangiopancreatography

For the basic diagnostic work-up of patients with postacute pancreatic pseudocysts, endoscopic retrograde cholangiopancreatography (ERCP) is not routinely necessary. However, if a symptomatic pancreatic pseudocyst requires treatment, ERCP has been shown to be an extremely helpful tool for selecting the appropriate management. Since pseudocyst–duct communications or pancreatic duct abnormalities due to underlying chronic pancreatitis have a significant impact on the choice and long-term outcome of treatment, ERCP is strongly recommended [11, 16, 23, 41]. It should be kept in mind, however, that ERCP carries the risk of inducing or exacerbating acute pancreatitis or infecting the pseudocyst. Therefore, it is recommended that ERCP should be performed only in patients for whom some kind of intervention is planned and who are being treated with broad-spectrum antibiotics [62]. Currently, magnetic resonance cholangiopancreatography is supplanting ERCP for assessing pancreatic and biliary duct morphology, because it also images adjacent structures, has similar diagnostic accuracy, and is noninvasive, but with the limitations already mentioned above [63].

Endoscopic Ultrasonography

Very recently endoscopic ultrasonography (EUS) is gaining increasing popularity in the diagnostic and therapeutic respect. EUS provides detailed information about cyst morphology such as septae or solid components, pancreatic ductal abnormalities, and topographic relationships between pseudocysts and neighboring organs. In addition, EUS is frequently used as a guide to obtain cyst fluid for further analysis [60] and for treatment such as stent-cystogastrostomy or cystoduodenostomy [64–66]. The sensitivity and specificity of EUS for diagnosing pancreatic pseudocysts has been reported to approach 100% in a recent report [59]. As with other approaches using ultrasonography, the main limitations of EUS are the demand for high personal experience and expensive technical equipment to achieve adequate diagnostic accuracy [67].

Indications for Treatment

An improved understanding of the natural course of postacute pseudocysts and the introduction of advanced imaging techniques has prompted substantial changes in management strategies away from surgery toward conservative or interventional approaches. At present, indications for treatment of pancreatic pseudocysts include:

1. Clinical symptoms.
2. Complications.
3. Ductal communication.
4. Cyst enlargement.
5. Persisting cyst size of >6 cm.
6. Suspected malignancy.

Because at least half of true postacute pancreatic pseudocysts resolve spontaneously, a selective algorithm to management is reasonable and safe. For the treatment of small (<4 cm), asymptomatic, and noninfected postacute pseudocysts, careful clinical and morphological follow-up is recommended [11, 20, 33, 34, 37, 38, 40, 48, 65]. In pseudocysts measuring 4–6 cm in diameter, management is more controversial. However, if a patient with a pancreatic pseudocyst remains asymptomatic after an episode of acute pancreatitis with a stable or decreasing cyst size upon follow-up, expectant treatment is still justified. In these patients, resolution is still possible beyond 6 weeks after initial diagnosis, and the risk of complications is less than 10% [40, 41, 62, 68]. Even in pseudocysts >6 cm conservative treatment can be successful [33, 34, 68], but resolution is less common and symptoms mandating some kind of treatment are the rule rather than the exception [6, 9, 37, 48]. The prior opinion that invasive treatment is mandatory in all patients with pancreatic pseudocysts that are present for more than 4–6 weeks is no longer justified [20]. Although there is literally no risk of malignancies in classic postacute pancreatic pseudocysts, there may be patients with postacute type II cysts due to underlying chronic pancreatitis, or patients with atypical presentation who ultimately require surgical treatment, if malignancy can otherwise not be ruled out.

Indications for Surgical Treatment

Improved diagnostic imaging and advanced percutaneous or endoscopic techniques along with new devices for drainage have challenged the previous dominating role of surgery in postacute pseudocysts during the past decade. Nowadays, nonoperative approaches are the first choice of treatment in the majority of postacute pancreatic pseudocysts. The most widely used techniques are percutaneous CT- or ultrasonographically guided drainage with or without lavage [69] and endoscopic transmural or transpapillary drainage with or without the use of EUS [70], which are discussed in detail in Chapter 24. Despite extremely favorable results of the interventional techniques in experienced hands, there is a subset of patients in whom surgery is still necessary to obtain satisfactory short- and long-term results. Indications for surgical treatment in postacute pancreatic pseudocysts include:

1. Ductal communication.
2. Lobulated cyst morphology.
3. Multiple pseudocysts.
4. Cyst location not accessible by other techniques.
5. Failure of interventional/endoscopic drainage.
6. Severe ductal changes (e.g., in chronic pancreatitis).
7. Suspected cystic neoplasm.

Surgical Strategies

Irrespective of the benefits of interventional treatment options, operative drainage still represents the "gold standard" against which other drainage procedures should be compared. To decide on the most appropriate surgical technique, several factors have to be reflected upon: (1) the presence of infection, (2) the age and wall thickness, (3) a pancreatic duct communication, (4) the size, number, and position of the cyst, and (5) underlying chronic or acute pancreatitis. For the management of postacute pseudocysts, three basic techniques are available: external drainage, internal drainage, and resection. Internal drainage modalities further include drainage into the stomach, the duodenum, or the jejunum. All operative strategies have been available for decades with well-documented morbidity, mortality, and recurrence rates (Table 23.4). Internal and external drainage are the most frequently used techniques in patients with postacute pseudocysts; resection modalities are usually limited to smaller cysts in chronic pancreatitis.

Internal Drainage

Internal drainage aims at creating a controlled fistula into the gastrointestinal tract and is the method of choice for all mature pseudocysts. Cystogastrostomy

Table 23.4. Results of open surgery for the treatment of postacute pancreatic pseudocysts. Review of series published since the 1990s. *n.r.* Not recorded

Author	*n*	Morbidity[a]	Mortality	Recurrence after follow-up (years)[a]	
Open surgery:					
Yeo et al. 1990 [33]	39	*n*=5 (13%)	*n*=0 (0%)	*n*=2 (5%)	n.r.
Newell et al. 1990 [75]	98	*n*=16 (16%)	*n*=4 (4%)	*n*=8 (8%)	0.3–6
Walt et al. 1990 [43][b]	233	n.r.	*n*=11 (5%)	*n*=21 (9%)	n.r.
Vitas et al. 1992 [34][b]	46	*n*=11 (24%)	*n*=0 (0%)	*n*=6 (13%)	3.3 (0.1–8)
Sanfey et al. 1994 [40][b]	46	n.r.	*n*=4 (9%)	*n*=8 (17%)	2.2 ± 2
Behrman et al. 1996 [45]	27	*n*=12 (44%)	*n*=4 (15%)	n.r.	n.r.
Spivak et al. 1998 [37]	32	*n*=9 (28%)	*n*=0 (0%)	*n*=3 (9%)	3 (0.5–9)
Heider et al. 1999 [48][b]	66	*n*=18 (27%)	*n*=0 (0%)	*n*=10 (15%)	n.r.
Rau and Beger et al. 2001 [9]	89	*n*=20 (22%)	*n*=3 (2%)	*n*=4 (4%)	6 (1–18)
Soliani et al. 2004 [15]	37	*n*=7 (19%)	*n*=0 (0%)	*n*=2 (5%)	n.r.
Nealon et al. 2005 [16]	100	*n*=6 (6%)	*n*=0 (0%)	*n*=0 (0%)	0.7
Total	813	*n*=104 (19%)	*n*=26 (3.2%)	*n*=64 (8%)	

[a] Follow-up presented as ranges, median (range), or as mean (standard deviation)
[b] Percentage of chronic pseudocysts between 27% and 54%

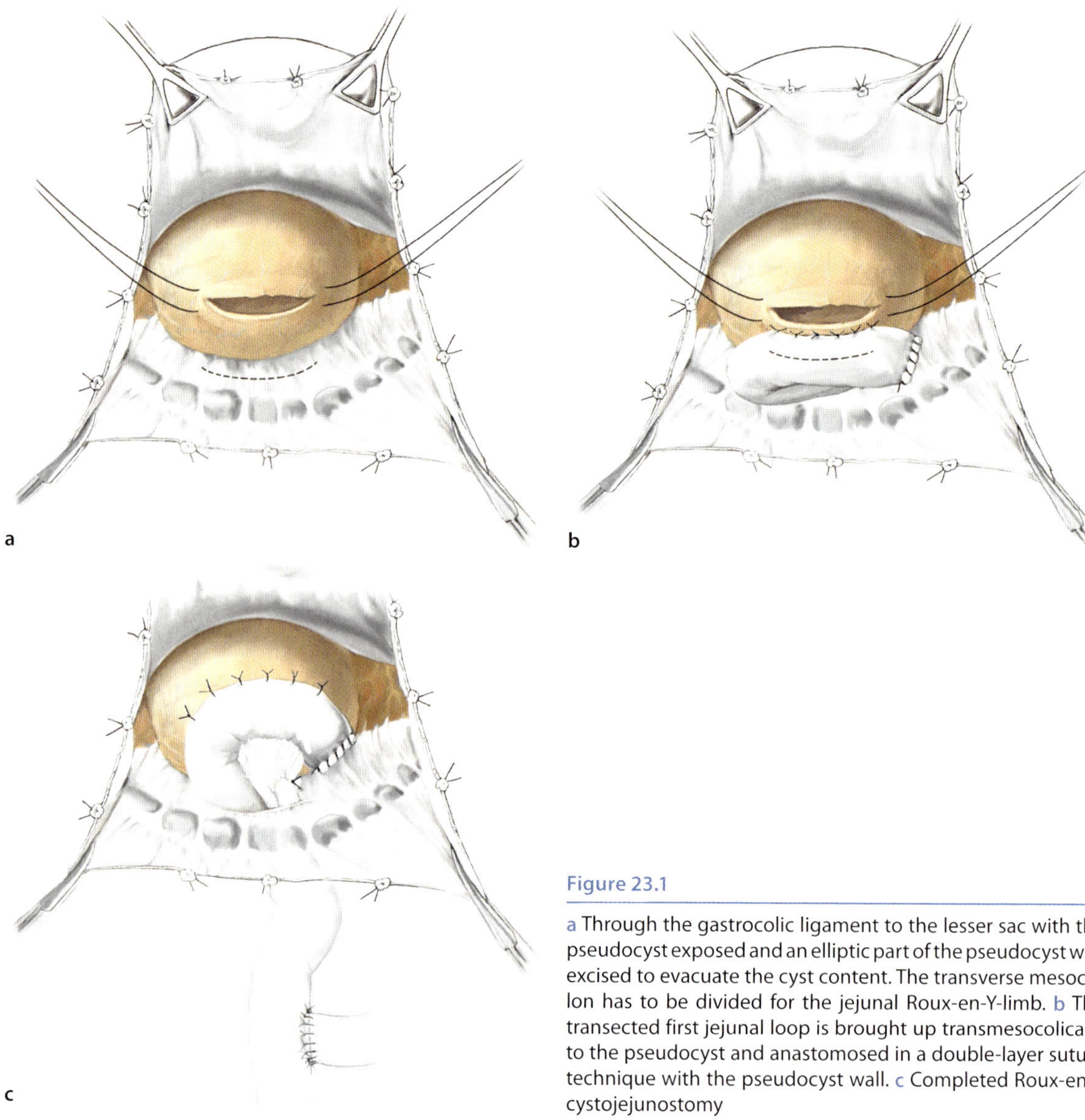

Figure 23.1

a Through the gastrocolic ligament to the lesser sac with the pseudocyst exposed and an elliptic part of the pseudocyst wall excised to evacuate the cyst content. The transverse mesocolon has to be divided for the jejunal Roux-en-Y-limb. b The transected first jejunal loop is brought up transmesocolically to the pseudocyst and anastomosed in a double-layer suture technique with the pseudocyst wall. c Completed Roux-en-Y cystojejunostomy

and cystojejunostomy are the most commonly performed methods for this purpose. Cystoduodenostomy is occasionally indicated for small cysts in the pancreatic head [44, 71, 72].

Transgastric cystogastrostomy is a relatively simple approach, which takes advantage of the observation that many mature pseudocysts are closely adherent to the posterior wall of the stomach. A cyst location remote from the lesser sac and the posterior wall of the stomach are objections to this technique. However, in large pseudocysts expanding below the greater curve of the stomach, this way of drainage may not be sufficient. In recent reports since the 1990s, cystogastrostomy was employed in about one-quarter of patients [7, 33, 34, 36, 37, 43–45, 48, 73, 74]. In a comparative analysis of 98 consecutive patients with pseudocysts, Newell et al. did not observe significant differences of both techniques [75], in contrast to previous reports from the 1880s [71]. In 1991, Johnson and colleagues noted that the complication rate of cystogastrostomy was directly proportional to the size of the pseudocyst [76].

Most reports in the literature favor cystojejunostomy [9, 33, 34, 36, 41, 44, 48, 73, 75, 77] in which the Roux-en Y loop is usually transmesocolically brought up and anastomosed to the lowest part of the cyst (Fig. 23.1). An argument that strongly supports this technique is the high versatility for most cysts even in locations remote from the lesser sac. Further arguments are a more dependent and effective drainage and fewer problems with postoperative bleeding. A meta-analysis of 1020 patients from the late 1960s reported a cyst recurrence rates of 4.5% after cystojejunostomy, compared with 2.5% after cystogastrostomy [78]. In our patient series, we employed cystojejunostomy as the surgical procedure of choice in 64 out of 97 (72%) cases of postacute pseudocysts, with an overall surgical complication rate of less than 6%.

Cystoduodenostomy is limited to few indications and is performed in an average of only 5% of patients with pseudocysts [33, 34, 36, 43, 44, 48, 72–74], with complication and recurrence rates of 5% each in reviewed series [78]. The main indications for this procedure are pseudocysts that are located in the head of the pancreas adjacent to the duodenum. A major concern in cystoduodenostomy is the injury of the intrapancreatic portion of the common bile duct [72].

External Drainage

External drainage is the most simple method of surgical cyst drainage and is performed in up to 18% of postacute pancreatic pseudocysts [9, 31, 33, 34, 36, 43, 45, 48, 68, 73]. Associated mortality is ranging between 0 and 6% and cyst recurrence is observed in up to 22%. These figures most likely reflect the severity of the preceding attack of acute pancreatitis rather than specific drawbacks of the technique itself. In most surgical series, external drainage is indicated mainly in grossly infected pseudocysts, in the presence of abundant necrotic content or where there is a friable pseudocyst wall that does not hold sutures, which is usually discovered intraoperatively in patients planned for internal drainage. Occasionally, external drainage is performed for hemorrhage or free rupture requiring emergency laparotomy. Persistent pancreatic fistulae are observed in about 10% of patients following this procedure [45] and may require further internal drainage.

Pancreatic Resection

Pancreatic resection is the prevailing surgical concept for patients suffering from chronic pancreatitis with or without associated small pseudocysts. In the treatment of postacute pseudocysts it is performed in less than 20% of all patients [33, 34, 41, 43, 73, 79], in our series in 18% (16/97) [9].

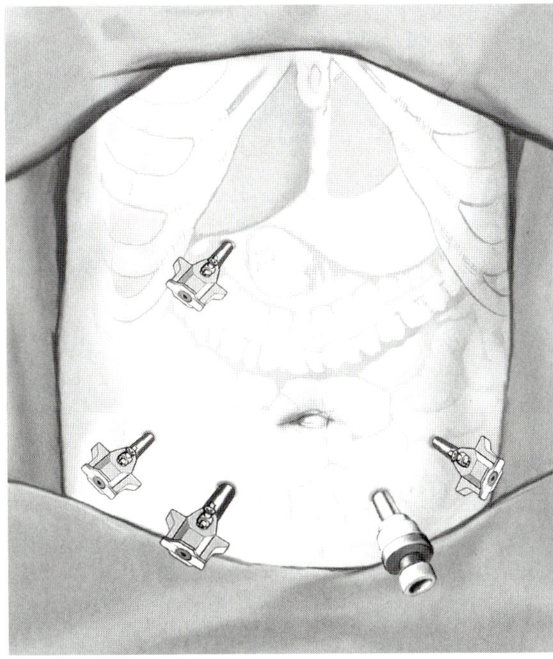

Figure 23.2

Placement of trocars for laparoscopic pseudocyst drainage (cystogastrostomy)

Laparoscopic Techniques

Increasing attention has been paid to laparoscopic techniques in the treatment of benign pancreatic disease recently [80]. Several reports have focused on different approaches to laparoscopic pseudocyst drainage, such as laparo-endoscopic cystogastrostomy [81–83], extra- and transgastric cystogastrostomy [81, 83–87], and Roux-en-Y cystojejunostomy [81, 84, 88]. By combining laparoscopic and endoscopic techniques, laparo-endoscopic drainage involves the laparoscopic-guided transabdominal placement of trocars into the stomach. This provides better visualization, access for instrumentation, and drainage of the pseudocyst into the stomach. Laparoscopic cystogastrostomy can be performed either transgastrically (anterior approach) or extragastrically (posterior approach) [89] and creates a side-to-side anastomosis between the stomach and the adjacent pseudocyst wall using sutures or staplers. In pseudocysts not located in the close vicinity of the stomach, laparoscopic cystojejunostomy is another approach reported in the literature, but is, however, technically more demanding than cystogastrostomy [83]. Figure 23.2 shows an example of the abdominal position of different trocars for laparoscopic cystojejunostomy. The majority of

Table 23.5. Results of laparoscopic surgery for the treatment of postacute pancreatic pseudocysts. Review of series published since the 1990s. *Suc* Successful

Author	Suc/ Total[a]	Conver- sion	Morbidity[b]	Mortality	Recurrence after follow-up (years)[c]	
Laparoscopic surgery:						
Mori et al. 2002 [86]	13/18	*n*=4 (22%)	*n*=1 (7%)	*n*=0 (0%)	*n*=0 (0%)	0.5–2.7
Park et al. 2002 [83]	28/29	*n*=0 (0%)	*n*=2 (7%)	*n*=0 (0%)	*n*=0 (0%)	0.1–3
Obermeyer et al. 2003 [87]	5/6	*n*=1 (17%)	*n*=0 (0%)	*n*=0 (0%)	*n*=0 (0%)	3.7 (0.3–4.9)
Texeira et al. 2003 [88]	8/8	*n*=0 (0%)	*n*=2 (25%)	*n*=0 (0%)	*n*=0 (0%)	2 (1–4)
Davila-Cervantes et al. 2004 [81]	9/10	*n*=0 (0%)	*n*=3 (30%)	*n*=0 (0%)	*n*=0 (0%)	1.8 (0.1–6)
Hauters et al. 2004 [84]	16/17	*n*=1 (6%)	*n*=2 (13%)	*n*=0 (0%)	*n*=0 (0%)	1 (0.5–3)
Hindmarsh et al. 2005 [85]	12/15	*n*=3 (20%)	*n*=1 (8%)	*n*=0 (0%)	*n*=2 (17%)	3.1 (0.3–6.8)
Barragan et al. 2005 [89]	8/ 8	*n*=0 (0%)	*n*=0 (0%)	*n*=0 (0%)	n.r.	n.r.
Total	99/111	*n*=9 (8%)	*n*=14 (14%)	*n*=0 (0%)	*n*=2 (2%)	

[a] Successfully completed laparoscopic procedures during the same hospital stay/total number of patients undergoing laparoscopy

[b] Morbidity in the laparoscopically completed procedures

[c] Follow-up presented as ranges, median (range) or mean (range)

the series on laparoscopic pseudocyst drainage comprise only small patient numbers and a highly selected patient subset, but carry favorable short- and long-term results, which compare well with the open approaches (Table 23.5). One of the largest series has been published by Park et al., employing various laparoscopic techniques that were successfully performed in 28 out of 29 patients with pancreatic pseudocysts [83]. Despite the known benefits of laparoscopic surgery, it has to be emphasized that laparoscopic interventions of the pancreas should be considered as an advanced laparoscopic procedure and require profound experience in pancreatic surgery by a team with advanced laparoscopic skills.

References

1. Bradley EL III (1993) A clinically based classification system for acute pancreatitis. Summary of the International Symposium on Acute Pancreatitis, Atlanta, Ga, September 11–13, 1992. Arch Surg 128:586–590
2. Kloppel G (2000) Pseudocysts and other non-neoplastic cysts of the pancreas. Semin Diagn Pathol 17:7–15
3. Brugge WR, Lewandrowski K, Lee-Lewandrowski E, Centeno BA, Szydlo T, Regan S, del Castillo CF, Warshaw AL (2004) Diagnosis of pancreatic cystic neoplasms: a report of the cooperative pancreatic cyst study. Gastroenterology 126:1330–1336
4. Baron TH, Morgan DE, Vickers SM, Lazenby AJ (1999) Organized pancreatic necrosis: endoscopic, radiologic, and pathologic features of a distinct clinical entity. Pancreas 19:105–108
5. Kourtesis G, Wilson SE, Williams RA (1990) The clinical significance of fluid collections in acute pancreatitis. Am Surg 56:796–799
6. London NJ, Neoptolemos JP, Lavelle J, Bailey I, James D (1989) Serial computed tomography scanning in acute pancreatitis: a prospective study. Gut 30:397–403
7. Schulze S, Baden H, Brandenhoff P, Larsen T, Burcharth F (1986) Pancreatic pseudocysts during first attack of acute pancreatitis. Scand J Gastroenterol 21:1221–1223
8. Maringhini A, Uomo G, Patti R, Rabitti P, Termini A, Cavallera A, Dardanoni G, Manes G, Ciambra M, Laccetti M, Biffarella P, Pagliaro L (1999) Pseudocysts in acute nonalcoholic pancreatitis: incidence and natural history. Dig Dis Sci 44:1669–1673
9. Rau B, Golling C, Beger HG (2001) Long-term follow-up after surgical and interventional management of postacute pancreatic pseudocysts: a 20 year single center experience. Pancreas 23:457 (abstract)
10. Stringer MD (2005) Pancreatitis and pancreatic trauma. Semin Pediatr Surg 14:239–246
11. D'Egidio A, Schein M (1991) Pancreatic pseudocysts: a proposed classification and its management implications. Br J Surg 78:981–984
12. Diculescu M, Ciocarlan M, Ciocarlan M, Stanescu D, Ciprut T, Marinescu T (2005) Predictive factors for pseudocysts and peripancreatic collections in acute pancreatitis. Rom J Gastroenterol 14:129–134
13. Kloppel G, Maillet B (1991) Pseudocysts in chronic pancreatitis: a morphological analysis of 57 resection specimens and 9 autopsy pancreata. Pancreas 6:266–274

14. Nguyen BL, Thompson JS, Edney JA, Bragg LE, Rikkers LF (1991) Influence of the etiology of pancreatitis on the natural history of pancreatic pseudocysts. Am J Surg 162:527–530; discussion 531
15. Soliani P, Franzini C, Ziegler S, Del Rio P, Dell'Abate P, Piccolo D, Japichino GG, Cavestro GM, Di Mario F, Sianesi M (2004) Pancreatic pseudocysts following acute pancreatitis: risk factors influencing therapeutic outcomes. JOP 5:338–347
16. Nealon WH, Walser E (2005) Surgical management of complications associated with percutaneous and/or endoscopic management of pseudocyst of the pancreas. Ann Surg 241:948–957; discussion 957–960
17. Neoptolemos JP, London NJ, Carr-Locke DL (1993) Assessment of main pancreatic duct integrity by endoscopic retrograde pancreatography in patients with acute pancreatitis. Br J Surg 80:94–99
18. Warren WD, Marsh WH, Muller WH Jr (1957) Experimental production of pseudocysts of the pancreas with preliminary observations on internal drainage. Surg Gynecol Obstet 105:385–392
19. Wallner RJ, Basara BE, Dadparvar S, Croll MN, Brady LW (1984) Subcapsular splenic hematoma vs intrasplenic pancreatic pseudocyst. Clin Nucl Med 9:348–351
20. Andren-Sandberg A, Dervenis C (2004) Pancreatic pseudocysts in the 21st century. Part I: classification, pathophysiology, anatomic considerations and treatment. JOP 5:8–24
21. Beauchamp RD, Winsett M, Nealon WH (1989) Operative strategies in the management of mediastinal pancreatic pseudocyst. Surgery 106:567–570
22. Heider R, Behrns KE (2001) Pancreatic pseudocysts complicated by splenic parenchymal involvement: results of operative and percutaneous management. Pancreas 23:20–25
23. Zhang AB, Zheng SS (2005) Treatment of pancreatic pseudocysts in line with D'Egidio's classification. World J Gastroenterol 11:729–732
24. Warshaw AL, Lee KH (1980) Aging changes of pancreatic isoamylases and the appearance of "old amylase" in the serum of patients with pancreatic pseudocysts. Gastroenterology 79:1246–1251
25. Lasson A, Goransson J, Ohlsson K (1989) Pancreatic pseudocyst fluid – a mixture of plasma proteins and pancreatic juice possessing a high proteolytic activity. Scand J Clin Lab Invest 49:403–412
26. Duvnjak M, Duvnjak L, Dodig M, Simicevic VN, Troskot B, Supanc V (1998) Factors predictive of the healing of pancreatic pseudocysts treated by percutaneous evacuation. Hepatogastroenterology 45:536–540
27. Sankaran S, Walt AJ (1975) The natural and unnatural history of pancreatic pseudocysts. Br J Surg 62:37–44
28. Pollak EW, Michas CA, Wolfman EF Jr (1978) Pancreatic pseudocyst: management in fifty-four patients. Am J Surg 135:199–201
29. Czaja AJ, Fisher M, Marin GA (1975) Spontaneous resolution of pancreatic masses (pseudocysts?) – Development and disappearance after acute alcoholic pancreatitis. Arch Intern Med 135:558–562
30. Bradley EL, Clements JL Jr, Gonzalez AC (1979) The natural history of pancreatic pseudocysts: a unified concept of management. Am J Surg 137:135–141
31. Martin EW Jr, Catalano P, Cooperman M, Hecht C, Carey LC (1979) Surgical decision-making in the treatment of pancreatic pseudocysts. Internal versus external drainage. Am J Surg 138:821–824
32. Warshaw AL, Rattner DW (1985) Timing of surgical drainage for pancreatic pseudocyst. Clinical and chemical criteria. Ann Surg 202:720–724
33. Yeo CJ, Bastidas JA, Lynch-Nyhan A, Fishman EK, Zinner MJ, Cameron JL (1990) The natural history of pancreatic pseudocysts documented by computed tomography. Surg Gynecol Obstet 170:411–417
34. Vitas GJ, Sarr MG (1992) Selected management of pancreatic pseudocysts: operative versus expectant management. Surgery 111:123–130
35. Mehta R, Suvarna D, Sadasivan S, John A, Raj V, Nair P, Balakrishnan V (2004) Natural course of asymptomatic pancreatic pseudocyst: a prospective study. Indian J Gastroenterol 23:140–102
36. Andersson R, Janzon M, Sundberg I, Bengmark S (1989) Management of pancreatic pseudocysts. Br J Surg 76:550–552
37. Spivak H, Galloway JR, Amerson JR, Fink AS, Branum GD, Redvanly RD, Richardson WS, Mauren SJ, Waring JP, Hunter JG (1998) Management of pancreatic pseudocysts. J Am Coll Surg 186:507–511
38. Naoum E, Zavos A, Goudis K, Sarros C, Pitsargiotis E, Karamouti M, Tsikrikis P, Karantanas A (2003) Pancreatic pseudocysts: 10 years of experience. J Hepatobiliary Pancreat Surg 10:373–376
39. Soliani P, Ziegler S, Franzini C, Dell'Abate P, Del Rio P, Di Mario F, Cavestro M, Sianesi M (2004) The size of pancreatic pseudocyst does not influence the outcome of invasive treatments. Dig Liver Dis 36:135–140
40. Sanfey H, Aguilar M, Jones RS (1994) Pseudocysts of the pancreas, a review of 97 cases. Am Surg 60:661–668
41. Nealon WH, Walser E (2002) Main pancreatic ductal anatomy can direct choice of modality for treating pancreatic pseudocysts (surgery versus percutaneous drainage). Ann Surg 235:751–758
42. Ephgrave K, Hunt JL (1986) Presentation of pancreatic pseudocysts: implications for timing of surgical intervention. Am J Surg 151:749–753
43. Walt AJ, Bouwman DL, Weaver DW, Sachs RJ (1990) The impact of technology on the management of pancreatic pseudocyst. Fifth annual Samuel Jason Mixter Lecture. Arch Surg 125:759–763
44. Yemos K, Laopodis B, Yemos J, Scouras K, Rissoti L, Lainas A, Patsalos C, Tzardis P, Tierris E (1999) Surgical management of pancreatic pseudocyst. Minerva Chir 54:395–402
45. Behrman SW, Melvin WS, Ellison EC (1996) Pancreatic pseudocysts following acute pancreatitis. Am J Surg 172:228–231
46. Grace RR, Jordan PH Jr (1976) Unresolved problems of pancreatic pseudocysts. Ann Surg 184:16–21
47. Criado E, De Stefano AA, Weiner TM, Jaques PF (1992) Long term results of percutaneous catheter drainage of pancreatic pseudocysts. Surg Gynecol Obstet 175:293–298
48. Heider R, Meyer AA, Galanko JA, Behrns KE (1999) Percutaneous drainage of pancreatic pseudocysts is associated with a higher failure rate than surgical treatment in unselected patients. Ann Surg 229:781–787; discussion 787–789
49. Cahen D, Rauws E, Fockens P, Weverling G, Huibregtse K, Bruno M (2005) Endoscopic drainage of pancreatic pseudocysts: long-term outcome and procedural factors associated with safe and successful treatment. Endoscopy 37:977–983
50. Lumsden A, Bradley EL III (1990) Secondary pancreatic infections. Surg Gynecol Obstet 170:459–467

51. Warshaw AL, Rattner DW (1980) Facts and fallacies of common bile duct obstruction by pancreatic pseudocysts. Ann Surg 192:33–37
52. Bradley EL III, Clements JL Jr (1976) Transenteric rupture of pancreatic pseudocysts: management of pseudocystenteric fistulas. Am Surg 42:827–837
53. Andren-Sandberg A, Dervenis C (2004) Pancreatic pseudocysts in the 21st century. Part II: natural history. JOP 5:64–70
54. Balachandra S, Siriwardena AK (2005) Systematic appraisal of the management of the major vascular complications of pancreatitis. Am J Surg 190:489–495
55. Yattoo GN, Khuroo MS, Wani NA, Wani KA, Bhat FA (1999) Haemosuccus pancreaticus: a clinical challenge. J Gastroenterol Hepatol 14:172–175
56. Lipsett PA, Cameron JL (1992) Internal pancreatic fistula. Am J Surg 163:216–220
57. Warshaw AL, Rutledge PL (1987) Cystic tumors mistaken for pancreatic pseudocysts. Ann Surg 205:393–398
58. van der Waaij LA, van Dullemen HM, Porte RJ (2005) Cyst fluid analysis in the differential diagnosis of pancreatic cystic lesions: a pooled analysis. Gastrointest Endosc 62:383–389
59. Frossard JL, Amouyal P, Amouyal G, Palazzo L, Amaris J, Soldan M, Giostra E, Spahr L, Hadengue A, Fabre M (2003) Performance of endosonography-guided fine needle aspiration and biopsy in the diagnosis of pancreatic cystic lesions. Am J Gastroenterol 98:1516–1524
60. Linder JD, Geenen JE, Catalano MF. Cyst fluid analysis obtained by EUS-guided FNA in the evaluation of discrete cystic neoplasms of the pancreas: a prospective single-center experience. Gastrointest Endosc 2006;64:697–702
61. Kim YH, Saini S, Sahani D, Hahn PF, Mueller PR, Auh YH (2005) Imaging diagnosis of cystic pancreatic lesions: pseudocyst versus nonpseudocyst. Radiographics 25:671–685
62. Lillemoe KD, Yeo CJ (1998) Management of complications of pancreatitis. Curr Probl Surg 35:1–98
63. Fayad LM, Kowalski T, Mitchell DG (2003) MR cholangiopancreatography: evaluation of common pancreatic diseases. Radiol Clin North Am 41:97–114
64. Kahaleh M, Shami VM, Conaway MR, Tokar J, Rockoff T, De La Rue SA, de Lange E, Bassignani M, Gay S, Adams RB, Yeaton P (2006) Endoscopic ultrasound drainage of pancreatic pseudocyst: a prospective comparison with conventional endoscopic drainage. Endoscopy 38:355–359
65. Brugge WR (2004) Approaches to the drainage of pancreatic pseudocysts. Curr Opin Gastroenterol 20:488–492
66. Will U, Wegener C, Graf KI, Wanzar I, Manger T, Meyer F (2006) Differential treatment and early outcome in the interventional endoscopic management of pancreatic pseudocysts in 27 patients. World J Gastroenterol 12:4175–4178
67. Yusuf TE, Baron TH (2006) Endoscopic transmural drainage of pancreatic pseudocysts: results of a national and an international survey of ASGE members. Gastrointest Endosc 63:223–227
68. Cheruvu CV, Clarke MG, Prentice M, Eyre-Brook IA (2003) Conservative treatment as an option in the management of pancreatic pseudocyst. Ann R Coll Surg Engl 85:313–316
69. Neff R (2001) Pancreatic pseudocysts and fluid collections: percutaneous approaches. Surg Clin North Am 81:399–403, xii
70. Fazel A (2005) An endoscopic perspective on pancreatic pseudocysts. Curr Gastroenterol Rep 7:107–113
71. Schattenkerk ME, De Vries JE, Bruining HA, Eggink WF, Obertop H (1982) Surgical treatment of pancreatic pseudocysts. Br J Surg 69:593–594
72. Altimari A, Aranha GV, Greenlee HB, Prinz RA (1986) Results of cystoduodenostomy for treatment of pancreatic pseudocysts. Am Surg 52:438–441
73. Imrie CW, Buist LJ, Shearer MG (1988) Importance of cause in the outcome of pancreatic pseudocysts. Am J Surg 156:159–162
74. Parks RW, Tzovaras G, Diamond T, Rowlands BJ (2000) Management of pancreatic pseudocysts. Ann R Coll Surg Engl 82:383–287
75. Newell KA, Liu T, Aranha GV, Prinz RA (1990) Are cystgastrostomy and cystjejunostomy equivalent operations for pancreatic pseudocysts? Surgery 108:635–639; discussion 639–640
76. Johnson LB, Rattner DW, Warshaw AL (1991) The effect of size of giant pancreatic pseudocysts on the outcome of internal drainage procedures. Surg Gynecol Obstet 173:171–174
77. O'Connor M, Kolars J, Ansel H, Silvis S, Vennes J (1986) Preoperative endoscopic retrograde cholangiopancreatography in the surgical management of pancreatic pseudocysts. Am J Surg 151:18–24
78. Becker WF, Pratt HS, Ganji H (1986) Pseudocysts of the pancreas. Surg Gynecol Obstet 127:744–747
79. Ahearne PM, Baillie JM, Cotton PB, Baker ME, Meyers WC, Pappas TN (1992) An endoscopic retrograde cholangiopancreatography (ERCP)-based algorithm for the management of pancreatic pseudocysts. Am J Surg 163:111–115; discussion 115–116
80. Fernandez-Cruz L, Cesar-Borges G, Lopez-Boado MA, Orduna D, Navarro S (2005) Minimally invasive surgery of the pancreas in progress. Langenbecks Arch Surg 390:342–354
81. Davila-Cervantes A, Gomez F, Chan C, Bezaury P, Robles-Diaz G, Uscanga LF, Herrera MF (2004) Laparoscopic drainage of pancreatic pseudocysts. Surg Endosc 18:1420–1426
82. Atabek U, Mayer D, Amin A, Camishion RC (1993) Pancreatic cystogastrostomy by combined upper endoscopy and percutaneous transgastric instrumentation. J Laparoendosc Surg 3:501–504
83. Park AE, Heniford BT (2002) Therapeutic laparoscopy of the pancreas. Ann Surg 236:149–158
84. Hauters P, Weerts J, Navez B, Champault G, Peillon C, Totte E, Barthelemy R, Siriser F (2004) Laparoscopic treatment of pancreatic pseudocysts. Surg Endosc 18:1645–1648
85. Hindmarsh A, Lewis MP, Rhodes M (2005) Stapled laparoscopic cystgastrostomy: a series with 15 cases. Surg Endosc 19:143–147
86. Mori T, Abe N, Sugiyama M, Atomi Y (2002) Laparoscopic pancreatic cystgastrostomy. J Hepatobiliary Pancreat Surg 9:548–554
87. Obermeyer RJ, Fisher WE, Salameh JR, Jeyapalan M, Sweeney JF, Brunicardi FC (2003) Laparoscopic pancreatic cystogastrostomy. Surg Laparosc Endosc Percutan Tech 13:250–253
88. Teixeira J, Gibbs KE, Vaimakis S, Rezayat C (2003) Laparoscopic Roux-en-Y pancreatic cyst-jejunostomy. Surg Endosc 17:1910–1913
89. Barragan B, Love L, Wachtel M, Griswold JA, Frezza EE (2005) A comparison of anterior and posterior approaches for the surgical treatment of pancreatic pseudocyst using laparoscopic cystogastrostomy. J Laparoendosc Adv Surg Tech A 15:596–600

Chapter 24

T. H. Baron

Interventional Management of Pancreatic Fluid Collections and Abscesses

Several types of pancreatic fluid collections (PFCs) may arise as a result of acute pancreatitis [1]. These include acute fluid collections, acute pancreatic pseudocysts, pancreatic abscesses, and organized pancreatic necrosis. Endoscopic and percutaneous (radiological) management are relatively new approaches to the management of these collections as compared to surgical therapy. Both approaches, however, which were developed in the 1980s and are frequently seen as adversarial to each other and to surgical therapy, are complementary. Their frequency of use is usually dictated by local expertise.

Types of Pancreatic Fluid Collections

The types of pancreatic fluid collection that occur as a result of acute pancreatitis are acute fluid collections, pancreatic necrosis, pancreatic abscess, and pancreatic pseudocysts.

Acute Fluid Collections

Acute fluid collections arise early in the course of acute pancreatitis, lack a well-defined wall, are usually peripancreatic in location, and usually resolve without sequelae, but may evolve into pancreatic pseudocysts or abscesses [1]. Acute fluid collections rarely require drainage.

Acute Pancreatic Pseudocyst

Acute pancreatic pseudocysts (APPs) arise as a sequela of acute pancreatitis, require at least 4 weeks to form, and are devoid of significant solid debris. APPs arise either as a result of pancreatic ductal injury and resultant ductal leak, or liquefaction of limited necrosis [2]. It is important to note that the 4-week time period does not imply that the collection has completely liquefied. Patients who initially had substantial pancreatic necrosis (≥30%) may evolve a collection at 4 weeks that resembles a pseudocyst radiographically, a term referred to as necroma or organized pancreatic necrosis (OPN) (described below). Applying pseudocyst drainage methods to OPN fails to evacuate solid debris, leading to infectious complications [3,4].

Organized Pancreatic Necrosis

Acute pancreatic necrosis is frequently accompanied by the development of major pancreatic ductal disruptions [5]. Over the course of several weeks, a collection of both liquid and solid debris may evolve and expand the initial area of necrosis. Some authors have used the term OPN to differentiate this process from the early (acute phase) of pancreatic necrosis that is seen in the first week [1,6]. The homogeneous computed tomography (CT) appearance of OPN is frequently similar to that of an acute pseudocyst because the underlying solid debris is frequently not discernible [7].

The distinction between an acute pseudocyst and organized necrosis can be made on clinical, radiologic, or endoscopic findings at the time of drainage. Patients with necrosis have frequently suffered a severe or complicated course of acute pancreatitis. A contrast-enhanced CT obtained during the initial bout of pancreatitis revealing significant glandular necrosis suggests that solid debris is present. The evolution of changes on serial CT scans can be traced from the original pancreatic and peripancreatic necrosis to the present collection. Magnetic resonance imaging (MRI) can delineate the solid debris within a collection [7]. CT after nonsurgical drainage depicts solid material once the liquid component has been removed [4]. Findings at the time of drainage that suggest the presence of necrotic debris include visualization of solid material or chocolate-brown/extremely turbid fluid (in the absence of clinical infection). The pancreatographic finding of complete ductal disruption also suggests underlying pancreatic necrosis.

Table 24.1. Types of pancreatic fluid collections complicating acute pancreatitis. *CECT* Contrast-enhanced computed tomography

Term	Definition
Acute fluid collection	A collection of enzyme-rich pancreatic juices occurring early (within 48 h) in the course of acute pancreatitis are located in or near the pancreas, and always lack a well-defined wall of granulation tissue or fibrous tissue
Acute pseudocyst	A collection of pancreatic juices enclosed by a wall of nonepithelialized granulation tissue, arising as a consequence of acute pancreatitis and requiring at least 4 weeks to form; it is devoid of significant solid debris
Pancreatic necrosis (early)	A diffuse or focal area of nonviable pancreatic parenchyma greater than 30% of the gland by CECT that is typically associated with peripancreatic fat necrosis
Organized pancreatic necrosis (late)	Evolution of acute necrosis to a partially encapsulated, well-defined collection of pancreatic juices and necrotic debris
Pancreatic abscess	A circumscribed intra-abdominal collection of pus, usually in proximity to the pancreas, containing little or no pancreatic necrosis, which arises as a consequence of acute pancreatitis or pancreatic trauma

Pancreatic Abscess

If a strict definition of pancreatic abscess is adhered to as a collection of pus in close proximity to the pancreas arising from liquefaction of limited pancreatic and/or peripancreatic fat necrosis, which becomes secondarily infected, then it is a rare entity [1]. However, some authors have also referred to infected pancreatic pseudocysts, late infected pancreatic necrosis, and infected postoperative collections as pancreatic abscesses.

Indications for Drainage of PFCs

In general, the indications for drainage of a PFC are symptom driven and/or infection. The specific indications for drainage of each collection will be discussed separately.

Acute Fluid Collections

Acute fluid collections almost always resolve without sequelae, and intervention is not indicated unless infection occurs. Percutaneous [8] and endoscopic drainage [9] for these collections has been described.

Acute Pancreatic Pseudocyst

Pseudocyst size alone is not an indication for drainage, although pseudocysts larger than 6 cm in maximal diameter tend to be symptomatic[10]. Pancreatic pseudocysts become symptomatic when they compress the stomach, duodenum, or bile duct, with resultant development of abdominal pain, gastric outlet obstruction, early satiety, weight loss, or jaundice. Progressive enlargement in an asymptomatic patient is considered by some authors to be an indication for drainage [11]. An infected pseudocyst is an absolute indication for drainage.

Pancreatic Necrosis

Nonsurgical drainage of pancreatic necrosis is controversial. Pancreatic necrosis is not amenable to endoscopic or percutaneous drainage until the process becomes organized, which usually occurs several weeks after the onset of pancreatitis. If the process remains sterile, the general indications for drainage are refractory abdominal pain, gastric outlet obstruction, or failure to thrive (continued systemic illness, anorexia, and weight loss) at 4 or more weeks after the onset of acute pancreatitis. The severity of CT scan findings alone is not an indication for drainage. Since drainage of these collections is more technically difficult, carries a higher rate of complications, and tends to involve a more severely ill patient group, the decision to proceed with nonsurgical intervention in OPN patients must be considered carefully, ideally in consultation with the surgical team.

Infected pancreatic necrosis is considered an indication for drainage. Infected necrosis may not be distinguishable clinically from sterile necrosis because of leukocytosis and fever. Percutaneous fine-needle aspiration may be required to determine the bacteriologic status of the necrosis.

Pancreatic Abscess

By definition, a pancreatic abscess is infected and is an indication for drainage.

Predainage Evaluation

Oral and Intravenous Contrast Abdominal CT Scan

This allows assessment of the precise location of the collection in relation to surrounding structures. Varices from the splenic vein, or portal vein thrombosis may also be visualized. The finding of inhomogeneity within the collection suggests the presence of underlying solid debris [7].

Coagulation Parameters

Consideration should be made for the following imaging studies prior to intervention:

1. Endoscopic ultrasound (EUS). EUS can be used to assess for the presence of significant solid debris, which may alter the approach, and to guide transmural drainage.
2. MRI to determine the presence of solid debris, in order to plan for irrigation methods or alternative drainage strategy [7].
3. Magnetic resonance cholangiopancreatography (MRCP) and/or endoscopic retrograde cholangiopancreatography) to define ductal anatomy. several studies suggest that the outcome of nonsurgical management of pseudocysts, particularly percutaneous therapy, is dependent on adequate identification of pancreatic duct communication and underlying ductal obstruction [12–14]. During the course of endoscopic therapy, pancreatic ductal anatomy is assessed [1].

Nonsurgical Methods of Drainage of PFCs

Endoscopic

The endoscopic management of OPN will be addressed separately. Pancreatic pseudocysts and abscesses can be drained by placing a stent into the main pancreatic duct (transpapillary) [15,16], placing drains through the gastric or duodenal wall (transmurally) [17], or both. [11,18] The decision to proceed with one approach over another is based upon the anatomic relationship of the collection to the stomach or duodenum, the presence of ductal communication, and the size of the collection. If the stomach or duodenum is not in close apposition to the wall of the collection (within 1 cm by CT), transmural drainage is not possible. If the collection is very large, transpapillary drainage alone may result in infection, since contrast injection introduces bacteria and/or fungal organisms into the collection and the drainage process is relatively slow because of the limited diameter prosthesis the pancreatic duct allows.

Transpapillary Approach

If the collection communicates with the main pancreatic duct, placement of a pancreatic endoprosthesis with or without pancreatic sphincterotomy is effective, especially for collections ≤6cm. If possible, the proximal end of the stent (toward the pancreatic tail) should completely bridge the leak (Fig. 24.1) [19]. The diameter of pancreatic stent used is dependent on the pancreatic ductal diameter, but is usually 7 Fr.

The advantage of the transpapillary approach over the transmural approach is the avoidance of bleeding or perforation that may occur with transmural drainage. The disadvantages of transpapillary drainage are scarring of the main pancreatic duct by the stent [20,21] and early occlusion of small-diameter stents, with resultant infection and/or pancreatitis.

Transmural Approach

Transmural drainage of PFCs is achieved by placing one or more large-bore (10 Fr) stents through the gastric or duodenal wall. Some endoscopic experts advocate EUS evaluation prior to transmural drainage [22,23].

EUS-Guided Transmural Drainage

Although EUS guidance may reduce the complications related to transmural entry, evidence-based studies are lacking. EUS guidance can be used two ways [24]. One use is for imaging alone to localize the collection in relationship to surrounding structures and to identify endoscopic landmarks. The echo endoscope is then removed and a standard non-EUS endoscope is used to perform the transmural drainage as described under non-EUS-guided drainage, below. The second way EUS can be used is to directly guide

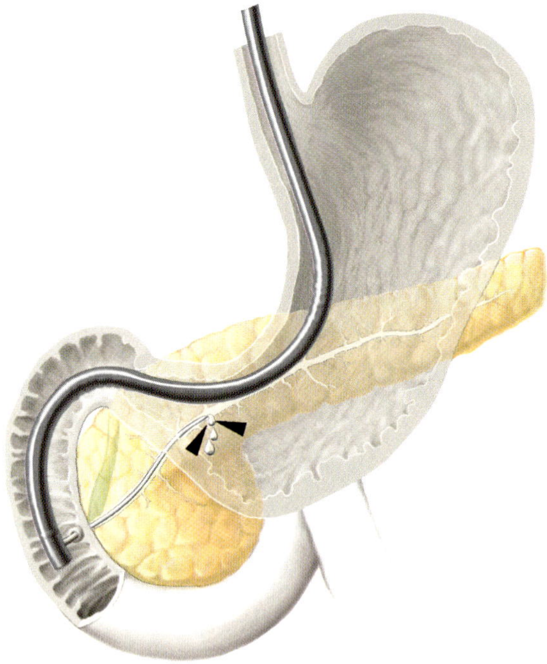

Figure 24.1

Illustration of endoscopic transpapillary drainage of a pancreatic pseudocyst. Note that the proximal end of the stent is proximal (tail) to the leak

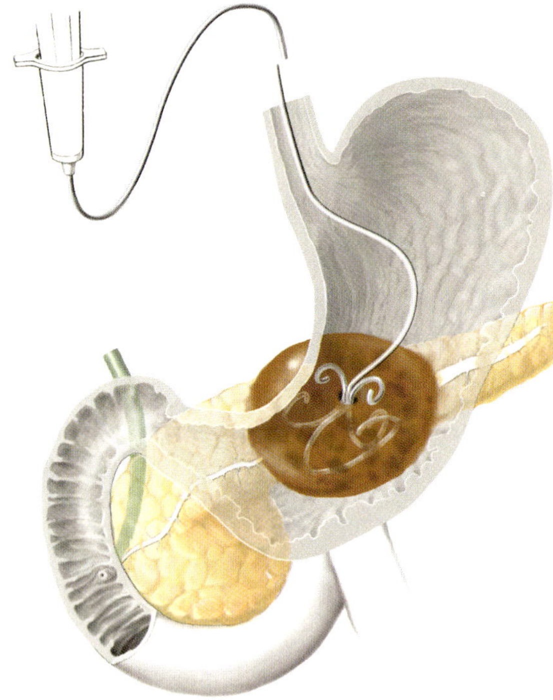

Figure 24.2

Illustration of endoscopic transmural drainage of organized pancreatic necrosis. A large transgastric tract is created. After placement of two 10-Fr, double-pigtail stents, an irrigation tube is passed through the channel of the endoscope, coiled in the collection, and transferred to exit the nose

and perform the transmural entry in order to minimize perforation and avoid vascular structures including varices [25,26].

Non-EUS-Guided Transmural Drainage

The collection is entered transgastrically or transduodenally at a point of endoscopically visible extrinsic compression using a needle or electrocautery [17]. After a guidewire is coiled within the collection, the transmural tract is enlarged with a dilating balloon. The practice of enlarging the transmural tract with a sphincterotome has been abandoned because of the risk of bleeding. One or more 10 F, double-pigtail stents are placed through into the collection.

Follow Up

Following uncomplicated endoscopic drainage of noninfected pancreatic pseudocysts, a short course of oral antibiotics is administered. Most outpatients do not require hospitalization [27,28]. In the absence of suspected complications or worsening clinical course, a follow up CT scan is obtained 4–6 weeks later to document radiographic resolution. The internal stents are then removed endoscopically and pancreatography performed, as indicated.

Endoscopic Drainage of OPN

Because of the need used to evacuate solid material, the endoscopic approach for the drainage of organized pancreatic necrosis differs from that used for drainage of pseudocysts. The transpapillary approach is usually not adequate to allow the removal of solid debris. Therefore, transmural drainage is the preferred approach. After transmural entry into the collection has been achieved, the gastric or duodenal wall is dilated by ≥15 mm on the initial endoscopy. This allows the egress of solid material around the endoprostheses. An irrigation system is required to lavage the solid debris. Thus, in addition to two 10-Fr stents, a 7-Fr irrigation tube is placed into the collection (standard nasobiliary tube) for aggressive irrigation (Fig. 24.2). Up to 200 ml of normal saline are forcefully and rapidly infused via the tube every 2–4 hours initially. In patients who are intolerant to nasocystic tubes and/or it is anticipated that irrigation may be required for many weeks, an alternative to nasocystic lavage is the placement of a percutaneous endoscopic gastrostomy tube (PEG) with placement of a "jejunal" extension tube into the collection [29]. More recently, an attempt to directly remove the necrotic material endoscopically using basket extraction has been described [30].

Patients undergoing attempted endoscopic drainage of OPN require preprocedural and postprocedural antibiotics. Outpatients are hospitalized for observation and institution of irrigation and discharged home after they are able to tolerate oral intake and care for the irrigation tube. Oral antibiotics and antifungal agents are administered, and irrigation is continued until the collection has resolved, as evidenced by follow-up CT. CT scans are obtained weekly or every other week. The internal drains are removed endoscopically several weeks after complete resolution of the collection.

Complications of Endoscopic Therapy of PFCs

Life-threatening complications (listed in Table 24.2) may occur after attempted endoscopic drainage of PFCs. Therefore, endoscopic drainage of PFCs is not recommended without the availability of surgical and interventional radiological support. The most serious complications of transmural drainage are bleeding and perforation. Bleeding after transmural drainage may be managed supportively, endoscopically, surgically, or with angiographic embolization. Perforations limited to the gastric wall that do not involve the collection can be managed nonsurgically, assuming a stent has not been placed through the perforation. Duodenal perforations are usually managed surgically [31]. Infectious complications usually occur from inadequate drainage of fluid and/or solid debris. If endoscopic drainage was performed on a liquefied collection by the transpapillary route, stent exchange and/or upsizing of the stent or conversion to a transmural approach may resolve the infection. Similarly, if solid material was present and unrecognized during the initial procedure, placement of irrigation tubes or converting to a transmural drainage approach may resolve the infection. Percutaneous drainage and/or irrigation catheters may be required to manage infectious complications and drain peripheral collections. Stent migration into the collection through the gastric or duodenal wall may occur during or after endoscopic stent placement.

Table 24.2. Complications of endoscopic therapy of pancreatic fluid collections

Bleeding
Perforation
Infection
Pancreatitis
Sedation complications
Aspiration
Stent migration/occlusion
Pancreatic ductal damage

Results of Endoscopic Therapy for PFCs

Pancreatic Pseudocysts

The success rates, recurrence rates, and complication rates following endoscopic drainage of pancreatic pseudocysts are variable. Successful endoscopic drainage is achieved in approximately 85% of cases, with complication rates occurring in 5–10% and recurrence rates of about ≤10%, especially in the absence of ongoing ductal leak or main pancreatic duct disconnection [1,11,28,32–34].

Pancreatic Abscesses

There are case reports and one series of successful endoscopic abscess drainage using transmural and transpapillary approaches, with overall success rates of about 90% [1,35–37].

Organized Pancreatic Necrosis

In the largest series to date, successful nonsurgical resolution of OPN was achieved in 31 out of 43 patients (72%) [27]. The rate of recurrent collections is high relative to the presence of severe residual ductal abnormalities, similar to what is seen after surgical intervention for necrosis [38].

Percutaneous (Radiological) Therapy

Percutaneous therapy is performed by accessing the collection under CT or ultrasound (US) guidance. CT is the preferred method of guidance because it provides superior visualization, especially of deeper col-

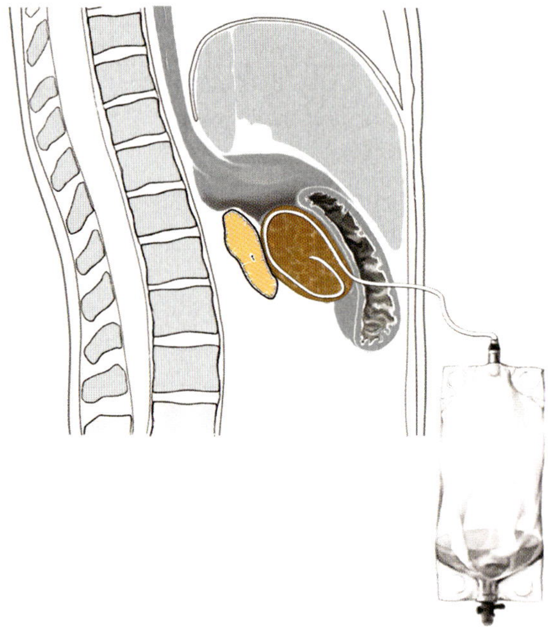

Figure 24.3

Percutaneous drainage of a pancreatic pseudocyst. A catheter has been passed percutaneously into a retrogastric collection

lections. US-guided drainage, however, can be performed at the bedside in the intensive care unit. The collection is entered with a needle while avoiding passage through vascular structures, luminal structures, and organs, although occasionally the transhepatic route may be required. A guidewire is passed into the collection and catheters subsequently passed over the guidewire. Locking internal loop catheters are used to secure the catheter internally (Fig. 24.3). Catheter sizes vary from as small as 7 Fr to as large as 30 Fr, although the larger-bore catheters are not placed at the initial drainage. Smaller catheters are adequate for pseudocyst drainage. Slightly larger catheters are needed for abscesses and the largest catheters are required for drainage of necrosis.

Results of Percutaneous Therapy for PFCs

Pancreatic Pseudocyst Drainage

Although needle aspiration alone has been described for the percutaneous treatment of pseudocysts, it is not effective because of the unacceptable recurrence rate. Thus drainage catheters are used and maintained until drainage ceases and a repeat CT scan documents resolution of the collection. High technical and clinical success rates for the resolution of pancreatic pseudocysts is achievable using the percutaneous approach, with the most recent series demonstrating an 80–90% success rate, particularly if there is no communication to the pancreatic ductal system [39,40]. However, if there is a communication with the pancreatic duct, a persistent pancreaticocutaneous fistula may occur, as suggested by high-output amylase-rich fluid from the drain despite collapse of the collection by imaging studies as well as by catheter injection or MRCP. Pancreaticocutaneous fistulae may respond to octreotide therapy with prolonged catheter drainage (weeks to months). The presence of pancreatic duct obstruction, uncommon as a sequela of mild acute pancreatitis, precludes the effectiveness of octreotide. Patients with pancreatic duct fistulae who do not respond to prolonged catheter drainage and octreotide can be managed effectively with endoscopic transpapillary stent placement [41]. A very small subset will require surgery. A percutaneous drainage approach that avoids the development of a pancreaticocutaneous fistula is transgastric placement of the catheter, an approach similar to endoscopic transgastric drainage. In this case, the catheters, which are internalized in the stomach, require endoscopic removal after collapse of the pseudocyst.

Pancreatic Abscess

The success rates for pancreatic abscess drainage are less than for pseudocyst drainage, with rates between 65 and 90% [39]. This is probably because some series included patients with infected necrosis rather than true abscesses [40].

Organized Pancreatic Necrosis

As in endoscopic therapy, the percutaneous approach to OPN differs from pseudocyst drainage. Successful percutaneous therapy for infected acute necrotizing pancreatitis has been described using large-bore percutaneous catheters up to 30 Fr in diameter in conjunction with aggressive irrigation [39,40,42,43]. Multiple catheter sites and frequent catheter exchanges with upsizing and repositioning are necessary to achieve successful resolution. Percutaneous therapy can be used as primary therapy, as a temporizing therapy, or to treat residual necrosis after surgical necrosectomy. Aggressive irrigation is performed and is paramount to enhancing the success. Frequent CT scans are needed to guide therapy. Solid debris can be removed percutaneously using basket extraction techniques [43]. In addition, there are now series describing endoscopic debridement of necrosis using baskets, performed through mature sinus tracts created percutaneously or surgically [44,45].

Similar to endoscopic therapy, the more liquefied the necrosis, the more likely percutaneous image-guided percutaneous drainage is likely to be effective. Percutaneous catheter drainage has been used to avoiding surgery or to temporize prior to necrosectomy. The overall success rate of percutaneous therapy for complete nonsurgical resolution as primary therapy in selected patients is widely variable, ranging from approximately 50% to 100%.

Complications of Percutaneous Therapy of PFCs

Introduction of infection into previously sterile PFCs may occur either from external or internal sources, such as during passage of a needle or catheter through a bowel lumen, and may occur after simple aspiration [46]. Likewise, fistula from the PFC to the skin or bowel lumen may occur. The latter may be a result of either passage of the catheter through the bowel during placement, or as result of catheter erosion after long-term placement [40]. Pseudoaneurysms rarely occur as a direct result of percutaneous therapy.

Surgical Implications of Complications following Interventional Therapy

Endoscopic and percutaneous therapy may be associated with complications and/or failures that require surgical management. It is possible that the outcome of surgical therapy may be adversely altered when compared to those patients undergoing primary surgical therapy [13].

Conclusion

Drainage options for patients with pancreatic necrosis are expanding. The experience using newer, nonsurgical drainage procedures is limited, and no interdisciplinary comparative data exist. When deciding on the timing or treatment modality to be employed in these complex patients, the expertise of the local surgeon, interventional endoscopist, and interventional radiologist must be considered. Nonsurgical drainage of pancreatic necrosis, whether performed acutely in the first weeks or subacutely at 1 month or more after pancreatitis onset should be undertaken only by expert interventional endoscopists or interventional radiologists familiar with the potential complications and time required for successful pancreatic drainage. It is important to emphasize that improperly drained sterile necrosis may lead to life-threatening infected necrosis. An upfront team approach in planning pancreatic interventions is useful, as some patients may benefit from multimodality drainage. The decision to intervene should be based on infection of the necrosis or, in the setting of sterile necrosis, severe clinical symptoms such as gastric outlet obstruction, intractable abdominal pain, or failure to thrive [47].

Summary

PFCs are amenable to nonsurgical drainage using either endoscopic or percutaneous therapy. With either approach, the management and success are dependent upon the degree of liquefaction; pseudocysts and abscesses are more likely to resolve than necrosis. Collections containing significant amounts of solid debris require placement of multiple drains and an irrigation system in order to evacuate solid debris. EUS-guided drainage may decrease the complications of bleeding and perforation during endoscopic transmural entry of PFCs. Refinement in nonsurgical techniques to improve the safety and efficacy of therapy as well as comparative studies between these methods and surgical drainage methods are needed.

References

1. Baron TH (2003) Endoscopic drainage of pancreatic fluid collections and pancreatic necrosis. Gastrointest Endosc Clin N Am 13:743–464
2. Kloppel G (1994) Pathology of severe acute pancreatitis. In: Bradley EL III (ed) Acute Pancreatitis: Diagnosis and Therapy. Raven, New York, pp 35–46
3. Hariri M, Slivka A, Carr-Locke DL, Banks PA (1994) Pseudocyst drainage predisposes to infection when pancreatic necrosis is unrecognized. Am J Gastroenterol 89:1781–1784
4. Kozarek RA (1996) Endotherapy for organized pancreatic necrosis: perspectives on skunk-poking. Gastroenterology 111:820–822
5. Uomo G, Molino D, Visconti M, Ragozzino A, Manes G, Rabitti PG (1998) The incidence of main pancreatic duct disruption in severe biliary pancreatitis. Am J Surg 176:49–52
6. Baron TH, Morgan DE, Vickers SM, Lazenby AJ (1999) Organized pancreatic necrosis: endoscopic, radiologic, and pathologic features of a distinct clinical entity. Pancreas 19:105–108

7. Morgan DE, Baron TH, Smith JK, Robbin ML, Kenney PJ (1997) Pancreatic fluid collections prior to intervention: evaluation with MR imaging compared with CT and US. Radiology 203:773–778
8. Baril NB, Ralls PW, Wren SM, Selby RR, Radin R, Parekh D, Jabbour N, Stain SC (2000) Does an infected peripancreatic fluid collection or abscess mandate operation? Ann Surg 231:361–367
9. Traverso LW, Kozarek RA (1999) Interventional management of peripancreatic fluid collections. Surg Clin North Am 79:745–757
10. Yeo CJ, Bastidas JA, Lynch-Nyhan A, Fishman EK, Zinner MJ, Cameron JL (1990) The natural history of pancreatic pseudocysts documented by computed tomography. Surg Gynecol Obstet 170:411–417
11. Libera ED, Siqueira ES, Morais M, Rohr MR, Brant CQ, Ardengh JC, Ferrari AP (2000) Pancreatic pseudocysts transpapillary and transmural drainage. HPB Surg 11:333–338
12. Nealon WH, Walser E (2002) Main pancreatic ductal anatomy can direct choice of modality for treating pancreatic pseudocysts (surgery versus percutaneous drainage). Ann Surg 235:751–8
13. Nealon WH, Walser E (2005) Surgical management of complications associated with percutaneous and/or endoscopic management of pseudocyst of the pancreas. Ann Surg 241:948–957
14. Zhang AB, Zheng SS (2005) Treatment of pancreatic pseudocysts in line with D'Egidio's classification. World J Gastroenterol 11:729–32
15. Barthet M, Sahel J, Bodiou-Bertei C Bernard JP (1995) Endoscopic transpapillary drainage of pancreatic pseudocysts. Gastrointest Endosc 42:208–213
16. Catalano MF, Geenen JE, Schmalz MJ, Johnson GK, Dean RS, Hogan WJ (1995) Treatment of pancreatic pseudocysts with ductal communication by transpapillary pancreatic duct endoprosthesis. Gastrointest Endosc 42:214–218
17. Monkemuller KE, Baron TH, Morgan DE (1998). Transmural drainage of pancreatic fluid collections without electrocautery using the Seldinger technique. Gastrointest Endosc 48:195–200
18. Binmoeller KF, Seifert H, Walter A, Soehendra N (1995) Transpapillary and transmural drainage of pancreatic psuedocysts. Gastrointest Endosc 42:219–224
19. Telford JJ, Farrell JJ, Saltzman JR, Shields SJ, Banks PA, Lichtenstein DR, Johannes RS, Kelsey PB, Carr-Locke DL (2002) Pancreatic stent placement for duct disruption. Gastrointest Endosc 56:18–24
20. Kozarek RA (1990) Pancreatic stents can induce ductal changes consistent with chronic pancreatitis. Gastrointest Endosc 36:93–95
21. Smith MT, Sherman S, Ikenberry SO, Hawes RH, Lehman GA (1996) Alterations in pancreatic ductal morphology following polyethylene pancreatic stent therapy. Gastrointest Endosc 44:268–275
22. Fockens P, Johnson TG, van Dullemen HM, Huibregtse K, Tytgat GN (1997) Endosonographic imaging of pancreatic pseudocysts before endoscopic transmural drainage. Gastrointest Endosc 46:412–416
23. Sedlack R, Affi A, Vazquez-Sequeiros E, Norton ID, Clain JE, Wiersema MJ (2002). Utility of EUS in the evaluation of cystic pancreatic lesions. Gastrointest Endosc 56:543–547
24. Chak A (2000) Endosonographic-guided therapy of pancreatic pseudocysts. Gastrointest Endosc 52:S23–S27
25. Giovannini M, Pesenti C, Rolland A-L, Moutardier V, Delpero JR (2001) Endoscopic ultrasound-guided drainage of pancreatic pseudocysts or pancreatic abscesses using a therapeutic echo endoscope. Endoscopy 33:473–477
26. Sriram PV, Kaffes AJ, Rao GV, Reddy DN (2005) Endoscopic ultrasound-guided drainage of pancreatic pseudocysts complicated by portal hypertension or by intervening vessels. Endoscopy 2005 37:231–235
27. Gibbs CM, Baron TH (2005) Outcome following endoscopic transmural drainage of pancreatic fluid collections in outpatients. J Clin Gastroenterol 39:634–637
28. Baron TH, Harewood GC, Morgan DE, Yates MR (2002) Outcome differences after endoscopic drainage of pancreatic necrosis, acute pancreatic pseudocysts, and chronic pancreatic pseudocysts. Gastrointest Endosc 56:7–17
29. Baron TH, Morgan DE (1999) Endoscopic transgastric irrigation tube placement via PEG for debridement of organized pancreatic necrosis. Gastrointest Endosc 50:574–577
30. Seewald S, Groth S, Omar S, Imazu H, Seitz U, de Weerth A, Soetikno R, Zhong Y, Sriram PV, Ponnudurai R, Sikka S, Thonke F, Soehendra N (2005). Aggressive endoscopic therapy for pancreatic necrosis and pancreatic abscess: a new safe and effective treatment algorithm (videos). Gastrointest Endosc 62:92–100
31. Beckingham IJ, Krige JE, Bornman PC, Terblanche J (1997) Endoscopic management of pancreatic pseudocysts. Br J Surg 84:1638–1645
32. Sharma SS, Bhargawa N, Govil A (2002) Endoscopic management of pancreatic pseudocysts: a long-term follow-up. Endoscopy 2002 3:203–207
33. Beckingham IJ, Krige JE, Bornman PC, Terblanche J (1999) Long term outcome of endoscopic drainage of pancreatic pseudocysts. Am J Gastroenterol 94:71–74
34. Cahen D, Rauws E, Fockens P, Weverling G, Huibregtse K, Bruno M (2005) Endoscopic drainage of pancreatic pseudocysts: long-term outcome and procedural factors associated with safe and successful treatment. Endoscopy 37:977–983
35. Park JJ, Kim SS, Koo YS, Choi DJ, Park HC, Kim JH, Kim JS, Hyun JH (2002) Definitive treatment of pancreatic abscess by endoscopic transmural drainage. Gastrointest Endosc 55:256–262
36. Giovannini M, Pesenti C, Rolland AL, Moutardier V, Delpero JR (2001) Endoscopic ultrasound-guided drainage of pancreatic pseudocysts or pancreatic abscesses using a therapeutic echo endoscope. Endoscopy 33:473–477
37. Venu RP, Brown RD, Marrero JA, Pastika BJ, Frakes JT (2000) Endoscopic transpapillary drainage of pancreatic abscess: technique and results. Gastrointest Endosc 51:391–395
38. Howard TJ, Moore SA, Saxena R, Matthews DE, Schmidt CM, Wiebke EA (2004) Pancreatic duct strictures are a common cause of recurrent pancreatitis after successful management of pancreatic necrosis. Surgery 136:909–916
39. Shankar S, vanSonnenberg E, Silverman SG, Tuncali K, Banks PA (2004) Imaging and percutaneous management of acute complicated pancreatitis. Cardiovasc Intervent Radiol 27:567–580
40. Maher MM, Lucey BC, Gervais DA, Mueller PR (2004) Acute pancreatitis: the role of imaging and interventional radiology. Cardiovasc Intervent Radiol 27:208–225
41. Kozarek RA, Ball TJ, Patterson DJ, Raltz SL, Traverso LW, Ryan JA, Thirlby RC (1997) Transpapillary stenting for pancreaticocutaneous fistulas. J Gastrointest Surg 1:357–361

42. Freeny PC, Hauptmann E, Althaus SJ, Traverso LW, Sinanan M (1998) Percutaneous CT-guided catheter drainage of infected acute necrotizing pancreatitis: techniques and results AJR Am J Roentgenol 170:969–975
43. Echenique AM, Sleeman D, Yrizarry J, Scagnelli T, Guerra JJ Jr, Casillas VJ, Huson H, Russell E (1998) Percutaneous catheter-directed debridement of infected pancreatic necrosis: results in 20 patients. J Vasc Interv Radiol 9:565–571
44. Mui LM, Wong SK, Ng EK, Chan AC, Chung SC (2005) Combined sinus tract endoscopy and endoscopic retrograde cholangiopancreatography in management of pancreatic necrosis and abscess. Surg Endosc 19:393–397
45. Carter CR, McKay CJ, Imrie CW (2000) Percutaneous necrosectomy and sinus tract endoscopy in the management of infected pancreatic necrosis: an initial experience. Ann Surg 232:175–180
46. Walser EM, Nealon WH, Marroquin S, Raza S, Hernandez JA, Vasek J (2005) Sterile fluid collections in acute pancreatitis: catheter drainage versus simple aspiration. Cardiovasc Intervent Radiol 29:102–107
47. Baron TH, Morgan DE (1999) Acute necrotizing pancreatitis. N Engl J Med 340:1412–141z

Chapter 25

G. Tsiotos · J. Tsiaoussis

Pancreatic and Intestinal Fistulas

Pancreatic fistulas (PFs) and intestinal fistulas (IFs) are troublesome, occasionally significant, and not uncommon sequelae of necrotizing pancreatitis (NP). They account for increased morbidity and sometimes mortality, and prolonged hospital stay, and they are costly both financially and with regard to resources.

Incidence varies between 5% and over 50% among published series, but there is a definite decreasing trend recently across the literature. The wide variation in incidence reflects not only different levels of expertise among the authors, but also the striking lack of a universally accepted and applied definition of PF specifically in the context of NP. Although recently a consensus definition and staging of *postoperative* PF was published [1], there has been no similar unifying attempt in the setting of NP, as is our topic. The decreased incidence of PF/IF in the recent literature, in addition to improved surgical expertise, certainly reflects in part the recent change in the overall management strategy of NP, as will be discussed below.

Higher imaging precision has led to more accurate diagnoses by the delineation of fine, but crucial anatomic details of both PF and IF. In addition, advanced technology and refined operative and interventional or minimally invasive techniques have contributed to an improved outcome in these patients.

In this chapter we will discuss the pathogenesis and management of PF and IF separately, but prior to this, it is essential to briefly outline a very significant change in the management scheme of NP that has taken place during the last decade, which has crucial implications in both the incidence and the treatment of PF and IF.

Modern Management of NP and its Implications

Since it has been recognized that the early peak of mortality in the biphasic mortality pattern of NP is due to the overwhelming systemic inflammatory response syndrome (SIRS; not sepsis), whereas the later second peak is due to sepsis, two major components of modern management have emerged: (1) very aggressive hemodynamic, ventilatory, metabolic, and nutritional support and avoiding operative treatment in the early phase, and (2) delayed operative treatment (where necessary) for as long as possible. This approach, which has been substantiated by cornerstone clinical studies [2,3] and is now the preferred management strategy in patients with NP [4], has led to optimized hemodynamics early after NP, much fewer reoperations for debridement (usually just one), essentially no gauze packing, and placement of fewer drains. As will be discussed in detail below, these factors have substantially decreased the incidence of NP/IF.

Pathogenesis

Although the pathogenesis of PF/IF is multifactorial, the most common factor in their development is the presence of pancreatic parenchymal necrosis, as this results in the disruption of small or large pancreatic ducts with subsequent extravasation of exocrine secretions into the retroperitoneum [5]. Operative necrosectomy and local drainage allow for external egress of these extravasated secretions and the potential for a pancreaticocutaneous fistula. The concurrent pancreatic and peripancreatic inflammatory process may also lead to stenosis of the pancreatic ducts, which represents a substantial element for the chronicity of fistulas. The importance of pancreatic parenchymal necrosis as the main risk factor in the pathogenesis of PF is stressed by the finding in one study that all patients who developed pancreaticocutaneous fistulas had proven pancreatic parenchymal necrosis, while none of the patients with peripancreatic retroperitoneal fat necrosis with an inflamed but viable pancreas developed a PF [6].

Compromised Blood Supply

Compromised blood supply (in the form of vascular thrombosis) to the colon and the duodenum has been postulated as a pathogenetic mechanism for the formation of gastrointestinal fistulas in particular. Enzyme-rich fluids and inflammatory products released or produced early in the course of the necrotizing process can dissect throughout the retroperitoneal tissues and into the transverse mesocolon to involve the vascular supply to the colon or duodenum, with consequent vascular thrombosis. The subsequent ischemia (if extensive enough) may lead to segmental colonic or duodenal necrosis and eventually the formation of a gastrointestinal fistula. Colonic ischemia may occur as a result of a low-flow state [7] caused by inadequate initial resuscitation or as a consequence of the hemodynamic response to the sepsis syndrome. This speculation would explain the tendency for fistulas to arise from the left transverse colon and the splenic flexure, where collateral flow is more compromised in low-flow states. However, the modern aggressive hemodynamic resuscitation in the early phase of NP (see above) has minimized a low-flow state as a cause of a fistula.

Autodigestion

Autodigestion of adjacent organs as a cause of IF in the course of NP has more of a theoretical background. According to this hypothesis, the extravasated exocrine secretions may result in transmural necrosis of the stomach and small intestine in a way similar to peripancreatic fat necrosis. This concept for the development of gastrointestinal tract fistulas seems much less likely because, unlike fat, the stomach and small intestine have a much better vascular supply and, thus, associated protective mechanisms [6].

Choice of Operative Technique

The development of fistulas may be related to the choice of operative technique, since repeated local trauma to the surface of an organ, as might occur with repeated open packing of the lesser sack or during "planned relaparotomies," may lead to intestinal wall erosions. To reduce this possibility, covering of the exposed viscera and major blood vessels with a form of nonadherent interface before applying the intra-abdominal gauze packing has been proposed [5]. In addition, recent studies indicate that necrosectomy followed by "closed packing" or by "closed continuous lavage" may lead to a lower incidence of PF/IF formation [8,9], as this approach requires fewer intra-abdominal interventions for the repeated removal of pancreatic necrotic material.

It is interesting, however, to note that the discussions about individual techniques and the comparisons among them tend to become obsolete, since today's management strategy of patients with NP consisting of aggressive nonoperative initial management followed by necrosectomy as late as possible (removal of well-demarcated necrotic tissue without compromising viable viscera usually 1 month after the onset of NP) leads to a more accurate distinction between viable and necrotic tissue and a more complete necrosectomy, with a lower risk of leaving nonviable infected debris behind. Thus, a much lower number of relaparotomies is required, with a lower incidence of adjacent organ injury and, as a result, a lower frequency of gastrointestinal fistulas.

Choice of Operative Approach to the Retroperitoneal Space

The choice of operative approach to the retroperitoneal space during necrosectomy could predispose to fistula development as a result of adjacent organ injury. The lesser sac can be approached through the transverse mesocolon, the gastrocolic omentum, or the gastrohepatic omentum. Because of the inflammatory process, the stomach and transverse colon may have been densely adherent to the inflammatory mass. Consequently, accessing the lesser sac through an avascular area of the mesocolon to the left of the ligament of Treitz seems quicker and safer, avoiding any inadvertent injury to the adjacent organs. Fernandez-del Castillo et al. recognized the fact that no colonic fistula developed in their series and attributed this to their preferred access via the mesocolon [3].

Pressure Necrosis

Another iatrogenic mechanism of fistula formation may be from pressure necrosis of a segment of bowel from an adjacent drain and such a mechanism could reflect the late development of certain colonic, small-bowel, or gastric fistulas. To avoid this, the peripancreatic drains should not be positioned directly on the duodenum or ascending colon when placed from the patient's right side, or on the descending colon when placed from the left side. The ideal placement of the drains is behind the splenic flexure of the colon and below the lower pole of the spleen, thereby exiting the abdominal wall in the left anterior axillary line. Also, large, hard, stiff sump drains should be avoided as an additional means of prevention of gastrointestinal fistula.

Minimally invasive techniques (percutaneous or endoscopic drainage) and minimally invasive surgery (retroperitoneoscopic debridement) are alternatives to open surgery in select cases, promising lower morbidity including lower incidence of PF [10]. These innovations have not been popularized yet and only a small number of series (with highly selected patients) have been published [11]. With the currently available experience, laparoscopy-assisted necrosectomy might be followed by a higher trend for significant injuries to intra-abdominal viscera including a higher incidence of PF/IF, as has been reported (20–60%) [9].

Pancreatic Fistulas

Definition and Incidence

The lack of a widely accepted definition of this complication in the setting of NP has contributed in part to the major discrepancy in its reported incidence among published series. Criteria such as amylase level in the excreted fluid, daily output of the fistula, and its duration vary among studies. Despite the varying definitions, a PF can be conceptualized anatomically as an abnormal communication between a pancreatic duct (major or minor) and the skin (pancreaticocutaneous fistula or external fistula), or between the pancreatic duct and peritoneal or pleural cavity, or another hollow viscus (internal fistula). Because of its clinical significance we will deal with external fistulas in this chapter. The presence of infected NP (versus sterile NP) seems to favor the development of PF, as PF is far more common (up to 76%) in the former group [6,12].

Diagnosis and Imaging

The diagnosis of the presence of a PF can be easily made by measuring the amylase activity of the fluid excreted through a drain tube; this is higher than 1000 IU/dl and usually up to a few thousands of IU/dl. Amylase activity levels of a few hundreds of IU/dl generally do not reflect a PF. The diagnosis of a PF should be followed by the precise delineation of its anatomic details. Complete mapping of the PF and its relationship to the pancreatic ductal system determines its prognosis and dictates the management options.

The two issues of paramount importance to be studied and looked for by imaging are:

1. Communication of the PF with the main pancreatic duct or one of its minor branches.
2. Integrity of the pancreatic duct downstream (i.e., between the ductal disruption and the sphincter of Oddi). The possibilities are the following:
   a. proximal stenosis (i.e., stenosis of the main pancreatic duct between its disruption and the sphincter of Oddi, in which case the PF is "fed" primarily, but not exclusively, by the portion of the pancreatic duct of the distal pancreas)
   b. disconnected pancreatic duct (i.e., no communication between the PF and the proximal pancreatic duct, in which case the PF is exclusively "fed" by the portion of the pancreatic duct of the distal pancreas. This distal portion of the pancreas is then an isolated pancreatic segment draining solely through the fistula)
   c. "normal" pancreatic duct (i.e., the PF is "fed" by a rather small disruption of the pancreatic duct, but its proximal and distal portions are in continuity and there is no stenosis along the length of the duct).

Imaging techniques that can be employed in order to extract this fine information include: (1) contrast sinogram, (2) contrast-enhanced computed tomography (CECT), (3) magnetic resonance cholangiopancreatography (MRCP), and (4) endoscopic retrograde cholangiopancreatography (ERCP).

The water-soluble contrast sinogram is the first imaging study that should be performed and it may well be the only one required. It is very easy to perform, dynamic, low-cost, and noninvasive. It may reveal a communication of the PF with the main or a side pancreatic duct. In cases of right or mid-body pancreatic necrosis, the sinogram may show filling of the distal pancreatic duct without opacification of the proximal pancreatic duct or the duodenum. A spiral CECT scan with thin cuts may also demonstrate the presence and anatomy of a PF, but there is no comparative study that favors CECT scan over sinogram.

MRCP has been utilized increasingly to demonstrate pancreatic ductal anatomy and certainly does have a role in the imaging of PF as they relate to the ductal system. It should be kept in mind, however, that although CECT and MRCP represent today the most modern modalities of cross-sectional anatomy and are readily available in most institutions, they may not necessarily provide more information pertinent to the precise anatomy of a PF compared to an expertly performed sinogram. Interestingly, it has been shown, for example, that although MRCP is capable of identifying major pancreatic ductal injuries, its reliability to discriminate subtle anomalies in anatomy or to demonstrate a communication between the pancreatic duct and a pseudocyst is not high [13]. ERCP is generally reserved when sinogram and cross-sectional modalities have not provided all of the necessary anatomic information, or when an endoscopic therapeutic procedure is contemplated after sinogram has precisely demonstrated the anatomy.

Management

PFs are quite often complicated by fluid and electrolyte abnormalities, malnutrition, skin erosion, and less often hemorrhage and sepsis. The initial management of PF is conservative and its fundamental principles are the following:

1. Provision of optimal drainage to avoid intra-abdominal fluid collections.
2. Maintenance of fluid and electrolyte balance.
3. Treatment of local infection.
4. Optimization of nutritional status by parenteral or preferably enteral feeding.
5. Skin care.

An additional appealing line of PF management is the reduction of pancreatic secretion (and thus PF output) by possible administration of octreotide. The role of octreotide in the prevention and the treatment of PF has been studied in the postpancreatectomy setting (for tumor or chronic pancreatitis), but not in the NP setting. It is fair to note that five of nine prospective randomized studies demonstrate a favorable effect of octreotide over placebo, whereas the remaining four did not [14]. Again, all nine studies included patients who had undergone an elective pancreatic operation and not patients with PF in the context of NP. Our experience with the use of octreotide in an effort to accelerate the closure of inflammatory PF has not been encouraging [6]. It seems unlikely that this issue will be definitively resolved in the near future; today, the use of octreotide in this setting is not evidence-based and should be reserved for use only within a clinical protocol.

Spontaneous closure of a PF should be the primary therapeutic goal. Compared to postoperative PF, post-NP PF tends to have less chances of spontaneous closure (53% vs 86%) and longer duration for those that do selfresolve (22 weeks vs 11 weeks) [15]. Although good nutritional status, optimal drainage, and absence of local and systemic infection certainly provide a favorable background for spontaneous PF closure, the single most important factor determining prognosis and dictating definitive management is the pattern of ductal disruption that has given rise to the development of the PF. Failure of spontaneous closure is generally due to anatomic factors such as downstream ductal obstruction and disconnected duct syndrome (isolated pancreatic tail). For example, recognition of an intact pancreatic duct without a downstream ductal obstruction indicates a high possibility of spontaneous closure. On the contrary, surgery is necessary when the PF is associated with a leak from the pancreatic duct that is not joined with the gastrointestinal tract. Indeed, no such PF closed after a mean of 26 weeks of aggressive medical therapy, and all of these patients required surgical intervention [15].

In general, when a PF persists for more than 2 weeks and its daily output remains essentially unchanged over this period (i.e., without significant, meaningful decrease), a sinogram should be performed, followed possibly by MRCP. The choice among further treatment options depends on the specific findings:

Communication of the PF with a Minor (Side) Pancreatic Duct

Nonoperative management is justified and the chances are that such a PF will eventually close, even after a few months, provided that the duct drains with no stenosis (stricture) toward the main pancreatic duct and to the duodenum.

Communication of the PF with the Main Pancreatic Duct that has a Proximal Stenosis

Spontaneous closure is unlikely because the pancreatic duct distal to the stricture is preferentially draining to the PF. These patients are ideal for endoscopic "bridging" of the proximal and distal parts of the pancreatic duct (traversing the stricture, as well as the ductal disruption "feeding" the PF) and stent placement. Small-diameter (5–7 mm) stents with variable length across the site of the ductal stricture and disruption may be used. Success rates are high (75–100%) [16,17]. Suboptimal stent placement, stent migration, or stent occlusion may require repetition of the technique to achieve complete closure of the PF (up to five stent placements in one patient have been reported for PF resolution). Interestingly, even when the stent only traverses the stricture, but does not bridge the site of ductal leakage, the outcome may be successful [18]. The duration of endoscopic therapy to close the PF varies from a few days to several weeks, and once it has been rendered, stents are retrieved after 10–14 days.

Communication of a PF with a Disconnected Pancreatic Duct

Nonoperative therapy is doomed to failure and endoscopic stent placement is highly unlikely to be successful since there is no communication between the proximal and the distal portions of the pancreatic duct; the distal "isolated" pancreatic segment is draining exclusively via the PF. Operative treatment should be planned after the surrounding inflammation has ceased and the general condition of the patient is improved (usually it is after several weeks or even a few months before operative treatment takes place). Surgical options include distal pancreatectomy with or without splenectomy (realistically, the latter is technically hard given the recent extensive retropancreatic inflammation and the fibrosis resulting from NP) and distal pancreaticojejunostomy using a defunctionalized Roux-en-Y loop. A more rarely utilized third option is a fistulojejunostomy, provided that the fistulous tract has well matured. Operative management, when indicated, is generally successful (>90%), but is associated with a not insignificant mortality (6%) [19]. Failures are due to inadequate resolution of the inflammatory process of the NP.

Communication of the PF with a "Normal" Main Pancreatic Duct

Although the main pancreatic duct has no strictures, it does have a disruption, but its portions proximal and distal to this disruption are in continuity. Enough time should be provided for spontaneous closure. If this does not take place, endoscopic stent placement should be performed and this is expected to be the definitive therapy.

Minimally invasive endoscopic techniques for stent placement today represent the definitive therapy of PF in the vast majority of patients with appropriately defined fistulas and pancreatic ductal anatomy. However, in the minority in whom this approach fails, an operation is mandatory. For patients with no disconnected pancreatic segment, a side-to-side pancreaticojejunostomy at the area of the origin of the fistulous tract is usually the optimal operative option.

Intestinal Fistulas

Definition and Incidence

As with PFs, the incidence of IFs varies widely among studies (1–43%) [10]. However, in the case of Ifs, this wide variation is not primarily due to variability of definition, but rather reflects differences in the technique of the initial necrosectomy and further operative debridements. It is especially with IFs where the changed management scheme of NP (i.e., delayed first necrosectomy with much lower number of subsequent debridements required) has resulted in a recent significant reduction in their incidence.

IFs should be conceptualized anatomically in upper-gut fistulas and colonic fistulas. This distinction is clinically relevant because the former have a generally milder course and tend to close nonoperatively, as opposed to the latter, which can be associated with significant morbidity and often require operative management. The pathogenesis of IF has been already discussed in detail earlier in this chapter.

The diagnosis of the presence of IF is easily suspected, solely by the nature of the fluid coming out via the drain tube (or the incision). Low-viscosity, bilious fluid, higher-viscosity, green-brownish fluid, and obvious fecal material obviously reflect duodenal/proximal jejunal, small intestinal, and colonic fistulas, respectively. Amylase activity level of the IF fluid is high, but certainly far lower than the levels associated with PFs; it is usually a few hundreds of IU/dl. When amylase activity level from an IF is in the range of thousands of IU/dl, one should suspect a coexisting PF draining through the same fistulous tract.

Imaging

Water-soluble contrast infusion through the fistulous tract under fluoroscopy (sinogram) is the first imaging modality to perform. This will show the length and width of the fistulous tract, it will "light up" the hollow viscous where the tract originates from (and thus define whether it is duodenum, proximal or distal small bowel, or colon), and will demonstrate the presence or absence of intestinal stenosis or obstruction distal to the intestinal disruption and the source of the fistula. A CECT scan should always be performed primarily to rule out an undrained fluid collection that often coexists at the time that the IF is first diagnosed.

Management

As with PF, the principles of IF management are: provision of excellent drainage, optimization of fluid, electrolyte, and nutritional status, treatment of local infection, and skin care. In patients with upper-gut fistulas, nutrition should be provided either parenterally or enterally distal to the site of the IF using a nasojejunal tube or a tube placed operatively.

A lot of the decision-making regarding further management depends upon the source of the fistula (upper gut versus colonic) and on the specific anatomic details of the IF:

1. Every undrained fluid collection seen in CECT should be well drained by percutaneously placed tubes under radiologic guidance. This will alleviate systemic infection and also "simplify" the fistulous tract by providing a direct communication between the intestine and the skin without pooling of intestinal content into the surrounding tissues.
2. The presence of a luminal obstruction or stenosis distal to the luminal disruption "feeding" the IF essentially guarantees failure of nonoperative management. On the contrary, absence of a distal stenosis justifies nonoperative management for long time.
3. The pattern of the fistulous tract is of paramount importance. Narrow and long fistulas are far more likely to close spontaneously compared to the wide and short ones. Prolonged nonoperative management is the preferred option for the former, whereas it is not justified for the latter.
4. The role of IF output is important and twofold. A high output (i.e., >200 ml/day persistently) may be first associated with hard-to-maintain electrolyte balance, and second with distal luminal stenosis and/or a wider and shorter fistulous tract. It is for these reasons that a persistently high-output IF is less likely to close spontaneously.

Provided that no absolute contraindication (i.e., distal luminal obstruction) is present for nonoperative management, the prognosis of IF is closely related to the part of the gastrointestinal tract that the IF originates from.

Duodenal Fistulas

Duodenal fistulas are very rare [20]. When present, they originate from the medial aspect of the duodenum as a result of extension of the pancreatic inflammatory process and duodenal wall necrosis. If well controlled, despite their potential for a high initial output, most close spontaneously. In patients where the duodenal fistula is diagnosed during the first or a subsequent necrosectomy, it is reasonable to proceed at that setting with pyloric exclusion (pyloric stapling with a noncutting device and gastrojejunostomy), or simple tube duodenostomy and excellent periduodenal drainage. Duodenal fistulas manifested and diagnosed prior to, or following necrosectomy should be controlled by interventional radiology means (percutaneous drainage). In patients where a duodenal fistula persists (longer than 2–3 months with essentially unchanged daily output) despite optimal nonoperative management, a Roux-en-Y duodenojejunostomy at the site of the duodenal wall defect is usually therapeutic. Needless to say, such a procedure should be delayed enough in relation to the time of onset of NP so that the inflammatory process has completely ceased and a safe operation can be performed.

Fistulas of the Small Intestine

In general, enteric fistulas tend to close spontaneously (more often than their duodenal counterparts). Plenty of time should be allowed (months) before the surgeon decides to proceed with an operation, provided (as previously emphasized) that the fistula and the intestine are well studied and there is no distal stenosis. In patients with a persisting high-output enteric fistula, operative management consists of resection of the fistulous tract, usually with the corresponding bowel segment and an anastomosis between the proximal and the distal bowel. Resection of the fistulous tract and oversewing of the bowel wall defect where the fistula originated from, although appealing, may be realistically more technically challenging and may in fact compromise the diameter of the bowel at that point.

Colonic Fistulas

Colonic fistulas are associated with more severe forms of NP, and the mortality of NP among patients with a concomitant colonic fistula is higher, highlighting the severity of this condition [21]. The portions of the colon more frequently involved in colonic fistulas are the transverse because of its close proximity to the lesser sac and the splenic flexure because of its vascular pattern and the subsequent suboptimal blood supply in low-flow states. Colonic fistulas not only reflect a more severe episode of NP, but also predispose patients to further comorbidity in and of themselves. This is why it has been highly recommended to proceed with immediate fecal diversion [12] as soon as a colonic fistula is diagnosed.

The increased morbidity due to a colonic fistula is usually secondary to undrained intra-abdominal fecal collections around the colonic wall defect; this may give rise to systemic sepsis. Sufficient and optimal percutaneous drainage cannot be always achieved due to the high viscosity and particulate nature of the fecal material. The combination of these factors usually dictate an urgent operation, during which proximal fecal diversion (loop ileostomy preferably, or loop colostomy) should be the first priority, followed by excellent debridement and some type of colectomy (depending on the site of the colonic defect and the extent of colonic wall necrosis).

It is important to realize, however, that it is not the mere presence of a colonic fistula that translates to operative treatment, but rather the concomitant presence of undrained fecal material pooled around the colonic necrosis and causing sepsis. If such conditions are proved by CECT scan not to be present and the patient is not septic, a colonic fistula may in fact be conceptualized as a colostomy and no immediate action needs to be taken. In such a setting, where colonic fistulas are clinically asymptomatic, well controlled, have a low output, and there is no distal colonic obstruction, they can be treated conservatively, and spontaneous closure may ensue.

Summary

PFs and IFs are notorious complications of NP, but their incidence has decreased due to the recent change of management scheme for NP consisting of aggressive initial hemodynamic support and delayed necrosectomy, which has led to a reduction in the number of reoperations required. Precise delineations of the fistulous tract in relation to the pancreatic ductal system and the pattern of pancreatic duct disruption dictate the prognosis and the appropriate management option for a PF. Many PFs close spontaneously, some require advanced endoscopic intrapancreatic procedures (ductal stent placement), and few require operative intervention. Most upper-gut fistulas close spontaneously provided that there is no distal intestinal stenosis, whereas colonic fistulas are generally troublesome, may lead to sepsis, and require urgent operative treatment.

References

1. Bassi C, Dervenis C, Butturini G, Fingerhut A, et al (2005) Postoperative pancreatic fistula: an international study group (ISGPF) definition. Surgery 138:8–13
2. Mier J, Luque-de Leon E, Castillo A, et al (1997) Early versus late necrosectomy in severe necrotizing pancreatitis. Am J Surg 173:71–75
3. Fernandez-Del Castillo C, Rattner DW, Makary MA, Mostafavi A, McGrath D, Warshaw AL (1998) Debridement and closed packing for the treatment of necrotizing pancreatitis. Ann Surg 228:676–684
4. Uhl W, Warshaw A, Imrie C, Bassi C, et al (2002) IAP Guidelines for the surgical management of acute pancreatitis. Pancreatology 2:565–573
5. Bradley EL III (1993) A clinically based classification system for acute pancreatitis. Arch Surg 128:586–590
6. Tsiotos GG, Smith CD, Sarr MG (1995) Incidence and management of pancreatic and enteric fistulas after surgical management of severe necrotizing pancreatitis. Arch Surg 130:48–52
7. Albridge MC, Francis ND, Glazer G, Dudley HAF (1989) Colonic complications of severe acute pancreatitis. Br J Surg 76:362–367
8. Buchler MW, Gloor B, Muller CA, et al (2000) Acute necrotizing pancreatitis: treatment strategy according to the status of infection. Ann Surg 232:619–626
9. Werner J, Feuerbach S, Uhl W, Buchler MW (2005) Management of acute pancreatitis: from surgery to interventional intensive care. Gut 54:426–436
10. Connor S, Alexakis N, Raraty MGT, et al (2005) Early and late complications after pancreatic necrosectomy. Surgery 137:499–505
11. Connor S, Ghaneh P, Raraty MGT, et al (2003) Minimally invasive retroperitoneal pancreatic necrosectomy. Dig Surg 20:270–277
12. Ho HS, Frey CF (1995) Gastrointestinal and pancreatic complications associated with severe pancreatitis. Arch Surg 130:817–823
13. Nealon WH, Walser E (2005) Surgical management of complications associated with percutaneous and/or endoscopic management of pseudocyst of the pancreas. Ann Surg 241:948–960
14. Alexakis N, Sutton R, Neoptolemos JP (2004) Surgical treatment of pancreatic fistula. Dig Surg 21:262–274
15. Howard TJ, Stonerock CE, Sarkar J, et al (1998) Contemporary treatment strategies for external pancreatic fistulas. Surgery 124:627–33
16. Boerma D, Rauws E, van Gulik T, Huibregtse K, Obertop H, Gouma D (2000) Endoscopic stent placement for pancreaticocutaneous fistula after surgical drainage of the pancreas. Br J Surg 87:1506–1509
17. Costamagna G, Mutignani M, Ingrosso M, et al (2001) Endoscopic treatment of postsurgical external pancreatic fistulas. Endoscopy 33:317–322

18. Kozarek R, Ball T, Patterson D, et al (1997) Transpapillary stenting for pancreaticocutaneous fistulas. J Gastrointest Surg 1:357–361
19. Voss M, Ali A, Eubanks E, Pappas T (2003) Surgical management of pancreaticocutaneous fistula. J Gastrointest Surg 7:542–546
20. Sakorafas GH, Tsiotos GG, Sarr MG (1999) Experience with duodenal necrosis: a rare complication of acute necrotizing pancreatitis. Int J Pancreatol 25:139–142
21. Kriwanek S, Gschwantler M, Beckerhinn P, et al (1999) Complications after surgery for necrotizing pancreatitis: risk factors and prognosis. Eur J Surg 165:952–957

Chapter 26

I.H. Nordback · J. Sand

Late Outcome after Necrosectomy

Long-term outcome after necrotizing pancreatitis is dependent on the severity of the disease, the method of treatment, and on the patient and his lifestyle after convalescence. Some data on these various circumstances exist.

Pancreatic Resection

Formal pancreatic resection was considered an important treatment option to remove the necrosis in acute necrotizing pancreatitis, especially during the 1970s and early 1980s. This form of therapy was abandoned not only due to the high early complication rate, but more due to the numerous late complications. The late results, however, are interesting since they offer a reference for comparison with the late results obtained after less radical removal of the necrosis.

Diabetes developed in virtually all of the patients, half requiring insulin therapy [1,2]. The mechanism of diabetes was not solely insulin deficiency, but also the decreased sensitivity of the tissues to insulin [3]. Severe exocrine pancreatic insufficiency, appearing as daily fatty diarrhea, affected the life of 20% of the patients [1]. The most disturbing complication was polyneuropathy. Numb extremeties with severe weaknesses appeared in up to 40% of the patients. Patients treated with pancreatic resection for acute necrotizing pancreatitis of alcoholic etiology appeared to be most vulnerable for this complication, later also known as "intensive care polyneuropathy" [1]. With achievements in nutrition and physical therapy during intensive care, this complication has become rare.

Necrosectomy

Recurring Disease

Overall, a substantial number of patients with acute pancreatitis of any severity will have a recurrent disease. These recurrencies concentrate on alcoholic acute pancreatitis, since the recurrence of biliary pancreatitis may well be prevented by adequate gallstone surgery performed immediately after recovery. Half of the patients who have recovered from the first acute alcohol-induced pancreatitis of any severity will develop a recurrent disease in a 10- to 20-year follow up. If the recurrency is going to take place, it will do so soon, usually within the first 3–4 years after convalescence from the first episode [4].

The major determinant of the recurrency is whether the patient continues alcohol consumption or not; the risk increases substantially along with increasing alcohol consumption. After acute necrotizing pancreatitis of alcoholic etiology, while one-third of patients will become total abstiners, one-third continue "some" drinking, and one-third remain heavy drinkers, who carry the highest risk of recurrence.

It is possible, that in addition to ongoing alcohol consumption, other factors have an effect on the development of recurrence. Metabolic disorders might be involved in the risk [5]. Also, the less severe the first attack of pancreatitis, the more likely is the development of multirecurring acute pancreatitis or chronic disease [4]. Necrotizing pancreatitis is the most severe form of pancreatitis, and recurrent acute pancreatitis is observed in only about 5% of patients after necrosectomy [6]. It has been postulated that the patients "learn their lession" better in the case of severe necrotizing pancreatitis, and withdraw from alcohol.

Table 26.1. Diabetes after necrosectomy

Reference	Number of patients	Follow up	Diabetes		
			Insulin	Oral medication/diet	Impaired glucose tolerance
van Goor et al. 1997 [11]	7	median 44 months	1 (14%)		6 (86%)
Tsiotos et al. 1998 [7]	44	mean 60 months	12 (27%)	4 (9%)	
Buscher et al. 1999 [10]	20	mean 63 months	5 (25%)		6 (30%)
Beattie et al. 2002 [8]	31	–	9 (29%)		
Endlicher et al. 2003 [16]	9	median 30 months			6 (67%)
Tzovaras et al. 2004 [6]	21	median 48 months	6 (29%)		4 (19%)
Connor et al. 2005 [9]	58	median 29 months	19 (33%)[a]		

[a] Insulin, oral medication, or diet only

Diabetes

Diabetes is less frequently observed after necrosectomy than after formal pancreatic resection, partly because with this method of treatment vital tissue may be better preserved. However, insulin-dependent diabetes is still observed in 15–30% of patients during the long-term follow up (Table 26.1) [7–10]. This diabetes is diagnosed not earlier than (median) 3 years after the necrosectomy, suggesting not only that it is an acute disease, but also that it is the surgical treatment that causes the diabetes [10]. In fact, another one-third of patients have impaired glucose tolerance [11–14], and a substantial number have increased fasting insulin levels and increased insulin resistance [10]. It is therefore obvious that after necrosectomy it is not only endocrine insufficiency that is responsible for the development of diabetes, but other factors are also important. Intrestingly, the risk for the development of late diabetes seems to be highest when there has been a question of post-endoscopic-retrograde-cholangiopancreatography (ERCP) pancreatitis [15].

Exocrine Insufficiency

Excorine insufficiency is observed in the long term in a quarter of the patients (Table 26.2) [7–9]. Half of these patients have also developed diabetes [7]. Intrestingly, most of the patients already have symptoms of excorine insufficiency during the initial hospitalization and some have observed that this insufficiency rather improved than deteriorated during the follow up [7]. Similar to diabetes, exocrine insufficiency also may be most common after post-ERCP pancreatitis [15].

In clinical practice, diarrhea may be easily considered as a sign of exocrine insufficiency after acute necrotizing pancreatitis treated with necrosectomy. This is not the case, because many other conditions besides exocrine insufficiency may also induce loose stools. It is therefore important to use an accepted diagnostic test to detect exocrine insufficiency. Measurement of fecal elastase-1 concentration is a much more simple test than measurement of fecal fat excretion for the detection of exocrine insufficiency, and is sensitive enough in most clinical settings.

Pseudocyst

Most of the local complications of acute necrotizing pancreatitis develop early in the course of the disease. Abscesses, acute fluid collections, and fistulae form the majority of these local complications. Some of the fluid collections may become encapsulated by a fibrous wall and thus form a pseudocyst. Pseudocysts may also develop as a result of closure of a pancreatic fistula. When a pseudocyst is detected late after convalescence from acute necrotizing pancreatitis treated with necrosectomy, it may remain open whether this pseudocyst has persisted from the early period or whether it has developed as a late complication. Independent of whether it is a persistent early complication or a true late complication, overall around 10% of patients have been detected as having a pseudocyst in a 2- to 4-year follow up (Table 26.3) [6,12,16]. The indications and preferred methods of treatment do not differ from those in chronic pancreatitis, as described in detail in Chap. 42.

Table 26.2. Exocrine insufficiency after necrosectomy

Reference	Number of patients	Follow up	Exocrine sufficiency	Definition of exocrine sufficiency
van Goor et al. 1997 [11]	7	Median 44 months	1 (14%)	Steatorrhea, supplementation therapy
Tsiotos et al. 1998 [7]	44	Mean 60 months	11 (25%)	Measurement of fecal fat excretion
Beattie et al. 2002 [8]	31	–	7 (23%)	Supplementation therapy
Endlicher et al. 2003 [16]	9	Median 30 months	5/8 (63%)	Abnormal pancreaolaryl test
			1/5 (20%)	Abnormal fecal elastase test
Tzovaras et al. 2004 [6]	21	Median 48 months	2 (10%)	Not known
Connor et al. 2005 [9]	63	Median 29 months	16 (25%)	Steatorrhea

Table 26.3. Pseudocyst after necrosectomy

Reference	Number of patients	Follow up	Pseudocyst
Bosscha et al. 1998 [12]	13	More than 12 months	1 (8%)
Beattie et al. 2002 [8]	31	?	4 (13%)
Endlicher et al. 2003 [16]	9	Median 30 months	1 (11%)
Tzovaras et al. 2004 [6]	21	Median 48 months	2 (10%)
Connor et al. 2005 [9]	63	Median 29 months	5 (8%)

Quality of Life

From the patient's perspective, the overall quality of life may be compromised by diabetes and its treatment, excocrine insufficiency appearing as diarrhea, and abdominal pain. Pain can be disturbing in 5–10% of patients late after necrosectomy [6,7,15]. However, when the quality of life was analyzed by stardardized SF-36 questionnaire, patients who have undergone necrosectomy do not differ significantly from the age-matched control population in this matter [17–19]. After a period of convalescence, which is often many months, most of the patients are able to return to their preillness activities, including work [7].

Conclusion

In the long term, patients who survive acute necrotizing pancreatitis after necrosetomy will gain a good overall quality of life and mostly return to predisease activities, including work. However, most of the patients have glucose intolerance.; half of these patients with those intolerance, up to one-third of all surviving patients, need exogenous insulin therapy for their diabetes. This diabetes is not only caused by absolute insulin deficiency, but also by insulin resistance. The late results of various methods of necrosectomies have not been prospectively compared. When comparing the various reports from these methods, it appears that one method is not clearly better than the other. Withdrawal from alcohol is one important target of therapy in alcoholic pancreatitis to prevent recurring and multirecurring disease with accompanying deteriorating gland function.

References

1. Nordback IH, Auvinen OA (1985) Long-term results after pancreas resection for acute necrotizing pacreatitis. Br J Surg 72:687–689
2. Doepel M, Eriksson J, Halme L, et al (1993) Good long-term results in patients surviving severe acute pancreatitis. Br J Surg 80:1583–1586
3. Erikson J, Doepel M, Widen E, et al (1992) Pancreatic surgery, not pancreatitis is the primary cause of diabetes after acute fulminant pancreatitis. Gut 33:843–847
4. Pelli H, Sand J, Laippala P, Nordback I (2000) Long-term follow-up after the first episode of acute alcoholic pancreatitis: time course and risk factors for recurrence. Scand J Gastroenterol 35:552–555
5. Pelli H, Lappalainen-Lehto R, Piironen A, et al. (2005) Continued abuse predicts recurrent acute alcoholic pancreatitis, but metabolic disordersmay be involved. Pancreatology 5(suppl 1):74
6. Tzovaras G, Parks RW, Diamond T, Rowlands BJ (2004) Early and Long-term results of surgery for severe necrotising pancreatitis. Dig Surg 21:41–47

7. Tsiotos GG, Luque-De Leon E, Sarr G (1988) Long-term outcome of necrotizing pancreatitis treated by necrosectomy. Br J Surg 85:1650–1653
8. Beattie GC, Mason J, Swan D, Madhavan KK, Siriwardena AK (2002) Outcome of necrosectomy in acute pancreatitis: the case for continued vigilance. Scand J Gastroenetrol 37:1449–1453
9. Connor S, Alexakis N, Raraty MGT et al (2005) Early and late complications after pancreatic necrosectomy. Surgery 137:499–505
10. Buscher HCJL, Jacobs ML, Ong GL, et al (1999) Beta-cell function of the pancreas after necrotizing pancreatitis. Dig Surg 16:496–500
11. Van Goor H, Sluiter WJ, Bleichrodt RP (1997) Early and long term results of necrosectomy and planned re-operations for infected pancreatic necrosis. Eur J Surg 163:611–618
12. Bosscha K, Hulstaert PF, Hennipman A, et al (1998) Fulminant acute pancreatitis and infected necrosis: results of open management of the abdomen and "planned" reoperations. J Am Coll Surg 187:255–262
13. Bosscha K, Reijnders K, Jacobs MH, et al (2001) Quality of life after severe bacterial peritonitis and infected necrotizing pancreatitis treated with open management of the abdomen and planned re-operations. Crit Care Med 29:1539–1543
14. Connor S, Alexakis N, Raraty MG, et al. (2005) Early and late complications after pancreatic necrosectomy. Surgery 137:499–505
15. Fung ASY, Tsiotos GG, Sarr MG (1997) ERCP-Induced acute necrotizing pancreatitis: is it a more severe disease? Pancreas 15:217–221
16. Endlicher E, Völk M, Schölmerich J, Schäffler A, Messmann H. (2003) Long-term follow-up of patients with necrotizing pancreatitis treated by percutaneous necrosectomy. Hepatogastroenterology 50:2225–2228
17. Broome AHRN, Eisen GM, Harland RC, et al (1996) Quality of life after treatment for pancraetitis. Ann Surg 223:665–672
18. Soran A, Chelluri L, Lee KKW, Tisherman SA (2000) Outcome and quality of life of pancraetitis with acute pancreatitis requiring intensive care. J Surg Res 91:89–94
19. Halonen KI, Pettilä V, Leppäniemi AK, et al (2003) Long-term health-related quality of life in survivors of severe acute pancreatitis. Intensive Care Med 29:782–786

Chronic Pancreatitis

Chapter 27 Mechanisms of Pain in Chronic Pancreatitis 295
P. Di Sebastiano, F. F. Di Mola

Chapter 28 Natural Course of Chronic Pancreatitis 301
J. Enrique Domínguez-Muñoz

Chapter 29 Chronic Pancreatitis: Inflammatory Mass in the Head of the Pancreas – Pacemaker of Chronic Pancreatitis 311
H. G. Beger, F. Gansauge, M. Schwarz, B. Poch

Chapter 30 Diagnosis: Functional Testing, Radiological Work-up of Chronic Pancreatitis 319
M. Kahl, J. Keller, P. Layer

Chapter 31 Medical Management of Chronic Pancreatitis 331
P. G. Lankisch, H. Lübbers, R. Mahlke

Chapter 32 Tropical Chronic Pancreatitis 349
H. Ramesh

Chapter 33 Hereditary Chronic Pancreatitis: Diagnosis and Management 361
N. Teich, V. Keim

Chapter 34 Endoscopic Interventional Treatment 373
R. Jakobs, J. F. Riemann

Chapter 35 Indication for Surgical Treatment in Chronic Pancreatitis 381
H. G. Beger, B. Poch

Chapter 36 Pancreatic Duct Drainage Procedures 387
R. A. Prinz, M. Gaffud, M. Edwards

Chapter 37 Duodenum-Preserving Pancreatic Head Resection 399
H. G. Beger, B. M. Rau, B. Poch

Chapter 38 Pancreaticoduodenctomy for Chronic Pancreatitis – With or Without Pylorus Preservation *413*
L. W. Traverso

Chapter 39 Central Pancreatectomy *425*
C. Iacono, L. Bortolasi, G. Serio

Chapter 40 Distal Pancreatectomy in Patients with Chronic Pancreatitis *441*
J. Lunger, K. Mair, M. Junger, M. H. Schoenberg

Chapter 41 Total Pancreatectomy *453*
I. Ihse

Chapter 42 Surgical Treatment of Pseudocysts in Chronic Pancreatitis *459*
R. Grützmann, H. D. Saeger

Chapter 43 Late Outcome After Medical and Surgical Treatment of Chronic Pancreatitis *477*
L. Gullo, R. Pezzilli

Chapter 27

Mechanisms of Pain in Chronic Pancreatitis

P. Di Sebastiano · F. F. Di Mola

Chronic pancreatitis (CP) is a disease that is found primarily in the civilized world, and is gaining more and more importance in our industrialized society. It is a disease of the exocrine pancreas, and is characterized by progressive destruction of the pancreatic parenchyma and remodeling processes leading to the replacement of the exocrine parenchyma by extensive fibrosis. The etiology of CP is probably multifactorial, with about 65–70% of the cases being attributed to alcohol abuse. The remaining cases are classified as idiopathic CP (ICP; 20–25%) or unusual causes including hereditary pancreatitis, cystic fibrosis (CF), and CP-associated metabolic and congenital factors, or autoimmune disorders [1,2]. However, the most clinically relevant feature of CP is recurrent upper abdominal pain. Pain can be so intense and long lasting that the follow-up care of patients is difficult and frustrating [3] and many patients become addicted to narcotics.

Three different typical pain profiles during the evolution of CP have been described: (1) acute intense pain associated with repeated episodes of acute pancreatitis (acinar necrosis) in the early stages, (2) spontaneous lasting pain relief in association with severe pancreatic dysfunction in the late stage of uncomplicated CP, and (3) persistent severe pain (or frequent recurrent episodes of pain) usually in association with local complications such as pseudocysts, ductal hypertension, or extrapancreatic complications such as partial obstruction of the common bile duct, peptic ulcer, and opiate addiction [4]. Several hypotheses have been advanced to explain pain genesis in CP, including pancreatic and extrapancreatic causes. In this short manuscript we will discuss different pain hypotheses in CP.

Extrapancreatic Pain

Bile duct stenosis and duodenal stenosis due to extensive pancreatic fibrosis and inflammation have been considered extrapancreatic causes of pain [5,6]. Becker and Mischke described, in 19.5% out of 600 patients with CP, a pathological condition named "groove pancreatitis" [7]. This is characterized by the formation of a scar plate between the head of the pancreas and the duodenum. A scar in the groove is said to lead to complications that are determined by the topography: disturbance in the motility of the duodenum, stenosis of the duodenum, and tubular stenosis of the common bile duct, occasionally leading to obstructive jaundice. These alterations are suggested to be responsible for several symptoms present in CP and for postprandial pain due to the compression of nerves and ganglia located between the pancreatic head and the duodenum [8].

Pancreatic Pain

Many investigators have related the origin of pain to increased pressure in the pancreatic ducts and tissue [9–12]. The ductal hypertension hypothesis as an explanation for pain in CP is supported by observations that decompression of a dilated pancreatic duct or pseudocyst frequently relieves pain [13]. According to this hypothesis, administration of pancreatic enzymes reduces pancreas juice production in patients with CP, producing lower intraductal pressure and thereby reducing pain. Interestingly, pancreatic insufficiency appearing in the late stage of the disease may be accompanied by reduction or complete relief of pain, thus suggesting that the disease can burn itself out [8]. Amman et al. [8] observed pain relief a median of 4.5 years after onset in association with a marked increase in pancreatic dysfunction and calcifications. However, the burn-out theory in CP has been questioned by epidemiological data, which show that pain in many patients with CP continues despite pancreatic insufficiency, the appearance of calcifications, alcohol withdrawal, or pancreatic surgery. In fact, it has been estimated that around 30% of the patients treated with decompressive surgery exhibit recurrent attacks of pain [14].

In addition, octreotide, a somatostatin analogue that strongly inhibits pancreatic secretion and therefore should interrupt this postulated pain cycle described above, failed to significantly reduce the pain syndrome in many patients with CP [15].

In addition, Manes et al. found no relationship between pain score and pancreatic pressure, although the intrapancreatic pressure was positively correlated with ductal changes, and they concluded that pancreatic parenchymal pressure is not closely related to pain in CP [13].

Another hypothesis suggests that pain is induced when increased pancreatic ductal and parenchymal pressure produce a compartment syndrome that causes ischemia [16]. This hypothesis is supported by experimental studies [17] that show that increased interstitial pressure is correlated with decreased blood flow in a feline model of CP. These abnormalities were reversed by surgical incision of the gland and draining the pancreatic duct, but were affected minimally by stenting the pancreatic duct. This would suggest that incision of the gland is more important in relieving pain than ductal drainage.

CP is characterized by the presence of intra- and perilobular fibrosis, which leads to irreversible scarring. The pathogenesis of pancreatic fibrogenesis is still unclear, but a common concept is that fibrosis leads to increased intraductal pressure in the chronically inflamed pancreas and thereby to pain during the course of CP [18]. However, different studies [19] revealed that the degree of pancreatic fibrosis has no significant influence on pain generation since no correlation between the degree of fibrosis and intensity of pain could be demonstrated.

Pseudocysts of the pancreas can cause intense pain in CP patients. In the majority of the cases (60%) treatment with octreotide results in a reduction in size and in the eventual disappearance of the pseudocysts together with reduction of pain [20]. Enlargement of pseudocysts, causing compression of adjacent structures, might be a mechanism for pain generation.

Several authors have described patients with CP associated with autoimmune diseases. Sarles et al. [21] described a type of CP that might be caused by an autoimmune mechanism and termed it “primary inflammatory sclerosis of the pancreas.” Yoshida and colleagues [22] reported a similar case and proposed that pancreatitis with these characteristics has to be considered as autoimmune pancreatitis. Current accepted terminology for this condition is lymphoplasmacytic sclerosing pancreatitis or autoimmune pancreatitis [22]. Autoimmune pancreatitis should be distinguished from alcoholic chronic pancreatitis because steroid therapy for the former type is effective, morphologic changes are reversible, and pancreatic function can return to normal levels. The incidence and prevalence of this disease are not well documented in the literature; however, 150 cases have been reported in the Japanese literature [23]. It has been defined as a special form of CP caused by an autoimmune disease mechanism or associated with autoimmune-related diseases. The presence of high IgG level (IgG4) and a history of autoimmune disease could guide the diagnosis and subsequently the medical therapy. Pain is often associated with this type of inflammation, although the genesis of this clinical symptom has not yet been investigated.

Neurogenic Inflammation

In many patients, recurrent attacks of acute inflammation lead to severe abdominal pain. The inflammatory process, involving activated enzymes and other injurious substances, could be responsible for pain generation. Various investigators have shown increased expression of the neurotrophin, nerve growth factor (NGF), during the course of experimental acute pancreatitis in the rat [24]. In human CP, neurotrophin gene expression is correlated with the intensity of pain [25]. By comparing these data we can speculate that similar pathogenetic mechanisms are operating. However, this possibility should be investigated further.

Keith et al. were the first to suggest that neural and perineural alterations might be important in pain pathogenesis in CP [26]. They concluded that pain severity was correlated with the duration of alcohol consumption, pancreatic calcification, and with the percentage of eosinophils in perineural inflammatory cell infiltrates, but not with duct dilatation.

A subsequent study demonstrated an increase in both the number and diameter of pancreatic nerve fibers in the course of CP [27]. In tissue specimens from patients suffering from CP, foci of chronic inflammatory cells were often found surrounding pancreatic nerves, which exhibit a damaged perineurium and invasion by lymphocytes (as evidenced by electron microscopy). The changed pattern of intrinsic and possibly extrinsic innervation of the pancreas in CP suggested that there could be an upregulation of neuropeptides that usually populate those enlarged nerves. In fact, a further study [28] showed that there were striking changes in peptidergic nerves in CP. The changes consisted of an intensification of immunostaining for calcitonin gene-related peptide (CGRP) and substance P (SP) in numerous nerve fibers. Because both of these peptides are generally regarded as pain neurotransmitters, these findings provide evidence for the direct involvement of pancreatic nerves in the long-lasting pain syndrome associated with CP. Subsequent reports [23,29] revealed that the presence of growth-associated-protein-43 (GAP-43), an established marker of neuronal plasticity, was directly correlated with the pain scores in patients with CP. GAP-43 is a neuronal protein that is known to be involved in the development of axonal growth cones and presynaptic terminals; mRNA and protein levels of GAP-43 are increased after neuronal lesions. In the chronically inflamed human pancreas, enzymatic and double fluorescence immunohistochemistry reveals a significant expression of GAP-43 in the majority of pancreatic nerve fibers. These immunohistochemical findings are correlated with clinical and pathological findings in CP patients, including the parenchyma–fibrosis ratio and the degree of perineural immune cell infiltration. Furthermore, a strong relationship with individual pain scores was present. The infiltration of pancreatic nerves by immune cells is significantly related to pain intensity, whereas pain scores do not correlate with the degree of pancreatic fibrosis or with the duration of the disease. The demonstration of a direct relationship between the degree of perineural inflammation and the clinical pain syndrome strongly supports the hypothesis of a "neuro-immune interaction" as an important, if not predominant, factor in pain generation in CP patients. An interesting question concerns the mechanisms that contribute to the enlargement of pancreatic nerves. A recent study analyzed the expression of NGF and one of its receptors (TrkA) in patients suffering from CP [25]. NGF belongs to the neurotrophin family and plays a role in neuroblast proliferation and neuronal maturation, affecting neuronal phenotype and maintaining neuronal survival. NGF signaling is mediated via binding high- and low-affinity receptors. TrkA is present in the dorsal root and peripheral ganglia cells of primary sensory nerves, and is involved in the signal transduction of noxious stimuli and tissue injury. Inflammation results in an elevation of NGF levels in different diseases. Interestingly, NGF may itself have cytokine-like functions; it can modify mast-cell, macrophage and B-cell functions, but may also activate TrkA located on sensory and sympathetic nerve fibers innervating the site of inflammation, thus modulating neuroimmune interactions. In CP tissue samples, NGF and TrkA mRNA expression are markedly increased and enhanced in pancreatic nerves and ganglia. Comparison of the molecular findings with clinical parameters reveals a significant relationship between NGF mRNA levels and pancreatic fibrosis and acinar cell damage, and between TrkA mRNA levels and pain intensity. These findings indicate that the NGF/TrkA pathway is activated in CP and that this activation might influence nerve growth and the pain syndrome, most probably by modulating the sensitivity of NGF-independent primary sensory neurons through increasing channel and receptor expression [25]. Similar results, showing positive correlation with pain intensity and frequency in patients suffering from CP, were reported for the gene expression of brain-derived neurotrophic factor, a member of the neurotrophin family [30]. In addition, upregulated NGF might influence the pain syndrome in CP patients by regulating the transcription and synthesis of SP and CGRP, as well as through the release of histamine. The neuropeptide SP is the main tachykinin involved in the neural transmission of sensory information, smooth muscle contraction, nociception, sexual behavior, and possibly wound healing and tissue regeneration [31–32]. SP has wide-ranging functional effects, including the crosstalk between nervous and immune systems by acting through its specific receptor, neurokinin 1 (NK-1R). A recent report by Shrikhande et al. [33] demonstrated a significant correlation between NK-1R and clinical-pathological findings in CP patients. In CP samples, mRNA and protein expression of NK-1R were localized mainly in nerves, ganglia, blood vessels, inflammatory cells, and occasionally in fibroblasts. A significant relationship between NK-1R mRNA levels and the intensity, frequency, and duration of pain in CP patients was reported. The expression of NK-1R in inflammatory cells and blood vessels also points to crosstalk between immunoreactive SP nerves and inflammatory cells and blood vessels, and further supports the existence of a neuroimmune interaction that probably influences the pain syndrome and chronic inflammatory changes in CP.

The exact mechanisms that are involved in the interaction between inflammatory cells and nerves and ganglia (neuroimmune cross-talk) are not yet fully clarified. Different cytokines have been shown to interact with SP in various paradigms for pain and inflammation. SP directly stimulates the release of interleukin-8 (IL-8) from macrophages. IL-8 release generates hyperalgesia by stimulation of postganglionic sympathetic neurons. A significant increase of IL-8 mRNA was reported in CP tissue samples [34]. IL-8 was present mainly in macrophages surrounding the enlarged pancreatic nerves, in remaining acinar

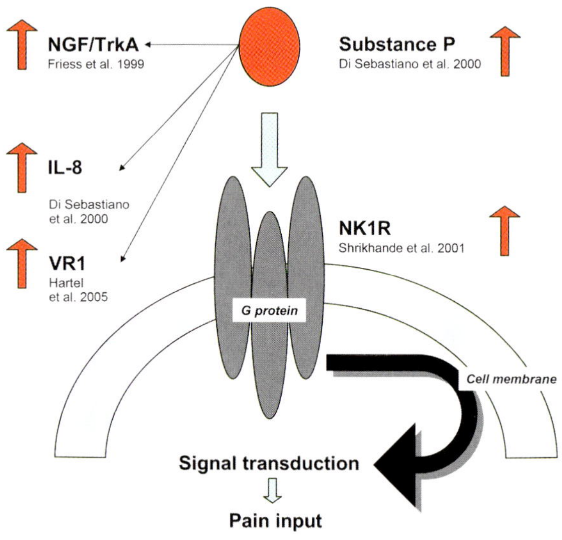

Figure 27.1

Neurogenic inflammation in chronic pancreatitis. *NGF* Nerve growth factor, *TrkA* an NGF receptor, *IL* interleukin, *VR1* vanilloid receptor subtype 1, *NK1R* neurokinin-1 receptor

cells and often in ductal cells. IL-8 mRNA expression was positively correlated with the inflammatory score and the presence of ductal metaplasia in CP tissue samples.

The reported findings in the literature on the interaction of SP and IL-8, in combination with what has reported regarding CP, suggests that the increased mRNA expression of IL-8 in CP is in part mediated by SP released from sensory pancreatic nerves. In addition, the release of IL-8 from the remaining exocrine pancreatic parenchyma suggests the fascinating hypothesis of an intrinsic maintenance of the inflammatory response after the initial damage to the pancreatic gland, thus sustaining the progression and evolution of the disease (Fig. 27.1). In addition, in a rat model it was demonstrated that repeated cerulein stimulation causes experimental pancreatitis that is mediated in part by stimulation of vanilloid receptor subtype 1 (VR1) on primary sensory neurons, resulting in endogenous SP release [35]. These results were confirmed in human pancreas in a recent study [36]. In fact, activation of the VR1 in pancreatic tissues from patients with pancreatic cancer and CP has recently been reported. This increase was correlated with pain score in those patients. The release of SP and neurokinin A from primary afferent (sensory) nerve endings to various stimuli is now considered to be induced by activation of the capsaicin (vanilloid) VR1 receptor (Fig. 27.1).

Conclusion

The pathophysiological mechanism underlying pain generation in CP remains a major clinical problem. The recent concept of neuropeptides released from enteric and afferent neurons, and their functional interactions with inflammatory cells, might play a key role. The most interesting finding in CP is the presence of a spatial relationship between peptidergic neurons and inflammatory cells. Furthermore, there is the intriguing possibility of functional interaction among neuropeptides, immune cells, cytokines, and nerve growth factors. A correlation between these molecular data and pain has been demonstrated in CP, and the present information provides evidence for neuroimmune crosstalk in the pathogenesis of pain and inflammation in CP.

References

1. Di Sebastiano P, di Mola FF, Büchler MW, Friess H (2004) Pathogenesis of pain in chronic pancreatitis. Dig Dis 22:267–272
2. Di Sebastiano P, di Mola FF, Friess H, Büchler MW (2003) Chronic pancreatitis: the perspective of pain generation by neuroimmune interaction. Gut 6:906–910
3. Warshaw AL, Banks PA, Fernandez-Del Castillo C (1998) AGA Technical review: treatment of pain in chronic pancreatitis. Gastroenterology 115:765–776
4. Jensen AR, Matzen P, Malchow-Moller A, Christoffersen I (1984) Pattern of pain, duct morphology and pancreatic function in chronic pancreatitis: a comparative study. Scand J Gastroenterol 19:334–338
5. Lankisch PG, Lohr-Happe A, Otto J, Creutzfieldt W (1993) Natural course of chronic pancreatitis. Pain, exocrine and endocrine pancreatic insufficiency and prognosis of the disease. Digestion 54:148–155
6. Levy P, Lesur G, Belghiti J, Fekete f, Bernades P (1993) Symptomatic duodenal stenosis in chronic pancreatitis: a study of 17 cases in a medical surgical series of 306 patients. Pancreas 8:563–567
7. Becker V, Mischke U (1991) Groove pancreatitis. Int J Pancreatol 10:173–182
8. Amman RW, Muellhaupt B, Zürich Pancreatitis Study Group (1999) The natural history of pain in alcoholic chronic pancreatitis. Gastroenterology 116:1132–1140
9. Manes G, Pieramico O, Uomo G (1992) Pain in chronic pancreatitis: recent pathogenetic findings Minerva Gastroenterol Dietol 38:137–43
10. Ebbehoj N (1992) Pancreatic tissue fluid pressure and pain in chronic pancreatitis. Dan Med Bull 39:128–133
11. Ebbehoj N, Borly L, Bulow J, Rasmussen SG, Madsen P, Matzen P, Owre A (1990) Pancreatic tissue fluid pressure in chronic pancreatitis. Relation to pain, morphology, and function. Scand J Gastroenterol 25:1046–1051
12. Manes G, Buchler M, Pieramico O, Di Sebastiano P, Malfertheiner P (1994) Is increased pancreatic pressure related to pain in chronic pancreatitis? Int J Pancreatol 15:113–117

13. Yin X (2005) The role of surgery in pancreatic pseudocyst. Hepatogastroenterology 52:1266–1273
14. Beger HG, Schlosser W, Friess HM, Buchler MW (1999) Duodenum-preserving head resection in chronic pancreatitis changes the natural course of the disease: a single-center 26-year experience. Ann Surg 230:512–519
15. Malfertheiner P, Mayer D, Buchler M, Dominguez-Munoz JE, Schiefer B, Ditschuneit H. Treatment of pain in chronic pancreatitis by inhibition of pancreatic secretion with octreotide. Gut 36:450–454
16. Reber HA, Karanjia ND, Alvarez C, Widdison AL, Leung FW, Ashley SW, Lutrin FJ (1992) Pancreatic blood flow in cats with chronic pancreatitis. Gastroenterology 103:652–659
17. Karanjia ND, Widdison AL, Leung F, Alvarez C, Lutrin FJ, Reber HA (1994) Compartment syndrome in experimental chronic obstructive pancreatitis: effect of decompressing the main pancreatic dust. Br J Surg 81:259–264
18. Monkemuller KE, Kahl S, Malfertheiner P (2004) Endoscopic therapy of chronic pancreatitis. Dig Dis 22:280–291
19. Di Sebastiano P, Fink T, Weihe E, Friess H, Innocenti P, Beger HG, Buchler MW (1997) Immune cell infiltration and growth-associated protein 43 expression correlate with pain in chronic pancreatitis. Gastroenterology 112:1648–1655
20. Gullo L, Barbara L (1991) Treatment of pancreatic pseudocysts with octreotide. Lancet 338:540–541
21. Sarles H, Sarles JC, Muratore R, et al (1961) Chronic inflammatory sclerosis of the pancreas: an autonomous pancreatic disease? Am J Dig Dis 6:688–698
22. Yoshida K, Toki F, Takeuchi T, et al (1995) Chronic pancreatitis caused by an autoimmune abnormality. Proposal of the concept of autoimmune pancreatitis. Dig Dis Sci 40:1561–1568
23. Okazaki K, Chiba T (2002) Autoimmune pancreatitis. Gut 51:1–4
24. Toma H, Winston J, Micci MA, Shenoy M, Pasricha PJ (2000) Nerve growth factor expression is up-regulated in the rat model of L-arginine-induced acute pancreatitis. Gastroenterology 119:1373–1381
25. Friess H, Zhu ZW, di Mola FF, Kulli C, Graber HU, Andren-Sandberg Å, Zimmermann A, Korc M, Reinshagen M, Büchler MW (1999) Nerve growth factor and its high affinity receptor in chronic pancreatitis. Ann Surg 230:615–624
26. Keith RG, Keshavjee SH, Kerenyi NR (1985) Neuropathology of chronic pancreatitis in humans. Can J Surg 28:207–211
27. Bockman DE, Buchler M, Malfertheiner P, Beger HG (1988) Analysis of nerves in chronic pancreatitis. Gastroenterology 94:1459–1469
28. Buchler M, Weihe E, Friess H, Malfertheiner P, Bockman E, Muller S, Nohr D, Beger HG (1992) Changes in peptidergic innervation in chronic pancreatitis. Pancreas 7:183–192
29. Fink T, Di Sebastiano P, Büchler M, Beger HG, Weihe E (1994) Growth associated protein-43 and protein gene product 9.5 innervation in human pancreas: changes in chronic pancreatitis. Neuroscience 63:249–266
30. Zhu ZW, Friess H, Wang L, Zimmermann A, Buchler MW (2001) Brain-derived neurotrophic factor (BDNF) is upregulated and associated with pain in chronic pancreatitis. Dig Dis Sci 46:1633–1639
31. Di Sebastiano P, Weihe E, di Mola FF, Fink T, Innocenti P, Friess H, Büchler MW (1999) Neuroimmune appendicitis. Lancet 354:461–466
32. Weihe E, Nohr D, Muller S, Buchler M, Friess H, Zentel HJ (1991) The tachykinin neuroimmune connection in inflammatory pain. Ann N Y Acad Sci 632:283–295
33. Shrikande S, Friess H, di Mola FF, Tempia A, Conejio-Garcia JR, Zhu Z, Zimmermann A, Büchler MW (2001) NK-1 receptor gene expression is related to pain in chronic pancreatitis. Pain 91:209–217
34. Di Sebastiano P, di Mola FF, Di Febbo C, Baccante G, Porreca E, Innocenti P, Friess H, Büchler MW (2000) Expression of Interleukin-8 (IL-8) and substance P in human chronic pancreatitis. Gut 47:423–428
35. Nathan JD, Patel AA, McVey DC, Thomas JE, Prpic V, Vigna SR Liddle RA (2001) Capsaicin vanilloid receptor-1 mediates substance P release in experimental pancreatitis. Am J Physiol Gastrointest Liver Physiol 281:G1322–G1328
36. Hartel M, di Mola FF, Salvaggi F, Mascetta G, Wente MN, Felix K, Giese NA, Hinz U, Di Sebastiano P, Buchler MW, Friess H (2006) Vanilloids in pancreas cancer: potential for chemotherapy and pain management. Gut 55:519–528

Chapter 28

J. Enrique Domínguez-Muñoz

Natural Course of Chronic Pancreatitis

Because histology is usually not available, diagnosis of chronic pancreatitis is based on the demonstration of the morphological and/or functional changes that typically develop over time within the gland in the course of the disease. Based on surgically obtained tissue specimens of the pancreas, it is known that chronic pancreatitis is characterized by the presence of a chronic inflammatory infiltration, interlobular fibrosis, loss of acinar cells, and relative conservation of endocrine islets [1]. However, histological observation of the pancreas is only possible late in the course of the disease, when chronic pain and/or complications have led to surgery. Therefore, if the available information regarding histology for the diagnosis of chronic pancreatitis is limited, reports on the pathological features of different stages of the disease and the natural course from the histological point of view are completely lacking. In this context, development of endoscopic ultrasound-guided biopsy techniques should be of help for acquiring a deeper morphological knowledge of the disease [2].

Chronic pancreatitis is a chronic inflammatory condition of the pancreas leading to the progressive substitution of viable exocrine and endocrine tissue by collagen and other fibrosis components. This explains the exocrine and endocrine functional impairment that develops over the natural course of the disease. Together with these functional abnormalities, inflammatory involvement of intrapancreatic nerves, increased intrapancreatic pressure, superimposed acute inflammation, and complications like pseudocysts or biliary and duodenal stenosis may occur, leading to abdominal pain. Since pain is the major and most limiting symptom of the disease, the study of the natural course of chronic pancreatitis is dominated by the natural history of pain. Last, but not least, different complications and associated diseases may develop over the course of chronic pancreatitis, which may strongly influence the prognosis of the disease (Table 28.1).

The clinical course of chronic pancreatitis is dependent mainly on the etiology of the disease. As our knowledge about the factors involved in the etiopathogenesis of chronic pancreatitis increases, a clearer concept of the prognosis and evolution of the disease is being established. Only little more than 10 years ago, chronic pancreatitis was still classified as alcoholic and early- and late-onset idiopathic disorder according to etiology [3]. Much has been investigated and reported over the last decade about the factors that play a causative or predisposing role in chronic pancreatitis, as well as about the pathogenetic mechanisms by which these factors are able to cause disease. The TIGAR-O (toxic-metabolic, idiopathic, genetic, autoimmune, recurrent and severe acute pancreatitis, or obstructive) system is probably the most relevant initiative in this context [4], which clearly recognizes the nowadays widely accepted concept of chronic pancreatitis as a complex disorder involving the variable interaction of several environmental, immune-inflammatory, metabolic, and genetic factors. It must be taken into account that any therapeutic or modifying action leading to the interruption or mod-

Table 28.1. Complications of chronic pancreatitis and potentially associated extrapancreatic diseases. Figures show the percentage of chronic pancreatitis patients developing each condition

Complication	Frequency
Pancreatic pseudocyst	25–30%
Bile duct stenosis	40–50%
Pancreatic cancer	1–3%
Splenic vein thrombosis	2–5%
Pseudoaneurysm	2–3%
Duodenal obstruction	4–5%
Pancreatic fistula	2–3%
Pancreatic abscess	2–3%
Extrapancreatic cancer	10–15%
Alcoholic liver disease	25–40%
Cardiovascular diseases	20–30%

ulation of any of these etiologic or predisposing factors has the potential of influencing the natural course of chronic pancreatitis.

It is easily understandable that talking about the natural course of chronic pancreatitis is a difficult task. First, patients with chronic pancreatitis are induced to abandon any toxic habits to try and modify the course of the disease. Second, more than half of patients with chronic pancreatitis are operated on at any time over the evolution of the disease, which has clear consequences on the course of pain, complications and, therefore, of the disease itself. Finally, other therapeutic measures are frequently applied, among them dietary and lifestyle modifications, analgesics, oral pancreatic enzymes, insulin, somatostatin analogues, antioxidants, and endoscopic procedures, which definitely influence the natural history of chronic pancreatitis. Most of the therapeutic studies on this disease lack a control group, and thus the effect of the therapy on the course of the disease is not clearly quantifiable. In conclusion, several features of the disease (i.e., etiology) and a wide variety of therapeutic and modifying actions influence the course of chronic pancreatitis, which may be carefully considered when talking about the "natural" history of the disease.

This chapter intends to summarize the present concepts on the course of chronic pancreatitis, taking into account the potential effect of the different etiologies and therapeutic measures applied. Most of the information provided here refers to alcoholic chronic pancreatitis, since this disease is the most deeply and widely studied. The natural course of other forms of the disease is thus presented using the alcoholic form as reference.

What is the Expected Evolution of Exocrine Pancreatic Insufficiency?

Exocrine pancreatic insufficiency with maldigestion is a major consequence of chronic pancreatitis. The probability of exocrine pancreatic insufficiency increases with time so that around 50% of patients with chronic pancreatitis develop exocrine pancreatic insufficiency at a median time of 10–12 years from onset of the disease [3]. Some confusion exists regarding the concept of exocrine pancreatic insufficiency in the medical literature [5]. Taking into account that insufficiency implies that an organ fails to maintain its function, the term exocrine pancreatic insufficiency should be reserved for those cases with maldigestion. This occurs only when pancreatic secretion decreases to values below 10% of normal [6]. Milder reduction of pancreatic secretion should be called dysfunction and not insufficiency [5].

Exocrine pancreatic function impairs progressively as the exocrine pancreatic tissue is destroyed and is replaced by fibrotic tissue [7]. Damage of pancreatic ducts may also play an important role in deteriorating exocrine function [8,9], probably by impairing the secretion of pancreatic juice. Taking into account that chronic pancreatitis develops over decades, studies evaluating the natural course of exocrine pancreatic function included an observation period that is too short for drawing definite conclusions. In addition, the methods applied to evaluate pancreatic function are variable, which may help to explain some diverging results.

Although long follow-up studies are lacking, it is accepted that exocrine pancreatic function deteriorates during the course of chronic pancreatitis [10]. Using fecal chymotrypsin as an indirect method to evaluate pancreatic secretion, Ammann et al. reported that severe exocrine pancreatic insufficiency develops within 5–6 years from onset of the disease [11]. This is strongly dependent on the cause of the disease, ranging from 13 years from onset of symptoms in alcoholic pancreatitis to 26 years in early-onset idiopathic disease [3]. Exocrine pancreatic function may also improve, mainly in patients with mild to moderate disease who stop drinking alcohol [10,12,13].

Exocrine pancreatic function and digestion clearly deteriorate after pancreatic surgery for chronic pancreatitis. The frequency of steatorrhea increases up to 16-fold after duodenopancreatectomy and 2-fold after pancreaticojejunostomy [14]. This is not only due to the removal of pancreatic parenchyma, but also to the changes in gastric physiology associated with partial gastrectomy, loss of the control mechanisms of gastric emptying and postprandial cholecystokinin release that occur after duodenectomy, bacterial overgrowth in cases of excluded intestinal loop, postprandial asynchrony between gastric emptying of nutrients and biliopancreatic secretion, and the negative feedback on pancreatic secretion mediated by unabsorbed nutrients reaching the ileal lumen. All of these changes, which cause exocrine pancreatic insufficiency and maldigestion after pancreatic surgery, are minimized in the case of duodenum-preserving pancreatic head resection [15,16], which appears to be the intervention preserving at best digestive function in chronic pancreatitis.

The clinical consequences of maldigestion are poorly studied. Because of that, some authors support the concept that exocrine pancreatic insufficiency does not play a major prognostic role. Enzyme substitution therapy is clearly indicated in patients with clinically relevant steatorrhea. However, since exocrine pancreatic insufficiency develops slowly over years, patients tend to adapt their diet progressively, so that steatorrhea is frequently not evident. In addition, we have previously shown that patients with exocrine pancreatic insufficiency may suffer from malnutrition, as shown by deficient levels of micronutrients, despite the absence of diarrhea and weight loss [17]. Plasma levels of high-density lipoprotein C, apolipoprotein A-I, and lipoprotein A are also reduced, which has been related to an increased risk of cardiovascular events in patients with chronic pancreatitis [18].

In conclusion, exocrine pancreatic insufficiency with maldigestion develops in most patients with chronic pancreatitis over time, which leads to a situation of malnutrition that may have an important prognostic impact. An optimal oral pancreatic enzyme substitution therapy is thus of major importance and not only a simple way to reduce diarrhea.

Natural Course of Endocrine Pancreatic Function During Chronic Pancreatitis

Studies on surgically obtained pancreas specimens have shown that Langerhans islets are preserved until the very end stages of chronic pancreatitis [1]. Based on that, it is expected that endocrine pancreatic insufficiency with diabetes mellitus requiring insulin develops late in the course of the disease as a consequence of islet destruction. Nevertheless, disturbance of carbohydrate metabolism in chronic pancreatitis is not as simple as it could seem to be.

Diabetes mellitus is a major late sequela of chronic pancreatitis, which plays an important prognostic role. In fact, diabetes mellitus is associated with life-threatening complications like severe hypoglycemia related to glucagon deficiency, together with the usual complications of diabetes like peripheral neuropathy and micro- and macroangiopathy. How frequent is diabetes mellitus in chronic pancreatitis and when does it develop in the course of the disease are questions awaiting a conclusive answer. The use of different diagnostic criteria for chronic pancreatitis, different definitions of onset of the disease, different severity criteria, different duration of follow up and different sources of patients (medical or surgical) in the studies reported on this topic may explain this uncertainty. In addition, different diagnostic criteria for glucose metabolism disturbance are also applied. Keeping all these confounders in mind, Lankisch et al. [19] reported moderate-to-severe endocrine pancreatic insufficiency in less than 10% of patients with chronic pancreatitis at onset. This figure increases up to 78% of patients after 10 years of follow up, and around half of them needed insulin therapy. Nevertheless, authors underlined that every fifth patient still had no diabetes even after this long observation period [19].

In a prospective cohort study of more than 400 chronic pancreatitis patients, Malka et al. [20] reported an annual rate of diabetes mellitus of 3.5%, and an annual rate of insulin requirement of 2.2%. Thus, and taking into account a prevalence of almost 10% at onset, around half of the patients are diabetic after 10 years of follow up, and almost 80% after 20 years. More than half of these diabetic patients require insulin therapy [20].

Regarding etiology, diabetes is found much more frequently at onset of the disease in patients with late-onset idiopathic chronic pancreatitis (22% of patients) than in those with early-onset idiopathic (0%) and alcoholic disease (8%) [3]. In fact, diabetes is the presenting symptom of chronic pancreatitis in almost every fourth patient with late-onset idiopathic disease. In addition, the time to diabetes development is also different in different etiologies. The expected median interval to diabetes is much longer in early-onset idiopathic pancreatitis (27.5 years) than in late-onset idiopathic (11.9 years) and alcoholic disease (19.8 years) [3]. Therefore, although with clear differences at onset, late-idiopathic and alcoholic pancreatitis behave similarly, and different from early-onset idiopathic disease, regarding endocrine pancreatic disturbance.

Although generally believed for years, pancreatic drainage and/or resection of the head of the pancreas neither prevent nor delay the development of diabetes mellitus in chronic pancreatitis [20]. Therefore, a risk reduction of endocrine pancreatic insufficiency cannot be expected after pancreatic surgery for chronic pancreatitis, and disease progression prevails in the risk of diabetes in these patients. On the contrary, and because of the anatomical distribution of endocrine cells, distal pancreatectomy is associated with a high prevalence of diabetes and insulin requirement in chronic pancreatitis, and around 60% of patients newly develop endocrine pancreatic insufficiency, half of them requiring insulin, within 5 years after this surgical intervention [20].

Islet destruction is, however, only the latest event in the natural history of chronic pancreatitis-related diabetes mellitus. The close correlation between en-

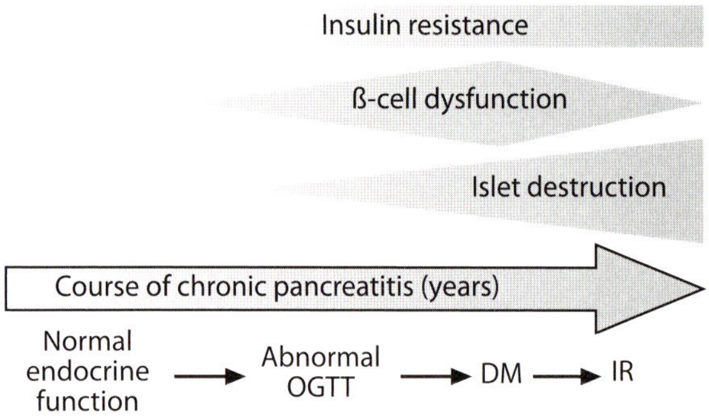

Figure 28.1

Natural history of diabetes mellitus in chronic pancreatitis based on pathophysiologic hypothesis. *OGTT* Oral glucose tolerance test, *DM* diabetes mellitus, *IR* insulin requirement

zyme secretion and insulin release at different stages of chronic pancreatitis [21], and the significant association between diabetes and the presence of pancreatic calcifications [20,21] support the concept that the development of diabetes is closely related to parenchyma destruction and fibrotic replacement. Nevertheless, features of patients with chronic pancreatitis and diabetes are far from homogeneous. Diabetic patients with calcifying pancreatitis have significantly lower levels of daily urinary C-peptide and fasting plasma glucagon than diabetics with noncalcifying disease [21]. It is easy to understand that only patients with abnormally low glucagon levels are at risk of severe hypoglycemia, and that they behave differently from diabetic patients with normal glucagon release.

At least in patients with tropical chronic pancreatitis, exocrine pancreatic function is similarly reduced in diabetics and nondiabetics [22]. As expected, diabetic patients have a significantly reduced insulin release after intravenous arginine infusion compared to nondiabetics; glucagon release is, however, similar in both groups of patients [22]. This supports the concept of a selective ß-cell dysfunction, instead of islet destruction, as the cause of diabetes in some patients with chronic pancreatitis. Peripheral insulin resistance has been also described in chronic pancreatitis [23]. In conclusion, the natural history of diabetes mellitus in chronic pancreatitis is not simply related to islet destruction. Diabetes can thus develop in earlier stages of the disease as a consequence of insulin resistance and/or ß-cell dysfunction (Fig. 28.1). This is of great clinical relevance with respect to therapy, insulin requirement, and tendency to hypoglycemia.

The frequency of complications of chronic pancreatitis-related diabetes mellitus is similar to that of type I diabetes. Although early reports showed a low frequency of microvascular complications, mainly retinopathy, in patients with diabetes secondary to chronic pancreatitis [24,25], more recent studies have consistently demonstrated that the duration of diabetes and not diabetes type is the main variable explaining the risk and severity of these complications [26,27]. Something similar can be said for macrovascular complications [28]. Thus, once diabetes appears in patients with chronic pancreatitis, evolution time and glycemic control are, similarly to type I diabetes, the main variables associated to the risk of diabetes-related complications. However, metabolic instability is more pronounced in pancreatic diabetes than in type I diabetes, and it is more difficult to achieve adequate glycemic control. Several factors are involved in this metabolic instability, among them glucagon deficiency, maldigestion secondary to exocrine pancreatic insufficiency, and lack of compliance of alcoholic patients with diet and therapy. An optimal patient education, a good nutritional status and alcohol abstinence, and probably an adequate oral enzyme substitution therapy are, together with the intensified insulin therapy, the therapeutic cornerstones to limit complications of diabetes mellitus in patients with chronic pancreatitis.

Behavior of Pain in the Course of Chronic Pancreatitis

Pain is without a doubt the main symptom in most patients with chronic pancreatitis, and that which characterizes best the natural course of the disease. Despite the vast majority of studies on chronic pancreatitis that have focused on pain, and pain in this context has been extensively reviewed [29–32], painful chronic pancreatitis remains poorly understood in terms of causes, natural history, and therapeutic approaches. Pain patterns differ among different patients with chronic pancreatitis, most probably related to different mechanisms of pain. In fact, there is no doubt that the natural history of pain depends mainly on its etiopathogenesis. Together with that, the etiology of chronic pancreatitis, persistence of risk factors, duration of the disease, lifestyle modifications, and therapeutic maneuvers may play a modifying role.

Pain Patterns in Chronic Pancreatitis

Patients with chronic pancreatitis may suffer from episodes of abdominal pain that last for few days, which are separated by pain-free intervals of months to years [33]. These same patients may have periods of persistent pain for some months. In addition, this pattern of prolonged periods of persistent pain may be the only pain pattern in some chronic pancreatitis patients. These two pain patterns, defined by Ammann [33] as type A and B, respectively, are probably due to different mechanisms and frequently lead to different therapeutic approaches, which in turn may modify the evolution of pain. In fact, complications like pseudocyst, biliary obstruction, or inflammatory mass are frequently associated to persistent pain, and surgical correction is usually followed by pain relief [33–36]. Short relapsing pain episodes are most probably related to relapsing inflammation, either associated or not with necrosis, which may require hospitalization but not surgery.

The prevalence of pain and pain patterns varies largely among different series [3,33,37–41]. This is most probably due to different mechanisms of pain as well as different risk factors and the etiological distribution of chronic pancreatitis patients. Thus, the persistence of risk factors like alcohol intake and cigarette smoking increases the number of pain episodes per year [38]. As mentioned above, persistent pain is mainly secondary to complications [33–36]. On the contrary, mutations in the cationic trypsinogen gene causing hereditary pancreatitis support the hypothesis of recurrent episodes of inflammation as a cause of relapsing pain [42]. Similarly, severe relapsing pain described in patients with early-onset idiopathic chronic pancreatitis may be at least partially related to cystic fibrosis transmembrane conductance regulator (CFTR) and/or serine protease inhibitor Kazal type 1 (SPINK1) gene mutations [4,43,44]. In fact, patients with idiopathic chronic pancreatitis associated to CFTR or SPINK1 gene mutations present usually with recurrent attacks of pancreatitis [45]. The presence of genetic anomalies also seems to be relevant in the pathogenesis of some cases of obstructive chronic pancreatitis and, therefore, in the origin of "obstructive" pain [46]. Inflammation also defines pain pattern in patients with autoimmune pancreatitis [47].

Natural History of Abdominal Pain

Taking into account all of the considerations mentioned above, the natural history of pain in chronic pancreatitis is expected to be highly variable depending on several different factors. Independent of that, and as a hypothesis, pain may be expected to decrease as the pancreatic parenchyma is destroyed and replaced by fibrotic tissue. In this situation, pancreatic secretion is markedly reduced, and this may be associated with a decreased intraductal pressure, and the parenchyma may respond to a lesser extent to toxic agents like alcohol or inflammatory relapses.

Ammann's theory of burning-out of the pancreas has been debated for years [7,11,33]. According to this theory, pain in chronic pancreatitis decreases and even disappears as exocrine and endocrine pancreatic function declines, and most patients become pain free in the late stages of the disease. Similar findings have been reported by other groups [48]. Nevertheless, this is far from being the rule, rather something that may occur in a proportion of patients with chronic pancreatitis. Actually, more than half of patients with chronic pancreatitis may still suffer from pain attacks despite having a severe exocrine pancreatic insufficiency after a long observation time [19,49]. Different methods of evaluating exocrine pancreatic function may partly explain this discrepancy, but no correlation can be found between pain and exocrine pancreatic function when direct intubation function tests are applied [19]. Something similar can be said with respect to endocrine pancreatic function, and more than half of patients with overt diabetes requiring insulin still suffer from pain attacks [19]. As a consequence of these findings, together with more recent reports from Ammann's group [33], the conclusion can be drawn that the character of pain and pain pattern are more important in predicting the natural history of pain than the degree of impairment of exocrine and endocrine pancreatic function [33]. Thus, the mechanism of pain is most probably the major determinant of the course of pain in chronic pancreatitis.

Whether pain decreases as severe morphological changes of the pancreas develop is controversial, although most reports do no support this association. Again, Ammann's group support a relationship between severe morphological abnormalities, namely pancreatic calcifications, and pain decrease [7,11]. Two further studies from Germany, however, found no correlation between the presence of calcifications and/or severe ductal changes and pain relief [19,50]. Most patients with pancreatic calcifications as detected by computed tomography scan still have abdominal pain [19,50], although complete pain relief is more frequent once calcifications develop [19]. The same two studies reported no significant correlation between pancreatic duct abnormalities detected by endoscopic retrograde cholangiopancreatography and frequency and intensity of pain [19,50].

Although the disappearance of pain with disease progression cannot be considered as a rule, pain decrease with the duration of chronic pancreatitis has been reported repeatedly [3,7,11,19,33,51], which, as discussed above, is most probably not related to morphological or functional pancreatic changes. More likely, factors like the etiology of chronic pancreatitis and abstinence from alcohol intake and cigarette smoking may play a role. As shown previously, patients previously classified as suffering from early-onset idiopathic chronic pancreatitis (most of whom are now considered as genetically determined [43,52]) have a long course of severe pain, whereas patients with a late-onset idiopathic pancreatitis, which is also genetically determined [53], often have a painless course [3]. Alcohol intake at different amounts probably determines the onset and severity of pain in patients who are genetically predisposed to late-onset pancreatitis.

Abstinence from alcohol intake and cigarette smoking probably contributes to pain relief in a relevant proportion of patients with chronic pancreatitis of different etiologies. Both factors are able to exert a toxic effect within the gland and to stimulate the local release of inflammatory mediators [54]. Although some authors reported no clear influence of alcohol abuse on pain profile once patients have advanced chronic pancreatitis [11,19,55], most other investigators found that alcohol abstinence is frequently associated with pain relief [38,51,56,57]. In fact, pain relief can be obtained in up to 60% of patients after alcohol abstinence, whereas this occurs in only 26% of patients who continue drinking [51]. Something similar can be said about smoking. Actually, smoking has been shown to be an important risk factor for chronic pancreatitis [38,58]. Regarding pain, patients who continue to smoke suffer from more pain episodes per year than those who do not smoke [38].

Effect of Endoscopic and Surgical Procedures on Natural History of Pain

Patients requiring surgery are usually those with severe and persistent pain. As mentioned above, pain in these patients is frequently related to complications like pseudocysts, biliary obstruction or inflammatory mass, which can be corrected by surgical procedures [33–36]. Problems related to analysis of the effect of endoscopic or surgical therapies on pain in chronic pancreatitis have been discussed in detail [59]. The natural history of pain, with frequent and prolonged periods of spontaneous relief, is an important confounder that needs to be controlled in randomized, placebo-controlled trials with stratification for different pain patterns. Since surgery is reserved mainly for patients with severe persistent pain, in whom noninvasive therapies have usually failed, the relapsing nature of pain is critical mainly in studies on endoscopic therapy. Actually, the best results after endoscopic therapy are obtained in patients with infrequent attacks of pain before therapy [60], who are actually those with the highest probability of having none or few further attacks of pain regardless of treatment. Whether and to what extent endoscopic therapy, either pancreatic stenting or stone removal, may influence the natural history of pain is therefore unknown. Supporting this idea is the fact that pain improves in an substantial proportion of patients even after an unsuccessful endoscopic attempt of clearing pancreatic stones [61,62].

It is also unclear to what extent the different surgical approaches to chronic pancreatitis influence the course of pain. This is mainly due to the variety of surgical procedures for the same indication depending on individual and local circumstances or preferences, the frequently vague definition and quantification of pain, the variable alcohol abstinence after surgery in different studies, the variety of duration of follow up, and the different causes and mechanisms of pain. Although because of all these factors, it is most probably inadequate to describe the effect of surgery on the course of pain in patients with chronic pancreatitis as a whole; the different surgical reports on this topic tend to show a significant pain relief in most patients over the first postoperative years, and a tendency to pain increase in longer follow up periods [10,63]. Again, randomized, controlled trials with stratification for potential causes of pain and pain patterns are needed.

Impact of Complications on Natural Course

Different pancreatic and extrapancreatic complications may develop in the course of chronic pancreatitis (Table 28.1). Among them, pseudocysts and biliary obstruction, together with alcohol-related diseases, are by far the most frequent ones. Pseudocysts influence the natural history of chronic pancreatitis in so far they can cause pain or develop complications (infection, bleeding), but they probably play no role as long as they remain asymptomatic. Chronic biliary obstruction causing persisting jaundice requires frequently a surgical decompression. Vascular complications like splenic vein thrombosis and pseudoaneurysm are rare and develop in around 2% of patients with chronic pancreatitis. Untreated pseudoaneurysms have a high mortality rate, whereas gastric variceal bleeding from pancreatitis-induced splenic vein thrombosis is a very rare event occurring in only 4% of these patients [64].

Patients with chronic pancreatitis are at risk of developing pancreatic cancer. Although it was classically believed that less than 5% of pancreatic carcinomas develop in the context of chronic pancreatitis, this figure should be revised based on the most recent knowledge on the genetic basis of both chronic pancreatitis and pancreatic cancer [65]. In an international historical cohort study involving more than 2,000 patients with chronic pancreatitis, the cumulative incidence of pancreatic cancer increases to 1.8% and 4% after 10 and 20 years from diagnosis of the disease, respectively [66]. Thus, the duration of exposure to inflammation seems to be the major factor involved in the transition from a benign to a malignant condition. Alcohol and, in particular, smoking seem to be important associated risks factors. According to case-control studies, the relative risk of developing pancreatic cancer in chronic pancreatitis ranges from 2.3 to 18.5 [67]. The risk of malignant transformation is much higher in cases of hereditary pancreatitis, in whom a standardized incidence ratio of 53 (95% confidence interval 23–105) has been described [68]. Patients with chronic pancreatitis also develop extrapancreatic cancer in up to 10–15% of cases, mainly of the respiratory and gastrointestinal tract [19,49,51,69,70]. As in pancreatic cancer, cigarette smoking and alcohol play an important role in the risk of extrapancreatic cancer in patients with chronic pancreatitis.

References

1. Klöppel G, Maillet B (1993) Pathology of acute and chronic pancreatitis. Pancreas 8:659–670
2. Iglesias García J, Abdulkader I, Lariño Noia J, Antúnez J, Forteza J, Domínguez Muñoz JE (2005) Diagnosis of chronic pancreatitis: which information may be obtained by fine needle biopsy. Pancreatology 5:599 (abstract)
3. Layer P, Yamamoto H, Kalthoff L, Clain JE, Bakken LJ, DiMagno EP (1994) The different courses of early- and late-onset idiopathic and alcoholic chronic pancreatitis. Gastroenterology 107:1481–1487
4. Etemad B, Whitcomb DC (2001) Chronic pancreatitis: diagnosis, classification, and new genetic developments. Gastroenterology 120:682–707
5. Domínguez-Muñoz JE (2005) Management of maldigestion in chronic pancreatitis: a practical protocol. In: Dominguez-Munoz JE (ed) Clinical Pancreatology for Practising Gastroenterologists and Surgeons. Blackwell, Oxford, pp 288–293
6. DiMagno EP, Go VLW, Summerskill WHJ (1973) Relations between pancreatic enzyme outputs and malabsorption in severe pancreatic insufficiency. N Engl J Med 288:813–815
7. Ammann RW, Heitz PU, Klöppel G (1996) Course of alcoholic chronic pancreatitis: a prospective clinico-morphological long-term study. Gastroenterology 111:224–231
8. Dominguez-Munoz JE, Manes G, Pieramico O, Buchler M, Malfertheiner P (1995) Effect of pancreatic ductal and parenchymal changes on exocrine function in chronic pancreatitis. Pancreas 10:31–35
9. Iglesias-García J, Vilariño-Insua M, Iglesias-Rey M, Sobrino-Faya M, Domínguez-Munoz JE (2004) Probability of exocrine pancreatic insufficiency in patients with severe chronic pancreatitis according to the findings on endoscopic ultrasonography. Gastroenterology 126:A231
10. Lankisch PG (2001) Natural course of chronic pancreatitis. Pancreatology 1:3–14
11. Ammann RW, Akovbiantz A, Largiader F, Schueler G (1984) Course and outcome of chronic pancreatitis: longitudinal study of a mixed medical-surgical series of 245 patients. Gastroenterology 86:820–828
12. Begley CG, Roberts-Thomson IC (1985) Spontaneous improvement in pancreatic function in chronic pancreatitis. Dig Dis Sci 30:1117–1120
13. García-Pugés AM, Navarro S, Ros E, Elena M, Ballesta A, Aused R, Vilar-Bonet J (1986) Reversibility of exocrine pancreatic failure in chronic pancreatitis. Gastroenterology 91:17–24
14. Iglesias-García J (2005) Management of exocrine pancreatic insufficiency associated to other clinical conditions: gastrointestinal surgery, diabetes mellitus, AIDS. In: Domínguez-Muñoz JE (ed) Clinical Pancreatology for Practising Gastroenterologists and Surgeons. Blackwell, Oxford, pp 299–305
15. Ito K (2005) Duodenum preservation in pancreatic head resection to maintain pancreatic exocrine function (determined by pancreatic function diagnostant test and cholecystokinin secretion). J Hepatobiliary Pancreat Surg 12:123–128
16. Yamaguchi K, Yokohata K, Nakano K, Ohtani K, Ogawa Y, Chijiiwa K, Tanaka M (2001) Which is a less invasive pancreatic head resection: PD, PPPD, or DPPHR? Dig Dis Sci 46:282–288
17. Iglesias-García J, Vilariño-Insua M, Iglesias-Rey M, Domínguez-Munoz JE (2003) Oral pancreatic enzyme supplementation in patients with exocrine pancreatic insufficiency: is it enough to evaluate clinical response? Gastroenterology 124: A632
18. Montalvo G, Zorreéis M, Carroccio A, et al (1994) Lipoproteins and chronic pancreatitis. Pancreas 9:137–138
19. Lankisch PG, Löhr-Happe A, Otto J, Creutzfeldt W (1993) Natural course in chronic pancreatitis: pain, exocrine and endocrine pancreatic insufficiency and prognosis of the disease. Digestion 54:148–155
20. Malka D, Hammel P, Sauvanet A, Rufat P, O'Toole D, Bardet P, et al (2000) Risk factors for diabetes mellitus in chronic pancreatitis. Gastroenterology 119:1324–1332
21. Nakamura T, Imamura K, Takebe K, Terada A, Arai Y, Tandoh Y, Yamada N, Ishii M, Machida K, Suda T (1996) Correlation between pancreatic endocrine and exocrine function and characteristics of pancreatic endocrine function in patients with diabetes mellitus owing to chronic pancreatitis. Int J Pancreatol 20:169–175
22. Rossi L, Parvin S, Hassan Z, Hildebrand P, Keller U, Ali L, et al (2004) Diabetes mellitus in tropical chronic pancreatitis is not just a secondary type of diabetes. Pancreatology 4:461–467

23. Cavallini G, Vaona B, Bovo P, Cigolini M, Rigo L, Rossi F, et al (1993) Diabetes in chronic alcoholic pancreatitis. Role of residual beta cell function and insulin resistance. Dig Dis Sci 38:497–501
24. Sevel D, Bristow JH, Bank S, Marks I, Jackson P (1971) Diabetic retinopathy in chronic pancreatitis. Arch Ophthalmol 86:245–250
25. Verdonk CA, Palumbo PJ, Gharib H, Bartholomew LG (1975) Diabetic microangiopathy in patients with pancreatic diabetes mellitus. Diabetologia 11:395–400
26. Gullo L, Parenti M, Monti L, Pezzilli R, Barbara L (1990) Diabetic retinopathy in chronic pancreatitis. Gastroenterology 98:1577–1581
27. Levitt NS, Adams G, Salmon J, Marks INS, Musson G, Swanepoel C, et al (1995) The prevalence and severity of microvascular complications in pancreatic diabetes and IDDM. Diabetes Care 18:971–974
28. Ziegler O, Candiloros H, Guerci B, Got I, Crea T, Drouin P (1994) Lower-extremity arterial disease in diabetes mellitus due to chronic pancreatitis. Diabete Metab 20:540–545
29. Adler G, Scmid RM (1997) Chronic pancreatitis: still puzzling? Gastroenterology 112:1762–1765
30. Warshaw AL, Banks PA, Fernández del Castillo C (1998) AGA Technical review on treatment of pain in chronic pancreatitis. Gastroenterology 115:765–776
31. Ihse I (1990) Pancreatic pain. Br J Surg 77:121–122
32. Leathy Al, Carter DC (1991) Pain and chronic pancreatitis. Eur J Gastroenterol Hepatol 3:425–433
33. Ammann RW, Muellhaupt B, and Zurich Pancreatitis Study Group (1999) The natural history of pain in alcoholic chronic pancreatitis. Gastroenterology 116:1132–1140
34. Büchler MW, Malfertheiner P, Friess H, Senn T, Beger HG (1993) Chronic pancreatitis with inflammatory mass in the head of the pancreas: a special entity? In: Beger HG, Büchler MW, Ditschuneit HH, Malfertheiner P (eds) Chronic Pancreatitis. Springer-Verlag, New York, pp 41–46
35. Beger HG, Schlosser W, Friess H, Büchler MW (1999) Duodenum-preserving head resection in chronic pancreatitis changes the normal course of the disease: a single-center 26-year experience. Ann Surg 230:512–519
36. Frey CF, Amikura K (1994) Local resection of the head of the pancreas combined with longitudinal pancreaticojejunostomy in the management of patients with chronic pancreatitis. Ann Surg 220:492–507
37. Lankisch PG, Seidensticker F, Lohr-Happe A, Otto J, Creutzfeldt W (1995) The course of pain is the same in alcohol- and nonalcohol-induced chronic pancreatitis. Pancreas 10:338–341
38. Talamini G, Bassi C, Falconi M, et al (1996) Pain relapses in the first 10 years of chronic pancreatitis. Am J Surg 171:565–569
39. Malfertheiner P, Mayer D, Buchler M, Dominguez-Munoz JE, Schiefer B, Ditschuneit H (1995) Treatment of pain in chronic pancreatitis by inhibition of pancreatic secretion with octreotide. Gut 36:450–454
40. Dumonceau JM, Deviere J, Le Moine O, Delhaye M, Vandermeeren A, Baize M, et al (1996) Endoscopic pancreatic drainage in chronic pancreatitis associated with ductal stones: long-term results. Gastrointest Endosc 43:547–555
41. Yadav D, Notahara K, Smyrk TC, Clain JE, Pearson RK, Farnell MB, Chari ST (2003) Idiopathic tumefactive chronic pancreatitis: clinical profile, histology and natural history alter resection. Clin Gastroenterol Hepatol 1:129–135
42. Gorry MC, Gabbaizedeh D, Furey W, Gates LK Jr, Preston RA, Aston CE, et al (1997) Mutations in the cationic trypsinogen gene are associated with recurrent acute and chronic pancreatitis. Gastroenterology 113:1063–1068
43. Cohn JA, Bornstein JD, Jowell PS (2000) Cystic fibrosis mutations and genetic predisposition to idiopathic chronic pancreatitis. Med Clin North Am 84:621–631
44. Witt H, Luck W, Hennies HC, et al (2000) Mutations in the gene encoding the serine protease inhibitor, Kazal type 1 are associated with chronic pancreatitis. Nat Genet 25:213–216
45. Frulloni L, Castellani C, Bovo P, Vaona B, Calore B, Liani C, et al (2003) Natural history of pancreatitis associated with cystic fibrosis gene mutations. Dig Liver Dis 35:179–185
46. Choudari CP, Imperiale TF, Sherman S, Fogel E, Lehman GA (2004) Risk of pancreatitis with mutation of the cystic fibrosis gene. Am J Gastroenterol 99:1358–1363
47. Ketikoglou I, Moulakakis A (2005) Autoimmune pancreatitis. Dig Liver Dis 37:211–215
48. Girdwood AH, Marks IN, Bornman PC, Kottler RE, Cohen M (1981) Does progressive pancreatic insufficiency limit pain in calcific pancreatitis with duct stricture or continued alcohol insult? J Clin Gastroenterol 3:241–245
49. Thorsgaard Pedersen N, Andersen BN, Pedersen G, Worning H (1982) Chronic pancreatitis in Copenhagen: a retrospective study of 64 consecutive patients. Scand J Gastroenterol 17:925–931
50. Malfertheiner P. Büchler M, Stanescu A, Ditschuneit H (1987) Pancreatic morphology and function in relationship to pain in chronic pancreatitis. Int J Pancreatol 2:59–66
51. Miyake H, Harada H, Kunichika K, Ochi K, Kimura I (1987) Clinical course and prognosis of chronic pancreatitis. Pancreas 2:378–385
52. Pfützer RH, Barmada MM, Brunskil APJ, Finch R, Hart PS, Neoptolemos J, et al (2000) SPINK1/PSTI polymorphisms act as disease modifiers in familial and idiopathic chronic pancreatitis. Gastroenterology 119:615–623
53. Tsiotos GG (2000) Natural history of idiopathic chronic pancreatitis. In: Büchler MW, Fries H, Uhl W, Malfertheiner P (eds) Chronic Pancreatitis: Novel Concepts in Biology and Therapy. Blackwell, Oxford, pp 316–324
54. Whitcomb DC (1999) Hereditary pancreatitis: new insights into acute and chronic pancreatitis. Gut 45:317–322
55. Girdwood AH, Marks IN, Bornman PC, Kottler RE, Cohen M (1981) Does progressive pancreatic insufficiency limit pain in calcific pancreatitis with duct stricture or continued alcohol insult? J Clin Gastroenterol 3:241–245
56. Sarles H, Sahel J (1976) Die chronische Pankreatitis. In : Forell M (ed) Handbuch der Inneren Medizin, vol 3/6: Pankreas, 5th edn. Springer, Berlin, pp 737–844
57. Trapnell JE (1979) Chronic relapsing pancreatitis: a review of 64 cases. Br J Surg 66:471–475
58. Imoto M, DiMagno EP (2000) Cigarette smoking increases the risk of pancreatic calcification in late-onset but not early-onset idiopathic chronic pancreatitis. Pancreas 21:115–119
59. DiMagno EP (1999) Toward understanding (and management) of painful chronic pancreatitis. Gastroenterology 116:1252–1257
60. Cremer M, Deviere J, Delhaye M, Vandermeeren A, Baize M (1990) Non-surgical management of severe chronic pancreatitis. Scand J Gastroenterol 175:77–84
61. Smits ME, Rauws AJ, Tytgat NJ, Huibregtse K (1996) Endoscopic treatment of pancreatic stones in patients with chronic pancreatitis. Gastrointest Endosc 43:556–560

62. Sherman S, Lehman GA, Hawes RH, Ponich T, Miller LS, Cohen LB, et al (1991) Pancreatic ductal stones: frequency of successful endoscopic removal and improvement in symptoms. Gastrointest Endosc 37:511–517
63. Taylor RH, Bagley FH, Braasch JW, Warren KW (1981) Ductal drainage or resection for chronic pancreatitis. Am J Surg 141:28–33
64. Heider TR, Azeem S, Galanko JA, Behrns KE (2004) The natural history of pancreatitis-induced splenic vein thrombosis. Ann Surg 239:876–880
65. Hruban RH, Goggins M, Parsons J, Kern SE (2000) **Progression model for pancreatic cancer.** Clin Cancer Res 6:2969–2972
66. Lowenfels AB, Maisonneuve P, Cavallini G, Ammann RW, LankischPG, Andersen JR, et al (1993) Pancreatitis and the risk of pancreatic cancer. N Engl J Med 328:1433–1437
67. Mössner J (2005) What is the epidemiologic impact of pancreatic cancer? In: Domínguez-Muñoz JE (ed) Clinical Pancreatology for Practicing Gastroenterologists and Surgeons. Blackwell, Oxford, pp 331–350
68. Lowenfels AB, Maisonneuve P, DiMagno EP, et al (1997) Hereditary pancreatitis and the risk of pancreatic cancer. International Hereditary Pancreatitis Study Group. J Natl Cancer Inst 89:442–446
69. Ammann RW, Knoblauc M, Möhr P, Deyhle P, Largiadèr F, Akovbiantz A, et al (1980) High incidence of extrapancreatic carcinoma in chronic pancreatitis. Scand J Gastroenterol 15:395–399
70. Rocca G, Gaia E, Iuliano R, Caselle MT, Rocca N, Calcamuggi G, Emmanuelli G (1987) Increased incidence of cancer in chronic pancreatitis. J Clin Gastroenterol 9:175–179

Chapter 29

H. G. Beger · F. Gansauge · M. Schwarz · B. Poch

Chronic Pancreatitis: Inflammatory Mass in the Head of the Pancreas – Pacemaker of Chronic Pancreatitis

Chronic pancreatitis, which is usually caused by chronic alcohol abuse, is primarily a disease of the exocrine compartment of the pancreas. Several pathological concepts have been proposed to explain the morphological changes that occur during the disease. The most widely accepted concept is based on the observation that overconsumption of alcohol leads to increasing formation of protein plaques [1, 2]. Protein plaques cause obstruction of the pancreatic ducts, resulting in the induction and perpetuation of local chronic inflammatory processes in the pancreas in addition to the alcohol damage imposed directly on the acinar and ductal cells.

In recent years, it has been hypothesized that chronic pancreatitis is the consequence of recurrent attacks of acute pancreatitis causing small areas of pancreatic necrosis, which lead to granulation tissue and fibrosis [3–5]. Periductal formation of fibrotic tissue after focal tissue necrosis and inflammatory areas lead to ductal obstruction, including the main pancreatic duct. However, none of these proposed concepts can conclusively explain the causal factors and the consequent local events leading to that disease. An additional factor that enhances chronic inflammatory pancreatitis is cigarette smoking, which has been shown in animal experiments to result in a specific type of chronic pancreatitis with tissue calcification [6].

Table 29.1. Etiology of chronic pancreatitis (*CP*). *FCPD* Fibrocalculus pancreatic diabetes

– Alcoholic CP (60–90%)
– Idiopathic CP (20%)
– Hereditary CP (<10%)
– Tropical CP (FCPD)
– CP associated with hyperparathyroidism
– Pancreas divisum (1%)

Table 29.2. Chronic pancreatitis with inflammatory mass in the head of the pancreas [8]. *CBD* Common bile duct, *MPD* main pancreatic duct

-30% of all patients with CP referred for surgical treatment
> 80% alcohol-induced
Predominantly men (70–90%)
Mean age <40 years at time of diagnosis
Clinical features
Severe, medically intractable pain: daily >75%
Stenosis of CBD: ~50%
Severe duodenal stenosis: 5–10%
Portal-vein/vascular obstruction: 18%
MPD – single stenosis in the head: ~ 40%

Inflammatory Mass in the Pancreatic Head: Clinical Factors

A subgroup of patients with chronic pancreatitis suffers from an inflammatory mass in the head of the pancreas (IMH) [6, 7]. IMH of the pancreas is observed in approximately 30–45% of all surgical patients suffering from chronic pancreatitis. Chronic alcohol misuse is the main cause of chronic pancreatitis in more than 80% of cases in Germany (Table 29.1). The clinical picture is dominated by severe medical, intractable pain, stenosis of the common bile duct, severe duodenal stenosis, or compression of the portal venous system. About 40% of patients suffer a single pancreatic main duct stenosis in the prepapillary duct of the pancreatic head (Table 29.2). The presence of pancreatic head enlargement in chronic pancreatitis does not appear to be influenced by the duration of alcohol misuse. However, when comparing patients with and without IMH, there are remarkable differences. Patients with pancreatic head enlargement have a higher pain score and, apart from the local complications, they show better-preserved pancreatic exocrine and endocrine function at the time of clini-

Table 29.3. Chronic pancreatitis with and without pancreatic head enlargement due to an inflammatory mass (Beger 2006, unpublished data)

	Head enlargement (138 patients) (%)	No head enlargement (141 patients) (%)
Slight to frequent pain	33	60
Daily severe pain	67	40
Cholestasis	46	11
Duodenal obstruction	30	7
Vascular involvement	15	8
Diabetes mellitus	18	30

Table 29.4. Common bile duct stenosis in chronic pancreatitis with an inflammatory mass (258 patients) [13]. *ERCP* Endoscopic retrograde cholangiopancreatography, *MRCP* magnetic resonance cholangiopancreatography, *γGT* Gamma glutamyl transferase, *AP* alkaline phosphatase, *Bili* bilirubin, *pts* patients

CBD stenosis (ERCP/MRCP)	129 pts	50%
Cholestasis (γGT, AP)	91 pts	35%
Jaundice (Bili, γGT, AP)	36 pts	14%
Previous episodes of jaundice	122/ 181 pts	67%

cal presentation than patients without pancreatic head enlargement (Table 29.3). These findings indicate that IMH is of clinical relevance early in the course of chronic pancreatitis [8].

IMH Causing Stenosis of the Common Bile Duct, Duodenum, and Portal Vein

The most important clinically relevant local complication in this subgroup of patients is common bile duct stenosis due to an inflammatory tumor, requiring diagnostic measures to discriminate a malignant lesion in the head from a benign compression. Common bile duct stenosis occurs frequently, as evidenced by endoscopic retrograde cholangiopancreatography. Biochemical analysis has shown that one-third of patients exhibit cholestasis and about 15% clinical jaundice (Table 29.4). Previous episodes of jaundice are observed in almost two-thirds of patients coming to surgical treatment [8, 9].

The Head of the Pancreas – Pacemaker of Chronic Pancreatitis?

The precise frequency and prevalence of pancreatic head enlargement in patients with chronic pancreatitis has yet to be established. Radiological diagnosis using contrast-enhanced computed tomography scanning has shown that approximately one-third to one-half of all patients hospitalized for treatment of chronic pancreatitis exhibit a pancreatic head enlargement. Radiological criteria of head enlargement is a pancreatic head diameter above 4 cm. Regarding the tissue mass of the normal pancreas, the pancreatic head including the neck up to the level of the portal vein covers approximately 40–55% of the pancreatic tissue. Embryologically, the head of the pancreas comprises two different parts: the dorsal and the ventral pancreas. This might influence the pathomorphology of chronic pancreatitis, at least with respect to the inflammatory process localized in the pancreatic head (Table 29.5). This is well known for pancreas divisum, different types of neoplastic lesions in the pancreatic head and the dorsal pancreas, and tumors located in the uncinate process [10, 11]. The double duct system in the pancreatic head, including the duct of Santorini and the duct of Wirsung is of clinical relevance for the pathomorphology of pancreatic inflammation, which has been observed in the pancreas divisum and in pancreaticobiliary maljunction in both children and adults. Experience with the management of recurrent acute and chronic pancreatitis in children caused by pancreas divisum reveals that duct anomalies in the pancreatic head can lead to an inflammatory process in the head due to obstruction of the ducts [11–13].

An additional weak point in the duct system is the papilla–duct connection within the ampulla of Vater and the separate entrance of the duct of Santorini in

Table 29.5. Head of the pancreas – pacemaker of the clinical course of chronic pancreatitis: factors and hypothesis. *IMH* Inflammatory mass of the pancreatic head

- Anatomy of the pancreatic head: 45–55% of pancreatic tissue
- Embryologically two parts: dorsal and ventral pancreas
- Two ductal systems with different drainage capacities: duct of Santorini, duct of Wirsung
- Pancreas divisum
- The development of IMH has been observed combined with marked changes of the ducts up to the confluence (knee)
- Papilla-duct connections
- Pancreaticobiliary maljunctions

Table 29.6. Chronic pancreatitis with inflammatory mass in the head of the pancreas – pathomorphological changes (380 patients; data obtained between November 1972 and April 1982 at the Department of Surgery, Free University of Berlin, and between May 1982 and September 1995 at Department of General Surgery, University of Ulm) [9]

	Patients	%
MPD stenosis in the head	149	39
Pseudocysts (~90% <2.0cm)	195	51
Focal necrosis (<0.5cm)	35	9
CBD stenosis	182	48
Duodenal stenosis (severe)	25	7
Portal-vein compression	49	13

the papilla minor. In most patients with pancreas divisum referred for surgical treatment, IMH is the leading pathomorphological sign of the disease [11]. The growing clinical experience in the management of patients with pancreaticobiliary disorder has demonstrated that a focal inflammatory process is frequently observed in the head of the pancreas.

Pathomorphological Changes

The continuous destruction of the pancreatic tissue during the course of chronic pancreatitis is characterized by a decrease in the number of pancreatic acinar cells and by a marked increase in connective tissue. Patients with IMH show pathomorphologically focal necrotic lesions, frequently small pseudocystic cavities, calcification of the pancreatic parenchyma, and duct stones in the head area (Table 29.6). In a series of patients operated on for chronic pancreatitis with IMH, pancreatic duct stones and calcifications has been observed in 20–30%, and main duct stenosis in the head was observed in almost half of patients. As a consequence of the inflammatory process in the enlarged head (because of inflammatory edema) and the increase in connective tissue, the common bile duct is narrowed, showing a stenosis [14].

Pain in chronic pancreatitis is thought to be caused by an increase in intraductal and intraparenchymal pressure [15]. However, recent pathomorphological studies have revealed morphological changes in the pancreatic nerves and in the interaction between the pancreatic nerves and the inflammatory cells [16, 17]. Foci of inflammatory cells often encircle pancreatic nerves. Electron microscope investigations have demonstrated the presence of nerve infiltration, resulting in perineural damage and invasion of granulocytes inside the nerves in the pancreas and in the nerve plexus. In comparison with normal pancreatic tissue, nerves with a significantly greater diameter have been described in chronic pancreatitis. In addition to these morphological alterations, increased levels of growth-associated protein 43, the pain-transmitting neuropeptide substance P, and calcitonin gene-related peptide have been measured (see Chapter 27). Pain generation in patients with chronic pancreatitis seems to be a mechanism with two components: increased ductal and tissue pressure in combination with hyperinnervation due to chronic-pancreatitis-associated neuritis [6, 8].

Molecular Aspects of the Development of an IMH

The mechanisms involved in the development of an IMH in chronic pancreatitis are unknown. The loss of exocrine tissue, mainly the acinar cell component of the pancreas, and the generation of extracellular matrix, including laminin, fibronectin, and collagens I and III are the main pathomorphological consequences of the chronic inflammation [5, 18, 19]. The molecular mechanism that contributes to these changes has recently been investigated. There is evidence that changes in the expression of growth factors and growth factor receptors are involved in chronic pancreatitis. Recent studies have revealed an overexpression of epidermal growth factor (EGF) receptor and the c-erB-2 protooncogene [20–23]. Operative tissue samples obtained from patients with chronic pancreatitis frequently exhibited a marked overexpression of transforming growth factor α (TGF-α, EGF-α) [23]. In one recently published study, enhancement of expression of c-erB-2 has been found to have a significant relationship to chronic pancreatitis with IMH [20]. In this study the tissue samples from patients with IMH were found to have significantly higher c-erB-2 mRNA levels than samples from patients with chronic pancreatitis without an IMH. These findings indicate that the overexpression of the EGF receptor and alterations in c-erB-2 expression in chronic pancreatitis might contribute to the pathophysiological process involved in the development of IMH [20, 22].

Inflammatory Tumor in the Head of the Pancreas – Is There an Increased Risk of the Development of a Malignant Lesion of the Pancreatic Head?

Epidemiological studies have shown that the risk of development of ductal pancreatic cancer is increased in patients with chronic pancreatitis (Table 29.7) [24, 25]. In the subset of patients suffering from chronic pancreatitis with IMH, ductal pancreatic cancer was found in the pancreatic head in 3.5–6.8% (Table 29.7). Histological examination does not allow a clear discrimination between cases with and without enlargement of the pancreatic head. However, molecular analysis at the mRNA level has revealed an increased expression of growth factor such as TGF-α and acidic and basic fibroblast growth factors as well as the EGF receptor in human pancreatic tissue with chronic pancreatitis, all of which are known to be overexpressed in pancreatic cancer [20, 21]. In pancreatic cancer, the EGF receptor and c-erB-2 are frequently overexpressed, whereas in chronic pancreatitis tissue an increased c-erB-2 expression was found only in cases with IMH. The expression of extracellular ma-

Table 29.7. Chronic pancreatitis: epidemiologic studies of pancreatic cancer risk

		Cohort pts	Follow-up time	Pancreatic cancer frequency/risk
Lowenfels [24]	1993	2015	7.4±6.3 years	16.5-fold, 4% 20 years
Beger [9]	1999	303	5.7 years	6.3%
Talamini [1]	1999	715		13- to 18-fold
Malka [35]	2002	373	9.2 years	26.7%

Table 29.8. Molecular biological changes in chronic pancreatitis. *EGF* Epidermal growth factor, *TGF* tissue growth factor, *FGF* fibroblast growth factor, *IMH* inflammatory mass of the pancreatic head

Gene	Alteration	Reference
K-ras	no mutations	Watanabe et al. [36]
p53	mutations in 3%	Gansauge et al. [33]
	polymorphisms in 8%	
p16 (MTS1)	no mutations	Caldas et al. [29]
EGF/TGF/EGF receptor	Overexpression in 30 – 60%	Korc et al. [37]
c-erbB-2	Overexpression in IMH	Friess et al. [21]
FGF	Overexpression in 30 – 60%	Friess et al. [23]
CD 44	Altered splice variants in 10%	Gansauge et al. [28]

Table 29.9. Gene mutations in chronic pancreatitis

Type CP	Gene	Location	Incidence of mutation/penetration	
Alcoholic CP	k-ras	12p13	0–60%	Yanagisawa 1993 [3]
	p 53	17p13	7.5/ 10%	Gansauge 1998 [34]
	p 16	9p21	95%	Hu 1992 [38]
	Smad 4	18q21	58%	Costentin 2002 [39]
	BRCA-1	17q12–21	downregulated	Beger 2004 [40]
Hereditary CP	PRSS1	78%	Whitcomb 1996 [26]	
	R122H			
	N297			
	SPINK-1			Whitcomb 1996 [26]
	N34S		PSTI gene	Witt 2000 [41]
	P55S		downregulated	
Idiopathic CP	SPINK-1 CFTR R117H		2–8%	Sharer 1998 [42]

Table 29.10. p53 Mutation in chronic pancreatitis. *SSCP* Single strand confirmation polymorphism, *RFLP* restriction fragment length polymorphism [33]

	SSCP of p53					RFLP of k-ras
	Exon 5	Exon 6	Exon 7	Exon 8	Exon 9	codon 12
Alterations (*n*=80)	2	4	2	0	0	0

trix molecules and their receptors was also slightly altered in chronic pancreatitis as compared to normal pancreatic tissue [18, 22].

These reports suggest a dysregulation of several genes, resulting in altered mRNA levels in chronic pancreatitis. Some of these changes, especially the overexpression of growth factors and their receptors, might contribute to ductal cell hyperplasia and pseudoductal cell formation (Table29.8) [23–25, 28]. The hypothesis of a sequential development of pancreatic cancer is supported by the observation of specimens of chronic pancreatitis in which these plastic structures are frequently found [21, 22, 29, 30]. A dysplasia-carcinoma sequence seems to be more likely than an single-step process. It is generally accepted that carcinogenesis is a multistep process including the activation of k-ras protooncogenes and inactivation of tumor suppressor genes, particularly the p-53 gene, as a genetic basis of carcinogenesis in the pancreas (Table 29.9) [19, 23, 25, 28, 31, 32].

Analysis of a large series of tissue specimens from patients with chronic pancreatitis demonstrated that p-53 mutations were occured in 3% of the cases, and polymorphism in the p-53 gene was found in 8% of the cases, whereas no k-ras mutations were detectable (Table 29.10). Corresponding to these findings, p-53 mutations are also found in precancerous lesions in other human tissues, such as hyperplastic prostatic epithelium, papillomatous hyperplasia, and fibroadenoma of the breast [33]. These data underline the hypothesis that p-53 mutations can occur at a very early stage of tumorigenesis and offer the possibility for an easily applicable molecular diagnostic tool for the detection of high-risk patients with chronic pancreatitis [33, 34].

References

1. Talamani G, Bassi C, Falconi M, Sartori N, Pasetto M, Salvia R, Di Francesco V, Frulloni L, Vaona B, Bovo P, Pederzoli P, Cavallini G (1999) Early detection of pancreatic cancer following the diagnosis of chronic pancreatitis. Digestion 60:554–561
2. Sarles H, Dagorn JC, Giorgi D, Bernard JP (1990) Remaining pancreatic stone protein as "lithostatin". Gastroenterology 99:900–905
3. Yanigasawa A, Ohtake K, Ohashi K, Hori M, Kitagawa T, Sugano H, Kato Y (1993) Frequent c-Ki-ras oncogene activation in mucous cell hyperplasias of pancreas suffering from chronic inflammation. Cancer Res 53:953–956
4. Klöppel G, Maillet B (1991) Pseudocysts in chronic pancreatitis: a morphological analysis of 57 resection specimens and 9 autopsy pancreata. Pancreas 6:266–274

5. D'Ardenne AJ, Kirkpatric P, Sykes BC (1984) Distribution of laminin, fibronectin, and interstitial collagen type III in soft tissue tumours. J Clin Pathol 37:895–904
6. Bordalo O, Bapista A, Dreiling D, Noronha M (1984) Early pathomorphological pancreatic changes in chronic alcoholism. In: Gyr KE, Singer MV, Sarles H (eds) Pancreatitis – Concepts and Classification. Elsevier/North-Holland, Amsterdam, p 642
7. Büchler M, Malfertheiner P, Friess H, Senn T, Beger HG (1990) Chronic pancreatitis with inflammatory mass in the head of the pancreas: a special entity? In: Beger HG, Büchler M, Ditschuneit H, Malfertheiner P (eds) Chronic Pancreatitis. Springer, Berlin, pp 41–46
8. Beger HG, Büchler M (1990) Duodenum-preserving resection of the head of the pancreas in chronic pancreatitis with inflammatory mass in the head. World J Surg 14:83–87
9. Beger HG, Büchler M, Bittner R, Oettinger W, Roscher R (1999) Duodenum-preserving resection of the head of the pancreas in severe chronic pancreatitis: early and late results. Ann Surg 209:273–278
10. Birk D, Schoenberg MH, Gansuge F, Formentini A, Fortnagel G, Beger HG (1998) Carcinoma of the head of the pancreas arising from the uncinate process – what makes the difference? Br J Surg 4:498–501
11. Warshaw AL: Pancreas divisum: a case for surgical treatment. Adv. Surg 1988; 21: 93–109
12. Widmaier U, Schmidt A, Schlosser W, Beger HG (1997) Die duodenumerhaltende Pankreaskopfresektion in der Therapie des Pancreas divisum. Chirurg 68:180–186
13. Schlosser W, Poch B, Beger HG (2002) Duodenum-preserving pancreatic head resection leads to relief of common bile duct stenosis. Am J Surg183:37–41
14. Oertel JE, Heffes CS, Oertel YC (1989) Pancreas. In: Sternberg SS (ed) Diagnostic Surgical Pathology. Raven Press, New York, pp 1057–1093
15. Ebbehoj N (1992) Pancreatic tissue fluid pressure and pain in chronic pancreatitis. Danish Med Bull 39:128–133
16. Bockmann DE, Büchler M, Malfertheiner P, Beger HG (1988) Analysis of nerves in chronic pancreatitis. Gastroenterology 94:1459–1469
17. Weihe E, Nohr D, Müller S, Büchler M, Friess H, Zentel HJ (1991) The tachykinin neuroimmune connection in inflammatory pain. Ann N Y Acad Sci 632:283–295
18. Gress TM, Müller-Pillasch F, Lerch MM, Friess H, Buchler M, Beger HG, Adler G (1994) Balance of expression of genes coding for extracellular matrix proteins and extracellular matrix degrading proteases in chronic pancreatitis. Z Gastroenterol 32:221–225
19. Shimoyama S, Gansauge F, Gansauge S, Oohara T, Beger HG (1995) Altered expression of extracellular matrix molecules and their receptors in chronic pancreatitis and adenomcarcinoma of the pancreas in comparison to normal pancreas. Int J Pancreatol 18:227–234
20. Friess H, Yamanka A, Büchler M, Hammer K, Kobrin MS, Beger HG, Korc M (1994) A subgroup of patients with chronic pancreatitis overexpress the c-erb-2 protooncogene. Ann Surg 220:183–192
21. Friess H, Yamanaka Y, Büchler M, Kobrin MS, Tahara E, Korc M (1994) Cripto, a member of the epidermal growth factor family, is overexpressed in human pancreatic cancer and chronic pancreatitis. Int J Cancer 56:668–674
22. van Laethem JL, Deviere J, Resibois A, Rickaert F, Vertongen P, Ohtani H, Cremer M, Miyazono K, Robberecht P (1995) Localization of transforming growth factor beta and its latent binding protein in human chronic pancreatitis. Gastroenterology 108:1873–1881
23. Friess H, Yamanaka Y, Buchler M, Beger HG, Do DA, Kobrin MS, Korc M (1994) Increased expression of acidic and basic fibroblast growth factors in chronic pancreatitis. Am J Pathol 144:117–128
24. Lowenfels AB, Maisonneuve P, Cavallini G, Ammann RW, Lankisch PG, Andersen JR, Dimagno EP, Andren-Sandberg A, Domellof L (1993) Pancreatitis and the risk of pancreatic cancer: International Pancreatitis Study Group. N Engl J Med 328:1433–1437
25. Schlosser W, Schoenberg MH, Siech M, Gansauge F, Beger HG (1996) Development of pancreatic cancer in chronic pancreatitis. Z Gastroenterol 34:3–8
26. Whitcomb DC, Gorry MC, Preston RA, Furey W, Sossenheimer MJ, Ulrich CD; Martin SP, Gates LK Jr, Amann ST, Toskes PP, Liddle R, McGrath K, Uomo G, Post JC, Ehrlich GD (1996) Hereditary pancreatitis is caused by a mutation in the cationic trypsinogen gene. Nat. Genet 14:141–145
27. Chen H, Jan Y, Chao T, Hwang T, Chen M (2003) Pancreaticoduodenectomy for chronic pancreatitis with an inflammatory mass of pancreatic head: preoperative and postoperative functional assessment. Hepatogastroenterology 50:2213–2217
28. Gansauge S, Gansuge F, Beger HG (1996) Molecular oncology in pancreatic cancer. J Mol Med 74:313–320
29. Caldas C, Hahn SA, da Costa LT, Redston MS, Schutte M, Seymour AB, Weinstein CL, Hruban RH, Yeo CJ, Kern SE (1994) Frequent somatic mutations and homozygous deletions of the p16 (MTSI) gene in pancreatic adenocarcinoma. Nature Genet 8:27–32
30. Muehling B, Kolb A, Ramadani M, Schmidt E, Gansauge F, Beger HG (2004) Comparative analysis of extracellular matrix proteins in chronic pancreatitis: differences between pancreatic head and tail. Pancreas 28:174–180
31. Matsubara T, Sakurai Y, Sasayama Y, Hori H, Ochiai M, Funabiki T, Matsumoto K, Hirono I (1996) K-ras point mutations in cancerous and noncancerous biliary epithelium in patients with pancreaticobiliary maljunction. Cancer 77:1752–1757
32. Barton CM, Hall PA, Hughes CM, Gullick WJ, Lemoine NR (1991) Transforming growth factor alpha and epidermal growth factor in human pancreatic cancer. J Pathol 163:111–116
33. Gansauge S, Schmid RM, Muller J, Adler G, Mattfeldt T, Beger HG (1998) Genetic alterations in chronic pancreatitis – evidence for early occurrence of p53 but not K-ras mutations. Br J Surg 85:337–340
34. Gansauge S, Schmid RM, Mueller J, Adler G, Mattfeldt T, Beger HG (1998) Genetic alterations in chronic pancreatitis: evidence for early occurrence of p53 but not K-ras mutations. Br J Surg 85:337–340
35. Malka D, Hammel P, Maire F, Rufat P, Madeira I, Pessione F, Levy P, Ruszniewski P (2002) Risk of pancreatic adenocarcinoma in chronic pancreatitis. Gut 51:849–852
36. Watanabe M, Tanaka J, Masauji N, Matsuura A, Kiyama Y, Morii K, Naohara T, Saitoh M, Higa T, Kasai M, et al (1993) Detection of point mutation of K-ras gene codon 12 in biliary tract and ampullary carcinoma by modified two-step polymerase chain reaction. Nippon Shokakibyo Gakkai Zasshi 90:789–794

37. Korc M, Friess H, Yamanaka Y, Kobrin MS, Büchler M, Beger HG (1994) Chronic pancreatitis is associated with increased concentrations of epidermal growth factor receptor, transforming growth factor α and phospholipase C-gamma. Gut 35:1468–1473
38. Hu CC, Skakura Y, Sasano Y, Shum L, Bringas P Jr, Werb Z, Slavkin HC (1992) Endogenous epidermal growth factor regulates the timing and pattern of embryonic mouse molar tooth morphogenesis. Int J Dev Biol 36:505–516
39. Costentin L, Pages P, Bouisson M, Berthelemy P, Buscail L, Escourrou J, Pradayrol L, Vaysse N (2002) Frequent deletions of tumor suppressor genes in pure pancreatic juice from patients with tumoral or nontumoral pancreatic diseases. Pancreatology 2:17–25
40. Beger C, Ramadani M, Meyer S, Leder G, Kruger M, Welte K, Gansauge F, Beger HG (2004) Down-regulation of BRCA1 in chronic pancreatitis and sporadic pancreatic adenocarcinoma. Clin Cancer Res 1:3780–3787
41. Witt H, Luck W, Hennies HC, Classen M, Kage A, Lass U, Landt O, Becker M (2000) Mutations in the gene encoding the serine protease inhibitor, Kazal type 1 are associated with chronic pancreatitis. Nat Genet 25:213–216
42. Sharer N, Schwarz M, Malone G, Howarth A, Painter J, Super M, Braganza J (1998) Mutations of the cystic fibrosis gene in patients with chronic pancreatitis. N Engl J Med 339:645–652

Chapter 30

M. Kahl · J. Keller · P. Layer

Diagnosis: Functional Testing, Radiological Work-up of Chronic Pancreatitis

Chronic pancreatitis is defined as a chronic inflammatory disease of the pancreas characterized by irreversible morphologic changes that typically are associated with pain and/or permanent loss of function. Diagnosis is usually simple in the late stages of the disease, because of the presence of manifest structural and functional alterations. However, the diagnosis of early or mild chronic pancreatitis prior to the development of detectable morphologic changes may be a much more difficult task; chronic pancreatitis is defined on a histopathologic basis, and histology is usually not available. Alternative classification systems have been proposed, which ideally should be simple, objective, precise, and relatively noninvasive, and should also incorporate etiology, pathogenesis, structure, function, and clinical status into one overall scheme.

The most widely used classification systems include the Marseille-Rome classification of 1988 [1] and the Cambridge classification of 1984 (Table 30.1) [2, 3]. The Cambridge classification uses imaging tests to provide a grading and severity system [2, 3], it also differentiates between acute and chronic pancreatitis, noting that a single episode of acute pancreatitis may have implications on pancreatic morphology and function [4]. However, these classification systems are based only on morphology and disregard clinical signs, functional abnormalities, and etiology. Thus, the Cambridge system proves more useful as a staging system once the diagnosis is made rather than a system for classifying the etiologies of chronic pancreatitis. Other systems such as clinically and/or etiologically based classifications [5, 6] are less widely accepted.

The Mayo Clinic score in its original [7, 8] or adapted version [9], which is based on functional and imaging results, has been widely accepted and used in several studies (Table 30.2).

Figure 30.1 presents the process of diagnosing, classifying, and staging chronic pancreatitis. There is limited consensus on these issues, especially on the interpretation and classification of abnormal function test results in the presence of normal imaging study results.

Table 30.1. Cambridge classification [68]. *ERCP* Endoscopic retrograde cholangiopancreatography, *CT* computed tomography, *US* ultrasound

Stage	Typical changes on ERCP	Typical changes on CT and US
Normal	Normal appearance of side branches and main pancreatic duct	Normal gland size, shape; homogeneous parenchyma
Equivocal	Dilatation/obstruction of less than three side branches; normal main pancreatic duct	Normal main pancreatic duct; heterogeneous parenchyma
Mild	Dilatation/obstruction of side branches (more than three); normal main pancreatic duct	Normal main pancreatic duct; heterogeneous parenchyma, side gland enlargement
Moderate	Additional stenosis and dilatation of main pancreatic duct	Small cysts (<10 mm in diameter), increased echogenicity of the main pancreatic duct wall, dilatation of the main pancreatic duct
Severe	Additional obstructions, cysts, stenosis of main pancreatic duct; calculi	Cysts (>10 mm in diameter), stenosis of main pancreatic duct with prestenotic dilatation; calculi

Table 30.2. Diagnosis of chronic pancreatitis by scoring systems [7, 9]. Four or more points: chronic pancreatitis. Three points: chronic pancreatitis possible, follow-up necessary. *In addition, two points were given for more than two previous attacks of acute pancreatitis and another point for diabetes mellitus

Parameter	Mayo Clinic score [7]*	Luneburg score [9]
Morphological examinations		
Postmortem diagnosis of chronic pancreatitis	4	4
Histology	4	4
Intraoperative findings characteristic of chronic pancreatitis	–	4
Exocrine pancreatic function tests		
Abnormal secretin pancreozymin test	2	3
Abormal pancreolauryl test	–	2
Abnormal fecal chymotrypsin level	–	2
Abnormal fecal elastase 1 level	–	2
Steatorrhea	2	1
Imaging procedures		
Abnormal ultrasound	–	3
Abnormal endoscopic ultrasound	–	3
Abnormal computed tomography	–	3
Abnormal ERCP	3	3
Pancreatic calcifications, shown by any imaging procedure	4	4

Functional Testing in the Evaluation of Chronic Pancreatitis

General Aspects

Pancreatic exocrine function tests should be specific for pancreatic insufficiency and should be sensitive enough to detect the early stages of impaired pancreatic exocrine function. The test should be able to define the level of insufficiency even in the absence of obvious malabsorption. It should be noninvasive, inexpensive, easily performed, reproducible, and able to monitor pancreatic function during the course of pancreatic disease. There is, of course, no such test available. All current tests have several disadvantages: sensitive tests are not only more invasive and unpleasant for the patient, but also expensive and not standardized among different laboratories. On the other hand, it is almost impossible to diagnose mild-to-moderate pancreatic insufficiency by noninvasive tests (Fig. 30.2). Thus, only patients with severe pancreatic exocrine insufficiency suffer from steatorrhea [10], which can be diagnosed visually with considerable accuracy only in cases where it is pronounced [11].

Pathophysiologic Basis

In chronic pancreatitis, enzyme synthesis and consequently enzyme output decreases by 60–90% within the first 5–10 years of alcoholic chronic pancreatitis [12]. This significant decrease in enzyme output is still associated with normal fecal fat excretion (compensated pancreatic insufficiency). Obvious steatorrhea occurs if enzyme output is less than 5–10% of normal lipase activity. This is usually reached after about 15 years [7].

Exocrine pancreatic function may be evaluated by means of direct tests or noninvasive indirect tests. The direct tests measure the secretory capacity of the pancreas during exogenous or endogenous stimulation and collection of duodenal juice via tubes, or estimate the fecal excretion of pancreatic enzymes. Indirect tests assess pancreatic function by measurement of a digestive function or malfunction.

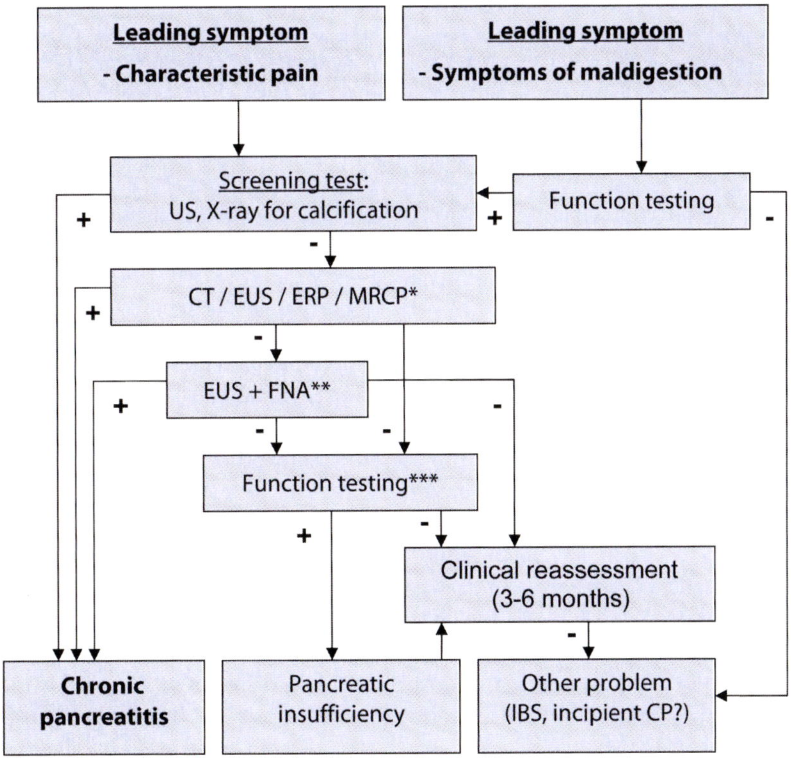

Figure 30.1

Diagnostic algorithm of suspected chronic pancreatitis (*CP*). The diagnostic algorithm is entered if characteristic pain or symptoms of maldigestion occur. If the leading symptom is pain, the evaluation should be started with a transabdominal ultrasound (*US*) examination (eventually combined with an abdominal x-ray). On a second step, if the diagnosis remains unclear *computed tomography (*CT*) is preferred to endoscopic retrograde pancreatography (*ERP*) at this stage. If available, endoscopic ultrasonography (*EUS*) is performed. **Biopsy is the gold standard [101], but is usually not available. In centers where EUS is not available, ERP is often used after nondiagnostic CT, especially if recurrent pancreatitis is also being considered. If the leading symptom is maldigestion, pancreatic function testing is performed as a first step. If the function test is abnormal, imaging procedures should be done. ***Pancreatic function testing in the presence of a normal imaging test result and/or biopsy represents pancreatic insufficiency until proven otherwise. Function testing may be used as supporting evidence of chronic pancreatitis (see Table 30.2). *MRCP* Magnetic resonance cholangiopancreatography, *IBS* irritable bowel syndrome

Figure 30.2

Sensitivity of pancreatic function tests in progressive pancreatic exocrine insufficiency. *fecal CT* Fecal chymotrypsin)

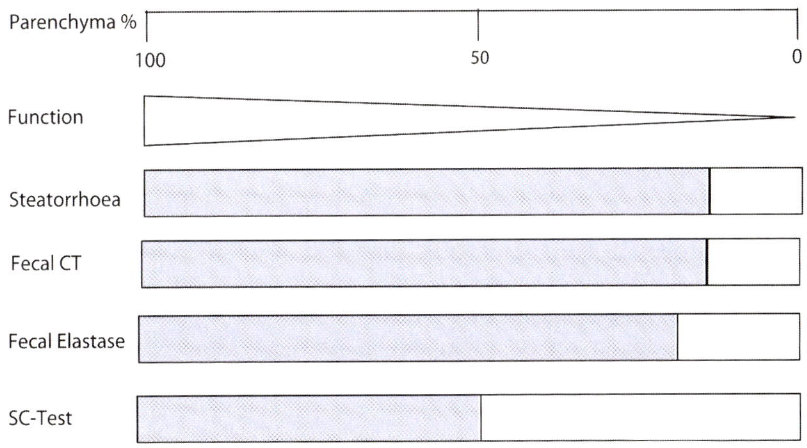

Table 30.3. Sensitivity and specificity of non-invasive pancreatic function tests [27]

	Sensitivity (%)			Specificity (%)
	Mild	Moderate	Severe	
Fecal chymotrypsin (cut-off = 6 U/g)	54	53	89	74
Pancreolauryl-test	63	76	94	85
Fecal elastase-1	54	75	95	85

Direct Pancreatic Function Tests

Secretin-Cerulein Test

The secretin-cerulein test is considered to be the gold standard for determining pancreatic exocrine function. The test measures pancreatic enzyme and bicarbonate output in response to a defined hormonal stimulus. To achieve this, a double-lumen nasoduodenal tube is placed for constant aspiration of gastric juice and collection of duodenal juice on ice, which is performed during basal conditions, during continuous intravenous infusion of secretin alone, and during infusion of secretin in combination with cholecystokinin (CCK) or an analogue such as cerulein. The sensitivity and specificity of this test for diagnosing chronic pancreatitis exceed 90% [10, 13–16] and it is the only means of reliably diagnosing mild-to-moderate pancreatic exocrine insufficiency. However, the test is invasive, costly, and not standardized among different centers. Incomplete collection of intestinal juice can be compensated by constant duodenal perfusion of a dilution marker, but this requires a triple-lumen tube and further complicates the performance of the test. On the other hand, endoscopic pancreatic function tests using collection of duodenal juice by upper gastrointestinal endoscopy and during stimulation with secretin or CCK may become valid alternatives for the diagnosis of pancreatic exocrine insufficiency [17–19]

Lundh Test

The Lundh test [20–22] also requires intestinal intubation for the direct measurement of enzyme output in duodenal juice. However, in contrast to the secretin test, pancreatic exocrine secretion is stimulated by a standardized test meal. The release of regulatory mediators from the intestinal mucosa is needed for stimulation of pancreatic secretion; as a consequence, false positive results may occur in intestinal diseases such as celiac sprue.

Fecal Tests

Individual enzymes measured in feces correlate with duodenal enzyme output [23]. Therefore, fecal excretion of certain pancreatic enzymes is used as a test of pancreatic exocrine function. Fecal chymotrypsin activity can be measured by a commercially available photometric test kit [24]. When this test is performed on three consecutive days, it detects severe pancreatic exocrine insufficiency with reasonable sensitivity, but sensitivity and specificity are poor in mild-to-moderate cases (Table 30.3) [24–27] . In addition, the test does not differentiate between porcine and human chymotrypsin, so that pancreatin preparations need to be discontinued at least 5 days in advance. On the other hand, fecal chymotrypsin can be used for monitoring compliance in patients who are refractory to enzyme treatment: patients who still suffer from steatorrhea even though they take the advised amount of pancreatin supplements are expected to have high fecal chymotrypsin activities, others, who fail to take (all) the medication, will have low chymotrypsin activities.

Measurement of fecal elastase-1 is offered as a commercial enzyme-linked immunosorbent assay, using an antibody highly specific for the human enzyme. Thus, in contrast to chymotrypsin, pancreatin supplements do not interfere with this pancreatic function test and do not have to be discontinued. Moreover, it does not require repeated performance on consecutive days or quantitative stool collection, but is usually done using a single stool sample. Measurement of fecal eastase-1 is the currently preferred pancreatic function test because it appears to be more sensitive and specific than measurement of fecal chymotrypsin (Table 30.3) [27–30]. However, since the test only assesses enzyme concentrations, there are numerous false positive results in patients with intestinal diseases and diarrhea. Moreover, mild-to-moderate stages of pancreatic exocrine insufficiency cannot be diagnosed reliably [27, 31, 32].

Indirect Tests

Stool Weight and Quantitative Fecal Fat Excretion

For this rather crude test, stool weight is measured on three consecutive days during ingestion of a normal, balanced diet. Pancreatic insufficiency is suspected if stool weight exceeds 200 g/day. Measurement of quantitative fecal fat excretion is the "gold standard" test for malabsorption, although it is an insensitive and nonspecific pancreatic function test because steatorrhea only occurs after loss of more than 90% of exocrine function [10]. In addition, other causes of malabsorption (e.g., celiac sprue or Crohn's disease) may also induce abnormal fecal fat excretion of more than 7 g/day or more than 5 g/100 g. However, in chronic pancreatitis, fecal fat concentration usually exceeds 10g/100g and steatorrhea occurs [33].

Fluorescein Dilaurate (Pancreolauryl Test) and the PABA Test

Neither the fluorescein dilaurate (pancreolauryl) test nor the NBT-PABA (N-benzoyl-L-tyrosyl-p-aminobenzoic acid) test are commercially available in Europe at present and, will therefore be discussed only briefly. For both tests, the patient is orally administered a substrate that is metabolized into two or more products by pancreatic enzymes. At least one of the metabolites is absorbed from the gut, conjugated, and excreted in the urine, where it can be measured. Thus, pancreatic exocrine insufficiency will lead to increased fecal excretion of the unsplit molecule and decreased absorption, blood levels, and urinary excretion of the metabolite. Because of interindividual variability of intermediary steps such as intestinal absorption and renal function, the fluorescein dilaurate test includes application of an absorbable metabolite (fluorescein) on a 2nd day and the results of the test are expressed as the ratio of excreted fluorescein on the test and the control day in percent. A ratio of less than 20% is abnormal, 20–30% is equivocal and more than 30% is considered normal. A modified serum test eliminates the need for a second test day, but does not increase sensitivity and specificity [27, 34, 35]. The fluorescein dilaurate test appears to be a little more sensitive for diagnosing mild exocrine insufficiency compared to the elastase-1 test [27], but still does not diagnose milder stages of pancreatic exocrine insufficiency reliably (Table 30.3) [27, 32].

Breath Tests

During recent years, several breath tests using ^{13}C-labeled substrates have been developed for measurement of pancreatic function. Of these, tests using ^{13}C-labeled lipids are most promising because lipase synthesis and secretion tend to be impaired earlier than those of other pancreatic enzymes in chronic pancreatitis [12]. The labeled lipids are ingested orally together with a test meal and need to be digested to monoglycerides and free fatty acids by pancreatic lipase prior to absorption. Hepatic metabolization of the absorbed lipids leads to production of $^{13}CO_2$, which is transported to the lung and exhaled. Thus, intestinal lipolysis by pancreatic lipase as the rate-limiting step of lipid absorption is reflected by the ratio of breath $^{13}CO_2/^{12}CO_2$ over time. Available substrates include 1,3 distearyl-2[^{13}C]-octanoate, which is the most commonly used, but uniformly labeled Hiolein (a mixture of long-chain triglycerides) and cholesteryl-^{13}C-octanoate are also used [36–39]. The sensitivity and specificity of certain test modifications have been reported to exceed 90% [40]. However, it has not been demonstrated, so far, that noninvasive ^{13}C-breath tests are able to diagnose mild-to-moderate pancreatic exocrine insufficiency.

Imaging Diagnosis of Chronic Pancreatitis

Transabdominal Ultrasound

Transabdominal ultrasound (TUS) is generally used as the first imaging method for patients with suspected chronic pancreatitis (Fig. 30.1). The sensitivity reported for TUS in chronic pancreatitis ranges from 49 to 96% [41–44]. This variation reflects the morphologic spectrum of chronic pancreatitis, ranging from normal in early or mild disease to grossly abnormal in severe disease. While the sensitivity of TUS is low for early lesions, it may detect more severe pancreatic changes as well as extrapancreatic alterations such as, for example, bile duct dilatation and fluid collections.

Computed Tomography

Abdominal computed tomography (CT) scanning has good sensitivity for diagnosing moderate-to-severe chronic pancreatitis (Fig. 30.1) [44–48]. However, the early changes associated with chronic pancreatitis are more difficult to identify on CT. Characteristic findings on CT include dilatation of the pancreatic duct and its side branches, focal and parenchymal atrophy, pancreatic calcification, focal parenchymal enlargement, bile duct dilatation, and alterations in peripancreatic fat or fascia, as shown in Table 30.1. Diagnostic criteria are similar as for TUS. Yet, compared with TUS, CT is less operator-dependent, not compromised by intervening bowel gas, and identifies sensitively pancreatic calcifications. As a rule, sensitivity of CT for chronic pancreatitis depends on the severity of the disease and ranges from <60% to 95% [42–44]. Yet, it should be kept in mind that in patients with early stages of chronic pancreatitis frequently have normal CT findings.

Moreover, CT will identify many local complications of chronic pancreatitis and is able to detect inflammatory masses or pseudocysts [49–51]. Abdominal CT is also useful for differential diagnosis of abdominal pain because CT may also help to identify peripancreatic and other abdominal abnormalities such as pancreatic cancer [51], and/or to exclude other intra-abdominal disorders [42–44].

Optimal evaluation of the pancreas requires helical CT scanning using a pancreas-optimized protocol [52–54]. This technology permits scanning of the complete pancreas during a single breath hold [51]. Whenever possible, an oral contrast agent should be used to maximize pancreatic visualization and especially the duodenal wall, the papilla, and the duodenal pancreatic boundaries [50, 51]. An initial scan without intravenous contrast will easily identify pancreatic calcifications. This should be followed by contrast infusion [50, 55, 56] to allow optimal enhancement of early tumors. A 150-ml bolus of nonionic contrast media is rapidly infused at a rate of 5 ml/s, followed by a rapid series of 3- to 5-mm scans taken after a 45-s delay (arterial phase) [56]. The scan is repeated after 70 s (dual-phase imaging) with 5- to 7-mm thick sections to identify venous obstruction and/or involvement, the biliary tree, and the liver parenchyma (liver/portal venous phase) [56].

Magnetic Resonance Imaging

Magnetic resonance imaging (MRI) and magnetic resonance cholangiopancreatography (MRCP) are increasingly used as additional imaging modality of patients suspected of having chronic pancreatitis [56–60]. MRI findings include atrophy of the gland, changes in signal intensity of pancreatic parenchyma, irregular dilatation of the pancreatic duct, pancreatic calcification, and pseudocysts. MRCP demonstrates pseudocysts in or near the pancreas and ductal abnormalities, including segmental dilatation, narrowing, ductal filling defects representing calculi, or mucinous casts in the pancreatic ducts [60–65]. Images can be acquired in only a few seconds during a single breath hold using a thick-slab (5 cm) acquisition or a multislice, thin-slice acquisition [56]. T1-weighted sequences with fat suppression images before and after gadolinium administration are the key sequences for evaluating the pancreatic parenchyma by MRI [66]. Morphologic findings of chronic pancreatitis on MRI are analogous to those seen on CT (Table 30.1). It has been emphasized that its sensitivity (81–100%), specificity (94–98%), positive (86–93%) and negative (94–98%) predictive values, and diagnostic accuracy (94–97%) are as high as those of endoscopic retrograde cholangiopancreatography (ERCP), which makes MRCP a promising alternative to diagnostic ERCP [60–65]. MRCP is noninvasive, avoids ionizing radiation and contrast administration, and does not routinely require sedation. Moreover, it can provide useful information on the parenchymatous organs in this region in combination with conventional cross-sectional magnetic resonance sequences.

Although it has advantages, MRCP also has certain drawbacks. Small duct changes and calcifications are not readily detected, and most importantly, it does not allow simultaneous therapeutic intervention. While ERCP offers a therapeutic option in the same session after the diagnosis is made (e.g., papillotomy, removal of choledocholithiasis, stenting of a biliary stricture), MRCP just offers the diagnosis. Clips, stents, pneumobilia, hemobilia, and ascites might result in artifacts and impede interpretation of the MRCP image. Despite the new technological advances in MRI, its resolution has remained lower than that of ERCP [67]. Maybe the innovative secretin-stimulated MRCP, which permits the detection of pancreatic flow dynamics and assessment of pancreatic exocrine function, will improve the sensitivity of MRCP in future [60].

Endoscopic Retrograde Pancreatography

Endoscopic retrograde pancreatography (ERP) is widely considered the gold standard for the morphologic diagnosis and staging of chronic pancreatitis. The most commonly used method for staging chronic pancreatitis is the Cambridge classification (Table 30.1) [68]. In mild or early disease, side-branch ectasia can be visualized. In more advanced disease, irregularity and dilatation of the main pancreatic duct, as well as strictures, calcifications and cysts may

Table 30.4. Sensitivity and specificity of radiological examinations for diagnosing chronic pancreatitis. *TUS* Transabdominal ultrasound

	Sensitivity				Specificity	
Author	TUS	CT	ERCP	EUS	EUS	Patients (n)
Wiersema et al. 1993 [71]			50%[a]	80%	86%	30
Giovannini and Seitz 1994 [72]			76%	93%	56%	17
Buscail et al. 1995 [44][b]	58%	75%	74%	88%	100%	81
Kahl et al. 2002 [73]			80.7%	100%	–[c]	130

[a] Sensitivity just for "early chronic pancreatitis" (sensitivity of EUS in patients with "early chronic pancreatitis": 86%

[b] Specificity: ERCP 100%, CT 95%, TUS 75%

[c] Patients without clinical suspicion for chronic pancreatitis were not included, therefore specificity cannot be assessed

be seen. In ERCP, slight changes (minimal disease) are often difficult to detect and variable to interpret. It has been reported that in 30% of patients with small duct disease who have had a normal or near-normal ERCP, an abnormal secretin stimulation test can be found [69].

ERP is considered to be the most accurate test for the diagnosis of chronic pancreatitis, with sensitivities of 70–90% and specificities of 90–100% (Table 30.4) [44, 70–73], dependent on disease and control populations studied and on the definition of a gold standard.

Overall, ERP is useful for those patients in whom other methods failed or are unavailable, in patients with a clinical pattern of recurrent acute pancreatitis, or when a therapeutic intervention is being considered [74]. The role of ERP in the evaluation of those patients suspected of having sphincter of Oddi dysfunction as a contributor to acute recurrent pancreatitis or chronic pancreatitis continues to be evaluated [75].

However, it should be noted that ERP is invasive and has a substantial risk of complications, in particular acute pancreatitis. In a recent multicenter survey, the overall complication rate was 4% and the procedure-related mortality rate was 0.4% [76].

Endoscopic Ultrasonography

EUS has an increasingly important role in diagnosing and evaluating patients with chronic pancreatitis. EUS was introduced in the early 1980s to image the pancreas. Its technique circumvents many of the limitations (abdominal gas and fat) of TUS in pancreatic diseases. EUS has a low risk of complications [76, 77] and is able to detect very small abnormalities of the pancreatic duct or parenchyma in patients with chronic pancreatitis that are not visible on any other imaging modality. The minimal changes in echotexture are difficult to interpret because there is no reference standard as a confirmatory test.

In standard EUS, the transducer is located at the tip of an endoscope. The pancreas can be examined transduodenally and transgastrally. Two different EUS systems are available. A rotating transducer makes a 360° ultrasound image possible. The other system offers 150° sector images. The latest sector scanning probes offer several additional features, like Doppler, color, and power Doppler tools, or the opportunity to take EUS-guided fine needle biopsy samples. Because of the small distance to the pancreas, without any interference (e.g., fat, bowel, or gas), high-frequency transducers (up to 20 MHz) can be used. This technique allows high-resolution images (1 mm) of the pancreatic parenchyma and duct structures.

The diagnosis of chronic pancreatitis at EUS is based on the finding of abnormalities in the pancreatic duct and parenchyma (Table 30.5) [71]. Most studies have used these nine sonographic features and defined the cut-off point for the diagnosis chronic pancreatitis when three or more features were seen. Several studies have compared the findings of EUS with ERCP (Table 30.3) [44, 46, 71, 73, 78–81] and pancreatic function tests [78, 82]. These studies suggest that EUS accurately diagnoses chronic pancreatitis in most patients with ERCP- or pancreatic-function-test-proven chronic pancreatitis. However, they also suggest that 25% of those patients with a normal ERCP and 40% of those with normal pancreatic function tests have an abnormal EUS [83]; at present it is unclear if these patients have chronic pancreatitis or if EUS produces false-positive results.

Table 30.5. Endosonographic criteria of chronic pancreatitis (*CP*) [71]

Ductular features (assessed in head, body, and tail)
Narrowing
Dilatation
Contour (irregular/regular)
Duct wall echogenicity (increased/normal)
Calculi (size if present)
Side branch dilatation
Parechymal features (assessed in head, body, and tail)
Gland size
Parenchyma echogenicity (focal regions of reduced echogenicity)
Echogenic foci (>3 mm in size)
Cysts (>3 mm in size)
Accentuation of lobular pattern

The threshold for diagnosing chronic pancreatitis based on EUS criteria can be variable (three or more, four or more, or five or more criteria); as a consequence, the sensitivity and specificity of EUS compared with ERCP depends on which threshold is chosen. If a low threshold is used (more than 1–2 criteria) the "sensitivity" (and negative predictive value) will be very high, but the "specificity" (and positive predictive value) will be low. If a higher threshold is used (more than 5–6 criteria) the "sensitivity" (and negative predictive value) will be low, but the "specificity" (and positive predictive value) will be high. Depending on the question, a different threshold can be used for diagnosing or excluding chronic pancreatitis. For example, a patient with only 0–1 criteria of chronic pancreatitis by EUS has a >90% chance of having a normal ERCP [82]. A high threshold (six or more EUS criteria) gives a positive predictive value of >80% of having an abnormal ERCP. Obviously, patients with an intermediate number of criteria may require further investigations to strengthen the diagnosis of chronic pancreatitis.

It must be noted that not all criteria are equally important. Calcification of the pancreas, for example, is highly predictive for chronic pancreatitis even in the absence of other criteria. Another aspect to consider is that age-related changes of the pancreas influence the diagnostic threshold. To date, there is no accepted scoring system that takes all of these effects into consideration. One common practice is to require a higher threshold (e.g., five or more criteria) for older patients and a lower threshold (e.g., four or more criteria) for younger patients [84]. In addition to this, EUS findings should be regarded in the whole clinical context. A scoring system (Table 30.2) can be used if additional factors are available [9]. According to our current understanding, a normal EUS should rule out the disease. Hence, to improve the usefulness of EUS in chronic pancreatitis, features of the normal pancreas also need to be defined and standardized, and yet there is a scarcity of data. Normal endosonographic findings of the pancreas have been described in only one series in healthy medical students [71].

EUS may also be used to obtain tissue and/or pancreatic juice during the examination. The potential to combine imaging with measures of pancreatic function, cytology/histology, and molecular markers may further increase the diagnostic importance of EUS in the future (Fig. 30.1).

Pancreatic Fine-Needle Aspiration

The main indication for EUS-guided fine-needle aspiration (FNA) in the pancreas is to obtain samples from an intrapancreatic mass [85–89]. EUS is able to detect and target abnormalities of the pancreas that cannot be seen by other imaging procedures [85]. Modern EUS-guided needles allow the histological analysis of tissue from the pancreas [90]. The Trucut needle is helpful for diagnosing benign parenchymal diseases of the pancreas, such as autoimmune pancreatitis [91]. Of particular importance is the potential to avoid unnecessary surgery [85].

Table 30.6. Endosonographic criteria and definitions of chronic pancreatits and presumed histologic correlates. *EUS* Endoscopic ultrasound, *MST* Minimum Standard Terminology version 1.0 [100]

EUS criteria for CP	MST definition	Histological correlate
Hyperechoic foci	Small distinct reflectors	Focal fibrosis
Hyperechoic strand	Small string-like hyperechoic structures	Bridging fibrosis
Lobular out gland margin	No MST definition	Fibrosis, glandular atrophy
Lobularity	Containing lobules-rounded homogeneous areas separated by strands of another echogenicity	Interlobular fibrosis
Cyst	Abnormal anechoic round or oval structure	Cysts/pseudocysts
Stone	Hyperechoic lesion with acoustic shadowing within a duct or gallbladder	Calcified stones
Calcification	Hyperechoic lesion with acoustic shadow within a parenchymal organ or a mass	Parenchymal calcification
Ductal dilatation	No MST definition	>3 mm in head, >2 mm in body, >1 mm in tail
Side branch dilatation	No MST definition	Side branch dilatation
Duct irregularity	Coarse, uneven outline of the duct	Focal dilatation/narrowing
Hyperechoic duct margins	No MST definition	Periductal fibrosis
Atrophy	No MST definition	Atrophy
Non-homogeneous echo pattern	No MST definition	Edema

FNA Techniques

A small-gauge needle is placed into the pancreatic mass and the needle is moved to and fro within the mass while applying suction to the syringe. The complication rate of EUS-FNA is considered to be very low (1–2%) [92–94]. The most common complication is bleeding, which is often selflimiting. Pancreatitis is also rare and usually mild and occurs more often after FNA of a cystic lesion than after FNA of a solid mass lesion (1.2%) [95].

The false-positive rate of FNA cytology is very rare when analyzed by specialized pathologists [96]. False-negative results occur at rates similar to other techniques. An on-site cytologist will improve the results of FNA cytology [97].

The following classification is used in clinical practice [98]:

Grade 0: No chronic pancreatitis (i.e., no relevant cellular infiltration, normal epithelial cells).

Grade 2: Mild chronic pancreatitis (mild-to-moderate lymphocytic/granulocytic infiltration, hyperplastic epithelial cells, presence of degenerated tissue, sparse protein precipitates).

Grade 3: Severe chronic pancreatitis (dense infiltration of lymphocytic cells/macrophages, massive epithelial degeneration, necrosis/cellular debris, numerous protein precipitates – plugs, calcifications).

In selected patients with normal or equivocal results from imaging studies, EUS combined with FNA cytology improves the negative predictive value, which may increase the sensibility of EUS in diagnosing mild-to-moderate chronic pancreatitis [99]. Cytology, however, cannot substantially increase the specificity of findings. The reasons for these limitations include: (1) the presence of residual inflammatory changes from a previous attack of acute pancreatitis, (2) the lack of an international standardized cytologic diagnosis and staging system for chronic pancreatitis, (3) differences in cytologic tissue processing techniques, and (4) problems with the interpretation of inconclusive cytology findings [99]. A summary of the reported EUS criteria of chronic pancreatitis and histologic correlates is shown in Table 30.6.

References

1. Sarles H, Adler G, Dani R, Frey C, Gullo L, Harada H, Martin E, Norohna M, Scuro LA (1989) The pancreatitis classification of Marseilles, Rome 1988. Scand J Gastroenterol 24:641–642
2. Sarner M, Cotton PB (1984) Definitions of acute and chronic pancreatitis. Clin Gastroenterol 13:865–870
3. Sarner M, Cotton PB (1984) Classification of pancreatitis. Gut 25:756–759
4. Lankisch PG (1999) Progression from acute to chronic pancreatitis: a physician's view. Surg Clin North Am 79:815–827
5. Ammann RW (1997) A clinically based classification system for alcoholic chronic pancreatitis: summary of an international workshop on chronic pancreatitis. Pancreas 14:215–221
6. Chari ST, Singer MV (1994) The problem of classification and staging of chronic pancreatitis: proposal based on current knowledge and its natural history. Scand J Gastroenterol 29:949–960
7. Layer P, Yamamoto H, Kalthoff L, Clain JE, Bakken LJ, Di Magno EP (1994) The different courses of early and late onset idiopathic and alcoholic chronic pancreatitis. Gastroenterology 107:1481–1487
8. Mahlke R, Lübbers H, Lankisch PG (2005) Diagnostik und Therapie der chronischen Pankreatitis. Internist (Berl) 46:145–156
9. Lankisch PG, Assmus C, Maisonneuve P, Lowenfels AB (2002) Epidemiology of pancreatic diseases in Lüneburg County. Pancreatology 2:469–477
10. DiMagno EP, Go VL, Summerskill WH (1973) Relations between pancreatic enzyme ouputs and malabsorption in severe pancreatic insufficiency. N Engl J Med 288: 813–815
11. Lankisch PG, Droge M, Hofses S, Konig H, Lembcke B (1996) Steatorrhoea: you cannot trust your eyes when it comes to diagnosis [letter] [see comments]. Lancet 347:1620–1621
12. DiMagno EP, Malagelada JR, Go VL (1975) Relationship between alcoholism and pancreatic insufficiency. Ann N Y Acad Sci 252:200–207
13. DiMagno EP, Malagelada JR, Go VL, Moertel CG (1977) Fate of orally ingested enzymes in pancreatic insufficiency. Comparison of two dosage schedules. N Engl J Med 296:1318–1322
14. DiMagno EP, Go WL, Summerskill WH (1972) Impaired cholecystokinin-pancreozymin secretion, intraluminal dilution, and maldigestion of fat in sprue. Gastroenterology 63:25–32
15. Lankisch PG, Schmidt I (1999) Exocrine pancreatic function tests, 1999: is the best we have good enough? [editorial]. Scand J Gastroenterol 34:945–947
16. Wormsley KG (1978) Tests of pancreatic secretion. Clin Gastroenterol 7:529–544
17. Conwell DL, Zuccaro G Jr, Vargo JJ, Trolli PA, Vanlente F, Obuchowski N, Dumot JA, O'laughlin C (2003) An endoscopic pancreatic function test with synthetic porcine secretin for the evaluation of chronic abdominal pain and suspected chronic pancreatitis. Gastrointest Endosc 57:37–40
18. Raimondo M, Imoto M, DiMagno EP (2003) Rapid endoscopic secretin stimulation test and discrimination of chronic pancreatitis and pancreatic cancer from disease controls. Clin Gastroenterol Hepatol 1:397–403
19. Conwell DL, Zuccaro G, Morrow JB, Van Lente F, Obuchowski N, Vargo JJ, Dumot JA, Trolli P, Shay SS (2002) Cholecystokinin-stimulated peak lipase concentration in duodenal drainage fluid: a new pancreatic function test. Am J Gastroenterol 97:1392–1397
20. Ihse I, Lilja P, Evander A, Skude G (1977) Time-related enzyme concentrations in duodenal aspirates after ingestion of a test meal. Scand J Gastroenterol 12:629–635
21. Moeller DD, Dunn GD, Klotz AP (1972) Comparison of the pancreozymin-secretin test and the Lundh test meal. Am J Dig Dis 17:799–805
22. James O (1973) The Lundh test. Gut 14:582–591
23. Katschinski M, Schirra J, Bross A, Goke B, Arnold R (1997) Duodenal secretion and fecal excretion of pancreatic elastase-1 in healthy humans and patients with chronic pancreatitis. Pancreas 15:191–200
24. Ammann RW, Akovbiantz A, Hacki W, Largiader F, Schmid M (1981) Diagnostic value of the fecal chymotrypsin test in pancreatic insufficiency, particularly chronic pancreatitis: correlation with the pancreozymin-secretin test, fecal fat excretion and final clinical diagnosis. Digestion 21:281–289
25. Bonin A, Roy CC, Lasalle R, Weber A, Morin CL (1973) Fecal chymotrypsin: a reliable index of exocrine pancreatic function in children. J Pediatr 83:594–600
26. Lankisch PG, Schreiber A, Otto J (1983) Pancreolauryl test. Evaluation of a tubeless pancreatic function test in comparison with other indirect and direct tests for exocrine pancreatic function. Dig Dis Sci 28:490–493
27. Siegmund E, Löhr JM, Schuff-Werner P (2004) Die diagnostische Validtät nichtinvasver Pankreasfunktionstests – Eine Metaanalyse. Z Gastroenterol 42:1117–1128
28. Dominguez-Munoz JE, Hieronymus C, Sauerbruch T, Malfertheiner P (1995) Fecal elastase test: evaluation of a new noninvasive pancreatic function test. Am J Gastroenterol 90:1834–1837
29. Glasbrenner B, Schon A, Klatt S, Beckh K, Adler G (1996) Clinical evaluation of the faecal elastase test in the diagnosis and staging of chronic pancreatitis. Eur J Gastroenterol Hepatol 8:1117–1120
30. Loser C, Mollgaard A, Folsch UR (1996) Faecal elastase 1: a novel, highly sensitive, and specific tubeless pancreatic function test [see comments]. Gut 39:580–586
31. Lankisch PG, Schmidt I, Konig H, Lehnick D, Knollmann R, Lohr M, Liebe S (1998) Faecal elastase 1: not helpful in diagnosing chronic pancreatitis associated with mild to moderate exocrine pancreatic insufficiency [see comments]. Gut 42:551–554
32. Lankisch PG, Schmidt I (2000) Fecal elastase 1 is not the indirect pancreatic function test we have been waiting for [letter; comment]. Dig Dis Sci 45:166–167
33. Bo-Linn GW, Fordtran JS (1984) Fecal fat concentration in patients with steatorrhea. Gastroenterology 87:319–322
34. Lock G, Kadow R, Messmann H, Zirngibl H, Scholmerich J, Holstege A (1997) Modified serum pancreolauryl test in chronic pancreatitis: evaluation in comparison to endoscopic retrograde pancreatography. Hepatogastroenterology 44:1110–1116
35. Malfertheiner P, Buchler M, Muller A, Ditschuneit H (1987) Fluorescein dilaurate serum test: a rapid tubeless pancreatic function test. Pancreas 2:53–60
36. Loser C, Brauer C, Aygen S, Hennemann O, Folsch UR (1998) Comparative clinical evaluation of the 13C-mixed triglyceride breath test as an indirect pancreatic function test [see comments]. Scand J Gastroenterol 33:327–334

37. Lembcke B, Braden B, Caspary WF (1996) Exocrine pancreatic insufficiency: accuracy and clinical value of the uniformly labelled 13C-Hiolein breath test. Gut 39:668–674
38. Lembcke B (1996) Current role of breath tests in gastroenterology. Z Gastroenterol 34:46–53
39. Wutzke KD, Radke M, Breuel K, Gurk S, Lafrenz JD, Heine WE (1999) Triglyceride oxidation in cystic fibrosis: a comparison between different 13C-labeled tracer substances. J Pediatr Gastroenterol Nutr 29:148–154
40. Dominguez-Munoz JE (2005) Pancreatic function tests for diagnosis and staging of chronic pancreatitis, cystic fibrosis, and exocrine pancreatic insufficiency of other etiologies. Clin Pancreatol pp 259–266
41. Villaba-Martin C, Dominguez-Munoz EJ (2005) Role of imaging methods in diagnosing, staging, and detecting complications of chronic pancreatitis in clinical practice: should MRCP and MRI replace ERCP and CT? Clin Pancreatol pp 236–245
42. Buscail L, Escourrou J, Moreau J, Delvaux M, Louvel D, Lapeyre F, Tregant P, Frexinos J (1995) Endoscopic ultrasonography in chronic pancreatitis: a comparative prospective study with conventional ultrasonography, computed tomography, and ERCP. Pancreas 10:251–257
43. Rosch T, Schusdziarra V, Born P, Bautz W, Baumgartner M, Ulm K, Lorenz R, Allescher HD, Gerhardt P, Siewert JR, Classen M (2000) Modern imaging methods versus clinical assessment in the evaluation of hospital in-patients with suspected pancreatic disease. Am J Gastroenterol 95:2261–2270
44. Buscail L, Escourrou J, Moreau J, et al (1995) Endoscopic ultrasonography in chronic pancreatitis: a comparative prospective study with conventional ultrasonography, computed tomography, and ERCP. Pancreas 10:251–257
45. Malfertheiner P, Buchler M (1989) Correlation of imaging and function in chronic pancreatitis. Radiol Clin North Am 27:51–64
46. Buscail L, Escourrou J, Moreau J, Delvaux M, Louvel D, Lapeyre F, Tregant P, Frexinos J (1995) Endoscopic ultrasonography in chronic pancreatitis: a comparative prospective study with conventional ultrasonography, computed tomography and ERCP. Pancreas 10:251–257
47. Malfertheiner P, Buchler M, Stanescu A, Ditschuneit H (1986) Exocrine pancreatic function in correlation to ductal and parenchymal morphology in chronic pancreatitis. Hepatogastroenterology 33:110–114
48. Fulcher AS, Turner MA (1999) Magnetic resonance pancreatography (MRP). Crit Rev Diagn Imaging 40:285–322
49. Clain JE, Pearson RK (1999) Diagnosis of chronic pancreatitis: is a gold standard necessary? Surg Clin North Am 79:829–845
50. Freeny PC, Marks WM, Ryan JA, Traverso LW (1988) Pancreatic ductal adenocarcinoma: diagnosis and staging with dynamic CT. Radiology 166:125–133
51. Thoeni RF, Blankenberg F (1993) Pancreatic imaging, computed tomography and magnetic resonance imaging. Radiol Clin North Am 31:1085–1113
52. Kusano S, Kaji T, Sugiura Y, Tamai S (1999) CT demonstration of fibrous stroma in chronic pancreatitis: pathologic correlation. J Comput Assist Tomogr 23:297–300
53. Hollett MD, Jorgensen MJ, Jeffrey RB Jr (1995) Quantitative evaluation of pancreatic enhancement during dual-phase helical CT. Radiology 195:359–361
54. Bonaldi VM, Bret PM, Atri M, Garcia P, Reinhold C (1996) A comparison of two injection protocols using helical and dynamic acquisitions in CT examinations of the pancreas. AJR Am J Roentgenol 167:49–55
55. Megibow AJ (1992) Pancreatic adenocarcinoma: designing the examination to evaluate the clinical questions. Radiology 183:297–303
56. Kalra MK, Maher MM, Sahani DV, Digmurthy S, Saini S (2002) Current status of imaging in pancreatic diseases. J Comput Assist Tomogr 26:661–675
57. Johnson PT, Outwater EK (1999) Pancreatic carcinoma versus chronic pancreatitis: dynamic MR imaging. Radiology 212:213–218
58. Sica GT, Braver J, Cooney MJ, Miller FH, Chai JL, Adams DF (1999) Comparison of endoscopic retrograde cholangiopancreatography with MR cholangiopancreatography in patients with pancreatitis. Radiology 210:605–610
59. Tamura R, Ishibashi T, Takahashi S (2006) Chronic pancreatitis: MRCP versus ERCP for quantitative caliber measurement and qualitative evaluation. Radiology 238:920–928
60. Merkle EM, Baillie J (2006) Exocrine pancreatic function: evaluation with MR imaging before and after secretin stimulation. Am J Gastroenterol 101:137–138
61. Lomanto D, Pavone P, Laghi A, Panebianco V, Mazzocchi P, Fiocca F, Lezoche E, Passariello R, Speranza V (1997) Magnetic resonance cholangiopancreatography in the diagnosis of biliopancreatic diseases. Am J Surg 174:33–38
62. Coakley FV, Schwartz LH (1999) Magnetic resonance cholangiopancreatography. J Magn Reson Imaging 9:157–162
63. Takehara Y (1998) Can MRCP replace ERCP? J Magn Reson Imaging 8:517–534
64. Soto JA, Barish MA, Yucel EK, Siegenberg D, Ferrucci JT, Chuttani R (1996) Magnetic resonance cholangiography: comparison with endoscopic retrograde cholangiopancreatography. Gastroenterology 110:589–597
65. Sahai AV, Devonshire D, Yeoh KG, Kay C, Feldman D, Willner I, Farber J, Patel R, Tamasky PR, Cunningham JT, Trus T, Hawes RH, Cotton PB (2001) The decision-making value of magnetic resonance cholangiopancreatography in patients seen in a referral center for suspected biliary and pancreatic disease. Am J Gastroenterol 96:2074–2080
66. Freeny PC (1999) Pancreatic imaging. New modalities. Gastroenterol Clin North Am 28:723–746
67. Keogan MT, Edelman RR (2001) Technologicl advances in abdominal MR imaging. Radiology 220:310–320
68. Kasugai T, Kuno N, Kizu M, Kobayashi S, Hattori K (1972) Endoscopic pancreatocholangiography. II. The pathological endoscopic pancreatocholangiogram. Gastroenterology 63:227–234
69. Gupta V, Toskes PP (2005) Diagnosis and management of chronic pancreatitis. Postgrad Med J 81:491–497
70. Caletti G, Brocchi E, Agostini D, Balduzzi A, Bolondi L, Labo G (1982) Sensitivity of endoscopic retrograde pancreatography in chronic pancreatitis. Br J Surg 69:507–509
71. Wiersema MJ, Hawes RH, Lehman GA, Kochman ML, Sherman S, Kopecky KK (1993) Prospective evaluation of endoscopic ultrasonography and endoscopic retrograde cholangiopancreatography in patients with chronic abdominal pain of suspected pancreatic origin [see comments]. Endoscopy 25:555–564
72. Giovannini M, Seitz JF (1994) Endoscopic ultrasonography with a linear-type echoendoscope in the evaluation of 94 patients with pancreatobiliary disease. Endoscopy 26:579–585

73. Kahl S, Glasbrenner B, Leodolter A, Pross M, Schulz HU, Malfertheiner P (2002) EUS in the diagnosis of early chronic pancreatitis: a prospective follow-up study. Gastrointest Endosc 55:507–511
74. Somogyi L, Martin SP, Venkatesan T, Ulrich CD II (2001) Recurrent acute pancreatitis: an algorithmic approach to identification and elimination of inciting factors. Gastroenterology 120:708–717
75. Venu RP, Brown RD, Halline AG (2002) The role of endoscopic retrograde cholangiopancreatography in acute and chronic pancreatitis. J Clin Gastroenterol 34:560–568
76. Bolan PJ, Fink AS. (2003) Endoscopic retrograde cholangiopancreatography in chronic pancreatitis. World J Surg 27:1183–1191
77. Williams DB, Hoffmann BJ (1999) Complications of interventional endoscopic ultrasonography. In: Bhutani M (ed) Interventional Endoscopic Ultrasonography. Harwood Academic, Amsteldijk, The Netherlands, pp 151–158
78. Catalano MF, Lahoti S, Geenen JE, Hogan WJ (1998) Prospective evaluation of endoscopic ultrasonography, endoscopic retrograde pancreatography, and secretin test in the diagnosis of chronic pancreatitis. Gastrointest Endosc 48:11–17
79. Nattermann C, Goldschmidt AJ, Dancygier H (1993) Endosonography in chronic pancreatitis – a comparison between endoscopic retrograde pancreatography and endoscopic ultrasonography. Endoscopy 25:565–570
80. Buscail L, Escourrou J, Moreau J, Delvaux M, Louvel D, Lapeyre F, Tregant P, Frexinos J (1995) Endoscopic ultrasonography in chronic pancreatitis: a comparative prospective study with conventional ultrasonography, computed tomography, and ERCP. Pancreas 10:251–257
81. Sahai AV, Zimmerman M, Aabakken L, Tarnasky PR, Cunningham JT, van Velse A, Hawes RH, Hoffman BJ (1998) Prospective assessment of the ability of endoscopic ultrasound to diagnose, exclude, or establish the severity of chronic pancreatitis found by endoscopic retrograde cholangiopancreatography. Gastrointest Endosc 48:18–25
82. Wiersema MJ, Hawes RH, Lehman GA, Kochman ML, Sherman S, Kopecky KK (1993) Prospective evaluation of endoscopic ultrasonography and endoscopic retrograde cholangiopancreatography in patients with chronic abdominal pain of suspected pancreatic origin. Endoscopy 25:555–564
83. Forsmark CE (2000) The diagnosis of chronic pancreatitis. Gastrointest Endosc 52:293–298
84. Jenssen C, Dietrich CF (2005) Endosonographie bei chronischer Pankreatitis. Z Gastroenterol 43:737–749
85. Chang KJ, Nguyen P, Erickson RA, Durbin TE, Katz KD (1997) The clinical utility of endoscopic ultrasoundguided fine-needle aspiration in the diagnosis and staging of pancreatic carcinoma. Gastrointest Endosc 45:387–393
86. Fritscher-Ravens A, Izbicki JR, Sriram PV, Krause C, Knoefel WT, Topalidis T, Jaeckle S, Thonke F, Soehendra N (2000) Endosonography guided, fine-needle aspiration cytology extending the indication for organ-preserving pancreatic surgery. Am J Gastroenterol 95:2255–2260
87. Harewood GC, Wiersema MJ (2002) Endosonography-guided fine needle aspiration biopsy in the evaluation of pancreatic masses. Am J Gastroenterol 97:1386–1391
88. Maire F, Couvelard A, Hammel P, Ponsot P, Palazzo L, Aubert A, Degott C, Dancour A, Felce-Dachez M, O'Toole D, Levy P, Ruszniewski P (2003) Intraductal papillary mucinous tumors of the pancreas: the preoperative value of cytologic and histopathologic diagnosis. Gastrointest Endosc 58:701–706
89. Brandwein SL, Farrell JJ, Centeno BA, Brugge WR (2001) Detection and tumor staging of malignancy in cystic, intraductal, and solid tumors of the pancreas by EUS. Gastrointest Endosc 53:722–727
90. Larghi A, Verna EC, Stavropoulos SN, Rotterdam H, Lightdale CJ, Stevens PD (2004) EUS-guided Trucut needle biopsies in patients with solid pancreatic masses: a prospective study. Gastrointest Endosc 59:185–190
91. Varadarajulu S, Fraig M, Schmulewitz N, Roberts S, Wildi S, Hawes RH, et al (2004) Comparison of EUS-guided 19-gauge Trucut needle biopsy with EUS-guided fine-needle aspiration. Endoscopy 36:397–401
92. Schadt ME, Kline TS, Neal HS, Scoma RS, Naryshkin S (1991) Intraoperative pancreatic fine needle aspiration biopsy. Results in 166 patients. Am Surg 57:73–75
93. Saez A, Catala I, Brossa R, Funes A, Jaurrieta E, Ferrer JE (1995) Intraoperative fine needle aspiration cytology of pancreatic lesions. A study of 90 cases. Acta Cytol 39:485–488
94. Gress FG, Hawes RH, Savides TJ, Ikenberry SO, Lehman GA (1997) Endoscopic ultrasound-guided fine-needle aspiration biopsy using linear array and radial scanning endosonography. Gastrointest Endosc 45:243–250
95. O'Toole D, Palazzo L, Arotcarena R, Dancour A, Aubert A, Hammel P, Amaris J, Ruszniewski P (2001) Assessment of complications of EUS-guided fine-needle aspiration. Gastrointest Endosc 53:470–474
96. Schwartz DA, Unni KK, Levy MJ, Clain JE, Wiersema MJ (2002) The rate of false-positive results with EUS-guided fine-needle aspiration. Gastrointest Endosc 56:868–872
97. Afify AM, al-Khafaji BM, Kim B, Scheiman JM (2003) Endoscopic ultrasound-guided fine needle aspiration of the pancreas. Diagnostic utility and accuracy. Acta Cytol 47:341–348
98. Nagai H, Ohtsubo K (1984) Pancreatic lithiasis in the aged. Its clinicopathology and pathogenesis. Gastroenterology 86:331–338
99. Hollerbach S, Klamann A, Topalidis T, Schmiegel WH (2001) Endoscopic ultrasonography (EUS) and fine-needle aspiration (FNA) cytology for diagnosis of chronic pancreatitis. Endoscopy 33:824–831
100. Lees WR (1986) Endoscopic ultrasonography of chronic pancreatitis and pancreatic pseudocysts. Scand J Gastroenterol Suppl 123:123–129
101. Bockmann DE (2005) Should histology and/ or catology be the gold standard for the diagnosis of chronic pancreatitis in clinical practise? Clin Pancreatol pp 253–258

Chapter 31

P.G. Lankisch · H. Lübbers · R. Mahlke

Medical Management of Chronic Pancreatitis

Abdominal pain, and exocrine and endocrine pancreatic insufficiency are the leading symptoms of chronic pancreatitis. For the majority of patients, however, pain is the decisive symptom, causing much discomfort in their daily lives. Thus, the medical management of chronic pancreatitis has three aims: treatment of pain as well as of exocrine and endocrine pancreatic insufficiency.

Pain in Chronic Pancreatitis

General

The cause of pain in chronic pancreatitis is uncertain. There are at least two, not necessarily mutually exclusive, hypotheses under investigation [1]. Bockman et al. [2] showed that in chronic pancreatitis perineural inflammation disrupted perineural neural sheaths, and hypothesized that the exposure of the unprotected nerves to bioactive substances triggers pain. A second hypothesis is that painful chronic pancreatitis is caused by increased pancreatic ductal and parenchymal pressure, producing a compartment syndrome that induces ischemia; this hypothesis is supported by experimental studies by Karanjia et al. [3, 4]. They showed increased interstitial and perfusion pressures and decreased blood flow in cases of feline chronic pancreatitis [3]. These abnormalities were reversed substantially by surgical incision of the gland and draining of the pancreatic duct, but were affected minimally by stenting the pancreatic duct [4]. Thus, incision of the gland rather than ductal drainage may be more important in relieving pain, and reducing pancreatic secretion will reduce pressure and alleviate pain [1]. Further studies are required.

More than three decades ago, Ammann [5] postulated a close correlation between pain relief and severe exocrine pancreatic insufficiency, the so-called burn-out of chronic pancreatitis. Since then, this hypothesis has been questioned in several studies. All groups agree that there is an inexorable march toward calcification and exocrine and endocrine pancreatic insufficiency. However, the association between the cessation of pain and onset of calcification and exocrine and endocrine pancreatic insufficiency is controversial.

Ammann's group has claimed that pain decreases with increasing duration of the disease [5–9]. In one long-term study, 85% of 145 patients with chronic pancreatitis felt no more pain after 4.5 years (median) duration of the disease [8]. In another series in which the interval between the onset of alcohol-induced chronic pancreatitis and pain relief was compared in a surgically and a nonsurgically treated patient group, the curves were virtually parallel: pain relief was obtained in about 50% within 6 years and in more than 80% within 10 years from the onset of illness [10].

The reports from Zürich are at variance with the studies from Japan and Germany. Miyake et al. [11] found that only 48.2% of patients with chronic pancreatitis became free of pain within 5 years, and 66–73% after more than 5 years. That meant that every third or fourth patient still suffered from relapsing pain attacks even after a longer observation time. Our group [12] reported that the incidence of relapsing pain attacks decreased during the observation period, but more than half of patients (53%) still suffered from relapsing pain attacks even after more than 10 years observation [12].

At present, the course of pain in alcoholic and idiopathic chronic pancreatitis remains to be clarified. Layer et al. [13] investigated a group of patients with idiopathic chronic pancreatitis who had never consumed alcoholic beverages during their lifetime. They found that patients with early-onset pancreatitis (onset at <35 years of age) have initially and thereafter a long course of severe pain, whereas patients with a late-onset pancreatitis (onset at >35 years) have a mild and often painless course. Both forms differ from alcoholic pancreatitis, with an equal gender distribution and a much slower rate of calcification. In contrast, our group found that the course of pain is the same in alcohol- and non-alcohol-induced chronic pancreatitis [14]. Even when we divided the nonalcoholic group into teetotalers and patients with little alcohol consumption, and compared separately their course of pain with that of alcoholics, there were no differences concerning pain relief among the three groups [15]. Further studies are required [16].

Pain Decrease and Progressing Exocrine and Endocrine Pancreatic Insufficiency

The Swiss group repeatedly observed a pain decrease as exocrine and endocrine pancreatic function declined [5–7, 9]. Similarly, Girdwood et al. [17] reported from South Africa that pain decreased as exocrine pancreatic function deteriorated.

On the contrary, groups from Denmark and Germany have reported the opposite. Thorsgaard Pedersen et al. [18] from Copenhagen found no correlation between pain and exocrine pancreatic function. Our group from Göttingen [12] used the secretin-pancreozymin test and fecal fat analysis to evaluate exocrine pancreatic insufficiency, whereas the Swiss group had used only indirect pancreatic function tests (i.e., chymotrypsin measurements) to evaluate exocrine pancreatic insufficiency [8]. We used a clear-cut grading of the severity of exocrine pancreatic insufficiency: mild impairment was defined as reduced enzyme output; moderate, as a decreased bicarbonate concentration along with reduced enzyme output but normal fecal fat excretion; and severe impairment was equated with an abnormal secretin-pancreozymin test plus steatorrhea. At the end of observation period, 141 (45%) of 311 patients with painful chronic pancreatitis had severe exocrine pancreatic insufficiency. The majority of them (81/144; 57%) still suffered from pain attacks.

We also studied the course of pain in correlation to endocrine pancreatic insufficiency. Endocrine pancreatic insufficiency was classified as absent, moderate (diabetes mellitus treated only by diet plus/minus oral medication), and severe (requiring insulin). At the end of the observation time, 117 (38%) patients were classified as having severe endocrine pancreatic insufficiency. The majority of them (69/117; 59%) still suffered from pain attacks [12, 19].

Thus, according to our results, the progression of exocrine and endocrine pancreatic insufficiency has limited influence, if any, on the course of pain in chronic pancreatitis.

Pain Decrease and Development of Morphological Changes of the Pancreas (Pancreatic Calcifications and/or Duct Abnormalities)

The Swiss group [7, 8] showed an increased the incidence of pancreatic calcifications, which in turn was associated with pain decrease. However, later on, the same group [20] reported a regression of pancreatic calcifications in a long-term study of patients with chronic pancreatitis. Thus, the prognostic role of pancreatic calcifications concerning the course of pain is unclear.

Furthermore, the Swiss results are at variance with those of two other studies. Malfertheiner et al. [21] found that 89% of patients had pain despite pancreatic calcifications (as observed using computed tomography), and 39% experienced very intense pain. In our study, freedom from pain was significantly higher among the calcification group as compared to the noncalcification group. However, the majority of patients with pancreatic calcifications (56%) still had relapsing pain attacks [12].

The correlation between pain and pancreatic duct changes or pressure in the duct system is also not clear. Ebbehøj et al. [22, 23] measured percutaneous or intraoperative pancreatic tissue fluid pressure and found a significant correlation with pain in patients with chronic pancreatitis but not with the endoscopic retrograde cholangiopancreatography (ERCP) results (i.e., the regional pressure tended to be highest in the region of the pancreas with the largest and not with the smallest duct diameter). Jensen et al. [24] found no correlation between pancreatic duct changes and pain. Warshaw et al. [25] found no pain relief in spite of a patent anastomosis detected by ERCP in two of ten of their patients, 1 year after a lateral pancreaticojejunostomy.

Two investigations have confirmed the nonparallel relationship between changes in the pancreatic duct and pain relief. Malfertheiner et al. [21] found severe pain in only 62% of patients who had advanced pancreatic duct changes, demonstrated by ERCP. We found no significant correlation between pancreatic duct abnormalities detected by ERCP and pain in 88 patients with chronic pancreatitis [12]. Severe pancreatic duct abnormalities – as defined by the Cambridge classification [26] – were present in 42 patients, but only 16 (31%) of these became free of pain. Despite a normal pancreatic duct in 14 patients, 10 (71%) of them suffered from persisting pain [12].

Thus, morphological changes such as pancreatic calcifications or pancreatic duct abnormalities are not necessarily helpful in making a prognosis of chronic pancreatitis or predicting the course of pain.

It has been shown recently that smoking has an effect on the natural course of the disease: it increases the risk of pancreatic calcification in late-onset but not early-onset idiopathic chronic pancreatitis [27].

Pain Decrease and Alcohol Abuse

Since alcoholism is the leading etiological factor in chronic pancreatitis, it has also been discussed whether alcohol abstinence influences pain or the progression of the disease. Sarles and Sahel [28] and Trapnell [29] reported pain relief in patients with chronic pancreatitis when alcohol abuse was discontinued in 50% and 75% of the cases, respectively.

Two other investigations confirmed that abstinence can be helpful: Miyake et al. [11] demonstrated pain relief in 60% of their patients who discontinued or reduced their alcohol intake, whereas in the group of patients who continued drinking, spontaneous pain relief was observed in only 26%. In another study [12], 66 (31%) of 214 patients with alcoholic chronic pancreatitis were motivated to stop drinking. Pain relief was obtained in only 52% of these patients, whereas the spontaneous relief in alcoholics was 37%. Thus, alcohol abstinence will probably lead in every second patient with chronic pancreatitis to some improvement of pain, but why exactly abstinence helps in some cases but not in others, remains to be investigated.

Treatment

General

The treatment of pain in chronic pancreatitis requires a correct evaluation of pain (Table 31.1) [30]. The treatment is either done by conservative or, if necessary, interventional and/or surgical procedures. Since the cause of pain is uncertain and the pathophysiological background not really known, there are only a few controlled studies for the treatment of pain in chronic pancreatitis, and none that compares the success of surgical with conservative treatment [30, 31]. The American Gastroenterological Association has worked out guidelines, which we suggest should be followed with the exception of a medication with high dosages of pancreatic enzyme preparations and endoscopic interventional therapy [30, 31].

Medical Treatment

In any case of relapsing or more or less constant pain in chronic pancreatitis, endoscopic or surgical removable causes of pain, such as strictures, pseudocysts, and stones in the pancreatic duct should be ruled out by imaging procedures. Medical pain treatment follows the suggestions of the World Health Organization initially designed for cancer pain relief [32].

Whereas a luminal, protease-dependent, negative feedback system is operative in humans, the possible contribution of this mechanism to the pathogenesis of pain is controversial [33–42]. Similarly, conflicting results have been reported from controlled therapeutic studies in patients with chronic pancreatitis [37, 43–46]. Experimental evidence suggests that hormone-induced inhibition of pancreatic secretion alone is ineffective in painful pancreatitis [47]. Rather, amelioration of pain following enzyme administration may originate from correction of pathologic maldigestion-induced ileal brake effects by increasing and accelerating digestion and thus reverting the luminal site of major nutrient exposure from the distal to the proximal intestine [48–53].

Table 31.1. Criteria for the evaluation of pain [30]

- Duration of pain dating back to the first episode
- Character of pain: intermittent vs. daily; frequency if intermittent
- Subjective estimation of intensity of pain: mild, moderate, or severe
- Objective measurement of pain: visual analogue or descriptor
- Use of narcotics and other medications to treat pain
- Evaluation of addiction to narcotics
- Documentation that other diseases have been excluded that could be causing abdominal pain
- Measurement of quality of life including work performance, social interaction, and family interaction

Interventional Procedures

There are unfortunately no controlled prospective studies proving the values [1, 54–57]. A long-time success is uncertain, and there are no safe predictors to say whether a patient will profit from such a procedure. An amelioration is mostly only transient and it is difficult to differentiate from the natural course of the disease. There are several procedure-induced complications, and it is also possible to overlook a pancreatic carcinoma on the basis of chronic pancreatitis. Nevertheless, the success of interventional and surgical procedures for the treatment of pain is discussed in other chapters herein.

Interventional procedures for pain treatment in chronic pancreatitis include fragmentation of stones by extracorporeal shock wave lithotripsy (ESWL), endoscopic stone extraction, and bridging of pancreatic strictures by stent applications. Reports of the effect of these procedures on pain are controversial and controlled studies are lacking. A large Japanese study collecting 555 patients who underwent ESWL for pancreatic stones reports a success rate of 92.4% (fragmentation of stones) and a complete stone clearance rate after ESWL alone or in combination with interventional endoscopy of 72.6%. Symptom relief was achieved in 91.1% of the patients. Complications developed in 6.3% of the patients including acute pancreatitis in 5.4%. A total of 504 patients could be followed up for a mean of 44.3 months, during which 122 (22%) suffered stone recurrence (mean time to recurrence, 25.1 months), and 22 (4.1%) required surgery [58]. In another series from Japan, a total of 117 patients with pancreatic stones underwent ESWL and endoscopic treatment. Immediate pain relief was achieved in 97%, and complete removal of stones in 56%. During a long-term follow-up over 3 years, 70% of the patients continued to be asymptomatic [59]. These results are at variance with a smaller German study in 80 patients with chronic pancreatitis, for example, ESWL was always followed by a further endoscopic procedure. Treatment success was defined as complete clearance of the main pancreatic duct or partial clearance that allowed implantation of a pancreatic stent. Successful treatment was more frequent in patients with solitary stones. The mean duration of follow-up was 40 months (range 24–92 months). Pain relief and necessity for further analgesia was independent of ESWL results (Table 31.2). Thus, in this study, pancreatic drainage by ESWL and endoscopy had almost no effect on pain in chronic pancreatitis in the long run [60].

The effect of pancreatic stents on pain in chronic pancreatitis is even more controversial. Patients undergoing pancreatic duct stent placement for disrupted ducts, isolated strictures, pancreas divisum, and hypertensive pancreatic sphincters, showed subsequent ductal changes consistent with chronic pancreatitis in 36% of all patients, but in 72% of these patients, the initial pancreatogram had been normal [61]. Furthermore, patients with preoperative endoscopic pancreatic stenting frequently had postoperative septic complications and a prolonged hospital stay [62].

Finally, a surgical review of pitfalls and limitations of stenting in chronic pancreatitis reported that the indication for surgery in patients with a pancreatic stent was severe abdominal pain in all of them, 77% had experienced relapsing pain attacks, and 14% necrotizing pancreatitis. Before being sent for surgery, patients underwent 4.5 ERCP procedures per patient and 3.7 stent exchanges per patient. Thus, from the surgical point of view, endoscopic pancreatic duct stenting in chronic pancreatitis seemed not to be indicated because of a low success rate and a substantial risk for complications [63].

The latter results are in sharp contrast to a long-term outcome study after pancreatic stenting in severe chronic pancreatitis in 100 patients from Belgium. The majority (70%) of patients who responded to pancreatic stenting remained pain free after definite stent removal. However, a significantly higher restenting rate was observed in patients with chronic pancreatitis and pancreas divisum [64].

Obviously, the results are different in special subgroups. Endoscopic stenting of biliary strictures in chronic pancreatitis provided an excellent shorter but only moderate long-term result in another study from Germany. Patients without calcifications of the pancreatic head benefit from biliary stenting. However, pa-

Table 31.2. Long-term effect on pain in 80 patients with chronic pancreatitis treated with extracorporeal shock wave lithotripsy [154]

Feature	Successful treatment of stones (*n*=43)	Unsuccessful treatment of stones (*n*=37)	p Value
Considerable or complete pain relief	34 (79%)	27 (73%)	0.75
No further analgesia necessary	27 (63%)	16 (43%)	0.23

Table 31.3. Five-year follow-up of pain in a prospective randomized trial comparing endoscopic and surgical treatment for chronic pancreatitis [66]

Feature	Endotherapy (*n*=64)	Surgery (*n*=76)	p Value
Abdominal pain			
Complete absence	14.3%	36.9%	0.002
Partial relief	50.8%	49.3%	n.s.
No success	34.9%	13.8%	n.s.

tients with calcifications have a 17-fold increased risk of failure during a 12-month course of follow-up [65].

Of special interest is a recent prospective randomized trial comparing endoscopic and surgical treatment of chronic pancreatitis. Endoscopic treatment included pancreatic sphincterotomy in all patients and additional stenting of the pancreatic duct in 33 (52%) patients. The mean duration of stent treatment was 16 months (range 12–27 months), and stents were exchanged six times (range 4–9). Surgical treatment included pancreatic resection in 61 (80%), and drainage procedures in 15 (20%) patients. Although the short-term effects were similar, the results after 5 years follow-up showed a comparatively low rate of patients with complete absence of abdominal pain (Table 31.3). However, the results for surgery were significantly better than for endotherapy [66]. The study has been criticized for the randomization, which was agreed to by only 51.4% of the patients.

For the time being, reports of treatment of chronic pancreatitis with ERCP by removal or destruction of stones, placement of stents, and dilation of strictures suggest that both immediate and long-term pain relief are possible. No controlled studies support the generalization of this finding or the merit of this approach compared to other management strategies. Studies of this area would be of value [67].

Celiac plexus block for control of pain in chronic pancreatitis has been shown to substantially reduce the severity of pain. About two-thirds of the patients showed long-term improvement of pain [68]. Gress et al. [69] showed that endoscopic ultrasound-guided celiac plexus block provided more persistent pain relief than computed-tomography-guided block and was the preferred technique among the subjects studied. Endoscopic ultrasound-guided celiac block appeared to be a safe, effective, and less costly method for controlling the abdominal pain in patients with chronic pancreatitis [69].

Finally, pancreatic denervation for pain relief is possible by performing transthoracic splanchnicectomy [70, 71]. Further studies are required. In contrast, neither electroacupuncture nor transcutaneous electric nerve stimulation brought about pain relief that could substitute for or supplement medical treatment [72].

Surgical Treatment

If pain cannot be managed by conservative or – if indicated – interventional procedures, and/or if imaging procedures show morphological changes that may be responsible for pain (pancreatic pseudocysts, duct irregularities) and can be operated, the indication for operation should be made early to avoid drug dependency. Surgical treatment is also indicated for several complications (Table 31.4) [73].

During the course of the disease, every second to fourth patient needs surgical treatment because of pain and/or organ complications, such as pancreatic pseudocysts [8, 12]. The choice of surgical procedure is definitely dependent on the particular circumstances of each patient. It is, unclear, however, to what extent surgical treatment influences the course of pain, since the different studies cannot be compared for the following reasons:

Table 31.4. Indications for surgical treatment in chronic pancreatitis. Modified according to Knoefel et al. 2002 [73]

Intractable pain (avoidance of drug dependency)
Suspicion of pancreatic carcinoma
Nonresolving common bile duct stenosis and/or duodenum
Symptomatic large pancreatic pseudocysts that cannot be treated endoscopically
Pseudoaneurysm or vascular erosions not controlled by radiological intervention (embolization)
Conservatively intractable internal pancreatic fistula

Table 31.5. Freedom from pain after different surgical procedures on the pancreas for chronic pancreatitis. Only reports of "total freedom from pain" are included. Further stages of postoperative improvement (e.g., partly free from pain) were not considered. Closure of literature research 12/2005

References	Surgical procedure	Median observation time (years)	*n*	Pain relief (%)
Way et al. [79]	Drainage/resection	ca. 5	37	64
Lankisch et al. [80]	Drainage/resection	$2^{1}/_{2}$	40	60
Mangold et al. [81]	Partial duodenopancreatectomy	$1^{8}/_{12}$	44	73
	Total duodenopancreatectomy	$2^{10}/_{12}$	18	91
	Partial left-sided resection	$3^{5}/_{12}$	37	60
	Subtotal left-sided resection	$2^{10}/_{12}$	17	83
Proctor et al. [82]	Pancreaticojejunostomy	$^{11}/_{12}$	22	50
Rosenberger et al. [83]	Resection	6	67	69
	Nonresective procedures	6	40	50
Lankisch et al. [84]	Pancreaticojejunostomy	$3^{1}/_{12}$	17	76
	Resection	$3^{1}/_{12}$	22	64
Prinz and Greenlee [85]	Pancreaticojejunostomy	$6^{1}/_{12}$–$7^{11}/_{12}$	91	35
Sato et al. [86]	Pancreaticojejunostomy	$6^{6}/_{12}$	38	68
	Left-sided resection	$6^{6}/_{12}$	14	79
	Whipple's operation	$6^{6}/_{12}$	9	67
Gall et al. [87]	Whipple's operation, pancreatic duct occlusion	>1	67	93
Morrow et al. [88]	Pancreatic duct drainage	4–13	46	46
	40–80% left-sided resection	4–13	21	33
	80–95% left-sided resection	4–13	8	100
	Drainage	6	46	80
	Subtotal pancreatectomy	7	21	24
Sato et al. [89]	Left-sided resection	$>^{6}/_{12}$	21	91
	Whipple's operation	$>^{6}/_{12}$	11	55
	Pancreaticojejunostomy	$>^{6}/_{12}$	43	91
Bradley [90]	Lateral pancreaticojejunostomy	$5^{9}/_{12}$	46	28
	Caudal pancreaticojejunostomy	$5^{9}/_{12}$	18	17
Cooper et al. [91]	Total pancreatectomy	$1^{6}/_{12}$	83	72
Frick et al. [92, 93]	Left-sided resection	$6^{6}/_{12}$	74	50
	Partial duodenopancreatectomy	$6^{6}/_{12}$	62	45
	Total duodenopancreatectomy	$6^{6}/_{12}$	22	55
	Drainage	$4^{7}/_{12}$	156	48
Lambert et al. [94]	Duodenum-preserving total pancreatectomy	$9^{5}/_{12}$	14	64
Rossi et al. [95]1	Whipple's operation	$^{6}/_{12}$	61	72
		2	44	61
		5	33	61
		10	18	61
		15	6	83
Mannell et al. [96]	Drainage/resection	$8^{6}/_{12}$	100	77
Stone et al. [97]	Whipple's operation	$6^{2}/_{12}$	15	53
	Total duodenopancreatectomy	$9^{1}/_{12}$	15	27
Beger et al. [98]	Duodenum-preserving pancreatic head resection	$3^{8}/_{12}$	128	77
Peiper and Köhler [99]	Resection	10	51	79
	Drainage	10	24	65

References	Surgical procedure	Median observation time (years)	n	Pain relief (%)
Beger and Büchler [100]	Duodenum-preserving pancreatic head resection	$3^{6}/_{12}$	141	77
Lankisch et al. [12]	Drainage/resection	6	70	57
Adams et al. [101]	Lateral pancreaticojejunostomy	$6^{4}/_{12}$	62	42
Frey and Amikura [102]	Local pancreatic head resection with longitudinal Pancreaticojejunostomy	$^{6}/_{12}$	50	34
Hakaim et al. [155]	Different operations – pancreatic duct drainage 56% – left-sided resection 20% – cyst drainage 24%	$5^{2}/_{12}$	50	30
Büchler et al. [103]	Duodenum-preserving pancreatic head resection	$^{6}/_{12}$	15	40
	Pylorus-preserving Whipple's operation	$^{6}/_{12}$	16	75
Fleming and Williamson [104]	Total pancreatectomy	$3^{6}/_{12}$	40	79
Izbicki et al. [105]	Duodenum-preserving pancreatic head resection			
	– Beger's procedure	$1^{6}/_{12}$	20	95
	– Frey's procedure	$1^{6}/_{12}$	22	94
Martin et al. [106]	Pylorus-preserving pancreaticoduodenectomy	$5^{3}/_{12}$	45	92
Stapleton and Williamson [107]	Proximal pancreaticoduodenectomy – pylorus-preserving (n=45) – Whipple's operation (n=7)	$4^{6}/_{12}$	52	80
Amikura et al. [156]	Pancreaticojejunostomy	$\geq^{6}/_{12}$	69	75
	Pancreaticojejunostomy plus pancreatic head resection	$\geq^{6}/_{12}$	11	90
	Left-sided resection	$\geq^{6}/_{12}$	37	80
	Whipple's operation	$\geq^{6}/_{12}$	13	65
Rumstadt et al. [108]	Whipple's operation	$8^{4}/_{12}$*	134	66
Traverso and Kozarek [109]	Whipple's operation	$3^{6}/_{12}$	47	76
	Total pancreatectomy	$3^{6}/_{12}$	10	76
Beger et al. [157]	Duodenum-preserving pancreatic head resection	$5^{8}/_{12}$*	303	88
Berney et al. [110]	Different procedures of pancreas resection	$6^{4}/_{12}$	68	62
Jimenez et al. [158]	Whipple's operation	$3^{5}/_{12}$	33	53
	Pylorus-preserving pancreatic head resection	$3^{5}/_{12}$	39	40
Sakofaras et al. [111]	Whipple's operation	$6^{7}/_{12}$	66	67
White et al. [112]	Total pancreatectomy	$^{6}/_{12}$	24	82
Nealon and Matin [159]	Pancreaticojejunostomy	$6^{9}/_{12}$	124	86
	Left-sided resection	$6^{9}/_{12}$	29	67
	Pancreatic head resection (duodenum-preserving or Pylorus-preserving pancreatic head resection)	$6^{9}/_{12}$	46	91
Sakoforas et al. [160]	Left-sided resection	$6^{8}/_{12}$	31	49
Hutchins et al. [161]	Left-sided resection	$2^{10}/_{12}$	84	48

1. The definition of freedom of pain is often vague; pain symptoms are usually not measured, for example on an analogue scale [19].
2. Not all patients received the same surgical treatment for the same indication. Several authors recommend not performing an indicated resection operation in alcoholics because of the postoperatively difficult treatment of diabetes mellitus in those patients [74, 75].
3. Although continued alcohol abuse distinctly worsens the effect of surgical treatment [76–78], it is still difficult to determine whether a postoperative deterioration results from chronic pancreatitis, from continued alcohol abuse, or from the surgical treatment.
4. Evaluation of pain differs very much with regard to the duration of the observation period. Postoperative results independent of the surgical procedure showed that freedom of pain will be obtained in up to 90% of

Table 31.6. Percentage of patients who became free of pain 6 months, 2 and 5 years after different surgical procedures because of chronic pancreatitis (113)

Follow-up	Whipple's operation	Pancreaticojejunostomy	Left-sided resection
Alcohol-induced pancreatitis			
6 months	82%	87%	60%
2 years	74%	53%	39%
5 years	71%	54%	26%
Idiopathic pancreatitis			
6 months	50%	80%	77%
2 years	50%	60%	46%
5 years	33%	60%	20%

patients over several years of follow-up (Table 31.5) [12, 79–112]. However, the persistence of freedom from pain has been differently reported. Taylor et al. [113]distinctly showed that in the course of a longer follow-up, pain increases (Table 31.6). In contrast, Martin et al. [106] showed that freedom from pain may persist over 5 years of follow-up after pylorus-preserving pancreaticoduodenectomy for chronic pancreatitis. Whether this difference is due to the different mode of operation remains to be clarified.

In a study including 207 patients with alcoholic chronic pancreatitis (91 without and 116 with surgical treatment for pain relief), Ammann et al. [10] discussed the pain pattern of chronic pancreatitis and its surgical implications. In their study, chronic pain was typically associated with local complications (mainly pseudocysts), relieved definitively by a single drainage procedure in approximately two-thirds of patients. Additional surgery was required for late pain recurrence in 39 patients, primarily symptomatic cholestasis. All patients with advanced chronic pancreatitis achieved complete pain relief. The authors conclude that in their experience, relief from chronic pain regularly follows selective surgery tailored to the presumptive pain cause, or occurs spontaneously in uncomplicated advanced chronic pancreatitis.

Exocrine Pancreatic Insufficiency

General

This overview is based on similar reviews [114–118]. Overt steatorrhea is the most important digestive feature of exocrine pancreatic insufficiency and may be associated with malabsorption of the lipid-soluble vitamins A, D, E, and K. Fat malabsorption usually develops prior to malabsorption of other nutrients [119], because protein digestion is induced by gastric proteolytic activity and intestinal brush-border peptidases, and is maintained even in the absence of pancreatic proteolytic activity [120]. Similarly, in those lacking pancreatic amylase, starch digestion reaches about 80% due to salivary amylase and brush-border oligosaccharidases [121]. Malabsorption of l ipids and proteins results in steatorrhea and creatorrhea. By contrast, fecal carbohydrate measurements do not represent the extent of starch malabsorption [122–125], because carbohydrates are metabolized by the intracolonic flora. Earlier fat (compared with protein and carbohydrate) malabsorption is caused by an interaction between several mechanisms [116]:

1. The synthesis and secretion of lipase decreases earlier and more markedly, compared with that of proteases [36, 42, 119].
2. Pancreatic bicarbonate secretion, which protects enzymes intraduodenally from denaturation by gastric acid, is diminished in exocrine pancreatic insufficiency. In consequence, intraluminal pH may decrease to below 4, which may result in lipase inactivation [36, 126].
3. Lipase is proteolyzed during small-intestinal transit more rapidly than are other enzymes [13, 41, 127, 128].
4. Extrapancreatic lipolysis (e.g., lingual and gastric lipase) contributes only marginally to cumulative fat digestion [129]

Hence, in progressive chronic pancreatitis, secretion of lipase decreases rapidly, its intraluminal survival is short, and its luminal digestive action is virtually uncompensated for by extrapancreatic enzymes. Therefore, steatorrhea is the earliest and most severe exocrine malfunction observed in chronic pancreatitis (Table 31.7) [116].

Table 31.7. Pathomechanisms explaining the pivotal role of lipase deficiency and lipase supplementation in exocrine pancreatic insufficiency due to chronic pancreatitis [117]

- Earlier and stronger impairment of lipase synthesis and secretion compared with other digestive enzymes
- Low intraduodenal pH because of impaired bicarbonate secretion and particular sensitivity of lipase to acidic destruction
- Particular susceptibility of lipase to proteolytic destruction within the intestinal lumen
- Lack of effective extrapancreatic lipolytic enzymes
- Additional inhibition of biliary secretion by malabsorbed nutrients and thereby additional impairment of lipid digestion and absorption

Treatment

General

Occasionally, endoscopic sphincterotomy or stenting of the main pancreatic duct in chronic pancreatitis may restore exocrine pancreatic function in some individuals with tumors or scars that are impairing pancreatic secretion into the duodenum. Similarly, exocrine pancreatic function in individual patients with tumors of the pancreatic head or the ampulla may benefit from a pancreaticojejunostomy. Exocrine pancreatic insufficiency may be improved in patients undergoing drainage operations [130, 131].

Although healthy humans may tolerate a more than 90% resection of the pancreas without developing steatorrhea [132], fat maldigestion usually worsens in chronic pancreatitis following far less extensive resection [133].

Enzymes for Steatorrhea

At present, the majority of patients with exocrine pancreatic insufficiency are treated with pH-sensitive pancreatin microspheres, which are taken with each meal. In order to reduce steatorrhea to less than 15 g/day of fat, a dosage of 25,000–40,000 IU of lipase per meal is required (Fig. 31.1). In many cases, these doses must be doubled because of insufficient lipolytic action.

Treatment effectiveness is checked clinically, mainly by monitoring body weight and consistency of feces. In cases of treatment failure, doses should be increased, and/or such patients should distribute their nutrient intake across five or six smaller meals [36]. If steatorrhea persists, the compliance of the patient needs to be checked by fecal chymotrypsin measurement. Low activity suggests insufficient intake of enzymes.

Whether pancreatin doses should be increased further in the compliant patient is controversial because ultrahigh doses have been associated with a dose-dependent risk of stenotic fibrosing colonopathy in patients with cystic fibrosis [134–136]. Recent evidence suggests that this risk is correlated directly with the dose of enzymes administered. There is no evidence that analogous complications may occur in chronic pancreatitis; nevertheless, we do not generally recommend dosages of more than 75,000 IU of lipase per meal. In refractory cases, pathophysiologic and therapeutic alternatives should be considered.

Addition of an acid blocker (proton pump inhibitor, H_2 blocker) may have beneficial effects when combined with an unprotected pancreatin preparation [42, 137–139]. After previous gastric and/or intestinal resection, bacterial overgrowth [140] or intestinal infections, such as infection with *Giardia lamblia* or other intestinal absorption disorders, may further compromise absorption and require specific medical or surgical intervention. Patients with accelerated gastric emptying due to gastric resection or gastroenterostomy should be treated with pancreatin granule or powder preparations. Achlorhydric patients, including those continuously receiving acid blockers, are treated successfully with conventional unprotected pancreatin preparations. In the presence of enzyme supplementation, medium-chain triglycerides do not further improve lipid absorption [141].

Pancreatic Enzyme Therapy Following Gastrointestinal Surgery

Postoperative indications for pancreatic enzyme therapy are frequently discussed in their context of surgical procedures in the gastrointestinal tract, especially after pancreatic, gastric, and small-intestinal resection [142]. It is difficult to recommend postoperative enzyme substitution because the number of studies demonstrating its usefulness after gastrointestinal procedures in general and after pancreatic surgery in particular is limited, and data on the kind of preparation that should be used are scarce (Table 31.8) [143].

Patients need enzyme replacement therapy after pancreatectomy. Enzyme replacement therapy is also necessary in most patients with partial pancreatic resection and pre-existing pancreatic disease (i.e., chronic pancreatitis). Further recommendations on pancreatic enzyme substitution following specific

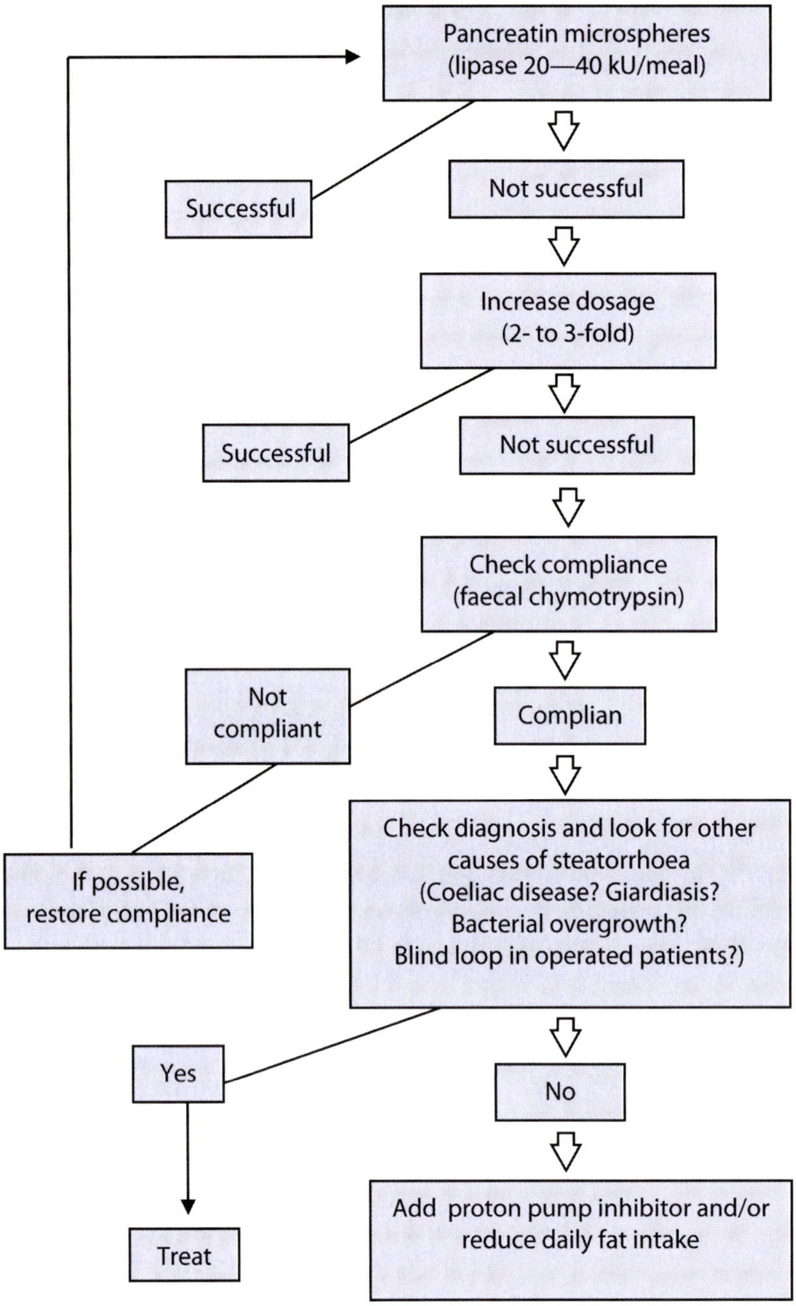

Figure 31.1

Treatment of exocrine pancreatic insufficiency. *kU* Kilounit)

pancreatic surgical procedures are given in Table 31.8.

Steatorrhea following gastrectomy has been discussed in relation to decreased exocrine pancreatic enzyme output. Gullo et al. [144] found a reduction of bicarbonate, lipase, and chymotrypsin output in a small number of patients after total gastrectomy. However, there was no correlation between decreased lipase and the degree of steatorrhea. The authors concluded that primary exocrine pancreatic insufficiency does not in itself play a major role in the pathogenesis of steatorrhea after total gastrectomy [144]. In contrast, Friess et al. [145] compared pre- and postoperative pancreatic function test results with total gastrectomy and found decreased trypsin, chymotrypsin, and amylase. Lipase was not measured. Nevertheless, the authors concluded that exocrine pancreatic insufficiency follows total gastrectomy [145]. Another hy-

Table 31.8. Recommended pancreatic enzyme substitution following pancreatic surgery

Surgical procedure	Recommendation
Right-sided resection with antrectomy	
Whipple operation	⇛ Enteric-coated enzyme microspheres (plus medication to reduce intestinal transit time)
Right-sided resection without antrectomy	
Duodenum-preserving resection of the head of the pancreas (Beger's procedure)	⇛ Enteric-coated enzyme microspheres plus proton pump inhibitor
Pylorus-preserving pancreaticoduodenectomy (Traverso and Longmire's procedure)	
Drainage operation	⇛ Enteric-coated enzyme microspheres
Distal resection	⇛ Enteric-coated enzyme microspheres
Total pancreatectomy	⇛ Enteric-coated enzyme microspheres

pothesis explaining steatorrhea after gastrectomy is the poor mixing of food and enzymes (postcibal asynchrony) or the bacterial degradation of pancreatic enzymes in the small intestine. The latter condition should be treated with antibiotics. Regardless of whether exocrine pancreatic insufficiency occurs after gastric resection or is caused by postcibal asynchrony, pancreatic enzyme substitution combined with a high-energy diet and distributed over six to eight meals per day should improve the postoperative nutrition status and nonspecific symptoms in these patients. Further studies are required [146]. There is little evidence that pancreatic enzyme substitution is beneficial in short-bowel syndrome [147].

Endocrine Pancreatic Insufficiency

General

Endocrine pancreatic insufficiency in chronic pancreatitis is a distinct form of clinical diabetes that is regarded as a secondary of type 1 diabetes [148]. Diabetes mellitus secondary to chronic pancreatitis accounts for <1% of all diabetes cases, which is probably the reason why it is not of much interest for most diabetologists. However, since about 80% of patients with chronic pancreatitis develop an overt diabetes mellitus in the long follow-up and diabetes mellitus is an independent risk factor for mortality in patients with chronic pancreatitis [8, 12, 149, 150], this form of diabetes mellitus is highly relevant to the gastroenterologist and especially to the pancreatologist.

It is generally believed that chronic pancreatitis progressively develops fibrosis and sclerosis, and thus alters pancreatic capillary circulation and thereby reduces islet perfusion. This results in an impaired function of the insulin-producing β-cells and the glucagon-producing α-cells [151]. The risk of diabetes mellitus manifestation in chronic pancreatitis is not influenced by elective surgical pancreatic procedures for the treatment of the disease, either than distal pancreatectomy [8]. This is in accordance with the heterogeneous distribution of Langerhans' islets along the pancreatic gland, prominently localized in the tail of the pancreas. Diabetes mellitus appearing after pancreaticoduodenectomy performed for chronic pancreatitis is almost always delayed for a minimum of 1 year after surgery, suggesting that disease progression prevails in the risk of diabetes mellitus as opposed to the surgery itself [151]. It is further supported by a strong correlation between the onset and the presence of pancreatic calcifications in endocrine pancreatic insufficiency [12, 150, 152].

The losses of exocrine and endocrine pancreatic function do not parallel each other. After 10 years, 22% of patients with exocrine pancreatic insufficiency due to chronic pancreatitis still had a normal glucose tolerance. More than half of the patients with severe exocrine pancreatic insufficiency requiring enzyme substitution had a normal glucose tolerance or did not need insulin therapy, even when they were diabetics. Vice versa, every second or third insulin-requiring diabetic did not need enzyme substitution for his exocrine pancreatic enzyme insufficiency [12, 153].

The diagnosis of diabetes mellitus in chronic pancreatitis is made similarly to that for other forms of diabetes, on the basis of fasting plasma glucose levels and/or 2-h glucose levels during an oral glucose tolerance test.

Table 31.9. Treatment of diabetes mellitus in chronic pancreatitis (modified according to Göke and Göke 2005 [151])

Basis of therapy Consider: Adequate nutritional status, sufficient enzyme substitution, alcohol abstinence, comorbidities and overall prognosis, age, and metabolic stability
Problem Consider: Severe hypoglycemia
Target HbA1c levels of 7–8%
Insulin requirement 0.30–0.45 IU insulin/kg body weight/day

Treatment

Several problems have to be taken into account for the treatment of diabetes in chronic pancreatitis (Table 31.9):

1. There may be a lack of appropriate compliance for an insulin treatment regimen, especially among alcoholics.
2. Pain after meals may lead to an inadequate eating and thus to an unpredictable consumption of carbohydrates.
3. There may be an accelerated intestinal transit following maldigestion if the enzyme replacement therapy is not effective. This may also have an impact on glucose metabolism.
4. A glucagon deficiency and/or blunted glucagon response may favor a reduced counterbalance in response to insulin injections, causing hypoglycemia.
5. Possibly due to a poorly controlled diabetes mellitus, neuropathic disease may lead to a disturbance of gastric emptying and intestinal transit that make dietary regimens hard to follow.
6. Insulin substitution with too high initial dosages may be too aggressive and lead to rapid severe hypoglycemia. HbA1c levels between 7% and 8% are often acceptable and are associated with the decreased risk of severe hypoglycemia;
7. All in all, therapy must be individually tailored based upon an adequate nutritional status of the patient, sufficient enzyme substitution, compensating exocrine pancreatic insufficiency and, if possible, alcohol abstinence. If there is a known incompliance, especially continuing alcohol consumption, insulin treatment is not indicated; 50% of patients with chronic pancreatitis can be treated by diet [151].
8. Oral antidiabetics are problematic: irregular oral intake and alcohol consumption may render the prescription of sulphonylureas inadvisable. Metformin is contraindicated in patients with alcohol consumption because of the risk of a lactic acidosis. Insulin sensitizers, such as glitazones are not indicated, since insulin deficiency rather than resistance is the key problem. α-Glucosidase inhibitors are not contraindicated but not advisable because the side effects, such as abdominal pain, meteorism, flatulence, and diarrhea, may worsen the symptoms of exocrine pancreatic insufficiency.
9. The patient is generally highly sensitive to insulin. To decrease the risk of hypoglycemia, blood glucose levels should be closely monitored. An intensified insulin treatment regimen with multiple injections of small amounts of short-acting insulin offers advantages, but requires compliance of the patients. In stable conditions, which are rare, a combination of normal and long-acting insulin may be used. The daily insulin requirement is low, ranging daily between 0.30 and 0.45 IU/kg body weight.
10. In highly motivated patients, insulin pump therapy may become an option. Basal infusion rates of the insulin pump amount, normally to 20–30% of the daily insulin needs, with meal-connected bolus infusions of 0.8–1.4 IU insulin/12 g carbohydrates. Insulin pumps are especially of interest for patients after total pancreatectomy [151].

References

1. DiMagno EP (1999) Toward understanding (and management) of painful chronic pancreatitis. Gastroenterology 116:1252–1257
2. Bockman DE, Buchler M, Malfertheiner P, Beger HG (1988) Analysis of nerves in chronic pancreatitis. Gastroenterology 94:1459–1469
3. Karanjia ND, Singh SM, Widdison AL, Lutrin FJ, Reber HA (1992) Pancreatic ductal and interstitial pressures in cats with chronic pancreatitis. Dig Dis Sci 37:268–273
4. Karanjia ND, Widdison AL, Leung F, Alvarez C, Lutrin FJ, Reber HA (1994) Compartment syndrome in experimental chronic obstructive pancreatitis: effect of decompressing the main pancreatic duct. Br J Surg 81:259–264
5. Ammann R (1970) Die chronische Pankreatitis. Zur Frage der Operationsindikation und Beitrag zum Spontanverlauf der chronisch-rezidivierenden Pankreatitis. Dtsch Med Wochenschr 95:1–7
6. Ammann R (1970) Die Behandlung der chronischen Pankreatitis. Dtsch Med Wochenschr 95:1234–1235
7. Ammann RW, Largiadèr F, Akovbiantz A (1979) Pain relief by surgery in chronic pancreatitis? Relationship between pain relief, pancreatic dysfunction, and alcohol withdrawal. Scand J Gastroenterol 14:209–215
8. Ammann RW, Akovbiantz A, Largiadèr F, Schueler G (1984) Course and outcome of chronic pancreatitis. Longitudinal study of a mixed medical-surgical series of 245 patients. Gastroenterology 86:820–828
9. Ammann R (1989) Klinik, Spontanverlauf und Therapie der chronischen Pankreatitis. Unter spezieller Berücksichtigung der Nomenklaturprobleme. Schweiz Med Wochenschr 119:696–706
10. Ammann RW, Muellhaupt B, Zurich Pancreatitis Study Group (1999) The natural history of pain in alcoholic chronic pancreatitis. Gastroenterology 116:1132–1140
11. Miyake H, Harada H, Kunichika K, Ochi K, Kimura I (1987) Clinical course and prognosis of chronic pancreatitis. Pancreas 2:378–385
12. Lankisch PG, Löhr-Happe A, Otto J, Creutzfeldt W (1993) Natural course in chronic pancreatitis. Pain, exocrine and endocrine pancreatic insufficiency and prognosis of the disease. Digestion 54:148–155
13. Layer P, Yamamoto H, Kalthoff L, Clain JE, Bakken LJ, DiMagno EP (1994) The different courses of early- and late-onset idiopathic and alcoholic chronic pancreatitis. Gastroenterology 107:1481–1487
14. Lankisch PG, Seidensticker F, Löhr-Happe A, Otto J, Creutzfeldt W (1995) The course of pain is the same in alcohol- and nonalcohol-induced chronic pancreatitis. Pancreas 10:338–341
15. Lankisch PG, Seidensticker F, Löhr-Happe A, Creutzfeldt W (1996) The course of pain is the same in alcoholics, alcohol consumers, and teetotalers (abstr). Pancreas 13:446
16. Müllhaupt B, Truninger K, Ammann R (2005) Impact of etiology on the painful early stages of chronic pancreatitis: a long-term prospective study. Z Gastroenterol 43:1293–1301
17. Girdwood AH, Marks IN, Bornman PC, Kottler RE, Cohen M (1981) Does progressive pancreatic insufficiency limit pain in calcific pancreatitis with duct stricture or continued alcohol insult? J Clin Gastroenterol 3:241–245
18. Thorsgaard Pedersen N, Andersen BN, Pedersen G, Worning H (1982) Chronic pancreatitis in Copenhagen. A retrospective study of 64 consecutive patients. Scand J Gastroenterol 17:925–931
19. Lankisch PG, Andrén-Sandberg Å (1993) Standards for the diagnosis of chronic pancreatitis and for the evaluation of treatment. Int J Pancreatol 14:205–212
20. Ammann RW, Muench R, Otto R, Buehler H, Freiburghaus AU, Siegenthaler W (1988) Evolution and regression of pancreatic calcification in chronic pancreatitis. A prospective long-term study of 107 patients. Gastroenterology 95:1018–1028
21. Malfertheiner P, Büchler M, Stanescu A, Ditschuneit H (1987) Pancreatic morphology and function in relationship to pain in chronic pancreatitis. Int J Pancreatol 2:59–66
22. Ebbehøj N, Borly L, Bülow J, Rasmussen SG, Madsen P (1990) Evaluation of pancreatic tissue fluid pressure and pain in chronic pancreatitis. A longitudinal study. Scand J Gastroenterol 25:462–466
23. Ebbehøj N, Borly L, Madsen P, Matzen P (1990) Comparison of regional pancreatic tissue fluid pressure and endoscopic retrograde pancreatographic morphology in chronic pancreatitis. Scand J Gastroenterol 25:756–760
24. Jensen AR, Matzen P, Malchow-Møller A, Christoffersen I, The Copenhagen Pancreatitis Study Group (1984) Pattern of pain, duct morphology, and pancreatic function in chronic pancreatitis. A comparative study. Scand J Gastroenterol 19:334–338
25. Warshaw AL, Popp JW Jr, Schapiro RH (1980) Long-term patency, pancreatic function, and pain relief after lateral pancreaticojejunostomy for chronic pancreatitis. Gastroenterology 79:289–293
26. Axon ATR, Classen M, Cotton PB, Cremer M, Freeny PC, Lees WR (1984) Pancreatography in chronic pancreatitis: international definitions. Gut 25:1107–1112
27. Imoto M, DiMagno EP (2000) Cigarette smoking increases the risk of pancreatic calcification in late-onset but not early-onset idiopathic chronic pancreatitis. Pancreas 21:115–119
28. Sarles H, Sahel J (1976) Die chronische Pankreatitis. In: Forell M (ed) Handbuch der Inneren Medizin, vol. 3/6, Pankreas, 5. Springer, Berlin-Heidelberg-New York, pp 737–844
29. Trapnell JE (1979) Chronic relapsing pancreatitis: a review of 64 cases. Br J Surg 66:471–475
30. American Gastroenterological Association (AGA) (1998) American Gastroenterological Association Technical Review. Treatment of pain in chronic pancreatitis. Gastroenterology 115:765–776
31. American Gastroenterological Association (AGA) (1998) American Gastroenterological Association Medical Position Statement Treatment of pain in chronic pancreatitis. Gastroenterology 115:763–764
32. World Health Organization (1996) Cancer pain relief. Geneva
33. Ihse I, Lilja P, Lundquist I (1977) Feedback regulation of pancreatic enzyme secretion by intestinal trypsin in man. Digestion 15:303–308
34. Krawisz BR, Miller LJ, DiMagno EP, Go VLW (1980) In the absence of nutrients, pancreatic-biliary secretions in the jejunum do not exert feedback control of human pancreatic or gastric function. J Lab Clin Med 95:13–18
35. Hotz J, Ho SB, Go VLW, DiMagno EP (1983) Short-term inhibition of duodenal tryptic activity does not affect human pancreatic, biliary, or gastric function. J Lab Clin Med 101:488–495
36. Read NW, McFarlane A, Kinsman RI, et al (1984) Effect of infusion of nutrient solutions into the ileum on gastrointestinal transit and plasma levels of neurotensin and enteroglucagon. Gastroenterology 86:274–280

37. Slaff J, Jacobson D, Tillman CR, Curington C, Toskes P (1984) Protease-specific suppression of pancreatic exocrine secretion. Gastroenterology 87:44–52
38. Owyang C, Louie DS, Tatum D (1986) Feedback regulation of pancreatic enzyme secretion. Suppression of cholecystokinin release by trypsin. J Clin Invest 77:2042–2047
39. Owyang C, May D, Louie DS (1986) Trypsin suppression of pancreatic enzyme secretion. Differential effect on cholecystokinin release and the enteropancreatic reflex. Gastroenterology 91:637–643
40. Adler G, Reinshagen M, Koop I, et al (1989) Differential effects of atropine and a cholecystokinin receptor antagonist on pancreatic secretion. Gastroenterology 96:1158–1164
41. Layer P, Jansen JBMJ, Cherian L, Lamers CBHW, Goebell H (1990) Feedback regulation of human pancreatic secretion. Effects of protease inhibition on duodenal delivery and small intestinal transit of pancreatic enzymes. Gastroenterology 98:1311–1319
42. DiMagno EP, Layer P, Clain JE (1993) Chronic pancreatitis. In: Go VLW, DiMagno EP, Gardner JD, Lebenthal E, Reber HA, Scheele GA (eds) The Pancreas: Biology, Pathobiology, and Disease, 2nd edn. Raven Press, New York, pp 665–706
43. Isaksson G, Ihse I (1983) Pain reduction by an oral pancreatic enzyme preparation in chronic pancreatitis. Dig Dis Sci 28:97–102
44. Halgreen H, Thorsgaard Pedersen N, Worning H (1986) Symptomatic effect of pancreatic enzyme therapy in patients with chronic pancreatitis. Scand J Gastroenterol 21:104–108
45. Mössner J, Stange JH, Ewald M, Kestel W, Fischbach W (1991) Influence of exogenous application of pancreatic extracts on endogenous pancreatic enzyme secretion. Pancreas 6:637–644
46. Mössner J, Secknus R, Meyer J, Niederau C, Adler G (1992) Treatment of pain with pancreatic extracts in chronic pancreatitis: results of a prospective placebo-controlled multicenter trial. Digestion 53:54–66
47. Malfertheiner P, Mayer D, Büchler M, Domínguez-Muñoz JE, Schiefer B, Ditschuneit H (1995) Treatment of pain in chronic pancreatitis by inhibition of pancreatic secretion with octreotide. Gut 36:450–454
48. Layer P, Peschel S, Schlesinger T, Goebell H (1990) Human pancreatic secretion and intestinal motility: effects of ileal nutrient perfusion. Am J Physiol 258:G196–G201
49. Layer P, Schlesinger T, Gröger G, Goebell H (1993) Modulation of human periodic interdigestive gastrointestinal motor and pancreatic function by the ileum. Pancreas 8:426–432
50. Keller J, Rünzi M, Goebell H, Layer P (1997) Duodenal and ileal nutrient deliveries regulate human intestinal motor and pancreatic responses to a meal. Am J Physiol 272:G632–G637
51. DiMagno EP, Layer P (1993) Human exocrine pancreatic enzyme secretion. In: Go VLW, DiMagno EP, Gardner JD, Lebenthal E, Reber HA, Scheele GA (eds) The Pancreas: Biology, Pathobiology, and Disease, 2nd edn. Raven Press, New York, pp 275–300
52. Layer P, Chan ATH, Go VLW, DiMagno EP (1988) Human pancreatic secretion during phase II antral motility of the interdigestive cycle. Am J Physiol 254:G249–G253
53. Layer P, von der Ohe MR, Holst JJ, et al (1997) Altered postprandial motility in chronic pancreatitis: role of malabsorption. Gastroenterology 112:1624–1634
54. Kozarek RA, Ball TJ, Patterson DJ (1992) Endoscopic approach to pancreatic duct calculi and obstructive pancreatitis. Am J Gastroenterol 87:600–603
55. Lankisch PG, Layer P (2000) Chronische Pankreatitis. Update: Diagnostik und Therapie 2000. Dtsch Ärztebl 97: a2169–2177
56. Laugier R, Grandval P (2002) Interventional treatment of chronic pancreatitis. Eur J Gastroenterol Hepatol 14:951–955
57. Hammarström L-E (2004) Endoscopic management of chronic and non-biliary recurrent pancreatitis. Scand J Gastroenterol 39:5–13
58. Inui K, Tazuma S, Yamaguchi T, et al (2005) Treatment of pancreatic stones with extracorporeal shock wave lithotripsy. Results of a multicenter survey. Pancreas 30:26–30
59. Tadenuma H, Ishihara T, Yamaguchi T, et al (2005) Long-term results of extracorporeal shockwave lithotripsy and endoscopic therapy for pancreatic stones. Clin Gastroenterol Hepatol 3:1128–1135
60. Carroccio A, Di Prima L, Di Grigoli C, et al (1999) Exocrine pancreatic function and fat malabsorption in human immunodeficiency virus-infected patients. Scand J Gastroenterol 34:729–734
61. Kozarek RA (1990) Pancreatic stents can induce ductal changes consistent with chronic pancreatitis. Gastrointest Endosc 36:93–95
62. Chaudhary A, Negi SS, Masood S, Thombare M (2004) Complications after Frey's procedure for chronic pancreatitis. Am J Surg 188:277–281
63. Schwarz M, Isenmann R, Beger HG (2000) Stenting bei chronischer Pankreatitis – Fehler und Limitationen. Z Gastroenterol 38:367–374
64. Eleftheriadis N, Dinu F, Delhaye M, et al (2005) Long-term outcome after pancreatic stenting in severe chronic pancreatitis. Endoscopy 37:223–230
65. Kahl S, Zimmermann S, Genz I, et al (2003) Risk factors for failure of endoscopic stenting of biliary strictures in chronic pancreatitis: a prospective follow-up study. Am J Gastroenterol 98:2448–2453
66. Díte P, Ruzicka M, Zboril V, Novotný I (2003) A prospective, randomized trial comparing endoscopic and surgical therapy for chronic pancreatitis. Endoscopy 35:553–558
67. Cohen S, Bacon BR, Berlin JA, et al (2002) National Institutes of Health State-of-the-Science Conference Statement: ERCP for diagnosis and therapy, January 14-16, Gastrointest Endosc 56:803–809
68. Bell SN, Cole R, Roberts-Thomson IC (1980) Coeliac plexus block for control of pain in chronic pancreatitis. Br Med J 281:1604
69. Gress F, Schmitt C, Sherman S, Ikenberry S, Lehman G (1999) A prospective randomized comparison of endoscopic ultrasound- and computed tomography-guided celiac plexus block for managing chronic pancreatitis pain. Am J Gastroenterol 94:900–905
70. Buscher HCJL, Jansen JBMJ, van Dongen R, Bleichrodt RP, van Goor H (2002) Long-term results of bilateral thoracoscopic splanchnicectomy in patients with chronic pancreatitis. Br J Surg 89:158–162
71. Maher JW, Johlin FC, Heitshusen D (2001) Long-term follow-up of thoracoscopic splanchnicectomy for chronic pancreatitis pain. Surg Endosc 15:706–709

72. Ballegaard S, Christophersen SJ, Dawids SG, Hesse J, Olsen NV (1985) Acupuncture and transcutaneous electric nerve stimulation in the treatment of pain associated with chronic pancreatitis. A randomized study. Scand J Gastroenterol 20:1249–1254
73. Knoefel WT, Eisenberger CF, Strate T, Izbicki JR (2002) Optimizing surgical therapy for chronic pancreatitis. Pancreatology 2:379–385
74. White TT, Keith RG (1973) Long term follow-up study of fifty patients with pancreaticojejunostomy. Surg Gynecol Obstet 136:353–358
75. Frey CF, Child III CG, Fry W (1976) Pancreatectomy for chronic pancreatitis. Ann Surg 184:403–414
76. Leger L, Lenriot JP, Lemaigre G (1974) Five to twenty year followup after surgery for chronic pancreatitis in 148 patients. Ann Surg 180:185–191
77. Holmberg JT, Isaksson G, Ihse I (1985) Long term results of pancreticojejunostomy in chronic pancreatitis. Surg Gynecol Obstet 160:339–346
78. Capitaine Y, Roche B, Wiesner L, Hahnloser P (1988) Pancréatite chronique: histoire naturelle et évolution en relation avec l'alcoolisme. Schweiz Med Wochenschr 118:817–820
79. Way LW, Gadacz T, Goldman L (1974) Surgical treatment of chronic pancreatitis. Am J Surg 127:202–209
80. Lankisch PG, Fuchs K, Schmidt H, Peiper H-J, Creutzfeldt W (1975) Ergebnisse der operativen Behandlung der chronischen Pankreatitis mit besonderer Berücksichtigung der exokrinen und endokrinen Funktion. Dtsch Med Wochenschr 100:1048–1060
81. Mangold G, Neher M, Oswald B, Wagner G (1977) Ergebnisse der Resektionsbehandlung der chronischen Pankreatitis. Dtsch Med Wochenschr 102:229–234
82. Proctor HJ, Mendes OC, Thomas CG Jr, Herbst CA (1979) Surgery for chronic pancreatitis. Drainage versus resection. Ann Surg; 189:664–671
83. Rosenberger J, Stock W, Altmann P, Pichlmaier H (1980) Spätergebnisse nach organerhaltenden und resezierenden Eingriffen wegen chronischer Pankreatitis. Leber Magen Darm 10:22–27
84. Lankisch PG, Fuchs K, Peiper H-J, Creutzfeldt W (1981) Pancreatic function after drainage or resection for chronic pancreatitis. In: Mitchell CJ, Kelleher J (eds) Pancreatic disease in clinical practice. Pitman Books, London, pp 362–369
85. Prinz RA, Greenlee HB (1981) Pancreatic duct drainage in 100 patients with chronic pancreatitis. Ann Surg 194:313–320
86. Sato T, Noto N, Matsuno S, Miyakawa K (1981) Follow-up results of surgical treatment for chronic pancreatitis. Present status in Japan. Am J Surg 142:317–323
87. Gall FP, Gebhardt C, Zirngibl H (1982) Chronic pancreatitis – results in 116 consecutive, partial duodenopancreatectomies combined with pancreatic duct occlusion. Hepatogastroenterology 29:115–119
88. Morrow CE, Cohen JI, Sutherland DER, Najarian JS (1984) Chronic pancreatitis: long-term surgical results of pancreatic duct drainage, pancreatic resection, and near-total pancreatectomy and islet autotransplantation. Surgery 96:608–616
89. Sato T, Miyashita E, Matsuno S, Yamauchi H (1986) The role of surgical treatment for chronic pancreatitis. Ann Surg 203:266–271
90. Bradley III EL (1987) Long-term results of pancreatojejunostomy in patients with chronic pancreatitis. Am J Surg 153:207–213
91. Cooper MJ, Williamson RCN, Benjamin IS, et al (1987) Total pancreatectomy for chronic pancreatitis. Br J Surg 74:912–915
92. Frick S, Jung K, Rückert K (1987) Chirurgie der chronischen Pankreatitis. I. Spätergebnisse nach Resektionsbehandlung. Dtsch Med Wochenschr 112:629–635
93. Frick S, Ebert M, Rückert K (1987) Chirurgie der chronischen Pankreatitis. II. Spätergebnisse nach nicht resezierenden Operationen. Dtsch Med Wochenschr 112:832–837
94. Lambert MA, Linehan IP, Russell RCG (1987) Duodenum-preserving total pancreatectomy for end stage chronic pancreatitis. Br J Surg 74:35–39
95. Rossi RL, Rothschild J, Braasch JW, Munson JL, ReMine SG (1987) Pancreatoduodenectomy in the management of chronic pancreatitis. Arch Surg 122:416–420
96. Mannell A, Adson MA, McIlrath DC, Ilstrup DM (1988) Surgical management of chronic pancreatitis: long-term results in 141 patients. Br J Surg 75:467–472
97. Stone WM, Sarr MG, Nagorney DM, Mellrath DC (1988) Chronic pancreatitis. Results of Whipple's resection and total pancreatectomy. Arch Surg 123:815–819
98. Beger HG, Büchler M, Bittner RR, Oettinger W, Roscher R (1989) Duodenum-preserving resection of the head of the pancreas in severe chronic pancreatitis. Early and late results. Ann Surg 209:273–278
99. Peiper H-J, Köhler H (1989) Chirurgische Therapie der chronischen Pankreatitis. Schweiz Med Wochenschr 119:712–716
100. Beger HG, Büchler M (1990) Duodenum-preserving resection of the head of the pancreas in chronic pancreatitis with inflammatory mass in the head. World J Surg 1990; 14:83–87
101. Adams DB, Ford MC, Anderson MC (1994) Outcome after lateral pancreaticojejunostomy for chronic pancreatitis. Ann Surg 219:481–489
102. Frey CF, Amikura K (1994) Local resection of the head of the pancreas combined with longitudinal pancreaticojejunostomy in the management of patients with chronic pancreatitis. Ann Surg 220:492–507
103. Büchler MW, Friess H, Müller MW, Wheatley AM, Beger HG (1995) Randomized trial of duodenum-preserving pancreatic head resection versus pylorus-preserving Whipple in chronic pancreatitis. Am J Surg 169:65–70
104. Fleming WR, Williamson RCN (1995) Role of total pancreatectomy in the treatment of patients with end-stage chronic pancreatitis. Br J Surg 82:1409–1412
105. Izbicki JR, Bloechle C, Knoefel WT, Kuechler T, Binmoeller KF, Broelsch CE (1995) Duodenum-preserving resection of the head of the pancreas in chronic pancreatitis. A prospective, randomized trial. Ann Surg 221:350–358
106. Martin RF, Rossi RL, Leslie KA (1996) Long-term results of pylorus-preserving pancreatoduodenectomy for chronic pancreatitis. Arch Surg 131:247–252
107. Stapleton GN, Williamson RCN (1996) Proximal pancreatoduodenectomy for chronic pancreatitis. Br J Surg 83:1433–1440
108. Rumstadt B, Forssmann K, Singer MV, Trede M (1997) The Whipple partial duodenopancreatectomy for the treatment of chronic pancreatitis. Hepatogastroenterology 44:1554–1559
109. Traverso LW, Kozarek RA (1997) Pancreatoduodenectomy for chronic pancreatitis. Anatomic selection criteria and subsequent long-term outcome analysis. Ann Surg 226:429–438

110. Berney T, Rüdisühli T, Oberholzer J, Caulfield A, Morel P (2000) Long-term metabolic results after pancreatic resection for severe chronic pancreatitis. Arch Surg 135:1106–1111
111. Sakorafas GH, Farnell MB, Nagorney DM, Sarr MG, Rowland CM (2000) Pancreatoduodenectomy for chronic pancreatitis. Long-term results in 105 patients. Arch Surg 135:517–524
112. White SA, Sutton CD, Weymss-Holden S, et al (2000) The feasibility of spleen-preserving pancreatectomy for end-stage chronic pancreatitis. Am J Surg 179:294–297
113. Taylor RH, Bagley FH, Braasch JW, Warren KW (1981) Ductal drainage or resection for chronic pancreatitis. Am J Surg 141:28–33
114. Lankisch PG, Banks PA (1998) Chronic pancreatitis: treatment. In: Lankisch PG, Banks PA (eds) Pancreatitis. Springer, Berlin-Heidelberg-New York, pp 303–336
115. Lankisch PG (2001) Natural course of chronic pancreatitis. Pancreatology 1:3–14
116. Layer P, Keller J, Lankisch PG (2001) Pancreatic enzyme replacement therapy. Curr Gastroenterol Reports 3:101–108
117. Keller J, Layer P (2003) Pancreatic enzyme supplementation therapy. Curr Treatment Options Gastroenterol 6:369–374
118. Mahlke R, Lübbers H, Lankisch PG (2005) Diagnostik und Therapie der chronischen Pankreatitis. Internist 46:145–156
119. DiMagno EP, Malagelada JR, Go VLW (1975) Relationship between alcoholism and pancreatic insufficiency. Ann N Y Acad Sci 252:200–207
120. Layer P, Baumann J, Hellmann C, Ohe M, Gröger G, Goebell H (1990) Effect of luminal protease-inhibition on prandial nutrient digestion during small intestinal chyme transit (abstr). Pancreas 5:718
121. Layer P, Zinsmeister AR, DiMagno EP (1986) Effects of decreasing intraluminal amylase activity on starch digestion and postprandial gastrointestinal function in humans. Gastroenterology 91:41–48
122. Bond JH, Levitt MD (1976) Fate of soluble carbohydrate in the colon of rats and man. J Clin Invest 57:1158–1164
123. Bond JH, Currier BE, Buchwald H, Levitt MD (1980) Colonic conservation of malabsorbed carbohydrate. Gastroenterology 78:444–447
124. Stephen AM, Haddad AC, Phillips SF (1983) Passage of carbohydrate into the colon. Direct measurements in humans. Gastroenterology 85:589–595
125. Flourie B, Florent C, Jouany J-P, Thivend P, Etanchaud F, Rambaud J-C (1986) Colonic metabolism of wheat starch in healthy humans. Effects on fecal outputs and clinical symptoms. Gastroenterology 1986; 90:111–119
126. DiMagno EP, Malagelada JR, Go VLW, Moertel CG (1977). Fate of orally ingested enzymes in pancreatic insufficiency. Comparison of two dosage schedules. N Engl J Med 296:1318–1322
127. Layer P, Go VLW, DiMagno EP (1986) Fate of pancreatic enzymes during small intestinal aboral transit in humans. Am J Physiol 251:G475–G480
128. Holtmann G, Kelly DG, Sternby B, DiMagno EP (1997) Survival of human pancreatic enzymes during small bowel transit: effect of nutrients, bile acids, and enzymes. Am J Physiol 273:G553–G558
129. Sternby B, Holtman G, Kelly DG, DiMagno EP (1992) Effect of gastric or duodenal nutrient infusion on gastric and pancreatic lipase secretion (abstr) Gastroenterology 102:a292
130. Nealon WH, Townsend CM Jr, Thompson JC (1988) Operative drainage of the pancreatic duct delays functional impairment in patients with chronic pancreatitis. A prospective analysis. Ann Surg 208:321–329
131. Nealon WH, Thompson JC (!993) Progressive loss of pancreatic function in chronic pancreatitis is delayed by main pancreatic duct decompression. A longitudinal prospective analysis of the modified Puestow procedure. Ann Surg 217:458–468
132. Dunger DB, Burns C, Ghale GK, et al (1988) Pancreatic exocrine and endocrine function after subtotal pancreatectomy for nesidioblastosis. J Pediatr Surg 23:112–115
133. Kodama M, Tanaka T (1984) Residual function of exocrine pancreas after operation for chronic pancreatitis by N-benzoyl-L-tyrosyl-p-aminobenzoic acid test (NBT–PABA test). Digestion 30:41–46
134. FitzSimmons SC, Burkhart GA, Borowitz D, et al (1997) High-dose pancreatic-enzyme supplements and fibrosing colonopathy in children with cystic fibrosis. N Engl J Med 336:1283–1289
135. Mac Sweeney EJ, Oades PJ, Buchdahl R, Rosenthal M, Bush A (1995) Relation of thickening of colon wall to pancreatic-enzyme treatment in cystic fibrosis. Lancet 345:752–756
136. Bansi DS, Price A, Russell C, Sarner M (2000) Fibrosing colonopathy in an adult owing to over use of pancreatic enzyme supplements. Gut 46:283–285
137. Regan PT, Malagelada J-R, DiMagno EP, Glanzman SL, Go VLW (1977) Comparative effects of antacids, cimetidine and enteric coating on the therapeutic response to oral enzymes in severe pancreatic insufficiency. N Engl J Med 297:854–858
138. Carroccio A, Pardo F, Montalto G, et al (1992) Use of famotidine in severe exocrine pancreatic insufficiency with persistent maldigestion on enzymatic replacement therapy. A long-term study in cystic fibrosis. Dig Dis Sci 37:1441–1446
139. Heijerman HG, Lamers CB, Bakker W (1991) Omeprazole enhances the efficacy of pancreatin (pancrease) in cystic fibrosis. Ann Intern Med 114:200–201
140. Casellas F, Guarner L, Vaquero E, Antolín M, de Gracia X, Malagelada J-R (1998) Hydrogen breath test with glucose in exocrine pancreatic insufficiency. Pancreas 16:481–486
141. Caliari S, Benini L, Sembenini C, Gregori B, Carnielli V, Vantini I (1996) Medium-chain triglyceride absorption in patients with pancreatic insufficiency. Scand J Gastroenterol 31:90–94
142. Lankisch PG (2001) Pancreatic enzyme therapy following surgical procedures in the gastrointestinal tract. Pancreatology 1:1–72
143. Lankisch PG (2001) Appropriate pancreatic function tests and indication for pancreatic enzyme therapy following surgical procedures on the pancreas. Pancreatology 1:14–26
144. Gullo L, Costa PL, Ventrucci M, Mattioli S, Viti G, Labò G (1979) Exocrine pancreatic function after total gastrectomy. Scand J Gastroenterol 14:401–407
145. Friess H, Böhm J, Müller MW, et al (1996) Maldigestion after total gastrectomy is associated with pancreatic insufficiency. Am J Gastroenterol 91:341–347
146. Friess H, Tempia-Caliera AA, Cammerer G, Büchler MW (2001) Indication for pancreatic enzyme substitution following gastric resection. Pancreatology 1:41–48
147. Layer P, Melle U (2001) Indication for pancreatic enzyme substitution following small intestinal resection (short bowel syndrome) Pancreatology 1:49–54

148. The Expert Committee on the Diagnosis and Classification of Diabetes Mellitus (2000) Report of the Expert Committee on the Diagnosis and Classification of Diabetes Mellitus. Diabetes Care 23:S4–S19
149. Levy P, Milan C, Pignon JP, Baetz A, Bernades P (1989) Mortality factors associated with chronic pancreatitis. Gastroenterology 96:1165–1172
150. Malka D, Hammel P, Sauvanet A, et al (2000) Risk factors for diabetes mellitus in chronic pancreatitis. Gastroenterology 119:1324–1332
151. Göke FJM, Göke B (2005) Optimal control of diabetes mellitus in pancreatitis. In: Ammann RW, Adler G, Büchler MW, DiMagno EP, Sarner M (eds) Pancreatitis: Advances in Pathobiology, Diagnosis and Treatment. Springer, Dordrecht, The Netherlands, pp 226–231
152. Löhr A (1990) Der natürliche Verlauf der chronischen Pankreatitis. Die Entwicklung der Leitsymptome Schmerzen, exokrine und endokrine Pankreasinsuffizienz und die Prognose der Erkrankung. Med. Dissertation. Medizinische Fakultät, Georg August Universität, Göttingen
153. Linde J, Nilsson LH, Bárány FR (1977) Diabetes and hypoglycemia in chronic pancreatitis. Scand J Gastroenterol 12:369–373
154. Adamek HE, Jakobs R, Buttmann A, Adamek MU, Schneider ARJ, Riemann JF (1999) Long term follow up of patients with chronic pancreatitis and pancreatic stones treated with extracorporeal shock wave lithotripsy. Gut 45:402–405
155. Hakaim AG, Broughan TA, Vogt DP, Hermann RE (1994) Long-term results of the surgical management of chronic pancreatitis. Am Surg 60:306–308
156. Amikura K, Arai K, Kobari M, Matsuno S (1997) Surgery for chronic pancreatitis – extended pancreaticojejunostomy. Hepatogastroenterology 44:1547–1553
157. Beger HG, Schlosser W, Friess HM, Büchler MW (1999) Duodenum-preserving head resection in chronic pancreatitis changes the natural course of the disease. A single-center 26-year experience. Ann Surg 230:512–523
158. Jimenez RE, Fernandez-del Castillo C, Rattner DW, Chang Y, Warshaw AL (2000) Outcome of pancreaticoduodenectomy with pylorus preservation or with antrectomy in the treatment of chronic pancreatitis. Ann Surg 231:293–300
159. Nealon WH, Matin S (2001) Analysis of surgical success in preventing recurrent acute exacerbations in chronic pancreatitis. Ann Surg 233:793–800
160. Sakorafas GH, Sarr MG, Rowland CM, Farnell MB (2001) Postobstructive chronic pancreatitis. Results with distal resection. Arch Surg 136:643–648
161. Hutchins RR, Hart RS, Pacifico M, Bradley NJ, Williamson RCN (2002) Long-term results of distal pancreatectomy for chronic pancreatitis in 90 patients. Ann Surg 236:612–618

Chapter 32

H. Ramesh

Tropical Chronic Pancreatitis

The terms "chronic calcifying pancreatitis of the tropics," "tropical pancreatitis," "tropical calcific pancreatitis," and "tropical chronic pancreatitis" (TCP) have been used to describe a disease that is characterized by abdominal pain, diabetes, and pancreatic calculi, which affects young nonalcoholic individuals in the tropics and subtropics. The first reports of this condition date back to the 1930s when Kini in Vishakapatnam, Southern India operated on a 39-year-old male patient with pancreatic calculi [1]. The pancreas was hard and nodular and the duct was dilated. External drainage was performed, but the patient died on the 3rd day following surgery. In 1955, Zuidema described 18 cases of disseminated pancreatic calcification in young nonalcoholic individuals in Indonesia [2]. In 1959, Mahadevan presented his experience with 17 cases of "pancreatic lithiasis" treated by surgery in the town of Munnar, in the western peninsular mountain ranges of India. External drainage of the pancreatic duct was performed in several patients, followed by washouts of calcareous material and stones for over 3 months. Pain relief lasting up to 14 years was obtained [3]!

In the 1960s and 1970s, there were reports of a similar syndrome from other countries in Asia (Bangladesh, Sri Lanka, Thailand, and Malaysia), Africa (Nigeria, Uganda, Burundi, Zaire, and Malawi), and South America (Brazil) [4–16]. Geevarghese et al. reported the single largest series of patients from the southwestern Indian state of Kerala, where this disease was found in endemic proportions [7]. The disease was relatively less common in the northern and western parts of India [15, 16]. TCP resembles chronic pancreatitis occurring due to alcohol abuse seen commonly in the western hemisphere except that patients were young and they did not consume alcohol. From the initial reports of "pain in childhood, diabetes in adolescence, and death in the prime of life," there have been many changes in the demographics with improved treatment of diabetes mellitus and its complications [17]. In this chapter, the epidemiology, etiology, distinctive clinical features, diagnosis, and management of TCP are described, and its features are compared with those of chronic pancreatitis secondary to alcohol abuse (Table 32.1).

Table 32.1. Comparison between alcoholic and tropical pancreatitis [83]. *TCP* Total chronic pancreatitis, *NS* not significant, *M:F* male to female ratio

Parameter	TCP	Alcoholic pancreatitis	P Value
Median age – benign	39 years	36.9 years	NS
Median age – malignant	46 years	-	
Sex M:F	1.7:1	All males	<0.001
Diabetes	56%	19%	<0.01
Jaundice	9%	1%	<0.01
Steatorrhea	36%	16%	<0.01
Biliary dilatation	18%	19%	NS
Calculi	96%	74%	<0.01
Dilated main pancreatic duct	94%	65%	<0.01
Mean diameter mm	8.5	5.2	<0.05
Cysts	12%	33%	<0.05
Malignancy	17%	Nil	<0.001
Pain relief with treatment	88%	89%	NS

Prevalence

Two population-based surveys were performed in Kerala during the past decade. In 1994, Balaji reported a prevalence of 1 in 793 among 28,567 individuals screened using clinical examination, abdominal x-ray, bentiromide test, and abdominal ultrasound [18]. Augustine and Ahuja screened 4000 persons in a geographic area using clinical examination and abdominal x-ray, and found 8 cases (1 in 500; unpublished data). Hospital data has revealed that 12–16% of diabetics presenting to two large teaching hospitals in Kerala had pancreatic calculi. A large diabetes center in Chennai on the southeastern coast of India has reported that 4% of all diabetics presenting before the age of 30 years had pancreatic calculi [19].

Etiology

Malnutrition

It is well known that malnutrition exerts a profound effect on pancreatic function. In addition, malnutrition can render the gland more susceptible to the effects of toxins. Most early reports of TCP came from developing countries and the lower socioeconomic stratum of society, and therefore malnutrition was regarded as a likely factor in etiology [20]. However, it is clear that the pancreatic changes due to protein malnutrition are reversible by protein supplementation. Although most patients may develop severe functional changes, only a minority develops diffuse fibrosis or atrophy, and virtually none develop pancreatic calculi. It is also not clear why the disease is most widely prevalent in the state of Kerala in India as compared to other states or countries where protein malnutrition is endemic [21]. In fact Kerala enjoys a 100% literacy rate, a low infant mortality rate, and high overall primary healthcare standards. Malnutrition may well be the result of long-standing pancreatic insufficiency and not its cause. This theory is supported by the observation of similar nutritional status in patients with fibrocalculous pancreatic diabetes and in other forms of insulin-dependent diabetes [22, 23]. The extreme emaciation seen in the early reports of the disease is no longer seen; this may reflect the fact that patients are now being diagnosed earlier in the course of the disease. There is some evidence that low fat intake may predispose to pancreatic calcification. It is well known that the diet in Kerala is extremely low in fat content [24]. A diet survey conducted among patients with tropical pancreatitis at our center revealed an average fat intake of 40.8±12.1 g/day, protein 52.8±9.7 g/day, and carbohydrates 279±7.7 g/day. This was not however different from controls (fat 34.5±11 g/day, protein 47.8±11.3 g/day, and carbohydrate 284±65 g/day) [25].

Food Toxins

The cyanogenic glycosides linnamarin and methyl linnamarin present in cassava, the tuber *Manihot esculenta*, have been thought to cause degenerative neurological disease, chronic pancreatitis, and endemic goiter [26]. When these glycosides react with gastric hydrochloric acid, hydrocyanic acid is liberated and this is highly toxic to cells. The enzyme rhodanese acts on hydrocyanic acid converting it into thiocyanates. This requires sulfur donors like methionine or cystine; the resultant depletion of methionine can cause pancreatic damage. Geevarghese et al. were the first to implicate cassava in the etiology of TCP [7]. Nwokolo and Oli attributed the high incidence of pancreatitis in the south of Nigeria compared to the north to higher consumption of cassava in the south [13]. Considerable evidence has now accumulated for a lack of association between cassava consumption and TCP. Fewer people in Kerala consume the tuber than before and the disease is widely seen among patients who have never consumed cassava. Narendranathan and Cheriyan published a case-control study to examine the association between cassava and pancreatitis and failed to find a relationship, despite controlling for the confounding effects of low socioeconomic status and vegetarian status [27, 28].

Micronutrient Deficiency

There have been some reports that isolated vitamin or micronutrient deficiency may cause pancreatic fibrosis. Selenium, copper, and vitamin A have been implicated [29]. Braganza and Mohan compared the antioxidant status of South Indian patients and controls with those in northwest England and found a lower biologic availability of beta carotene and ascorbic acid in South Indian patients [30]. They suggested that culinary practices eroded the bioavailability of these antioxidants, causing pancreatitis at an early age. However, there is no clear-cut evidence that antioxidant deficiency causes TCP.

Genetic Factors

In the 1980s, there were reports of familial clustering of the disease in association with the human leukocyte antigen (HLA) phenotype. However, in 1996 it was discovered that mutations in the cationic trypsinogen gene (PRSS1) caused hereditary pancreatitis [31]. This opened new possibilities for a likely genetic basis for TCP, given that it was present in an endemic area. In 1998, Rossi et al. excluded mutations of the cationic trypsinogen gene in TCP [32]. Chandak et al. suggested that the SPINK1 N34S variant (serum protease inhibitor, Kazal type 1) might be a cause. The N34S variant was found in 7 out of 24 subjects with fibrocalculous pancreatic diabetes and in 16 out of 44 patients with TCP without diabetes [33]. Hassan et al. studied SPINK1 mutations in 180 subjects with TCP and diabetes and found the N34S variant in 33.6% of subjects, as compared to 3.7% of those with type 2 diabetes and 10.6% of those with early-onset diabetes [34]. Similar findings were reported by Bhatia et al. [35]. A recent multicenter study demonstrated that the G 191R variant of PRSS2 mitigates intrapancreatic trypsin activity and protects against chronic pancreatitis. This variant was present in 3.4% of controls but in only 1.3% of affected individuals [36]. Other circumstantial evidence in favor of a genetic basis are: (1) the occurrence of TCP among the people of Kerala origin who settled abroad, and (2) a low incidence among populations who had migrated to Cochin several generations before, such as those from South Canara, in neighboring Karnataka. Studies of keratin 8 expression in pancreatitis and pancreatic cancer did not, however, establish any relationship [37].

Pathology

Macroscopically, the pancreas is small in size and firm to touch. The changes may be focal or diffuse; the gland may feel normal in the early stages. As the disease becomes more advanced, three types are recognized, (1) a fibrotic type, where the gland undergoes atrophy with a fibrotic texture, (2) an adipose type where the overall size of the gland is maintained, but the parenchyma is replaced by fat, and (3) an inflammatory, phlegmonous type, where the gland is enlarged, woody in consistency, and the parenchyma is friable rather than fibrotic. It is regarded that the phlegmonous type may represent cases encountered earlier in the disease process, whereas types (1) and (2) may occur at the late stages.

On microscopic examination, the following features are seen: the presence of calculi, a patchy lobular distribution of lesions, and canalicular regression or tubular complexes (the existence in damaged lobules of dilated cavities surrounded by the cuboidal epithelium). Eventually there is extensive atrophy of acini with replacement by fibrous tissue. Balaraman et al. observed that despite severe atrophy of the acinar cells, the islets are spared. In fact, they found hypertrophy and hyperplasia of islets, in many cases amounting to a pseudonesidioblastosis [38]. Necrosis or parenchymal calcifications are absent and inflammatory cell infiltration is unusual. There is ductal dilatation in most cases, but the ductal epithelium is preserved and a paucity of protein plugs is seen. The chief differences between TCP and Western alcoholic pancreatitis are the absence of ductal disruption, necrosis, and inflammatory cell infiltrates in the former [25].

Clinical Features

The natural history of TCP was succinctly described by Geevarghese in 1968 as "recurrent pain in childhood, diabetes in adolescence, and death in the prime of life" [39]. Most patients in his early reports had marked emaciation, a peculiar cyanotic hue of the lips, bilateral parotid gland enlargement, and a distended upper abdomen. Nearly 40 years later, we hardly ever encounter a patient with marked emaciation or other evidence of malnutrition. Body mass index and other anthropometric measurements showed no difference between patients with TCP and controls [22]. In fact, field studies indicate that the disease is milder, affects females more than males, and the onset of disease is at an older age. Balaji et al. suggested that previous hospital-based reports of a severe illness with male preponderance might be due to the fact that males and seriously ill patients tended to report to hospital more frequently [18].

There has also been a gradual increase in the age of presentation to hospitals. While the average age of death in Geevarghese's series was 26.6 years, the average age at presentation to most hospitals in Kerala is now between 30 and 40 years (median age among patients with TCP in our unit was 39 years, and among those with TCP and associated cancer, 46 years) [39–41]. Many patients have now been diagnosed as having the disease for the first time in the sixth and seventh decades of their life, and the oldest patient to undergo surgery in this unit is 79 years. On the other hand, the disease can also appear in infancy [42].

The male to female ratio of cases is 1.7:1 in Kerala, 2:1 in Nigeria, and 5:1 in the Congo [20]. However, in field studies, the ratio was 1:1.8 [18]. This discrepancy may be explained by the fact that fewer women reported to hospital for treatment.

The main symptoms were abdominal pain (35%), diabetes mellitus (55%), weight loss (60%), obstructive jaundice (<10%), and steatorrhea in one-third of the patients. Other rare symptoms include abdominal mass, ascites, pleural effusion, and gastrointestinal bleeding. However these figures pertained to a gastroenterology unit specializing in pancreatic surgery. Data from diabetes centers, on the other hand, showed that the chief presenting symptom was uncontrolled diabetes, and abdominal pain was not a feature. Abdominal pain was typically pancreatic in character and episodic (type A pain). Some patients, however, had unrelenting pain (type B) that was not relieved by drugs and warranted therapy. On the other hand, patients may experience pain-free episodes for years. There is very little data regarding the natural history of pain in TCP. Data from the author's center indicate that about 15% of asymptomatic patients develop symptoms over a 3-year period. In 1956, Mohan Rao reported complete disappearance of calcification in a patient who had extensive calculi and who had undergone a laparotomy alone [43]. Stones may pass into the duodenum or into the jejunum following a pancreatic enteric anastomosis. However, there is no convincing evidence of a "burn out" resulting in pain relief and regression of calcification similar to that described among patients with alcoholic pancreatitis [44].

Pain may be classified into four grades: (1) no pain, (2) mild pain that is easily controlled by medication with no interference with work, (3) severe pain interfering with work but responding to medication, and (4) severe unrelieved pain. Other centers have used the visual analog scale, but it has the disadvantage of being too subjective and depends heavily on whether the description is being made during the episode or during pain-free intervals. It was observed that patients generally exaggerated the pain during its occurrence [41].

Diabetes in TCP presents most frequently in the third decade of life. A family history of diabetes in parents is seen in 20% of cases [45]. In about half of patients, their diabetes is controlled by using oral hypoglycemic agents, but the remainder require insulin. Insulin resistance leading to a very high dosage requirement occurs in less than 10% [46]. Of the TCP diabetics attending our clinic, 26% required purified or human insulin. Such treatment is expensive in the absence of a national health service. Despite these findings, ketosis is relatively uncommon due to a higher fasting and post-gluconic-C-peptide response than in patients with insulin-dependent diabetes mellitus [47]. The higher C-peptide response may in turn reflect an intact islet cell mass. Pathological studies have shown that patients with TCP may have a normal or even increased islet cell mass. Stimulation with enteroglucagon results in insulin release. Yet, a relative or absolute deficiency of insulin exists in many cases, the cause of which is not clear. One hypothesis has been that there is poor islet circulation and insulin absorption due to surrounding fibrosis, and this was thought to account for the improvement in diabetic status seen in some patients after surgery. Another feature of TCP diabetics is the low level of glucagons, which may predispose the patient to dangerous hypoglycemia [48]. TCP diabetes has the same potential for causing vascular complications. Metabolic alterations in the elderly may pose difficult problems when patients require surgery. There has been dramatic improvement in the treatment of diabetes mellitus over the past five decades, and this may be responsible for the improved survival of patients now as compared with those in Geevarghese's original series.

Steatorrhea occurs in about 35% of cases, but is severe only in 5%, probably due to poor dietary fat intake. However, studies on fecal fat excretion revealed exocrine deficiency in over 75% of patients. Other semiquantitative and quantitative tests of pancreatic exocrine function include estimation of fecal chymotrypsin and fecal elastase, and the bentiromide test (n-benzoyl-L-tyrosyl-p-amino-benzoic acid, NBT-PABA). However, Gagee et al. reported that the recovery of p-amino-benzoic acid (PABA) from Indian patients was lower than that in English patients. By calculating a percentage PABA/p-aminosalicylic acid excretion index, exocrine assessment could be achieved with 75% sensitivity, 92% specificity, and an overall efficiency of 86% [49].

Diagnosis

A diagnosis of TCP would require the following criteria:

1. Absence of alcohol intake.
2. Absence of hyperparathyroidism.
3. Two out of the following:
   a. Calculi on abdominal x-ray.
   b. Dilated main pancreatic duct on ultrasound or computed tomography (CT) scan.

c. Pancreatographic (endoscopic retrograde cholangiopancreatography, ERCP, or magnetic resonance cholangiopancratography, MRCP) evidence of ductal changes of chronic pancreatitis.
d. Endoscopic ultrasound changes of chronic pancreatitis.

These criteria allow patients with acalculous disease and with nondilated ducts to be identified [50].

Grading

There has long been recognized a serious need for a simple, widely applicable staging/grading system that would describe the disease accurately and would allow data from patients in different series to be compared. The widely used Cambridge classification may well identify two patients with severe pancreatitis, as evidenced by the extent of ductal dilatation, but one of these may be asymptomatic and not require any treatment other than follow up, whereas the other may experience severe intractable pain with or without complications. Therapy is directed against patient symptoms and asymptomatic patients merely require follow up. In 1993, the author proposed an ABC system that is based on clinical observations. There seems little doubt that patient symptoms dictate treatment pathways. Thus, the presence of symptomatic steatorrhea or diabetes is more significant from a therapeutic point of view than laboratory estimation.

The ABC system is as follows [50]:

A: No pain.
B: Pain, but no complications.
C: Complications present, pain may or may not be present.

Each grade is subdivided into:

0: no diabetes mellitus or symptomatic steatorrhea.
1. Diabetes mellitus only.
2. Steatorrhea only.
3. Diabetes and steatorrhea.

Thus a patient, who belongs to A0, requires only follow up as he has no pain and no functional deficiency, whereas a patient in C3 requires treatment for complications, and also exocrine and endocrine replacement.

Complications of TCP

The complications associated with TCP are as follows:

1. Cysts and abscesses.
2. Biliary obstruction.
3. Pancreatic ascites and pleural effusion.
4. Gastrointestinal bleeding.
5. Gastric varices due to splenic vein thrombosis.
6. Erosion of vessels (gastroduodenal, splenic), which results in hemosuccus pancreaticus.
7. Malignancy.

Several retrospective and prospective studies have reported a high association between tropical pancreatitis and carcinoma of the pancreas [41, 51–55]. In most cases, the calculi have existed for several years prior to the development of the malignancy. The presence of changes of chronic pancreatitis in the ductal system downstream from the tumor establishes that these cases do not have tumor-induced obstructive pancreatitis. According to tumor registries, Southern India, which has the highest incidence of tropical pancreatitis, has a relatively low incidence of carcinoma of the pancreas. The largest reports have come from Kerala. In 1992, Augustine and Ramesh reported a high incidence of cancer among patients with TCP [41]. Cancers occurring in cases of TCP were different in their characteristics from de novo cancers. It appeared that pancreatic cancer occurred in TCP 15 years earlier (mean age 46 years) than those with a normal pancreas (mean 61 years). They also reported the presence of dysplasia and cancer in the same histological specimen suggesting an etiologic relationship [41]. Detection of cancer in TCP is a difficult task in many situations. Fine-needle biopsy may have a poor yield due to the extreme fibrosis of the gland and the lack of cellular material aspirated through the syringe. High CA 19-9 levels, the presence of a main pancreatic duct block on endoscopic pancreatography, the presence of biliary obstruction with deep jaundice, and a heterogeneous mass on CT scanning are all suggestive of cancer, but no single diagnostic test has been identified.

Investigations for TCP [56]

These include:
1. Plain x-ray.
2. Abdominal ultrasonography.
3. CT and magnetic resonance imaging (MRI) scan.

4. Pancreatography:
   a. Magnetic resonance.
   b. Endoscopic retrograde.
   c. Operative:
      i. Prograde (after distal pancreatectomy).
      ii. Retrograde (through papilla after duodenotomy).
      iii. Ambigrade (by puncture of the main pancreatic duct).
      iv. Cyst puncture.
   d. Percutaneous pancreatography [57].
5. Exocrine function tests:
   a. Stool fat excretion.
   b. Fecal chymotrypsin.
   c. Fecal elastase-2.
   d. NBT-PABA test (research value)
6. Endocrine function tests:
   a. Fasting and postprandial blood sugar.
   b. Glucose tolerance test.
   c. Glycosylated hemoglobin.
   d. Serum insulin and C-peptide levels (research value).
7. Mass lesions:
   a. Markers: CA 19-9.
   b. Fine-needle aspiration biopsy.
8. Screening of family members.
9. Screening for genetic mutations.

Imaging establishes the morphology of the pancreas and the ductal system so that treatment may be tailored to the individual case.

Management

Steatorrhea

Steatorrhea is not often a prominent symptom at presentation because the patient's food intake may be poor as a result of pain. Following surgery, patients may change to a higher fat intake in order to improve their general health, and may then develop steatorrhea, which can be controlled by the use of pancreatic enzymes.

Diabetes Mellitus

Two-thirds to three-quarters of patients presenting to a general hospital with TCP may have diabetes; nearly one-third are controlled by diet alone, another third by oral hypoglycemic agents, and only one-third may require insulin. Vascular complications including ophthalmic problems must be looked for and managed promptly. Although some patients develop diabetic nephropathy and end-stage renal failure, there have been no reports of combined renal-pancreas transplantation in TCP.

Pain

This is the most distressing symptom, which may lead to absence from work and loss of income at the prime of life, and contribute to addiction to alcohol or narcotic drugs. Type A pain is episodic, with long pain-free intervals, and can be treated by analgesics. Pancreatic enzyme preparations with high protease may help to relieve pain. Patients with type B pain may need intervention, either by endotherapy or surgery. Indications for intervention are intractable pain and complications.

Intractable Pain

Does early treatment delay the onset of pancreatic insufficiency? In 1988, Nealon et al. described the results of pancreatic function assessment in 83 Western patients with chronic pancreatitis, 47 of who underwent pancreatic drainage by surgery, while 36 did not [58]. Pancreatic function was preserved in 87% of operated versus only 22% of nonoperated patients. By 1993, Nealon and Thompson published a second paper emphasizing the lack of progression to severe pancreatitis after surgery and recommended early surgery, even if disabling pain did not exist [59]. Sidhu et al. have also reported improvement in diabetic status after drainage procedures in TCP patients [60].

Complications

Complications associated with pain include:

1. Pancreatic pseudocysts.
2. Abscesses.
3. Biliary obstruction.
4. Duodenal obstruction.
5. Pancreatic ascites and pleural effusion.
6. Pancreatic mass.
7. Cancer.
8. Gastrointestinal bleed:
   i. Pancreatic pseudoaneurysm.
   ii. Splenic vein thrombosis and gastric varices.
9. Doubt or proof of malignancy in an "inflammatory mass."

Endoscopy in TCP

Endotherapy has several potential advantages: it offers an appealing alternative to surgery with diminished morbidity and mortality; it does not, however, preclude surgery later. In fact, it is believed that the positive response to endotherapy could be used as a predictor of successful surgical outcome [61].

Endotherapy is applicable to four situations: (1) pancreatic ductal disruptions (pseudocysts, ascites or pleural effusion, (2) pancreatic ductal strictures, (3) pancreatic ductal stones, and (4) biliary obstruction. Endoscopic therapy may be divided into three groups depending upon its applicability [62]:

1. High yield: pancreas divisum with TCP affecting the dorsal anlage, pancreatic ductal disruptions, pseudocysts, ascites, and pleural effusion.
2. Medium yield: biliary obstruction, dominant head stricture, head calculi.
3. Low yield: body and tail disease, mass lesions, diffuse disease with chain-of-lakes appearance.

There is however, a paucity of published data on endotherapy in TCP [63, 64]. While a consensus meeting on chronic pancreatitis in the Asia Pacific region concluded that endotherapy was the first-choice procedure when medical treatment failed, there has been a surprising lack of published literature on endotherapy in TCP from India [65]. The only publication from Hyderabad in Southern India came several years later and described the role of extracorporeal shock-wave lithotripsy (ESWL) and endoscopic clearance of stones in 250 consecutive patients with TCP (mean±SD age 35.2±11.9 years; 66% men), 86.8% of whom had multiple radio-opaque stones. Complete clearance of pancreatic calculi was achieved in 149 (59.6%) patients and partial clearance in 59 (23.6%). Main pancreatic ductal decompression was achieved in 70.0% (175/250) of patients. Complications occurred in 5.6% (14/250) during ESWL and in 1.2% (3/250) during ERCP. A mean of 1.3 sessions, with mean±SD 5.5±0.7 intensity setting, 85.8±13.5 pulses/min and 3862±1426 shocks per session were required. The paper failed to correlate stone clearance with relief of symptoms, and no follow up was available [66].

Surgical Treatment

The aims of surgery are [67]:

1. To relieve pain.
2. To forestall complications or treat them.
3. Minimize operative morbidity and mortality or prevent them altogether.
4. Provide good quality of life, for which preservation of the pancreatic parenchyma is crucial [62].

The technical approaches of surgery can be summarized as follows:

1. Clearance of stones and strictures from the main pancreatic duct and main side branches, biopsy sampling when required. The rationale of achieving stone clearance is based on the premise that stones occur where the maximum areas of stasis exist, and clearance of stones would automatically ensure drainage of the areas of maximum stasis.
2. Anastomosis of pancreatic duct/gland from the tail to the head (within 0.5 cm of the medial border of the duodenum).
3. Addition of head coring or subtotal resection of the head when there is an inflammatory mass in the head.
4. If the disease is more advanced, a head resection may be considered, but the duodenum should be preserved.
5. A Whipple resection is reserved only for patients who have large head masses with or without pseudocysts, and biliary and duodenal obstruction or if malignancy is suspected, and who cannot be satisfactorily drained.

Patients may be grouped as:

1. Large-duct disease (main pancreatic duct 6 mm or greater in diameter).
2. Small-duct disease (main pancreatic duct less than 6 mm diameter).
3. Inflammatory masses.
4. Complications as listed above.

Large-Duct Disease

The Partington-Rochelle modification of the Puestow-Gillesby procedure is the optimum procedure [68]. Initial results reveal a pain relief of 85–90% of cases. Data has shown that failures occur within the first 48 months and are most likely due to technical reasons [69]. The pancreatic parenchyma is preserved and postoperative pancreatic function does not deteriorate in the majority of patients.

In patients with bulky heads, the ductotomy cannot be carried over to the head as the duct dips deep into the parenchyma. In such cases, decompression of the head ducts including the duct of Santorini and uncinate process ducts is not satisfactory, and this may be responsible for the development of inflammatory masses in the head after drainage operations. It has been calculated that in a 5-cm head, at a point 3 cm from the medial border of the duodenum, the distance between the duct and the ampulla of Vater is 6 cm [70]. In a multivariate analysis of risk factors correlating with pain relief after surgery, incomplete stone clearance and ductotomy stopping short of the head were associated with early recurrence of pain [40]. Hence, an additional procedure to achieve good drainage of head ducts is necessary. This can be achieved by head coring (the Frey procedure). The advantage of this operation is that it enables the surgeon to tailor the extent of the coring to the extent of the disease and the size of the mass. Patients with an atrophic gland and little or no mass in the head required minimal coring, if at all. On the other hand, large inflammatory masses may require coring out of as much as 50 g of pancreatic tissue to achieve good drainage.

Small-Duct Disease

Pancreatic resection is indicated when the disease predominantly involves one portion of the gland, in cases where effective drainage cannot be achieved (especially in the head), and in patients with normal-sized ducts or recurrent pain following earlier drainage procedures. The benefits of resection must be weighed against the problems due to exocrine and endocrine deficiency, which invariably occur. Total pancreatectomy is also not a satisfactory alternative. Chacko Valayil (personal communication) performed four total pancreatectomies for chronic pancreatitis; all patients were dead within 6 months of the operation.

Ductal drainage in small-duct disease has not been extensively studied. The results were poor in one series, but excellent in another [71, 72]. A good explanation for such contrasting results is not available. A major problem in these patients is to locate the main pancreatic duct at surgery. The duct may occupy an eccentric location inside the parenchyma, and attempts to palpate the duct may be hampered by an enlarged woody gland. Surgical experience, the use of intraoperative ultrasound and radiographic C-arm-guided puncture of the main duct help in duct location at surgery. Recent data suggests the successful application of lateral drainage, with head coring in 45 patients; 94% pain relief over a median follow up of greater than 30 months was accompanied by preservation of pancreatic function in the majority [73]. There are no reports of the longitudinal V-shaped excision of the pancreas as describe by Izbicki in patients with TCP [74].

Mass Lesions

Mass lesions, particularly in the pancreatic head, present great diagnostic and therapeutic problems. Cancer needs to be ruled out with certainty. While a positive biopsy is useful, a negative biopsy does not rule out cancer. Pancreaticoduodenectomy may allow removal of the maximally involved gland, but runs the risk of loss of parenchyma and resulting pancreatic insufficiency. Among 168 patients with pancreatic head mass in chronic pancreatitis, 123 had head coring plus drainage, and 45 underwent resections. There was excellent pain relief following both operations; patients in the resection group, however, had a significantly higher deterioration in exocrine and endocrine function, and this deterioration was responsible for a poor quality of life. Only 47% felt healthy after resection, whereas 78 did so after head coring with lateral drainage. These findings are similar to observations in Western series [75–79].

Other Procedures

There have been only two reports of nerve interruption procedures in TCP. In 1976, Bahuleyan reported excellent early results following splanchnicectomy in 12 patients, but there was no long-term follow up [80]. In another report, Venkatesh Rao reported good or fair results in 11 of 15 patients undergoing postceliac neurectomy; this operation was combined with a pancreaticogastrostomy [81].

Functional Results

In a series of 14 patients who underwent surgical or endoscopic treatment for pain due to chronic pancreatitis, Agarwal et al. found that beta-cell function and exocrine status remained unchanged after surgery, although pain and elevated serum trypsin levels returned to normal. In a long-term follow-up study, nearly two-thirds of patients had stable pancreatic function; there was improvement in 15% and deterioration in 18% of patients [82].

Controversies

Many aspects of the disease are as yet poorly understood. There is still a strong suggestion of a genetic predisposition; the etiology may in fact be multifactorial. Although most (96%) of patients have calculi at presentation; it is clear that a precalculous disease does exist. The disease may have a long latent period and actually present first with a complication such as cancer. There is strong evidence that TCP is premalignant, but the natural history of its causation remains to be unraveled. Identification of an animal model may help in this process.

The future goals in TCP lie in efforts at disease prevention by the precise determination of causative factors; improved methods of treatment for exocrine and endocrine deficiency, judicious use of nonoperative and operative modalities in relief of pain, and prevention or at the very least early identification of life threatening complications such as pancreatic cancer.

References

1. Kini MG (1937) Multiple pancreatic calculi with chronic pancreatitis. Br J Surg 25:705
2. Zuidema PJ (1955) Calcification and cirrhosis of the pancreas in patients with deficient nutrition. Doc Med Geograph Trop Amsterdam 5:229–251
3. Mahadevan R (1961) Pancreatic lithiasis. A follow up study of 17 cases. Br Med J 5226:626–629
4. Nagarathnam N, Gunawardane KRW (1972) Aetiological factors in pancreatic calcifications in Ceylon. Digestion 5:9–16
5. Chandraprasert S, Samranvej P, Arthachinta S, Isarasena S (1976) Diabetes mellitus and tropical form of chronic calcific pancreatitis in Thailand. Aust NZ J Med 6:316–320
6. Balasegaram M (1987) Pancreatitis in the tropics. In: Howard JM, Jordan GL Jr, Reber HA (eds) Surgical Diseases of the Pancreas. Lea Febiger, Philadelphia, p 257
7. Geevarghese PJ, Kumarapillai V, Joseph MP, Pitchumoni CS (1962) The diagnosis of pancreatogenous diabetes (a clinicopathological study of one hundred cases of pancreatic calculi associated with diabetes mellitus). J Assoc Physicians India 10:173
8. Kinnear TW (1963) The pattern of diabetes in a Nigerian teaching hospital. East Afr Med J 40:288–294
9. Shaper AG (1960) Chronic pancreatic disease and protein malnutrition. Lancet i:1223–1224
10. Goodall JW, Pilbeam ST (1964) Diabetes in Nyasaland. Trans R Soc Trop Med Hyg 58:575–578
11. Sonnet J, Brisbois P, Bastin JP (1966) Chronic pancreatitis with calcifications n Congolese Bantus. Trop Geogr Med 18:97–113
12. Olurin EO, Olurin O (1969) Pancreatic calcification: a report of 45 cases. Br Med J 4:534–539
13. Nwokolo C, Oli J (1980) Pathogenesis of juvenile tropical pancreatitis syndrome. Lancet i:456–459
14. Dani R, Nogueira CE (1976) [Chronic calcifying pancreatitis in Brazil: analysis of 92 cases]. Leber Magen Darm 6:272–275
15. Balakrishnan V (1987) Tropical pancreatitis: epidemiology, pathology and etiology. In: Balakrishnan V, Thankappan KR (eds) Chronic Pancreatitis in India. St Joseph's Press, Trivandrum, pp 79–87
16. Rai RR, Acharya SK, Nundy S, Vashisht S, Tandon RK (1988) Chronic calcific pancreatitis. Clinical profile in northern India. Gastroenterol Jpn 23:195–200
17. Thomas PG, Augustine P, Ramesh H, Rangabashyam N (1990) Observations and surgical management of tropical pancreatitis in Kerala and Southern India. World J Surg 14:32–42
18. Balaji LN, Tandon RK, Tandon BN, Banks PA (1994) Prevalence and clinical features of chronic pancreatitis in southern India. Int J Pancreatol 15:29–34
19. Ramachandran A, Mohan V, Snehalatha C, Bharani G, Chinnakrishnudu M, Mohan R, Viswanathan M (1988) Clinical features of diabetes in the young as seen at a diabetes centre. Diabetes Res Clin Pract 4:117–125
20. Pitchumoni CS (1984) Special problems of tropical pancreatitis. Clin Gastroenterol 13:941–959
21. Barbezat GO, Hansen JD (1968) The exocrine pancreas and protein-calorie malnutrition. Pediatrics 42:77–92
22. Padmalayam I, John S, Mohan V, Ramachandran A, Viswanathan M (1991) Anthropometric studies in diabetics in the tropics. Acta Diabetol Lat 28:55–60
23. Mohan V, Snehalatha C, Bhattacharyya PK, Ramachandran A, Viswanathan M (1991) Nutrition profile of fibrocalculous pancreatic diabetes and primary forms of diabetes seen in southern India. Diabetes Res Clin Pract 11:203–207
24. Balakrishnan V, Sauniere JF, Haritharan M, Sarles H (1988) Diet, pancreatic function and chronic pancreatitis in South India and France. Pancreas 3:30–35
25. Sarles H, Augustine P, Laugier R, Mathew S, Dupuy P (1984) Pancreatic lesions and modifications of pancreatic juice in tropical chronic pancreatitis (tropical calcific diabetes). Dig Dis Sci 39:1337–1344
26. Pitchumoni CS, Thomas E (1973) Chronic cassava toxicity: possible relationship to chronic pancreatitis disease in malnourished populations. Lancet i:1397–1398
27. Narendranathan M, Cheriyan A (1994) Lack of association between cassava consumption and tropical pancreatitis syndrome. J Gastroenterol Hepatol 9:282–285
28. Mori M, Hariharan M, Anandakumar M, Tsutsumi M, Ishikawa O, Konishi Y, Chellam VG, John M, Praseeda I, Priya R, Narendranathan M (1999) A case-control study on risk factors for pancreatic diseases in Kerala, India. Hepatogastroenterology 46:25–30
29. Narendranathan M, Sharma KN, Sosamma PI (1989) Serum rhodanese in goiter and calcific pancreatitis of tropics. J Assoc Physicians India 37:648–649
30. Braganza JM, Schofield D, Snehalatha C, Mohan V (1993) Micronutrient antioxidant status in tropical compared with temperate zone chronic pancreatic. Scand J Gastroenterol 28:1098–1104
31. Whitcomb DC, Gorry MC, Preston RA, Furey W, Sossenheimer MJ, Ulrich CD, Martin SP, Gates Jr LK, Amann ST, Toskes PP, Liddle R, McGrath K, Uomo G, Post JC, Ehrlich GD (1996) Hereditary pancreatitis is caused by a mutation in the cationic trypsinogen gene. Nat Genet 14:141–45

32. Rossi L, Whitcomb DC, Ehrlich GD, Gorry MC, Parvin S, Sattar S, Ali L, Azad Khan AK, Gyr N (1998) Lack of R117H mutation in the cationic trypsinogen gene in patients with tropical calcific pancreatitis from Bangladesh. Pancreas 17:278–280
33. Chandak GR, Idris MM, Reddy DN, Bhaskar S, Sriram PVJ, Singh L (2002) Mutations in the pancreatic secretory trypsin inhibitor gene (PSTI/ SPINK1) rather than the cationic trypsinogen gene (PRSS1) are significantly associated with tropical calcific pancreatitis. J Med Genet 39:347–351
34. Hassan Z, Mohan V, Ali L, Allotey R, Barakat K, Faruque MO, Deepa R, McDermott MF, Jackson AE, Cassell P, Curtis D, Gelding SV, Vijayaravaghan S, Gyr N, Whitcomb DC, Khan AK, Hitman GA (2002) SPINK1 is a susceptibility gene for fibrocalculous pancreatic diabetes in subjects from the Indian subcontinent. Am J Hum Genet 71:964–968
35. Bhatia E, Choudhuri G, Sikora SS, Landt O, Kage A, Becker M, Witt H (2002) Tropical calcific pancreatitis: strong association with SPINK1 trypsin inhibitor mutations. Gastroenterology 123:1020–1025
36. Witt H, Sahin-Toth M, Landt O, Chen JM, Kahne T, Drenth JP, Kukor Z, Szepessy E, Halangk W, Dahm S, Rohde K, Schulz HU, Le Marechal C, Akar N, Ammann RW, Truninger K, Bargetzi M, Bhatia E, Castellani C, Cavestro GM, Cerny M, Destro-Bisol G, Spedini G, Eiberg H, Jansen JB, Koudova M, Rausova E, Macek M Jr, Malats N, Real FX, Menzel HJ, Moral P, Galavotti R, Pignatti PF, Rickards O, Spicak J, Zarnescu NO, Bock W, Gress TM, Friess H, Ockenga J, Schmidt H, Pfutzer R, Lohr M, Simon P, Weiss FU, Lerch MM, Teich N, Keim V, Berg T, Wiedenmann B, Luck W, Groneberg DA, Becker M, Keil T, Kage A, Bernardova J, Braun M, Guldner C, Halangk J, Rosendahl J, Witt U, Treiber M, Nickel R, Ferec C (2006) A degradation-sensitive anionic trypsinogen (PRSS2) variant protects against chronic pancreatitis. Nat Genet 38:668–673
37. Choudhuri G, Singh D (2005) Molecular mechanisms of pancreatic cancer. Trop Gastroenterol 26:111–114
38. Balaraman Nair M, Latha P (1987) Pancreas in chronic calcifying pancreatitis In: Balakrishnan V, Thankappan KR (eds) Chronic Pancreatitis in India. St Joseph's Press, Trivandrum, pp 113–120
39. Geevarghese PJ (1968) Pancreatic Diabetes: a Clinicopathological Study of Growth Onset Diabetes with Pancreatic Calculi. Popular Prakashan, Bombay, p 96
40. Ramesh H, Augustine P (1992) Surgery in tropical pancreatitis: analysis of risk factors. Br J Surg 79:544–549
41. Augustine P, Ramesh H (1992) Is tropical pancreatitis premalignant? Am J Gastroenterol 87:1005–1008
42. Premalatha G, Mohan V (1994)Fibrocalculous pancreatic diabetes in infancy – two case reports. Diabetes Res Clin Pract 25:137–140
43. Mohan Rao U (1956) Spontaneous resorption of pancreatic calcification. Indian J Surg 18:471
44. Amman RW, Akovbiantz A, Largiader F, Shueler G (1984) Course and outcome of chronic pancreatitis. Longitudinal study of a mixed medical-surgical series of 245 patients. Gastroenterology 86:820–828
45. Mohan V, Chari ST, Hitman GA, Suresh S, Madanagopalan N, Ramachandran A, Viswanathan M (1989) Familial aggregation in tropical fibocalculous pancreatic diabetes. Pancreas 6:690–693
46. Mohan V, Ramachandran A, Vijaya Kumar G, Snehalatha C, Viswanathan M (1988) Insulin resistance in fibrocalculous pancreatic diabetes. Horm Metab Res 20:746–748
47. Mohan V, Snehalatha C, Ramachandran A, Jayshree R, Viswanathan M (1983) Pancreatic beta cell function in tropical pancreatic diabetes. Metabolism 32:1091–1092
48. Mohan V, Snehalatha C, Ramachandran A, Chari S, Madanagopalan N, Viswanathan M (1990) Plasma glucagon responses in fibrocalculous pancreatic diabetes. Diabetes Res Clin Pract 9:97–101
49. Gagee P, Pemberton P, Lobely R, Chaloner C, Snehalatha C, Mohan V, Braganza JM (1992) The BT-PABA/PAS test in tropical diabetes. Clin Chim Acta 212:103–111
50. Ramesh H (2002) Proposal for a new grading system for chronic pancreatitis: the ABC system. J Clin Gastroenterol 35:67–70
51. Chari S, Mohan V, Snehalatha C, Pitchumoni CS, Madanagopalan N, Viswanathan M (1992) Pancreatic carcinoma complicating tropical chronic pancreatitis – a follow-up study. Gastroenterology 102:a260
52. Narendranathan M (1981) Chronic pancreatitis of the tropics. Trop Gastroenterol 2:40
53. Thomas PG, Augustine P (1987) Pancreatic cancer in siblings with tropical pancreatitis. Ind J Gastroenterol 6:185–187
54. Chari ST, Mohan V, Pitchumoni CS, Viswanathan M, Madanagopalan N, Lowenfels AB (1994) Risk of pancreatic carcinoma in tropical calcifying pancreatitis: an epidemiological study. Pancreas 9:62–66
55. Shenoy KT, Narendranathan M, Hariharan M (1986) Tropical pancreatitis – sequelae and complications: a prospective study. In: Balakrishnan V, Thankappan KR (eds). Proceedings of the Annual Conference of the Indian Society of Pancreatology, Trivandrum, Medical College Trivandrum, p 16
56. Augustine P, Tharakan A (2001) Diagnostic approaches in chronic pancreatitis. Asian J Surg 24:93–102
57. Augustine P, Jose J (1991) Percutaneous pancreatography in tropical pancreatitis. Indian J Gastroenterol 10:114
58. Nealon WH, Townsend CM Jr, Thompson JC (1988) Operative drainage of the pancreatic duct delays functional impairment in patients with chronic pancreatitis: a prospective study. Ann Surg 208:321–329
59. Nealon WH, Thompson JC (1993) Progressive loss of pancreatic function in chronic pancreatitis is delayed by main pancreatic duct decompression. A longitudinal prospective analysis of the modified Puestow procedure. Ann Surg 217:458–466
60. Sidhu SS, Nundy S, Tandon RK (2001) The effect of the modified Peustow procedure on diabetes in patients with tropical chronic pancreatitis – a prospective study. Am J Gastroenterol 96:107–111
61. Huibregtse K, Smits ME (1994) Endoscopic management of diseases of the pancreas. Am J Gastroenterol 89:S66–77
62. Ramesh H, Jacob G (2002) Management of pain in chronic pancreatitis: has anything changed in the past twenty years? In: Jagannath P (ed) Hepatopancreatobiliary Surgery – Current Concepts. Churchill Livingstone, New Delhi, pp 149–157
63. Reddy DN, Rao GV, Kumar PV, Reddy GJ (1991) Endoscopic stenting relieves pain in tropical pancreatitis. Proceedings of the 6th International Workshop on Therapeutic Endoscopy, Hong Kong, p 101
64. Reddy DN, Sriram PVJ, Das G, Rao GV (2001) Endoscopic treatment of pancreatic disorders. Trop Gastroenterol 22:149–154
65. Garg PK, Tandon RK (2004) Survey on chronic pancreatitis in the Asia-Pacific region. J Gastroenterol Hepatol 19:998–1004

66. Ong WC, Tandan M, Reddy V, Rao GV, Reddy DN (2006) Multiple main pancreatic duct stones in tropical pancreatitis: Safe clearance with extracorporeal shockwave lithotripsy. J Gastroent Hepatol 21:1514–1518
67. Moossa AR (1987) Surgical treatment of chronic pancreatitis; an overview. Br J Surg 74:661–667
68. Partington PF, Rochelle REL (1960) Modified Puestow procedure for retrograde drainage of the pancreatic duct. Ann Surg 152:1037–1043
69. Ramesh H, Varghese CJ (1994) Tropical Pancreatitis: long-term results of surgery. In: Proceeding of the 10th World Congress of Gastroenterology, Los Angeles, p 44
70. Frey CF, Smith GJ (1987) Description and rationale of a new operation for chronic pancreatitis. Pancreas 2:701–707
71. Rios GA, Adams DB, Yeoh KG, Tarnasky PR, Cunningham JT (1988) Outcome of lateral pancreaticojejunostomy in the management of pancreatitis with non dilated ducts. J Gastrointest Surg 2:222–229
72. Delcore R, Rodriguez FJ, Thomas JH, Foster J, Hermreck AS (1994) The role of pancreaticojejunostomy in patients without dilated pancreatic ducts. Am J Surg 168:598–602
73. Ramesh H, Jacob G, Lekha V, Venugopal A (2003) Ductal drainage with head coring in chronic pancreatitis with small-duct disease. J Hepatobiliary Pancreat Surg 10:366–372
74. Izbicki JR, Bloechle C, Broering DC, Kuechler T, Broelsch CE (1998) Longitudinal V-shaped excision of the ventral pancreas for small duct disease in severe chronic pancreatitis: prospective evaluation of a new surgical procedure. Ann Surg 227:213–219
75. Traverso LW, Kozarek RA (1997) Pancreaticoduodenectomy for chronic pancreatitis: anatomic selection criteria and subsequent long term outcome analysis. Ann Surg 226:429–438
76. Eddes EH, Masclee AA, Lamers CB, Gooszen HG (1996) Duodenum preserving head of the pancreas in painful chronic pancreatitis. Eur J Surg 162:545–549
77. Buechler MW, Friess H, Muller MW, Wheatley AM, Beger HG (1995) Randomised trial of duodenum-preserving pancreatic head resection versus pylorus-preserving Whipple in chronic pancreatitis. Am J Surg 169:65–69
78. Izbicki JR, Bloechle C, Broering DC, Knoefel WT, Kuechler T, Broelsch CE (1998) Extended drainage versus resection in surgery for chronic pancreatitis: a prospective randomized trial comparing the longitudinal pancreaticojejunostomy combined with local pancreatic head excision with the pylorus preserving Pancreaticoduodenectomy. Ann Surg 228:771–779
79. Izbicki JR, Bloechle C, Knoefel WT, Kuechler T, Binmoeller KF, Broelsch CE (1995) Duodenum-preserving resection of the head of pancreas. A prospective randomized trial. Ann Surg 221:350–358
80. Bahuleyan CK (1976) Splanchnicectomy for pancreatic calculi. Indian J Gastroenterol 38:188–192
81. Venkatesh Rao PS (1983) The role of post-celiac neurectomy and surgical drainage in management of chronic pancreatitis. MS (General Surgery) Thesis, Christian Medical College, Vellore
82. Agrawal G, Sikora SS, Choudhuri G, Bhatia E (2002) Prospective study of pancreatic beta cell and exocrine function following duct decompression in tropical calcific pancreatitis. World J Surg 26:171–175
83. Ramesh H (1996) Tropical pancreatitis. In: Gupta RL (ed) Recent Advances in Surgery, Volume 5. Jaypee Brothers, Delhi, pp 147–166

Chapter 33

N. Teich · V. Keim

Hereditary Chronic Pancreatitis: Diagnosis and Management

Hereditary chronic pancreatitis (HCP) is a very rare form of early-onset chronic pancreatitis. With the exception of the young age at diagnosis and a slower progression, the clinical course, morphological features and laboratory findings of HCP do not differ from those of patients with alcoholic chronic pancreatitis. In addition, the diagnostic criteria and treatment of HCP resemble that of chronic pancreatitis of other causes. The clinical presentation is highly variable and includes chronic abdominal pain, impairment of endocrine and exocrine pancreatic function, nausea and vomiting, maldigestion, diabetes, pseudocysts, bile duct and duodenal obstruction, and rarely pancreatic cancer. Fortunately, most patients have a mild disease. Mutations in the PRSS1 gene, encoding cationic trypsinogen, play a causative role in chronic pancreatitis. It has been shown that cationic trypsinogen gene (*PRSS1*) mutations increase the autocatalytic conversion of trypsinogen to active trypsin, and thus probably cause premature, intrapancreatic trypsinogen activation disturbing the intrapancreatic balance of proteases and their inhibitors. Other genes, such as anionic trypsinogen (*PRSS2*), the serine protease inhibitor, Kazal type 1 (*SPINK1*) and cystic fibrosis transmembrane conductance regulator (*CFTR*) have also been found to be associated with chronic pancreatitis (idiopathic and hereditary). Genetic testing should only be performed in carefully selected patients by direct DNA sequencing, and antenatal diagnosis should not be encouraged. Treatment focuses on enzyme and nutritional supplementation, pain management, pancreatic diabetes, and local organ complications, such as pseudocysts, or bile duct or duodenal obstruction. The disease course and prognosis of patients with HCP is unpredictable. Pancreatic cancer risk is elevated. Therefore, HCP patients should strongly avoid environmental risk factors for pancreatic cancer.

Definition

Already in 1952, Comfort and Steinberg were the first to recognize that chronic pancreatitis may accumulate in selected families, suggesting a genetic background [1]. Thereafter, HCP was defined as an autosomal dominant disease with a penetrance of approximately 80%. However, in the daily clinical setting, the inheritance pattern cannot be determined in some cases. In 1996, several groups mapped a gene for HCP to chromosome 7 [2–4]. In the same year, Whitcomb and colleagues identified an R122H mutation in the cationic trypsinogen gene (*PRSS1*) [5]. Several other mutations were described subsequently (A16V, D22G, K23R, N29I, N29T, R122C) [6–12]. Until now, the R122H and N29I mutations of the PRSS1 gene have been identified as the most common disease-associated mutations [5–7].

In the last decade, several authors identified associations of chronic pancreatitis (idiopathic and hereditary) to other genes, such as *PRSS2*, *SPINK1*, and *CFTR* [13–16]. On the other hand, environmental factors as smoking, alcohol consumption, or the lack of antioxidants were assumed to be important manifestation factors, even in HCP (Fig. 33.1) [17–20].

The definition of HCP as a classic autosomal dominant disorder represents the current knowledge. However, the criteria of the diagnosis of HCP have been changing throughout the years and are currently different in the various clinical centers. In the recently published Europac study, the diagnosis of hereditary pancreatitis was made on the basis of two first-degree relatives or three or more second-degree relatives, in two or more generations with recurrent acute pancreatitis, and/or chronic pancreatitis for which there were no precipitating factors. Cases in which these strict criteria were not met, but more than one affected family member was identified, mostly within the same generation, were classified as familial chronic pancreatitis [21]. However, the diagnostic value of this classification is questionable. Therefore, we define HCP if the patient has no other detectable cause of chronic pancreatitis and if he/she has one first-or second-de-

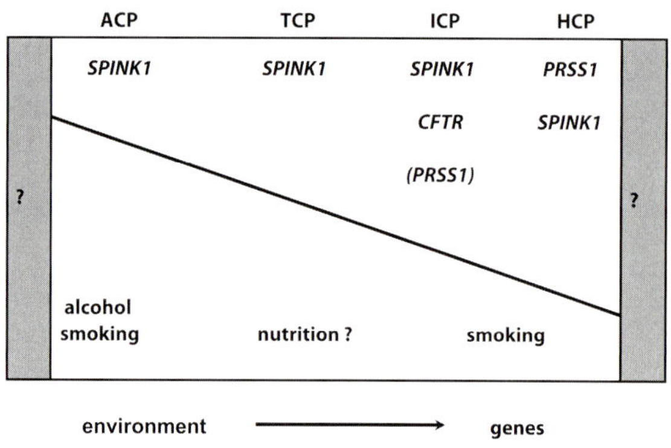

Figure 33.1

Diagrammatic illustration of genetic and environmental factors with their suspected influences on the pathogenesis of chronic pancreatitis [85]. *ACP* Alcoholic chronic pancreatitis, *TCP* tropical calcific chronic pancreatitis, *ICP* idiopathic chronic pancreatitis, *HCP* hereditary chronic pancreatitis, *CFTR* cystic fibrosis transmembrane conductance regulator gene, *SPINK1* serine protease inhibitor, Kazal type 1 gene, *PRSS1* protease, serine, 1 (trypsin 1), cationic trypsinogen gene

gree relative with proven chronic pancreatitis. An international consensus is needed in the near future to classify affected families unambiguously.

Clinical Definition

Chronic pancreatitis in adults is defined as a relapsing or continuing inflammatory disease of the pancreas characterized by irreversible morphological changes, upper abdominal pain and, in some patients, permanent impairment of exocrine function, endocrine function, or both [22]. The clinical course during an acute attack may range from mild edematous to severe necrotizing inflammation of the pancreas. The resulting morphological changes can be summarized as irregular sclerosis with focal, segmental, or diffuse destruction of the parenchyma. Frequently, dilatations, strictures, or intraductal plugs can be seen in the pancreatic duct system. Initially, chronic pancreatitis is characterized by a recurrent stage of acute pancreatitis (early-stage chronic pancreatitis) passing over to progressive pancreatic dysfunction and/or pancreatic calcification (late stage chronic pancreatitis).

Noteworthy in children, the cardinal symptom is recurring, suddenly appearing epigastric pain. Contrary to adults, enduring pain is not a common clinical finding in children. Other symptoms are nausea, vomiting, and abdominal pressure pain. Children partially develop pancreatic insufficiency with steatorrhea and insulin-dependent diabetes, but these complications normally occur later than in patients with chronic alcoholic pancreatitis.

Diagnostic Criteria

Diagnosis of chronic pancreatitis is made by clinical findings, a typical medical and family history, imaging methods, and pancreatic function tests. The use of invasive function tests (secretin test, pancreozymin-secretin test) has been declining over recent years. In recent reviews it was stated that invasive function tests in combination with pancreatic calcification are still the gold standard in the diagnosis of chronic pancreatitis, but these tests are laborious and costly [23–26]. Noninvasive tests (fecal chymotrypsin, para-aminobenzoic acid, pancreolauryl, and fecal elastase tests) are insufficient for the detection of minor or moderate insufficiency as a result of their restricted sensitivity compared to the pancreozymin-secretin test. As a consequence, function tests are of restricted value, particularly in early-stage chronic pancreatitis [26,27]. A pragmatic and reasonable treatment is the supplementation of pancreatic enzymes *ex juvantibus* in patients with chronic pancreatitis and suspected exocrine insufficiency.

No imaging test has been established thus far for the diagnosis of early-stage chronic pancreatitis. In patients with late-stage chronic pancreatitis, several imaging methods (endoscopic retrograde cholangiopancreatography, magnetic resonance imaging, magnetic resonance cholangiopancreatography, enteroscopy, computed tomography, ultrasound, abdominal x-ray) are sufficient to detect typical morphological changes (e.g., duct alterations, calcification).

Epidemiology

There are no data regarding the incidence or prevalence of chronic hereditary pancreatitis or of chronic pancreatitis in children. The incidence of chronic pancreatitis of any cause is expected to be about 3.5–10 per 100,000 inhabitants per year in Europe and the USA [28,29].

Clinical Characteristics

Alcoholic chronic pancreatitis and HCP exhibit essentially identical clinical laboratory results and histopathological or morphological features. Remarkably, HCP manifests typically at an earlier age, and pancreatic calcification and diabetes mellitus are less frequent complications in comparison to chronic alcoholic pancreatitis. Certainly estimable is the fact that most investigated subjects with the N29I or R122H *PRSS1* mutation had mild disease or were asymptomatic [17,30].

Our investigations revealed no difference in the age of onset between carriers of the these mutations. The median age of onset was 11 years in the N29I and 10 years in the R122H group. Only 4% of our patients had severe chronic pancreatitis with exocrine and endocrine insufficiency, pancreatic calcification, and duct dilatation as well as hospitalizations due to pancreatitis. In general, half of the mutation carriers had little or no complaints or complications [17]. A European study revealed a mean age of onset of 10 years and 14.5 years for affected carriers of the *PRSS1* mutations R122H and N29I, respectively, but showed no mutation-dependent differences in complications such as exocrine or endocrine insufficiency or increased pancreatic cancer risk [21]. Data on the frequencies of acute pancreatitis attacks and pain in patients with HCP are not available to date. Chronic pancreatitis presents with a wide range of pain from mild to severe and from intermittent to persistent. Interestingly, endocrine insufficiency can regress over time, which is in contrast to current belief, that pancreatic diabetes is an irreversible sign of pancreatic failure [31]. However, prospective investigations of the course of diabetes in patients with HCP are lacking so far.

Hereditary Chronic Pancreatitis and Pancreatic Cancer

As shown in an investigation of 8 patients with pancreatic cancer in a cohort of 246 HCP patients, the lifetime risk of pancreatic cancer is about 50-fold higher than in the control population and corresponds to 1 per 1066 person-years. It is only 20-fold elevated in patients with chronic alcoholic pancreatitis [32,33]. In our cohort of 101 HCP patients (25 N29I carrier, 76 R122H carrier), pancreatic cancer was diagnosed in 3 patients with the R122H mutation with a median of 23 years after the onset of pancreatitis. This corresponds to a rate of about 1 per 1200 person-years among affected R122H carriers [17]. Obviously, the data basis for the estimation of the pancreatic cancer risk in patients with *PRSS1*-associated HCP is small. The largest clinical investigation in the pregenetic era, however, revealed no pancreatic cancer in 72 patients from 7 families [19]. Taken together, the pancreatic cancer risk in HCP patients with a *PRSS1* mutation seems to be elevated 2 with an uncertain relative risk increase. Today, there is no generally accepted protocol for screening HCP patients for early pancreatic cancer. However, affected mutation carriers should be strongly advised to stop smoking, as it is an additional risk factor for pancreatic cancer [34].

Other Genes Associated with Chronic Pancreatitis

SPINK1 Mutations in Chronic Pancreatitis

Witt and colleagues were the first to describe an association between *SPINK1*mutations and chronic pancreatitis [14]. SPINK1 is a potent protease inhibitor that is thought to be a specific inactivation factor of intrapancreatic trypsin activity. During incubation of equimolar quantities of trypsin and SPINK1, the formation of a covalent bond between the catalytic serine residue of trypsin and the lysine carboxyl group of the reactive site of SPINK1 is carried out. After prolonged incubation, trypsin activity reappears over time. This is explainable by the fact that SPINK1 is degraded by trypsin [35]. The most frequently found *SPINK1* mutation is N34S. This mutation was found predominantly in patients with idiopathic chronic pancreatitis. Further investigations showed an association of *SPINK1* mutations and alcoholic chronic pancreatitis as well as tropical chronic pancreatitis [36–41]. Since 1–2% of controls carry the N34S mutation, this mutation alone seems to be insufficient to explain the pathogenesis of chronic pancreatitis in mutation carriers. Moreover, a functional analysis of recombinant SPINK1 with the N34S mutation showed an unchanged function of N34S SPINK1 as well as an unchanged trypsin susceptibility [42]. This indicates that mechanisms other than the conformational change of N34S might underlie the predisposition to chronic pancreatitis in mutation carriers.

CFTR Mutations in Chronic Pancreatitis

Cystic fibrosis (*OMIM 219700*) is an autosomal recessive disorder with an incidence in whites of approximately 1 in 2500 live births. In 1989, *CFTR* (*OMIM 602421*) was identified as the underlying gene. In 1998, Sharer et al. and Cohn et al. were able to show an association of *CFTR* mutations with chronic pancreatitis [15,16]. This association is pathophysiologically comprehensible since 1–2% of patients with cystic fibrosis suffer from chronic pancreatitis [43,44]. The variety of pancreatic disorders in cystic fibrosis range from complete loss of exocrine and endocrine function to almost normal pancreatic function. So far, more than 1500 mutations of the *CFTR* gene have been described [45]. According to their effect, the mutations are split up into five or six classes (I–V/VI) [46,47]. In cystic fibrosis, the most common mutation is F508del, accounting for approximately 66% of all mutated alleles [48]. Interestingly, the clinical course of cystic fibrosis can be variable in patients carrying the same mutations, indicating the influence of environmental and maybe other genetic factors.

Recently published studies have confirmed the association between chronic pancreatitis and *CFTR* mutations, but until now the underlying mechanisms leading to the development of chronic pancreatitis have been poorly understood [49–54]. One of the main findings in all investigations is the detection of mostly rare *CFTR* mutations showing a different spectrum of detected mutations than in cystic fibrosis and congenital bilateral aplasia of the vas deferens. Some authors state that compound heterozygous *CFTR* carriers have a distinct elevated risk for the development of chronic pancreatitis, which is even higher when an additional *SPINK1* mutation is present [51,54].

However, the role of some *CFTR* mutations has to be reconsidered, since Rohlfs et al. demonstrated that the mutation I148T in exon 4, which was classified as a severe cystic-fibrosis-causing mutation, is not associated with cystic fibrosis. According to their data, the complex allele 3199del6, and I148T seem to be the relevant factors [55]. In summary, *CFTR* mutations alone are not sufficient for the pathogenesis of chronic pancreatitis in most patients and further studies are needed to elucidate the role of CFTR in the pathogenesis of chronic pancreatitis.

PRSS2 Mutations in Chronic Pancreatitis

In an actual study of 2466 patients with chronic pancreatitis (including 1857 with hereditary or idiopathic pancreatitis) and 6459 controls by Witt et al., the G191R variant of the anionic trypsinogen was overrepresented in controls (32 vs. 220, odds ratio 0.37; $P=1.1\times10^{-8}$). The analysis of the recombinantly expressed G191R variant revealed a complete loss of trypsin activity due to the introduction of a novel tryptic cleavage site that renders the enzyme hypersensitive to autocatalytic proteolysis. Taken together, the G191R variant of PRSS2 mitigates intrapancreatic

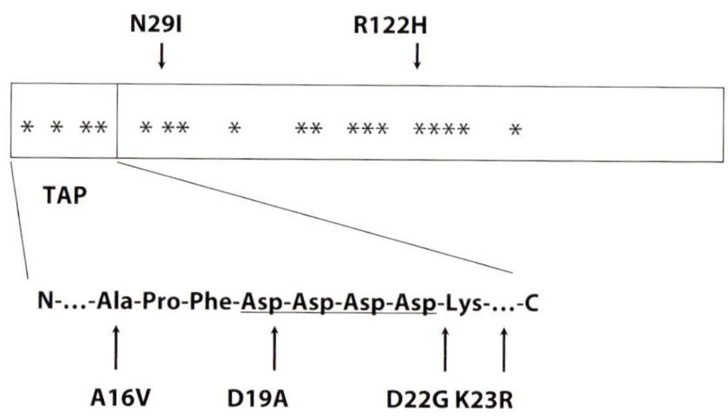

Figure 33.2

Linear map of pancreatitis associated mutations (*red*) within the primary structure of the human cationic trypsinogen. The amino-acid positions affected by the pancreatitis-associated *PRSS1* mutations are denoted by asterisks (*). The positions of the most frequent *N29I* and *R122H* mutations are indicated. The blue call-out demonstrates the sequence of the trypsinogen activation peptide (*TAP*) and the mutations found in this region. The highly conserved tetra-aspartate motif in the activation peptide is *underlined* and *bold*

trypsin activity and thereby plays a protective role against chronic pancreatitis [13]. This is the first study demonstrating a mutation with a protective effect in chronic pancreatitis.

Etiology and Biochemical Analysis of Disease-Associated PRSS1 Mutations

Classic HCP seems to follow an autosomal dominant inheritance with incomplete penetrance and highly variable disease expression. As stated above, the results of research done within the last decade implicate a more complex inheritance pattern.

The *PRSS1* mutations are located in three clusters within the trypsinogen sequence: in the trypsinogen activation peptide (TAP), in the N-terminal part of trypsin, or in the longest peptide segment not stabilized by disulfide bonds between Cys64 and Cys139 (Fig. 33.2). Thus far, all pancreatitis-associated *PRSS1* mutations discovered to date seem to cluster in the N-terminal half of the molecule encoded by exons 2 and 3. It is important to note, however, that investigation of the *PRSS1* gene in patients with suspected genetically determined chronic pancreatitis is restricted to these exons in most laboratories, and possible C-terminal mutations may have been missed.

The discovery of pancreatitis-associated cationic trypsinogen mutations in 1996 demonstrated that trypsinogen plays a central role in the pathogenesis of human pancreatitis. These mutations seem to disturb

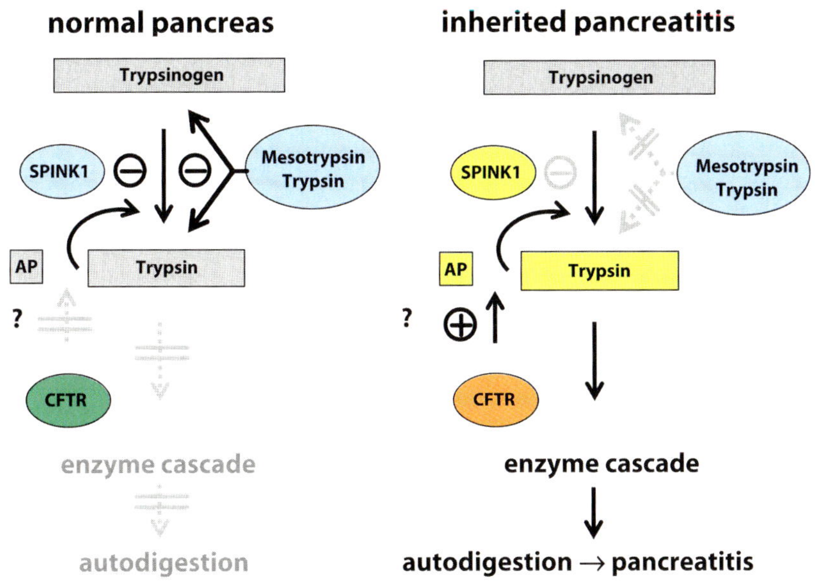

Figure 33.3

Model of inherited pancreatitis [87]. In the normal pancreas (*left*) trypsin that is prematurely activated within the pancreas is inhibited by SPINK1 and in the second line by trypsin and mesotrypsin, preventing autodigestion. In inherited pancreatitis (*right*) mutations in *PRSS1* or *SPINK1* lead to an imbalance of proteases and their inhibitors, resulting in autodigestion. Until now, the role of CFTR was poorly understood. *AP* activation peptide

the balance of proteases and their inhibitors within the pancreas, leading to autodigestion of the organ (Fig. 33.3).

The R122H and the N29I mutations are the most common *PRSS1* mutations worldwide. They have been frequently reported from Europe, North America, and Asia [56], and R122H was also recently found in a family of Aboriginal descent in Australia [57]. Neither mutation was detected in two hereditary pancreatitis families from Brazil [58] and no hereditary pancreatitis cases have been reported from Africa. Hereafter we summarize the most important genetic and biochemical data of the two common HCP-associated *PRSS1* mutations, N29I and R122H. These data are discussed more extensively in an actual review by our group [59].

R122H and Increased Trypsin Stability

David Whitcomb proposed that the Arg122–Val123 autolytic peptide bond in trypsin plays an important role in the degradation of prematurely activated trypsin in the pancreas. Disruption of this "failsafe mechanism" by the R122H mutation would increase intrapancreatic trypsin activity and disturb the protease–antiprotease equilibrium and eventually provoke pancreatitis [5]. Biochemical evidence supports the notion that Arg122 is important for autolysis of trypsin and mutations of this amino acid result in increased trypsin stability [60–63]. A study using cerulein-induced zymogen activation in isolated rat acini demonstrated that autodegradation of trypsin mitigates cathepsin-B-mediated trypsinogen activation, suggesting that a failsafe mechanism might be indeed operational in the mammalian pancreas [64]. The Whitcomb model in its original form has remained very popular over the years, even though a more detailed biochemical analysis indicated that the R122H mutation results not only in increased trypsin stability, but also in increased zymogen stability and increased autoactivation [62,63]. A weak trypsin-inhibitory activity associated with the Arg122 site is also lost in the R122H mutant [63]. Thus, the pleiotropic biochemical effect of R122H raises the possibility that the pathogenic alteration is unrelated to trypsin stability. More importantly, the model fails to explain how the other pancreatitis-associated *PRSS1* mutations might work, as the majority of these do not affect trypsin stability.

N29I and Enhanced Trypsinogen Autoactivation

Biochemical characterization of the N29I mutation using recombinant trypsinogen found no effect on trypsin or trypsinogen stability. On the other hand, two independent have laboratories observed moderately increased autoactivation in four studies [62,65–

67]. The N29T mutant, first described by Pfützer et al. in 2002, exhibited a phenotype similar to that of R122H, whereby both increased trypsin stability and enhanced autoactivation were documented [11,64]. Since increased autoactivation was observed with the R122H, N29I, and N29T mutations, whereas N29I had no effect on trypsin stability, the logical conclusion was put forth that enhanced autoactivation is the common pathogenic mechanism of hereditary pancreatitis-associated *PRSS1* mutations [62].

Animal Models

Genetically engineered animals offer the opportunity to study the effects of the aforementioned mutations in vivo. Transgenic expression of rat SPINK1 in mice reduced the severity of experimental secretagogue-induced pancreatitis [68]. The transgenic animals had 190% increased endogenous trypsin inhibition capacity. Transgenic expression of SPINK1 did not hinder trypsinogen activation, but reduced trypsin activity after supramaximal stimulation with cerulein. These in vivo results underline the hypothesis that enhanced inhibitory capacity of trypsin protects against pancreatitis.

Results from a mouse with targeted disruption of the pancreatic secretory trypsin inhibitor are puzzling [69]. A knockout (–/–) of the mouse homolog of human SPINK1, murine Spink3, is lethal within 2 weeks after birth. Spink3 –/– embryos developed normally until day 15.5 after conception. Subsequently, autophagic degeneration of the pancreatic acinar cells started, interestingly without significant inflammatory cell infiltration. In this study, the authors were not able to detect enhanced trypsin activity in the acinar cells of the SPINK –/– animals. However, in a further study, enhanced tryptic activity was found in pancreatic acini prepared 1 day after birth using a more sensitive assay [70]. Therefore, these data indicate that the total loss of SPINK3 function leads to a strong imbalance in favor of trypsin activity, resulting in acinar cell death and involution of the whole gland, and finally leading to the lethal phenotype.

Two recent publications describe transgenic animals expressing R122H-mutated trypsinogen [71,72]. Our group developed a mouse expressing R122H human trypsinogen in the exocrine pancreas by using the rat elastase-2 promoter [71]. The animals showed slightly elevated serum levels of lipase without any significant histological alteration, suggesting a subtle acinar damage. After repetitive induction of experimental pancreatitis, pancreata of transgenic animals showed a higher inflammatory reaction than controls. The mild phenotype in these animals is probably caused by a low expression level of R122H-mutated trypsinogen.

Transgenic expression of the R122H mutation of murine trypsin 4 in mouse pancreas led to progressive fibrosis and chronic inflammation of the pancreas [72]. Repetitive inductions of experimental pancreatitis with supramaximal doses of cerulein resulted in extensive deposition of collagen in periacinar and perilobular spaces of the transgenic animals. Thus, this animal model, which gives a significant expression level of R122H-mutated trypsinogen, seems to recapitulate the human disease.

In summary, the animal studies indicate that disarranging the balance between trypsin and its inhibitors in favor of a higher intra-acinar tryptic activity contributes to the development of pancreatitis.

The Trypsinogen and SPINK1 Mutation Database

Since the first description of a trypsinogen mutation in hereditary pancreatitis, the experimental and clinical information on genetic alterations in chronic pancreatitis has been growing rapidly, resulting in a more and more complex data set. To address this issue, we implemented a continuously updated database in early 2001, which contains all genetic variants of the PRSS and SPINK1 genes [73]. In addition to exact genetic data, this database contains links to the clinical characterization of patients with different mutations and to in vitro studies with mutant molecules.

Molecular Diagnostic Methods

The recommended "gold standard" method is direct DNA sequencing of both strands. Most laboratories have focused their studies on *PRSS1* exons 2 and 3, and until now no unambiguous disease-associated mutation has been identified in the other exons. However, it is still possible that new variants will be identified in exons 1, 4, and 5, or in the intronic and promoter regions. Interestingly, the triplication of a segment containing the *PRSS1* gene was found recently in patients with HCP. This triplication seems to result in a gain of trypsin through a gene dosage effect and represents a previously unknown mechanism causing HCP [74].

There are several more methods to detect *PRSS1* mutations, such as single-strand conformation polymorphism analysis, restriction fragment length polymorphism analysis (RFLP) or denaturing high performance liquid chromatography. These methods are limited by a lack of sensitivity and specificity, and since the nucleotide sequence is not detected, subsequent sequencing of the altered probe is necessary in most cases. Above all Howes et al. showed that false negative results may be obtained regarding the R122H mutation if RFLP is used with the restriction endonuclease *Afl III*, when a neutral polymorphism is present within the restriction site [75]. Melting curve analysis using fluorescence resonance energy transfer probes is a highly efficient method with a very high sensitivity and specificity; however, this only detects the defined mutation and only partly other mutations located under the probes.

Therefore, since DNA sequencing has become more affordable within the last years and is also able to detect further mutations within the amplified fragment, sequencing of both strands should be performed.

Differential Diagnosis

Well-recognized causative factors of chronic pancreatitis are anatomic anomalies, metabolic disorders, trauma, cystic fibrosis, and inflammatory bowel disease. Since HCP manifests predominantly in childhood or early adulthood, alcohol abuse as the most common predisposing condition can nearly be ruled out. One of the most important differential diagnoses is cystic fibrosis. Therefore, all patients with onset of the disease in childhood and early adulthood should be screened for a pathological sweat chloride test and subsequently for the most common *CFTR* mutations of their population. Other rare differential diagnoses are hyperlipidemia type I, familiar (hypocalciuric) hypercalcemia, hereditary hyperparathyroidism, and autoimmune pancreatitis, the latter usually manifesting in late adulthood [76–80].

Genetic Counseling and Testing

First of all, genetic counseling should be performed in an experienced multidisciplinary clinic that can address the resulting issues. Before genetic testing is performed, the implications of finding HCP-related mutations in the *PRSS1* gene for the health and the medical care of the patients should be discussed. Moreover, the elevated pancreatic cancer risk and the possible adverse effects for the patient regarding health and life insurance and employment should be brought up. Before performing the test, the form of communicating the test result should be assessed. Genetic testing should only be performed after informed consent is obtained.

The indication for *PRSS1* and *SPINK1* mutation testing in symptomatic patients should be one of the following:

1. Recurrent unexplained attacks of acute pancreatitis and a positive family history.
2. Unexplained chronic pancreatitis and a positive family history.
3. Unexplained chronic pancreatitis without a positive family history after exclusion of other causes (see differential diagnoses).
4. Unexplained pancreatitis episode in children.

Worthy of note is that genetic testing in children is a complex issue, since (depending on their age) children cannot always be included in the process of decision-making of whether genetic testing should be performed. Therefore, extensive genetic counseling illuminating the aforementioned aspects is necessary. Another important facet may be the information for anxious parents that genetic testing cannot predict the age of onset or the severity of the disease, and that the findings of the analysis do not change the management of the disease today.

Beyond the hitherto discussed aspects, the detection of *PRSS1* and *SPINK1* mutations will lead to a correct classification of the disease, helping the affected individual to better understand their disease and clearing up misclassifications (e.g., alcoholic chronic pancreatitis).

Predictive genetic testing should only be offered by a recognized service with pretest counseling, posttest support, and clinical follow-up. The persons eligible for testing should have a first-degree relative with a defined HCP gene mutation, should be able to understand the different aforementioned aspects, and the request for genetic testing should have been consistently stated [81].

We want to emphasize anew that all HCP patients or potential *PRSS1* mutation carriers should be informed that the finding of a disease-associated mutation neither predicts the onset or course of the disease nor bears specific diagnostic or therapeutic consequences.

Antenatal Diagnosis

As the penetrance of inherited *PRSS1* mutations is incomplete, and a highly variable disease manifestation occurs within most affected families, no antenatal diagnosis should be encouraged. Even in recently published guidelines concerning genetic testing in HCP the authors had reservations against antenatal diagnosis, but highlight that they cannot be so prescriptive as to refuse molecular genetic testing in an age of patient autonomy and informed consent [81]. Requesting parents should be informed that even a painful course of the disease is self-limited to only a few years in the most cases. No patients in our cohort find their life not livable due to disease-associated health limitations.

Management

No prospective randomized trial has been published for any medical or surgical problem of the management of HCP. Several case reports, but few systematic studies, have addressed the medical and surgical treatment of HCP. Generally, treatment does not differ from that for common forms of chronic pancreatitis.

In most instances treatment of chronic pancreatitis focuses on pain management, maldigestion, diabetes, pseudocysts, bile duct obstruction, duodenal obstruction, and pancreatic cancer [27,82–84]. Regarding pain management, amenable causes like pseudocysts, biliary and duodenal obstruction, and coincident peptic ulceration should be ruled out before an adequate pain therapy is started.

In order to prevent disease progression, alcohol drinking should be kept infrequent, whereas smoking should be avoided completely. In the context of pancreatic insufficiency, frequent small meals with a low fat content may help to limit pancreatic stimulation while maintaining caloric intake. Maldigestion should be treated with supplementation of pancreatic enzymes in sufficient dosage. Management of endocrine failure is carried out according to the guidelines of approved diabetes societies.

A widely accepted indication for surgery in patients with HCP is chronic pain in the presence of a persistent dilatation of the main pancreatic duct. Many surgeons favor a longitudinal pancreaticojejunostomy (Puestow procedure modified by Partington and Rochelle) with good early results.

However, in patients without pancreatic duct dilatation, the operation seems not to be beneficial for the further course of pancreatitis or for the quality of life [85]. In addition, surgical interventions should be discussed with caution in children, as periods of only a few or even no symptoms frequently extend into adulthood. For these reasons, a decision to "wait and see" might be more appropriate than early operation in pediatric patients with HCP. In adults, surgical decisions on the basis of the guidelines concerning indications for surgical treatment of patients with chronic pancreatitis of the more common underlying causes seem to be as effective in patients with HCP as in patients with chronic pancreatitis of other origins [86]. Unfortunately, there are no data regarding endoscopic procedures in the management of chronic pancreatitis patients. Therefore, prospective studies are needed to further elucidate the role of surgical and endoscopic management in chronic pancreatitis.

Prognosis

Today, the individual outcome of HCP is unpredictable. It is not yet possible to predict further episodes of acute pancreatitis, chronic bile duct obstruction, exocrine or endocrine pancreatic insufficiency, or the occurrence of pancreatic cancer.

Future Perspectives

From a genetic aspect, a most interesting quest in the near future will be for modifier genes that might explain the incomplete penetrance, for example why some carriers of *PRSS1* mutations remain healthy, whereas their relatives with the same mutation exhibit severe disease. Despite intensive research, the disease mechanism remains poorly understood. Although the biochemical alterations caused by the mutations have been largely clarified in vitro, their phenotypic effect in vivo remains unclear in most instances. In this respect, future development of cellular and animal models of HCP will be particularly valuable.

References

1. Comfort MW, Steinberg AG (1992) Pedigree of a family with hereditary chronic relapsing pancreatitis. Gastroenterology 21:54–63
2. Whitcomb DC, Preston RA, Aston CE, Sossenheimer MJ, Barua PS, Zhang Y, Wong-Chong A, White GJ, Wood PG, Gates LK Jr, Ulrich C, Martin SP, Post JC, Ehrlich GD (1996) A gene for hereditary pancreatitis maps to chromosome 7q35. Gastroenterology 110:1975–1980
3. Le Bodic L, Bignon JD, Raguenes O, Mercier B, Georgelin T, Schnee M, Soulard F, Gagne K, Bonneville F, Muller JY, Bachner L, Ferec C (1996) The hereditary pancreatitis gene maps to long arm of chromosome 7. Hum Mol Genet 5:549–554

4. Pandya A, Blanton SH, Landa B, Javaheri R, Melvin E, Nance WE, Markello T (1996) Linkage studies in a large kindred with hereditary pancreatitis confirms mapping of the gene to a 16-cM region on 7q. Genomics 1996, 38:227–230
5. Whitcomb DC, Gorry MC, Preston RA, Furey W, Sossenheimer MJ, Ulrich CD, Martin SP, Gates LK Jr, Amann ST, Toskes PP, Liddle R, McGrath K, Uomo G, Post JC, Ehrlich GD (1996) Hereditary pancreatitis is caused by a mutation in the cationic trypsinogen gene. Nat Genet 14:141–145
6. Gorry MC, Gabbaizedeh D, Furey W, Gates LK Jr, Preston RA, Aston CE, Zhang Y, Ulrich C, Ehrlich GD, Whitcomb DC (1997) Mutations in the cationic trypsinogen gene are associated with recurrent acute and chronic pancreatitis. Gastroenterology 113:1063–1068
7. Teich N, Mössner J, Keim V (1998) Mutations of the cationic trypsinogen in hereditary pancreatitis. Hum Mutat 12:39–43
8. Ferec C, Raguenes O, Salomon R, Roche C, Bernard JP, Guillot M, Quere I, Faure C, Mercier B, Audrezet MP, Guillausseau PJ, Dupont C, Munnich A, Bignon JD, Le Bodic L (1999) Mutations in the cationic trypsinogen gene and evidence for genetic heterogeneity in hereditary pancreatitis. J Med Genet 36:228–232
9. Witt H, Luck W, Becker M (1999) A signal peptide cleavage site mutation in the cationic trypsinogen gene is strongly associated with chronic pancreatitis. Gastroenterology 117: 7–10
10. Le Marechal C, Chen JM, Quere I, Raguenes O, Ferec C, Auroux J (2001) Discrimination of three mutational events that result in a disruption of the R122 primary autolysis site of the human cationic trypsinogen (PRSS1) by denaturing high performance liquid chromatography. BMC Genet 2001, 2:19
11. Pfutzer R, Myers E, Applebaum-Shapiro S, Finch R, Ellis I, Neoptolemos J, Kant JA, Whitcomb DC (2002) Novel cationic trypsinogen (PRSS1) N29T and R122C mutations cause autosomal dominant hereditary pancreatitis. Gut 50:271–272
12. Simon P, Weiss FU, Sahin-Toth M, Parry M, Nayler O, Lenfers B, Schnekenburger J, Mayerle J, Domschke W, Lerch MM (2002) Hereditary pancreatitis caused by a novel PRSS1 mutation (Arg-122->Cys) that alters autoactivation and autodegradation of cationic trypsinogen. J Biol Chem 277:5404–5410
13. Witt H, Sahin-Toth M, Landt O, Chen JM, Kahne T, Drenth JP, Kukor Z, Szepessy E, Halangk W, Dahm S, Rohde K, Schulz HU, Le Marechal C, Akar N, Ammann RW, Truninger K, Bargetzi M, Bhatia E, Castellani C, Cavestro GM, Cerny M, Destro-Bisol G, Spedini G, Eiberg H, Jansen JB, Koudova M, Rausova E, Macek M Jr, Malats N, Real FX, Menzel HJ, Moral P, Galavotti R, Pignatti PF, Rickards O, Spicak J, Zarnescu NO, Bock W, Gress TM, Friess H, Ockenga J, Schmidt H, Pfutzer R, Lohr M, Simon P, Weiss FU, Lerch MM, Teich N, Keim V, Berg T, Wiedenmann B, Luck W, Groneberg DA, Becker M, Keil T, Kage A, Bernardova J, Braun M, Guldner C, Halangk J, Rosendahl J, Witt U, Treiber M, Nickel R, Ferec C (2006) A degradation-sensitive anionic trypsinogen (PRSS2) variant protects against chronic pancreatitis. Nat Genet 38:668–673
14. Witt H, Luck W, Hennies HC, Classen M, Kage A, Lass U, Landt O, Becker M (2000) Mutations in the gene encoding the serine protease inhibitor, Kazal type 1 are associated with chronic pancreatitis. Nat Genet 25:213–216
15. Sharer N, Schwarz M, Malone G, Howarth A, Painter J, Super M, Braganza J (1998) Mutations of the cystic fibrosis gene in patients with chronic pancreatitis. N Engl J Med 339:645–652
16. Cohn JA, Friedman KJ, Noone PG, Knowles MR, Silverman LM, Jowell PS (1998) Relation between mutations of the cystic fibrosis gene and idiopathic pancreatitis. New Engl J Med 339:653–658
17. Keim V, Bauer N, Teich N, Simon P, Lerch MM, Mossner J (2001) Clinical characterization of patients with hereditary pancreatitis and mutations in the cationic trypsinogen gene. Am J Med 111:622–626
18. Sossenheimer MJ, Aston CE, Preston RA, Gates LK Jr, Ulrich CD, Martin SP, Zhang Y, Gorry MC, Ehrlich GD, Whitcomb DC (1997) Clinical characteristics of hereditary pancreatitis in a large family, based on high-risk haplotype. The Midwest Multicenter Pancreatic Study Group (MMPSG) Am J Gastroenterol 92:1113–1116
19. Sibert JR (1978) Hereditary pancreatitis in England and Wales. J Med Genet 15:189–201
20. Amann ST, Gates LK, Aston CE, Pandya A, Whitcomb DC (2001) Expression and penetrance of the hereditary pancreatitis phenotype in monozygotic twins. Gut 48:542–547
21. Howes N, Lerch MM, Greenhalf W, Stocken DD, Ellis I, Simon P, Truninger K, Ammann R, Cavallini G, Charnley RM, Uomo G, Delhaye M, Spicak J, Drumm B, Jansen J, Mountford R, Whitcomb DC, Neoptolemos JP; European Registry of Hereditary Pancreatitis and Pancreatic Cancer (EUROPAC: European Registry of Hereditary Pancreatitis and Pancreatic Cancer (2004) Clinical and genetic characteristics of hereditary pancreatitis in Europe. Clin Gastroenterol Hepatol 2:252–261
22. Singer MV, Gyr K, Sarles H (1985) Report of the Second International Symposium on the Classification of Pancreatitis in Marseille, France, March 28–30, 1984. Gastroenterology 89:683–685
23. Boeck WG, Adler G, Gress TM (2001) Pancreatic function tests: when to choose, what to use. Curr Gastroenterol Rep 3:95–100
24. Choudhurry RS, Forsmark E (2003) Review article: pancreatic function testing. Aliment Pharmacol Ther 17:733–750
25. Siegmund E, Löhr JM, Schuff-Werner P (2004) Die diagnostische Validität nicht-invasiver Pankreasfunktionstests – eine Metaanalyse. Z Gastroenterol 42:1117–1128
26. Ammann RW (2006) Diagnosis and management of chronic pancreatitis: current knowledge. Swiss Med Wkly 136:166–174
27. Etemad B, Whitcomb DC (2001) Chronic pancreatitis: diagnosis, classification, and new genetic developments. Gastroenterology 120:682–707
28. Andersen BN, Pedersen NT, Scheel J, Worning H (1982) Incidence of alcoholic chronic pancreatitis in Copenhagen. Scand J Gastroenterol 17:247–252
29. Barkin JS, Fayne SD (1986) Chronic pancreatitis: update 1986. Mt Sinai J Med 53:404–408
30. Keim V, Witt H, Bauer N, Bodeker H, Rosendahl J, Teich N, Mossner J (2003) The course of genetically determined chronic pancreatitis. JOP 4:146–154
31. Uhlig HH, Galler A, Keim V, Mossner J, Kiess W, Caca K, Teich N (2006) Regression of pancreatic diabetes in chronic hereditary pancreatitis. Diabetes Care 29:1981–1982

32. Lowenfels AB, Maisonneuve P, DiMagno EP, Elitsur Y, Gates LK Jr, Perrault J, Whitcomb DC (1997) Hereditary pancreatitis and the risk of pancreatic cancer. International Hereditary Pancreatitis Study Group. J Natl Cancer Inst 89:442–446
33. Malka D, Hammel P, Maire F, Rufat P, Madeira I, Pessione F, Levy P, Ruszniewski P (2002) Risk of pancreatic adenocarcinoma in chronic pancreatitis. Gut 51:849–852
34. Lowenfels AB, Maisonneuve P, Whitcomb DC (2000) Risk factors for cancer in hereditary pancreatitis. International Hereditary Pancreatitis Study Group. Med Clin North Am 84:565–573
35. Laskowski M, Wu FC (1953) Temporary inhibition of trypsin. J Biol Chem 204:797–805
36. Witt H, Luck W, Becker M, Bohmig M, Kage A, Truninger K, Ammann RW, O'Reilly D, Kingsnorth A, Schulz HU, Halangk W, Kielstein V, Knoefel WT, Teich N, Keim V (2001) Mutation in the SPINK1 trypsin inhibitor gene, alcohol use, and chronic pancreatitis. JAMA 285:2716–2717
37. Drenth JP, te Morsche R, Jansen JB (2002) Mutations in serine protease inhibitor Kazal type 1 are strongly associated with chronic pancreatitis. Gut 50:687–692
38. Chandak GR, Idris MM, Reddy DN, Bhaskar S, Sriram PV, Singh L (2002) Mutations in the pancreatic secretory trypsin inhibitor gene (PST1/SPINK1) rather than the cationic trypsinogen gene (PRSS1) are significantly associated with tropical calcific pancreatitis. J Med Genet 39:347–351
39. Hassan Z, Mohan V, Ali L, Allotey R, Barakat K, Faruque MO, Deepa R, McDermott MF, Jackson AE, Cassell P, Curtis D, Gelding SV, Vijayaravaghan S, Gyr N, Whitcomb DC, Khan AK, Hitman GA (2002) SPINK1 is a susceptibility gene for fibrocalculous pancreatic diabetes in subjects from the Indian subcontinent. Am J Hum Genet 71:964–968
40. Bhatia E, Choudhuri G, Sikora SS, Landt O, Kage A, Becker M, Witt H (2002) Tropical calcific pancreatitis: strong association with SPINK1 trypsin inhibitor mutations. Gastroenterology 123:1020–1025
41. Schneider A, Suman A, Rossi L, Barmada MM, Beglinger C, Parvin S, Sattar S, Ali L, Khan AK, Gyr N, Whitcomb DC (2002) SPINK1/PST1 mutations are associated with tropical pancreatitis and type II diabetes mellitus in Bangladesh. Gastroenterology 123:1026–1030
42. Kuwata K, Hirota M, Shimizu H, Nakae M, Nishihara S, Takimoto A, Mitsushima K, Kikuchi N, Endo K, Inoue M, Ogawa M (2002) Functional analysis of recombinant pancreatic secretory trypsin inhibitor protein with amino-acid substitution. J Gastroenterol 37:928–934
43. Shwachman H, Lebenthal E, Khaw W (1975) Recurrent acute pancreatitis in patients with cystic fibrosis with normal pancreatic enzymes. Pediatrics 55:86–94
44. Atlas AB, Orenstein SR, Orenstein DM (1992) Pancreatitis in young children with cystic fibrosis. J Pediatr 120:756–759
45. Cystic Fibrosis Mutation Database [http://www.genet.sickkids.on.ca/cftr]
46. Welsh M, Smith A (1993) Molecular mechanisms of CFTR chloride channel dysfunction in cystic fibrosis. Cell 73:1251–1254
47. Wilschanski M, Zielenski J, Markiewicz D, Tsui LC, Corey M, Levison H, Durie PR (1995) Correlation of sweat chloride concentration with classes of the cystic fibrosis transmembrane conductance regulator gene mutations. J Pediatr 127:705–710
48. The Cystic Fibrosis Genetic Analysis Consortium (1994) Population variation of common cystic fibrosis mutations. Hum Mutat 4:167–177
49. Castellani C, Bonizzato A, Rolfini R, Frulloni L, Cavallini GC, Mastella G (1999) Increased prevalence of mutations of the cystic fibrosis gene in idiopathic chronic and recurrent pancreatitis (letter) Am J Gastroenterol 94:1993–1995
50. Castellani C, Gomez Lira M, Frulloni L, Delmarco A, Marzari M, Bonizzato A, Cavallini G, Pignatti P, Mastella G (2001) Analysis of the entire coding region of the cystic fibrosis transmembrane regulator gene in idiopathic pancreatitis. Hum Mutat 18:166
51. Noone PG, Zhou Z, Silverman LM, Jowell PS, Knowles MR, Cohn JA (2001) Cystic fibrosis gene mutations and pancreatitis risk: relation to epithelial ion transport and trypsin inhibitor gene mutations. Gastroenterology 121:1310–1319
52. Audrezet MP, Chen JM, Le Marechal C, Ruszniewski P, Robaszkiewicz M, Raguenes O, Quere I, Scotet V, Ferec C (2002) Determination of the relative contribution of three genes – the cystic fibrosis transmembrane conductance regulator gene, the cationic trypsinogen gene, and the pancreatic secretory trypsin inhibitor gene – to the etiology of idiopathic chronic pancreatitis. Eur J Hum Genet 10:100–106
53. Weiss FU, Simon P, Bogdanova N, Mayerle J, Dworniczak B, Horst J, Lerch MM (2005) Complete cystic fibrosis transmembrane conductance regulator gene sequencing in patients with idiopathic chronic pancreatitis and controls. Gut 54:1456–1460
54. Cohn JA, Neoptolemos JP, Feng J, Yan J, Jiang Z, Greenhalf W, McFaul C, Mountford R, Sommer SS (2005) Increased risk of idiopathic chronic pancreatitis in cystic fibrosis carriers. Hum Mutat 26:303–307
55. Rohlfs EM, Zhou Z, Sugarman EA, Heim RA, Pace RG, Knowles MR, Silverman LM, Allitto BA (2002) The I148T CFTR allele occurs on multiple haplotypes: a complex allele is associated with cystic fibrosis. Genet Med 4:319–323
56. Nishimori I, Kamakura M, Fujikawa-Adachi K, Morita M, Onishi S, Yokoyama K, Makino I, Ishida H, Yamamoto M, Watanabe S, Ogawa M (1999) Mutations in exons 2 and 3 of the cationic trypsinogen gene in Japanese families with hereditary pancreatitis. Gut 44:259–263
57. McGaughran JM, Kimble R, Upton J, George P (2004) Hereditary pancreatitis in a family of Aboriginal descent. J Paediatr Child Health 40:487–489
58. Bernardino AL, Guarita DR, Mott CB, Pedroso MR, Machado MC, Laudanna AA, Tani CM, Almeida FL, Zatz M (2003) CFTR, PRSS1 and SPINK1 mutations in the development of pancreatitis in Brazilian patients. JOP 4:169–177
59. Teich N, Rosendahl J, Toth M, Mossner J, Sahin-Toth M (2006) Mutations of human cationic trypsinogen and chronic pancreatitis. Hum Mutat 27:721–730
60. Higaki JN, Light A (1986) Independent refolding of domains in the pancreatic serine proteinases. J Biol Chem 261:10606–10609
61. Gaboriaud C, Serre L, Guy-Crotte O, Forest E, Fontecilla-Camps JC (1996) Crystal structure of human trypsin 1: unexpected phosphorylation of Tyr151. J Mol Biol 259:995–1010
62. Sahin-Tóth M, Tóth M (2000) Gain-of-function mutations associated with hereditary pancreatitis enhance autoactivation of human cationic trypsinogen. Biochem Biophys Res Commun 278:286–289
63. Kukor Z, Toth M, Pal G, Sahin-Toth M (2002) Human cationic trypsinogen. Arg(117) is the reactive site of an inhibitory surface loop that controls spontaneous zymogen activation. J Biol Chem 277:6111–6117

64. Halangk W, Lerch MM, Brandt-Nedelev B, Roth W, Ruthenbuerger M, Reinheckel T, Domschke W, Lippert H, Peters C, Deussing J (2000) Role of cathepsin B in intracellular trypsinogen activation and the onset of acute pancreatitis. J Clin Invest 106:773–781
65. Sahin-Tóth M (2000) Human cationic trypsinogen. Role of Asn-21 in zymogen activation and implications in hereditary pancreatitis. J Biol Chem 275:22750–22755
66. Szilagyi L, Kenesi E, Katona G, Kaslik G, Juhasz G, Graf L (2001) Comparative in vitro studies on native and recombinant human cationic trypsins. Cathepsin B is a possible pathological activator of trypsinogen in pancreatitis. J Biol Chem 276:24574–24580
67. Teich N, Nemoda Z, Kohler H, Heinritz W, Mossner J, Keim V, Sahin-Toth M (2005) Gene conversion between functional trypsinogen genes PRSS1 and PRSS2 associated with chronic pancreatitis in a six-year-old girl. Hum Mutat 25:343–347
68. Nathan JD, Romac J, Peng RY, Peyton M, Macdonald RJ, Liddle RA (2005) Transgenic expression of pancreatic secretory trypsin inhibitor-I ameliorates secretagogue-induced pancreatitis in mice. Gastroenterology 128:717–727
69. Ohmuraya M, Hirota M, Araki M, Mizushima N, Matsui M, Mizumoto T, Haruna K, Kume S, Takeya M, Ogawa M, Araki K, Yamamura K (2005) Autophagic cell death of pancreatic acinar cells in serine protease inhibitor Kazal type 3-deficient mice. Gastroenterology 129:696–705
70. Ohmuraya M, Hirota M, Araki K, Baba H, Yamamura K (2006) Enhanced trypsin activity in pancreatic acinar cells deficient for serine protease inhibitor kazal type 3. Pancreas 33:104–106
71. Selig L, Sack U, Gaiser S, Kloppel G, Savkovic V, Mossner J, Keim V, Bodeker H (2006) Characterisation of a transgenic mouse expressing R122H human cationic trypsinogen. BMC Gastroenterology 6:30
72. Archer H, Jura N, Keller J, Jacobson M, Bar-Sagi D (2006) A mouse model of hereditary pancreatitis generated by transgenic expression of R122H trypsinogen. Gastroenterology 131:1844–55
73. Database of Genetic Variants in Patients with Chronic Pancreatitis [www.uni–leipzig.de/pancreasmutation]
74. Le Marechal C, Masson E, Chen JM, Morel F, Ruszniewski P, Levy P, Ferec C (2006) Hereditary pancreatitis caused by triplication of the trypsinogen locus. Nat Genet 38:1372–1374
75. Howes N, Greenhalf W, Rutherford S, O'Donnell M, Mountford R, Ellis I, Whitcomb D, Imrie C, Drumm B, Neoptolemos JP (2001) A new polymorphism for the R122H mutation in hereditary pancreatitis. Gut 48:247–250
76. Wilson DE (1993) Mutations in exon 3 of the lipoprotein lipase gene segregating in a family with hypertriglyceridemia, pancreatitis, and non-insulin-dependent diabetes. J Clin Invest 92:203–211
77. Trump D, Whyte MP, Wooding C, Pang JT, Pearce SH, Kocher DB, Thakker RV (1995) Linkage studies in a kindred from Oklahoma, with familial benign (hypocalciuric) hypercalcaemia (FBH) and developmental elevations in serum parathyroid hormone levels, indicate a third locus for FBH. Hum Genet 96:183–187
78. Jackson CE (1958) Hereditary hyperparathyroidism associated with recurrent pancreatitis. Ann Intern Med 49:829–836
79. Kamisawa T, Egawa N, Nakajima H, Tsuruta K, Okamoto A, Kamata N (2003) Clinical difficulties in the differentiation of autoimmune pancreatitis and pancreatic carcinoma. Am J Gastroenterol 98:2694–2699
80. Sarles H, Sarles JC, Muratore R, Guien C (1961) Chronic inflammatory sclerosis of the pancreas: an autoimmune pancreatic disease? Am J Dig Dis 6:688–698
81. Ellis I, Lerch MM, Whitcomb DC (2001) Genetic testing for hereditary pancreatitis: Guidelines for indications, counselling, consent and privacy issues. Pancreatology 1:405–415
82. Lankisch PG, Lohr-Happe A, Otto J, Creutzfeldt W (1993) Natural course in chronic pancreatitis. Pain, exocrine and endocrine pancreatic insufficiency and prognosis of the disease. Digestion 54:148–155
83. Lankisch PG, Seidensticker F, Lohr-Happe A, Otto J, Creutzfeldt W (1995) The course of pain is the same in alcohol- and non-alcohol-induced chronic pancreatitis. Pancreas 10:338–341
84. Layer P, Yamamoto H, Kalthoff L, Clain JE, Bakken LJ, DiMagno EP (1994) The different courses of early- and late-onset idiopathic and alcoholic chronic pancreatitis. Gastroenterology 107:1481–1487
85. Moir CR, Konzen KM, Perrault J (1992) Surgical therapy and long-term follow-up of childhood hereditary pancreatitis. J Pediatr Surg 27:282–286
86. Miller AR, Nagorney DM, Sarr MG (1992) The surgical spectrum of hereditary pancreatitis in adults. Ann Surg 215:39–43
87. Witt H (2003) Chronic pancreatitis and cystic fibrosis. Gut 52(Suppl II):ii34–ii41

Chapter 34

R. Jakobs · J. F. Riemann

Endoscopic Interventional Treatment

Chronic pancreatitis is an inflammatory process of the pancreas that is characterized by fibrotic and calcific changes of the gland tissue. Pain is the leading symptom and affects more than two-third of patients. The treatment of patients with symptomatic chronic pancreatitis remains a challenge for all physicians involved in their care.

Since the introduction of endoscopic retrograde cholangiopancreatography (ERCP) and endoscopic sphincterotomy endoscopic techniques rapidly advanced and are now used for the diagnosis and treatment of biliary disorders and chronic pancreatitis. Although therapeutic endoscopy is well-established for the treatment of biliary diseases, its role in the treatment of pancreatic disorders is still evolving. The limited number of prospective randomized trials and concerns over serious complications have restricted the acceptance of endoscopic techniques for pancreatic disorders in parts of the medical community. On the other hand some therapeutic options like the endoscopic drainage of pancreatic pseudocysts have gained worldwide acceptance because of their high efficacy and low complication rate.

1. Three main complications of chronic pancreatitis are indications for endoscopic interventional therapy and with will be discussed in this chapter: (1) pancreatic duct strictures and stones, (2) pancreatic pseudocysts, and (3) distal common bile-duct strictures.

Pancreatic Duct Strictures and Stones

Many of the patients with chronic pancreatitis have several changes of the pancreatic duct and its side branches. In a subgroup of patients, strictures or pancreatic duct stones obstruct the main pancreatic duct and lead to upstream dilatation. These patients may benefit from endoscopic intervention like stone removal and duct drainage (Table 34.1).

Rationale for Therapy

1. Pancreatic ductal and interstitial pressures in patients with chronic pancreatitis and a dilated duct are elevated compared with controls [1,2,3].
2. Ductal and interstitial pressure in patients with chronic pancreatitis and pain is higher than in CP patients without pain [1,4,5].
3. Elevated interstitial pancreatic pressures fall after surgical pancreatic duct drainage [6].

Table 34.1. Results of endoscopic pancreatic duct drainage in patients with chronic pancreatitis and a dominant stricture. *n.m.* Not mentioned

Author (year) [reference]	Patients (n)	Follow-up period	Clinically improved (%)
Cremer et al. 1991 [33]	75	37	94
Binmoeller et al. 1995 [34]	93	39	74
Ponchon et al. 1995 [8]	23	26	61
Smits et al. 1995 [35]	49	34	82
Boerma et al. 2000 [18]	16	51	69
Morgan et al. 2002 [36]	25	n.m.	71
Rösch et al. 2002[a] [9]	1,018	59	88
Gabrielli et al. 2005 [10]	22	72	55

[a] Multicenter survey; patients with pancreatic duct strictures and stones

4. In patients with recurrent pain, interstitial pressures are again elevated [4].
5. Endoscopic stent placement results in ductal decompression similar to what occurs after lateral pancreaticojejunostomy [4,6].
6. Compared to drainage operations, endoscopic interventions can easily be repeated if pain occurs again.

The indication for endoscopic intervention for pancreatic duct stones and strictures are [7,8]:

1. Obstruction of the main pancreatic duct in the proximal (duodenal) part of the pancreas with prestenotic (upstream) dilatation.
2. Stones or strictures in the main pancreatic duct, not only in side branches.
3. Symptomatic patient with recurrent or chronic abdominal pain not explained by extrapancreatic reason.

Procedure-Relevant Preparation

Before endoscopic intervention is performed on the pancreatic duct, other reasons for pain should be disclosed. The diagnostic work-up before intervention consists of: (1) esophagogastroduodenoscopy (EGD) to disclose a gastroduodenal ulcer, (2) imaging techniques like computed tomography (CT) scan or magnetoresonance tomography, (3) ERCP to visualize the duct morphology and to check if the stricture/stone is amenable to endoscopy, and (4) laboratory testing, including the tumor markers CA 19-9 and CEA, thrombocyte count, and coagulation parameters. If the diagnostic work-up raises the suspicion for pancreatic cancer, pancreatic resection should be discussed instead of endoscopic intervention.

Procedural Technique

The main steps are pancreatic endoscopic sphincterotomy, insertion of a pancreatic endoprosthesis, stone extraction, and lithotripsy, if required. Endoscopic intervention on the pancreas is usually performed under conscious sedation using midazolam and/or pethidine. Recently, the use of propofol has gained acceptance in many endoscopy units. Antibiotics are not generally recommended.

Endoscopic Pancreatic Sphincterotomy

This procedure is performed using a standard sphincterotome or a needle-knife sphincterotome. For safe access to the pancreatic duct, a guide wire could be introduced in the pancreatic duct via the papilla. A guide-wire sphincterotome is passed into the papilla and then the orifice of the papilla of Vater is cut for a length of about 4–8 mm in the 1- to 2-o'clock position. Some endoscopists prefer the use of pure cutting current at the pancreatic duct to reduce the risk of pancreatitis (due to swelling of the papillary tissue).

Pancreatic Duct Endoprosthesis

Dominant strictures are drained by insertion of a pancreatic endoprosthesis. Endoprosthesis insertion is performed in the standard fashion, similar to biliary stent placement. A guide wire is introduced in the major pancreatic duct through the stenosis and then a plastic prosthesis is placed for drainage by advancing a pushing catheter. Most of the study groups publishing on pancreatic duct intervention prefer a programmed prosthesis placement therapy. Endoprostheses are changed every 3rd month and the complete treatment duration is about 12–18 months [8,9]. In a recently published trial on endoscopic treatment for chronic pancreatitis, plastic stents were changed on-demand only with good clinical results [10].

Bougienage

If the stricture is very tight, bougienage is performed before endoprosthesis placement as an ancillary therapy. Dilatation catheters are passed through the stenosis over a guide wire. The outer diameter of the dilation catheters is 5–10 Fr, depending on the stenosis. A technical alternative is the use of a stent retriever for stricture ablation, which is turned through the stenosis, thereby removing the stricture tissue [11].

Removal of Stones in the Pancreas

If stones are located in the pancreatic head or proximal body of the pancreas they can be removed with the aid of baskets or balloons. Specially designed dormia baskets – smaller diameter than for biliary stone removal – are introduced into the pancreatic duct after sphincterotomy. The basket is opened in the duct, the stone is entrapped and then pulled out. The baskets used should be ready for mechanical lithotripsy to allow fragmentation of the stone if it could not pass through a stenosis or the papillary orifice. The best treatment results are reported for single stones with a maximal outer diameter below 10 mm.

If stones are larger or multiple, the extraction is more difficult, and more sophisticated lithotripsy techniques are mandatory. Extracorporeal shock wave lithotripsy (ESWL) is successful for stone fragmentation in 55–99% of cases and results in a stone-free duct in about 42–75% of patients (in combination with endoscopic stone removal) [12,13].

Lithotripsy

Many of the patients with symptomatic chronic pancreatitis have a complex duct morphology with strictures and stones. In these patients a combination of lithotripsy techniques, stone removal and drainage procedures using plastic stents are needed.

Early Postinterventional Course

After pancreatic sphincterotomy and intervention on duct patients, severe complications are not frequent. Bleeding after sphincterotomy can usually be stopped by means of endoscopy. Intervention on the pancreatic duct in patients with chronic pancreatitis can result in an acute bout of pancreatitis. The risk of acute pancreatitis in this special setting, however, is reported to be lower than the risk after endoscopic sphincterotomy in patients without chronic pancreatitis, and severe pancreatitis with systemic response is rare [14,15]. If the postinterventional course is free of complications, patients can usually eat and drink on the same day and are discharged from hospital on the same or following day.

Long-Term Outcome After Endoscopic Intervention for Pancreatic Duct Strictures and Stones

A lot of retrospective series and several prospective nonrandomized studies on endoscopic pancreatic duct drainage and stone removal have been published in the past 10 years. In several series with a follow-up period ranging from 37 to 72 months 55–88% of the patients had a significant improvement of pain. Pain relapses can be treated successfully by recurrent endoscopic interventions [8–10,16–18].

The first and only randomized study comparing surgery and endoscopy for the treatment of chronic pancreatitis was published recently from Dite et al. [19]. They randomized 72 patients for surgical intervention (80% pancreatic resection; 20% drainage operation) or endoscopy (sphincterotomy; 52%endosocpic duct drainage and 23%stone extraction). After 5 years of follow up in the randomized subgroup, results were similar (complete pain relief: 34% in the surgical cohort and 15% in the endoscopic cohort; partial pain relief in 52% vs. 46%, respectively). This study demonstrates a (nonsignificant) advantage for complete pain relief after surgery, but in the patients treated by means of endoscopy, repeat endoscopic interventions were not allowed and ESWL was not part of the treatment plan for pancreatic duct stones.

Learning from these data we have to keep in mind that the proper selection of patients for endoscopic intervention is demanding and the possible need and option for repeated intervention should be a topic of discussion with the patient preceding commencement of the treatment. Surgery, however, remains an option after endoscopic intervention.

On the other hand, the data for the surgical candidates in the study published by Dite et al. [19] demonstrate that only one-third of the patients were completely pain-free after 5 years. In addition, for patients with pain recurrence after pancreatic head resection, endoscopic intervention is impossible due to the postoperative anatomy.

Endoscopic Drainage of Pancreatic Pseudocysts

Pancreatic pseudocysts are diagnosed in 20–40% of patients with chronic pancreatitis. Most of these pseudocysts are asymptomatic and do not require therapy [20]. Endoscopic pseudocyst drainage is indicated if patients suffer from complications like abdominal pain, jaundice due to compression of the bile duct, or enteric obstruction, depending on the size and location of the pseudocyst [20,21].

Endoscopic drainage of pancreatic pseudocyst is contraindicated if larger vessels are in the drainage site and cannot safely be passed. If a pseudocyst is not creating an obvious bulge, transmural drainage should not be performed without endoscopic ultrasound (EUS) for safety reasons. Complex pseudocysts that are multiseptated, associated with necrosis, or associated with totally disrupted main pancreatic duct are less amenable to endoscopic drainage. Infection of a pseudocyst is not a contraindication to endoscopy [22].

Procedure-Relevant Preparation

Laboratory testing should contain blood cell count (required thrombocyte count >50,000/μl) and coagulation check (international normalized ratio>1.5). The following endoscopic/imaging procedures are recommended before endoscopic treatment.

Abdominal ultrasound or CT scan should demonstrate the diameter and localization of the fluid containing cavity and its relation to neighboring structures. A Doppler scan of the pseudocyst lumen should be performed to exclude a vascular malformation (e. g., pseudoaneurysm of the splenic artery), which might be misinterpreted as a pseudocyst.

EGD should diagnose if the pseudocyst bulges into the gastric or duodenal lumen, and an ERCP is performed to exclude/diagnose a connection between the pseudocyst lumen and the pancreatic duct and to check if there is a stricture in the main pancreatic duct as the cause of pseudocyst formation

EUS is strongly recommended before transmural drainage. It gives the option for a more precise delineation of the anatomic structure and may reduce the risk of bleeding by excluding larger vascular structures in the intended way for drainage [23].

Technique of Pseudocyst Drainage

Endoscopic drainage of pseudocysts can be performed transpapillary or transmurally from the stomach or proximal duodenum. Transpapillary drainage of a pancreatic pseudocyst is intended if the cavity communicates with the pancreatic duct. For this type of drainage, pancreatic endoscopic sphincterotomy is performed and than a pancreatic duct endoprosthesis is placed via a pancreatic duct stricture to alleviate outflow of the content from the pseudocyst. The plastic stent can be removed after some weeks in most of the patients depending on the size of the pseudocyst. Transpapillary placement of a nasocystic drainage is an alternative preferred by some authors. A small-caliber (5 or 6 Fr) catheter is placed in the pseudocyst over a guide wire via the papilla and left in situ for 2 days to 2 weeks depending on the regression of the cavity. Via the nasocystic drain it is possible to suck the content from the cyst lumen and to perform a lavage. At the end of treatment the nasocystic drain is removed easily without additional endoscopy.

If the pseudocyst lumen is not communicating with the pancreatic duct and/or bulges the gastric or duodenal lumen transmural endoscopic cystoenterostomy is performed.

Transmural drainage can be performed via a standard endoscope or a therapeutic EUS-scope with a large working channel (Fig. 34.1). After disclosure of vessels in the planned drainage way a modified needle-knife catheter is used to create a fistula between the stomach/duodenum and the pseudocyst. A guide wire is introduced into the pseudocyst to maintain access immediately after puncture. Once the access is assured (e.g., endosonographically) a catheter can be advanced to inject contrast media into the pseudocyst lumen. If the proper placement of the catheter is proven, the fistula tract can be dilated by using a balloon dilator. The use of a needle knife or a standard sphincterotome to extend the small opening is under debate because of the risk of hemorrhage.

After creating a large fistula, the contents of the pseudocyst egress from the cavity. One or (typically) two double-pigtail-prostheses with an outer diameter of 7 Fr or preferably 10 Fr are placed via the guide wire. One end of the stent is allowed to deploy in the cavity, while the other end pigtails in the lumen of the stomach or duodenum. If a pseudoycst is infected or contains a large amount of debris, a nasocystic drain can be placed additionally alongside the pigtail in the cavity to allow lavage.

The duration of stenting depends on the size and the location of pseudocyst, the presence of infection, and the underlying pancreatic duct morphology. Typically, the pigtail stents are left in situ for 4–6 weeks until an abdominal ultrasound scan has demonstrated that the pseudocyst has resolved [24].

Early Postinterventional Course

Pre- and postprocedural application of a broad-spectrum antibiotic is recommended to decrease the risk of pseudocyst infection, especially if pancreatic necrosis is present. If the drainage is working well, the risk of cavity infection seems to be low. The main risks of pseudocyst drainage are hemorrhage from the fistula tract, perforation of the enteric wall, and infection of the pseudocyst cavity in case of endoprosthesis occlusion.

Long-Term Outcome of Pseudocyst Drainage

Complete resolution of pancreatic pseudocysts was demonstrated in 81–97% of the patients in several clinical studies with medium- to long-term follow up [20,24,25]. The reported recurrence rate after pseudo-

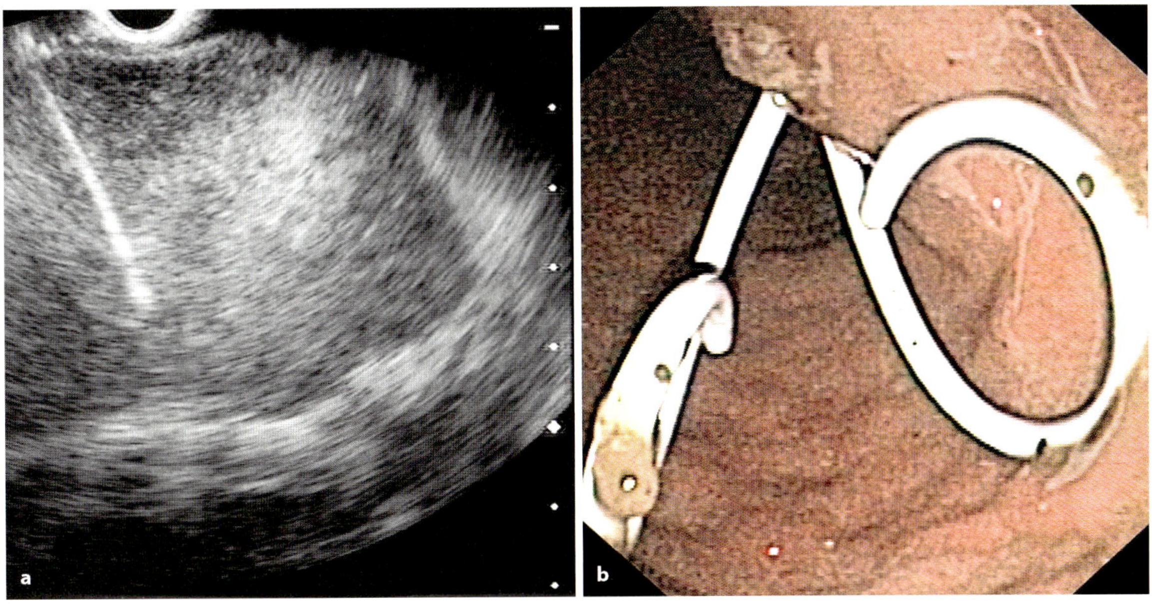

Figure 34.1

Endosonography-guided drainage of a large infected pseudocyst. a Placement of the guide wire into the pseudocyst. b After transmural insertion of two pigtail-endoprostheses

cyst drainage ranged from 6% to 16%. Most of the symptomatic pseudocyst recurrences were treated successfully by means of repeated endoscopy.

Treatment of Bile-Duct Strictures due to Chronic Pancreatitis

The incidence of common bile duct obstruction among patients hospitalized with chronic pancreatitis ranges from 3 to 23% with a mean of 6%, if the pancreatic head is involved in the inflammatory process the incidence of bile duct stricture is reported to be about 60% [7]. After the first successful insertion of a biliary endoprosthesis by Reynders-Frederix and Soehendra in 1978, this technique emerged worldwide as a standard therapy in endoscopy units for malignant bile duct obstruction.

The long-term data for endoscopic drainage of bile duct strictures due to chronic pancreatitis are disappointing, with a reported success rate of 10–30%. The long-term success rate of surgical drainage compares favorably with the results of endoscopy, therefore surgery is recommended as the treatment of first choice for surgical candidates [26,27].

Possible Indications for Endoscopic Bile Duct Drainage

1. Cholangitis evidenced by symptoms or infected bile.
2. Persistent jaundice.
3. Elevation of cholestasis parameters (alkaline phosphatase, three times normal levels or more) and biopsy evidence of biliary cirrhosis.
4. Presence of associated common bile duct stones.

Preprocedural Diagnostic Work-up

Abdominal ultrasound to demonstrate the dilatation of the extrahepatically (and intraheptically) located bile ducts, the stenosis in the distal common bile duct, do disclose bile duct stones and liver cirrhosis. Laboratory testing should include serum bilirubin level, alkaline phosphatase, alanine aminotransferase and aspartate aminotransferase, blood cell count and coagulation parameters.

If endoscopic drainage is planned, retrograde cholangiography should be performed, followed by endoprosthesis insertion during the same session. If endoscopic drainage is under discussion only, magnetic resonance cholangiography (MRC) is preferred, to minimize the risk for cholangitis.

Endoscopic biliary drainage is performed by placing a polyethylene or Teflon endoprosthesis into the bile duct to bypass the stricture. Prior to drainage a endoscopic biliary sphincterotomy is recommended to alleviate the introduction of the stent. Placement of a bile duct endoprosthesis is performed in a standard fashion via a guide wire (see Pancreatic Duct Strictures and Stones). Straight Amsterdam-type endoprostheses are preferred for stenting. The outer diameter of the biliary endoprostheses 7–11.5 Fr. In general, a programmed exchange every 3rd month is recommended to prevent acute cholangitis due to stent clogging.

Early Postinterventional Course

Early complications are in most cases sequelae of endoscopic sphincterotomy (bleeding, acute pancreatitis, and perforation). Early stent clogging may lead to acute cholangitis or recurrence of jaundice during the first days after the procedure. Complications due to stent exchanges without endoscopic sphincterotomy are rare. If the endoscopic intervention is performed without complications the patient can start to drink and eat on the same day and is discharged on the same evening or after one night in the hospital.

Long-Term Results of Endoscopic Biliary Drainage in Chronic Pancreatitis

The short-term results of biliary endoprosthesis placement are excellent. The insertion of a biliary stent will result in normalization of the cholestasis parameters in almost all patients within days. An acute cholangitis is treated very effectively.

Long-term results of biliary drainage are less favorable. Occlusion or dislocation of endoprostheses were frequently seen in several studies in up to 30% of patients. Normalization of the bile duct stricture itself is rare, with a reported rate of 10–23% of the patients. Therefore, most of the patients would be candidates for a lifelong stent-exchange program.

The compliance of patients is one of the limiting factors for this treatment. Many patients with chronic pancreatitis have alcohol consumption problems. If they were enrolled in a scheduled stent-exchange program they often miss the day of exchange, and the risk of stent occlusion and septic cholangitis rises with the stent duration. In one study, a mortality rate of up to 10% is reported due to septic cholangitis [27].

Metal stent placement has a significantly lower occlusion rate in short- and medium-term follow up. In the long-run, most of the stents will occlude due to mucosal hyperplasia in the stent and then placement of a biliary plastic stent in the metal stent is necessary to overcome the stent stenosis [28].

Three recently published studies on plastic stent placement for common bile duct strictures due to chronic pancreatitis demonstrate favorable results if multiple plastic stents (up to six stents) are inserted and drainage therapy is performed over a 12- to 18-month period, with stent exchanges every 3rd month. This multistenting approach resulted in a sufficient dilatation of the bile duct stricture in up to 60% of patients. The long-term results of this approach have only recently been presented, and therefore multistenting cannot be recommended in general [29–36]. To conclude, drainage of distal bile duct strictures should be considered for surgical intervention. In patients who are not candidates for surgery, endoscopic drainage is the method of choice, and has a very high short-term success rate. Long-term results for biliary drainage are less favorable due to stent occlusion and septic cholangitis.

References

1. Bradley EL (1982) Pancreatic duct pressure in chronic pancreatitis. Am J Surg 144:313–316
2. Ebbehoj N, Borly L, Bulow J, Rasmussen SG, Madsen P (1990) Evaluation of pancreatic tissue fluid pressure and pain in chronic pancreatitis. A longitudinal study. Scand J Gastroenterol 25:462–464
3. Madsen P, Winkler K (1982) The intraductal pancreatic pressure in chronic obstructive pancreatitis. Scand J Gastroenterol 17:553–554
4. Ebbehoj N, Borly L, Bulow J, Rasmussen SG, Madsen P, Matzen P, et al (1990) Pancreatic tissue fluid pressure in chronic pancreatitis. Relation to pain, morphology, and function. Scand J Gastroenterol 25:1046–1051
5. Novis BH, Bormann PC, Girdwood AW, Marks IN (1985) Endoscopic manometry of the main pancreatic duct and sphincter zone in patients with chronic pancreatitis. Dig Dis Sci 30:225–228
6. Karanija ND, Widdison AL, Alvarez C, Lutrin FJ, Reber HA (1994) Compartment syndrome in experimental chronic obstructive pancreatitis: effect of decompressing the main pancreatic duct. Br J Surg 81:259–264
7. Vijungco JD, Prinz RA (2003) Management of biliary and duodenal complications of chronic pancreatitis. World J Surg 27:1258–1270
8. Ponchon T, Bory RM, Hedelius F, Roubein LD, Paliard P, Napoleon B, et al (1995) Endoscopic stenting for pain relief in chronic pancreatitis: results of a standardized protocol. Gastrointest Endosc 42:452–456

9. Rösch T, Daniel S, Scholz M, Huibregtse K, Smits S, Schneider T, et al (2002) Endoscopic treatment of chronic pancreatitis: a multicenter study of 1000 patients with long-term follow-up. Endoscopy 34:756–761
10. Gabrielli A, Pandolfi M, Mutignani M, Spada C, Perri V, Petruzziello L, Costamagna G (2005) Efficacy of main pancreatic-duct endoscopic drainage in patients with chronic pancreatitis and pain. Gastrointest Endosc 61:576–581
11. Ziebert JJ, DiSario JA (1999) Dilation of refractory pancreatic duct strictures: the turn of the screw. Gastrointest Endosc 49:632–635
12. Guda NM, Partington S, Freeman ML (2005) Extracorporeal shock wave lithotripsy in the management of chronic calcific pancreatitis: a meta-analysis. JOP 6:6–12
13. Kozarek RA, Brandabur JJ, Ball TJ,Gluck M, Patterson DJ, Attia F, France R, Traverso W, Koslowski P, Gibbons RP (2002)Clinical outcomes in patients who undergo extracorporeal shockwave lithotripsy for chronic calcific pancreatitis. Gastrointest Endosc 56:496–500
14. Ell C, Rabenstein T, Schneider HT, Ruppert T, Nicklas M, Bulling D (1998) Safety and efficacy of pancreatic sphincterotomy in chronic pancreatitis. Gastrointest Endosc 48:244–249
15. Jakobs R, Benz C, Leonhardt A, Schilling D, Pereira-Lima JC, Riemann JF (2002) Pancreatic endoscopic sphincterotomy in patients with chronic pancreatitis: a single-center experience in 171 consecutive patients. Endoscopy 34:551–554
16. Hammarström LE, Stridbeck H, Ihse I (1997) Endoscopic drainage in benign pancreatic disease: immediate and medium term outcome. Br J Surg 163:577–589
17. Delhaye M, Arvanitakis M, Verset G, Cremer M, Deviere J (2004) Long-term clinical outcome after endoscopic pancreatic ductal drainage for patients with painful chronic pancreatitis. Clin Gastroenterol Hepatol 2:96–106
18. Boerma D, Huibregtse K, Gulik TM, Rauws EA, Obertop H, Gouma DJ (2000) Long-term outcome of endoscopic stent placement for chronic pancreatitis associated with pancreas divisum. Endoscopy 32:452–456
19. Dite P, Ruzicka M, Zboril V, Novotny I (2003) A prospective randomised trial comparing endoscopic with surgical therapy for chronic pancreatitis. Endoscopy 35:553–558
20. Andren-Sandberg A, Dervenis C (2004) Pancreatic pseudocysts in the 21st century. Part II: natural history. JOP 5:64–70
21. Baillie J (2004) Pancreatic pseudocysts (Part II). Gastrointest Endosc 60:105–113
22. Lehman GA (2002) Role of ERCP and other endoscopic modalities in chronic pancreatitis. Gastrointest Endosc 56(Suppl):S237–240
23. Giovannini M (2005) Endoscopic ultrasound-guided pancreatic pseudocyst drainage. Gastrointest Endosc Clin N Am 15:179–188
24. Baillie J (2004) Pancreatic pseudocysts (Part I). Gastrointest Endosc 59:873–879
25. Vetter S, Weickert U, Jakobs R, Schilling D, Siegel E, Riemann JF (2003) Endoscopic drainage of symptomatic pancreatic pseudocysts. An efficient and safe therapy in the clinical routine? Dtsch Med Wochenschr 128:2355–2359
26. Eickhoff A, Jakobs R, Leonhardt A, Eickhoff JC, Riemann JF (2001) Endoscopic stenting for common bile duct stenoses in chronic pancreatitis: results and impact on long-term outcome. Eur J Gastroenterol Hepatol13:1161–1167
27. Kiehne K, Folsch UR, Nitsche R (2000) High complication rate of bile duct stents in patients with chronic alcoholic pancreatitis due to noncompliance. Endoscopy 32:377–380
28. Cahen DL, van Berkel AM, Oskam D, Rauws EA, Weverling GJ, Huibregtse K, Bruno MJ (2005) Long-term results of endoscopic drainage of common bile duct strictures in chronic pancreatitis. Eur J Gastroenterol Hepatol 17:103–108
29. Eickhoff A, Jakobs R, Leonhardt A, Eickhoff JC, Riemann JF (2003) Self-expandable metal mesh stents for common bile duct stenosis in chronic pancreatitis: retrospective evaluation of long-term follow-up and clinical outcome pilot study. Z Gastroenterol 41:649–654
30. Draganov P, Hoffman B, Marsh W, Cotton P, Cunningham J (2002) Long-term outcome in patients with benign biliary strictures treated endoscopically with multiple stents. Gastrointest Endosc 55:680–686
31. Catalano MF, Linder JD, George S, Alcocer E, Geenen JE (2004) Treatment of symptomatic distal common bile duct stenosis secondary to chronic pancreatitis: comparison of single vs. multiple simultaneous stents. Gastrointest Endosc 60:945–952
32. Pozsar J, Sahin P, Laszlo F, Forro G, Topa L (2004) Medium-term results of endoscopic treatment of common bile duct strictures in chronic calcifying pancreatitis with increasing numbers of stents. J Clin Gastroenterol 38:118–123
33. Cremer M, Deviere J, Delhaye M, Baize M, Vandermeeren A (1991) Stenting in severe chronic pancreatitis; results of medium term follow-up in 76 patients. Endoscopy 23:171–176
34. Binmoeller KF, Jue P, Seifert H, Nam WC, Izbicki J, Soehendra N (1995) Endoscopic pancreatic stent drainage in chronic pancreatitis and a dominant stricture: long term results. Endoscopy 27:638–644
35. Smits M, Badiga SM, Rauws EAJ, Tytgat GNJ, Huibregtse K (1995) Long term results of pancreatic stents in chronic pancreatitis. Gastrointest Endosc 42:461–467
36. Morgan DE, Smith JK, Kidaday M, Wilcox CM (2003) Endoscopic stent therapy in advanced chronic pancreatitis: relationships between ductal changes, clinical response, and stent patency. Am J Gastroenterol 98:821–826

Chapter 35

H. G. Beger · B. Poch

Indication to Surgical Treatment of Chronic Pancreatitis

In industrialized countries, two-thirds of patients suffer from chronic alcoholic pancreatitis, 20% from idiopathic chronic pancreatitis, and <10% from hereditary chronic pancreatitis. It is believed that chronic alcoholic pancreatitis is a consequence of recurrent attacks of acute pancreatitis causing small areas of pancreatic necrosis, which lead to tissue granulation and fibrosis [1]. Chronic pancreatitis is a disease of the exocrine pancreatic tissue compartment, which, in the late course, extends to the endocrine tissue. In the majority of patients it develops after a preclinical period of 3–12 years, with upper abdominal pain being the first sign of disease. Continuous alcohol consumption and cigarette smoking enhances the progression of chronic pancreatitis. In the late stage, local complications are caused by a progressive inflammatory process. In addition to severe medically intractable upper abdominal pain, morbidity is characterized in about 30–50% by the development of an inflammatory mass in the head of the pancreas, by common bile duct stenosis in 30%, and by the development of large pseudocysts, severe stenosis of the duodenum, portal vein compression, portal vein and splenic vein occlusion/thrombosis, and most frequently by pancreatic main duct and side branch stenoses (Table 35.1) [2].

Table 35.1. Frequency of local complications of chronic pancreatitis

Pancreatic pseudocysts (>4–6 cm)	15–25%
Common bile duct stenosis	30–50%
Severe stenosis of the duodenum	7%
Compression/occlusion of portal/superior mesenteric vein	8–15%
Splenic vein thrombosis	3–5%
Pancreatic fistula	<5%
Pancreatic abscess	3%
Chronic pancreatitis + pancreatic cancer	3–6%
Pancreatic tissue necrosis	<5%

The Head of the Pancreas – Pacemaker of Chronic Pancreatitis?

In 30–50% of hospitalized patients with chronic pancreatitis, radiological data (contrast-enhanced computed tomography) reveal an inflammatory tumor in the pancreatic head. The inflammatory mass in the head of the pancreas causes stenosis of the common bile duct, the duodenum, and the portal vein [3]. For details of the natural course of chronic pancreatitis, please refer to Chap. 28.

Indication to Surgical Treatment

Surgery of the pancreas is in any case a palliative treatment; the aims of surgical treatment of chronic pancreatitis are pain relief and the control of pancreatitis-associated complications of adherent tissues and organs. Preservation of exocrine and endocrine pancreatic functions is a major goal of surgical treatment. Since most of the patients with chronic pancreatitis are relatively young and professionally active, social and occupational rehabilitation and improve-

Table 35.2. Indication to surgical treatment for chronic pancreatitis

1.	Upper abdominal pain refractory to medical treatment (daily pain)
2.	Inflammatory mass of the pancreatic head
3.	Stenosis of the intrapancreatic common bile duct
4.	Multiple narrowing of the pancreatic main duct
5.	Compression of the portal and/ or superior mesenteric vein
6.	Severe stenosis of the peripapillary duodenum
7.	Large persisting pancreatic/peripancreatic pseudocyst after interventional/ endoscopic treatment
8.	Inflammatory process suspected to be associated with a malignant process

ment of quality of life are long-term goals. Most of the patients decide to change from medical pain management to surgical treatment because of severe pain in spite of strong analgesic medication. Upper abdominal pain refractory to medical treatment in combination with local complications is most frequently suggestive for surgical treatment (Table 35.2).

Surgical Procedures

Table 35.3 lists the current established surgical techniques. Patients who suffer from chronic pancreatitis with dilatation of the pancreatic main duct to >7 mm without side-duct stenosis are candidates for a duct drainage procedure using a pancreatic-duct-to-jejunum anastomosis or the coring out technique of the pancreatic head in combination with the duct drainage procedure introduced by Frey. However, the long-term pain relief achieved after pancreatic duct drainage by pancreaticojejunostomosis is disappointing. About 25–45% of patients who undergo pancreatic duct drainage procedures have unsatisfactory long-term results with recurrence of abdominal pain associated with reoccurrence of a severe abdominal pain pattern (Table 35.4). Experience with repeated surgery after failure to control pain following pancreatic duct drainage surgery has revealed that an inflammatory mass in the head of the pancreas is the source of the pain recurrence, head resection has resulted in a pain-free status. Pain recurrence after the coring out technique of Frey has been reported to occur in 15–20% of cases [22–24]. Surgical main duct drainage in case with highly established side branch stenosis do not lead to a complete decompression of the ductal system with emptying of pancreatic juice into the jejunal loop.

Duodenum-preserving pancreatic head resection has become a standard surgical procedure in patients who have an inflammatory mass in the head of the pancreas. The major advantage of duodenum-preserving pancreatic head resection are the maintenance of duodenum, stomach, biliary tree, and endocrine function [25–30]. However, in cases in which an association exists between inflammatory mass of the head of the pancreas and a ductal pancreatic adeno-

Table 35.3. Surgical procedures for the treatment of chronic pancreatitis

Duct drainage	**Partington-Rochelle procedure [4]**
	Coring out procedure of Frey [5]
	Pseudocystojejunostomy
Organ preserving resection	**Duodenum preserving pancreatic head resection [6]**
	Spleen preserving left resection
	Middle segment resection [7]
Major resection	**Pylorus-preserving pancreatic head resection (Traverso-Longmayr) [8]**
	(Total duodenum preserving pancreatectomy)
	Splanchnicectomy (thoracal)
Historical	Whipple resection
	Puestov procedure
	Total duodenopancreatectomy
	Bypass procedure

Table 35.4. Pain relief and failure of pain treatment after pancreatic duct drainage by pancreaticojejunostomy: long-term results (>5-year follow up). Experience from 13 publications (*n*=582 patients in total) [9–21]

	Complete pain relief	Pain but improved	Failure of pain control	Unsatisfactory long-term results
582 patients	55%	25%	20%	45%

Table 35.5. Application of surgical procedures in chronic pancreatitis – experience of the Departments of Surgery at the University of Ulm (May 1982–September 2001) and the Free University of Berlin (November 1972–April 1982). *DPPHR* Duodenum-preserving pancreatic head resection, *PPPHR* pylorus-preserving pancreatic head resection

Duct Drainage[b] (*n*)	Left resection[b] (*n*)	DPPHR[a] (*n*)	PPPHR[b] (*n*)	Others[b] (*n*)	Kausch Whipple[b]
121	83	548	78	12	63
13%	9%	61%	9%	1%	7%

[a] November 1972–April 1982 Free University Berlin
[b] 05/ 82 – 09/ 01 Dep. of General Surgery, University of Ulm

Table 35.6. Surgery for chronic pancreatitis – selection of procedures determined by pathomorphological criteria of the pancreas. *CP* Chronic pancreatitis, *IMH* inflammatory mass in the head of the pancreas, *PMD* pancreatic main duct

CP + PMD dilatation without side-branch stenoses absence of IMH	Duct drainage procedure: Partington-Rochelle: Frey modification
CP + IMH	Duodenum-preserving pancreatic head resection
CP + IMH suspected to be malignant lesion	Pylorus preserving pancreatoduodenectomy
Pancreas divisum + CP	Duodenum-preserving pancreatic head resection

carcinoma, which has been described to develop in 4–6% of patients, a duodenum-preserving pancreatic head resection will lead to unsatisfactory late results. In patients with a tumor in the pancreatic head suspected to be a malignant lesion, an oncological resection using the pylorus-preserving pancreatic head resection has to be used [31]. A total duodenum- and spleen-preserving pancreatectomy is rarely indicated; only patients suffering medically refractory, abdominal pain episodes and are diabetic will have a long-term benefit. The application of a classical Whipple procedure is a rather historical procedure. For patients with chronic pancreatitis, the Whipple procedure is a superfluous treatment since the preservation of the duodenum, the biliary tree, and the stomach can be performed using duodenum-preserving pancreatic head resection. Furthermore, in about 20% of cases, the Whipple resection results in a status of diabetes mellitus in the immediate early postoperative period. The frequency of the surgical procedures used in the Departments of General Surgery in Ulm and Berlin over a period of 28 years is given in Table 35.5. The indication to a surgical procedure for chronic pancreatitis is determined by the specific pathomorphological changes of the pancreas. As displayed in Table 35.6, the duct pathomorphology and the presence or absence of an inflammatory mass of the head of the pancreas are the main criteria for the use of a duct drainage or a resective procedure.

Endotherapy or Surgery in Chronic Pancreatitis?

Endotherapy for obstructive chronic pancreatitis has been reported by several recent studies with good results. However, these studies are retrospective, including a selected group of patients with chronic pancreatitis. With regard to the long-term treatment of the pain syndrome in chronic pancreatitis, only a very few retrospective data have been published [23–36]. Data from a retrospective multicenter analysis have been reported long-term pain improvement; however a decreasing number of pain-free patients have been observed [32]. Sphincterectomy and stenting of the pancreatic main duct is a temporary treatment with a high risk for stent occlusion and the need for restenting [35]. Surgical reports of duct pathomorphology after periods of duct stenting of chronic pancreatitis documented an enhancement of the chronic inflammatory process in the stent region of the pancreatic duct [37]. Endoscopic extraction of pancreatic duct stones entails fragmentation of the tissue-anchored stones and results mostly in an incomplete recanalization. Disappointing results are reported using extracorporeal shock-wave treatment of pancreatic main duct stones.

Data from two prospective, randomized, single-institution trial in which endotherapy and surgical therapy were compared has been published recently

[38, 39]. The short-term pain relief was similar in both groups. However, in terms of the long-term outcome, significant differences between both treatment modalities have been found. After a 5-year follow up, complete absence of pain was observed significant more frequently in the surgical group than in the endotherapy group (34% vs. 15%). The increase in body weight was greater by 20–25% in the surgical group. New onset of diabetes developed in 34% of the surgical group and in 43% of the endotherapy group.

In patients with chronic pancreatitis, dilatation of the pancreatic main duct, and absence of multiple stenosis of the main duct and the side branches of the duct system, stenting can be regarded as the first choice. However, after recurrence of pain or duct occlusion, a surgical procedure is more effective to control local complications and the level of pancreatitis-induced abdominal pain. The long-term results in regard to pain control favors surgical treatment but not endless restenting. Surgical treatment of chronic pancreatitis, using duodenum-preserving pancreatic head resection, has been reported to result in a high percentage of patients with a pain-free status after 5 years. The pain-free status of patients who underwent a surgical duct drainage procedure using the Partington-Rochelle procedure or the Frey modification was disappointing, since about 40–50% of the patients regained a pain syndrome, and about 20–25% of the failures had reoccurrence of the same level of abdominal pain that they had experienced prior to surgical treatment. Duct drainage, whether performed by surgical technique or duct stenting, is ineffective for half of the patients with advanced chronic pancreatitis and severe pain.

References

1. Klöppel G, Maillet B (1991) Chronic pancreatitis: evolution of the disease. Hepatogastroenterology 38:408–412
2. Beger HG, Büchler M, Bittner R, Oettinger W, Roscher R (1989) Duodenum-preserving resection of the head of the pancreas in severe chronic pancreatitis. Early and late results. Ann Surg 209:273–278
3. Beger HG, Schlosser W, Poch B, Gansauge F (1998) Inflammatory mass in the head of pancreas. In: Beger HG, Warshaw AL, Carr-Locke D, Russell C, Buchler MW, Neoptolemos JP, Starr MG (eds) The Pancreas. Blackwell Science, Oxford, pp 757–760
4. Partington PF, Rochelle REL (1960) Modified Puestow procedure for retrograde drainage of the pancreatic duct. Ann Surg 152:1037–1043
5. Frey CF, Smith GJ (1987) Description and rationale of a new operation for chronic pancreatitis. Pancreas 2:701–707
6. Beger HG, Witte C, Krautzberger W, Bittner R (1980) Erfahrung mit einer das Duodenum erhaltenden Pankreaskopfresektion bei chronischer Pankreatitis. Chirurg 51:303–307
7. Warshaw AL, Papp JW Jr, Schapiro RH (1980) Long-term patency, pancreatic function, and pain relief after lateral pancreaticojejunostomy. Gastroenterology 79: 289–293
8. Traverso LW, Tompkins RK, Urrea PT, Longmire WP Jr (1979) Surgical treatment of chronic pancreatitis: twenty two years experience. Ann Surg 190:312–319
9. Leger L, Lenriot JP, Lemaigre G (1974) Five- to 20-year follow up after surgery for chronic pancreatitis in 148 patients. Ann Surg 180:185–191
10. White TT, Slavotinek AH (1979) Results of surgical treatment of chronic pancreatitis. Report of 142 cases. Ann Surg 189:217–224
11. Prinz RA, Greenlee HB (1981) Pancreatic duct drainage in 100 patients with chronic pancreatitis. Ann Surg 194:313–320
12. Morrow CE, Cohen JI, Sutherland DER, Najarian JS (1984) Chronic pancreatitis: long-term surgical results of pancreatic duct drainage, pancreatic resection, and near-total pancreatectomy and islet autotransplantation. Surgery 96:608–615
13. Bradley EL III (1987) Long-term results of pancreaticojejunostomy in patients with chronic pancreatitis. Am J Surg 153:207–213
14. Drake DH, Fry WJ (1989) Ductal drainage for chronic pancreatitis. Surgery 105:131–140
15. Greenlee HB, Prinz RA, Aranha GV (1990) Long-term result of side-to-side pancreaticojejunostomy. World J Surg 14:70–76
16. Wilson C, Auld CD, Schlinkert R, Hasan AH, Imrie CW, MacSween RNM, Carter DC (1989) Hepatobiliary complications in chronic pancreatitis. Gut 30:520–527
17. Adams DB, Ford MC, Anderson MC (1994) Outcome after lateral pancreaticojejunostomy for chronic pancreatitis. Ann Surg 219:481–489
18. Kestens PJ, Gigot JF, Foxius A, Collard A, Gianello P (1996) Surgical treatment of chronic pancreatitis with predominant cephalic involvement by double Wirsung duct diversion and restoration of permeability of the cephalic duct. Ann Chir 10:853–860
19. Gonzales M, Herrera MF, Laguna M, Gamino R, Uscanga L Robles-Diaz G, Moran MA, Campuzano M (1997) Pain relief in chronic pancreatitis by pancreatico-jejunostomy. An institutional experience. Arch Med Res 3:387–390
20. Sharma AK, Pande GK, Sahni P, Nundy S (1998) Surgery for non-alcoholic chronic pancreatitis. World J Surg 3:236–239
21. Sidhu SS, Nundy S, Tandon RK (2001) The effect of the modified Puestow procedure on diabetes in patients with tropical chronic pancreatitis – a prospective study. Am J Gastroenterol 96:107–111
22. Apelund G, Topazian M, Lee JH, Andersen DK (2005) Improved outcome for benign disease with limited pancreatic head resection. J Gastrointest Surg 9:400–409
23. Schnelldorfer T, Lewin DN, Adams DB (2006) Reoperative surgery for chronic pancreatitis: is it safe? World J Surg 7:1321–1328
24. Chaudhary A, Negi SS, Masood S, Thombare M (2004) Complications after Frey's procedure for chronic pancreatitis. Am J Surg 188:277–281
25. Büchler MW, Friess H, Müller MM, Beger HG (1995) Randomized trial of duodenum-preserving pancreatic head resection versus pylorus-preserving Whipple in chronic pancreatitis. Am J Surg 169:65–70

26. Klempa I, Spatny M, Menzel J, Baca I, Nustede R, Stockmann F, Arnold W (1995) Pancreatic function and quality of life after resection of the head of the pancreas in chronic pancreatitis. A prospective, randomized comparative study after duodenum-preserving resection of the head of the pancreas versus Whipple's operation. Chirurg 66:350–359
27. Itzbicki JR, Bloechle C, Knoefel WT, Kuechler T, Binmoeller KF, Broelsch CE (1995) Duodenum-preserving resection of the head of the pancreas in chronic pancreatitis. A prospective, randomized trial. Ann Surg 221:350–358
28. Itzbicki JR, Bloechle C. Broering DC, Knoefel WT, Kuechler T, Broelsch CE (1998) Extended drainage versus resection in surgery for chronic pancreatitis: a prospective randomized trial comparing the longitudinal pancreatico-jejunostomy combined with local pancreatic head excision with the pylorus-preserving pancreatoduodenectomy. Ann Surg 228:771–779
29. Witzigman H, Max D, Uhlmann D, Geissler F, Schwarz R, Ludwig S, Lohmann T, Caca K, Keim V, Tannapfel A, Hauss J (2003) Outcome after duodenum-preserving pancreatic head resection is improved compared with classic Whipple procedure in the treatment of chronic pancreatitis. Surgery 134:53–62
30. Kimura W, Nagai N (1995) Study of the surgical anatomy for duodenum preserving resection of the head of the pancreas. Ann Surg 221:359–363
31. Löwenfels AB, Maisonneuve P, Cavallini G, Ammann RW, Lankisch PG, Andersen JR, Dimagno EP, Andren-Sandberg A, Domellof L (1993) Pancreatitis and the risk of pancreatic cancer. International Pancreatitis Study Group. N Engl J Med 328:1433–1437
32. Rösch T, Daniel S, Scholz M, Huibregtse K, Smits M, Schneider T, Ell C, Haber G, Riemann JF, Jakobs R, Hintze R, Adler A, Neuhaus H, Zavoral M, Zavada F, Schusdziarra V, Soehendra N (2002) endoscopic treatment of chronic pancreatitis: a multicenter study of 1000 patients with long-term follow up. European Society of Gastrointestinal Endoscopy Research Group. Endoscopy 34:765–771
33. Cremer M, Devière J, Delhaye M, Balze M, Vandermeeren A (1991) Stenting in severe chronic pancreatitis: results of medium-term follow-up in seventy-six patients. Endoscopy 23:171–176
34. Bittencourt PL, Delhaye M, Devière J, Lemoine O, Baize M, Matos C, Vandermeeren, A, Cremer M (1996) Immediate and long-term results of pancreatic ductal drainage in severe painful chronic pancreatitis. Gut 39:A99
35. Provansal-Cheylan M, Bernard JP, Mariani A, Soehendra N, Cremer M, Sahel J, Sarles H (1989) Occluded pancreatic endoprostheses: analysis of the clogging material. Endoscopy 21:63–69
36. Sherman S, Alvarez C, Robert M, Ashley SW, Reber HA, Lehman GA (1993) Polyethylene pancreatic duct stent-induced changes in the normal dog pancreas. Gastrointest Endosc 39:658–664
37. Kozarek RA, Patterson DJ, Ball TJ, Traverso LW (1989) Endoscopic placement of pancreatic stents and drains in the management of pancreatitis. Ann Surg 209:638–644
38. Dite P, Ruzicka M, V Zboril, Novotny I (2003) A prospective, randomized trial comparing endoscopic and surgical therapy for chronic pancreatitis. Endoscopy 35:553–558
39. Cahen DL, Gouma DJ, Nio Y et al. (2007) Endoscopic versus surgical drainage of the pancreatic duct in chronic pancreatitis. N Engl J Med 356:676–684

Chapter 36

R. A. Prinz · M. Gaffud · M. Edwards

Pancreatic Duct Drainage Procedures

Chronic Pancreatitis is an inflammatory disease that is characterized by permanent alteration of the anatomic structure of the pancreas and by progressive loss of pancreatic function. Clinically, its most notable and reported symptom is severe abdominal pain. Other signs and symptoms of progressive exocrine and endocrine deficiency such as diarrhea, fatty stools, and loss of glucose homeostasis from diabetes mellitus are also common. The initial treatment is medical and comprises pain control, oral supplementation of pancreatic enzymes, and diabetes management with oral hypoglycemic agents and insulin as needed. The most common indication for surgery is to relieve intractable abdominal or back pain. Surgical intervention is also indicated for suspicion of malignancy, presence of pseudocysts, and associated obstruction of the common bile duct or duodenum. The ideal surgical intervention would provide lasting pain relief and preserve exocrine and endocrine function. Despite the innovations and technical advances of the past century, no single procedure can achieve this goal because of the multiple facets and variations of this disease. Surgical therapy must be individually tailored to each patient.

The most common cause of chronic pancreatitis is alcohol abuse, which is the etiologic agent in 80% of all patients in the United States. Alcohol has a direct toxic effect on acinar cells and induces a microcirculatory perfusion change that alters epithelial permeability. This causes changes in acinar protein secretion and leads to protein plug and ductal stone formation. There are multiple causes of non-alcohol-induced chronic pancreatitis. Tropical chronic pancreatitis is common in areas of malnutrition. The disease is associated with inadequate protein and trace element nutrition, and intake of dietary toxins, tapioca, and cassava. Hereditary pancreatitis is associated with mutations in trypsinogen. Other causes include hypercalcemia, autoimmune diseases, and chronic obstruction of the pancreatic duct system due to tumors, stictures, or aberrant anatomy. As many as 20% of patients in some series have an unclear etiology and are categorized as idiopathic chronic pancreatitis [1].

The etiology of the pain of chronic pancreatitis is most likely multifactorial. One possible explanation for the severe pain of chronic pancreatitis is ductal hypertension and dilation due to progressive fibrosis and obstruction. Intraoperative ductal manometry has demonstrated pressures greater than 30 mmHg in chronic pancreatitis, whereas normal pancreatic duct pressure is 10–15 mmHg [2]. Elevations in pancreatic tissue pressure, much like a compartment syndrome, are another potential etiology. In chronic pancreatitis, pancreatic tissue pressure is elevated throughout the pancreas and is greater in areas of calcification. The increased parenchymal pressure will decrease tissue perfusion. The associated localized tissue acidosis may be a potential cause of pain [3]. Damage to pancreatic nerves is also a likely explanation for the pain in chronic pancreatitis. Inflammatory cell infiltration of the nerves within and around the pancreas and release of cytokines has been shown in this disease and occurs in patients with and without dilation of their pancreatic duct [4].

Historical Perspective

Goethe Link reported the first pancreatic duct drainage operation for chronic pancreatitis in 1911. After he inserted a catheter into the duct of Wirsung to drain the exocrine fluid out through the skin, the patient reported pain relief and return to normal weight [5]. Two procedures were developed in the 1950s. Duval reported a distal pancreatectomy, splenectomy, and caudal pancreaticojejunostomy in 1954. The caudal pancreaticojejunostomy was performed end-to-end and theoretically decompressed the pancreatic duct retrogradely [6]. However, if strictures were present throughout the ductal system, the entire duct would not be decompressed. Puestow and Gillesby introduced the lateral pancreaticojejunostomy, which was a longitudinal incision of the pancreatic duct and implantation of the tail of the gland into the Roux-en-Y limb of the jejunum [7]. This decompressed a greater length of pancreatic duct, but involved a splenectomy and did not decompress the pancreatic head because the jejunal limb was not able to be brought to the right of the superior mesenteric vessels. Partington and Rochelle modified the Puestow-Gillesby pancreaticojejunostomy by creating an anastomosis between a longitudinally incised anterior surface of the pancreas and a longitudinally incised Roux-en-Y jejunal limb [8]. Their modification did not require caudal pancreatectomy, splenectomy, or mobilization of the pancreas from its retroperitoneal attachments. Anastomosis to the opened anterior surface of the pancreas allowed decompression of the pancreatic duct from the tail to the head of the pancreas.

Patient Evaluation and Selection

A successful result with the lateral pancreaticojejunostomy begins with appropriate patient selection. Preoperative assessment confirms the diagnosis and establishes the extent of disease, the severity of pain, the amount of exocrine and endocrine insufficiency, and the morphology of the gland. A complete history establishes the nature of the pain and the degree of disability. The severity of the pain should be quantified as objectively as possible using an analog scale. The patient's need for narcotic pain control and the severity of alcohol abuse need to be established. If the patient is still consuming alcohol, the likelihood of postoperative pain relief decreases. Patients who are working, not drinking alcohol, and who have a supportive family structure fare well. Less favorable outcomes can be expected in patients who cannot be rehabilitated from alcohol or drug use. Other potential sources of pain, such as peptic ulcer and calculous biliary tract disease, should be considered and treated. Malnutrition and weight loss are common features due to alcohol abuse, malabsorption, and pain induced by eating. In addition to routine laboratory studies, nutritional studies and tumor markers should also be evaluated. Hypoalbuminemia is present in approximately 30% of patients before pancreaticojejunostomy. Although tumor markers can be elevated in patients with chronic pancreatitis, CA 19-9 and carcinoembryonic antigen should be obtained preoperatively because of the possible presence of pancreatic cancer. If elevated, pancreatic cancer must be considered and ruled out before a diagnosis of chronic pancreatitis is accepted, even in an alcoholic patient.

Review of appropriate imaging studies ultimately indicates whether lateral pancreaticojejunostomy should be the procedure of choice. Patients with nondilated pancreatic ducts are unlikely to experience the benefits of lateral pancreaticojejunostomy. Recommendations for the minimum duct caliber for satisfactory decompression vary from 5 mm to 10 mm. We consider lateral pancreaticojejunostomy to be acceptable for patients with ducts larger than 5 mm.

Computed tomography (CT) and endoscopic retrograde cholangiopancreatography (ERCP) have been the most informative studies for the assessment of the ductal anatomy in chronic pancreatitis. We obtain a dynamic CT scan with 3-mm cuts through the pancreas as part of our preoperative evaluation. This study usually provides sufficient anatomic information for surgical decision-making. This imaging modality can demonstrate dilation of the pancreatic duct and is the most accurate method for detecting ductal and parenchymal calcifications. CT can also identify other abnormalities such as pseudocysts, mass lesions, and stricture or dilation of the bile ducts.

Due to its risk of acute pancreatitis or introduction of infection in the setting of established chronic pancreatitis, ERCP is no longer routinely performed before lateral pancreaticojejunostomy. Information regarding duct size and anatomy that an ERCP provides can often be obtained from the CT scan. ERCP may fail to visualize a dilated pancreatic duct when there is complete or tight ductal obstruction at or near the duodenum. ERCP can clarify biliary pathology in patients with bile duct strictures or choledocholithiasis that are not easily visible with CT scans. The "double duct sign," localized obstruction of the common bile duct and the pancreatic duct, is suggestive of pancreatic cancer when seen with ERCP. In addition to its diagnostic use, interventions such as brush biopsy sampling, sphincterotomy, and stent placement can be performed during ERCP.

Magnetic resonance cholangiopancreatography (MRCP) and endoscopic ultrasound (EUS) are being used more frequently to evaluate the pancreas and the anatomy of the pancreatic duct. Both diagnostic modalities are less invasive than ERCP. While the aforementioned interventions are not needed, we rely on MRCP and EUS to clarify or give added information about the anatomy of the pancreas if needed after the initial CT scan. ERCP is used when a question remains about the ductal anatomy despite the use of the other noninvasive modalities, or when there is a need for its potential interventions.

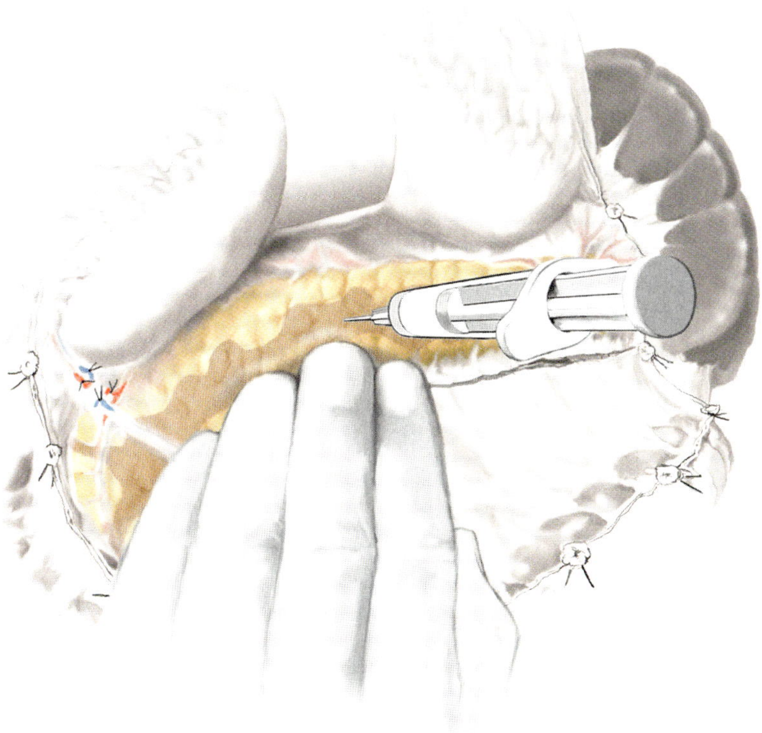

Figure 36.1

After exposition of the pancreas, the lesser sack is opened by dissection of the gastrocolic ligament, and the pancreatic duct is identified by puncture and aspiration

Operative Technique

The technical performance of the Partington-Rochelle modified Puestow Procedure has a substantial impact on the long-term results achieved with pancreatic duct decompression. Antibiotic prophylaxis is prudent. We recommend preoperative administration of a broad-spectrum antibiotic with adequate coverage against Gram-negative enteric organisms. We administer a mechanical bowel preparation in all patients because the transverse colon may be firmly adherent to the retroperitoneal process and there is a small, but real risk of possible colotomy. The operating room should have fluoroscopic equipment available for possible intraoperative pancreatography or cholangiography.

Either a bilateral subcostal chevron incision or midline incision may be used to enter the peritoneal cavity depending on the patient's body habitus. We prefer the chevron incision, which allows better exposure of the pancreatic tail in patients with a more vertical orientation of the pancreas. Initial exploration confirms the finding of chronic pancreatitis and evaluates for possible malignancy. The diseased pancreas should have a uniform, firm fibrotic texture. Localized hard areas or masses palpated in the pancreas should be aspirated with an 18-gauge needle and immediately evaluated for cytology. An incisional biopsy procedure is also appropriate if the lesion is located away from the pancreatic duct. Suspicious lesions on the surface of the gland or infiltrating along the root of the mesentery should be sampled by biopsy. The mesenteric, peritoneal, and hepatic surfaces should be thoroughly inspected and any suspicious lesions should be biopsied for frozen section. One must not neglect a thorough exploration because large series of patients with chronic pancreatitis undergoing surgery for relief of pain have shown that the presence of malignancy is possible.

After thorough exploration, complete exposure of the entire surface of the pancreas is obtained. Sparing the gastroepiploic vessels, the lesser sac is accessed by ligation and division of the gastrocolic omentum. The gastrocolic ligament should be divided as far to the

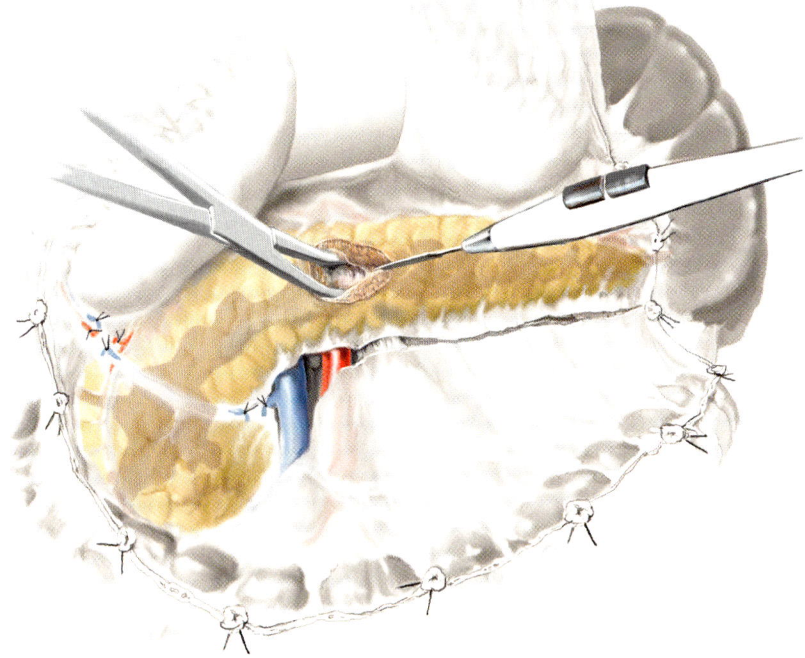

Figure 36.2

After identification of the pancreatic main duct, a ductotomy is performed in the body section. The incision is extended to the tail and into the duct of Wirsung and duct of Santorini up to the prepapillary duct segments

left as possible in order to expose completely the pancreatic tail. The transverse colon and hepatic and splenic flexures should be fully mobilized and retracted inferiorly. In chronic pancreatitis, the tail is frequently retracted away from the splenic hilum. Fibrous adhesions between the posterior wall of the stomach and the anterior surface of the pancreas are taken down by cautery or sharp dissection. Care must be taken to avoid injury to the blood vessels and vagus nerves along the lesser curvature that may be contained within dense adhesions. Additional time spent at this stage clearing the anterior surface of the pancreas will facilitate suture placement during the subsequent anastomosis.

A wide Kocher maneuver is performed from the common bile duct to the superior mesenteric vein. To avoid avulsion of vessels, sharp dissection should be performed to raise the duodenum and pancreas from their retroperitoneal attachments. Special attention should be made to identify the superior mesenteric vein within the fibrosed adhesions and to avoid avulsion of the branches of this vessel. Following the path of the middle colic vein helps pinpoint the location of the superior mesenteric vein. Anterior pancreaticoduodenal and gastroepiploic veins may be suture ligated and divided if necessary for full exposure of the head of the gland. Having freed the pancreatic head, it should be palpated for masses and any suspicious lesions should be biopsied and sent for frozen section. Posterior dissection of the body and tail of the pancreas is unnecessary and not advised due to the potential for vessel avulsion when dissecting in an area with so much inflammation and fibrosis.

After adequate exposure of the pancreas has been achieved, the pancreatic duct is identified (Fig. 36.1). Within the mid to distal body of the gland, the dilated duct can be palpated as a soft and compressible area in an otherwise firm pancreas. To confirm the location, aspiration with a 20-guage needle on a 10-ml syringe should yield clear exocrine fluid. A pancreatogram can be obtained if necessary with gentle injection of 2–5 ml of full-strength radiopaque contrast and fluoroscopic imaging. Usually, preoperative imaging has provided sufficient anatomic information

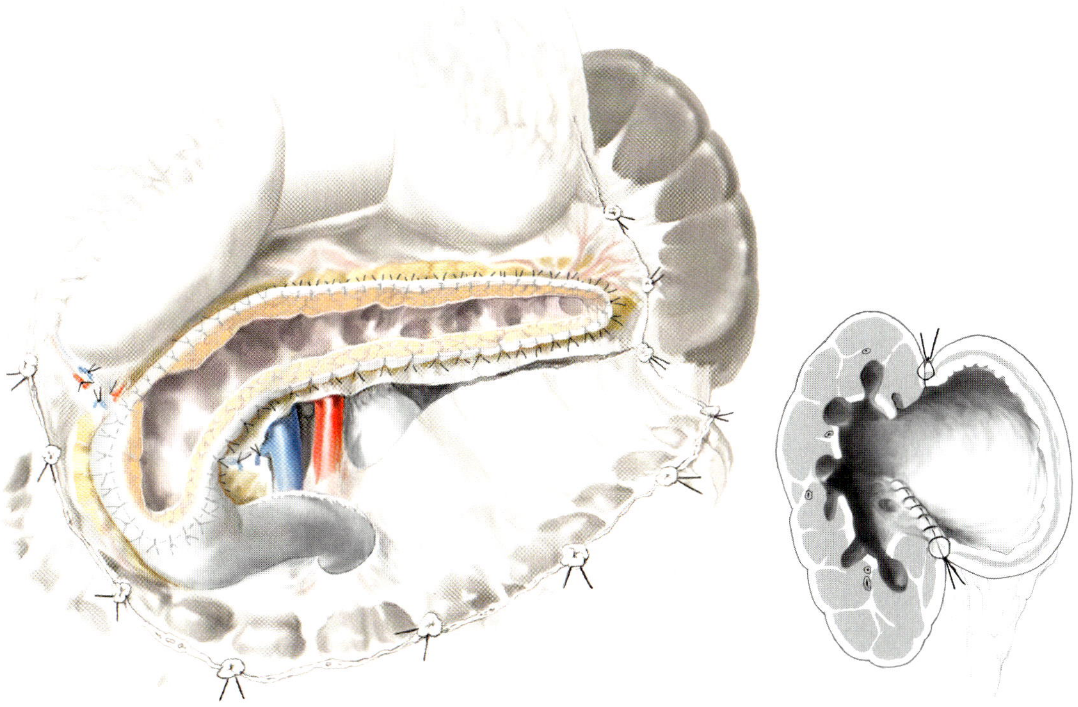

Figure 36.3

A side-to-side anastomosis between the excluded jejunal loop and the wall of the ventral pancreas is sutured using a single-layer continuous anastomosis with an absorbable monofilament suture material

and a pancreatogram is not needed. If the duct is difficult to locate, intraoperative ultrasound may be used or a vertical incision into the parenchyma at the level of mid body to the left of the mesenteric vein can be made and carried down until the duct is entered.

The ductotomy is extended by incising the overlying parenchyma with cautery. A dissecting clamp or metal probe is placed in the duct to identify its course within the gland. The extent of the ductal incision does not have a set length; rather, the duct should be incised as far as possible to ensure full decompression. To the left, the duct should be incised to within 1 cm of the tip of the pancreatic tail. Decompression of the head is more complex and more critical. Inadequate drainage here can account for failure and the need for reoperation. The gland is often bulky in this region and the course of the duct as it travels posterior and inferior to the right of the superior mesenteric vein can make adequate decompression difficult. The ductotomy on the main and accessory ducts should be carried to within 1 cm of the ampulla of Vater and the duodenum (Fig. 36.2). It may be necessary to place a probe or catheter into the common bile duct via the cystic duct or a choledochotomy to help identify the common bile duct as it courses through the pancreatic head to reduce its risk of injury. If adequate drainage is not possible with ductotomy alone, consider local resection or "coring out" of the pancreatic head as described by Frey [9]. This debulks the area of overlying tissue to enhance exposure and obtain thorough drainage of the proximal main pancreatic duct. With the left hand placed behind the head of the gland, the anterior capsule of the gland and the underlying pancreatic tissue to the level of the main pancreatic duct can be removed using cautery. Approximately 5 mm of parenchyma should be left intact for suture placement. Resected parenchyma should be sent for frozen section to rule out the presence of occult carcinoma. All ductal calculi and concretions that can be safely removed should be. Concretions of calcium carbonate can extend into the parenchyma and must be firmly extracted. Pancreatic bleeding can be controlled with cautery, suture ligature, or topical hemostatic agents.

A 50- to 60-cm Roux-en-Y limb is constructed after dividing the jejunum 20–30 cm distal to the ligament of Treitz. An intestinal stapler can be used and the staple line can be reinforced with a layer of nonabsorbable sutures if there is any concern about the security of the stapled end of jejunum. The Roux-en-Y limb is passed retrocolically through a mesenteric window between the right and middle colic vessels. An enterotomy is made along the antimesenteric border of the jejunal loop. The enterotomy length should be slightly shorter than the length of the duct incision, as the intestine will stretch.

There are various techniques for performing a pancreaticojejunal anastomosis; no single method has proven to be superior. The technique should be adapted to the size of the duct and the thickness of the parenchyma. We recommend a single-layer, continuous anastomosis of an absorbable, long-lasting monofilament suture. Starting at the most difficult area to suture, the pancreatic tail, the anastomosis proceeds along the superior and inferior borders by taking full-thickness bites of jejunum and pancreatic capsule until it is completed at the head of the pancreas (Fig. 36.3). The pancreatic stitch may include a small portion of the transected parenchymal edge. We do not attempt to sew directly to the mucosa of the pancreatic duct, although this may be done toward the tail, where the parenchyma often becomes thin. Sutures placed deep into the gland in an attempt to reach the ductal mucosa may occlude side branches and lead to a postoperative leak of pancreatic fluid or limit pancreatic decompression. Intestinal continuity is re-established by an end-to-side stapled or sutured jejunojejunostomy. The mesocolon is carefully closed around the Roux limb to prevent future internal hernias.

Cholecystectomy is traditionally performed during lateral pancreaticojejunostomy. A feeding jejunostomy may be necessary if the patient is malnourished or if an unusually long period of bowel recovery is anticipated. Drains are not usually needed, but closed suction drains may be used if there is a concern about leakage of bile or pancreatic secretions. Nasogastric decompression is continued postoperatively until bowel function resumes. Oral intake is resumed as after any major abdominal procedure.

Results

Chronic pancreatitis is a debilitating and progressive disease. In the presence of ductal obstruction and dilation, the Partington-Rochelle modified Puestow procedure is the operation of choice. This procedure has low mortality and morbidity rates compared with resection-type operations (Table 36.1).

Relief of pain, freedom from narcotics, and return to activities of normal living are the ultimate desired results for patients who have this procedure. Methods of measuring pain relief vary according to studies, but relief or reduction of pain is reported in up to 85% of patients (Table 36.2) [10–17]. Continued use of alcohol is associated with ongoing postoperative pain despite successful decompression. In one study, substantial symptomatic improvement followed decompression in 91% of patients who refrained from alcohol, and minimal improvement in pain relief was reported in 88% of patients who continued to consume alcohol [10]. In addition to relieving chronic pain, lateral pancreaticojejunostomy decreases the incidences of acute exacerbations of pain. Defining acute exacerbations as pain requiring hospital admission or cessation of oral intake for greater than 48 h, 90% of patients who experienced acute exacerbations preoperatively did not have these episodes after surgery [18].

Although pain relief is likely after lateral pancreaticojejunostomy, the status of pancreatic function after surgery varies. Ultimately, there is no evidence that pancreatic function worsens due to lateral pancreaticojejunostomy. With a drainage operation, potential metabolic problems caused by removal of functional pancreatic tissue are avoided. However, chronic pancreatitis is a progressive inflammatory process that more than likely continues despite operative intervention. Nealon and Thompson noted that a group of patients with mild or moderate disease (based on their morphology/function grading) benefited from early pancreatic duct drainage when compared to their nonoperative counterparts. Nonoperated patients advanced to severe disease and had progressive weight loss. Early pancreatic duct drainage can prevent or reduce the need for pancreatic enzyme replacement after surgery [19]. Sielezneff and coworkers reported a significant decrease in enzyme requirements after surgery [11]. Prinz and Greenlee reported an increase in the number of patients who required enzyme replacement; however, the majority of their patients never required enzyme therapy [10].

Diabetes is the most common complication throughout the natural history of chronic pancreatitis. Surgical drainage involves minimal loss of remaining islet cells. On long-term follow up, Prinz and Greenlee reported that less than half of their patients became diabetic. Only 30% of their patients eventually required insulin. Of their patients who were non-

Table 36.1. Complications of pancreatic duct drainage

Author/Year	Patients	Complications	Mortality
Boerma et al. 2002 [13]	50	14%	0
Kalady et al. 2000 [16]	60	40%	0
Adams et al. 1994 [12]	85	5.9%	0
Sielezneff et al. 2000 [11]	57	30%	0
Prinz and Greenlee 1981 [10]	100	21%	3.8%
Cahen et al. 2007 [14]	20	35%	0
Frey and Mayer 2003 [15]	0	22%	0

Table 36.2. Long-term results of pancreatic duct drainage

Author/Year	Patients *n*	Mean follow up	Pain improved	Reoperations	Survival
Boerma et al. 2002 [13]	44	27 months (3–156 months)	78%	7%	90%
Adams et al. 1994 [12]	62	6.3 years	68%	6%	74%
Sielezneff et al. 2000 [11]	57	65 months (8–206 mo)	75%	25%	79%
Lucas et al. 1999 [17]	78	36.1 months (5–138 months)	94%	–	–
Prinz and Greenlee 1981 [10]	87	7.9 years (1–25 years)	82%	9%	47%
Cahen et al. 2007 [14]	20	24 months	75%	5%	100%
Frey and Mayer 2003 [15]	50	37 months	87%	10%	90%

diabetic preoperatively, only 20% developed diabetes during follow up [10]. Maartense compared resection and drainage procedures with respect to pancreatic endocrine function. Glucose tolerance improved after lateral pancreaticojejunostomy compared to resection procedures. Despite this improvement in glucose tolerance, diabetes and insulin dependence did develop in some of their patients after pancreatic duct drainage [20].

Managing Associated Problems

Many patients undergoing lateral pancreaticojejunostomy also have other complications of chronic pancreatitis that require operative intervention. These are pseudocysts, biliary obstruction, and duodenal obstruction. Pseudocysts can present with the same symptoms as chronic pancreatitis. This can divert attention from the underlying chronic pancreatitis and can lead to incomplete treatment. Pseudocysts are present in up to 40% of patients with chronic pancreatitis and should be managed at the time of pancreatic duct decompression by drainage or aspiration. Combined drainage with the pancreatic duct is a safe and effective treatment of the pseudocyst. Intrapancreatic pseudocyst drainage can be performed by extending the pancreatic ductal incision into the pseudocyst and incorporating it into the jejunal limb (Fig. 36.4). Extrapancreatic pseudocyst drainage can be performed by anastomosing the free end of the jejunal limb to the dependent portion of the cyst (Fig. 36.5) [21]. An alternative to drainage into the jejunum is aspiration. For easily accessible small cysts, aspiration combined with duct drainage can be effective. Nealon and Walsner proposed the concept of a fistula between the main pancreatic duct and the pseudocyst. With decompression of the pseudocyst into the jejunum, pancreatic fluid flows into the bowel instead of the pseudocyst. Aspiration allows immediate decompression and the lateral pancreaticojejunostomy provides prolonged drainage so it does not recur. Potential advantages of aspiration are decreased dissection and operative time [22].

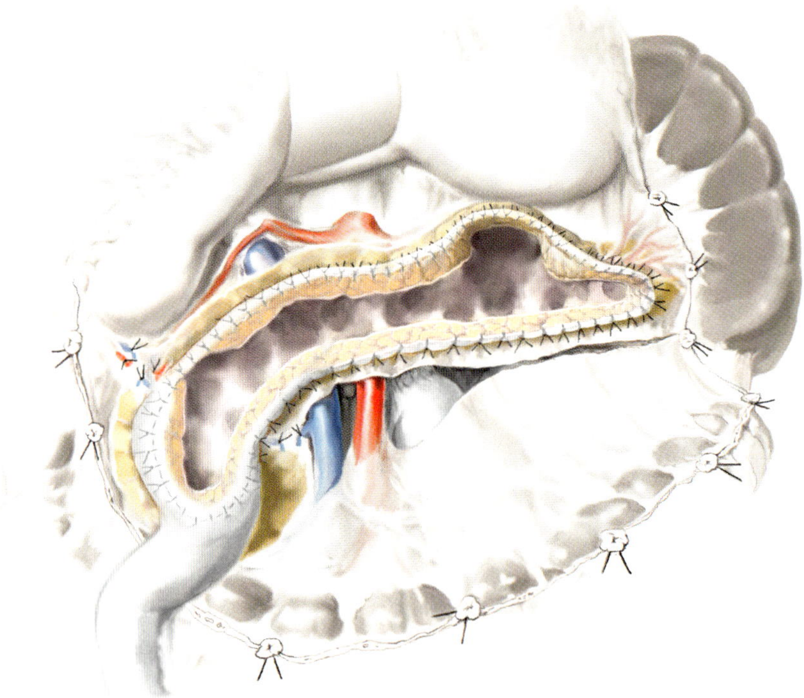

Figure 36.4

Combined drainage of the pancreatic duct including an intrapancreatic pseudocystic lesion in the body or tail of the pancreas

Biliary obstruction or stricture occurs in up to 30% of patients with chronic pancreatitis undergoing pancreatic duct drainage. While some patients may be asymptomatic, others will have progressive jaundice or even life-threatening cholangitis. Both choledochoduodenostomy and choledochojejunostomy are acceptable methods for achieving biliary drainage (Fig. 36.6).

Duodenal obstruction occurs in 10–15% of patients with chronic pancreatitis undergoing pancreatic duct decompression. Obstruction may be due to inflammation alone and resolve without operative intervention. Fixed obstruction requires operative therapy. When performing a lateral pancreaticojejunostomy, lysis of adhesions or drainage of a concomitant pseudocyst can relieve some obstructions. If bypass is required, a side-to-side gastrojejunostomy proximal to the jejunojejunostomy can be constructed (Fig. 36.7). Pancreaticoduodenectomy or simultaneous bypass with pancreaticojejunostomy, gastrojejunostomy, and choledochoduodenostomy are appropriate for patients with chronic pancreatitis and obstruction of the common bile duct and duodenum [23].

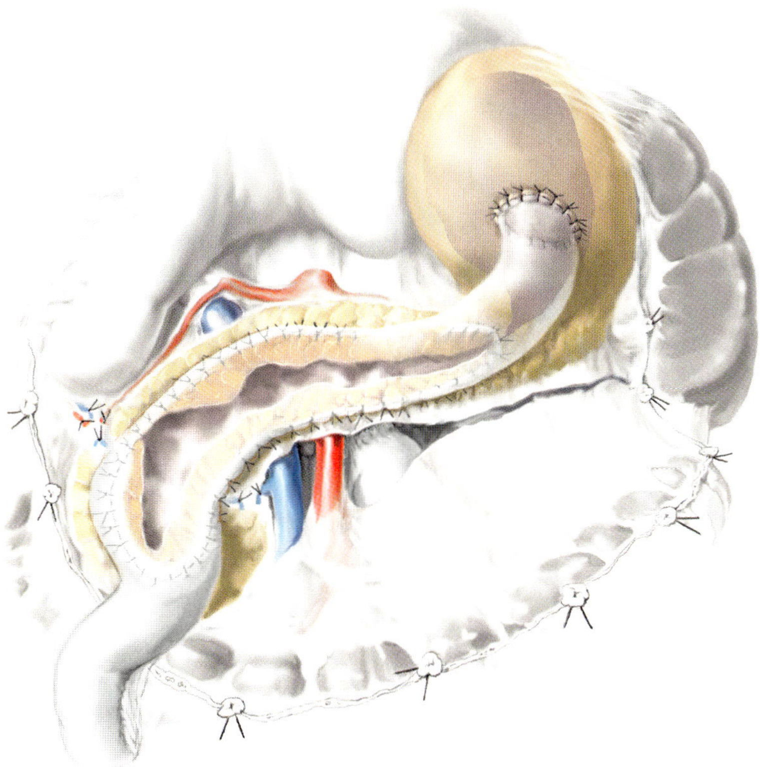

Figure 36.5

Extrapancreatic pseudocysts can be drained by anastomosing the free end of the jejunal loop that häs been used to drain the pancreatic duct to the dependent portion of the cyst

Persistent Pain

Persistent pain after lateral pancreaticojejunostomy requires thorough re-evaluation. The initial diagnosis of chronic pancreatitis must be reassessed and other possible etiologies of pain such as pancreatic cancer, peptic ulcer disease, biliary tract disease, or upper gastrointestinal obstruction should also be considered. The adequacy of drainage at the initial operation must be evaluated by reimaging the pancreas; usually ERCP is required for this. The presence of a nonfilling Roux-Y loop, undrained segments of the pancreatic duct containing strictures or dilations, or new pseudocysts require reoperation. Redrainage is the operation of choice with these abnormal ERCP findings. Pain relief after redrainage is comparable with the results of pain relief after the initial operation, and the development of endocrine and exocrine insufficiency as a result of the surgery is avoided [24].

If all other causes of pain have been ruled out and ERCP demonstrates a patent anastomosis with adequate decompression of the pancreatic duct, a resection may be the only possible option. A pylorus-preserving Whipple procedure is the usual resection performed in North America, while a duodenal-preserving resection of the pancreatic head, the Beger procedure, is often performed in Europe. This is a very difficult group of patients and the results in terms of achieving pain relief are not as good as with the initial procedure. Nevertheless, patients can benefit from these resections. Total pancreatectomy is best avoided because of the nutritional deficits and difficulties managing diabetes that result in these often poorly compliant patients.

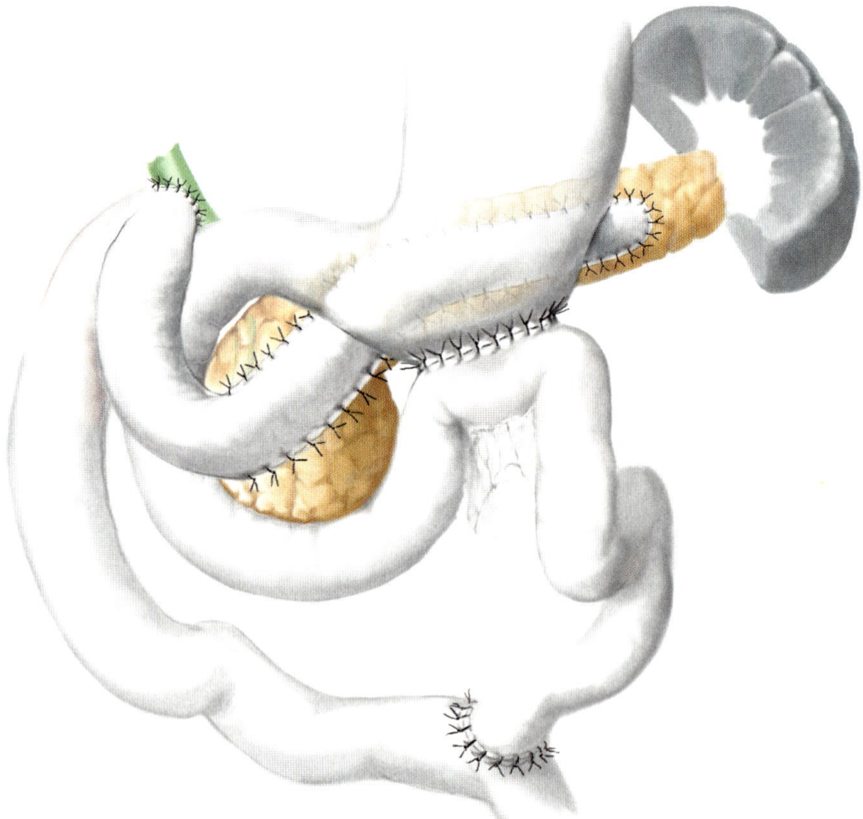

Figure 36.6

Biliary obstruction is relieved by a side-to-side-anastomosis between the supraduodenal common bile duct and the excluded jejunal loop. The suture technique is single stitches but a continuous technique may also be used

Pancreatic Duct Drainage for Small-Duct Disease

Patients with small-duct chronic pancreatitis are typically candidates for resection instead of drainage procedures. New methods may potentially allow these patients to be considered for drainage instead of resection and thereby avoid sacrifice of a functional pancreas. Madura et al. reported the use of lateral pancreaticojejunostomy after small ducts were enlarged by insertion of a wall stent. The pancreatic duct was progressively dilated with plastic stents and then a 10-mm expandable metal stent was placed. Two weeks after the metal stent was inserted, a mucosa-to-mucosa lateral pancreaticojejunostomy was performed with removal of the stent. Postoperative ERCP confirmed patency in all patients undergoing the procedure. Patients reported improvement of their pain, but the majority still required narcotics for pain control [25].

Izbicki et al. have modified the lateral pancreaticojejunostomy to a longitudinal V-shaped excision of the ventral pancreas for patients with small-duct chronic pancreatitis. The wedge resection not only decompresses the main pancreatic duct, but also the secondary and tertiary duct branches. The pain relief and preservation of endocrine and exocrine function that were present during the follow-up period were comparable to those reported in studies of lateral pancreaticojejunostomy in patients with a dilated pancreatic duct. The operation has similar morbidity and mortality in comparison to the traditional lateral pancreaticojejunostomy [26].

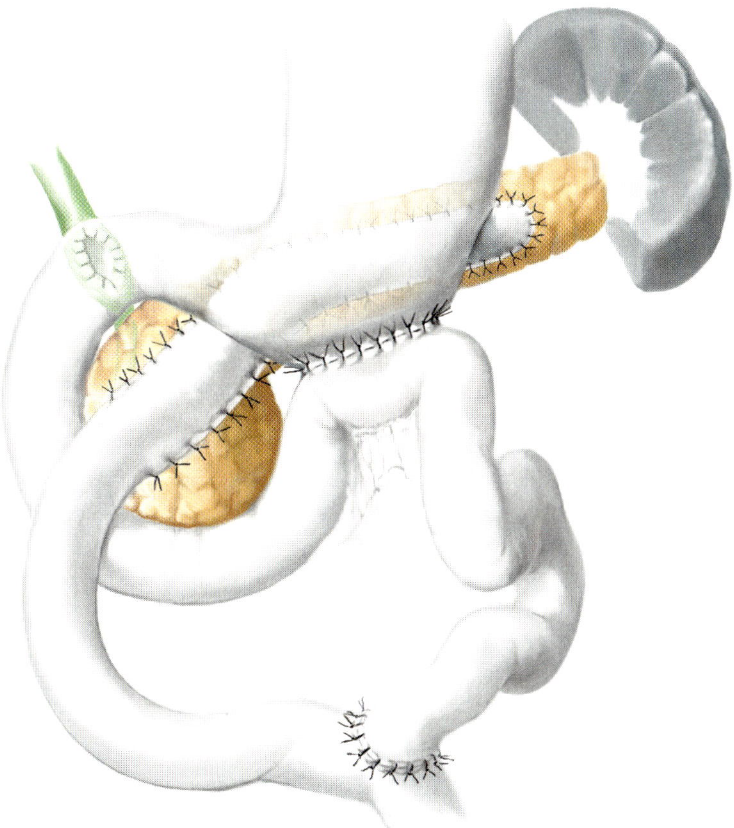

Figure 36.7

Chronic pancreatitis can cause severe duodenal obstruction. To relieve gastric stasis, a gastrojejunostomosis is performed together with the duct drainage. A choledochoduodenostomy can be performed to relieve concommitant biliary construction

Operations that Combine Drainage and Resection

Frey has developed a procedure that combines both resection and drainage to achieve better pain relief without sacrificing much endocrine or exocrine function. The Frey procedure incorporates a limited excision of the pancreatic head in combination with a Partington-Rochelle lateral pancreaticojejunostomy. The procedure addresses the most troublesome area of pancreatic duct drainage, the fibrosed pancreatic head [10].

Conclusion

Surgery for chronic pancreatitis should be regarded as a palliative intervention. Surgery treats the complications of the disease process and may slow its progression in some patients. Continued alcohol abuse increases the mortality of the disease. Patients who continue to drink are unlikely to experience pain relief despite surgery and are likely to die from the complications of alcoholism and tobacco use. Lateral pancreaticojejunostomy benefits patients who are committed to abstaining from alcohol and determined to resume their activities of daily living.

References

1. Strate T, Yekebas E, Knoefel WT, Bloechle C, Izbicki JR (2002) Pathogenesis and the natural course of chronic pancreatitis. Eur J Gastroenterol Hepatol 14:929–934
2. Jalleh RP, Aslam M, Williamson RCN (1991) Pancreatic tissue and ductal pressures in chronic pancreatitis. Br J Surg 78:1235–1237
3. Karanjia ND, Widdison AL, Leung F, Alvarez C, Lutrin FJ, Reber HA (1994) Compartment syndrome in experimental chronic obstructive pancreatitis: effect of decompressing the main pancreatic duct. Br J Surg 81:259–264
4. DiSebastiano P, diMola FF, Bockman DE, Freiss H, Buchler MW (2003) Chronic pancreatitis: the perspective of pain generation by neuroimmune interaction. Gut 52:907–911
5. Link G (1953) The treatment of chronic pancreatitis by pancreatostomy. Ann Surg 138:287–288
6. DuVal MK (1954) Caudal Pancreaticojejunostomy for chronic relapsing pancreatitis. Ann Surg 140:775–785
7. Puestow CB, Gillesby WJ (1958) Retrograde surgical drainage of pancreas for chronic relapsing pancreatitis. Arch Surg 76:898–907
8. Partington PF, Rochelle RE (1960) Modified Puestow Procedure for Retrograde Drainage of the Pancreatic Duct. Ann Surg 152:1037–1043
9. Ho HS, Frey CF (2001) The Frey procedure. Arch Surg 136:1353–1358
10. Prinz RA, Greenlee H (1981) Pancreatic duct drainage in 100 patients with chronic pancreatitis. Ann Surg 1194:313–320
11. Sielezneff I, Malouf A, Salle E, Brunet C, Thirion X, Sastre B (2000) Long term results of lateral pancreaticojejunostomy for chronic alcoholic pancreatitis. Eur J Surg 166:58–64
12. Adams DB, Ford MC, Anderson MC (1994) Outcome after lateral pancreaticojejunostomy for chronic pancreatitis. Ann Surg 219:481–487
13. Boerma D, van Gulik TM, Rauws EA, Obertop H, Gouma DJ (2002) Outcome of pancreaticojejunostomy after previous endoscopic stenting in patients with chronic pancreatitis. Eur J Surg 168:223–228
14. Cahen DL, Gouma DJ, Nio Y, Rauws EA, Boermeester MA, Busch OR, Stoker J, Lameris JS, Dijkgraaf MG, Huibregtse K, Bruno MJ (2007) Endoscopic versus surgical drainage of the pancreatic duct in chronic pancreatitis. N Engl J Med 356:676–684
15. Frey CF, Mayer KL (2003) Comparison of local resection of the head of the pancreas combined with longitudinal pancreaticojejunostomy (Frey procedure) and duodenum-preserving resection of the pancreatic head (Beger procedure). World J Surg 27:1217–1230
16. Kalady MF, Broome AH, Meyers WC, Pappas TN (2001) Immediate and long-term outcomes after lateral pancreaticojejunostomy for chronic pancreatitis. Am Surg 67:478–483
17. Lucas CE, McIntosh B, Paley D, Ledgerwood AM, Vlahos A (1999) Surgical decompression of ductal obstruction in patients with chronic pancreatitis. Surgery 126:790–797
18. Nealon WH, Matin S (2001) Analysis of surgical success in preventing recurrent acute exacerbations in chronic pancreatitis. Ann Surg 233:793–800
19. Nealon WH, Thompson JC (1993) Progressive loss of pancreatic function in chronic pancreatitis is delayed by main pancreatic duct decompression. Ann Surg 217:458–468
20. Maartense S, Ledeboer M, Bemelman WA, Ringers J, Frolich M, Masclee AM (2004) Effect of surgery for chronic pancreatitis on pancreatic function: pancreaticojejunostomy and duodenum-preserving resection of the head of the pancreas. Surgery 135:125–130
21. Munn JS, Aranha GV, Greenlee HB, Prinz RA (1987) Simultaneous treatment of chronic pancreatitis and pancreatic pseudocyst. Arch Surg 122:662–667
22. Nealon WH, Walsner E (2002) Duct drainage alone is sufficient in the operative management of pancreatic pseudocyst in patients with chronic pancreatitis. Ann Surg 237:614–622
23. Vijungco JD, Prinz RA (2003) Management of biliary and duodenal complications of chronic pancreatitis. World J Surg 27:1258–1270
24. Prinz RA, Aranha GV, Greenlee HB (1986) Redrainage of the pancreatic duct in chronic pancreatitis. Am J Surg 151:150–156
25. Madura JA, Canal DF, Lehman GA (2003) Wall stent-enhanced lateral pancreaticojejunostomy for small-duct pancreatitis. Arch Surg 138:644–650
26. Izbicki JR, Bloechle C, Broering DC, Kuechler T, Broelsch CE (1998) Longitudinal v-shaped excision of the ventral pancreas for small duct disease in severe chronic pancreatitis. Ann Surg 227:213–219

Chapter 37

H. G. Beger · B. M. Rau · B. Poch

Duodenum-Preserving Pancreatic Head Resection

Duodenum-preserving pancreatic head resection (DPPHR) was introduced in clinical practice in 1972 after experimentation on dogs to elucidate the technique of a segmental resection of pancreatic tissue with regard to early and late histology of the two pancreaticojejunostomoses and maintenance of adequate vascularization of the pancreatic head rest along the duodenum.

The Head of the Pancreas – Pacemaker of Chronic Pancreatitis?

The development of an inflammatory mass in the head (IMH) and the prevalence of pancreatic head enlargement in patients with chronic pancreatitis (CP) regarding the epidemiology of the disease are not precisely known. In terms of radiologic diagnosis, using angio contrast-enhanced computed tomography (CECT) scanning of the pancreas, approximately 30–50% of all patients referred for surgical treatment demonstrate pancreatic head enlargement (size >3–4 cm). The double-duct system in the pancreatic head – the duct of Santorini and duct of Wirsung – is of clinical relevance for the pathomorphogenesis of IMH, and in patients suffering from complete pancreas divisum [1]. Pathomorphologically, patients with IMH frequently show focal necrotic lesions, small but rarely large pseudocystic cavities, calcifications of the pancreatic parenchyma, or duct stones in the main duct [2]. The loss of exocrine tissue, mainly the acinar-cell component, and the generation of extracellular matrix proteins, including laminin, fibronectin, and collagens, are the main pathomorphological consequences of the chronic inflammation [3]. The molecular mechanisms that contribute to these changes have been investigated. Overexpression of epidermal growth factor receptor and the c-erb-B2 proto-oncogene as well as overexpression of transforming growth factor α are identified as factors influencing the inflammatory process in the pancreatic head [1, 3–8].

Rationale for Pancreatic Head Resection, and DPPHR

1. Major pathomorphological changes during the course of CP [based on imaging investigations (CECT, magnetic resonance imaging, MRI) or surgical specimen (histology)] are observed in the pancreatic head: head enlargement, pancreatic duct pathomorphology, common bile duct (CBD) obstruction, duct stones, pancreatic main duct (PMD) stones, pseudocystic cavities, compression of the portal vein (PV) and superior mesenteric vein (SMV), calcifications of parenchyma.
2. Duct drainage procedures are indicated in a small subgroup of patients with PMD dilatation and absence of side-branch stenoses or obstructions. Regarding long-term pain control, duct drainage procedures have unsatisfactory results with reappearance of pain syndrome after 5 years in about 30% of patients.
3. Epidemiological studies indicate that CP may be associated with the development of pancreatic cancer, with prevalent location in the pancreatic head. The estimated cumulative risk in patients with hereditary CP was found to be increased for patients aged 40–70 years [9]. Regarding alcoholic CP, the risk of developing pancreatic cancer in conjunction with CP is believed to be related to the duration of CP and cigarette smoking. In the subset of patients suffering from alcoholic CP after 3–20 years of the disease, ductal pancreatic cancer can be found in 2–5% in Western countries. Cancer develops in 30–80% of patients with tropical CP.
4. Rationale for DPPHR. DPPHR results in a 95% resection of the pancreatic head, leaving a small rim of pancreatic tissue along the duodenal wall. Preservation of the duodenum and the biliary system has major advantages for patients regarding short- and long-term outcome in comparison to Kausch-Whipple resection and the pylorus-preserving resection.

Indications to DPPHR:

1. CP with an IMH.
2. CP with an intrapancreatic CBD stenosis causing cholestasis or jaundice.
3. Pancreas divisum causing CP.
4. Cystic neoplasia of the pancreatic head causing occlusion or compression of the PMD and/or the CBD
5. Adenomatous endocrine neoplasia of the pancreatic head complicating the duct systems.
6. CP causing PV/SMV compression
7. CP causing stenosis of the duodenum

In CP with an IMH of the pancreas 70–90% are men, mostly in the age below 40 years at the time of diagnosis. The clinical features are characterized by severe medically intractable pain; about 75% of the patients suffer from daily severe pain. A stenosis of the CBD is observed in 40–55% of patients; a severe duodenum stenosis is observed in 5–10% [10].

A single stenosis of the PMD using endoscopic retrograde cholangiopancreatography (ERCP) or MRI investigation is present in about 40%; the PV system is involved in about 12–18% of cases.

Diagnostic Work-up

The rationale for DPPHR in CP is the removal of the main inflammatory process, which is considered to be the pacemaker of the disease, while preserving the upper gastrointestinal tract. The surgical procedure preserves the stomach, duodenum and biliary tree. The clinical evaluation is directed to objectify the nutritional status, level of cholestasis (i.e., jaundice), signs of portal hypertension, and presence of ascites. For each patient, the knowledge of the endocrine function: fasting glucose level, and oral glucose tolerance test (OGTT) is mandatory. Regarding exocrine function, the most appropriate is the measurement of the fecal elastase, but the pancreolauryl serum test is also sufficient. The laboratory testing has to include the tumor markers CEA and CA 19-9 as well as the biochemistry of pancreatic and liver functions. Regarding invasive, instrumental, and radiological investigations, an upper gastrointestinal endoscopy as well as an ERCP or MRI with reconstruction of the intrapancreatic ducts has to be done. Pathomorphological changes of the pancreas are objectified by an angio-CECT.

Surgical Technique Includes Two Major Steps

1. Subtotal resection of the mass of the head between the PV and the intrapancreatic segment of the CBD [11,12].
2. Reconstruction with an excluded jejunal loop. Two pancreatic anastomoses have to be performed [11,12].

The head of the pancreas is exposed by dividing the gastrocolic ligament, preserving the gastroepiploic vessels. After transection of the duodenocolic ligament, a Kocher maneuver is performed. The exposition of the surgically relevant structures starts with the identification of the SMV below the pancreatic head. The common hepatic artery as well as the CBD are identified and looped. Starting at the SMV, the groove of the PV on the dorsal surface of the pancreatic head is dissected. In most patients it is possible to transect this space between the anterior surface of the PV and the posterior capsule of the pancreatic head by blunt dissection without difficulty. In the case of an inflammatory process with adhesions to the PV, a step-by-step mobilization of the vein from the pancreatic head tissue is to be performed, avoiding a lesion of the PV or the splenic vein. The SMV below and the PV above the pancreatic head is looped to control any possible bleeding. After finishing the dissection of the PV from the dorsal pancreatic tissue, a silk ribbon is positioned around the neck of the pancreas, which is then temporarily ligated, resulting in compression of the vessels; the loops are then used to lift the neck of the pancreas. Before transecting the pancreatic neck, the anterior gastroduodenal artery is identified and ligated near the common hepatic artery. Subtotal resection of the pancreatic head takes place by transecting the neck of the gland, starting at the uncinate edge of the SMV/PV. Bleeding vessels are immediately sutured. After identification of the PMD, the transection is completed (Fig. 37.1).

A blunt dissection of the tissue dorsal to the PV towards the dorsal pancreatic head capsule eases the exposition of the pancreatic head. Small branches entering the PV directly from the head must be ligated and divided. Subtotal resection of the pancreatic head starts after rotation of the head by 90° into a ventral/dorsal position.

Subtotal resection of the pancreatic head starts on the dorsal surface of the head after placement of single-stitch sutures along the resection line (Fig. 37.2). The resection along the duodenal wall takes place for a distance of 5 mm (Fig. 37.3). The transection is finished by dividing the head tissue along the wall of the

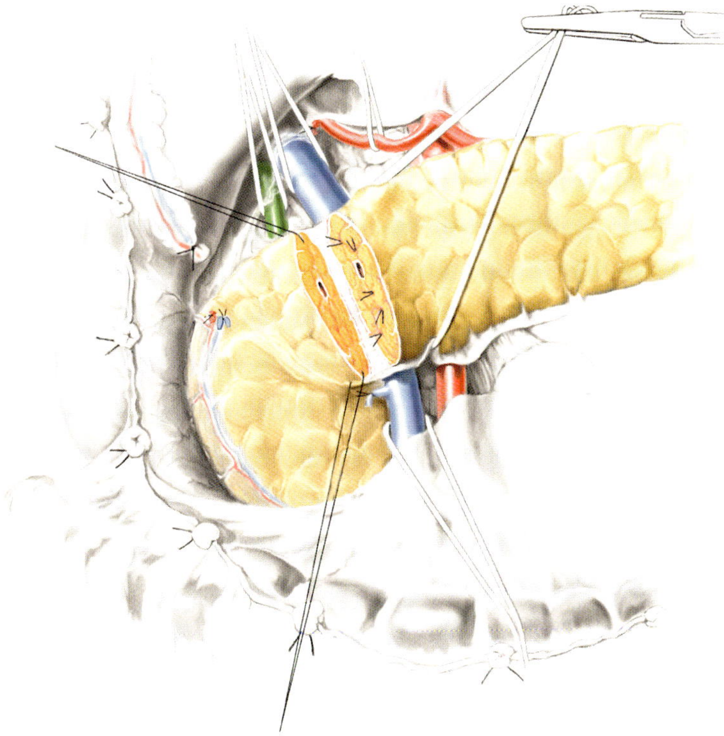

Figure 37.1

Duodenum-preserving pancreatic head resection (DPPHR): after tunneling of the portal vein behind the pancreas, transection of the pancreatic neck at the level of the duodenal side of the portal vein is performed

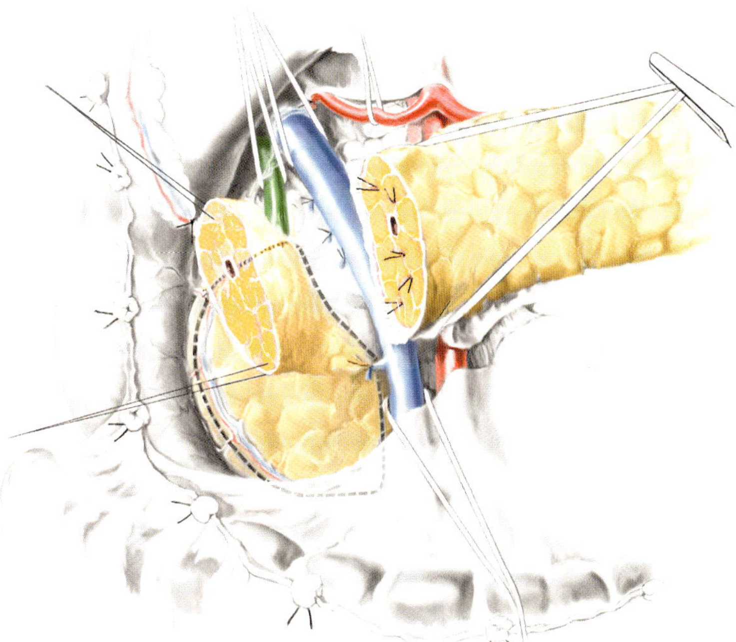

Figure 37.2

After hemostasis, using single stitches (5x0 nonresorbable monofilament sutures) on the transection surface of the left pancreas, the pancreatic head is rotated by 90° in a ventral/dorsal position

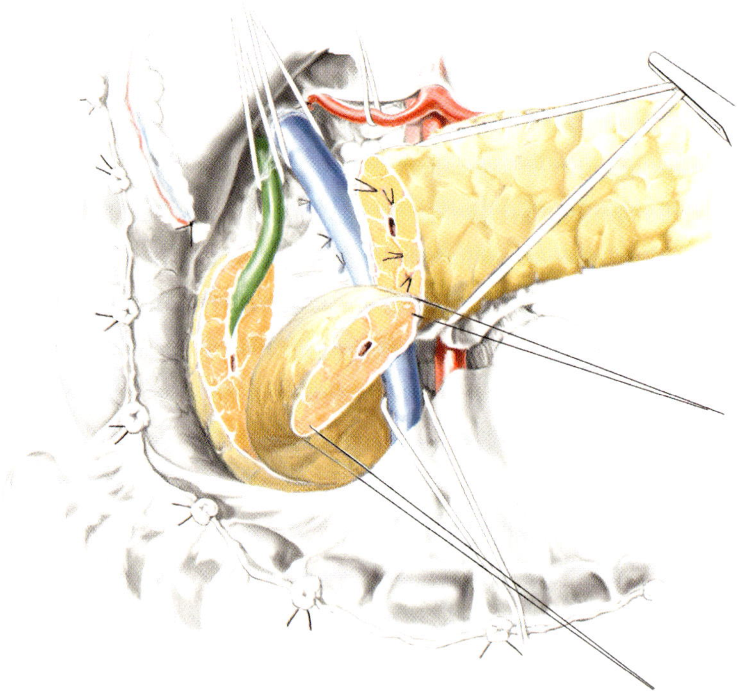

Figure 37.3

Resection of the pancreatic head starts after rotation on the dorsal surface of the pancreatic head toward the level of the intrapancreatic common bile duct. The common bile duct is identified at the level of the hepatoduodenal ligament. The transection follows the wall of the intrapancreatic common bile duct toward the prepapillary level

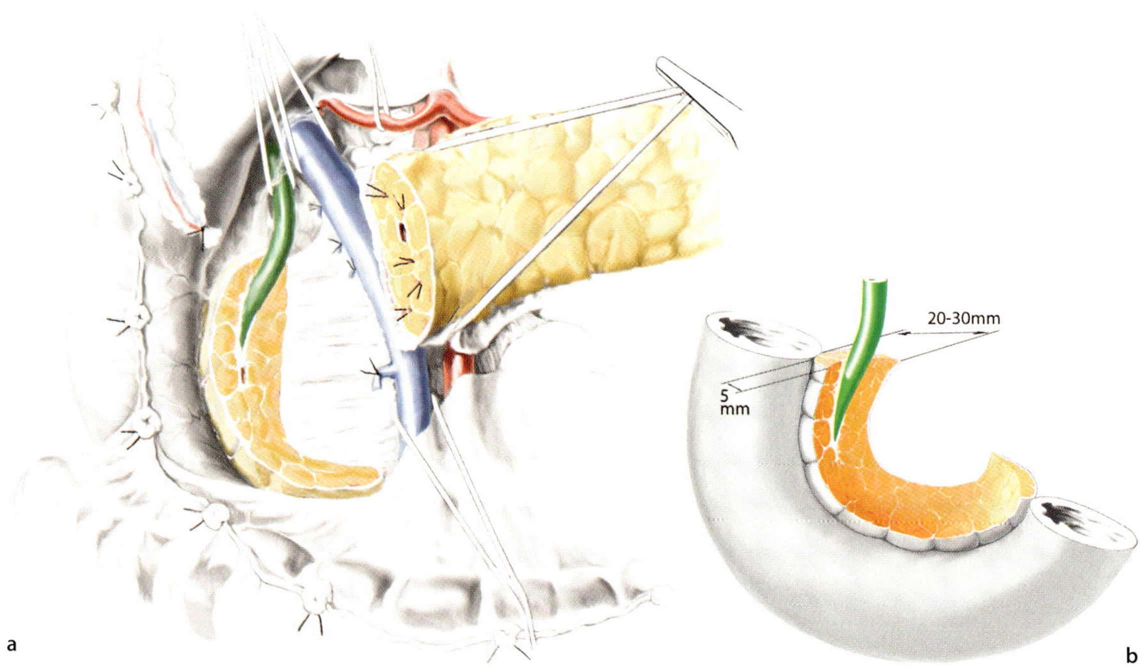

Figure 37.4 a, b

a The distance of the resection line of the pancreas to the duodenal wall is 5 mm ventrally and 2–3 cm dorsally. b The shell-like rest of the pancreatic head has a much longer distance to the duodenal wall behind and dorsal from the intrapancreatic common bile duct intrapancreatic portion of the CBD toward the papilla (Fig. 37.3). The distance of the cut-line of the pancreas to the duodenal wall is ventral 5 mm and dorsal 2–3 cm (Fig. 37.4).

In some cases the identification of the intrapancreatic CBD is difficult; in these cases a Kehr sonde is placed toward the papilla in the CBD via a small incision of the duct in the hepatoduodenal ligament. It is not necessary to preserve the anterior gastroduodenal artery for adequate blood supply to the duodenum. The supraduodenal vessels as well as the vessels arising from the superior mesenteric artery dorsal to the pancreatic head maintain sufficient perfusion of the duodenal wall (Fig. 37.5). Removal of the fibrotic tissue along the CBD results frequently in decompression of the duct. If there is an inflammation in the wall of the CBD, the duct is opened by an incision in the prepapillary duct segment [11]. Finally a shell-like remnant of the pancreatic head between the CBD and the duodenal wall remains.

The aboral jejunal loop, about 20 cm distal to the ligament of Treitz, is transected for reconstruction. The jejunal loop is transpositioned through a retrocolic mesenteric cleft to the right of the middle colic artery to the level of the pancreatic head. Reconstruction starts with a side-to-end anastomosis between the jejunal loop and the left pancreas (Fig. 37.6).

A side-to-end anastomosis is made between the jejunal loop about 8 cm distal of the left pancreatic anastomosis with the shell-like rest of the head. The jejunal incision is 4–5 cm in length. The inner layer of the anastomosis between the jejunum and the pancreas along the incision line is sutured continuously; the second layer is sutured between the pancreatic capsule and the seromuscularis of the jejunum using mostly interrupted single stitches (Fig. 37.7). For restoration of the intestinal tract continuity an entero-entero-anastomosis (Roux-en-Y) is carried out 20 cm distal to the pancreatic head anastomosis.

In patients with a prepapillary CBD stenosis that persists after subtotal resection of the pancreatic head, an additional anastomosis between the suprastenotic portion of the CBD and the jejunal loop is created (Fig. 37.7). It is not necessary to perform an additional side-to-side suturing between the duct and the jejunal wall; the prepapillary incision of the intrapancreatic CBD is included in the anastomosis [12].

In patients with a dilated pancreatic duct who shows multiple stenoses of the PMD and an absence of side-branch duct obstructions, the PMD is opened longitudinally on its ventral surface extending toward

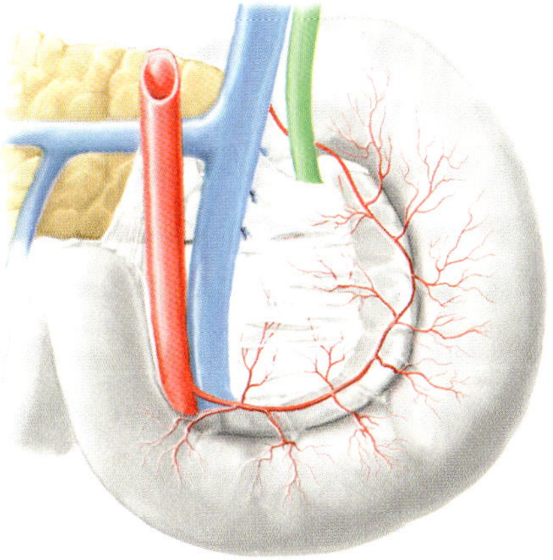

Figure 37.5

The dorsal capsule of the pancreatic head is preserved. To maintain the blood flow to and from the duodenal wall, the dorsal pancreaticoduodenal arcades and the inferior anterior pancreaticoduodenal artery are maintained

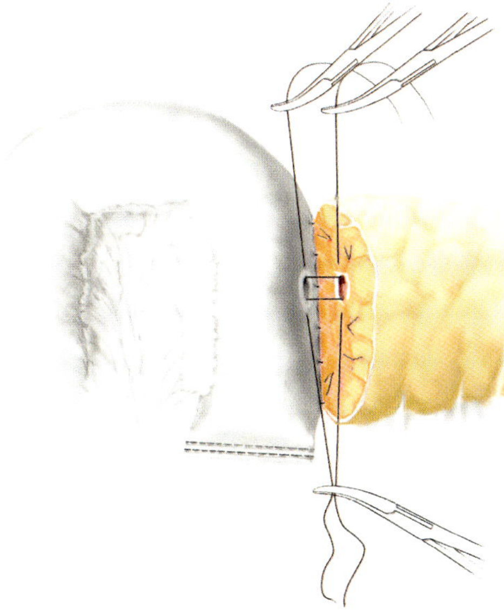

Figure 37.6

Reconstruction after the subtotal pancreatic head resection is performed with the upper jejunal loop. A mucosa-to-mucosa anastomosis with the left pancreas is made, the mucosa layer is sutured with 6x0 resorbable material; the autolayer between the pancreatic tissue and seromuscularis of the jejunal loop is sutured with 4x0 resorbable material

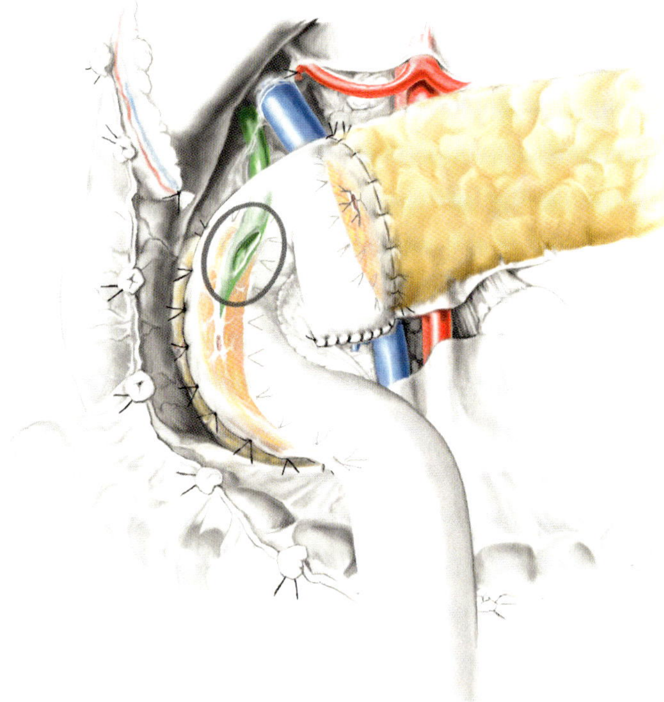

Figure 37.7

In cases of severe common bile duct stenosis, the wall of the common bile duct is opened in the prepapillary segment. The bile flow is maintained via the jejunal loop; the jejunal loop in the roof is sutured between the seromuscularis and the ventral part of the common bile duct using single stitches with 4x0 or 5x0 resorbable sutures

the tail of the pancreas. A side-to-side anastomosis using the Partington-Rochelle technique for duct-jejunostomosis is made (Figs. 37.8).

Postoperative Testing

After finishing the early postoperative period with restoration of oral food intake, the patient should be checked for the level of the glucose metabolism with the aid of an OGTT, and the level of exocrine function measured using fecal elastase estimation.

Early Postoperative Course

In many patients a surprising observation can be made because they are, even in the first postoperative days, completely free of CP-induced pain. In the early postoperative period local complications are not frequent; local bleeding, which appears as intestinal blood loss, anastomotic leakage, which is mostly evidenced by the appearance of intestinal content in the drainage fluid, and the development of a pancreatic fistula (evacuation of amylase-rich fluid after the 6th postoperative day through the drain near the pancreatic head) are observed. Mild laboratory signs of pancreatitis are frequent and last only 1–3 postoperative days. Systemic complications with regard to pulmonary dysfunction occur in around 10% of cases. The patients are usually on the 3rd to the 5th postoperative day on regular oral nutrition (Table 37.1).

Regarding the long-term outcome and the quality of life of these patients, the success of the surgical treatment is determined by the state of being free of pain and the level of endocrine insufficiency.

Long-Term Outcome After DPPHR

Preservation of the duodenum using DPPHR is superior to the classical duodenopancreatectomy (Kausch-Whipple resection) in CP. The most important benefit is the preservation of the duodenum because of the high capacity of the endocrine part of the duodenum in the regulation of the glucose metabolism. Further-

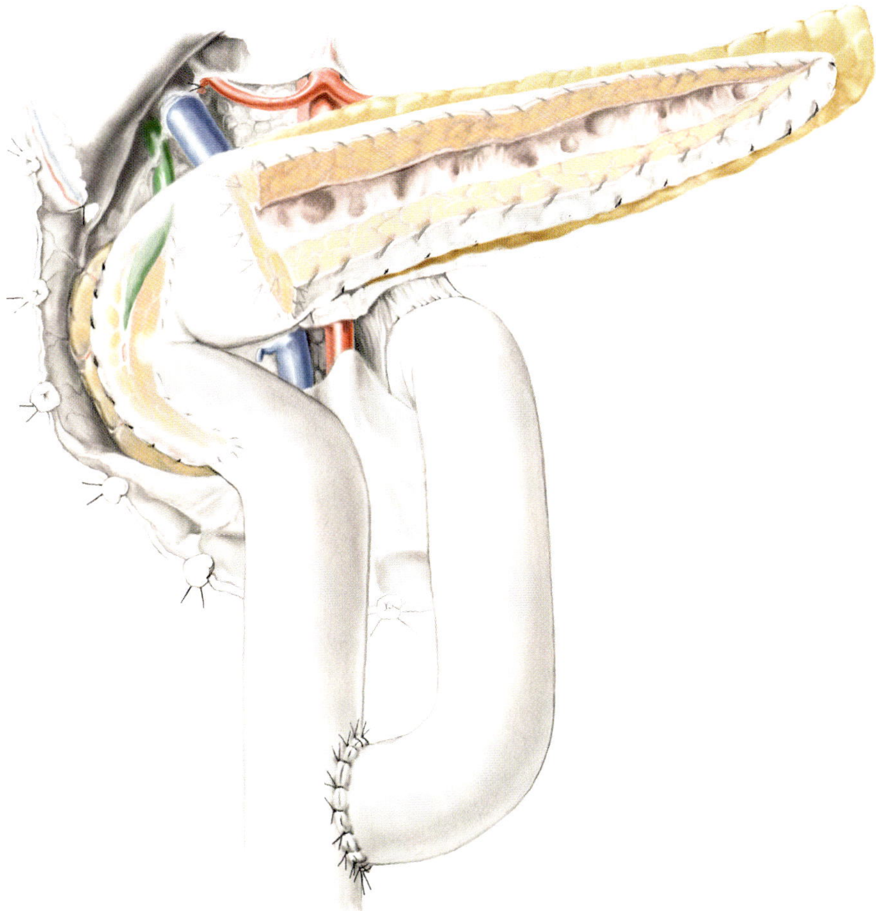

Figure 37.8

In cases of multiple stenosis of the pancreatic main duct and absence of side branch duct obstructions, a side-to-side pancreaticojejunostomosis is performed. The pancreatic main duct is opened by incision up to the tail of the pancreas. The jejunal loop is sutured by a two-layer suture technique, side to side, including the pancreatic tissue. This modification of pancreatic anastomosis with opening of the pancreatic main duct was first published in a series of patients in 1985 [10]

Table 37.1. Duodenum-preserving pancreatic head resection (DPPHR): early postoperative results in 603 patients[a]

Preoperative condition		No of patients
Pancreatic fistula	3.3%	20
Lreakage of pancreaticojejunostomy	1.5%	9
Intra-abdominal abscess	2.8%	17
Delay of gastric emptying	1.5%	9
Hospitalization (postop.)	14.5 (7–87) days	
	11.6 (6–33) days[b]	
Relaparotomy	4.6%	28
Hospital mortality	0.7%	4

[a] December 1972 to October 2001, Department of Surgery, Free University Berlin (May 1982) Department of General Surgery, University of Ulm (5/1982–9/2001)

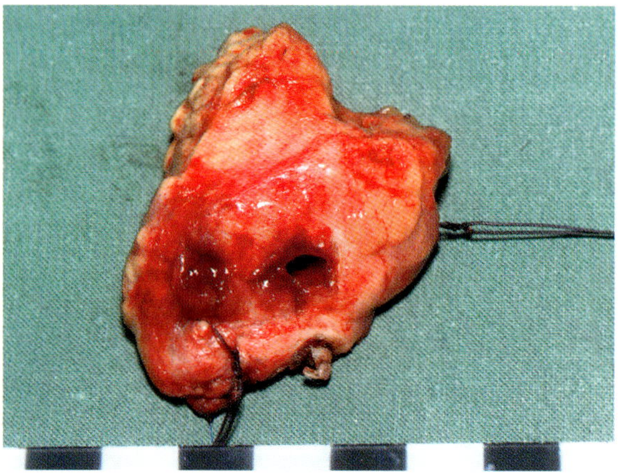

Figure 37.9

Operative specimen after subtotal, DPPHR. The wet weight of the operative specimen is between 25 and 45 g

Table 37.2. Late outcome after DPPHR in 388 patients, post-operative follow up in 94% of patients after median 5.7 years (range 0.3–14 years). *IDDM* Insulin-dependent diabetes mellitus

Patient condition	Patients
Pain free	91.3%
Continuing abdominal pain	8.7%
Complaints lower abdomen	12.0%
Hospitalization due to pancreatitis	12.5%
Professional rehabilitation[a]	69%
Glucose metabolism normal	39%
IDDM	44%
Quality of life (Karnofsky) >80	72%

[a] After follow up of (median) 5.7 years (range 0.3–14 years) Annals of Surgery 1999 [14]

Table 37.3. Pancreatic head resection in chronic pancreatitis. DPPHR versus Whipple resection. Results of randomized trials. PP Pylorus-preserving duodenopancreatectomy, *postop.* postoperative

Trials compared	Significant (>) or equal (=) differences	References
DPPHR >>>> PP Whipple	>postop. morbidity	Büchler et al. Am J Surg 1995 [16]
	>glucose metabolism	
	>gastric emptying	
	>frequency of rehospitalization	
DPPHR >>> Whipple	>postop. morbidity	Klempa et al. Chirurg 1995 [17]
	>glucose metabolism	
	>frequency of rehospitalization	
DPPHR = Frey[a]	= pain control	Itzbicki et al. Annals Surg 1995 [19]
	= glucose metabolism	
	= postop. morbidity	
	< quality of life	
Frey[a] >>> PP Whipple	>postop. morbidity	Itzbicki et al. Annals Surg 1998 [20]
	>gastric emptying	
	>quality of life	
DPPHR>>>>PP Whipple	>postop. morbidity	Witzigmann et al. Surgery 2003 [21]
	>maintenance of endocrine functions	
	>frequency of rehospitalization	
	>quality of life	

[a] Frey, modified by Itzbicki (coring-out-technique of Frey results in a tissue loss of 5 g (wet weight [18]). After subtotal DPPHR, the weight of the operative specimen is 25–45 g [14]

more, the duodenum regulates the gastric emptying of solid and liquid food. Due to the preservation of the duodenum, the endocrine function of the pancreas is maintained after DPPHR. The hormones with anti-insulin effects (e.g., glucagon and somatostatin) are reduced in the circulation after removal of the pancreatic head [13]. The observed improvement of endocrine functions in the postoperative period after DPPHR in some patients is the result of diminishing the glucagon- and somatostatin-cell compartment.

After a median observation period of 5.7 years and a follow up of 94%, the control of pancreatic pain is complete and long lasting in about 90% of the patients [14]. The combination of DPPHR with PMD drainage was only used in cases with multiple PMD stenoses, but there was an absence of side-duct obstructions. The use of the side-to-side anastomosis between the PMD and the jejunal loop has been shown to be unsatisfactory in almost 30% of the patients with regard to long-term outcome, because of side-duct obstructions and persistence of the IMH [22,23]. Subtotal resection of the pancreatic head results in the removal of 25–45 g of pancreatic tissue (Fig. 37.9). Around 70% of the patients experience a complete professional rehabilitation even in the long-term (Table 37.2) [15].

Comparing DPPHR with the Kausch-Whipple procedure (pylorus-preserving pancreatic head resection) and the Frey-Itzbicki modification of duct-drainage procedure in CP, the results of five randomized prospective controlled clinical trials have been published (Table 37.3). In comparison to the Whipple type of pancreatic head resection, DPPHR was superior in terms of postoperative morbidity, maintenance of glucose metabolism, frequency of delay of gastric emptying, and frequency of rehospitalization. Regarding the Frey procedure as performed by Itzbicki [19,20], the level of pain control, maintenance of glucose metabolism, frequency of postoperative morbidity, and quality of life were almost equal to those of DPPHR [14, 15].

DPPHR for Neoplastic Cystic Lesions

In the last 10 years modifications of the DPPHR procedure have been applied in patients suffering cystic neoplastic lesions located in the pancreatic head (Fig. 37.10). Cystic neoplastic lesions include intraductal papillary mucinous tumor (IPMT), mucinous cystic tumor (MCT), serous cyst adenoma, cystic forms of solid pseudopapillary tumors, acinar cell carcinomas, and endocrine and neurocrine neoplasms (Table 37.4). The most frequently diagnosed cystic neoplasia is the IPMT, with about 60% of the patients developing a lesion in the pancreatic head. The work-up for diagnosis of cystic neoplastic lesions includes: EUS, ERCP, CECT, and OGTT. The application of a DPPHR is

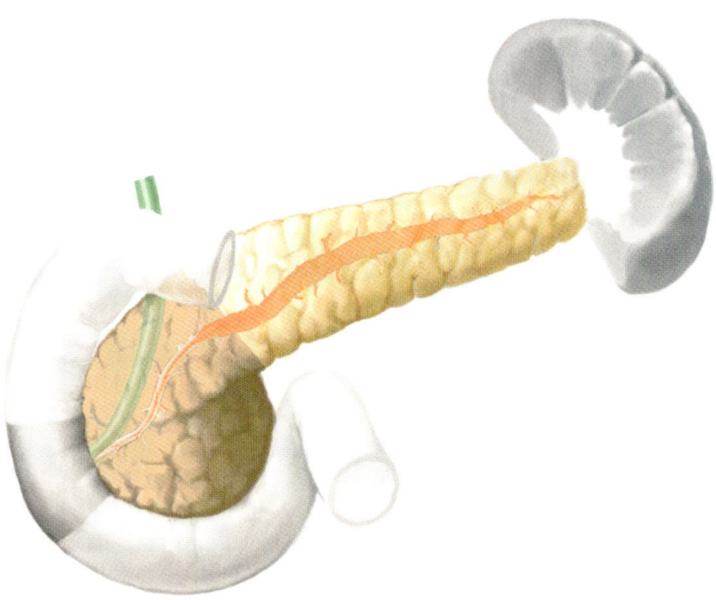

Figure 37.10

A cystic neoplastic lesion located in the pancreatic head with close connection to the peripapillary wall of the duodenum necessitates a duodenum-preserving total pancreatic head resection (DPPHRt) in the modification, which includes a segmental resection of the peripapillary duodenum

Table 37.4. Cystic neoplasm of the pancreas. *IPMT* Intraductal papillary mucinous tumor, *MCT* mucinous cystic tumor

IPMTs (head 58%, body 21%, elderly, males)
MCTs (body and tail, 70%, women)
Serous cystadenoma
Cystic forms of solid pseudopapillary tumors
acinar cell carcinomas
endocrine/ neuroendocrine neoplasms

Table 37.5. DPPHR Modifications. *CBD* Common bile duct, *PMD* pancreatic main duct, *e–s* End-to-side anastomosis, *s–s* side-to-side anastomosis, *e–e* entero-to entero anastomosis

DPPHR
+ biliary (CBD) anastomosis (e–s)
+ PMD drainage using jejunal loop (s–s)
Duodenum-preserving total pancreatic head resection (DPPHRE)
+ segmental resection of peripapillary duodenum (e–e)
Duodenum-preserving total pancreatectomy (DPTP)
with conservation of spleen
Duodenum-preserving resection of uncinate process (DPPHRu)
with segmental resection of postpapillary duodenum (e–e)

Table 37.6. Indications for DPPHR. *IPMT* Intraductal papillary mucinous Tumor, *MCT* Mucinous cystic tumor, *SCA* Serous cyst adenoma

1.	IPMT localized in pancreatic head >2 cm
	main and combined duct type
2.	MCT with compression of CBD and PMD
3.	Pancreatic endocrine or neuroendocrine neoplastic lesion with adhesion to the duodenum
4.	SCA growing, compression of CBD and PMD

Table 37.7. Indications for DPPHR. *DPPHRs* Duodenum-preserving subtotal pancreatic head resection, *DPPHRt* duodenum-preserving total pancreatic head resection, *DPTP* duodenum-preserving total pancreatectomy, *SP* spleen-preserving, *CP* chronic pancreatitis, *AP* acute recurrent pancreatitis, *SD* segment resection of duodenum

DPPHRs	Chronic pancreatitis
	Pancreas divisum + CP/ +AP
DPPHRt	IPMT (adenoma, borderline lesion, carcinoma in situ
	MCT (head localization of lesion)
	SCA
DPPHRu + SD	IPMT uncinate location Endocrine neoplasia
DPTP + SP	IPMT lesion in head, body and tail

Table 37.8. DPPHR for neoplastic lesion [24–29]. *Pts* Patients, *Neopl* neoplasm, *Endocr.* endocrine, *TM* tumor, *S* duodenum-preserving subtotal pancreatic head resection, *T* duodenum-preserving total pancreatic head resection, *Recur.* recurrences [24–29]

	Pts *N*	Cystic Neopl	Endocr. TM	Others	DPPHR S	T+SD	DPTP	Hospital mortality	Recur.
1993–2005	61	34	7	20	20	38	3	0%	3,3%

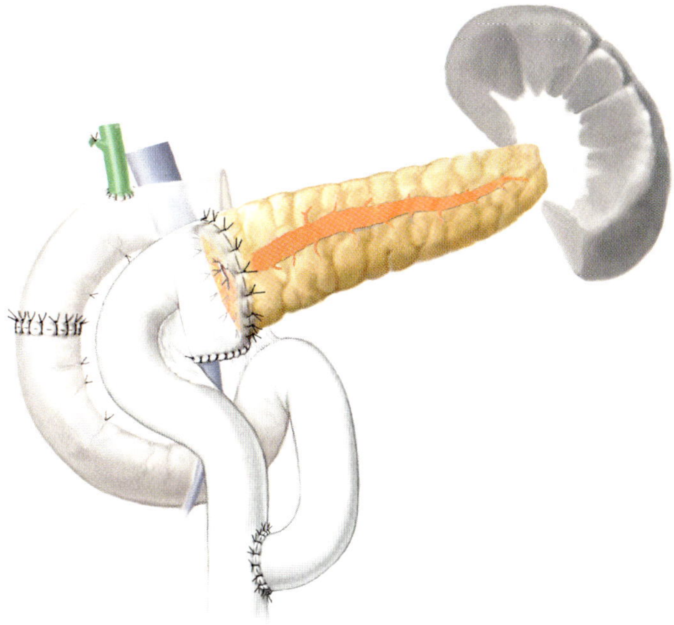

Figure 37.11

A DPPHRt with a segmental resection of the duodenum reduces the risk of recurrence of an IPMT or an MCT, or an endocrine neoplasia. For reconstruction, three anastomoses are necessary

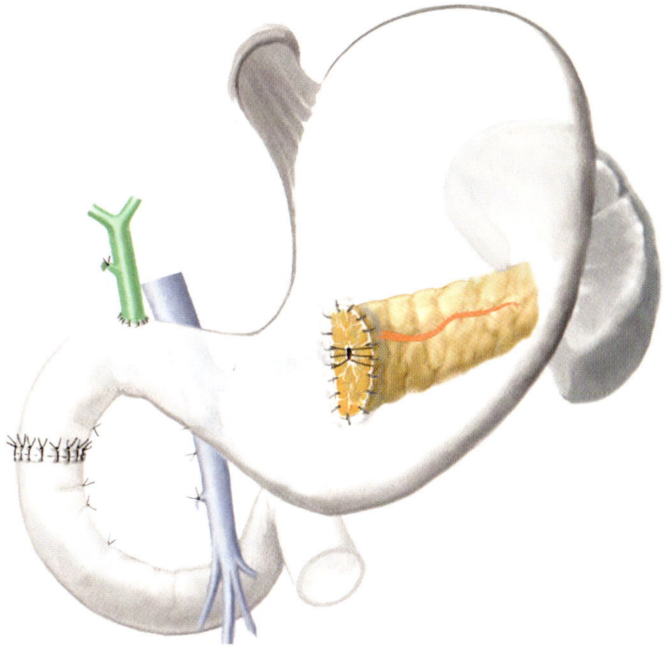

Figure 37.12

DPPHRt with implantation of the pancreatic stump into the dorsal wall of the stomach

more beneficial than a Whipple type of pancreatic head resection. DPPHR preserves endocrine function and most of the exocrine function of the pancreas and restores the patient's quality of life. It has been found that DPPHR lowers total hospital costs in comparison to the Whipple-type resection [22].

Three modifications of the classical duodenum-preserving subtotal pancreatic head resection have

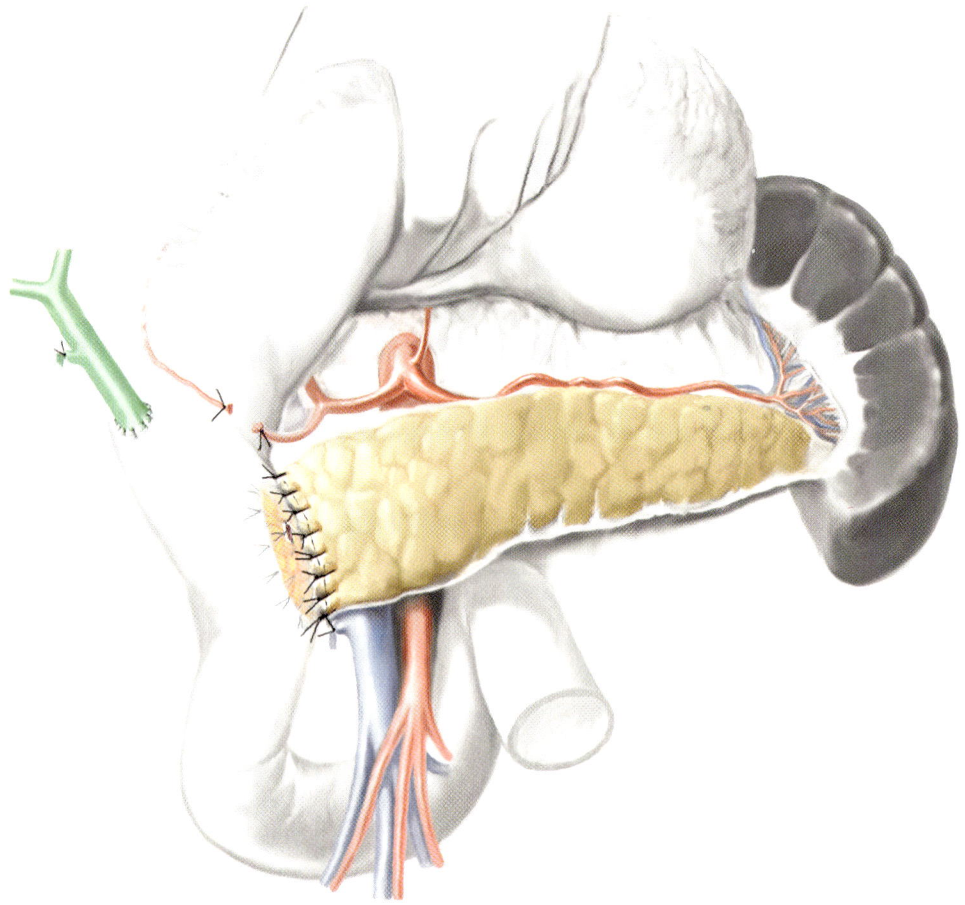

Figure 37.13

DPPHRt with anastomosis to the duodenum. Preservation of the spleen, biliary anastomosis of the common bile duct with the proximal duodenum (Imaizumi [25]

been applied (Table 37.5) [24–30]. Duodenum-preserving total pancreatic head resection, including a segmental resection of the peripapillary duodenum and duodenum-preserving total pancreatectomy with conservation of the spleen (Figs. 37.11–37.13). The application of the type of DPPHR is determined by the nature and extent of the neoplastic cystic lesion. Regarding the intraoperative criteria for the application of a DPPHR, it is recommended that the lesion is completely extirpated. To ensure completeness, a frozen section of the resection margins (the pancreas and the duodenum) has to be performed. In terms of IPMT, the indication for application of DPPHR exists in the case of a benign adenoma borderline lesion or carsinoma in situ (Table 37.6). In the case of a combination of a cystic adenoma and advanced carcinoma, which are observed in about 40% of cases, an oncological resection using the pylorus-preserving pancreatic head resection as a standard in addition to lymph-node dissection has to be done. To maintain the blood supply to the peripapillary segment of the duodenum it is mandatory to protect the dorsal pancreaticoduodenal arteries. In the case of an infiltration of the inflammatory cystic neoplastic process into the wall of the duodenum or an ischemic change of the wall of the duodenum, a segmental resection of the duodenum of the peripapillary area must also be carried out. The reconstruction of the duodenum takes place by an end-to-end anastomosis (Fig. 37.14). In the case of IPMT extension into the body and tail of the pancreas, a duodenum-preserving total pancreatectomy preserving the spleen has been applied (Fig. 37.15).

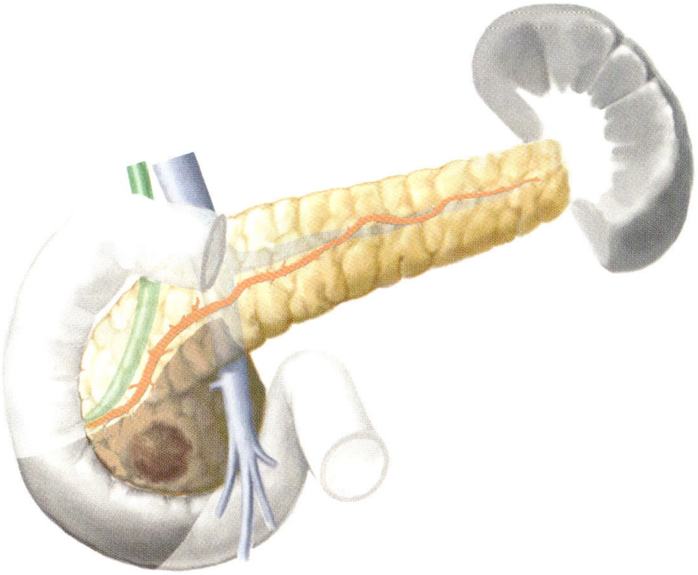

Figure 37.14

Cystic neoplastic lesions or endocrine neoplasia located in the uncinate process of the pancreas are treated with duodenum-preserving partial head resection. The uncinate process is resected along with a segment of the postpapillary duodenum. The common bile duct and the pancreatic main duct are maintained

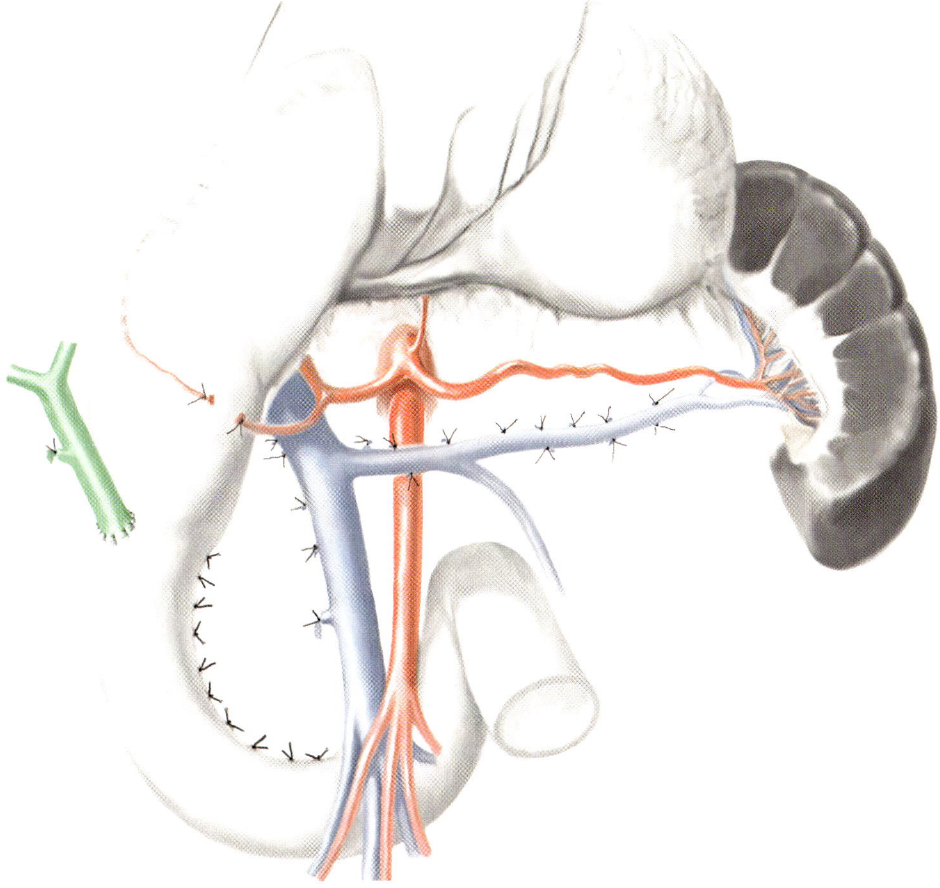

Figure 37.15

Duodenum-preserving total pancreatectomy with spleen preservation. A biliary anastomosis between the common bile duct and the proximal duodenum has to be carried out

References

1. Beger HG, Schlosser W, Poch B, Gansauge F (1998) Inflammatory mass in the head of pancreas. In: Beger HG, et al. (ed) The Pancreas. Blackwell Science, London, pp 757–760
2. Beger HG, Büchler M, Bittner R, et al (1989) Duodenum preserving resection of the head of the pancreas in severe chronic pancreatitis. Early and late results. Ann Surg 209:273–278
3. Friess H, Yamanaka Y, Büchler M, et al (1994) Cripto, a member of the epidermal growth factor family, is overexpressed in human pancreatic cancer and chronic pancreatitis. Int J Cancer 56:668–674
4. Korc M, Friess H, Yamanaka Y, et al (1994) Chronic pancreatitis is associated with increased concentrations of epidermal growth factor receptor, transforming growth factor, and phospholipase C. Gut 35:1468–1473
5. Gress TM, Menke A, Bachem M, et al (1998) Role of extracellular matrix in pancreatic diseases. Digestion 59:625–637
6. Bockman DE, Büchler MW, Malfertheiner P, Beger HG (1988) Analysis of nerves in chronic pancreatitis. Gastroenterology 94:1459–1469
7. Di Sebastiano P, Fink T, Weihe E, et al (1997) Immune cell infiltration and growth-associated protein. Gastroenterology 112:1648–1655
8. Miyake H, Harada H, Kunichika K, Ochi K, Kimura I (1987) Clinical course and prognosis of chronic pancreatitis. Pancreas 2:378–385
9. Löwenfels AB, Maisonneuve P, Cavallini G, et al (1993) Pancreatitis and the risk of pancreatic cancer. N Engl J Med 328:1433–1437
10. Beger HG, Krautzberger W, Bittner R, et al (1985) Duodenum-preserving resection of the head of the pancreas in patients with severe chronic pancreatitis. Surgery 97:467–473
11. Beger HG, Krautzberger W, Gögler H (1981) Résection de la tête du pancréas (pancréatectomie céphalique) avec conservation du duodénum dans les pancréatites chroniques, les tumeurs de la tête du pancréas et la compression du canal choledoque. Chirurg 107:597–604
12. Beger HG, Witte C, Krautzberger W, Bittner R (1980) Erfahrung mit einer das Duodenum erhaltenden Pankreaskopfresektion bei chronischer Pankreatitis. Chirurg 51:303–307
13. Bittner R, Butters M, Büchler M, et al (1994) Glucose homeostasis and endocrine pancreatic function in patients with chronic pancreatitis before and after surgical therapy. Pancreas 9:47–53
14. Beger HG, Schlosser W, Friess HM, Büchler MW (1999) Duodenum-preserving head resection in chronic pancreatitis changes the natural course of the disease. A single-center 26-year experience. Ann Surg 230:512–523
15. Büchler MW, Firess H, Bittner R, et al (1997) Duodenum-preserving pancreatic head resection: long-term results. J Gastrointest Surg 1:13–19
16. Büchler MW, Friess H, Müller MM, Beger HG (1995) Randomized trial of duodenum-preserving pancreatic head resection versus pylorus-preserving Whipple in chronic pancreatitis. Am J Surg 169:65–70
17. Klempa I, Spatny M, Menzel J, et al (1995) Pancreatic function and quality of life after resection of the head of the pancreas in chronic pancreatitis. A prospective, randomized comparative study after duodenum-preserving resection of the head of the pancreas versus Whipple's operation. Chirurg 66:350–359
18. Frey CF, Smith GJ (1987) Description and rationale of a new operation for chronic pancreatitis. Pancreas 2:701–707
19. Itzbicki JR, Bloechle C, Knoefel WT, Kuechler T, Binmoeller KF, Broelsch CE (1995) Duodenum-preserving resection of the head of the pancreas in chronic pancreatitis. A prospective, randomized trial. Ann Surg 221:350–358
20. Itzbicki JR, Bloechle C. Broering DC, Knoefel WT, Kuechler T, Broelsch CE (1998) Extended drainage versus resection in surgery for chronic pancreatitis: a prospective randomized trial comparing the longitudinal pancreatico-jejunostomy combined with local pancreatic head excision with the pylorus-preserving pancreatoduodenectomy. Ann Surg 228:771–779
21. Witzigman H, Max D, Uhlmann D, Geissler F, Schwarz R, Ludwig S, Lohmann T, Caca K, Keim V, Tannapfel A, Hauss J (2003) Outcome after duodenum-preserving pancreatic head resection is improved compared with classic Whipple procedure in the treatment of chronic pancreatitis. Surgery 134:53–62
22. Aspelund G, Topazian M, Lee JH, Andersen DK (2005) Improved outcome for benign disease with limited pancreatic head resection. J Gastrointest Surg 9:400–409
23. Howard TJ, Jones JW, Sherman S, Fogel E, Lehman GA (2001) Impact on pancreatic head resection on direct medical costs in patients with chronic pancreatitis. Ann Surg 234:661–667
24. Takada T, Yasuda H, Uchiyama K, Hasegawa H (1993) Duodenum preserving pancreatoduodenostomy. A new technique for complete excision of the head of the pancreas with preservation of biliary and alimentary integrity. Hepatogastroenterology 40:356–359
25. Imaizumi T, Hanyu F, Suzuki M, Nakasako T, Harada N, Hatori T (1995) Clinical experience with duodenum-preserving total resection of the head of the pancreas with pancreaticocholedochoduodenostomy. J Hepatobil Pancreat Surg 2:38–44
26. Nagakawa T, Ohta T, Kayahara M, Ueno K (1997) Total resection of the head of the pancreas preserving the duodenum, bile duct and papilla with end-to-end anastomosis of the pancreatic duct. Am J Surg 173:210–212
27. Pedrazzoli S, Sperti C, Pasquali C (2001) Pancreatic head resection for noninflammatory benign lesions of the head of the pancreas. Pancreas 23:309–315
28. Murakami Y, Uemura K, Yokoyama Y, Sasaki M, Morifuji M, Hayashidami Y, Sudo T, Sueda T (2004) Pancreatic head resection with segmental duodenectomy for intraductal papillary mucinous tumors of the pancreas. J Gastrointest Surg 8:713–718
29. M Siech, SU Thuenmayer, D Henne-Bruns, HG Beger (2004) Die Behandlung zystischer Tumoren des Pankreas, radikal oder organsparend? Chirurg 75:615–621
30. Kimura W (2003) IHPBA in Tokyo 2002; surgical treatment of IPMT vs MCT: a Japanese experience. J Hepatobil Pancreat Surg 10:156–162

Chapter 38

L. W. Traverso

Pancreaticoduodenctomy for Chronic Pancreatitis – With or Without Pylorus Preservation

Removing the head of the pancreas for chronic pancreatitis can be very effective in relieving disabling abdominal pain. The principles of successful treatment of chronic pancreatitis by head resection are based on two observations. First, the main reason for head resection is the disabling abdominal pain. This clinical syndrome is always associated with severe anatomic defects in the pancreas. Second, the locations of these anatomic defects are centered in the head of the pancreas; the "pacemaker" of chronic pancreatitis is in the head of the gland. William P. Longmire Jr, taught this concept to me during residency in the 1970s; others described it later in the 1980s. The pacemaker concept is so reliable that if the epicenter of the inflammation is not in the head of the pancreas then some other etiology should be considered, such as autoimmune pancreatitis, neoplasm, or continued occult alcohol use.

Rationale for Pancreatic Head Resection

The main goal of head resection is therefore pain relief. The following indications for resection have been developed to guide surgeons toward designing surgical resections that will result in pain relief. After long-term follow-up of almost 5 years, we have observed the postresection disappearance of disabling pain in virtually everyone after applying these strict indications for head resection. A pain-free state was achieved in three-quarters of the group.

A note about endotherapy here will make our discussion complete. Endotherapy is the transampullary dilatation of main pancreatic duct stricture or strictures and, if present, removal of pancreatic duct calculi, with or without extracorporeal shock-wave lithotripsy. For those institutions that have an experienced cross-specialty team for chronic pancreatitis, consider endotherapy before surgical resection. At least half of our patients have been able to avoid surgery with these new techniques. The anatomic selection criteria for head resection also apply to endotherapy.

The excellent pain relief achieved after head resection in our institution is a tribute to the efficacy of surgical resection because head resection was not employed until all other interventional and endoscopic treatments had failed.

A recent review using evidence-based medicine examined a variety of reports that listed pain relief and sequelae after all types of head resection for chronic pancreatitis [1]. Major relief from pain was observed in 70–100% of patients after the standard pancreaticoduodenectomy (PD), pylorus-preserving pancreaticoduodenectomy (PPPD), duodenum-preserving head resection (Beger procedure), or the ventral head resection with upstream ductal drainage (Frey procedure). These studies were difficult to compare, although many of them were randomized controlled trials. The reason for this difficulty was the lack of standard selection criteria for head resection. The criteria listed in the current chapter are based on imaging studies and would be a great opportunity for the surgical community to standardize. For example, many head resections in Europe are performed just for an inflammatory "pseudotumor" of the head without mention of ductal anatomy. Currently the trend in Europe and North America is to use the less time-consuming and less complex Frey procedure. However, a recent paper from eight German universities that perform pancreatic resections in high-volume centers shows that pancreaticoduodenectomy is still the preferred operation for head resection [2]. The advantages of PPPD for head resection include: (1) minimal pancreatic parenchyma has to be cut, resulting in little blood loss, (2) the procedure is familiar to all general surgeons, and (3) the entire stomach and duodenum are preserved.

Indications for Surgery

After completing a long-term follow-up study that averaged almost 5 years postresection [3], we believe that all of the following indications must be met in order to achieve pain relief with head resection:

Table 38.1. Cambridge classification of image severity for chronic pancreatitis. Summarized from Axon et al. (1984) [5]

Cambridge class	Main pancreatic duct	Abnormal side branches
1. Normal	Normal	None
2. Equivocal	Normal	<3
3. Mild	Normal	>3
4. Moderate	Abnormal	>3
5. Marked	Abnormal[a]	>3

[a] Any one of the following anatomic findings will place the case into the "marked" category:
1. Main pancreatic duct (MPD) terminates prematurely (abrupt, tapering, irregular).
2. Multiple MPD strictures.
3. MPD dilated >10 mm.
4. Ductal-filling defects (stones).
5. Intra- or extrapancreatic "cavities," also known as pseudocysts.
6. Contiguous organ involvement in or around the pancreas (common bile duct stricture, duodenal stenosis, or arterial venous fistula).

1. Chronic pancreatitis is documented using the 1963 Marseille definition of "residual pancreatic damage, either anatomical or functional, that persists even if the primary cause or factors are eliminated" [4]. This irreversible change in the pancreas is usually fibrosis.
2. The etiology of the chronic pancreatitis must have been remedied or eliminated (e.g., gallstones, autoimmune pancreatitis, or current use of alcohol). The patient usually denies the latter until pain persists after head resection due to smoldering pancreatitis in the pancreatic remnant.
3. Imaging studies must show anatomical defects that meet the criteria of "marked" in the Cambridge image severity score [5] (e.g., at least a main pancreatic duct stricture with or without stones; Table 38.1). Resection is designed to address this anatomy, which is almost always in the pancreatic head. As mentioned earlier, the surgeon should use caution if the epicenter of the disease is not in the head of the gland. Consider then other causes such as neoplasm, autoimmune, or occult alcohol use. One clue to the presence of continued alcohol abuse is "small duct pancreatitis." Resection is contraindicated as the process is still in evolution, excessive parenchyma might be removed and without pain relief.

Diagnostic Work-up

The Cambridge image severity score has proven very useful. To gain this anatomic information we depend on several types of modern imaging. In a patient with chronic pancreatitis more will be known preoperatively about their pancreatic anatomy than in the patients thought to have cancer. The workup requires a computed axial tomogram (CT) of the "pancreas protocol" variety and endoscopic retrograde cholangiopancreatography (ERCP). The latter provides unparalleled fine anatomical details and brush cytology of any stricture that is potentially malignant. The result of these imaging studies is a picture of the "composite pancreas." Endoscopic ultrasound may be helpful in some of these patients when CT does not provide enough information. This is particularly true when CT shows a prominent head that is isodense (no low-density mass but neoplasm is still suspected). Magnetic resonance cholangiopancreatography has not been practical to obtain fine detail of ductal anatomy unless the institution has a dedicated magnetic resonance radiologist willing to spend hours with the image software.

Finally, the anatomic criteria must be correlated with the clinical presentation. The surgeon should always consider the possibility that an occult neoplasm is present. Blood tumor markers such as CA 19-9 should be obtained.

On the day before surgery the patient undergoes mechanical bowel preparation. Antibiotics are administered at the induction of anesthesia. A single does of intravenous cephalosporin and metronidazole is administered. Since almost every patient has or has had biliary or pancreatic duct stents, this method has made abdominal abscess or wound infection an uncommon postoperative occurrence.

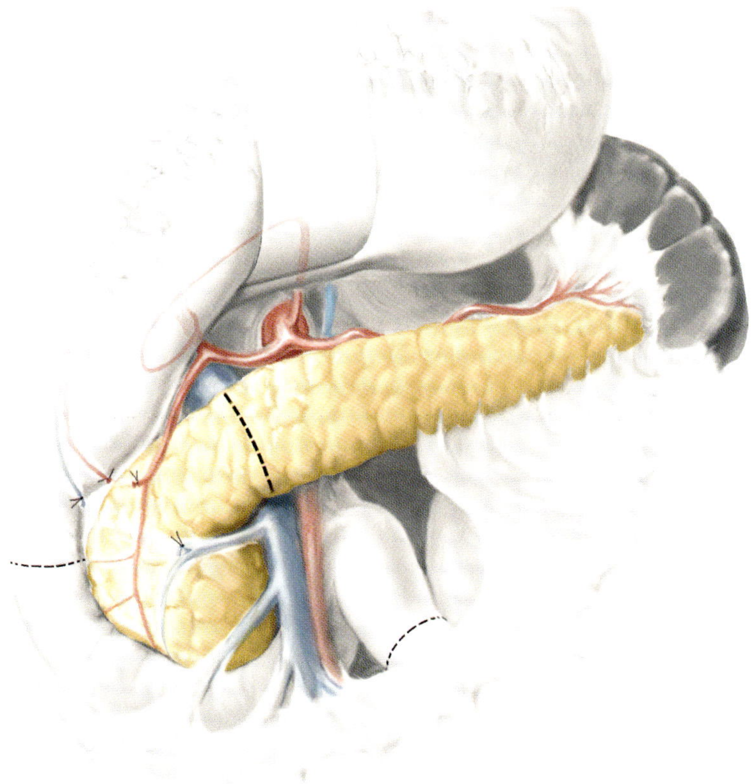

Figure 38.1

The areas to be resected with the pylorus-preserving pancreaticoduodenectomy are depicted: head of pancreas, duodenum (parts 2, 3, and 4), and segment of the proximal jejunum. The entire head of the gland is removed. Note that the duodenum, in this noncancer operation, is divided at the "angle" where the pancreas and duodenum become intimately associated. The right gastroepiploic vessels are divided near their origins. The right gastric artery is divided away from the stomach near its origin. This allows the neurovascular supply of the antrum and pylorus to be preserved and may minimize the incidence of delayed gastric emptying. Reprinted with permission from Traverso (1993) [9]

Surgical Technique

Type of Operation

No matter what type of head resection is chosen, if the patient meets the strict selection criteria listed they will benefit by modern and safe pancreatic resection. Like the German study [2], I have preferentially used PD (see Long-Term Outcomes). More specifically, I use PPPD for head resection in an attempt to accrue a 20-year follow-up after the same type of head resection and using the same selection criteria based on the Cambridge severity score. This effort should prove complimentary and supportive of the resections that remove less of the pancreatic head such as the Beger procedure, the Frey procedure, and their hybrids. If the premise is correct that the head of the pancreas is the pacemaker of chronic pancreatitis, then removal of the entire head should produce the best pain relief. Since PPPD by itself cannot cause disabling abdominal pain, the incidence of relief of disabling pain after PPPD should be the benchmark that the less extensive head resection procedures should strive to achieve.

Technique of Pylorus-Preserving Pancreaticoduodenctomy

This procedure removes all of the head of the pancreas and the duodenum (except the duodenal bulb), as is shown in Fig. 38.1. Reconstruction in our institution is depicted in Fig. 38.2. The duodenojejunostomy is in an antecolic position, a location that minimizes delayed gastric emptying (DGE). This concept has recently been demonstrated in a prospective randomized trial [6]. The incidence of DGE after the PPPD with this antecolic position should be <10%. When DGE occurs, it will most often be associated with an occult or obvious pancreatic anastomotic leak.

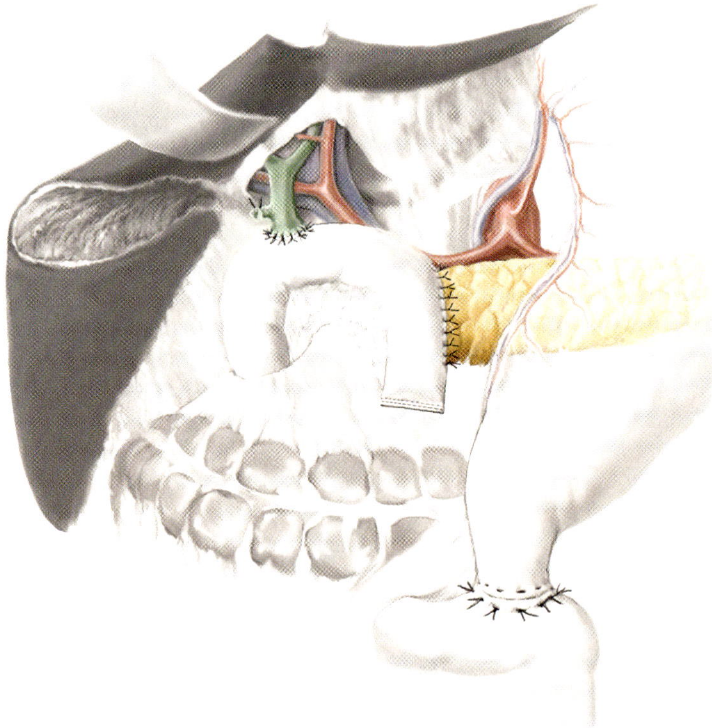

Figure 38.2

Reconstruction of the pancreatic duct and bile duct is via a retrocolic jejunal limb. The end-duodeno-to-side-jejunostomy is in an antecolic position to isolate the duodenal anastomosis from the pancreatic anastomosis and minimize delayed gastric emptying. Modified and reprinted after permission from Traverso (1999) [10]

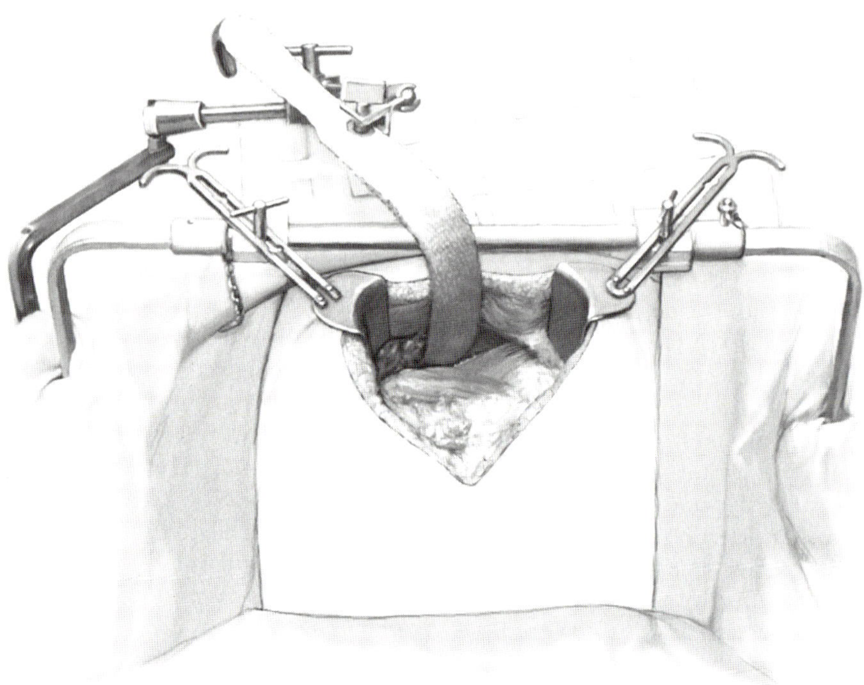

Figure 38.3

The retractor setup is depicted with the patient's head at the top. The Upper Hand system's retractor blades hold the costal margin up and out, while the multiarticulated Martin Arm can hold the liver or stomach back at any angle depending on the dissection task. The system allows sufficient exposure of the pancreatic head through the midline incision

The Smallest Incision Made Possible by Retractors

I use the smallest incision possible to provide the least morbidity and earliest patient mobilization. This is achieved with postoperative epidural analgesia and a short upper midline incision. The latter is made from the xiphoid to just above or below the umbilicus. Compared to the bilateral subcostal variety, the midline incision avoids cutting abdominal wall muscle and improves recovery in the postoperative period. When the upper midline incision is combined with epidural anesthesia, the incidence of postoperative pneumonia should be close to zero. Great exposure allows for better hemostasis. Great exposure with the upper midline incision is obtained with the Upper Hand system (Fowler retractor, Pilling Surgical, Horsham, PA, USA; Fig. 38.3). With the duodenum mobilized to the midline, this retractor system allows superb exposure as it elevates and retracts the costal margins. Also useful is the articulating Martin Arm retractor (Elmed, Addison, IL, USA) to retract the liver off the hepatoduodenal ligament or hold the antrum back while dissecting under the duodenal bulb on the right gastroepiploic vessels and superior mesenteric vein (SMV).

Mobilization of Structures

A wide Kocher maneuver mobilizes the duodenum to the midline and down to the level of the inferior mesenteric artery. The lesser sac is opened widely by removing the entire greater omentum off the transverse colon. Every attempt is made to preserve the greater omentum. The omentum is left attached to the stomach as this "watchdog of the abdomen" may have some ameliorative intra-abdominal properties to promote healing and prevent infection [7].

Next, the superior portion of the duodenal bulb and pylorus are mobilized for preservation with the stomach. Wide dissection is required to preserve the neurovascular supply to the pylorus. The preserved pylorus must be a functional pylorus. In order to accomplish wide dissection, the following blood vessels are divided at their origins away from the pylorus: the right gastric artery (if present, there usually is not one major vessel) and the supraduodenal vessels of Wilkie. The vessels are more easily dissected by starting at their parent vessels. I find the ultrasonic scissors to be very useful here, allowing for zero blood loss. Ultimately, the superior portion of the duodenal bulb and the pylorus are detached from their neurovascular connections in the hepatoduodenal ligament.

Now the inferior surface of the duodenal bulb is detached from the head of the pancreas, right gastroepiploic artery (RGEA), and the nest of right gastroepiploic vein branches. The latter have a huge anatomic variation as one to three right gastroepiploic veins may enter the SMV and/or the middle colic vein from the medial surface of the pancreatic head. Experience allows the surgeon to avoid losing blood in this area, as each individual vein needs to be divided near the SMV or middle colic vein. The RGEA is divided at the inferior border of the pancreas where it emerges off the surface of the pancreatic head. The ultrasonic scissors should never be used for the RGEA, but they are very useful for the veins in this area.

The retropyloric dissection continues along the duodenal bulb until it merges with the pancreas, forming an "angle" (Fig. 38.1). Here there are several tiny blood vessels shared by the pancreas and duodenum. They are best divided using an ultrasonic dissection instrument. About 3–5 cm of duodenum is now preserved with the stomach. A stapling device is used to divide the duodenum at the "angle." The stomach with the preserved duodenal bulb and omentum are placed in the left upper quadrant.

Excision of the Pancreatic Head, Remaining Duodenum, and Distal Common Bile Duct

The hepatoduodenal ligament is now dissected by first dividing the gastroduodenal artery (GDA) near but not at its origin. Since major postoperative bleeding from this vessel has resulted in sudden mortality, the GDA is triply ligated with nonabsorbable 2/0 silk suture well out onto the head of the pancreas. Once the GDA is divided, the plane behind the GDA provides easy access to the grove between the common bile duct (CBD) and the portal vein (PV). Now the neck of the pancreas can be more easily isolated from the underlying PV and divided. Even though electrocautery or ultrasonic scissors are useful in dividing the pancreatic parenchyma while facilitating hemostasis, the pancreatic duct itself should be "cold-cut" with a scalpel to avoid devascularizing the duct wall and promoting a pancreatic anastomotic leak.

The pancreatic neck is rolled up and to the right. Blunt dissection separates the lateral wall of the PV from the dorsal pancreatic head. Then the CBD is encircled with a vascular loop and divided over a bulldog clamp. Caution should be exerted here, as about one in four people will have a large vessel in the retro-CBD area. These are easily palpated before division of the CBD. Always palpate for them! These anomalous

Table 38.2. Benchmarks for single-surgeon pancreaticoduodenectomy. Modified with permission from Traverso et al. (2004) [8]. *ASA* American Society of Anesthesiologists, *OR* operation room

Outcome	Virginia Mason *N* = 232 1996–2002	Literature *N* = 2,730 1997–2003
ASA classification	I = 0% II = 56% III = 42% IV = 2%	Not stated
Mortality	0%	1.9%
OR time	450 min	431 min
Estimated blood loss	382 ml	1,183 ml
Transfusion required	3.0%	Not stated
Length of stay postoperative	11.2 days	17.8 days
Pancreatic anastomotic leak		9.9%
"Broad"[a]	12.9%	
"Clinically relevant"[b]	6.5%	
Biliary leak	0.4%	Not stated
Delayed gastric emptying at 10/14 days	9.5%/6.0%	13.9%
Postoperative percutaneous drainage	5.6%	Not stated
Reoperation	0.4%	3.8%
Readmission	4.3%	Not stated

[a] Amylase 5× elevated in drain fluid, >5 days postoperative, and >30 ml/day
[b] Criteria met but did not have delay in discharge

vessels can represent a replaced-right, accessory-right, or replaced-common hepatic artery. Division of a replaced artery will result in a devascularized upstream CBD and subsequent bile anastomotic breakdown.

Next, the attachments of the dorsal pancreatic head to the superior mesenteric artery (SMA) have to be divided. The potential problem areas for venous blood loss in the previous dissection was the right gastroepiploic vein system, but in the current dissection we will encounter the posterior superior pancreaticoduodenal vein and the first jejunal vein (posterior and inferior) as it courses over the SMA in the inferior retropancreatic head area. The former is usually a single large vessel that will be encountered during dissection of the dorsal superior pancreatic head just caudal to where the CBD is usually divided. This vein requires suture ligation on the PV side. The first jejunal vein does not have to be divided and can be controlled during the dissection described below.

Other than these veins there are potential areas for blood loss within the dorsal pancreatic head attachments. The lymph nodes do not have to be removed in this noncancer operation, but staying directly on the SMA can facilitate a hemostatic dissection. Unless the surgeon is prepared the dissection can be bloody because of the variation in the location of veins and arteries in this area. Surgeons should note that the blood supply to the pancreas has the highest variability in the location of its named arteries. Every patient is different! The surgeon should know the problem areas and develop a method that works best for them to ensure that no blood is lost during dissection in this SMA area. Blood loss during a Whipple operation should be minimal (<400 ml, Table 38.2) and will usually occur during parenchymal division of the pancreatic neck.

A method that works for me to avoid any blood loss as the dissection proceeds along the SMA is as follows. The bridge of tissue between the SMA and the dorsal pancreatic head is made up of dense matted lymph nodes, a variety of arteries including the inferior pancreaticoduodenal artery (IPDA), and a variety of small veins returning blood to the PV. I begin at the superior head and divide the retro-SMA tissue in small sections by dissecting caudally towards the uncinate process. Each division is accomplished by placing a single long Collar clamp over the tissue close to the SMA. The tissue is divided between the clamp and

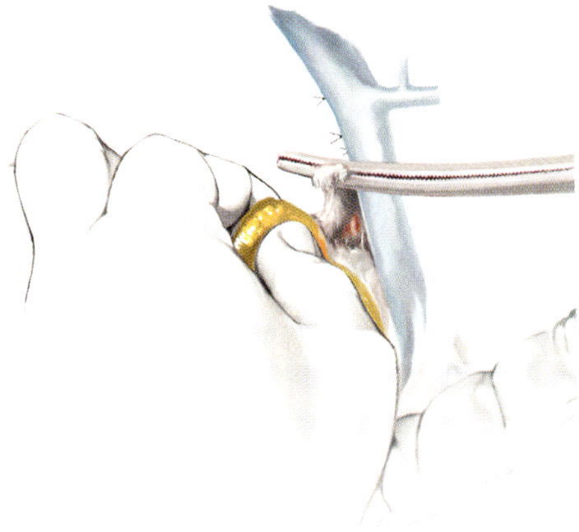

Figure 38.4

Hand compression of the specimen is used to control blood loss while the retroperitoneal attachments of the dorsal medial pancreatic head and uncinate process are divided from the superior mesenteric artery (SMA). The surgeon on the left side of the patient places their left hand on the lymph node-laden mesentery attaching the dorsal head and uncinate process to the SMA area. As this "mesentery" is divided sequentially from cephalad to caudad along the SMA, the hand pressure controls bleeding from the specimen and the clamps control bleeding from the SMA side

the specimen. The left hand of the left-sided surgeon nicely controls blood loss from the specimen as the surgeon on the patient's right side ties the sutures behind the clamp (Fig. 38.4). The clamp is removed after a 2/0 silk suture is tied between the clamp and the SMA. Large bleeders from the specimen are controlled by compression with the surgeon's left hand. These can be sutured and ligated later after the pancreatic head is mobilized out of its bed.

As the division continues in a caudal fashion, the surgeon will notice that after several clampings the SMA becomes closer to the dissection. This is usually the point where one encounters the IPDA, a vessel that is not seen well because it is buried in dense lymphatic tissue. The IPDA is controlled and ligated in the same manner. Once the IPDA is divided the SMA seems to fall away from the dissection. The first jejunal branch does not have to be divided; rather divide just the branches from the uncinate process before they enter this large vein. The same clamp technique with left-hand vascular control is used to divide the last of the uncinate attachments directly on the surface on the uncinate process, while preserving the first jejunal vein. Much blood can be lost in this area. Proceed slowly, with caution, and with profound knowledge of the anatomical variations.

The following point should be emphasized in order to locate the area of the IPDA. After the surgeon has divided about two-thirds of the attachments in a caudal direction from the CBD area then the surgeon will be very near the IPDA; it lies inside dense lymphatic tissue just before the first jejunal branch. The latter can be seen entering the back of the SMV (i.e., the IPDA is in the area just cephalad to the first jejunal vein).

To remove the PPPD specimen, all that remains is to divide the jejunum using the gastrointestinal stapling device, about 6 cm below the ligament of Trietz. The mesenteric vascular attachments can be very easily divided with ultrasonic scissors here. Sutures do not have to be employed. Then the defect in the ligament of Trietz created by removing the jejunum and fourth part of the duodenum is closed with interrupted sutures to avoid internal hernia.

Prereconstruction Pancreatography

An intraoperative fluoroscopic pancreatogram may be useful to visualize the ductal system in the pancreatic remnant if the duct has not been visualized by ERCP. This ensures that the main cause of persistent pain (smoldering remnant pancreatitis) is minimized by complete main duct decompression. A partial longitudinal incision and lateral pancreaticojejunostomy to the body and tail may be indicated if there are significant chain-of-lake strictures seen on pancreatogram (Fig. 38.5).

Reconstruction - Pancreatic Anastomosis

The avascular window in the transverse mesocolon is located and incised just to the left of the middle colic vein and the stump of the jejunal limb is brought into the lesser sac area. The pancreatic and biliary anastomoses will be retrocolic, while the duodenal anastomosis will be antecolic (Figs. 38.2 and 38.5). The anastomoses are positioned in this way to isolate potential leakage of the bile and pancreatic duct connections from the duodenojejunostomy. This maneuver has minimized DGE to 8% in the last 215 cases. The stomach, with preserved pylorus and duodenal bulb, is brought antecolic to the left transverse colon, allowing for an easy duodenojejunostomy remote from the other anastomoses.

As stated earlier, if a chain-of-lakes-type ductal dilatation is present in the remnant with significant strictures, then a longitudinal side-to-side technique

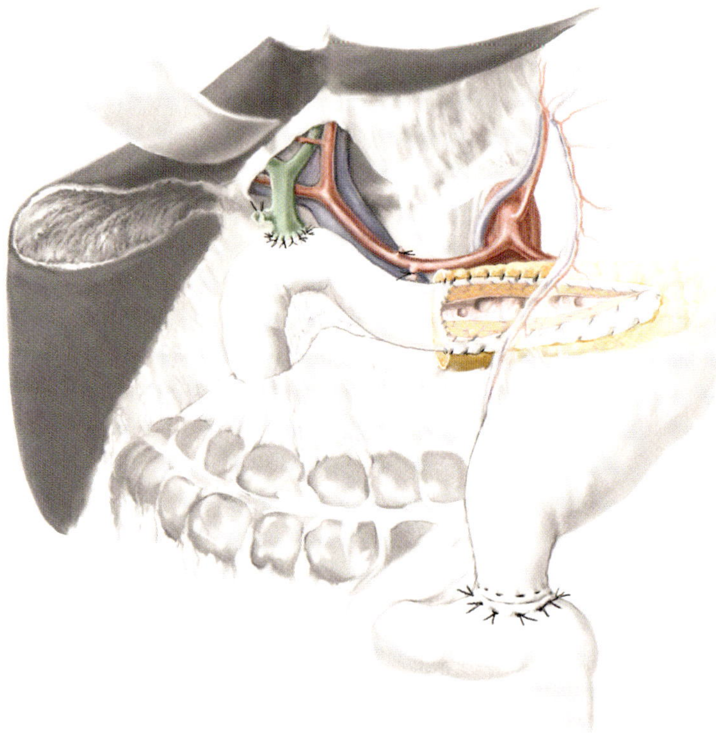

Figure 38.5

If multiple strictures from chronic pancreatitis are present in the pancreatic remnant, then the duct must be decompressed using a lateral pancreaticojejunostomy much like with the Puestow lateral drainage procedure

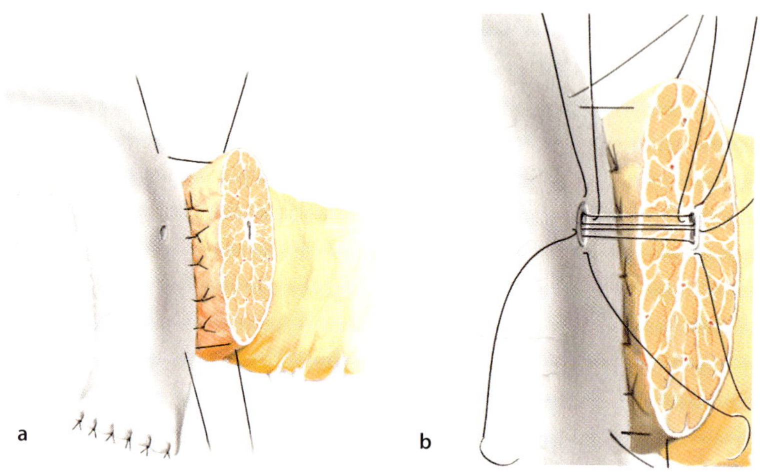

Figure 38.6

a The back wall of the pancreatic anastomosis has been created with interrupted sutures. These knots have been tied anteriorly. b The illustration depicts four quadrant tacking of the jejunal wall on the left to the pancreatic duct wall on the right. The first suture is the most dorsal and is placed "outside-in" through the jejunal wall and then "inside-out" through the pancreatic duct wall. This knot will be tied outside the new lumen, but first the superior and inferior sutures are placed. These sutures are also placed so that their knots can be tied on the outside of the new lumen. After the second and third sutures are placed, then the first suture's knot is tied. The stent is introduced and the fourth and final suture is placed. The knots of the second, third, and fourth sutures are then tied in that order. Modified with permission from Traverso (2006) [11]

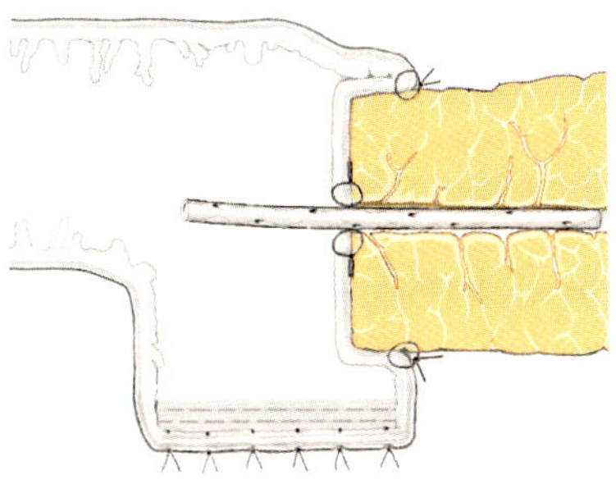

Figure 38.7

The final end-to-side stented pancreaticojejunostomy is depicted with the knots on the outside of the new lumen and the outer seromuscular envelope. Modified with permission from Traverso (2006) [11]

is used, but many patients will have a normal duct in the pancreatic remnant with a diameter of 2–3 mm. These small pancreatic ducts are more prone to leakage after pancreaticojejunostomy, although chronic pancreatitis and fibrosis make the incidence of leakage minimal. After a pancreatic-duct-to-jejunal-mucosa anastomosis, an outer layer or "seromuscular envelope" is constructed containing a stented end-to-side, duct-to-mucosa pancreaticojejunostomy.

First the back wall of the outer layer is constructed using interrupted 3/0 silk sutures. These knots are tied anteriorly (Fig. 38.6A). Then a tiny hole is made in the jejunal mucosa opposite the pancreatic duct. The mucosa-to-mucosa anastomosis is created with interrupted 6/0 Vicryl suture on an RB3 needle (Ethicon, Somerville, New Jersey, USA). Note that all knots are tied on the outside of the new lumen to avoid sludge and stone formation (Fig. 38.6B). If the pancreatic parenchyma is rock hard then 5/0 PDS suture with an RB1 needle will be required as the smaller RB3 needle cannot penetrate a fibrotic pancreas. For small ducts of ≤3 mm the task is to place exact mucosal sutures to tack the pancreatic duct wall to the jejunal wall while not crossing these tiny sutures. This four-quadrant apposition is the key to success during pancreaticojejunostomy (Fig. 38.6B). The visual cues available using the surgical microscope at ×12.5 to ×16.0 power have lowered the leakage rate to almost zero when a small duct is present. The microscope is particularly useful when a soft gland with a small duct is present, as with ampullary of duodenal carcinoma.

A 3-Fr polytetrafluoroethylene radio-dense stent also helps avoid crossing the sutures. The "Geenan" stent is used because it has multiple holes throughout the stent (Wilson-Cook Medical, Winston-Salem, North Carolina, USA). This stent is cut to be about 4 cm long and inserted into the duct just before placement of the last (anterior) mucosa-to-mucosa stitch. The stent is loosely attached in its midportion to the jejunal mucosa near the last anterior stitch with a single 6/0 Vicryl suture. The stent ensures adequate apposition of the mucosa and decompresses the pancreatic duct upstream from the swollen mucosa due to sutures. It passes spontaneously in about 10–14 days. Its presence can be checked with an abdominal x-ray. The anterior outer layer of interrupted 3/0 silk Lembert sutures is now placed to complete the anastomosis (Fig. 38.7).

Reconstruction – Biliary Anastomosis

The goal of the biliary anastomosis is to place the interrupted sutures so that all of the knots are tied on the outside. The technique begins with placing several sutures "outside-in" on the anterior (ventral) aspect of the bile duct stump. The needles are not removed from the sutures. These sutures are then elevated with clamps that stabilize the bile duct into position. Then an opening that is smaller than the bile duct lumen is cut in the jejunal limb just downstream from the pancreatic anastomosis. An end-choledocho-to-side-jejunal anastomosis is created with a single layer of interrupted absorbable 5/0 PDS (Ethicon). Once again, all of the knots are placed so that they can be tied on the outside (to prevent stone formation on knots of this delayed-absorbable suture). A T-tube is not used. At the point of exit from the transverse mesocolon the jejunal limb is tacked to the mesenteric exit site with 3/0 silk sutures.

Reconstruction – Antecolic Duodenojejunostomy

The stomach, first part of duodenum, and the omentum are brought over the left side of the transverse colon. Although the duodenal stump may look cyanotic, this is due to venous spasm. I have never had a duodenojejunostomy leak. Vascular supply can be assured by examining for mucosal integrity inside the lumen of the duodenal bulb when the staple line is excised after the backside of the outer layer has been finished. The anastomosis is made in two layers. The inner layer is of running 3/0 Vicryl and the outer layer is interrupted 3/0 silk. The location of the end-duodeno-to-side-jejunostomy on the jejunal limb is downstream from the biliary and pancreatic anastomoses and about 10–15 cm below the exit site of the jejunal limb from the transverse mesocolon.

Abdominal Wall Closure

A closed-suction, round, 15-Fr silicone rubber drainage catheter is placed under the biliary and pancreatic anastomoses from a right upper quadrant stab wound. The midline fascia is closed with figure-of-eight 0 PDS interrupted sutures, but nonabsorbable monofilament suture is used if the patient is at risk for nonhealing, for example if they suffer from malnutrition or obesity, or have been administered preoperative steroids.

Early Postoperative Course, Benchmarks, and Milestones

During and after the surgery, several outcomes are created for each patient. These can be compared to national benchmarks to see how well the hospital compares for this complex operation. Some of these outcomes occur during the postoperative recovery and might better be termed milestones. All of the outcomes will culminate in discharge from the hospital. A list of these milestones is termed a "critical pathway." Examples of milestones include the period required for nasogastric suction (3–5 days), return to unlimited oral intake (5–7 days), the absence of DGE (DGE rate 4–9%), and the length of hospital stay (9–11 days) after the operation. The nursing staff then use milestones to assess patient progress after the Whipple procedure by using the average values obtained by patients who have previously undergone this operation in our high-volume center. In this way an experienced health-care team can monitor and improve the outcomes of high-volume complex operations. A list of these intraoperative and postoperative outcomes compared to benchmarks from a literature review is provided in Table 38.2. Note that collected outcomes after a Whipple operation need to be standardized just like the indications for head resection based on anatomy. In Table 38.2, four items were not collected well in the literature, for example blood transfusion rates or need for postoperative percutaneous drainage. Specific benchmarks have been suggested for the Whipple operation [8].

Postoperative Testing

All patients at 3 months after resection are interviewed to ensure they are taking pancreatic enzyme supplements if fecal elastase indicates they are required. Fecal elastase measurements are obtained at 3 months and 1 year after surgery. Many patients will have a low fecal elastase at 3 months postoperative, but this returns to normal levels at 1 year. Since patients are at a mild risk for marginal ulceration (said to be 6%), all patients are asked to take a proton pump inhibitor in the morning before eating. A letter is sent to the primary care provider explaining that any person after a Whipple procedure requires an annual physical that includes testing for anemia, vitamin deficiency, fasting blood sugar, and fecal elastase. Imaging studies are not required unless the patient develops recurrent symptoms.

Long-Term Outcome After Pylorus-Preserving Pancreaticoduodenctomy

Over the last decade and a half we have noticed less need for resection due to the improved results of endotherapy. The cases reaching the surgeon are therefore more complicated, but using the selection criteria presented in Table 38.1 we observed great outcomes for pain relief. In 1997, we reported the short- and long-term outcomes (mean 55 months) from 57 patients who had undergone pancreaticoduodenectomy for chronic pancreatitis. Since then we have extended the experience to over 120 patients. In the original report the indications for head resection were as listed in Table 38.1. All patients had the Cambridge image severity score of "marked," but to be more specific, 96% had main pancreatic duct obstruction and the 4% who did not were patients with intrapancreatic pseudocysts in the pancreatic head. All patients had multiple other elements of the Cambridge classification to support head resection as listed in the footer of Table 38.1.

The progressive role of endotherapy was prominent in these patients. CBD obstruction was observed in 65% of patients, and therefore 47% of them had undergone prior CBD stenting. Pancreatic duct obstruction was seen in 96% of patients, with 39% of them with a documented upstream main pancreatic duct disruption (blow-out). Pancreatic duct stenting had been used in 35% of patients and these treatments had failed to achieve pain relief. In addition, 19% had required percutaneous drainage of peripancreatic fluid collections. The surgery was safe. There was no hospital or 30-day mortality. PPPD was used in 97%, since 3% already had an anterectomy from previous ulcer surgery.

The onset of new diabetes was interesting. We did not see a predisposition for diabetes due to PPPD, as has been suggested by others. In those who were not diabetic preoperatively ($n = 37$), the actual 5-year diabetic occurrence rate was 32%. This diabetes was not a consequence of the resection because no patient became diabetic sooner than 12 months after the resection, indicating that the criteria for surgery had been accurate enough to ensure that only nonfunctional pancreatic tissue had been excised. These data supported the concept that diabetes was a result of continued fibrosis in the pancreatic remnant.

Patients that were at least 1 year after their Whipple operation ($n = 43$) were then questioned after a mean follow-up period of 55 months. In the patients who originally had disabling pain as an indication for surgery, every patient indicated that they had a good response to surgery and that their pain was no longer disabling. In addition, 76% of the patients indicated that they were pain free. The origin of residual pain was progressive disease in the pancreatic remnant, but the pain was not disabling. All patients were able to maintain their preoperative weight and there were no patients who complained of dumping or significant diarrhea. However, 77% of the patients were taking exocrine enzymes and 14% indicated that they had diarrhea if they didn't take them. Another surprising finding was the incidence of marginal ulceration in 6% of those with PPPD, but in 44% of those with total pancreatectomy. Since the time of this report we have avoided total pancreatectomy regardless of their diabetic status and placed patients on chronic daily proton pump inhibitors.

A cautionary note is provided about those patients thought to have small-duct pancreatitis. The often-discussed need for total pancreatectomy for small-duct pancreatitis has not been necessary in our practice. The vast majority of patients we have seen for small ductal pancreatitis were found to either not have chronic pancreatitis or were currently drinking alcohol and, therefore, not candidates for resective surgery (see indication no. 2 of Indications for Surgery, above).

Summary

After long-term follow up of almost 5 years after PPPD the benchmark for relief of disabling pain should approach 100% provided patients are selected using strict anatomic selection criteria. It is hoped that this benchmark for pain relief could be equaled by a variety of promising operations using a more limited head resection, such as the Frey or Beger operations. The results of PPPD should be complimentary and support attempting lesser resective procedures. Of utmost importance for comparison studies is that the patients must be selected with a standard list of reliable clinical and anatomic imaging criteria such as those suggested in this chapter. Specific anatomic criteria for limited head resection have not been used in studies for these other operations. The specific benchmarks listed in this paper for a Whipple operation would make series more comparable. If the premise is correct that the head of the pancreas is the pacemaker of chronic pancreatitis in most cases, then limited head resections should approach or equal the pain relief that we have observed after PPPD.

References

1. Schafer M, Mullhaupt B, Clavien PA (2002) Evidence-based pancreatic head resection for pancreatic cancer and chronic pancreatitis. Ann Surg 236:137–148
2. Makowiecz F, Hopt UT, and GAST Study Group (2005) Current techniques and complication rates in pancreatic surgery: results of a multi-institutional survey of 6 German centers with 1,083 pancreatic head resections (GAST Study Group). J Gastrointest Surg 9:1080–1087
3. Traverso LW, Kozarek RA (1997) Pancreaticoduodenectomy for chronic pancreatitis. Anatomic selection criteria and subsequent long-term outcome analysis. Ann Surg 226:429–438
4. Sarles H (1963) Proposal adopted unanimously by the participants of the symposium. In: Sarles H (ed) Pancreatitis Symposium, Marseilles, April 25 and 26, 1963. Karger, Basel pp VII–VIII
5. Axon ATR, Classen M, Cotton PB, et al (1984) Pancreatography in chronic pancreatitis: international definitions. Gut 25:1107–1112
6. Tani M, Terasawa, H, Kawai M, Ina, S, Hirono S, Uchiyama K, Yamaue H (2006) Improvement of delayed gastric emptying in pylorus-preserving pancreaticoduodenectomy: results of a prospective, randomized, controlled trial. Ann Surg 243:316–320
7. Traverso LW, MacFarlane SK (1987) Pancreatic juice in the peritoneal cavity: antibiotics or omental preservation prevent mortality. J Surg Res 43:220–225
8. Traverso LW, Shinchi H, Low DE (2004) Useful benchmarks to evaluate outcomes after esophagectomy and pancreaticoduodenectomy. Am J Surg 187:604–608
9. Traverso LW (1993) The pylorus-preserving Whipple procedure for severe complications of chronic pancreatitis. In: Beger HG, Buchler MW, Malfertheimer P (eds) Standards of Pancreatic Surgery. Springer-Verlag, Heidelberg, p 397
10. Traverso LW (1999) The surgical management of chronic pancreatitis: the Whipple procedure. In: Cameron JL (ed) Advances in Surgery, vol. 32, Mosby, St. Louis, pp 23–39
11. Traverso LW (2006) Pylorus-preserving pancreaticoduodenectomy for chronic pancreatitis. In: Clavien PA, Sarr M, Fong Y (eds) Atlas of Upper Abdominal Surgery. Springer Verlag, Heidelberg pp 849–884

Chapter 39

Central Pancreatectomy

C. Iacono · L. Bortolasi · G. Serio

Central pancreatectomy (CP) is a segmental resection of the pancreas that is indicated to remove benign or low-grade malignant tumors located in the isthmus and proximal part of the body. It allows to the functional parenchyma to be saved with no risk of exocrine or endocrine insufficiency, it also spares the spleen and the upper digestive and biliary tract, which is not possible with splenopancreatectomy and pancreaticoduodenectomy, respectively.

History

Central pancreatectomy was first performed by Dagradi and Serio in 1982 to resect an insulinoma of the pancreatic isthmus, it was published in 1984 in Enciclopedia Medica Italiana [1]. Other authors subsequently reported this technique [2–5]. Some authors believe that this technique was described for the first time in 1957 by Guillemin and Bessot [6], others by Letton and Wilson in 1959 [7]. Nevertheless, these two operations dealt only with the reconstructive aspect of central pancreatectomy. In fact, the French authors [6] carried out only a transection of the isthmus followed by a double digestive anastomosis of the two pancreatic stumps to a jejunal loop. Letton and Wilson [7] performed only the reconstructive part after burying the cephalic stump and carrying out a pancreaticojejunostomy to the distal stump after a traumatic transection of the neck.

From the technical point of view, central pancreatectomy requires a first stage for the resection of the central segment, isthmus, and proximal body, followed by the reconstructive part, which comprises suturing the cephalic stump and the digestive anastomosis of the distal stump [1].

A description of the complete operation was reported for the first time by the head of our school [1] in 1984 and subsequently brought to the attention of a wider audience, with many reports in the national and international literature as well as congress with oral presentations and videos [8, 9]. However, the first description of a segmental pancreatic resection was given by Beger [10], as in 1980 he reported the technique of duodenum-sparing pancreas head resection (Beger procedure); nevertheless, this operation is similar to central pancreatectomy, differing because of the site of resection.

We therefore believe that this technique should be called the Dagradi-Serio-Iacono operation, according to the names of the surgeons who first performed it (Dagradi and Serio), and the names of the surgeons responsible for reporting it worldwide (Iacono and Serio). In fact, in the last two decades Serio and Iacono have made great efforts to popularize the technique of central pancreatectomy with the correct indications [8, 9].

Rationale for Central Pancreatectomy

The rationale for central pancreatectomy is to remove the tumor-preserving functional parenchyma, avoiding major procedures such as pancreaticoduodenectomy or left splenopancreatectomy. This assures no risk of diabetes and exocrine insufficiency compared to standard operations; other major advantages are preservation of upper digestive and biliary tract functions (not possible with pancreaticoduodenectomy) and of infective, immunologic, and coagulative balance (not possible with left splenopancreatectomy).

Indications

Basic conditions that have to be fulfilled are:

1. Tumor size between 2 and 5 cm. In fact in this case a simple enucleation entails a high risk of lesion of the main pancreatic duct, and a high risk of non-radical resection.
2. Small tumors that are deeply located in the gland and therefore not eligible for enucleation (functioning endocrine tumors such as insulinoma).
3. Benign or low grade malignant tumors allowing a conservative resection with disease free margins: endocrine tumors, serous and mucinous cystade-

nomas, noninvasive intraductal mucinous producing tumors (IMPT), solid pseudopapillary tumors, and other less-frequently occurring lesions.
4. Non-neoplastic cystic lesions such as lymphoepithelial, dermoid, and hydatid cysts.
5. It is indicated for resection of solitary metastases of pancreatic neck (especially renal metastasis) and in pancreatic endocrine tumors with metastases in a multimodal treatment.
6. Focal chronic pancreatitis with isolated and short stenosis of Wirsung's duct, cystic inflammatory lesion, or pancreatic duct lithiasis.

Contraindications

Contraindications are represented by:

1. Large lesions for which it is not possible to preserve at least 5 cm distal to the pancreatic stump.
2. Distal body–tail atrophy.
3. Malignant tumors (especially ductal carcinoma).
4. Neoplastic involvement from other organs (stomach, transverse colon).
5. Diffuse chronic pancreatitis or focal pancreatitis not involving the central part of the gland.
6. Central pancreatectomy is contraindicated when the body–tail of the pancreas receives its arterial blood supply exclusively from the transverse pancreatic artery (left branch of the dorsal pancreatic artery; Fig. 39.1); this anatomical variation of vascularization, which can be clearly seen on angiography, angio-computed tomography (CT) or angio-magnetic resonance (MR), is defined by Mellière and Moullé [11] as type III and was present in about 25% of their cases.

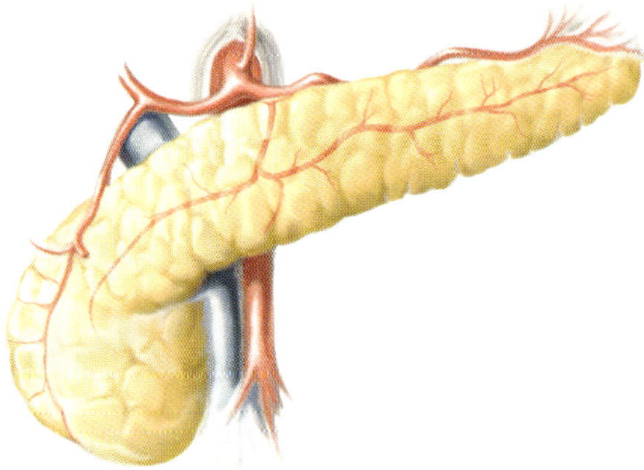

Figure 39.1

Pancreatic body–tail vascularization supported exclusively by the transverse pancreatic artery, left branch of the dorsal pancreatic artery (type III according to Mellière and Moullé), contraindicates central pancreatectomy

Diagnostic Work-Up

Preoperative functional studies are directed to assess the nutritional status of the patient with complete laboratory tests. Serum carcinoembryonic antigen, CA 19-9, neuron-specific enolase, and α-chromogranin are determined. In case of suspected endocrine neoplasm, specific hormone dosages are assessed.

Radiologic investigations as ultrasonography (US), CT, MR scanning and endoscopic retrograde cholangiopancreatography (ERCP) provide important information about the characteristics of the lesion. In particular, dynamic CT scanning and MR pancreatography give useful details regarding the blood supply of the neoplasm and its relationship with vessel and pancreatic duct.

In the case of differential diagnosis, fine-needle aspiration cytology under US control can be performed percutaneously or endoscopically.

Exocrine and endocrine function studies are evaluated preoperatively to diagnose possible insufficiencies and to compare with postoperative results. Endocrine function is evaluated by measuring serum levels of glucose, glycosylated hemoglobin, insulinemia, and C-peptide, and with the oral glucose tolerance test (OGTT). Exocrine function is assessed using the pancreo-lauryl test and assaying fecal fat excretion and/or determination of fecal elastase-1.

Preoperative Preparation

Antibiotic and antithrombotic prophylaxis is given. Some authors advise prophylaxis with somatostatin analogs to prevent pancreatic fistulae; however, randomized studies on major pancreatic resections have not show any benefits. We do not use any somatostatin or analogs.

Surgical Technique

The surgical technique includes the following major steps: (1) first stage for resection of the central segment, isthmus, and proximal body (Fig. 39.2a–d); (2) reconstructive part, which comprises burying the cephalic stump and performing the digestive anastomosis on the distal stump (Fig. 39.2e).

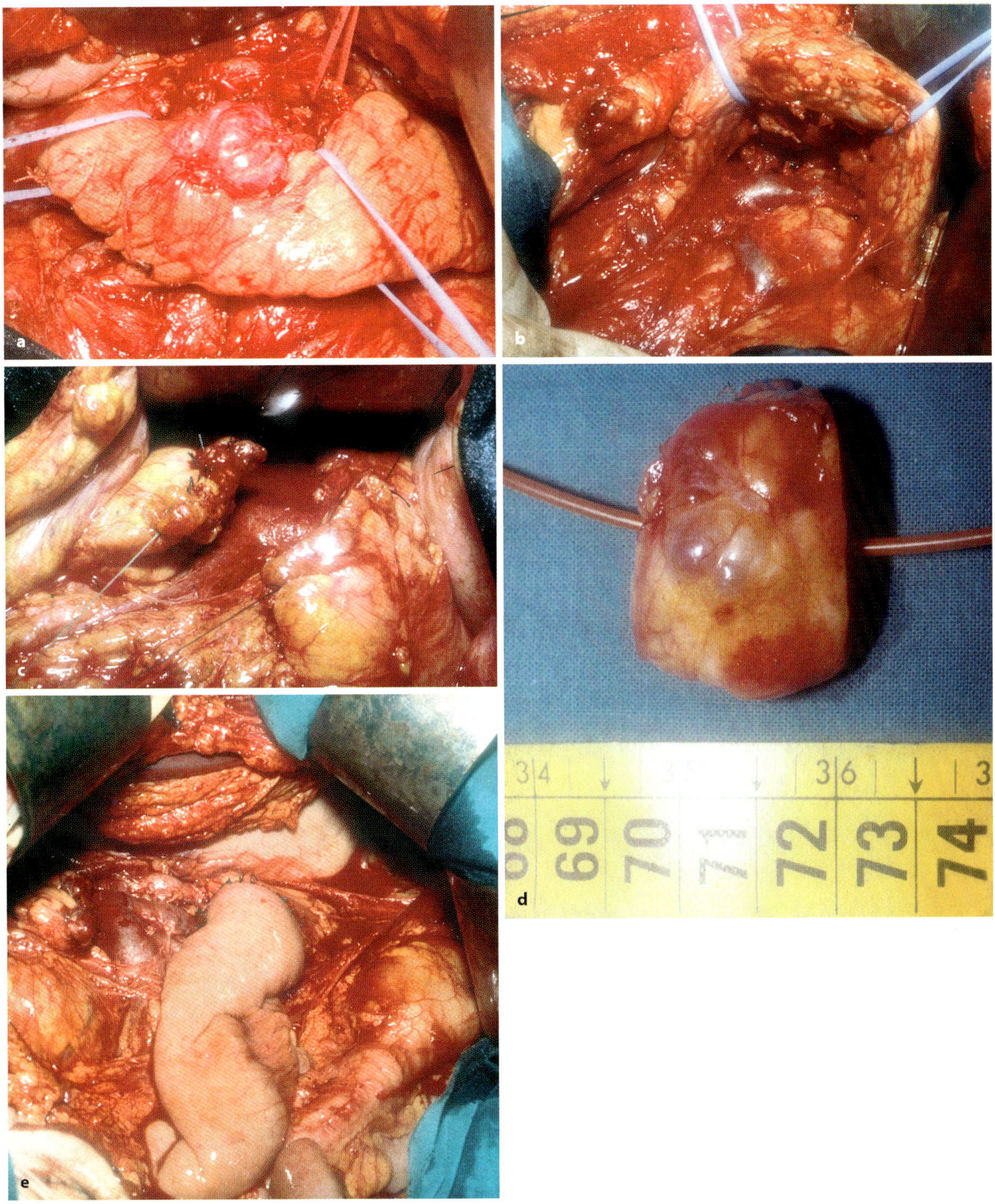

Figure 39.2

a The pancreas is mobilized after incision of posterior peritoneum along the superior and inferior margins. b Pancreatic segment harboring the lesion is dissected from the portomesenteric axis and splenic vessels and is suspended with loops. c Proximal and distal stumps after the resection of the isthmus. d Pancreatic specimen with a stent showing Wirsung's duct. e The proximal stump and the end-to-end invaginated pancreaticojejunostomy (reproduced with permission from Iacono et al. 2005 [9]

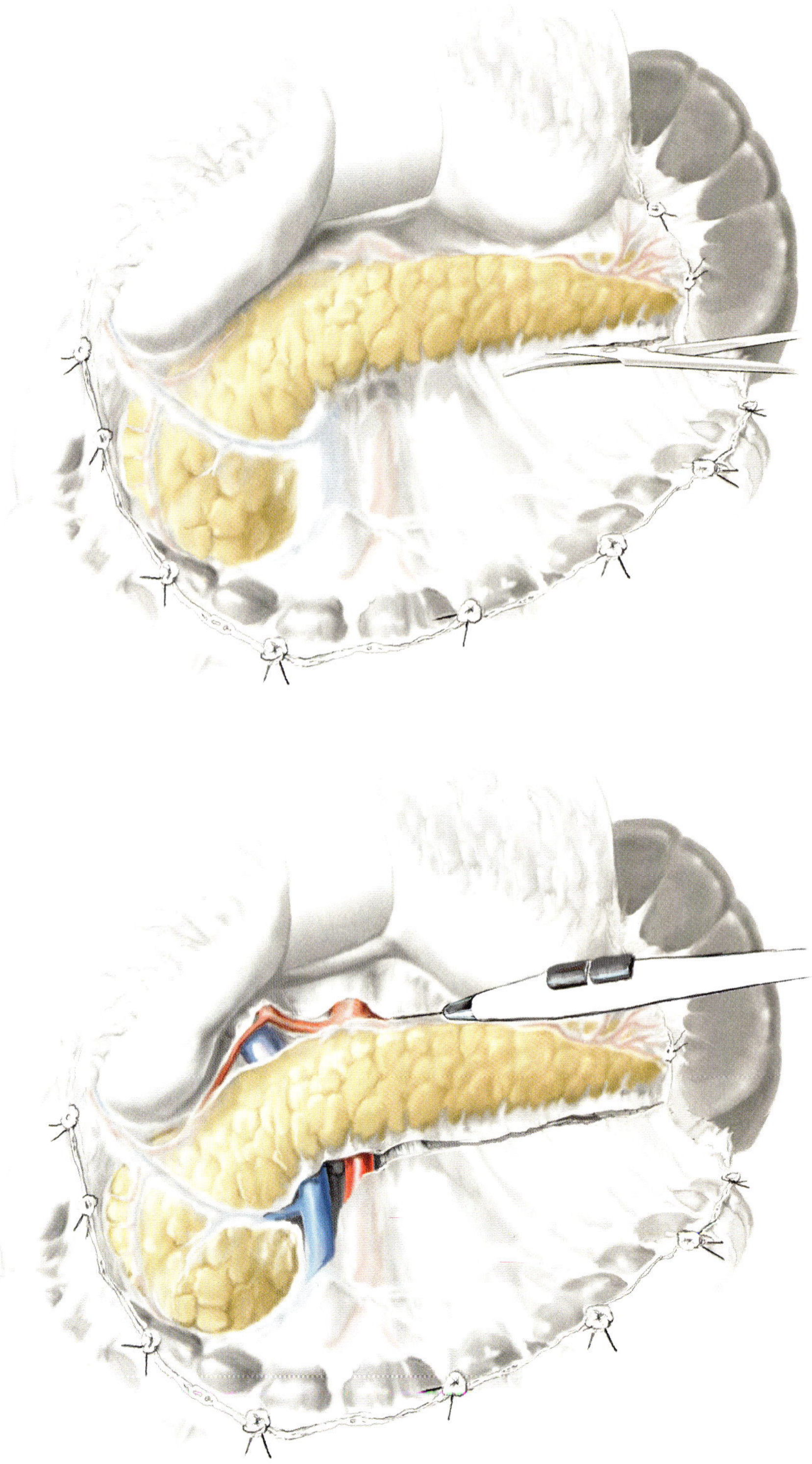

Figure 39.3

After entering the lesser sac, the posterior peritoneum is incised along the superior and inferior margins of the pancreas

Incision and Surgical Exposure

The patient is placed the supine position with the feet slightly lower than the head. A midline incision from over the xiphoid to below the umbilicus can provide excellent exposure, or else a bilateral subcostal incision with a midline extension to the xiphoid in obese or brevilineal patients.

Exploration Time

The lesser sac is entered through dissection of the transverse colon from the omentum, or by transection of the gastrocolic ligament. The pancreas is exposed and the intraoperative diagnostic work up can be completed with:

1. Ultrasonography, which allows identification of the lesion, its relationship with vascular structures and the main pancreatic duct, and multifocal lesions, particularly in endocrine neoplasm.
2. Fine-needle aspiration cytology to achieve a correct diagnosis in the case of uncertain lesions, and to rule out adenocarcinoma.
3. Pancreatography to evaluate Wirsung's duct distal to a stenosis.
4. Pancreatoscopy after resection in case of IMPT.

Resection Time

An incision is made in the posterior peritoneum along the superior and inferior margins (Figs. 39.2a and 39.3) of the segment of the pancreas (Fig. 39.4). The splenomesenteric axis is dissected carefully from the posterior surface of the gland with blunt dissection; sometimes, a better exposure is obtained by ligating and dividing the middle colic vein. To complete the dissection of the pancreatic body from the portal vein, a vessel loop is passed around the isthmus to facilitate the ligature and division of some pancreatic veins (Figs. 39.2b and 39.5). Attention must be paid at this time to the prevention of tearing of the splenic vein, which requires accurate hemostatic sutures lest stenosis and thrombosis of the vessel occur.

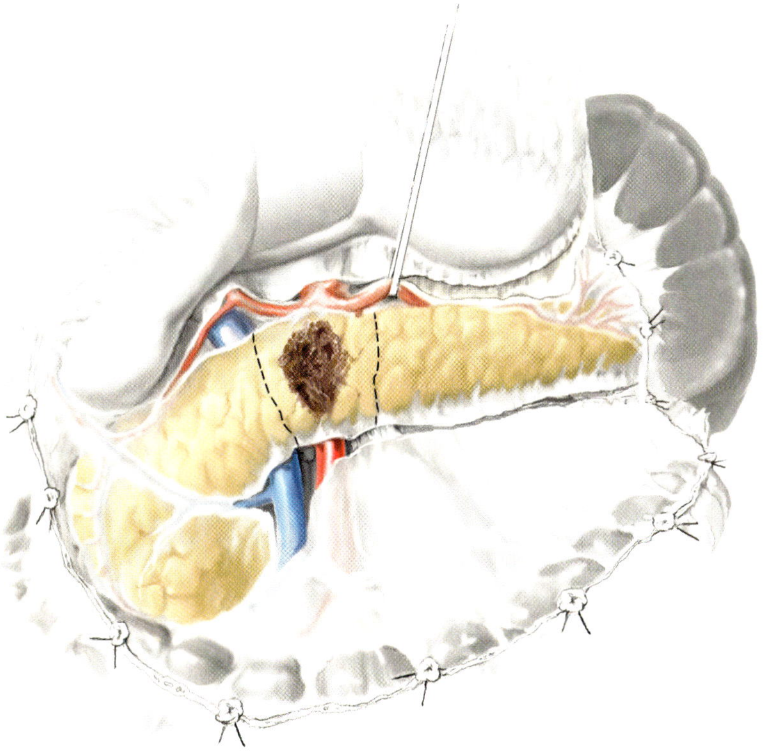

Figure 39.4

Usually 1 cm margin from the tumor is adequate for benign and low-grade malignant tumor. The limits of central pancreatectomy (gastroduodenal artery on the cephalic side and a minimum length of 5 cm of distal stump) are marked with *dotted lines*. The splenic artery is passed around with a vessel loop to allow identification and ligature of the dorsal pancreatic artery and other collaterals

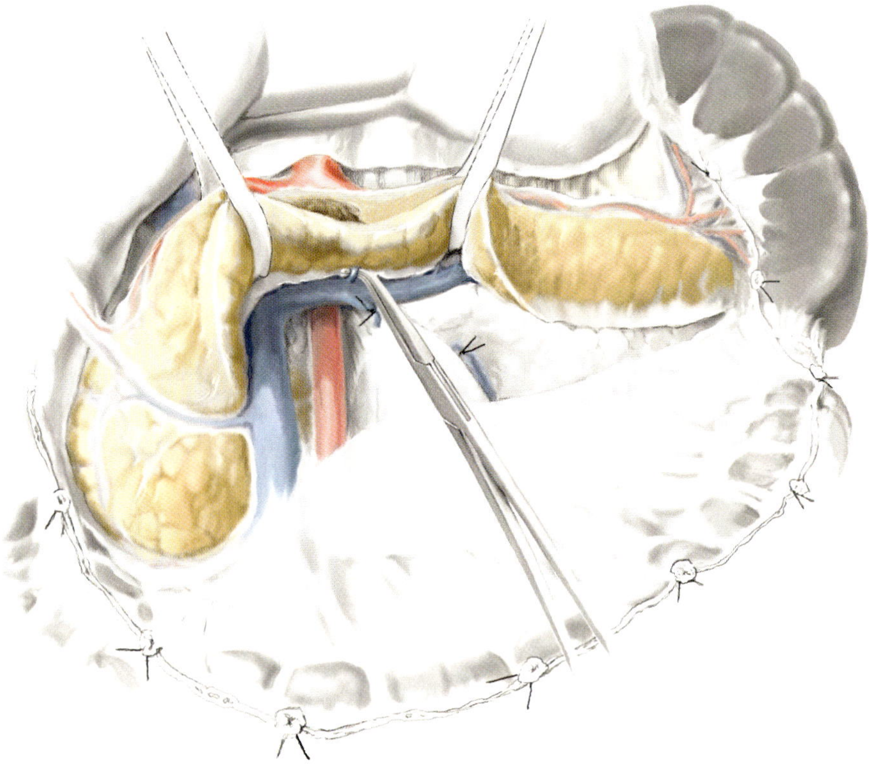

Figure 39.5

The pancreatic segment harboring the lesion is suspended with two surgical loops to allows easier dissection of the pancreatic veins from the splenic vein and better mobilization of the pancreatic body

To ease this phase of the operation, transection of the pancreas on the cephalic side can be performed in order to mobilize the pancreatic stump toward the left, exposing all of the slim pancreatic veins, which can be easily severed. Another vessel loop is passed around the splenic artery, and its collaterals are divided, including dorsal pancreatic artery (Fig. 39.4). If this artery is particularly large, this raises the suspicion of vascularization of the left pancreas maintained only by the transverse pancreatic artery, which is the left branch of dorsal artery (Fig. 39.1). This variant represents a contraindication to central pancreatectomy, as division of this vessel may induce necrosis of the left pancreas, and therefore distal pancreatectomy with splenic preservation has to be performed. Other useful criteria to identify this variant are the absence of collaterals from the splenic artery and the lack of bleeding after pancreatic section on the cephalic side. Occasionally the common hepatic artery has to be freed as it runs along the superior border of the pancreas, and some collaterals to the isthmus need to be tied as possible candidates for the dorsal pancreatic artery.

After the pancreatic dissection is accomplished with 1 cm margin on both side from the lesion, transection of the gland can be carried out. On the cephalic side the limit of CP is the gastroduodenal artery, and on the caudal side is a minimum length of 5 cm of remaining distal pancreas. Two hemostatic stitches are positioned on the margins of both sides of the section: the transection is performed with a knife (Figs. 39.2c and 39.6). The cephalic stump can be stapled. The two raw surfaces are inspected to ensure patent vascularization, particularly on the distal stump – if this has to be anastomosed differently, the resection must be extended for 2–3 cm.

The specimen is then sent to the pathologist for frozen section to confirm the diagnosis (benign or borderline) and clear resection margins (Figs. 39.2d and 39.7). In the presence of malignant disease, the operation has to switch to pancreaticoduodenectomy or left splenopancreatectomy with extended lymphadenectomy, according to the extension of the lesion toward the head or the body–tail.

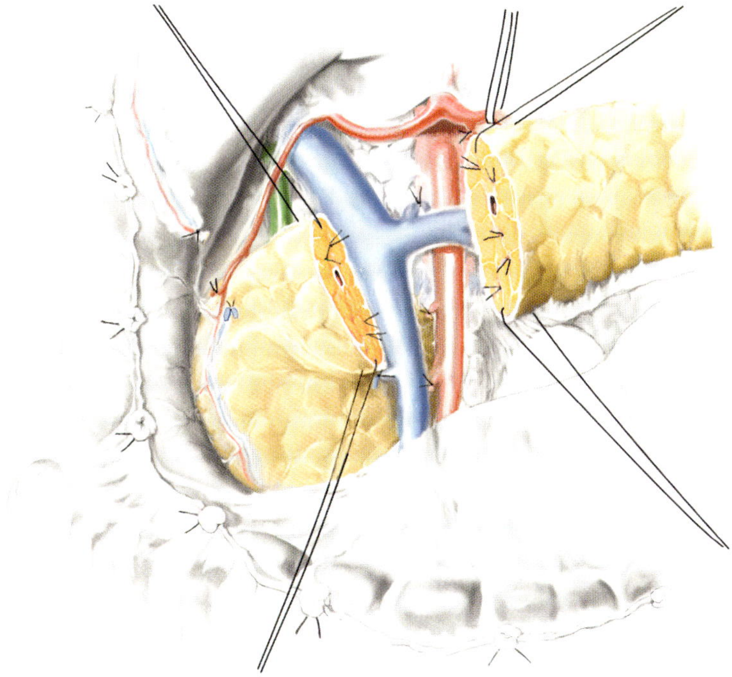

Figure 39.6

Proximal and distal pancreatic stumps after resection of the isthmus and elective hemostasis of bleeding vessels with interrupted stitches.

Figure 39.7

a Macroscopic view of a central pancreatectomy specimen with a serous cystadenoma. b Macroscopic view of a central pancreatectomy specimen with a solid cystic papillary tumor (reproduced with permission from Iacono et al. 2005 [9]

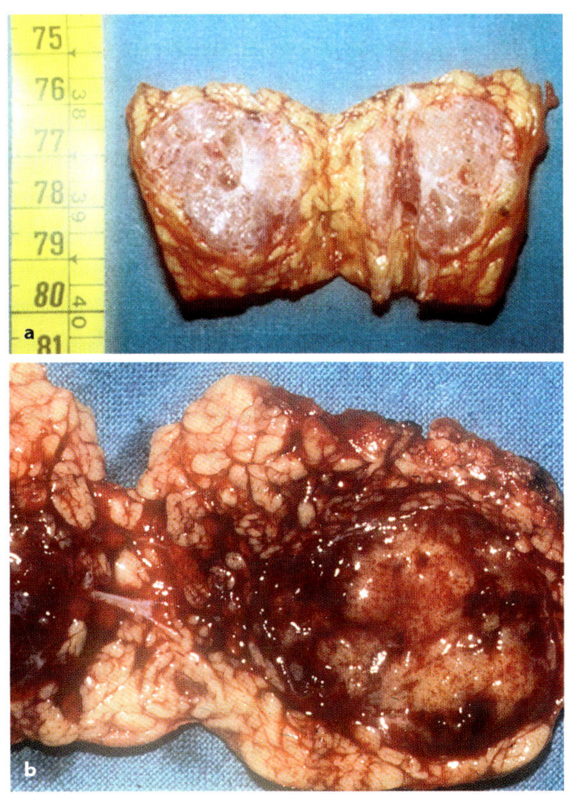

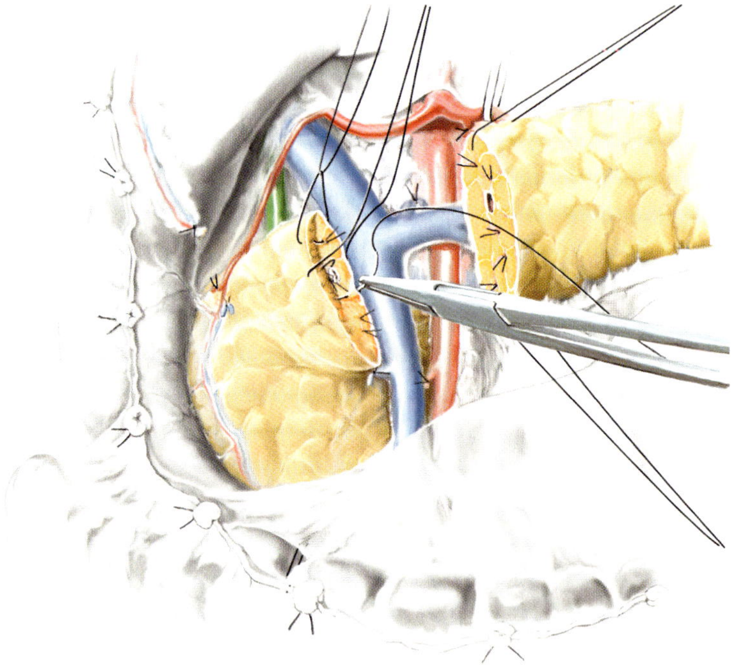

Figure 39.8

The Wirsung duct is ligated electively and mattress stitches are passed through the entire gland to suture the cephalic stump

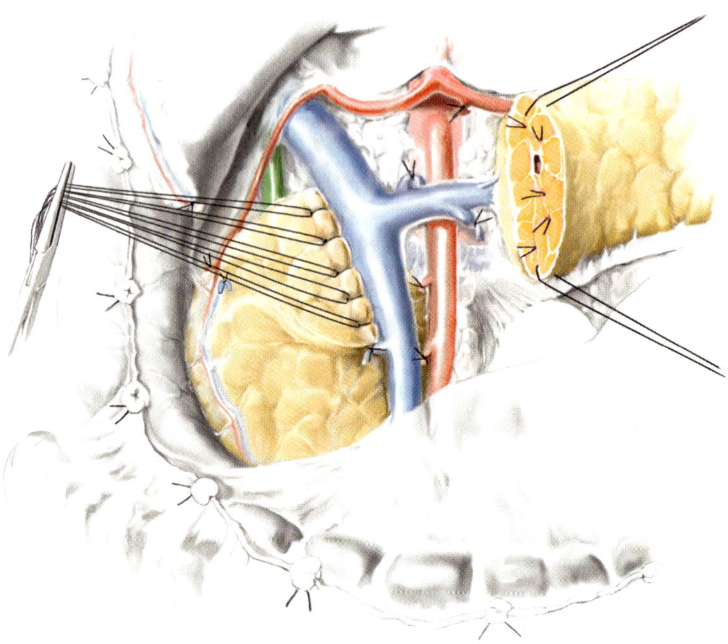

Figure 39.9

The pancreatic stump has been sutured and the body–tail stump is mobilized so that it can be anastomosed

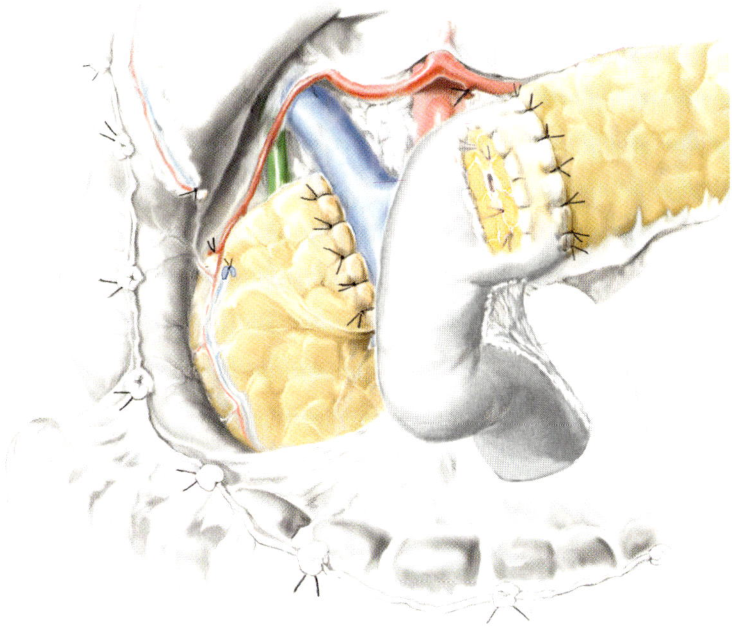

Figure 39.10

Pancreaticojejunostomy on Roux-en-Y jejunal loop is constructed in a single or double layer and brought up through an opening in the mesocolon

In the presence of IMPT, pancreatoscopy is performed just after resection through the main pancreatic duct in both stumps to rule out other ductal lesions.

Reconstruction Time

Accurate hemostasis is completed with 4–5/0 monofilament selective stitches (Fig. 39.6); the cephalic stump is sutured with mattress stitches after elective closure of the main pancreatic duct with a figure-of-eight stitch (Figs. 39.8 and 39.9). Some authors prefer to carry out an anastomosis also on the cephalic stump using the same jejunal loop of the distal stump anastomosis.

Dissection of the splenic vessels, as described, allows freeing of the distal pancreatic stump for 15–20 mm in order to carry out easily the anastomosis with the jejunal loop or stomach. The jejunal loop is isolated 15–20 cm distal to Treitz's ligament and brought up through an opening in the mesocolon to the right of the middle colic vessels.

Pancreaticojejunostomy

Pancreaticojejunostomy can be carried out in different ways: (1) end-to-end, (2) end-to-side, (3) duct–mucosa, (4) side-to-side, or (5) double pancreaticojejunostomy.

End-to-End

End-to-end jejunostomy techniques can be: simple, simple invagination, or telescopic invagination (Figs. 39.2e and 39.10). The first method is the easier but less utilized; it is carried out with a single layer of interrupted stitches between the pancreatic parenchyma and the capsule, and all layers of the bowel. For the simple invagination technique, the pancreatic stump is invaginated into the jejunal loop for 15–20 mm and sutured all around with interrupted stitches to the bowel. The telescopic method requires two layers: the first suture line, the outer, of interrupted stitches is between the pancreatic capsule and seromuscular coat of the bowel in the posterior surface at 2 cm from the pancreatic resection surface and the free margin of the jejunal loop. The posterior aspect is completed with the second suture line, the inner, between the pancreatic capsule at the margin of resec-

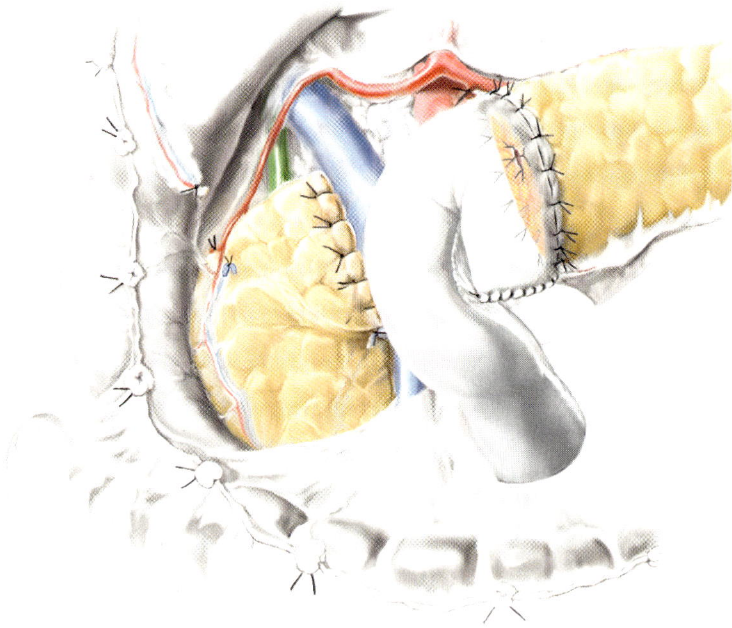

Figure 39.11

End-to-side pancreaticojejunostomy for the distal stump

tion and the free margin of the bowel; this suture line continues along the anterior aspect to complete the inner layer of the anastomoses all around the stump. Eventually, the outer suture line is completed on the anterior surface, again at 2 cm from the free margin, as behind. A useful suggestion is to tie two or three stitches temporarily to avoid tension on a single point.

End-to-Side

End-to-side pancreaticojejunostomy is performed a few centimeters proximal to the stapled end of the jejunal loop: as with the end-to-end technique, it can be carried out in a single or double layer (Fig. 39.11). It is considered the best choice by some authors; we recommend it in case of a discrepancy between the size of the pancreatic stump and the jejunal loop.

Duct–Mucosa

The anastomosis is carried out with 5/0 interrupted absorbable stitches between a lateral 5-mm opening on the bowel and the Wirsung duct (Fig. 39.12). Some authors advise the use of a stent to provide support for the anastomosis.

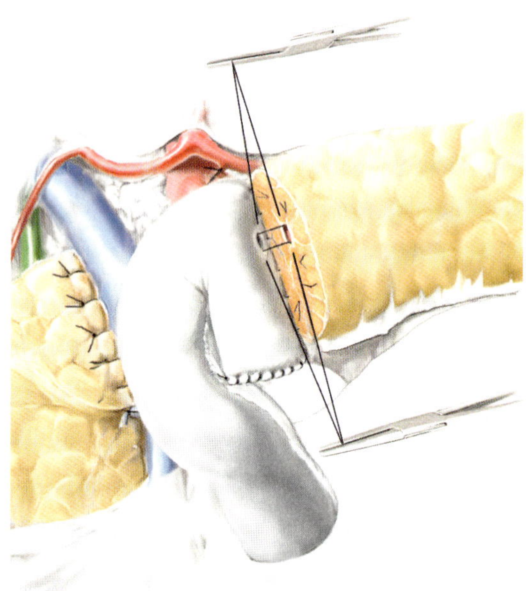

Figure 39.12

Duct–mucosa pancreaticojejunostomy for the distal stump

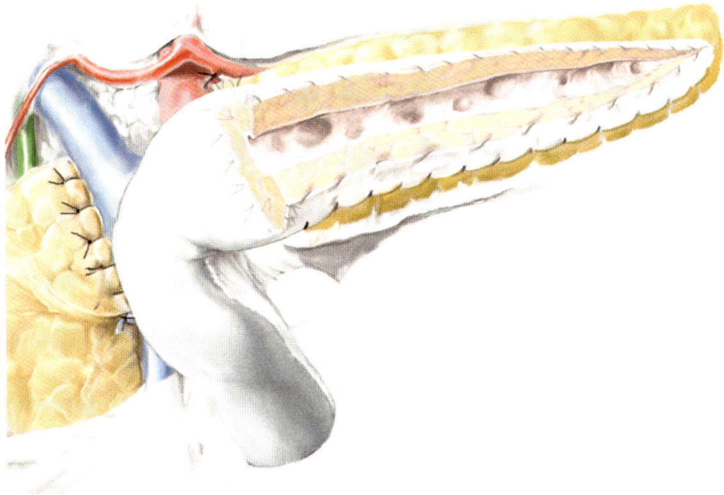

Figure 39.13

Side-to-side pancreaticojejunostomy according to Partington-Rochelle after opening of Wirsung's duct on the distal stump in patients with chronic pancreatitis and a dilated duct

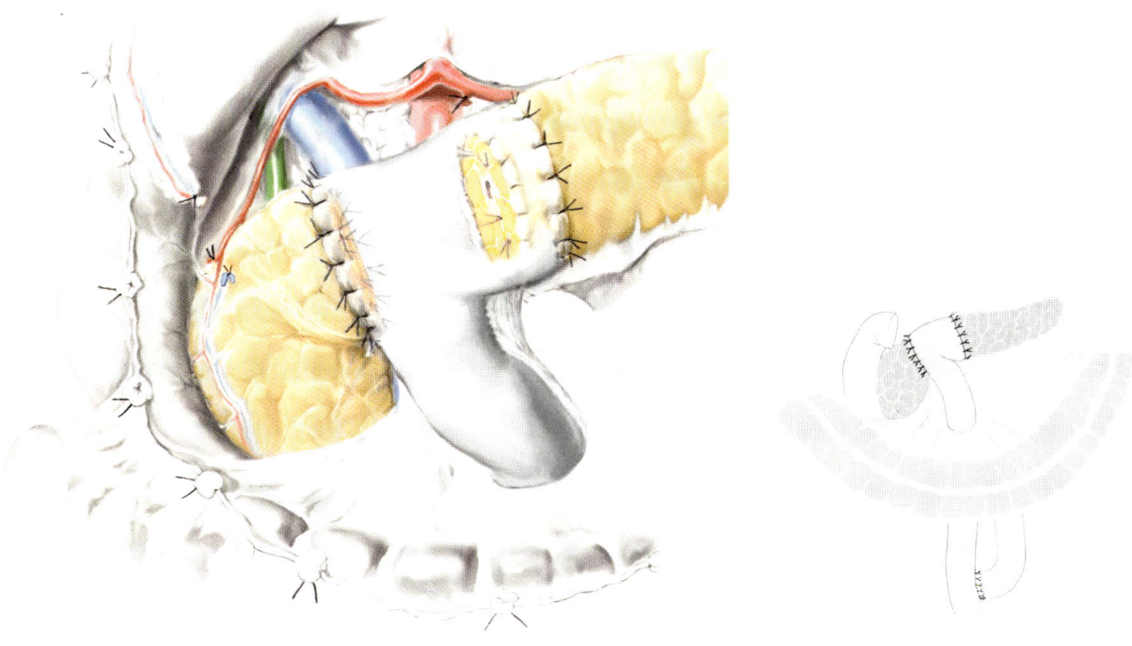

Figure 39.14

Reconstruction with a double jejunal loop anastomosed to both of the stumps

Side-to-Side

This technique is used when there is focal chronic pancreatitis with a dilated Wirsung duct (Fig. 39.13). The distal pancreas is opened longitudinally along its ventral surface from the margin of resection to the tail, and a side-to-side anastomosis is performed, as in the Puestow or Partington-Rochelle technique.

Double Pancreaticojejunostomy

A Double pancreaticojejunostomy can be either end-to side and end-to-end (Fig. 39.14), or both end-to-side.

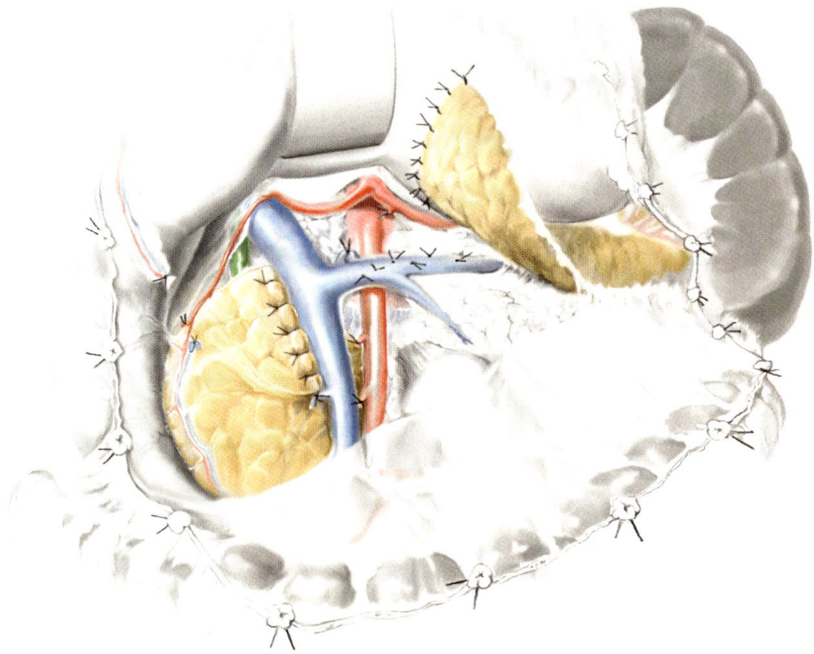

Figure 39.15

Reconstruction of the distal stump with a pancreaticogastrostomy

Pancreaticogastrostomy

Different variants have been described; nevertheless, the most often used entails implantation of the open end of the pancreas directly into the gastric pouch through a 2- to 3-cm opening in its posterior surface (Fig. 39.15). The anastomosis can be carried out in a single or double layer. This technique is the most used by French [12–14] and, more recently, American authors [15, 16]. Among the advantages of this technique, the most important are, according some authors, the very low or absence of pancreatic fistula and the chance to examine the anastomosis directly by endoscopy; the disadvantages are mainly related to the alteration of digestive enzymes, particularly lipase, caused by gastric juice, which result in impairment of exocrine function. Considering the good outcome of these patients, the low risk of development of a pancreatic fistula may be less important than the normal postoperative pancreatic function achieved with this technique.

In exceptional cases (e.g., atrophic pancreatic stump, pancreatic duct not evident), the pancreatic stump is buried and good care is taken to place drains. Some prefer to seal the main pancreatic duct on distal stump by injecting synthetic glue [17]; however this technique results in pancreatic atrophy and diabetes.

A end-to-side jejunojejunostomy is then constructed 40–50 cm distal to the pancreatic anastomosis. One or two soft, closed drains are placed and brought out on the right abdominal side or on the right and left side.

Early Postoperative Course

The nasogastric tube is removed after 24 h and the patient is on clear diet on postoperative day 2, and a solid diet on day 3. The fluid collected from the drains is checked for amylase levels on postoperative days 3, 5, and 7; if the level is low or absent, the drains are removed on postoperative days 6–8.

Postoperative Complications and Management

The morbidity rate ranges from 0 to 75% [1–5, 8, 9, 12–28], while the reported mortality amounts to only one case due to a pancreatic fistula complication on

Table 39.1. Postoperative morbidity and mortality rates of central pancreatectomy (CP). Values in parentheses are the reported number of patients with pancreaticogastrostomy

First author	Year	No. of cases	Morbidity rate	No. cases of local complications	No. cases of systemic complications	Reoperation (no. of cases)	Mortality rate
Fagniez [2]	1988	2	0%	0	0	0	0
Asanuma [4]	1993	2	0%	0	0	0	0
Rotman [3]	1993	14	29%	4	1	3[a]	0
Ikeda [18]	1995	24	12.5%	3	0	0	0
Fernandez-Cruz [22]	1997	3	0%	0	0	0	0
Iacono [8]	1998	13	30%	3	1	0	0
Partensky [13]	1998	10 (10)	40%	4	0	1	0
Warshaw [5]	1998	12	25%	3	0	0	0
Takeyoshi [19]	1999	3	0%	0	0	0	0
Sperti [20]	2000	10	40%	3	1	0	0
Yamaguchi [26]	2000	10	40%	4	–	–	0
Celis [24]	2001	6	0%	0	0	0	0
De Clavier [12]	2002	11 (9)	63%	6	1	2	0
Sauvanet [14]	2002	53(25)[b]	41%	22	2	3	2%
Shibata [27]	2002	10	50%	4	1	0	0
Su [25]	2002	4	75%	3	0	0	0
Christein [21]	2003	3	0%	0	0	0	0
Goldstein [21]	2004	12 (12)	25%	0	3	0	0
Efron-Yeo [16]	2004	14 (14)	50%	5	2	2[c]	0
Siech-Beger [23]	2004	6	–	–	–	–	–
Iacono [9]	2004	20	35%	5	2	0	0

[a] One patient has been reoperated for infiltrated margin
[b] Multicentric report
[c] For gastrointestinal bleeding, one immediately postoperatively and one 10 days after CP

postoperative day 18, which resulted in massive gastrointestinal bleeding (Table 39.1). At the reoperation, leakage of the pancreaticojejunostomy was confirmed and splenoportal confluence thrombosis was observed [14]. The patient underwent removal of the pancreaticojejunostomy and distal pancreatectomy with portal thrombectomy. The patient died after surgery from multiple organ failure. The more frequently occurring and troublesome complication is pancreatic fistula, with a frequency that ranges in literature between 0 and 54% [1–5, 8, 9, 12–28]; this wide difference is due to the small series of cases reported and to the fact that the groups are not homogeneous. Nevertheless, after a broad evaluation, it seems that its frequency is slightly higher than that reported after pancreaticoduodenectomy. The pancreatic fistulas that come from the proximal stump are pure, while those that come from pancreaticojejunostomy are mixed; however as they are not exposed to the enzymatic activation of bile, as after pancreaticoduodenectomy, and usually heal spontaneously with maintenance of the drains, parenteral nutrition, and administration of a somatostatin-analog.

Other reported surgical complications are intraperitoneal abscess and fluid collections that are often related to pancreatic fistulae, splenic vein thrombosis with secondary infarction of the spleen, abscess, pancreatitis, delayed gastric emptying, wound infection, and intestinal obstruction.

The treatment of choice for fluid collection and abscess is percutaneous drainage with CT or US control and, if these are not feasible, with a surgical approach. Complications of the spleen are frequently treated with splenectomy, but in selected cases lienal abscesses can be drained percutaneously.

Table 39.2. Late outcome of CP

First author	Year	No. of cases	No. cases of endocrine insufficiency	No. cases of exocrine insufficiency	Recurrence rate (%)
Fagniez [2]	1988	2	0	0	0
Asanuma [4]	1993	2	1[a]	0	0
Rotman [3]	1993	14	0	1	0
Ikeda [18]	1995	24	0	2[b]	0
Fernandez-Cruz [22]	1997	3	0	0	0
Iacono [8]	1998	13	0	0	0
Partensky [13]	1998	10	0	0	0
Warshaw [5]	1998	12	0	0	0
Takeyoshi [19]	1999	3	0	0	0
Sperti [20]	2000	10	0	0	0
Yamaguchi [26]	2000	10	0	0	0
Celis [24]	2001	6	0	0	0
De Clavier [12]	2002	11	1	1	0
Sauvanet [14]	2002	53[c]	2[d]	3[d]	8[e]
Shibata [27]	2002	10	1	0	0
Su [25]	2002	4	0	0	0
Christein [21]	2003	3	0	0	0
Goldstein [21]	2004	12	2	0	0
Efron-Yeo [16]	2004	14	0	0	0
Siech-Beger [23]	2004	6	–	–	–
Iacono [9]	2004	20	0	0	0

[a] The patient returns to normal value 36 months after operation
[b] Two patients with chronic pancreatitis
[c] Multicentric report
[d] One patient had a wide CP (15 cm) and another patient developed exocrine insufficiency 104 months after CP for fibrotic stenosis of Wirsung duct after severe pancreatitis
[e] Four patients: one gastric cancer invading the pancreas, one renal metastasis and two intraductal mucinous producing tumors

Digestive and intra-abdominal bleeding is reported as early or late complications secondary to vascular erosion or pseudoaneurysm of a peripancreatic artery. Early hemorrhage requires immediate reoperation, while late hemorrhage can be treated either with embolization or, if this fails, reoperation.

The more frequent medical complications are pleuropulmonary and urinary tract infections.

Long-Term Outcome After Central Pancreatectomy

Our experience and that of other authors confirms that this technique preserves completely exocrine and endocrine functions: in the literature only six cases of exocrine insufficiency have been reported, onc by Rotman [3], two by Ikeda [18] who underwent central pancreatectomy for chronic pancreatitis, and three by Sauvanet [14] (Table 39.2).

Diabetes or impaired glucose tolerance has never been observed either in our own experience or in that reported in the literature, except in six cases, two reported by Glodstein [15] and by Sauvanet [14], one by de Clavière [12], and one by Asanuma [4]. In this last case the immediate postoperative alterations returned to normal within 36 months of the operation (Table 39.2).

The question of diabetes is still open to debate, based on the fact that the incidence of diabetes after left pancreatectomy is very low when the resected volume of the gland is less than 70%. Data in the literature are contradictory and there have been no studies comparing pancreatic function tests (exocrine and endocrine) before and after left pancreatectomy. This

Table 39.3. CP for chronic focal (segmental) pancreatitis and pseudocysts of the pancreatic neck or proximal portion of body of the pancreas

First author	Year	No. of cases of focal pancreatitis	No. of cases of pseudocyst
Rotman [3]	1993	–	1
Ikeda [18]	1995	7	–
Fernandez-Cruz [22]	1997	1	2
De Clavier [12]	2002	1	–
Sauvanet [14]	2002	4	3
Efron-Yeo [16]	2004	1	1
Muller-Buchler [28]	2005	12	–

gap has now been filled by the study of Kendall et al. [29] at the Minneapolis Transplantation Center. In fact they show that at 1 year, 25% of pancreatic transplant donors who underwent left pancreatectomy presented with glucose intolerance.

Central pancreatectomy preserves all normal pancreatic tissue and especially the body–tail where insular cells seem to be more numerous, thus avoiding the risk of diabetes associated with left resections. In our previous report [8], we evaluated preoperative and postoperative exocrine function by means of the pancreo-lauryl test and assay of fecal fat excretion, while endocrine function was assessed by the OGTT; no functional impairment was observed.

Some authors [25–27] have compared the results after central pancreatectomy with those following distal pancreatectomy and conclude that with distal pancreatectomy, the incidence of diabetes is statistically significantly higher than that after central pancreatectomy.

When the indication is correct, the local recurrence rate is nil. In the literature [14] four cases have been reported: two cases of IMPT, a case of gastric cancer involving the pancreas, and another case of pancreatic metastasis from renal cancer. Facing IMPT, the decision to perform a central pancreatectomy must be taken very carefully; in one of the two cases of local recurrence reported by Sauvanet [14] after 40 and 48 months, intraoperative frozen sectioning was not performed and in the other the intraoperative and final pathology showed moderate dysplasia in the proximal portion, which is where the recurrence developed (Table 39.2). In three cases epithelial hyperplasia was present and no recurrence was observed, as in the Johns Hopkins experience [16].

To lower the risk of local recurrence, Japanese authors have stated that intraoperative pancreatoscopy can be useful. However a careful and close follow up is mandatory.

Central pancreatectomy in chronic pancreatitis has little space as focal localization on isthmus is rare [3, 12, 14, 16, 18, 22, 28] (Tab. 3). Nevertheless, surgical indication is taken when imaging techniques (Wirsung-MR or ERCP) show an unclear focal stenosis in the central portion of the gland, the nature of which is doubtful.

Conclusions

Central pancreatectomy is, in the presence of precise anatomic and pathological indications, a reliable and correct technique from the oncology stand-point. It assures that as much of the functional parenchyma is saved as is possible, and avoids the infective and thrombotic complications associated with splenectomy.

References

1. Dagradi A, Serio G (1984) Pancreatectomia intermedia. In: Enciclopedia Medica Italiana. Pancreas, vol XI. USES Edizioni Scientifiche, Firenze, pp 850
2. Fagniez PL, Kracht M, Rotman N (1988) Limited conservative pancreatectomy for benign tumours: a new technical approach. Br J Surg 75:719
3. Rotman N, Sastre B, Fagniez P (1993) Medial pancreatectomy for tumors of the neck of the pancreas. Surgery 113:532–535
4. Asanuma Y, Koyama K, Saito K, Tanaka J (1993) An appraisal of segmental pancreatectomy for benign tumors of the pancreatic body: a report of two cases. Surg Today 23:733–736
5. Warshaw AL, Rattner DW, Fernandez del Castillo C, Z'graggen K (1998) Middle segment pancreatectomy. A novel technique for conserving pancreatic tissue. Arch Surg 133:327–331
6. Guillemin P, Bessot M (1957) Pancreatite cronique calcificante chez un tuberculeux renal: pancreato-jejunostomie selon un tecnique originale. Mem Acad Chirurg (Paris) 83:869–871

7. Letton AH, Wilson JP (1959) Traumatic severance of pancreas treated by Roux-Y anastomosis. Surg Gynecol Obstet 109:473–478
8. Iacono C, Bortolasi L, Serio G (1998) Is there a place for central pancreatectomy in pancreatic surgery? J Gastrointest Surg 2:509–517
9. Iacono C, Bortolasi L, Serio G (2005) Indications and technique of central pancreatectomy – early and late results. Langenbeks Arch Surg 390:266–271
10. Beger HG, Witte C, Krautzberger W, Bittner (1980) Erfahrung mit einer das Duodenum erhaltenden Pancreaskopfresektion bei chronischer Pankreatitis. Chirurg 51:303–307
11. Mellière MM, Moulle P (1968) Variations des arteries hepatiques et du carrefour pancreatique. J Chir 95:5–42
12. De Clavière G, Paye F, Fteriche S, et al (2002) Pancreatectomie mediane: resultats d'une serie de 11 patients. Ann Chir 127:48–54
13. Partensky C, Apa D, Marchal F, et al (1998) Pancreatectomie mediane avec anastomose pancreatogastrique pour neoformation pancreatique. Chirurgie 123:363–367
14. Sauvanet A, Partensky C, Sastre B, et al (2000) Medial pancreatectomy: a multi-institutional retrospective study of 53 patients by the French Pancreas Club. Surgery 132:836–843
15. Goldstein MJ, Toman J, Chabot JA (2004) Pancreaticogastrostomy: a novel application after central pancreatectomy. J Am Coll Surg 198: 871–6
16. Efron DT, Lillemoe KD, Cameron JL, Yeo CJ 82004) Central pancreatectomy with pancreaticogastrostomy for benign pancreatic pathology. J Gastrointest Surg 8:532–538
17. Balzano G, Zerbi A, Veronesi P, Di Carlo V (2003) Surgical treatment of benign and borderline neoplasms of the pancreatic body. Dig Surg 20:506–510
18. Ikeda S, Matsumoto S, Maeshiro K, et al (1995) Segmental pancreatectomy for the diagnosis and treatment of small lesions in the neck or body of the pancreas. Hepatogastroenterology 42:730–733
19. Takeyoshi I, Ohwada S, Nakamura S, et al (1999) Segmental pancreatectomy for mucin-producing pancreatic tumors. Hepatogastroenterology 46:2585–2588
20. Sperti C, Pasquali C, Ferronato A, et al (2000) Median pancreatectomy for tumors of the neck and body of the pancreas. J Am Coll Surg 190:711–716
21. Christein JD, Kim AW, Golshan MA, et al (2003) Central pancreatectomy for the resection for the benign or low malignant potential neoplasms. World J Surg 27:595–598
22. Fernadez-Cruz L, Sabater l, Pera M, et al (1997) Conservative pancreatic resection in patients with obstructive chronic pancreatitis. Hepatogastroenterology 44:1023–1028
23. Siech M, Thumerer SU, Henne-Bruns D, Beger HG (2004) Die behandlung zystischer tumoren des pancreas. Radikal oder organsparened? Chirurg 75:615–621
24. Celis J, Berrospi F, Ruiz E, et al (2001) Central pancreatectomy for tumors of the neck and body of the pancreas. J Surg Oncol 77:132–135
25. Su CH, Shyr YM, Lui WY, P'eng FK (2004) Surgical treatment for serous cystadenoma of the pancreas. Segmental pancreaticectomy or conventional resection? Hepatogastroenterology 51:595–598
26. Yamaguchi K, Yokohata K, Ohkido M, et al (2000) Which is less invasive – distal pancreatectomy or segmental resection? Int Surg 85:297–302
27. Shibata S, Sato T, Andoh H, et al (2004) Outcomes and indications of segmental pancreatectomy. Comparison with distal pancreatectomy. Dig Surg 21:48–53
28. Muller MW, Friess H, Henning R, et al (2005) Segmental pancreatic resection has developed into a standard operation. Abstracts 39th Meeting of the Pancreas Club. Chicago, Il, May 15, 2005; p 100 (poster n.20)
29. Kendall DM, Sutherland D, Najarian JS, et al (1990) Effects of hemipancreatectomy on insulin secretion and glucose tolerance in healthy humans. New Engl J Med 29:898–903

Chapter 40

J. Lunger · K. Mair · M. Junger · M.H. Schoenberg

Distal Pancreatectomy in Patients with Chronic Pancreatitis

Surgical therapy of chronic pancreatitis will probably increase in the future since: (1) the incidence of this disease has significantly increased in the Western world [1]; (2) early surgical treatment seems to influence the course of disease in a positive way [2, 3]; (3) it has been shown that there seems to be a relationship between chronic alcoholic pancreatitis and pancreatic carcinoma [4, 5]; (4) the perioperative morbidity and mortality of pancreatic resection is acceptably low today [6].

Definition and Classification

Chronic pancreatitis of the pancreatic corpus and tail is defined as a recurrent chronic inflammation of the pancreas limited to the left mesentericoportal part of the pancreatic gland. Concomitant to the overall definition of chronic pancreatitis, chronic inflammation of the corpus and tail of the pancreas is classified according to the Marseille-Rome Conference 1988 [7, 8] and is depicted in Table 40.1 and based mainly on the morphological characteristics.

Table 40.1. Classification according to the Marseille-Rome Conference 1988 [75]

Acute pancreatitis	
Chronic pancreatitis	Chronic calcifying pancreatitis
	Chronic inflammatory pancreatitis
	Chronic obstructive pancreatitis

Epidemiology

The prevalence of chronic pancreatitis amounts to 26 cases per 1,000,000 inhabitants in Western industrial countries (USA and Western Europe). The yearly incidence is 8 newly diagnosed patiens of this disease per 1,000,000 inhabitants [9]. The percentage of patients suffering from chronic inflammation of the pancreatic tail is not explicitly described in the literature.

Etiology

In the Western industrialized countries, chronic intake of alcohol is the main reason for chronic pancreatitis, followed by biliary diseases [10]. In China and other Asian countries, biliary alterations are the primary cause of the chronic inflammation of the gland [11]. Other reasons such as pancreas divisum, pancreas anulare, stenosis of the papilla of Vater, and stenosis of the ductus Wirsungianus as well as diverticula of the duodenum, for example, seldom occur. In these cases the concomitant "downstream obstruction" of the pancreatic duct and other anomalies situated in the pancreatic head and/or corpus lead to a chronic inflammation in the distal part of the pancreas.

Medical History and Clinical Symptoms

In most cases the patients suffer from recurrent severe chronic pain on the upper left side of the abdomen reaching up to the vertebral region. These patients have a long medical history with numerous consultations and examinations. Often the patients are stigmatized as chronic pain patients with an excessive use of analgesics for years. Mainly male patients admit a long history of alcohol abuse [10].

Besides pain, often the symptoms are due to displacement of other organs, stenosis of the biliary and pancreatic duct, and alterations as well as occlusion of neighboring arterial and venous blood vessels because of pseudocysts and an inflammatory tumor of the pancreatic tail. The compression and thrombosis, especially of the veins in this region, lead to splenomegaly, which is often palpable during physical examination.

As a sign of endocrine and exocrine insufficiency, patients inflicted with chronic inflammation of the pancreas tail also suffer from diabetes mellitus due to an increased destruction of the islet cells in the pancreatic corpus and tail, and fatty stools accompanied by weight loss.

Diagnostics

Despite the unspecific clinical symptoms, the medical history and physical examination often reveal important facts that are indicative of chronic inflammation of the pancreatic tail. This is even more likely if risk factors such as drinking habits are conceded.

The physical examination often reveals pathological alterations such as palpable resistances in the upper abdomen in the case of pancreatic pseudocysts, pain in the upper gastrointestinal tract extending to the vertebra, and distention of the upper abdomen.

The standard laboratory data often are normal and any changes are inconclusive. Even the serum lipase/amylase concentrations may be increased, decreased, or in the normal range. Therefore, different tests of pancreatic function such as secretin/cholecystokinin test have been suggested and are performed to assess exocrine function. These tests, however, are often very invasive, sometimes not specific, and have been replaced by other less invasive methods for "first-line" diagnostic procedures.

The first diagnostic step to determine the exocrine pancreatic functions is to measure the fecal elastase concentration [12–14]. Furthermore, the patients' endocrine function can be tested with the aid of an oral glucose tolerance test [9].

More indicative of the diagnosis of chronic pancreatitis are imaging procedures such as computed tomography (CT), magnetic resonance imaging (MRI), and the concomitant magnetic resonance cholangiopancreatography (MRCP; "one-stop shopping"). With this technique, possible alterations of the pancreatic gland, and especially the pancreatic ducts, can be visualized reliably. In particular, MRCP has proven to be of extraordinary significance. In accordance with the Cambridge classification, patients with chronic pancreatitis were examined by ERCP and by MRCP (see Table 40.2). It has been shown that MRCP is able to replace ERCP as a diagnostic procedure in most patients. Therefore, the possible complications induced by ERCP can be avoided.

Table 40.2. Magnetic resonance cholangiopancreatography (*MRCP*) grades [15]. *ERCP* Endoscopic retrograde cholangiopancreatography

MRCP grade	ERCP grade (Cambridge)		
	Mild (*n*=8)	Moderate (*n*=17)	Severe (*n*=16)
Normal	5	3	
Equivocal	1		
Mild	1	1	
Moderate	1	10	3
Severe		3	13

Sugiyama et al. [15] showed that the enlargement of the pancreatic duct was detected using MRCP in 94% of 41 patients with chronic pancreatitis. In the same study, duct stenoses were detected in 82% and pseudocysts in 100% of all patients. Alterations of the small pancreatic ducts, however, were only seen using MRCP in 74% of the cases, amounting to a sensitivity of only 25%. Moderate changes in the pancreatic duct could only be detected in 82%, severe alterations, however, in 100% as compared to ERCP.

The main advantages of MRI is the simultaneous imaging of neighboring vessels such as, for example, the portal vein, splenic vein, celiac trunk, splenic artery, and common hepatic artery. It was shown previously that possible alterations of the vessels can be visualized with a sensitivity comparative to that of invasive techniques such as angiography.

ERCP remains a valuable diagnostic and interventional tool; the sensitivity of small and moderate duct changes as early signs of inflammation can be enhanced by ERCP combined with secretin stimulation [15]. Moreover, the combination of ERCP with endoscopic ultrasound (EUS) can improve the specificity and sensitivity of early pancreatic changes. Kahl et al. [16] showed that in all of their patients, the early alterations due to chronic pancreatitis that were visible using ERCP (*n*=92) were also observed using EUS. Moreover, in patients with a normal ERCP but a pathological EUS, a later follow-up study revealed that 68.8% of these patients suffered from clinically apparent chronic pancreatitis. Therefore, EUS, regardless of its inherent limitations, is one of the most sensitive diagnostic methods for chronic pancreatitis at an early stage of disease. As a screening method, however, it does not seem to be suitable because it is rather invasive.

Indications for Surgery

Chronic pancreatitis is a progressive inflammatory disease that should normally be treated conservatively. Surgical treatment of chronic pancreatitis is only indicated if the patients suffer from persistent severe abdominal pain and local complications due to the disease, as well as the suspicion of malignancy [11, 17–21]. Little valid data are available concerning indications for surgery specifically for chronic pancreatitis of the tail. Between 1982 and 1995 we examined 74 patients who had undergone pancreatic left resection for chronic pancreatitis; 97.2% of the patients had severe recurrent pain in the upper abdomen extending to the back [22]. Furthermore, over half of the patients were suffering from local complications induced by large pseudocysts (51%) or benign pancreatic tumors (56.8%), often leading to a displacement of other neighboring organs or vessels. Only one-quarter of the patients suffered from a stenosis and a consecutive "downstream obstruction" in the pancreatic duct. One-quarter of the patients had a tumor, although it was difficult to determine whether it was a benign or malignant lesion. Table 40.3 depicts the indications for surgery in this group of patients.

A large variety of resective procedures are suggested for chronic pancreatitis. The extent of the operative procedure depends on preoperative diagnostics and the intraoperative situation. Nevertheless, resective procedures in chronic pancreatitis should be tailored according to the principle "as much as necessary – as little as possible." Consequently, left resection is only indicated if the inflammatory disease and complications resulting from inflammation in this region are localized to the left side of the gland (corpus and tail) [23]. The pancreatic head should appear to be morphologically normal.

Table 40.3. Operation indications by patients undergoing pancreatic left resection [22]

Operation indication	Patients (n=74)%
Pain	97.2
Tumor of the corpus and cauda	56.8
Pseudocysts	54.1
Suspicion of malignancy	24.3
Stenosis of the pancreatic duct	5.4
Stenosis of the common bile duct	25.7
Pancreaticolithiasis	10.8
Duodenum stenosis	4.1
Stenosis of the vessels	5.4
Various indications	29.2

Therapy

In general, operative treatment of chronic pancreatitis can be subdivided into two types: pancreatic duct drainage and resection of the diseased segments of the pancreas [24–26]. In the past, surgeons regarded a dilatation of the duct of Wirsungianus of more than 7 mm to be suitable for a drainage procedure [10]. Local complications due to the enlargement of the inflammatory process and smaller ducts rather require a resection [27].

Pancreatic Duct Drainage

The first pancreaticojejunostomy was performed by DuVal and Zollinger in 1954, as a caudal pancreaticojejunostomy that drained the distal part of the pancreatic gland. This procedure had a success rate of only about 50% and it was therefore highly questionable as to whether this procedure, also taking into account the possible complications, was really a reasonable therapeutic option [27].

Later, Puestow and Gillesby [28] defined specific duct alterations in chronic pancreatitis as a "chain of lakes" and performed a retrograde surgical drainage. This drainage opened the pancreatic duct longitudinally from the transected tail to the right of the mesenteric vessels and anastomosed the opened body and tail into an open end of the Roux-en-Y loop of the jejunum. Partington and Rochelle followed with a lateral, or side-to-side, pancreaticojejunostomy without sacrificing pancreatic tissue [29]. Later, Frey and Amikura [30] observed that inflammation in the pancreatic head requires "extended drainage." He introduced a local pancreatic head resection with longitudinal pancreaticojejunostomy in order to provide drainage of all three main ducts of the pancreas by extending the Roux limb to the duodenum. In this procedure, after opening the gastrocolic ligament, hepatic flexure mobilization, and Kocher maneuver, the pancreatic duct is identified by needle aspiration through the anterior pancreatic parenchyma [31]. A longitudinal incision is followed by the extraction of all ductal calculi. Creating a retrocolic window, a Roux-en-Y jejunal limb, about 30–40 cm distal from Treitz's ligament, is brought parallel to the opened pancreatic duct [31]. Anastomosis is performed along the antimesenteric aspect of the intestine, proceeding from the pancreatic tail to its head [31].

The exposition of the pancreatic corpus and tail may sometimes be quite demanding due to the presence of inflammatory adhesions to the posterior gastric wall. This difficulty, however, is common to all pancreatic procedures in chronic pancreatitis.

Five long-term follow-up studies including a total of 264 patients treated with a drainage operation, mainly according to the Partington-Rochelle procedure, showed that long-term pain relief was achieved in only 46% of the treated patients. Interestingly, pain relief decreased to 28–42% with increasing observation time [32]. Therefore, if pain is the main reason for surgical treatment, drainage procedures are, in most cases, not the first choice. Nevertheless, as shown in a recent study by Cahen et al. [33], surgical drainage of the pancreatic duct is more efficient than the endoscopic treatment.

Pancreatic Resection

Nowadays, distal resection of the pancreas for chronic pancreatitis is considered by all authors as a safe and effective procedure [27, 34–36]. It can be performed as either: (1) resection with splenectomy, (2) resection while preserving the spleen, or (3) a spleen-preserving procedure with ligation of the splenic vein and artery.

Distal resection is indicated in patients who suffer from intractable pain and who also have complications resulting from the inflammatory disease localized on the left side of the gland (tail) [23]. The pancreatic head should appear to be morphologically normal. These specific alterations are seen in 5–15% of all patients with chronic pancreatitis [23, 27]. Pain relief after distal resection varies between 31% [37] and 90% [23] for this selected group of patients. Schoenberg et al. observed significant long-term pain relief in 72% of the 58 treated patients after an observation interval of 58 months [22]. Similarly, a recent study by Sakorafas and Zobolas (n=40) demonstrated pain relief in 81% of the patients after median follow up of 6.7 years (Table 40.4) [44]. These results suggest that resective procedures lead to significant and long lasting reduction of pain.

Resection Technique and its Problems

As laparoscopic procedures are advancing in almost all surgical fields, surgeons also perform pancreatic resections with and without splenectomy laparoscopically [38]. The experienced surgeon has to make several decisions. First he has to choose either the conventional open or a laparoscopic approach. Additionally, he decides whether he wants to preserve the spleen or not. Furthermore, he has to choose between different techniques for dissecting the pancreas tissue (conventional scalpel, harmonic scalpel) [39, 40] and also closing the pancreas remnant (stapler, suture, fibrin glue as well as combinations [41]).

Open Resection with Splenectomy

The incision is made in the upper-midline or left-subcostal line. The lesser sac is entered through the gastrocolic omentum outside of the gastroepiploic arcade [42]. After the gastrosplenic ligament and the splenic flexure of the colon have been dissected, the splenic artery and vein are ligated. The retroperitoneum is opened along the inferior margin of the pancreas. The pancreas is mobilized from the retroperitoneal space toward the spleen, taking care of the capsula of the left adrenal gland, which is often affected by chronic inflammation [42]. Now the pancreas tissue is dissected anterior of the portal vein, near to the first ligated branches of the splenic artery and vein. This important step in the procedure ensures that these vessels supply the end tip of the pancreas remnant. If the dissection of the pancreas tissue is performed too far apart from the previously ligated vessels, the remnant's tip may become ischemic and may result in pancreatic leakage [43].

Table 40.4. Distal pancreatectomy in chronic pancreatitis patients and its long-term effect on pain relief. N.d. Not done

Authors	*n*	Distal pancreatectomy in chronic pancreatitis patients	Pain relief (%) at follow up	Median follow up (months)
Schoenberg et al. 1999 [22]	74	74	72	58
Sohn et al. 2000 [36]	255	67	n.d.	33
Sakorafas and Zobolas 2001 [44]	40	38	81	80
Hutchins et al. 2002 [48]	90	90	57	34

Closure of the Pancreas Remnant

Since fistulas from the pancreatic remnant are a major complication after distal pancreatectomy, techniques dissecting the pancreas tissue by scalpel or ultrasonic dissector, and closure of the pancreas remnant with stapler, suture, fibrin glue, and combinations of these methods have been studied [43]. Recent studies favor separate and selective closure of the pancreatic duct in order to prevent a pancreatic leak [39, 45–47]. Although some techniques are advertised as "the solution to this issue," the evidence is highly questionable [47].

In a meta-analysis including 262 studies concerning the closure of the pancreatic remnant after a distal pancreatectomy, Knaebel et al. [46] identified only 10 studies of suitable quantity and quality, including a total of 1080 patients. The indication for surgery was chronic pancreatitis in only 24% of the patients included in these studies. In these studies, stapler versus hand-sutured closure was compared without showing any significant difference. Apparently in patients with chronic pancreatitis, due to its firm and fibrotic tissue, the remnant exhibits a lower leakage rate per se as compared to the "soft pancreas" [48, 49]. It seems that the surgeon him/herself seems to represent the most relevant risk factor for fistulas and therefore should employ the techniques he/she is most familiar with.

Splenectomy versus Spleen Preservation

Spleen preservation can be performed in two different ways, one of which was described by Mallet-Guy in 1943. This procedure requires the division of the pancreas and short splenic vessels, which are difficult to identify and to ligate. In particular in patients with a chronic inflammatory situation, the identification and preservation of the splenic vessels is difficult to achieve due to adhesions and subsequent alterations of the splenic artery and vein [22]. Therefore, this procedure can be technically demanding. Moreover, uncontrolled bleeding, especially from the splenic vein, may make a splenectomy necessary.

An alternative method is ligation of the splenic artery and vein leaving the spleen supplied by short gastric and gastroepiploic vessels as described by Warshaw et al. [50]. This procedure is especially noteworthy for spleen preservation in laparoscopic procedures. Most patients exhibit severe inflammatory adhesions around the tail of pancreas and the hilum of the spleen, making spleen preservation under these conditions very difficult, if not impossible [38].

Data concerning the actual rate of spleen preservation in distal pancreatectomy for chronic pancreatitis are few. Carrere et al. [35] describe an overall preservation rate of 95% out of 36 patients after resection, with only 3 patients suffering from chronic pancreatitis. Lillemoe et al. [34] could only preserve the spleen in 15% of 54 patients with chronic pancreatitis. In their study, Schoenberg et al. could preserve the spleen in 34% of 74 patients with chronic pancreatitis [22]. Similarly, Sakorafas and Zobolas [44] provided data on 40 chronic pancreatitis patients with a distal pancreas resection. In this study, 29 patients underwent splenectomy; the spleen was preserved in 9 patients. Nevertheless, all authors agree that in case of splenic thromboses a concomitant splenectomy should be performed.

Little is known about the effect of spleen preservation in patients undergoing distal resection for chronic pancreatitis [35, 42, 51, 52]. In the literature only a small number of studies with few patients [50, 52, 53] deal with this issue explicitly. In their study on 74 patients with chronic pancreatitis, Schoenberg et al. [32] found no differences in pain improvement or early postoperative complications in patients with and without spleen preservation [22]. The overall blood loss was 1220±350 cm^3 and did not differ between the patients with and without splenectomy. Similarly, the rate of early postoperative complications did not differ between the spleen-preservation and splenectomy groups. Carrere et al. [35] examined the particular aspect of spleen preservation with ligation of the splenic artery and vein in a matched study, but included only six patients with chronic pancreatitis in this evaluation. According to this recent study by Carrere et al. [35], spleen preservation reduces the number of postoperative complications – especially intra-abdominal infections, but does not differ from distal pancreas resection with splenectomy in terms of transfusions needed and mortality. In contrast, an earlier study by Lillemoe et al. [34], 8 years ago, saw quite a significant difference in hospital stay between a spleen-preservation (13 days) and splenectomy (21 days) group. In the study of Carrere et al. [35], the overall complication rate of patients with a distal resection in the splenectomy group was 34% (13 out of 38 patients); in the spleen-preservation group the rate was only at 13% (5 out of 38 patients). In addition, the incidence of intra-abdominal infections was higher in the splenectomy group (18%, seven cases) than in the spleen-preservation group (3%, one case). In contrast, only Benoist et al. [52] report a higher postoperative fistula rate with spleen preservation (40% vs. 12%) and a higher rate of subphrenic abscesses (27% vs. 4%) in a group of 40 patients with a distal pancreatectomy.

Preserving the spleen is a difficult operation demanding careful ligation of little branches of the splenic artery and vein that enter the pancreas tissue. In addition, firm adhesions can make spleen preservation difficult to accomplish. Nevertheless, spleen preservation means maintaining the immunologic function of the spleen. On the other hand, distal resection with splenectomy is the easier procedure with acceptable mortality and morbidity. Mellemkjaer et al. reported about 20 years ago an interesting aspect in this matter; they found a significantly higher risk for malignancies in later life for patients with splenectomy [54]. There have been no further studies on this topic.

At the present time, due to lack of sufficient data, the issue of for versus against splenectomy has not yet been settled and certainly warrants further research.

Laparoscopic Approach

The laparoscopic approach holds on to the same structures as the open procedure. In laparoscopic "chopstick surgery," however, surgery is performed in a very vulnerable area of chronic inflammation, which is already difficult to operate for the experienced surgeon with his/her sensitive and trained hand. Even gentle handling of the pancreas tissue by graspers may disrupt the parenchyma and cause bleeding. While laparoscopic resection of the pancreas has been performed fairly often in some institutions [55], there is very little data concerning this procedure in chronic pancreatitis. Table 40.5 provides a summary of studies on this particular topic.

In most patients, laparoscopic resections of the corpus and tail were performed for benign or cystic tumors in this region [43, 51, 56]. In 1994, Cuschieri et al. [57] described laparoscopic pancreatic surgery in detail. The handling of the "soft pancreas" tissue is generally still discussed by many surgeons performing a laparoscopic approach. This issue is, however, different in the fibrotic pancreatic tissue of patients with chronic pancreatitis. In 21 laparoscopic left resections, Dulucq et al. [58] operated only 3 times on patients suffering from chronic pancreatitis. Velanovich et al. [56] performed the minimally invasive procedure only on two patients with chronic pancreatitis.

The operation time for a laparoscopic pancreas resection ranges from 3.1 h [55] to 4.7 h [59], and is comparable to that for open procedures (Schoenberg et al. [22], n=74 t=3.4 h; Lillemoe et al. [34], n=235, t=4.3 h). The conversion rate ranges between 14 and 18% [57, 60] and the mean hospital stay is around 7 days [55], slightly shorter as compared to that for open procedures [34].

In laparoscopic procedures, the spleen preservation rate varies between 62% [55] and 76% [61]. The higher rate of spleen preservation in this technique is probably due to the magnification of the site during the operation and selection of patients with less severe inflammatory alterations. Moreover, blood loss is limited and less than with an open procedure (Dulucq et al. [58], 150 ml; Schoenberg et al. [22], 1220 ml). It is not clear whether this is due to the advantages of the laparoscopic strategy or to the fact that more demanding operations would not be planned as laparoscopic procedures. Again, these are general observations for laparoscopic surgery in the pancreas, since the subgroup of patients with chronic pancreatitis undergoing laparoscopy is still too small to be conclusive (Table 40.5).

Technique

Laparoscopic resection can be performed with the patient in a 45° right lateral decubitus position, flexing the operating table to open the space between the patient's costal margin and iliac crest [61]. Another approach is the supine position with the legs apart [58]. Ports can be placed in the epigastrium and left of the axillary line with a 12-mm port in the left midclavicular line, or on the right side of the mammarian line,

Table 40.5. Current literature on laparoscopic distal pancreatectomy in chronic pancreatitis

Authors	n	Laparoscopic distal pancreatectomy	Laparoscopic distal pancreatectomy in patients with chronic pancreatitis
Fabre et al. 2002 [38]	13	13	1
Edwin et al. 2004 [60]	32	17	0
Dulucq et al. 2005 [58]	32	21	3
Mabrut et al. 2005 [55]	127	82	11
Velanovich 2006 [56]	11	11	2

2 cm above the umbilical level and midclavicular line, subcostally [58]. Dulucq et al. [58] also describe a laparoscopic procedure with a retroperitoneal approach, since the patient had undergone previously multiple operations and adhesions in this region were suspected. The gastrocolic ligament is divided from the right gastroepiploic vessels to the gastric fundus. Manipulations on the pancreas itself have a high risk for potential damage of the tissue. New techniques, such as Velanovich's lasso [56], try to ensure careful handling of the vulnerable pancreas. The retroperitoneum is dissected along the inferior border of the pancreas. While carefully handling the splenic artery and vein, the pancreas is explored to the right side above the portal vein. If the splenic artery and vein are supposed to be saved, careful dissection using clips is needed to ligate the splenic vessels [58].

Spleen Preservation in Laparoscopic Surgery of the Pancreas

In laparoscopic surgery of the pancreas surgeons try to save the spleen as far as possible. During the preparation and dissection of the spleen, however, small vessels originating from the splenic artery and vein, which supply the pancreas, are difficult to detect and are dissected securely. This is especially difficult to perform in an area of chronic inflammation, adhesions, or occurrence of a splenic thrombosis. The conventional technique gives the surgeon more space to act and provides a better view at the entire situs. Nevertheless, some surgeons argue in favor of laparoscopic resection, as they postulate that these small vessels are much easier to detect and securely ligated in laparoscopy, where the operative field is magnified by optics [61].

In fact preservation or control of these vessels appears to be the key aspect of spleen preservation in laparoscopic surgery. If there is bleeding from these vessels, the advantages of laparoscopic approach may turn to disadvantage as the surgeon does not have good visualization of the area, but still needs to settle the bleeding. This is a point when conversion to an open technique may be necessary. As described previously, if the splenic artery cannot be preserved, Warshaw's strategy [50] of ligating the splenic artery and vein while leaving the small gastric arteries intact, can be used and provides enough of a blood supply to the spleen to avoid splenic ischemia and splenectomy. Whether this aspect leads to lower postoperative morbidity remains subject to be established; further study is required to resolve this issue.

The conversion rates of recent studies are reported generally to range between approximately 5% (Dulucq et al. 2005, [58]) and 14% (Mabrut et al. [55]) in laparoscopic distal pancreatectomies. As Table 40.5 shows, due to the small number of patients, it is not possible to draw a conclusion on conversion rates in patients with chronic pancreatitis. This rate may decrease as the use of laparoscopic pancreas surgery increases.

Pancreatic Remnant in Laparoscopic Surgery

As discussed earlier in the text, closure of the pancreas remnant is very important with respect to postoperative complications as fistulas. The same applies to laparoscopic procedures. Laparoscopically, the distal pancreas is resected by an endo-gastrointestinal anastomosis stapler with vascular staples or by another dissecting method (e.g., harmonic scalpel) as mentioned above with the open operation technique [58]. The pancreas remnant is controlled for bleeding and additional stitches may be applied. Some surgeons favor fibrin glue in order to minimize the incidence of pancreatic fistulas [46]. The advantage of this procedure, however, has not been proven so far. There is only one aspect that implies a trend toward fewer complications – the additional suture of the pancreas remnant after stapling resection in an open procedure [46]. Again, this issue is remains unsettled. Several different operative techniques are suggested in order to avoid a pancreas fistula. This, as often in surgery, is a sign that the adequate technique is still under debate and more relevant studies are necessary in order to draw any conclusions on this topic.

Postoperative Complications after Distal Pancreatectomy for Chronic Pancreatitis

Distal pancreatic resection for chronic pancreatitis, regardless of its etiology, is associated with a very low postoperative mortality rate, which ranges from 0 to 9%. In high-volume centers it is significantly lower and does not exceed 4% [40, 43, 51, 62, 63]. The late mortality, however, is with 10% significantly higher and mostly due to the fact that these patients do not stop drinking [34, 48]. Regardless of the low early postoperative mortality rate, the early postoperative morbidity, however, ranges from 9 to 47% [34, 64–66]. Thereby, pancreatic fistula and sequelae are thought to be the main cause of the high morbidity rate [41, 63].

The most common postoperative complications after pancreatic left resections are pancreatic fistulas, intra-abdominal fluid collection, abscess, exo- and endocrine disturbances, or loss of function. Concomitant acute pancreatitis and immunological problems are often seen.

According to the literature, fistulas of the pancreas occur in 3–26% of all patients and are therefore the most frequent postoperative complication (see Table 40.6) [34, 41, 45, 66]. This large variation is most likely due to different definitions of pancreatic fistulas in the literature. Pancreatic fistulas are normally defined according to three criteria: increased amylase or lipase concentration in the pancreatic fluid, the volume of pancreatic fluid secreted, and its duration [43]. Principally, pancreatic fistulas and the concomitant secretions can be very dangerous and lead to sepsis and septic hemorrhage, especially if the fluid is activated by enterokinesis, thus enhancing the proteolytic and lipolytic capacity of the pancreatic juice [67, 68].

What are the predisposing factors for the pancreatic fistulas after left resection of the pancreatic gland? Two factors seem to be evident. Firstly, inadequate closure of the pancreatic duct, which should be performed by ligature with a monofil unresorbable suture. The second factor is resection of the segment of the pancreatic corpus. Both factors increase the risk of pancreatic fistulas significantly.

Pannegeon et al. [43] showed that 29% of patients (18 of 61 patients) without a sufficient ligature of the pancreatic duct suffered from a pancreatic fistula as compared to 19% (22 of 114 patients) with sufficient closure. Moreover, 35% of the patients (13 of 37 patients) developed a pancreatic fistula after resection in the pancreatic corpus segment, whereas this occurred in only 20% (27 of 138 patients) of those patients in who the resection was extended to the pancreatic isthmus. These data were recently confirmed by Frey et al. [69] (17% fistula rate after resections extending to 40–80% of distal pancreas versus 8% in which 80–95% of the distal pancreas was resected) and Bilimoria et al. [45] (9.6% fistula rate after ligature of the main pancreatic duct versus 34% fistula rate in absence of the ligature).

The role of somatostatin and its analogs in the prevention of postoperative fistulas after distal pancreatic resections is still not clear. Although 12 randomized studies have evaluated the therapeutic effect of this treatment, only 3 dealt with this therapeutic regime after pancreatic left resections. No significant benefit was seen in any of these three studies (see Table 40.7) [43, 70–72].

Table 40.6. Pancreatic fistulas: incidence after pancreatic left resection

Author	Year of publication	Patients	Frequency of fistulas *n* (%)
Suzuki et al. [39]	1999	56	16 (28%)
Schoenberg et al. [22]	1999	74	4 (16%)
Lillemoe et al. [34]	1999	235	12 (5%)
Sohn et al. [36]	2000	52	4 (8%)
Balcom et al. [64]	2001	190	27 (14%)
Fahy et al. [41]	2002	51	13 (26%)
Sheehan et al. [47]	2002	85	12 (14%)
Hutchins et al. [48]	2002	90	3 (12%)
Pratt et al. [76]	2006	66	8 (12%)
Σ		899	99 (11%)

Table 40.7. Prevention of pancreatic fistulas: octreotide in randomized studies

Author	Year	Group	Patient *n*	Dosage	Complications *n* (%)	Fistulas *n* (%)
Montorsi et al. [70]	1995	Octreotide	111	100 µg/3×daily	24 (22%)	10 (9%)
		Placebo	107		39 (36%)	21 (20%)
Sarr et al. [71]	2003	Vapreotide	135	600 µg/2×daily	40%	30.4%
		Placebo	140		42%	26.4%
Suc et al. [72]	2004	Octreotide	122	100 µg/3×daily	27 (22%)	21 (17%)
		Placebo	108		35 (32%)	20 (19%)

Pancreatic fistulas are accompanied by long-term percutaneous drainage therapy with increased risk for infections and abscess formation. In particular, the latter can result in very severe life-threatening intra-abdominal bleeding [73]. Fortunately, most patients with pancreatic fistulas after distal pancreatectomy can be treated successfully by percutaneous drainage. Persistent intra-abdominal fluid collections can be treated easily by CT-guided interventions. Moreover, comparing pancreatic fistulas derived from pancreatic head resections, the pancreatic secretion resulting from left resection is generally not activated by enterokinases of the intestinal mucosa, and is therefore less dangerous.

Endocrine and Exocrine Function

Resections of the distal pancreas do not significantly impair the exocrine function [48, 74]. In a study by Hutchins et al. [48] it was shown that exocrine failure was present in two-thirds of patients suffering from chronic pancreatitis preoperatively and was unchanged at follow-up assessment. The endocrine function, however, is problematic. In fact, the main argument against the segmental resective therapy in chronic pancreatitis is the development of diabetes mellitus. In contrast to inflammatory tumors localized in the pancreatic head, which nowadays are resected preserving the duodenum, distal pancreatectomy may often lead to a deterioration of endocrine function, as a significant number of the islet cells are localized in the pancreatic corpus and tail.

Interestingly, in our study we showed, with a medium follow-up time of 4.8 years, that only one-quarter of all patients developed impairment of endocrine function. Manifest diabetes mellitus developed during the observation period in 14.4% of our cases who did not previously suffer from the condition. Consequently, after almost 5 years, nearly half of the patients suffered from latent or manifest diabetes mellitus. On the other hand despite operation and distal pancreatectomy leading to a significant pain reduction, endocrine function remained unchanged in 75.5% of the patients. Similar good results were observed after 6.5 and 10 years. In these studies, postoperative deterioration was seen in 29 and 34.4%, respectively [22].

Conclusion

The indications for a resective procedure in chronic pancreatitis are severe pain and local complications with displacement of the neighboring organs or vessels. Drainage procedures save pancreatic tissue; however, as shown in longer follow-up studies, they do not lead to a long-lasting pain relief. Pancreatic resection can be performed nowadays with little preoperative morbidity and an acceptably low mortality rate. A large variety of resective procedures are suggested for chronic pancreatitis; however, these resective procedures should be tailored according to the principal: "as much as necessary – as little as possible." Keeping this overriding principal in mind, the operative treatment of chronic pancreatitis has significant advantages, such as early pain relief without severe impairment of endocrine or exocrine function. Due to the important function of the spleen, both immunologically and hematologically, distal pancreatectomy should be performed while preserving the spleen if possible. Various techniques are described herein. The possibility of laparoscopic distal pancreatectomy has emerged recently and although the results are interesting, they are inconclusive and warrant further research.

References

1. Jaakkola M, Nordback I (1993) Pancreatitis in Finland between 1970 and 1989. Gut 34:1255–1260
2. Nealon WH, Townsend CM Jr, Thompson JC (1988) Operative drainage of the pancreatic duct delays functional impairment in patients with chronic pancreatitis: a prospective analysis. Ann Surg 208:321–329
3. Nealon WH, Thompson JC (1993) Progressive loss of pancreatic function in chronic pancreatitis is delayed by main pancreatic duct decompression: a longitudinal prospective analysis of the modified Puestow procedure. Ann Surg 217:458–466
4. Lowntrefels AB, Maisonneuve P, Cavallini G, Ammann RW, Lankisch PG, Anderson JR, Dimagno EP, Andren-Sandberg A, Domellof L (1993) Pancreatitis and the risk of pancreatic cancer. N Engl J Med 328:1433–1437
5. Schlosser W, Schoenberg MH, Rhein E, Siech M, Gansauge F, Beger HG (1996) Pancreatic carcinoma in chronic pancreatitis with inflammatory tumor of the head of the pancreas. Z Gastroenterol 34:3–8
6. Pederzoli P, Bassi C, Falconi M, Camboni MG (1994) Efficacy of octreotide in the prevention of complications of elective pancreatitis surgery. Br J Surg 81:265–269
7. Sarles H, Adler G, Dani R, Frey C, Gullo L, Harada H, Martin E, Norohna M, Scuro LA (1989) The pancreatitis classification of Marseilles-Rome 1988. Scand J Gastroenterol 24:641–642
8. Banks PA (2007) Classification and diagnosis of chronic pancreatitis. J Gastroenterol 42:148–151

9. Becker H, Encke A, Röher HD (2006) Viszeralchirurgie, 2nd edition. Urban and Fischer, München, pp 742–743
10. Duffy PD, Reber HA (2002) Surgical treatment of chronic pancreatitis. J Hepatobiliary Pancreat Surg 9:659–668
11. Liao Q, Wu WW, Li BL, Zhang T-P, Zhao Y-P (2002) Surgical treatment of chronic pancreatitis. Hepatobiliary Pancreat Dis Int 1:462–464
12. Krechler T, Kocna P, Vanickova Z, Svestka T, Lukas M, Dosedel J, Kohout P, Zak A (2006) Faecal elastase I – its use in diagnosis of chronic pancreatitis. Cas Lek Cesk 145:480–483
13. Luth S, Teyssen S, Forssmann K, Kolbel C, Krummenauer F, Singer MV (2001) Fecal elastase-1 determination: "gold standard" of indirect pancreatic function tests? Scand J Gastroenterol 36:1092–1099
14. Molinari I, Souare K, Lamireau T, Fayon M, Lemieux C, Cassaigne A, Mountaudon D (2004) Fecal chymotrypsin and elastase-1 determination on one single stool collected at random: diagnostic value for exocrine pancreatic status. Clin Biochem 37:758–763
15. Sugiyama M, Haradome H, Yutaka A (2007) Magnetic resonance imaging for diagnosing chronic pancreatitis. J Gastroenterol 42:108–112
16. Kahl S, Glasbrenner B, Leodolter A, Pross M, Schulz HU, Malfertheiner P (2002) EUS in the diagnosis of early chronic pancreatitis: a prospective follow-up study. Gastrointest Endosc 55:507–511
17. Falconi M, Valerio A, Caldiron E, Salvia R, Sartori N, Talamini G, Bassi C, Pederzoli P (2000) Changes in pancreatic resection for chronic pancreatitis over 28 years in a single institution. Br J Surg 87:428–433
18. Reber HA (1997) Chronic pancreatitis. In: Zinner MJ (ed) Maingot's Abdominal Operations, 10th edn. Appleton Lange, Stanford, pp 1941–1960
19. Stapleton GN, Williamson RCN (1996) Proximal pancreatoduodenectomy for chronic pancreatitis. Br J Surg 83:1433–1440
20. Heise JW, Katoh M, Luthen R, Roher H-D (2001) Long-term results following different extent of resection in chronic pancreatitis. Hepatogastroenterology 48:864–868
21. Vickers SM, Chan C, Heslin MJ, Bartolucci A, Aldrete JS (1999) The role of pancreatectomy in the treatment of severe chronic pancreatitis. Am Surg 65:1108–1111
22. Schoenberg MH, Schlosser W, Rück W, Beger HG (1999) Distal pancreatectomy in chronic pancreatitis. Dig Surg 16:130–136
23. Sawyer R, Frey F (1994) Is there still a role for distal pancreatectomy in surgery for chronic pancreatitis? Am J Surg 168:6–9
24. Ho HS, Frey CF (1997) Current approach to the surgical management of chronic pancreatitis. Gastroenterologist 5:128–136
25. Sarr MG (1999) Treatment of cancer of the exocrine pancreas. Am J Surg 178:435–436
26. Wong GY, Sakorafas GH, Tsiotos GG, Sarr MG (1999) Palliation of pain in chronic pancreatitis. Use of neural blocks and neurotomy. Surg Clin North Am 79:873–893
27. Duffy JP, Delano MJ, Reber HA (2002) Pancreatic surgery. Curr Opin Gastroenterol 18:568–573
28. Puestow CB, Gillesby WJ (1958) Retrograde surgical drainage of pancreas for chronic relapsing pancreatitis. AMA Arch Surg 76:898–907
29. Partington PF, Rochelle RE (1960) Modified Puestow procedure for retrograde drainage of the pancreatic duct. Ann Surg 152:1037–1043
30. Frey CF, Amikura K (1994) Local resection of the head of the pancreas combined with longitudinal pancreaticojejunostomy in the management of patients with chronic pancreatitis. Ann Surg 220:492–504; discussion 504–507
31. Howard J, Idezuki Y, Ihrese I, Prinz R (eds) (1998) Surgical Diseases of the Pancreas, 3rd edn. Williams and Wilkins, Baltimore
32. Schoenberg MH, Schlosser W, Beger HG (1999) Surgical treatment of chronic pancreatitis. Dtsch Ärztebl 96:625–631
33. Cahen DL, Gouma DJ, Nio Y, Rauws EA, Boermeester MA, Busch OR, Stoker J, Lameris JS, Dijkgraaf MG, Huibregtse K, Bruno MJ (2007) Endoscopic versus surgical drainage of the pancreatic duct in chronic pancreatitis. N Engl J Med 356:676–684
34. Lillemoe KD, Kaushal S, Cameron JL, Sohn TA, Pitt HA, Yeo CJ (1999) Distal pancreatectomy: indications and outcomes in 235 patients. Ann Surg 229:693–6988; discussion 698–700
35. Carrere N, Abid S, Julio CH, Bloom E, Pradere B (2007) Spleen-preserving distal pancreatectomy with excision of splenic artery and vein: a case-matched comparison with conventional distal pancreatectomy with splenectomy. World J Surg 31:375–382
36. Sohn TA, Campbell KA, Pitt HA, Sauter PK, Coleman JA, Lillemoe KD, Yeo CJ, Cameron JL (2000) Quality of life and long-term survival after surgery for chronic pancreatitis. J Gastroenterol Surg 4:355–364
37. Rattner DW, Fernandez-del Castillo C, Warshaw AL (1996) Pitfalls of distal pancreatectomy for relief of pain in chronic pancreatitis. Am J Surg 171:142–145; discussion 145–146
38. Fabre JM, Dulucq JL, Vacher C, Lemoine MC, Wintringer P, Nocca D, Burgel JS, Domergue J (2002) Is laparoscopic left pancreatic resection justified? Surg Endosc 16:1358–1361
39. Suzuki Y, Fujino Y, Tanioka Y, Hori Y, Ueda T, Takeyama Y, Tominaga M, Ku Y, Yamamoto YM, Kuroda Y (1999) Randomized clinical trial of ultrasonic dissector or conventional division in distal pancreatectomy for non-fibrotic pancreas. Br J Surg 86:608–611
40. Sugo H, Mikami Y, Matsumoto F, Tsumura H, Watanabe Y, Futagawa S (2000) Distal pancreatectomy using the harmonic scalpel. Surgery 128:490–491
41. Fahy BN, Frey CF, Ho HS, Beckett L, Bold RJ (2002) Morbidity, mortality, and technical factors of distal pancreatectomy. Am J Surg 183:237–241
42. Uranues S, Grossman D, Ludwig L, Bergamaschi R (2007) Laparoscopic partial splenectomy. Surg Endosc 21:57–60
43. Pannegeon V, Pessaux P, Sauvanet A, Vullierme MP, Kianmanesh R, Belghiti J (2006) Pancreatic fistula after distal pancreatectomy: predictive risk factors and value of conservative treatment. Arch Surg 141:1071–1076; discussion 1076
44. Sakorafas GH, Zobolas B (2001) Lateral pancreatojejunostomy in the surgical management of chronic pancreatitis. Current concepts and future perspectives. Dig Liver Dis 33:187–191
45. Bilimoria MM, Cormier JN, Mun Y, Lee JE, Evans DB, Pisters PW (2003) Pancreatic leak after left pancreatectomy is reduced following main pancreatic duct ligation. Br J Surg 90:190–196
46. Knaebel HP, Diener MK, Wente MN, Buchler MW, Seiler CM (2005) Systematic review and meta-analysis of technique for closure of the pancreatic remnant after distal pancreatectomy. Br J Surg 92:539–546

47. Sheehan MK, Beck K, Creech S, Pickleman J, Aranha GV (2002) Distal pancreatectomy: does the method of closure influence fistula formation? Am Surg 68:264–267
48. Hutchins RR, Hart RS, Pacifico M, Bradley NJ, Williamson RC (2002) Long-term results of distal pancreatectomy for chronic pancreatitis in 90 patients. Ann Surg 236:612–618
49. Andren-Sandberg A, Wagner M, Tihanyi T, Lofgren P, Friess H (1999) Technical aspects of left-sided pancreatic resection for cancer. Dig Surg 16:305–312
50. Warshaw AL (1988) Conservation of the spleen with distal pancreatectomy. Arch Surg 123:550–553
51. Richardson DQ, Scott Conner CE (1989) Distal pancreatectomy with and without splenectomy: a comparative study. Am Surg 55:21–25
52. Benoist S, Dugue L, Sauvanet A, Valverde A, Mauvais F, Paye F, Farges O, Belghiti J (1999) Is there a role of preservation of the spleen in distal pancreatectomy? J Am Coll Surg 188:255–260
53. Shoup M, Brennan MF, McWhite K, Leung DHY, Klimstra D, Conlon KC (2002) The value of splenic preservation with distal pancreatectomy. Arch Surg 137:164–168
54. Mellemkjaer L, Olsen JH, Linet MS, Gridley G, McLaughlin JK (1995) [Cancer risk after splenectomy]. Ugeskr Laeger 157:5097–5100
55. Mabrut JY, Fernandez-Cruz L, Azagra JS, Bassi C, Delvaux G, Weerts J, Fabre JM, Boulez J, Baulieux J, Peix JL, Gigot JF; Hepatobiliary and Pancreatic Section (HBPS) of the Royal Belgian Society of Surgery; Belgian Group for Endoscopic Surgery (BGES); Club Coelio (2005) Laparoscopic pancreatic resection: results of a multicenter European study of 127 patients. Surgery 137:597–605
56. Velanovich V (2006) The lasso technique for laparoscopic distal pancreatectomy. Surg Endosc 20:1766–1771
57. Cuschieri A (1994) Laparoscopic surgery of the pancreas. J R Coll Surg Edinb 39:178–184
58. Dulucq JL, Wintringer P, Stabilini C, Feryn T, Perissat J, Mahajna A (2005) Are major laparoscopic pancreatic resections worthwhile? A prospective study of 32 patients in a single institution. Surg Endosc 19:1028–1034
59. Fernandez-Cruz L, Martinez I, Gilabert R, Cesar-Borges G, Astudillo E, Navarro S (2004) Laparoscopic distal pancreatectomy combined with preservation of the spleen for cystic neoplasms of the pancreas. J Gastrointest Surg 8:493–501
60. Edwin B, Skattum X, Rader J, Trondsen E, Buanes T (2004) Outpatient laparoscopic splenectomy: patient safety and satisfaction. Surg Endosc 18:1331–1334
61. Tagaya N, Kasama K, Suzuki N, Taketsuka S, Horie K, Furihata M, Kubota K (2003) Laparoscopic resection of the pancreas and review of the literature. Surg Endosc 17:201–206
62. Aldrige MC, Williamson RCN (1991) Distal pancreatectomy with and without splenectomy. Br J Surg 78:976–979
63. Wisner DH, Wold RL, Frey CF (1990) Diagnosis and treatment of pancreatic injuries. Arch Surg 125:1109–1113
64. Balcom JH, Rattner DW, Warshaw AL, Chang Y, Fernandez-del Castillo C (2001) Ten-year experience with 733 pancreatic resections: changing indications, older patients, and decreasing length of hospitalization. Arch Surg 136:391–398
65. Brennan MF, Moccia RD, Klimstra D (1996) Management of adenocarcinoma of the body and tail of the pancreas. Ann Surg 223:506–512
66. Fabre JM, Houry S, Manderscheid JC, Huguier M, Baumel H (1996) Surgery for left-sided pancreatic cancer. Br J Surg 83:1065–1070
67. Kukor Z, Toth M, Sahin-Toth M (2003) Human anionic trypsinogen: properties of autocatalytic activation and degradation and implications in pancreatic diseases. Eur J Biochem 270:2047–2058
68. Suzuki S, Kanai S, Miyasaka K, Jimi A, Funakoshi A (2000) Regulation of pancreas secretion by vagal nerve during short-term duct occlusion in conscious rats. Pancreas 20:94–101
69. Frey CF, Child CG, Fry W (1976) Pancreatectomy for chronic pancreatitis. Ann Surg 184:403–414
70. Montorsi M, Zago M, Mosca F, et al (1995) Efficacy of octreotide in the prevention of pancreatic fistula after elective pancreatic resections: a prospective, controlled, randomized clinical trial. Surgery 117:26–31
71. Sarr MG; Pancreatic Surgery Group (2003) The potent somatostatin analogue vapreotide does not decrease pancreas-specific complications after elective pancreatectomy: a prospective, multicenter, double-blinded, randomized, placebo-controlled trial. J Am Coll Surg 196:556–565
72. Suc B, Msika S, Piccinini M, Fourtanier G, Hay JM, Flamant Y, Fingerhut A, Fagniez PL, Chipponi J; French Associations for Surgical Research (2004) Octreotide in the prevention of intra-abdominal complications following elective pancreatic resection: a prospective, multicenter randomized controlled trial. Arch Surg 139:288–294
73. Ohwada S, Ogawa T, Tanahashi Y, Nakamura S, Takeyoshi I, Ohya T, Ikeya T, Kawashima K, Kawashima Y, Morishita Y (1998) Fibrin glue sandwich prevents pancreatic fistula following distal pancreatectomy. World J Surg 22:494–498
74. Jalleh RP, Williamson RCN (1992) Pancreatic exocrine and endocrine function after operations for chronic pancreatitis. Ann Surg 216:656–662
75. Klöppel G (2007) Toward a new classification of chronic pancreatitis. J Gastroenterol 42:55–57
76. Pratt W, Maithel SK, Vanounou T, Callery MP, Vollmer CM Jr (2006) Postoperative pancreatic fistulas are not equivalent after proximal, distal, and central pancreatectomy. J Gastrointest Surg 10:1264–1279

Chapter 41

Total Pancreatectomy

I. Ihse

Debilitating abdominal and back pain remains the most common indication for surgery in patients with chronic pancreatitis. Even if there have been substantial advances in understanding of the natural history [1,2] and pathogenesis [2–4] of chronic pancreatitis, the cause of pain continues to be obscure. The two most common hypotheses are the duct-tissue-hypertension theory [5] and the inflammatory mass theory [6]. Accordingly, surgical procedures as a rule are directed at duct decompression and/or resection of the pancreas. Reportedly, up to one-third of patients, however, continue to suffer pain after surgery [7,8]. This might reflect a lack in concordance between the causes of pain and the objectives of the surgical procedure chosen in such unsuccessful cases. What is more, even if the whole gland is ablated, half of the patients will have no or only slight pain relief [9]. However, excellent results are now reported from specialty centers after different kinds of surgical procedures emphasizing the importance of the volume–outcome association for the experience and skill of the surgeon and treatment team [10] and of proper selection of the right patient for the right operation at the right time [11–13]. In this chapter, the role, if any, of total pancreatectomy in the management of patients with chronic pancreatitis will be discussed.

Rationale and Indications

Chronic pancreatitis normally affects the whole gland. This is true in cases where the pancreas is small and atrophic. It is also true when there are local inflammatory masses in the pancreatic head, body, or tail as the rest of the gland also shows signs of pancreatitis. Therefore, the rationale for total pancreatectomy was originally that elimination of all inflammatory tissue required removal of the whole gland.

During the 1960s and 1970s the operation was practiced in some centers in Europe and USA. The disappointing results, however, gave it a questionable reputation and the indications for its use quickly became narrowed. Today, total pancreatectomy may be warranted in patients with disabling pain due to advanced chronic pancreatitis in whom medical therapy and partial resection or duct-drainage procedures have failed and who suffer end-stage pancreatic function.

In patients with previous partial resection, removal of the remaining part of the gland (head or tail/body) is sometimes necessary in case of delayed complications to the disease such as abscess or fistulas. Completion pancreatectomy may also be indicated when complications (e.g., leakage of anastomoses or abscess) develop in the immediate period following a pancreaticoduodenectomy.

There is a small group of patients with no or minimal duct abnormalities who have repeated periods of pancreatic pain and who do not respond to partial resection. They can be appropriately managed by total pancreatectomy if carefully assessed and selected by an experienced treatment team. Thus, the principle today underlying total pancreatectomy for chronic pancreatitis is that it is a last-resort operation.

Preoperative Preparation

Before embarking on a total pancreatectomy, the case should be carefully discussed by an experienced treatment team of pancreatic surgeons, gastroenterologists, diagnostic radiologists, anesthesiologists, psychiatrists, and others. They should analyze and try to answer the question as to why the previous operation/treatment failed. The patient should be given full information on the chances of success and the risks and sequelae, and alcoholic and narcotic abuse must preferably be stopped preoperatively. Ongoing abuse is to be regarded as a contraindication to the operation. It should also be agreed that the treatment team is prepared to take responsibility for the care of the patient for a long time postoperatively.

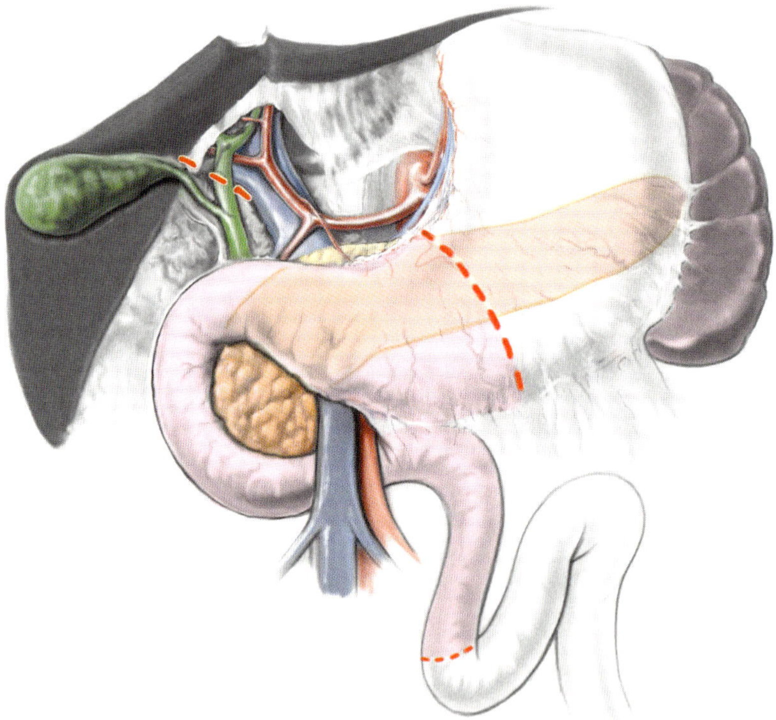

Figure 41.1

The extent of resection. The broken red lines show lines of resecton of jejunum, stomach and bile duct. The standard operation includes removal of the whole pancreas and the spleen

The Operation and its Modifications

A bilateral subcostal incision carried further to the left is recommended since good exposure of the spleen and pancreatic tail is essential. An inflatable pillow that elevates the lower parts of the thorax further improves the access to the retroperitoneal area.

Standard total pancreatectomy comprises removal of the entire gland, duodenum, distal half of the bile duct, gallbladder, antrum, and spleen. The extent of resection is illustrated in Fig.41.1. The steps of mobilization of the duodenum, pancreatic head and neck, the gallbladder, and the dissection of the hepatoduodenal ligament are followed as described in Chap. 38.

Before mobilizing the spleen and the left pancreas, blood loss is minimized by ligating the splenic artery at its origin. The left flexure of the colon is reflected downward and the spleen is mobilized and its diaphragmatic attachments severed. The avascular plane behind the spleen and pancreatic tail is identified: the spleen and pancreatic tail are usually easy to lift out of the retroperitoneum (Fig. 41.2). The splenic vein is divided at its confluence with the superior mesenteric vein. After dissection of the vessels running from the portal vein and the mesenteric root into the pancreatic head and uncinate process, the pancreas is fully mobilized. As the partial gastrectomy and the division of jejunum have already been performed (see Chap. 38), the specimen can now be discarded en bloc.

As the operation is performed for a benign disease there are no reasons to proceed to a lymphadenectomy. The reconstructions after a standard total pancreatectomy are illustrated in Fig. 41.3. As the disease, again, is benign, a retrocolic gastrojejunostomy is preferable. The operative field is drained for 2–3 days by two passive, soft tubes, one subhepatically and one in the left hypochondrium.

Total pancreatectomy can, like the partial resection, be combined with sparing of the pylorus (see Chap. 38) [14]. The operation has also been performed with preservation of the duodenum, the spleen, or both the duodenum and spleen [15–17].

Total pancreatectomy has been combined with intraportal islet autotransplantation in patients with chronic pancreatitis in order to counteract the severe diabetic control problems seen after this operation. Even if most patients continue to be insulin-depen-

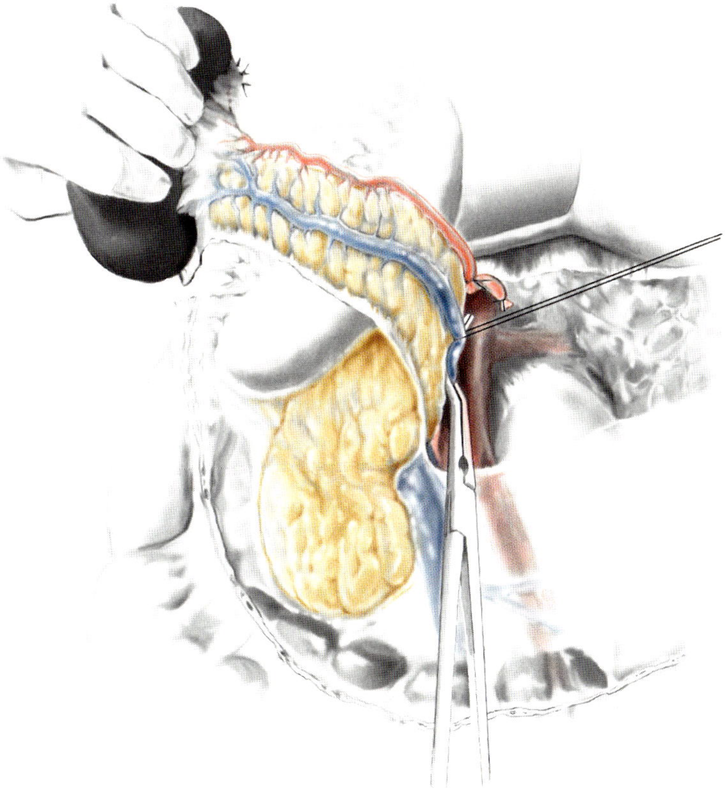

Figure 41.2

Mobilization of the spleen and pancreatic tail

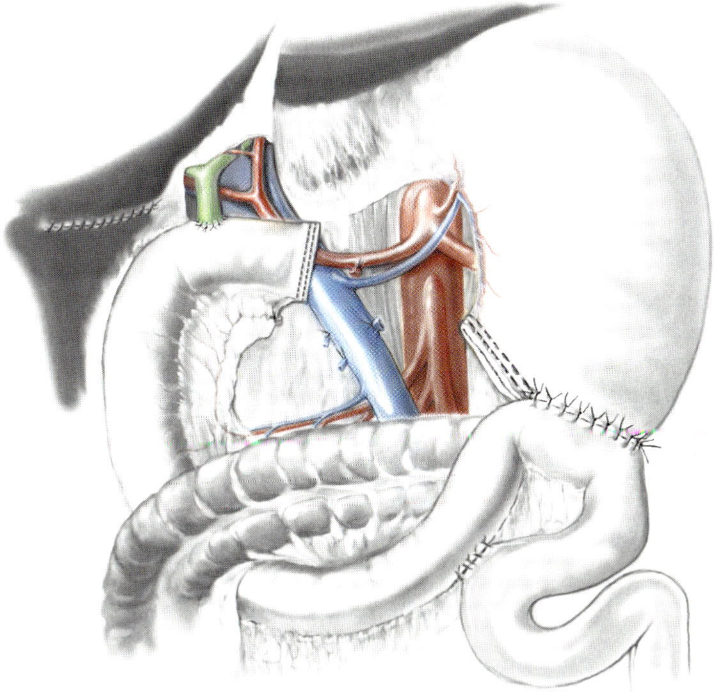

Figure 41.3

Reconstruction after standard total pancreatectomy

dent, they have decreased daily insulin requirements and glycosylated hemoglobin (HbA1C) levels compared with patients undergoing total pancreatectomy alone [18–20].

Postoperative Care

The patients stay overnight in a postoperative unit and go the next day to their ordinary ward. Modern precise operative techniques with decreased blood loss and improved monitoring and correction of aberrations in vital parameters throughout the procedure have more or less abolished the need for postoperative intensive care of the patients. Sips of water are allowed from the first postoperative day and food intake can normally start on day 3 or 4. Delayed gastric emptying is, however, relatively frequent following such extensive retroperitoneal dissection. If so a nasogastric tube is required, as is parenteral nutrition, until duodenal mobility returns. As infection prophylaxis, 1.5 g cefuroxim and 1.5 g metronidazol is given at the start of the operation and another dose of cefuroxim after 8 h. Low-molecular-weight heparin is used for prophylaxis of thromboembolism.

Due to the propensity for hypoglycemic attacks, meticulous management of the patient's diabetes is mandatory. On the first postoperative day, S-glucose is measured every 2nd h and then every 4th h until the patient has resumed full oral food intake. Initially, regular (short-acting) insulin is used for about 1 week, followed by neutral protamine Hagedorn (NPH) insulin. Pancreatic enzyme substitution is started as soon as food is introduced.

For management of pain, epidural opioid anesthesia in combination with nonsteroidal anti-inflammatory drugs is helpful in the immediate postoperative period. It is advisable to switch to oral analgesics as early as possible after the patient has started to eat. The patients should be kept in hospital until they are off narcotics and it is also important that they are competent in managing their diabetes before they are discharged. Finally, as mentioned above, they must be followed up regularly by an experienced pancreatic treatment team.

Early Postoperative Course

Data on total pancreatectomy for chronic pancreatitis are sparse and often based on small retrospective patient series. The hospital mortality rate remains significant even if there seems to have been an improvement with time, as for the Whipple operation. In a series of 63 total pancreatectomies performed for chronic pancreatitis between 1972 and 1977, Gall reported a mortality of 21% [21]. Frey published in 1989 a collective review of 324 patients among whom the average mortality was found to be 9.6% [22], and in more recent series the figure has dropped to 6% or lower [23–26]. Still, hospital mortality continues to be higher than that after pancreaticoduodenectomy or other modifications of resections used to treat chronic pancreatitis [27].

The complication rate following total pancreatectomy is as high as 40% [24]. As with the pancreaticoduodenectomy, there has been no reduction in the risk of postoperative morbidity over the years. Thus, the decreased hospital mortality rate after the two types of operations is not explained by the lower complication rate; however, it seems as if we have learned to handle the complications in a better way. One rationale of total pancreatectomy was originally that elimination of the pancreaticojejunal anastomoses could diminish the risk of abdominal sepsis and make the development of pancreatic fistulas impossible. In our own experience, abdominal sepsis, abscesses, and abdominal fistulas, surprisingly, are equally common after total and partial pancreatectomy [28].

Long-Term Outcome and Management

Whereas pain is the main indication for operation in patients with chronic pancreatitis, it is also the most important parameter when assessing outcome of the surgical treatment. In recent studies between 50% and 80% of the patients are reported to experience long-lasting pain relief after total pancreatectomy [9,16,23,27,29]. Thus, the results appear inferior to those after different types of partial resections. As total pancreatectomy is associated with greater perioperative mortality, higher late morbidity, and shorter survival [27], it should be chosen only in highly selected patients after careful assessment by an experienced pancreatic treatment term.

Total pancreatectomy inevitably leads to diabetes mellitus, which, as mentioned above, is saddled with a substantial risk of hypoglycemic attacks. There have even been late deaths reported due to hypoglycemia [30,31]. That the diabetes in many of these patients is brittle and difficult to control is another reason for them to be managed at well-organized joint clinics of surgeons and gastroenterologists/diabetologists and to have regular access to liaison nurses.

The ensuing malabsorption following total pancreatectomy is easily treated by oral pancreatic enzyme administration. The requirements vary among patients, which is why the appropriate dose has to be tested out individually. Supplementation with vitamins A, D, E, and K is given routinely in order to counteract osteopenia, coagulopathia, and night blindness.

References

1. Ammann RW, Heitz PU, Klöppel G (1996) Course of alcoholic chronic pancreatitis: a prospective clinicomorphological long-term study. Gastroenterology 111:224–231
2. Layer P, Yamamoto H, Kalthoff L, Clain JE, Bakken LJ, et al (1994) The different courses of early- and late-onset idiopathic and alcoholic chronic pancreatitis. Gastroenterology 107:1481–1487
3. Bockman DE, Büchler MW, Malfertheiner P, Beger HG (1988) Analysis of nerves in chronic pancreatitis. Gastroenterology 94:1459–1469
4. Etemad B, Whitcomb DC (2001) Chronic pancreatitis: diagnosis, classification, and new genetic developments. Gastroenterology 120:682–707
5. Ihse I (1990) Pancreatic pain. Br J Surg 77:121–122
6. Beger HG, Schlosser W, Poch B, Gansauge F (1998) Inflammatory mass in the head of the pancreas. In: Beger HG, Warshaw AL, Büchler MW, Carr-Locke D, Neoptolemos JP, Russel C, Sarr MG (eds) The Pancreas. Blackwell Science, Oxford, pp 757–760
7. Ihse I, Borch K, Larsson J (1990) Chronic pancreatitis: results of operations for pain. World J Surg 14:53–58
8. Frey CF (1995) Current management of chronic pancreatitis. Adv Surg 82:337–370
9. Russell RCG (1998) Total pancreatectomy and its modifications. In: Howard JM, Idezuki Y, Ihse I, Prinz R (eds) Surgical diseases of the pancreas. Williams & Wilkins, Baltimore, pp 393–397
10. Ihse I (2003) The volume outcome relationship in cancer surgery – a hard sell. Ann Surg 238:777–781
11. Izbicki JR, Bloechle C, Broering DC, Knoefel WT, Broelsch CE (1998) Extended resection versus resection in surgery for chronic pancreatitis: a prospective, randomized trial comparing longitudinal pancreaticojejunostomy combined with local pancreatic head excision with pylorus-preserving pancreaticoduodenectomy. Ann Surg 228:771–779
12. Sohn TA, Campbell KA, Pitt HA, Sauter PK, Coleman JA, et al (2000) Quality of life and long-term survival after surgery for chronic pancreatitis. J Gastrointest Surg 4:355–364
13. Beger HG, Schlosser W, Friess HM, Büchler MW (1999) Duodenum-preserving head resection in chronic pancreatitis changes the natural course of the disease; a single-center 26-year experience. Ann Surg 230:512–519
14. Wagner M, Z´graggen K, Vagianoss C, Redaelli C, Holziger F, Sadowski C, et al (2001) Pylorus-preserving total pancreatectomy. Early and late results. Dig Surg 18:188–195
15. Lamberg MA, Linehan IP, Russell RC (1987) Duodenum-preserving total pancreatectomy for end stage chronic pancreatitis. Br J Surg 47:35–39
16. White SA, Sutton CD, Weymss-Holden S, Berry DP, Pollard C, et al (2000) The feasibility of spleen-preserving pancreatectomy for end-stage pancreatitis. Am J Surg 179:294–297
17. Alexakis N, Ghaneh P, Conner S, Raraty M, Sutton R, et al (2003) Duodenum- and spleen-preserving total pancreatitis for end-stage chronic pancreatitis. Br J Surg 90:1401–1408
18. White SA, Davies JE, Pollard C, Swift SM, Clayton HA, et al (2001) Pancreas resection and islet autotransplantation for endstage chronic pancreatitis. Ann Surg 233:423–431
19. Clayton HA, Davies JE, Pollard CA, White SA, Musto PP, et al (2003) Pancreatectomy with islet autotransplantation for the treatment severe chronic pancreatitis: the first 40 patients at Leicester General Hospital. Transplantation 76:92–98
20. Gruessner RW, Sutherland DE, Dumm DL, Najarian JS, Jie T, et al (2004) Transplant options for patients undergoing total pancreatectomy for chronic pancreatitis. J Am Coll Surg 199:516
21. Gall FP, Mühe E, Gebhardt C (1981) Results of partial and total pancreticoduodenectomy in 117 patients with chronic pancreatitis. World J Surg 5:269–275
22. Frey CF, Suzuki M, Isaji S, Zhu Y (1985) Pancreatic resection for chronic pancreatitis. Surg Clin North Am 69:499–528
23. Cooper MJ, Wiliamson RCN, Benjamin JS, Carter DC, Cushieri A, et al (1987) Total pancreatectomy for chronic pancreatitis. Br J Surg 74:912–915
24. Kiviluotu T, Schröder T, Lempinen M (1985) Total pancreatectomy for chronic pancreatitis. Surg Gynecol Obstet 160:223–227
25. Keith RG, Saibil FG, Sheppard RH (1989) Treatment of chronic pancreatitis by pancreatic resection. Am J Surg 157:156–162
26. Stone WM, Sarr MG, Nagorney DM, McIllrath DC (1988) Chronic pancreatitis – result of Whipple´s resection and total pancreatectomy. Arch Surg 123:815–819
27. Sakorafas GH, Farnell lMB, Farley DR, Rowland CM, Sarr MG (2000) Long-term results after surgery for chronic pancreatitis. Int J Pancreatol 27:131–142
28. Ihse I, Andersson H, Andrén-Sandberg Å (1996) Total pancreatectomy for cancer of the pancreas – is it appropriate. Word J Surg 20:288–294
29. Fleming WR, Williamson RCN (1995) Role of total pancreatectomy in the treatment of patients with end-stage chronic pancreatitis. Br J Surg 82:1409–1412
30. Ihse I, Lilja P, Arnesjö B, Bengmark S (1977) Total pancreatectomy for cancer: an appraisal of 65 cases. Ann Surg 186:675–680
31. McCullagh EP, Cook JR, Shirley EK (1958) Diabetes following total pancreatectomy: clinical observations of ten cases. Diabetes 7:298–307

Chapter 42

R. Grützmann · H.D. Saeger

Surgical Treatment of Pseudocysts in Chronic Pancreatitis

Pancreatic pseudocysts are one of the most frequent complications (20–60%) of chronic pancreatitis [1]. A pancreatic pseudocyst is a localized collection of pancreatic-enzyme-rich fluid, originating in or adjacent to the pancreas and enclosed in a wall of granulation and/or fibrous tissue lacking an epithelial lining [2].

The principle mechanism leading to the formation of a pancreatic pseudocyst is believed to involve disruption of the main pancreatic duct and/or peripheral ductules causing leakage and activation of pancreatic enzymes, which in turn leads to localized autodigestion and necrosis of the pancreatic parenchyma. This causes an inflammatory response and thereby the formation of a distinct pseudocyst wall composed of granulation tissue and blood vessels. In the further course it organizes with more connective tissue and fibrosis [1]. Histological findings show that pseudocysts complicating chronic pancreatitis are identical to those complicating acute pancreatitis, although they have a different natural history [3].

Only less than 10% of pseudocysts larger than 6 cm will resolve without treatment, whereas the majority of pseudocysts associated with acute pancreatitis will resorb spontaneously. Moreover, the incidence of complications in chronic pancreatitis pseudocysts can be as high as 55% [4].

The treatment of pancreatic pseudocysts has traditionally been surgical. The history of pancreatic surgery started with pseudocyst surgery in 1879, when Thiersch drained, in two stages, a fluctuating tumor of the pancreas, evacuating 3 l of chocolate-colored liquid. The first pseudocystogastrostomy was performed 1921 by Jedlicka [5]. Formerly, traditional management of pseudocysts included observation for 6 weeks, followed by surgical therapy for persistent pseudocysts [6]. Recent studies about the natural history demonstrate that observation is a safe option for small asymptomatic pseudocysts [7–10]. There are several options for the operative management of pancreatic pseudocysts in chronic pancreatitis. These include internal drainage, external drainage, and resection. With the first two of these surgical options, a generous biopsy of the pseudocyst wall has always to be performed, as well as visual examination of the internal surface of the pseudocyst cavity, to exclude the presence of a cystic pancreatic neoplasm (i.e., intraductal papillary mucinous neoplasm).

Recently, various interventional therapeutic procedures like transmural (gastric or duodenal) cystic drainage or transpapillary stent application have been introduced [11]. These endoscopic techniques are limited to patients with cystic adherence to the stomach/duodenum or communication of the cyst with the duct system, whereas in patients with chronic pancreatitis, pseudocysts are commonly associated with ductal obstruction from stones or strictures, which are not suitable for interventional drainage. The treatment of pseudocysts by transcutaneous catheter drainage has been reported, with encouraging results. However, other studies have shown increased persistence and complications following external drainage [8]. These techniques are described in Chapter 34. So far, there have been no prospective, randomized trials that have evaluated the results of the three major modalities of therapy (percutaneous, endoscopic, and surgical). Before one can definitely recommend percutaneous drainage or endoscopic approach as the preferred initial mode of therapy, further studies are necessary.

Despite the development of nonsurgical invasive techniques for dealing with pancreatic pseudocysts in chronic pancreatitis, there remains a clear role for operative treatment. The advantages of surgical treatment are that any associated underlying pathology may be dealt with and that the drainage of the pseudocyst itself may be regarded as definitive. Moreover, it allows concomitant drainage of the main pancreatic duct or an obstructed common bile duct, or resection of adjacent unhealthy pancreatic tissue.

Rationale for Surgical Treatment of Pseudocysts in Chronic Pancreatitis

1. Pain is the leading clinical symptom in the majority of patients with chronic pancreatitis and pseudocysts. One of the favored pathophysiological concepts concerning pain in chronic pancreatitis is increased intraductal and intraparenchymatous pressure within the pancreas. A reduction of tissue pressure in patients undergoing a drainage procedure was followed by a substantial relief of pain [12]. Moreover, changes in the pancreatic nerves themselves might be responsible for the long-lasting pain syndrome in chronic pancreatitis [13].
2. Many chronic pancreatitis patients with pseudocysts in the pancreatic head suffer from pain even if the pancreatic duct is not dilated. Resection of the pancreatic head, obviously representing a pacemaker of chronic pancreatitis and pain, can make these patients free of symptoms.
3. Pancreatic pseudocyst may regress spontaneously, persist with or without symptoms, or progress and lead to complications. Factors associated with failure to resolve are, according to Warshaw and Rattner: chronic pancreatitis, persistence >6 weeks, and a thick wall on imaging [14].
4. The size of the pseudocyst seems to be a predictive factor for pseudocyst resolution, but there is no definable threshold [7]. Most authors suggest 6 cm as the limit for surgical treatment [2].
5. The risk of life-threatening complications of pancreatic pseudocysts is about 10% and includes: biliary duct compression, duodenal stenosis, rupture, compression of larger vessels (portal vein, superior mesenteric or splenic vein) with formation of collateral veins, pseudoaneurysms, hemorrhage, pancreatic ascites, and infection [6].
6. The operative results in different retrospective series concerning mortality, morbidity, and cyst recurrence rate justify surgical treatment [4].

Clinical Data Leading to Surgical Treatment of Pseudocysts in Chronic Pancreatitis

The commonest symptoms are abdominal pain (76–94%), early satiety, nausea, vomiting (50%), and weight loss (20–51%). Obstructive jaundice (up to 20%) and duodenal obstruction may result from compression of the adjacent duodenum or bile duct. A period of observation should be included in the therapy to permit spontaneous resolution of the pseudocyst. For most pseudocysts associated with chronic pancreatitis, the best time for surgical intervention is upon diagnosis, in the confident expectation of finding a mature cyst capable of holding sutures [4]. Formerly, the traditional management of pseudocysts included observation for 6 weeks, followed by surgical therapy for persistent pseudocysts [6]. Recent studies regarding the natural history demonstrate that observation is a safe option for small asymptomatic pseudocysts [7–10]. Therefore, only symptomatic pseudocysts should be treated surgically, unless cystic neoplasm has been suspected.

Indications for Surgical Treatment of Pseudocysts in Chronic Pancreatitis

The indications for surgical treatment of pseudocysts in chronic pancreatitis are:

1. Symptoms like pain, early satiety, and compression of the stomach or duodenum causing obstruction, compression of the bile duct causing jaundice, or liver function abnormalities.
2. Contraindication or failure of endoscopic or percutaneous methods (ultrasound or radiologically guided).
3. Pseudocyst with complex or multiple main pancreatic duct strictures.
4. Associated complex pathology like inflammatory mass in the head of the pancreas.
5. Pseudocysts with a main bile duct stricture.
6. Multiple pseudocysts.
7. Most pseudocysts of the pancreatic tail.
8. Hemorrhage not adequately controlled by angiographic embolization.
9. Suspicion of a neoplastic cyst.

Absolute Contraindications for Surgery for Pseudocysts in Chronic Pancreatitis

The only general absolute contraindication is the patient's general condition being too poor for general anesthesia and abdominal surgery.

Diagnostic Work-up Before Surgery for Pseudocysts in Chronic Pancreatitis

Clinical examination and taking the patient's history are the first steps in diagnosing pseudocysts in chronic pancreatitis. Special attention is to be paid to the history of pain and of chronic pancreatitis. The preoperative assessment of cardiovascular and respiratory function is mandatory.

Preoperative imaging should include ultrasonography, computed tomography (CT) or magnetic resonance imaging (MRI), and endoscopic retrograde cholangiopancreatography (ERCP) or magnetic resonance cholangiopancreatography (MRCP). In addition, the mapping of the arterial and venous vessels by CT or MRI, or in some cases by conventional angiography, might be helpful. These techniques are used to provide information about size, location, number of cysts, the thickness of the cystic wall, the extent of parenchymal disease, the size and shape of the main pancreatic duct and its relationship to the cyst, and finally the presence of portal hypertension, venous occlusion, arterial abnormalities and pseudoaneurysms.

ERCP usually demonstrates duct abnormalities typical for chronic pancreatitis. It may be helpful for determining the appropriate surgical strategy, including concomitant pancreatic duct or biliary drainage into the jejunum [15]. Nealon et al. introduced a classification of ductal abnormalities seen in patients with pseudocysts [15]. Type VI is seen in chronic pancreatitis, without duct–cyst communication, whereas type VII includes chronic pancreatitis with duct–cyst communication. Recently, MRCP has become widely available and today has mostly replaced ERCP in the preoperative assessment of chronic pancreatitis unless therapeutic intervention, like stent implantation, is planned.

In patients with suspected portal hypertension and history of ulcers of the stomach, an upper gastrointestinal endoscopy is performed.

A full blood count, serum biochemical analysis, including albumin and liver function tests, and tests for common bile duct obstruction (alkaline phosphatase, gamma glutamyl transferase, total bilirubin), as well as coagulation tests are important. Lipase and amylase may be elevated due to an acute inflammatory episode of the underlying chronic pancreatitis. The same is true for a higher c-reactive protein or elevated white blood count, which can also be elevated as a result of the pseudocyst itself. Serum tumor markers, such as carcinoembryonic antigen (CEA) or carbohydrate antigen 19-9 (CA 19-9), may be useful if the question of malignancy arises, even if they are not specific or sensitive.

Pancreatic cyst fluid analysis includes staining of epithelial cells, mucin, evaluation of viscosity, lipase level, and analysis of tumor markers such as CEA and CA19-9. This can be used for differentiation of pancreatic neoplastic cysts and pancreatic pseudocysts, although the results are not convincing [16]. If a tumor marker analysis of the cystic fluid is performed, CEA seems to be the only indicator as to the nature of the cyst.

Preparation Prior to Surgery for Pseudocysts in Chronic Pancreatitis

Since all pancreatic operations bear substantial risks, general preoperative precautions are important. Correction of anemia, nutritional support in patients with malnutrition, and physiotherapy should be performed to improve the general condition of the patient. Crossmatched blood should be available. All patients should receive single-shot antibiotic prophylaxis. In case splenectomy is needed, preoperative immunization of the patient against *Pneumococcus*, *Hemophilus influenzae* type B, and *Meningococcus* is advisable. If possible, the vaccines should be given at least 2 weeks before operation. Otherwise it has to be given 3 weeks postoperatively.

Surgical Standard Procedures for Pseudocysts in Chronic Pancreatitis

For the individualized selection of the most appropriate operation, several factors have to be considered. For most of the larger pseudocysts in the head, body, and tail the Roux-en-Y pseudocystojejunostomy is the easiest operation. If the pseudocyst is located in the head of the pancreas and is adherent to the duodenum (distant to the ampulla of Vater and the common bile duct) a pseudocystoduodenostomy can easily be done. For smaller intrapancreatic pseudocysts within the pancreatic head, a pancreatic head resection (duodenum-preserving if possible, or pylorus preserving) may be appropriate. If the pseudocyst is small and located in the tail of the pancreas, distal pancreatectomy (if possible without splenectomy) is recommended.

Internal Drainage

The preferred operative procedure for the management of most pseudocysts in chronic pancreatitis is internal pseudocystoenteric drainage. The three standard operations include drainage into a defunctionalized (Roux-en-Y) jejunal limb (pseudocystojejunostomy), drainage into the stomach (pseudocystogastrostomy), and drainage into the duodenum (pseudocystoduodenostomy). Those operations can be performed with or without drainage of the pancreatic duct (pancreaticojejunostomy).

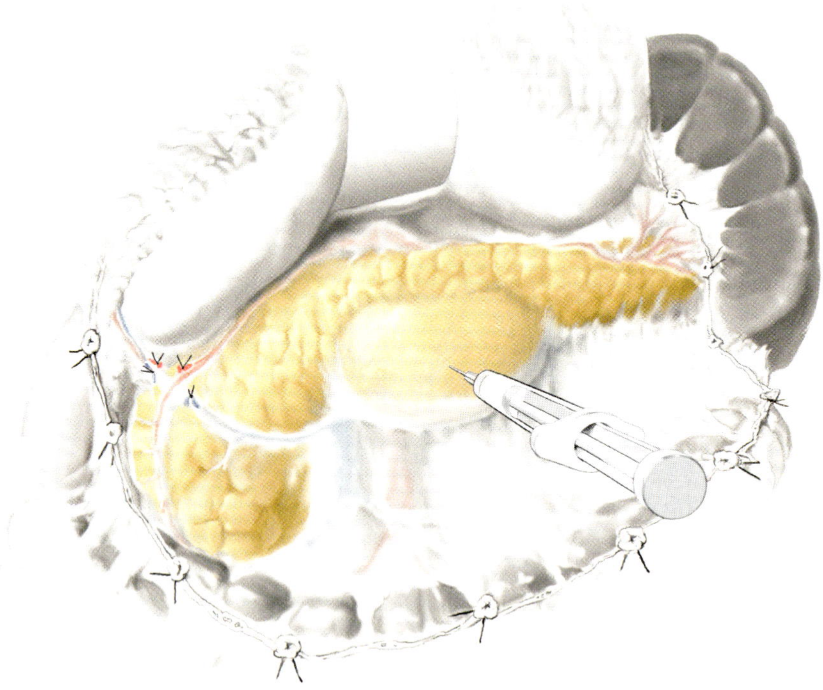

Figure 42.1

Exploration of the intra-abdominal situs. Identifying and exposing the lowest part of the cystic wall. Aspiration of cyst contents

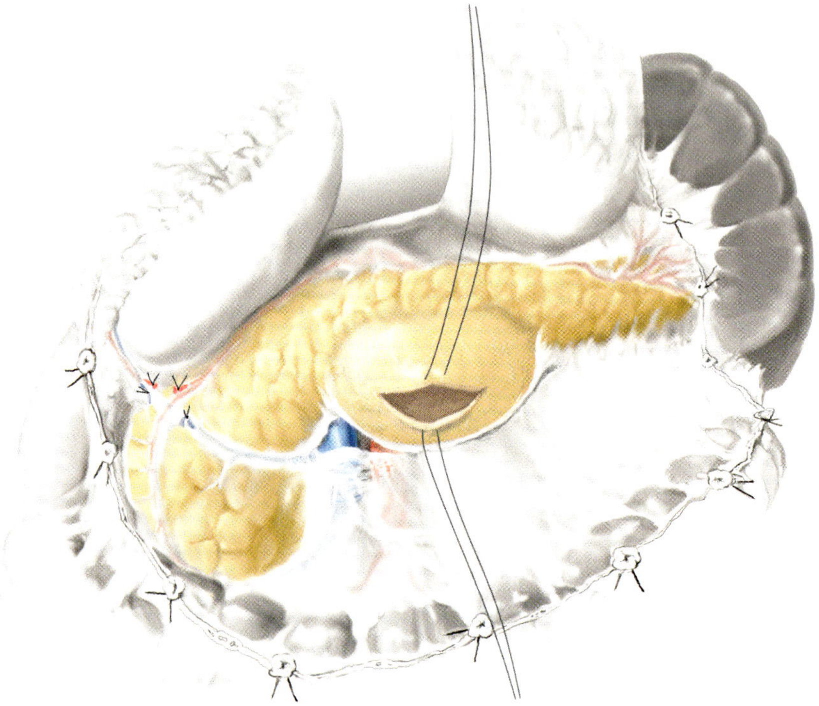

Figure 42.2

Opening of the pseudocyst. Frozen section of the wall

Pseudocystojejunostomy

Pseudocystojejunostomy is the most common method for pseudocyst drainage. The operation can be combined with simultaneous drainage of the biliary tract, if necessary. The same jejunal limb can be used for both biliary and the pseudocyst drainage. The surgical technique includes the following major steps (Figs. 42.1–42.3):

1. Exploration of the intra-abdominal situs.
2. Identifying and exposing the lowest part of the cystic wall.
3. Aspiration of cyst content. Excision of the free lower part of the cystic wall and frozen section of a part of the pseudocyst wall.
4. Dissection of the proximal jejunum for construction of a Roux-en-Y loop.
5. Anastomosis of the jejunum to the pseudocyst with an all-layer running suture using absorbable material.

Pseudocystojejunostomy can be performed from a median laparotomy or bilateral transverse subcostal incision. The incision chosen depends on the patient's build, presence of scars from previous operations, and on the expected location of the pseudocyst.

After exploration of the abdomen, the palpable cyst is located. Aspiration of the cystic fluid can help to identify the lesion. Only a small aliquot of the pseudocyst contents is aspirated, as complete evacuation of the cyst will result in a more difficult entry into the pseudocyst. Aspiration is also useful to exclude hemorrhage into the cyst from an arterial pseudoaneurysm. If the size of the pseudocyst that is palpated during surgery is different from the expected size from preoperative imaging, intraoperative ultrasonography should be performed. If the operative finding is smaller than expected, a second or a loculated pseudocyst may be present.

Another reason could be recent spontaneous rupture. After having verified the pseudocyst, a Roux-en-Y loop of the proximal jejunum is constructed. The segment of intestine excluded from small bowel continuity usually prevents from intestinal reflux into

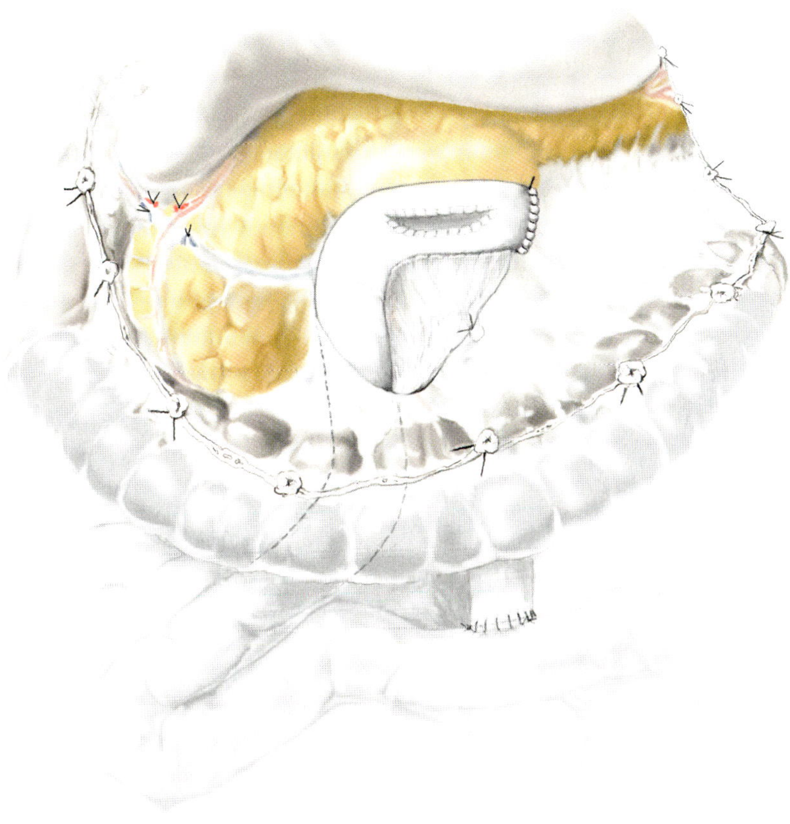

Figure 42.3

Anastomosis of the Roux-en-Y loop to the pseudocyst with an all-layer running suture using absorbable material the pseudocyst and pancreatic duct. The Roux-en-Y jejunal loop is placed in position adjacent to the pseudocyst, followed by a cystic wall excision as wide as possible, usually using electrocautery. Once the cyst is open, the contents are fully aspirated. The excised section of the pseudocyst wall is sent to the pathologist for frozen section, to eliminate concern about the cystic lesion being a cystic neoplasm. The posterior row is than placed, using a continuous all-layer suture of 3/0 monofilament and absorbable material (e.g., polydioxanone), and continued anteriorly.

After completion, the anastomosis can be easily palpated. The abdomen is usually drained with one abdominal drain, which can be removed in the early postoperative period.

If there is a concomitant biliary stenosis, the Roux-en-Y jejunal loop used for pseudocyst drainage can also be used for bilioenteric anastomosis [17].

Pseudocystogastrostomy

When the pseudocyst is located high up in the abdominal cavity and is not palpable through the transverse mesocolon, it is often found to be adherent to the posterior wall of the stomach. In these cases, internal drainage of the pseudocyst can be performed through the stomach as pseudocystogastrostomy. The surgical technique includes the following major steps (Figs. 42.4–42.6):

1. Exploration of the intra-abdominal situs and identifying the pseudocyst behind the stomach, if necessary guided by ultrasound sonography.
2. Opening of the anterior gastric wall.
3. Transgastric aspiration of the cyst content.
4. Opening of the pseudocyst through the posterior wall of the stomach.
5. Frozen section of a part of the pseudocyst wall.
6. Anastomosis with an all-layer running suture, with absorbable material.
7. Closure of the anterior gastric wall.

After placing of stay sutures in the anterior wall of the stomach, a 5- to 7-cm anterior gastrostomy is performed. Then, the location of the pseudocyst is confirmed by aspiration of cystic fluid through the posterior gastric wall.

Only a part of the pseudocyst contents are aspirated, as complete aspiration of the contents will result in a more difficult entry into the pseudocyst. If there is a discrepancy between the intraoperatively detected size and preoperative findings, an intraoperative ultrasonography should be performed. If the operative finding is smaller than expected, concern should arise that a second or a lobulated pseudocyst may be present.

After confirmation of the size and position of the pseudocyst, the pseudocyst is opened through the posterior wall of the stomach using electrocautery or a scalpel. Once the cyst is open, the contents are fully

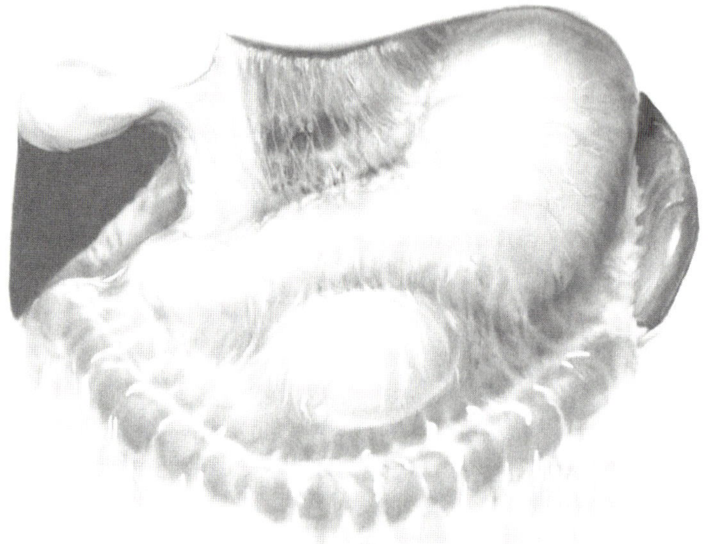

Figure 42.4

Exploration of the intra-abdominal situs. Identification of the pseudocyst behind the stomach, if necessary guided by ultrasound sonography

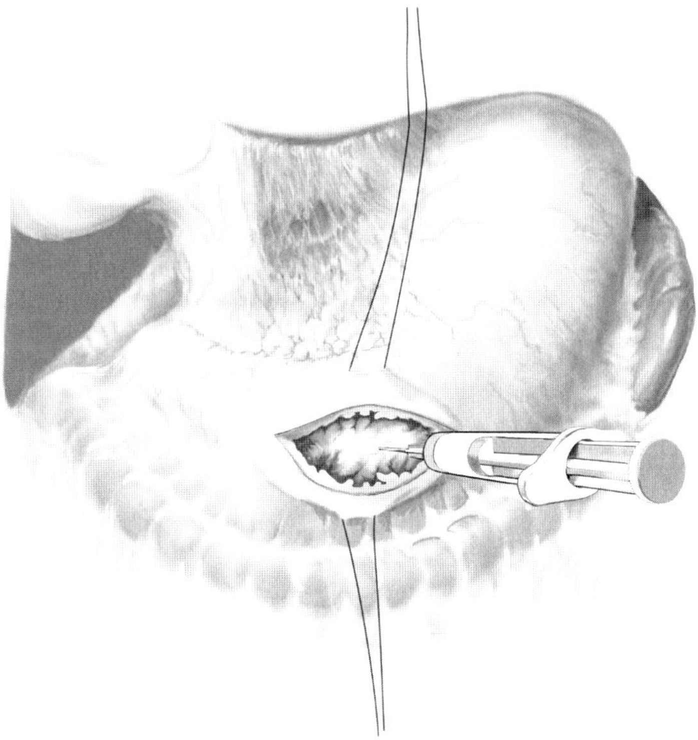

Figure 42.5

Anterior gastrotomy. Aspiration of cyst contents

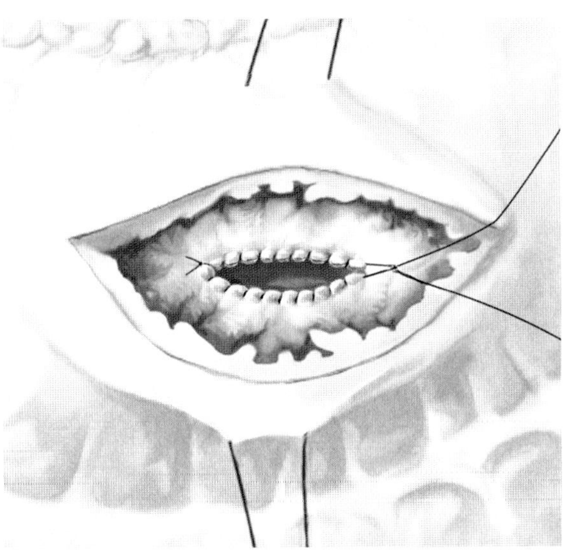

Figure 42.6

Opening of the pseudocyst. Frozen section of the wall. All-layer running suture using absorbable material of the posterior gastric wall and the pseudocyst wall

aspirated, and a section of the pseudocyst wall is excised for frozen section, to exclude a cystic neoplasm of the pancreas. A visual inspection of the inner wall of the pseudocyst should always be performed.

The opening between the stomach and the pseudocyst should be as wide as possible. Both edges are sutured together with a running 3/0 synthetic absorbable suture including all layers to ensure hemostasis and to keep the communication between the pseudocyst and the stomach open until the pseudocyst can resolve. The anterior gastrostomy is closed by a running suture with 3/0 synthetic absorbable material. Drainage of the abdomen is normally not necessary.

Pseudocystoduodenostomy

If the pseudocyst is located in the head of the pancreas, the cyst can be drained directly into the duodenum. This operation is rarely conducted because it is only applicable in pseudocysts of the infra-ampullary pancreatic head or the uncinate process, which have close contact to the duodenum. The possibility of duodenal leakage or duodenal fistula makes this operation the least attractive for internal drainage of pancreatic pseudocysts. The surgical technique includes the following major steps (Figs. 42.7–42.9:

1. Exploration of the intra-abdominal situs and identifying the pseudocyst in the infrapancreatic pancreatic head or uncinate process with close contact to the duodenum, if necessary guided by ultrasound sonography.
2. Kocher maneuver: the lateral duodenal wall is opened longitudinally, followed by transduodenal aspiration of the cyst content.
3. Opening of the pseudocyst through the medial wall of the infrapapillary duodenum. Frozen section of a part of the pseudocyst wall. Anastomosis with an all-layer running suture, with absorbable material.
4. Closure of the anterior duodenal wall.

The technique is similar to that of pseudocystogastrostomy. After confirmation of location and size of the pseudocyst the Kocher maneuver is performed. After positioning of stay sutures, the duodenal wall is opened longitudinally. After an exact definition of the extension of the common wall, a direct communication between the pseudocyst and the duodenum through a medial duodenotomy is created. Injury to the periampullary region has to be avoided. A part of the pseudocyst wall is sent to frozen section. The opening between the duodenum and the pseudocyst should be at least 3 cm. Both edges are anastomosed with a running 3/0 synthetic absorbable suture to ensure hemostasis and to keep the communication between the pseudocyst and the duodenum open until the pseudocyst can resolve. The lateral duodenotomy is closed by a single row, running suture with 3/0 synthetic absorbable material. Drainage of the abdomen is normally not necessary.

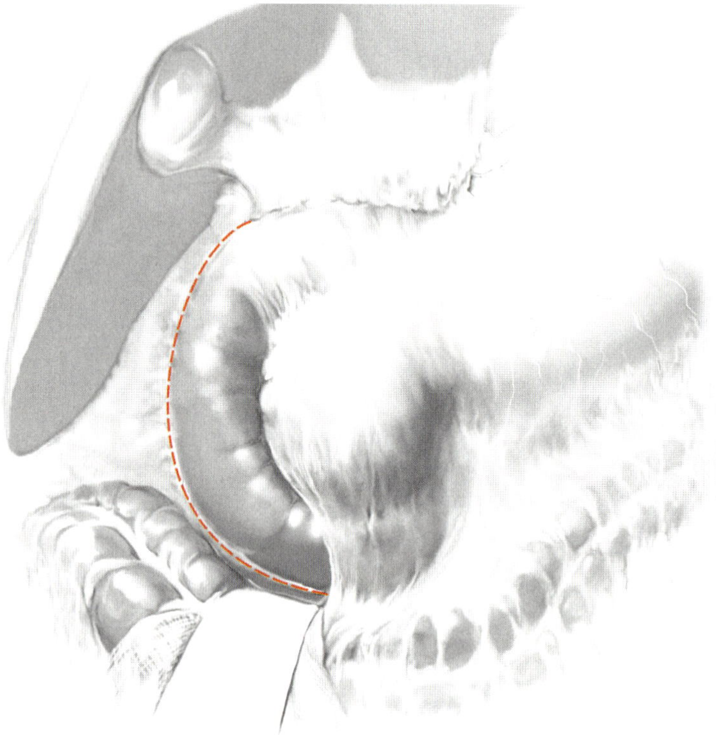

Figure 42.7

Exploration of the intra-abdominal situs. Identification of the pseudocyst, if necessary guided by ultrasound sonography.The red dotted line indicates the retroperitoneal incision for Kocher´s maneuver

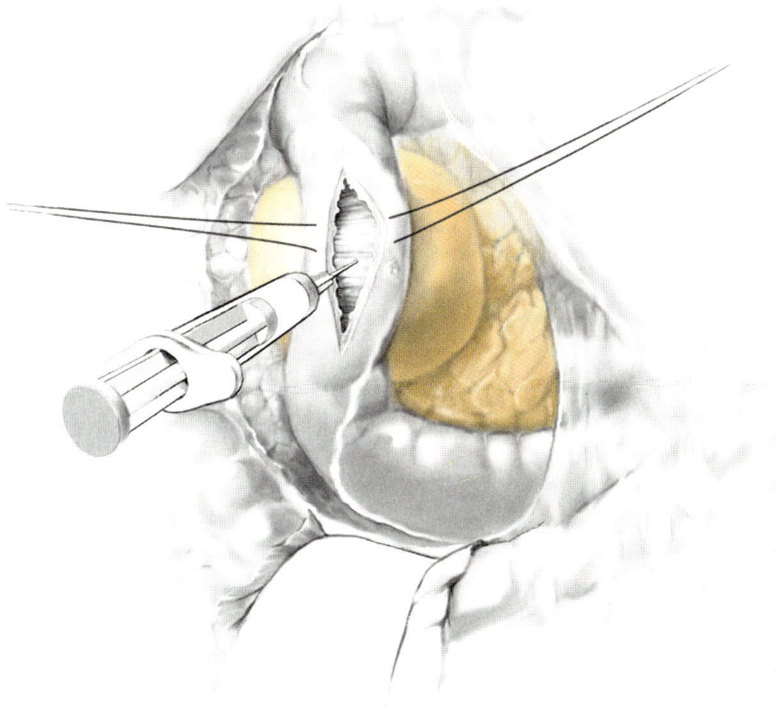

Figure 42.8

Kocher maneuver. The lateral duodenal wall is opened longitudinally. Transduodenal aspiration of the cyst contents

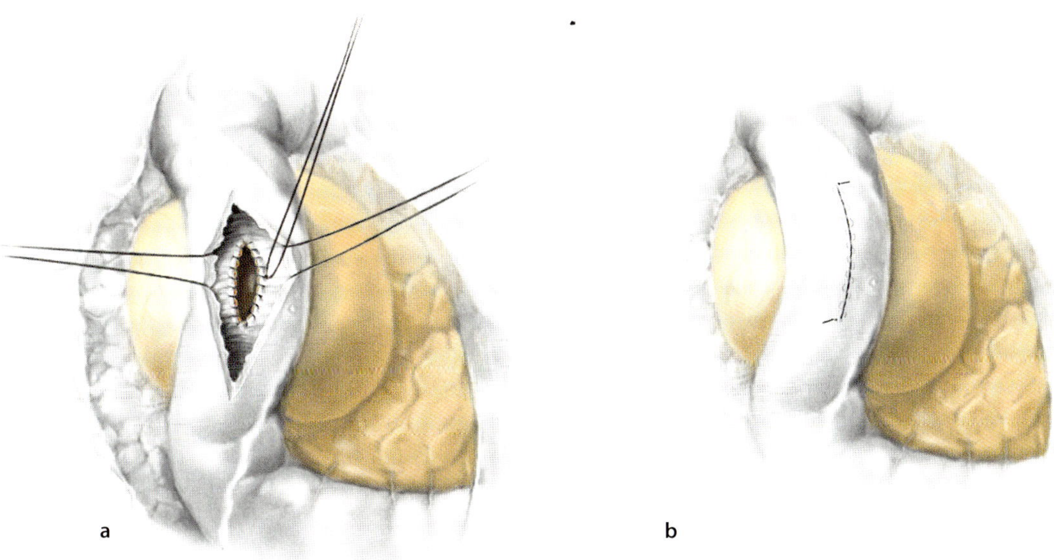
a b

Figure 42.9 a, b

Opening of the pseudocyst. Frozen section of the wall. All-layer running suture using absorbable material of the medial duodenal wall and the pseudocyst wall. Closing the duodenotomy by a longitudinal running

Pancreaticojejunostomy (Partington-Rochelle)

In patients with chronic pancreatitis associated pseudocysts, multiple strictures of the otherwise dilated pancreatic duct are often present. Side-to-side pancreaticojejunostomy has evolved to be the operation of choice, permitting an excellent drainage of the entire pancreatic ductal system [18]. Removal of the spleen is not necessary in every case. Moreover, the pancreatic tissue can be completely preserved.

The operation might be combined with pseudocystojejunostomy and/or simultaneous drainage of the biliary tree, if necessary. The same jejunal limb can be used for the biliary, the pancreatic duct, and the pseudocyst drainage. While most authors prefer pseudocystojejunostomy in chronic pancreatitis patients with pseudocysts, Nealon and colleagues stated that ductal drainage alone is sufficient and effective in completely resolving associated pseudocysts [19]. The surgical technique includes the following major steps (Figs. 42.10–42.13):

1. Exploration of the pancreas and identifying the pancreatic duct.
2. Opening of the pancreatic duct.
3. Frozen section of a part of pancreatic tissue.
4. Side-to-side pancreatojejunal anastomosis with interrupted suture, between the gastroduodenal artery and the splenic hilus.
5. End-to-side jejunojejunostomy.

After entering the abdomen by transverse or upper-abdominal incision, an exploration of the abdomen is performed. The anterior surface of the pancreas is then exposed widely by dividing the gastrocolic omentum extensively and opening the lesser sac. The anterior surface of the pancreas is palpated to determine whether the enlarged duct can be felt. Intraoperative ultrasonography and puncture might be useful in many cases.

The pancreatic duct is opened longitudinal in an easily accessible part of the pancreas. The incision is then completed by electrocautery to the left, including the head and the uncinate process as well as to the right to the body and the tail. A piece of the pancreatic tissue is sent for histological examination. The Roux-en-Y loop is prepared after the entire pancreatic duct system has been unroofed by scalpel or electrocautery. The jejunum is divided at a distance of 10–15 cm from the ligament of Treitz, where the mesentery is mobile enough to reach the pancreas without tension. The jejunum is dissected using a stapling device and the stapler line is oversewn in the distal seg-

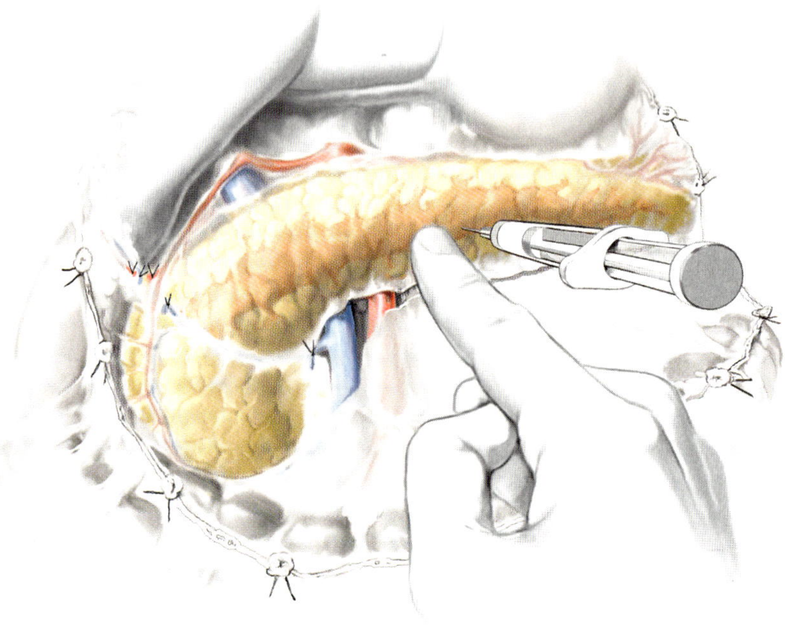

Figure 42.10

Exploration of the pancreas and identifying the pancreatic duct

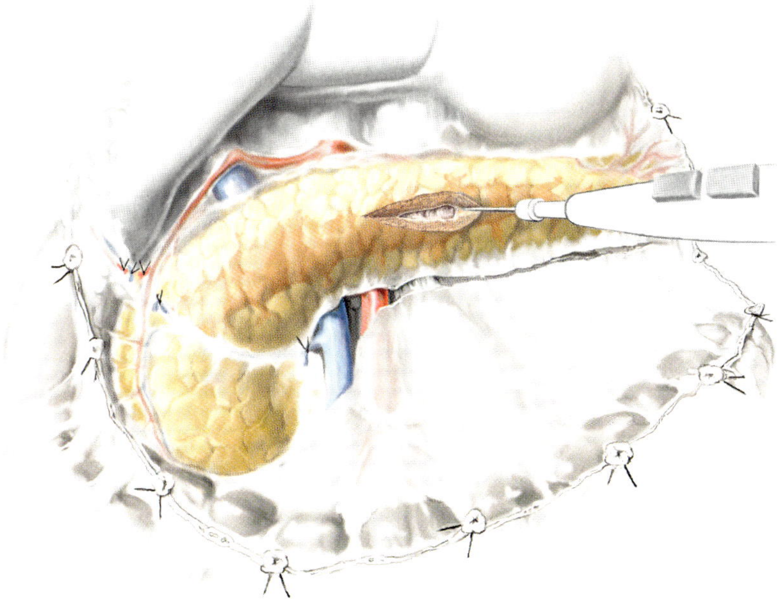

Figure 42.11

Opening of the pancreatic duct. Frozen section of a part of pancreatic tissue

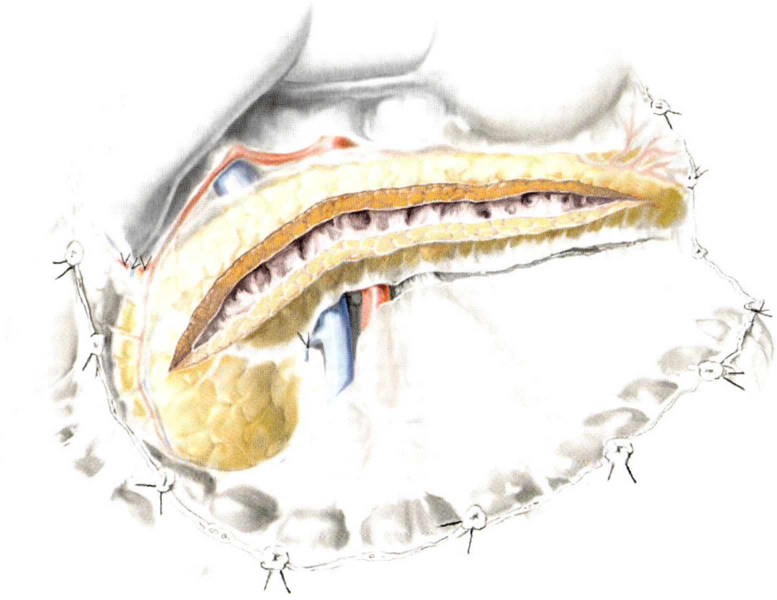

Figure 42.12

Complete opening of the pancreatic duct between the gastroduodenal artery and the splenic hilus

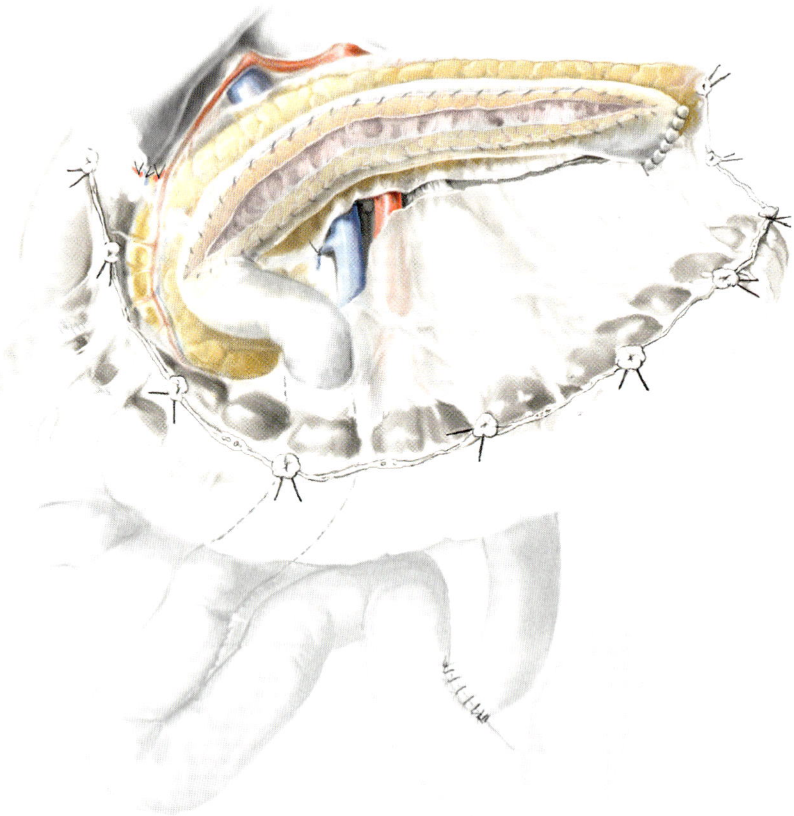

Figure 42.13

Side-to-side pancreatojejunal anastomosis with a running suture between the antimesenteric surface of the jejunum (Roux-en-Y loop) and the pancreatic tissue including the fibrous capsule of the pancreas

ment. This efferent jejunal limb is brought through an avascular area of the transverse mesocolon to the anterior surface of the pancreas, the closed limb positioned in the splenic hilus. A side-to-side pancreatojejunal anastomosis is then created with a running suture between the antimesenteric surface of the jejunum and the fibrotic pancreatic tissue including the fibrous capsule of the pancreas. The best technique is to start at the posterior border from the middle of the incision, around the edges, to the center of the anterior incision margin, where both ends of the suture (double-needle) are tied together. The sutures are passing through the full thickness of the jejunal wall. Intestinal continuity is re-established with an end-to-side jejunojejunostomy placed approximately 40 cm distal to the pancreaticojejunostomy. The most suitable suture material is probably monofilament and resorbable. Defects in the mesentery of the small and large intestine are closed. External drainage is usually not required.

Laparoscopic Approaches

The application of minimally invasive surgery allows laparoscopic management of pancreatic pseudocysts, but to date the data is preliminary and therefore not comparable to the aforementioned standard internal drainage operations [20].

External Drainage

External drainage, or marsupialization, of the pseudocyst is rarely indicated in pseudocyst in chronic pancreatitis, because the cystic wall in most cases is strong enough to hold the sutures of an anastomosis. External drainage is only performed if the cyst wall at the time of operation is friable and unsuitable for anastomosis, or if the pseudocyst is grossly infected. The drainage catheter is inserted into the cyst and exteriorized through the abdominal wall. The external drainage procedure carries with it a higher morbidity and mortality, largely due to urgent circumstances when this method is applied. Due to stricture or obstruction of the main duct, inhibiting sufficient secretion into the duodenum, recurrence and persistent pancreatic fistula are often seen. External drainage is therefore not definitive, and the subsequent surgery of underlying pancreatic pathology will be necessary in most cases [21].

Pancreatic Resection for the Treatment of Pancreatic Pseudocysts in Chronic Pancreatitis

Pancreatic resection for the treatment of pancreatic pseudocysts in chronic pancreatitis is only performed in a minority of patients. The resection typically involves distal pancreatectomy for pseudocysts of the body or of the tail of the pancreas, or resection of the pancreatic head in the case of pseudocysts localized there. Resections are more frequently performed for multiple small pseudocysts, biliary and pancreatic duct strictures, duodenal obstruction, hemorrhage, and underlying extensive chronic pancreatitis with severe symptoms. Recurrent pancreatic pseudocysts, true cystic lesions or cystic neoplasms discovered at the time of operation by frozen section of the wall are also indications for resection. Pancreatic cystic lesions that are septated and those containing mucinous fluid with elevated CEA levels are generally treated by resection because of the possibility that they represent a cystic neoplasm [22]. In rare cases, hemorrhage, mostly due to pseudoaneurysms, can enforce a pancreatic resection, if angiographic intervention fails. In chronic pancreatitis patients with pseudocysts and concomitant bile duct or duodenal obstruction proximal pancreatectomy (Kausch-Whipple operation, pylorus-preserving pancreatoduodenectomy or duodenum-preserving pancreatic head resection) might be indicated. Total pancreatectomy is only very rarely performed any more in chronic pancreatitis.

Distal Pancreatectomy

Smaller pseudocysts in the tail or the body of the pancreas may be optimally controlled by distal pancreatic resection, if possible with conservation of the spleen [23]. Synchronous concomitant splenectomy can be necessary in cases of splenic vein thrombosis or encasement of splenic vessels within inflammatory scar tissue. After distal pancreatectomy, if there is evidence for an obstructed proximal pancreatic duct, enteric drainage of the pancreatic duct by Roux-en-Y pancreatojejunostomy is indicated. Distal pancreatectomy is described in Chapter 40.

Pancreatic Head Resection

In only a few patients with pseudocysts in the head of the pancreas is pancreaticoduodenectomy required. In most of these cases, symptomatic pseudocysts are associated with an inflammatory mass in the head of the pancreas. The operation performed depends on the findings and may require duodenum-preserving pancreatic head resection, pylorus-preserving pancreaticoduodenectomy, or Kausch-Whipple operation. The principle surgical steps for these standard operations are described in Chapters 37, 38, and 51, respectively.

Surgery for Complications of Pseudocysts in Chronic Pancreatitis

Infection

Infection of a pancreatic pseudocyst in chronic pancreatitis is rare. Although bacteria might be present in a pseudocyst at the time of treatment, they are often of no clinical significance. In the absence of pus, these pseudocysts are considered as contaminated or colonized and should be treated like the "normal" pseudocyst. In the case of suspected pus, a percutaneous diagnostic puncture is indicated and, when pus is found, subsequent percutaneous drainage. Retrospective studies comparing interventional percutaneous and operative external drainage of infected pseudocysts showed comparable success rates with lower mortality for the interventional group. Careful clinical and imaging follow up is needed in all cases to ensure complete pseudocyst resolution. Primary or repeated operative drainage should be performed, when clinical deterioration occurs or the pseudocyst does not resolve [24].

Hemorrhage

Pancreatic pseudocysts have a high risk of bleeding due to numerous vessels in the vicinity, especially if the walls of the vessels are weakened by the pseudocyst or its aggressive fluid. A review of pseudocystic hemorrhage showed predominantly male patients with alcoholic pancreatitis. The bleeding arose most commonly from the splenic (45%), gastroduodenal (18%), and pancreaticoduodenal (18%) arteries. Arteriography is the diagnostic and therapeutic procedure (i.e., embolization of wire coils or sponge pledgets; stenting) of choice in stable patients. Surgical therapy is only indicated if angiographic techniques fail or if the patient needs urgent surgery. Surgical treatments typically performed in these cases are splenic-artery ligation with distal pancreatectomy and splenectomy, transpseudocystic arterial ligation, and in rare cases emergency pancreatic resections [25].

Obstruction

Pseudocysts may cause mechanical obstruction of different parts of the gastrointestinal tract from the esophagus to the colon, most commonly the duodenum, the biliary tract, and the portal-venous system. In most of these cases, appropriate intervention can solve the problem, at least as a preliminary treatment.

Rupture

Spontaneous rupture is an uncommon complication of pancreatic pseudocysts. The patients present with or without abdominal pain, followed by the development of pancreatic ascites or pleural effusion. The therapy typically starts noninvasively with parenteral therapy and symptomatic pain medication. Approximately 50% of all patients with a ruptured pancreatic pseudocyst can be treated successfully without surgery. Patients who fail to improve should undergo ERCP or MRCP to document the anatomy of the pancreatic duct, followed by surgical intervention according to the site of the ductal leak by pancreaticojejunostomy or distal pancreatectomy.

Postoperative Management after Surgery of Pseudocysts in Chronic Pancreatitis

Postoperative care is similar to any other involving anastomosis of the small intestine. A nasogastric tube can usually be removed just after the operation. Oral food intake may be started with tea 5 h after the drainage operation and is as quickly advanced as tolerated. It seems likely that these patients should be treated with the concept of fast-track rehabilitation, as shown in a recent small study [26].

Bowel movement can be activated by a suppository or clyster on the 3rd postoperative day unless is has already started spontaneously. The drainage tubes can be removed on the 2nd postoperative day if no signs of insufficiency of the anastomosis are found. If a highly elevated level of lipase is found in the secretion, the drainage stays until the value drops to normal.

Early Postoperative Course after Surgery for Pseudocysts in Chronic Pancreatitis

The reported results of surgical treatment of pseudocysts in chronic pancreatitis are often difficult to interpret because of incomplete follow up, lack of objective assessment by independent observers, different inclusion criteria, and patient selection. Major postoperative complications include: bleeding, postoperative ileus, and insufficiency of anastomosis. Most of these can be treated nonsurgically.

The drainage procedures have an appreciably lower operation mortality and morbidity compared to pancreatic resection. In the case of resection or pancreaticojejunostomy, the thickened fibrosed pancreas holds sutures well and leakage from these anastomoses is unusual in skilled hands. Bleeding complication is rarely seen in drainage operations in the absence of splenic-vein thrombosis or portal hypertension.

Operative mortality and the complication rates reported in many recent published series are shown in Table 42.1. Operative mortality in most series is as low as 0–5% [2]. A recent population-based study reported a 2.8% mortality for surgical treatment of chronic and acute pancreatic pseudocysts [10]. Significant differences in complications, length of stay (15±15 days versus 21±22 days, $P<0.0001$), and inpatient mortality (5.9% versus 2.8%, $P<0.0001$) favored the surgical approach. In addition, ERCP use had a protective effect on mortality (odds ratio, 0.7), whereas percutaneous drainage had an increased risk of mortality (odds ratio, 1.4). This population-based study suggests that surgical drainage of pancreatic pseudocysts, particularly when coupled with use of ERCP, leads to decreased complications, length of stay, and mortality in comparison with percutaneous drainage. Results of pseudocystojejunostomy and pseudocystogastrostomy concerning mortality and morbidity are comparable [27]. Pseudocystojejunostomy seems to be more popular and perhaps leads to somewhat better results than pseudocystogastrostomy.

Table 42.1. Early results after operative therapy of pancreatic pseudocysts in chronic pancreatitis. *NR* Not reported, *PJ* pancreaticojejunostomy

Therapy	No. of patients	Mortality (%)	Complications (%)	Reference
Internal drainage	22	0	18	[28]
External drainage	39	5	38	
Resection	41	12		
Internal drainage	30	0	NR	[7]
External drainage	7	0	NR	
Resection	1	0	NR	
Pseudocystojejunostomy	59	3	NR	[27]
Pseudocystogastrostomy	39		NR	
Internal drainage	48	2	46	[4]
Resection	56	0		
Pseudocystojejunostomy	54			[31]
PJ	47	0	16	[19]
PJ and pseudocystojejunostomy	56	0	11	
Internal drainage	37	3	22	[1]
Resection	169	0	28	
Internal drainage	43	0	16	[29]

The complication rate was highest after external drainage of the pseudocysts and ranges from 25 to 50% [28].

Concerning pancreatic resection, morbidity and mortality have decreased to 15% and <5%, respectively. Recurrence rates are low; however, resection of the pancreatic parenchyma may result in pancreatic insufficiency, both endocrine and exocrine [29].

Late Outcome after Surgery for Pseudocysts in Chronic Pancreatitis

There are only few studies concerning late results after surgery of pseudocysts in chronic pancreatitis. No prospective randomized studies have been performed on this topic. The main factors of late outcome are pain relief, recurrence of pseudocysts, and exocrine and endocrine pancreatic insufficiency (Table 42.2).

Most chronic pancreatitis patients with pseudocysts are pain free immediately after the operation, irrespective of the type of operation (internal drainage or resection) [30]. Long-term pain relief was achieved in 53–90% of patients [1, 19, 30]. The recurrence of pain in many patients during follow up may reflect the progression of the disease or the continuation of alcohol abuse as the main underlying factor, or both. In the long-term follow-up studies on the course of operated pancreatic pseudocysts, pain relief was considered to be poor in up to 43% [30]. In a study of the group of Beger, resection compared to drainage alone was found to have a higher rate of pain-free patients after a follow-up period of 7.3 years (94% vs. 75%); however, the risk for diabetes was increased in the resection group [1].

After drainage operation, Schlosser et al. [1] found a significant higher rate of recurrence of pseudocysts compared to resection (8% vs. 2%), whereas Nealon and Walser [19] observed only 2 recurrences in 153 patients (1.3%) treated with drainage operation only. The recurrence rate of pseudocysts may indicate the true reappearance of pseudocysts. However, development of newly formed pseudocysts due to a progression of the chronic pancreatitis is also possible.

Endocrine pancreatic insufficiency in patients with chronic pancreatitis appears, deteriorates, or remains unchanged, but does not show improvement. This was also reported in a series of operated pancreatic pseudocysts in chronic pancreatitis patients [30].

There are no studies about the quality of life after surgical treatment of pseudocysts in chronic pancreatitis.

Table 42.2. Late results after operative therapy of pancreatic pseudocysts in chronic pancreatitis

Therapy	No. of patients	Follow up (months)	Pain (%)	Recurrence (%)	Reference
Internal drainage	22	NR	32	0	[28]
External drainage	39	NR	23	15	
Resection	41	NR	32	13	
Internal drainage	30	NR	0	NR	[7]
External drainage	7	NR	0	NR	
Resection	1	NR	0	NR	
Pseudocystojejunostomy	59	NR	NR	7	[27]
Pseudocystogastrostomy	39	NR	NR	10	
Internal drainage	48	NR	26	0	[4]
Resection	56	NR		5	
PJ	47	61	13	0	[19]
PJ and pseudocystojejunostomy	56	89	12	4	
Pseudocystojejunostomy	54	156		5	[31]
Internal drainage	24	77	25	8	[1]
Resection	115	88	93	2	
Pseudocystojejunostomy	42	132	53	NR	[30]
Resection	13			NR	
Internal drainage	43	88			[29]

References

1. Schlosser W, Siech M, Beger HG (2005) Pseudocyst treatment in chronic pancreatitis – surgical treatment of the underlying disease increases the long-term success. Dig Surg 22:340–345
2. Rosso E, Alexakis N, Ghaneh P, Lombard M, Smart HL, Evans J, Neoptolemos JP (2003) Pancreatic pseudocyst in chronic pancreatitis: endoscopic and surgical treatment. Dig Surg 20:397–406
3. Crass RA, Way LW (1981) Acute and chronic pancreatic pseudocysts are different. Am J Surg 142:660–663
4. Usatoff V, Brancatisano R, Williamson RC (2000) Operative treatment of pseudocysts in patients with chronic pancreatitis. Br J Surg 87:1494–1499
5. Jedlicka R (1923) Eine Nervenoperationsmethode der Pancreaspseudozysten (Pancreato-gastrostomie). Zentralb Chir 184:80–84
6. Bradley EL, Clements JL Jr, Gonzalez AC (1979) The natural history of pancreatic pseudocysts: a unified concept of management. Am J Surg 137:135–141
7. Yeo CJ, Bastidas JA, Lynch-Nyhan A, Fishman EK, Zinner MJ, Cameron JL (1990) The natural history of pancreatic pseudocysts documented by computed tomography. Surg Gynecol Obstet 170:411–417
8. Heider R, Meyer AA, Galanko JA, Behrns KE (1999) Percutaneous drainage of pancreatic pseudocysts is associated with a higher failure rate than surgical treatment in unselected patients. Ann Surg 229:781–787; discussion 787–789
9. Nealon WH, Walser E (2002) Main pancreatic ductal anatomy can direct choice of modality for treating pancreatic pseudocysts (surgery versus percutaneous drainage). Ann Surg 235:751–758
10. Morton JM, Brown A, Galanko JA, Norton JA, Grimm IS, Behrns KE (2005) A national comparison of surgical versus percutaneous drainage of pancreatic pseudocysts: 1997–2001. J Gastrointest Surg 9:15–20; discussion 20–11
11. Byrne MF, Mitchell RM, Baillie J (2002) Pancreatic Pseudocysts. Curr Treat Options Gastroenterol 5:331–338
12. Ebbehoj N, Borly L, Bulow J, Rasmussen SG, Madsen P, Matzen P, Owre A (1990) Pancreatic tissue fluid pressure in chronic pancreatitis. Relation to pain, morphology, and function. Scand J Gastroenterol 25:1046–1051
13. Buchler M, Weihe E, Friess H, Malfertheiner P, Bockman E, Muller S, Nohr D, Beger HG (1992) Changes in peptidergic innervation in chronic pancreatitis. Pancreas 7:183–192
14. Warshaw AL, Rattner DW (1985) Timing of surgical drainage for pancreatic pseudocyst. Clinical and chemical criteria. Ann Surg 202:720–724
15. Nealon WH, Townsend CM Jr, Thompson JC (1989) Preoperative endoscopic retrograde cholangiopancreatography (ERCP) in patients with pancreatic pseudocyst associated with resolving acute and chronic pancreatitis. Ann Surg 209:532–538; discussion 538–540
16. Sand J, Nordback I (2005) The differentiation between pancreatic neoplastic cysts and pancreatic pseudocyst. Scand J Surg 94:161–164
17. Munn JS, Aranha GV, Greenlee HB, Prinz RA (1987) Simultaneous treatment of chronic pancreatitis and pancreatic pseudocyst. Arch Surg 122:662–667

18. Greenlee HB, Prinz RA, Aranha GV (1990) Long-term results of side-to-side pancreaticojejunostomy. World J Surg 14:70–76
19. Nealon WH, Walser E (2003) Duct drainage alone is sufficient in the operative management of pancreatic pseudocyst in patients with chronic pancreatitis. Ann Surg 237:614–620; discussion 620–612
20. Fernandez-Cruz L, Cesar-Borges G, Lopez-Boado MA, Orduna D, Navarro S (2005) Minimally invasive surgery of the pancreas in progress. Langenbecks Arch Surg 390:342–354
21. Adams DB, Srinivasan A (2000) Failure of percutaneous catheter drainage of pancreatic pseudocyst. Am Surg 66:256–261
22. Lewandrowski KB, Southern JF, Pins MR, Compton CC, Warshaw AL (1993) Cyst fluid analysis in the differential diagnosis of pancreatic cysts. A comparison of pseudocysts, serous cystadenomas, mucinous cystic neoplasms, and mucinous cystadenocarcinoma. Ann Surg 217:41–47
23. Warshaw AL (1989) Pancreatic cysts and pseudocysts: new rules for a new game. Br J Surg 76:533–534
24. Adams DB, Anderson MC (1992) Percutaneous catheter drainage compared with internal drainage in the management of pancreatic pseudocyst. Ann Surg 215:571–576; discussion 576–578
25. Balachandra S, Siriwardena AK (2005) Systematic appraisal of the management of the major vascular complications of pancreatitis. Am J Surg 190:489–495
26. Wichmann MW, Roth M, Jauch KW, Bruns CJ (2006) A prospective clinical feasibility study for multimodal "fast track" rehabilitation in elective pancreatic cancer surgery. Rozhl Chir 85:169–175
27. Newell KA, Liu T, Aranha GV, Prinz RA (1990) Are cystgastrostomy and cystjejunostomy equivalent operations for pancreatic pseudocysts? Surgery 108:635–639; discussion 639–640
28. Kiviluoto T, Kivisaari L, Kivilaakso E, Lempinen M (1989) Pseudocysts in chronic pancreatitis. Surgical results in 102 consecutive patients. Arch Surg 124:240–243
29. Boerma D, Obertop H, Gouma DJ (2000) Pancreatic pseudocysts in chronic pancreatitis. Surgical or interventional drainage? Ann Ital Chir 71:43–50
30. Lohr-Happe A, Peiper M, Lankisch PG (1994) Natural course of operated pseudocysts in chronic pancreatitis. Gut 35:1479–1482
31. Kohler H, Schafmayer A, Ludtke FE, Lepsien G, Peiper HJ (1987) Surgical treatment of pancreatic pseudocysts. Br J Surg 74:813–815

Chapter 43

L. Gullo · R. Pezzilli

Late Outcome After Medical and Surgical Treatment of Chronic Pancreatitis

Chronic pancreatitis is a progressive inflammatory disorder that is characterized by recurrent episodes of upper abdominal pain and progressive loss of exocrine and endocrine function [1,2]. The disease is more frequently attributable to chronic alcohol abuse, even if other etiological factors, such as cystic fibrosis transmembrane conductance regulator gene mutations, cationic trypsinogen gene mutations, autoimmunity, and obstruction, have recently been postulated [3]. Alcohol abuse remains, however, the main etiological factor of chronic pancreatitis throughout the years, as can be seen in Table 43.1. Even if the interval between the first and the second study cited in this table is of about 30 years, more than 70% of patients enrolled into both studies are heavy drinkers [4,5]. In this chapter, we will discuss the late outcome of this disease.

Complications of the Advanced Stages of Chronic Pancreatitis

The clinical onset of chronic pancreatitis most commonly occurs when the patient is in his thirties or forties [4, 6–9]. A typical patient with chronic pancreatitis is a male who is employed in a job that requires heavy labor and who generally (70–80% of cases) drinks alcohol in excess [4,6–11]. In Italy, alcohol is by far the most frequent etiologic factor, present in 75–80% of patients with chronic pancreatitis who have an average daily consumption of 120–140 g of pure alcohol [4]. Thus, the first and most important task for the physician is to convince the patient to stop drinking alcohol, informing him that if he does not do so there is little or no chance that his condition will improve, and that he may well also develop unpleasant complications. It should also be explained that if he ceases to drink, the attacks may become less frequent and eventually disappear. Unfortunately, not all patients quit drinking, and of those who do, some resume once a painful attack has subsided (Table 43.2). A majority of individuals with chronic pancreatitis also smoke, and so another duty of the physician is to persuade the patient to quit this habit as well.

Pain, the most important symptom in chronic pancreatitis, particularly in its initial stage [4,6–9], must be carefully assessed and monitored in each patient. If the frequency and intensity of the painful attacks are reduced by cessation of alcohol ingestion, the attacks are likely to eventually disappear, generally within the first 5 or 6 years of the disease; for these patients, surgical intervention is not indicated. Among our patients, roughly 50% fall into this category [4]. If, on the contrary, the frequency and inten-

Table 43.1. Etiology of chronic pancreatitis in Italy in two series of patients studied in 1977 [4] and in 2005 [5]

1977 Causative condition	% of cases	2005 Causative condition	% of cases
Alcohol abuse	75.1%	Alcohol abuse	77.4%
Other causes	3.6%	Other causes	5.8%
Hereditary pancreatitis		Hereditary pancreatitis	
Cholelithiasis		Pancreas divisum	
		Cystic dystrophy of duodenal wall	
		CFTR gene mutations	
		Autoimmune pancreatitis	
Idiopathic	21.3%	Idiopathic	16.8%

Table 43.2. What to do in follow-up

1.	Ascertain whether the patient has stopped drinking.
2.	In nonalcoholic forms, determine the cause and eliminate it.
3.	Evaluate pain; if the attacks are frequent, consider surgery or in selected patients, endoscopy.
4.	Assess exocrine and endocrine pancreatic function; if impaired, treat accordingly.
5.	Assess for complications and treat accordingly.
6.	Activity limitations and dietetic rules: this is pertinent mainly to patients with severe steatorrhea or advanced diabetes with complications.
7.	Arrange for check-up visits at least every 6–12 months, when possible, with a specialist in pancreatic diseases.

sity of the painful attacks increase or remain high, surgery or, for a few selected patients, endoscopic intervention should certainly be considered, which is the case for about 50% of our patients [4]. For most of the patients who undergo surgery, this generally occurs within 5 or 6 years of clinical onset [4,7,8,12,13].

It is important to study exocrine and endocrine pancreatic function from the initial stages of the disease, both to support the clinical diagnosis of chronic pancreatitis and to guide its treatment. In studies that utilized duodenal intubation and prolonged maximal pancreatic stimulation [1,14], we showed that exocrine pancreatic function is impaired in almost all patients with chronic pancreatitis, starting in the initial stages of the disease, at which point the functional impairment is generally mild or moderate. Although duodenal intubation is the more sensitive means of assessing exocrine pancreatic function, it is time-consuming and troublesome and is no longer used in clinical practice. At present, it has been substituted by indirect tests of pancreatic function that often show normal results when the chronic pancreatitis is mild. We now use the fecal elastase test, which has good sensitivity, particularly in patients who have moderate or severe pancreatic insufficiency [15].

Patients who have mild or moderate pancreatic insufficiency do not have steatorrhea and therefore do not require the use of pancreatic extracts. However, some authors [16,17] have advocated the use of the extracts in patients with mild to moderate insufficiency as well, for the purpose of preventing attacks of pain. In this regard, various studies [16–20] have been carried out, but the results have been conflicting, possibly due to the different types of enzyme preparations that have been used [16,17]. The preparations that seemed to be useful in preventing attacks of pain were those administered in tablet form.

Endocrine pancreatic function is generally normal in the initial phases of chronic pancreatitis, and clinically evident diabetes usually appears in the advanced stages of the disease, generally 8–10 years after onset [4,7]. Thus, in the early stages of the disease, blood glucose determination and a glucose tolerance test every 6–12 months are generally sufficient for monitoring endocrine function.

For optimal management of patients with chronic pancreatitis it is essential to have frequent follow-up visits, at least once every 6 or 12 months. This serves to monitor the frequency of episodes of pain as well as the appearance of other disturbances, and especially to determine whether the patient has stopped drinking. Many patients quit drinking alcohol and these same individuals generally keep their appointments for follow-up visits. Others, who are typically heavier drinkers and who do not stop drinking, often do not keep their scheduled appointments but may show up only after an attack of severe pain.

In the nonalcoholic forms of chronic pancreatitis (about 20–30% of cases) [4,6–8], the most important measure is to determine the cause of the disease and to eliminate it, which usually leads to improvement in the clinical picture. With regard to the follow-up, the measures are essentially the same as those for alcoholic pancreatitis.

The patient with advanced chronic pancreatitis, who has had the disease for longer than 8–10 years, generally presents with different clinical problems. In the majority of studies on chronic pancreatitis [4,6–8,11–13], it is reported that pain, the principal clinical manifestation in the early stages of the disease, is generally no longer present in the more advanced stages. The patient may have had surgery for the pancreatitis, or the pain may have resolved on its own. Those for whom pain continues to be a significant problem are generally either those who continue to drink, and for these patients it is difficult to find a definitive solution for the pain, or they are patients who have developed a complication, most often a pseudocyst. We should mention, however, that in one study pain has been reported to be frequent even in the advanced stages of the disease [10].

In the advanced stages of chronic pancreatitis, generally after 8–10 years from clinical onset, exocrine pancreatic insufficiency may become severe (<10% of normal enzyme production) and steatorrhea develops, necessitating the administration of pancreatic extracts. It is very important to establish the correct daily dose of the extracts, which must be adequate to prevent the loss of fat in the feces; a dose of 30,000 U per meal should be sufficient. If steatorrhea does not disappear completely, this dose can be increased. In patients with gastric acid hypersecretion it can be helpful to administer H_2 blocking agents or proton pump inhibitors with the extracts in order to prevent their inactivation by gastric acid. Steatorrhea develops in about 50–60% of patients with advanced chronic pancreatitis [4].

In advanced stages of chronic pancreatitis, diabetes can develop as a result of the destruction of islet cells by pancreatic fibrosis. It usually starts in a mild form that is treatable with oral antidiabetic agents or low doses of insulin, but often progresses to a more severe form with higher insulin requirements. The complications of diabetes due to chronic pancreatitis are similar to those of primary diabetes. In particular, we studied [21] the frequency of diabetic retinopathy in chronic pancreatitis and found that it is similar to that of patients with type I diabetes. Diabetes develops in about 60–70% of patients with advanced chronic pancreatitis [4,6].

Complications

Of the various complications that can develop in the course of chronic pancreatitis, pseudocysts and stenosis (generally mild) of the retropancreatic portion of the common bile duct are the most frequent. Several less common ones can also be encountered (Table 43.3).

Pancreatic Pseudocysts

Pseudocysts most commonly develop during the initial stages of chronic pancreatitis; their reported frequency varies from study to study, but they are fairly frequent, occurring in about 30% of cases [4,7]. In surgical series their frequency is higher (about 50%) [4,6]. Most often, pseudocysts present as a single lesion, but sometimes two or more can be seen; their size is variable, they are often symptomatic (persistent pain being the most frequent symptom), and they are occasionally complicated by rupture or infection. In our experience [4], in the great majority of cases the pseudocysts derive from dilated ducts, and thus are true cysts; as they dilate, the epithelial lining can be lost, at which point they no longer appear to be true cysts. Among our patients with chronic pancreatitis, postnecrotic pseudocysts are rare, the main reason being that we see few patients (about 10%) who have had an acute necrotic attack.

Table 43.3. Complications, associated diseases, and mortality associated with chronic pancreatitis

Pancreatic pseudocysts	25–30%
Stenosis (usually mild) of the retropancreatic common bile duct	40–50%
Pancreatic cancer	1–3%
Extrapancreatic cancer	10–15%
Splenic vein thrombosis	2–5%
Pancreatic pseudoaneurysm	2–3%
Duodenal obstruction	4–5%
Pancreatic fistula	2–3%
Pancreatic abscess	2–3%
Alcoholic liver diseases	25–40%
Cardiovascular diseases	20–30%
Mortality	20–35%

As far as treatment is concerned, if the pseudocysts are asymptomatic and without complications they can be left untreated, but repeat ultrasound is recommended every 6 months to control their size. If they become painful or develop a complication, treatment becomes obligatory. Years ago the only treatment available was surgery; more recently this has been abandoned in favor of endoscopic intervention.

Another possibility in the treatment of painful pseudocysts in chronic pancreatitis is the administration of octreotide, a synthetic analog of somatostatin, which causes the cysts to shrink and eventually disappear. We have shown [22,23] that this treatment (100 μg every 8 h) is effective mainly when the cysts do not communicate with the Wirsung duct and if the drug is administered when their size is increasing. When these criteria are met, the pain disappears completely and definitively after 3–4 days of octreotide treatment, as the cysts begin to shrink in size; the cysts then disappear completely after 6–8 weeks of treatment [22,23].

We would like to point out that size alone is not an indication for treatment. Although it has been a guiding principle that cysts of greater than 5–6 cm in diameter should be treated, we feel that if the cysts are asymptomatic treatment is not necessary, regardless of their size. We have followed several patients whose cysts have been larger than 5 or 6 cm and stable in size for many years, during which they have also been pain-free; we believe that intervention is not necessary in these cases. Generally speaking, once cysts are treated they are no longer problematic.

Stenosis of the Retropancreatic Common Bile Duct

Stenosis of the distal portion of the common bile duct can be observed in up to 40–50% of cases [4]; it is generally mild and does not obstruct the flow of bile. The stenosis is caused by pancreatic fibrosis in the area of the duct. It can contribute to a generally mild and transient (lasting 3–10 days) form of jaundice that can occur during attacks of pain, when the already stenotic bile duct is compressed by pancreatic edema.

In about 5–10% of the patients with chronic pancreatitis the jaundice persists and requires treatment [4]. It is due to complete obstruction of the retropancreatic common bile duct, most often by pancreatic fibrosis, although sometimes it is due to compression of the duct by a cyst of the pancreatic head or, more rarely, by cancers of the pancreatic head, which can complicate chronic pancreatitis. In these cases, it is necessary to perform a choledochojejunostomy. A stent is sometimes placed endoscopically, but these tend to become occluded, and the procedure is often complicated by the development of cholangitis; for this reason, it should only be used in carefully selected cases, such as in patients awaiting surgery or in those who present a high surgical risk.

Pancreatic Cancer

Many studies have been published on the risk of pancreatic cancer in patients with chronic pancreatitis, but results have been conflicting: some have concluded that there is a risk [24,25], others that there is not or that it is very low [26–28]. We believe that chronic pancreatitis is a risk factor for pancreatic cancer, but that this risk is low, in the order of 2–3% [8,28]. Lowenfels et al. [24] reported a cumulative risk of pancreatic cancer in subjects with chronic pancreatitis who were followed for 10 and 20 years after the diagnosis of pancreatitis of 1.8 and 4%, respectively.

The risk of pancreatic cancer has been reported to be very much higher in patients with hereditary chronic pancreatitis. Lowenfels et al. [29] have shown that the estimated cumulative risk of pancreatic cancer to age 70 years in patients with this disease approaches 40%.

Extrapancreatic Cancer

Patients with chronic pancreatitis have a high incidence (10–15%) of extrapancreatic cancer, the commonest sites being the upper and lower airways as well as the gastrointestinal tract [8,11,13,30]. The reason for this increased incidence is not clear, but the abuse of tobacco and alcohol in these patients is thought to be responsible.

Splenic Vein Thrombosis

While splenic vein thrombosis is well known as a complication of chronic pancreatitis, its incidence is not. Bradley [31] reported an incidence of 2% among his patients with this disease. It can result in the development of gastric or esophageal varices; although there are no precise data regarding the frequency with which these varices bleed, the percentage is generally low.

Pseudoaneurysm

This is a rare complication of chronic pancreatitis, seen in about 2–3% of cases. It usually occurs in association with pancreatic pseudocysts, the mechanism of formation being erosion of an expanding pseudocyst into a nearby artery. The vessels most commonly involved are the splenic, gastroduodenal, pancreaticoduodenal, and hepatic arteries. Pancreatic pseudoaneurysms cause bleeding that may be slow and intermittent or acute and massive. Treatment is necessary even if they are not actively bleeding because untreated pseudoaneurysms have a very high mortality rate [32,33]. Bleeding can be successfully controlled by arteriographic transcatheter embolization or surgery.

Duodenal Obstruction

This complication occurs in about 4–5% of patients with chronic pancreatitis. It is generally due to marked fibrosis of the head of the pancreas that involves the duodenum or to a pseudocyst; treatment consists of surgery for the former and endoscopic drainage or surgical treatment for the latter.

Pancreatic Fistula

Pancreatic fistulas are a rare complication of chronic pancreatitis (2–3%). External fistulas generally develop after surgical procedures on the pancreas or after attacks of necrotic pancreatitis. Internal pancreatic fistulas are generally due to rupture of the main pancreatic duct or leakage from a pseudocyst. The main complications of internal fistulas are pancreatic ascites or pleural effusions. Treatment consists of fasting, parenteral nutrition, octreotide (100 µg every 8 h), or endoscopic stent placement [34,35]; if the fistula persists, surgery is indicated.

Pancreatic Abscess

This is a rare complication that involves only about 2–3% of patients with chronic pancreatitis. The abscess often develops at the site of a previous pseudocyst. Treatment with antibiotics is generally unsuccessful, leaving surgery as the only viable alternative.

Alcoholic Liver Disease

In a study [36] done on surgical biopsies samples of the liver taken from 50 patients with chronic alcoholic pancreatitis undergoing surgery for pancreatitis, we showed that 22 (44%) had associated alcoholic liver disease; of these 22, 13 had alcoholic hepatitis, 7 cirrhosis, and 2 steatosis. The percentage of alcoholic liver disease in this series of patients was similar to that found in the general alcoholic population [37].

We have seen that patients with chronic alcoholic pancreatitis who develop hepatic disease are most often those who drink larger quantities of alcohol (>200 g of pure alcohol daily) and for a longer period of time (>20 years). It is therefore important that patients with chronic alcoholic pancreatitis, especially those whose alcohol consumption is to the aforementioned extent, are monitored periodically with liver function and imaging tests for early recognition and timely treatment of any associated liver disease.

Cardiovascular Lesions

Several investigators have reported an increased frequency of vascular lesions in patients with chronic pancreatitis [38,39], but while some have assumed that this was simply a coincidence, others have suggested that a causal relationship may exist [40,41]. In a study of 54 patients with chronic pancreatitis (mean age 44 years, range 26–66 years) [42], we found evidence of vascular involvement in 18 (33%) of the patients and in 5 (9%) of the controls. In particular, we found electrocardiographic signs of coronary artery disease in 8 patients, as well as peripheral signs and symptoms of obliterative atherosclerotic disease in the lower extremities in 12 patients. No significant differences in the prevalence of the major vascular risk factors were noted between patients with vascular lesions and those without, or between the patients and the control subjects.

In another study [43], we showed that in 57 patients with chronic pancreatitis there was radiologic evidence of aortic calcification in 35 (41.4%), but only in 12 of 40 (30%) smoker controls. Interestingly, these patients had a mean age of 44 years (range 26–59 years), whereas in the general population aortic calcifications are rarely seen in persons under the age of 50–60 years. None of these patients with chronic pancreatitis had conditions associated with atherosclerosis, such as diabetes, arterial hypertension, obesity, or hyperlipidemia. It should be mentioned that aortic calcification is associated with a marked increase in the risk of death by cardiovascular disease [44]. These two studies indicate that, compared with the general population, patients with chronic pancreatitis have more frequent cardiovascular lesions and the lesions tend to develop at an earlier age; the reason for these findings is not clear.

Mortality

All of the studies published on mortality in chronic pancreatitis have concluded that it is high. Ammann et al. [8], in their study of 245 patients with chronic pancreatitis, reported that 86 (35%) died; the mean age at death was 54 years in 54 patients with alcoholic chronic pancreatitis and 66 years in 32 with nonalcoholic pancreatitis. In patients with alcoholic chronic pancreatitis the survival times after medical or surgical treatment were similar (Fig. 43.1). In a study by Levy et al. [45] of 240 patients with chronic pancreatitis, of whom 210 were drinkers, it was reported that after a mean of 20 years from the clinical onset of the disease, 57 patients (23.7%) were dead and that the average age at the time of death was 52 years; in this study, the factors associated with late mortality were the presence of previous elective surgery and hepatopathy.

Regarding pancreatic surgery, there are several studies evaluating late death in this field. In Table 43.4 the rate of late mortality and the relative causes are reported; the rates of late deaths are similar among the various surgical procedures [46].

The mortality rate for chronic alcoholic pancreatitis is higher than it is for idiopathic or other forms of chronic pancreatitis; as would be expected, among patients with alcoholic pancreatitis the mortality rate

Table 43.4. Comparison of causes of late deaths after operations for chronic pancreatitis (modified from [46])

Operation	Late deaths *n* (%)	Alcohol, accidents, nonpancreatic cancer (%)	Pancreatic cancer (%)	Suicide, pancreatitis (%)	Diabetes (%)	Unrelated causes (%)	Unknown causes (%)
Longitudinal pancreaticojejunostomy	16 (16.26)	16.3	9.8	37.7	9.8	26	
Total pancreatectomy	25 (16.3)	4.7	0	62	14	14	
Pancreaticoduodenectomy	73 (16.5)	15.2	0	51.3	11.1	22	
Duodenal preservation and local resection	12 (5.8)	8.3	0	83.3	8.3	0	
Distal pancreatectomy (less than 80%)	10 (11)	8	1.35	36.4	1.35	30	23

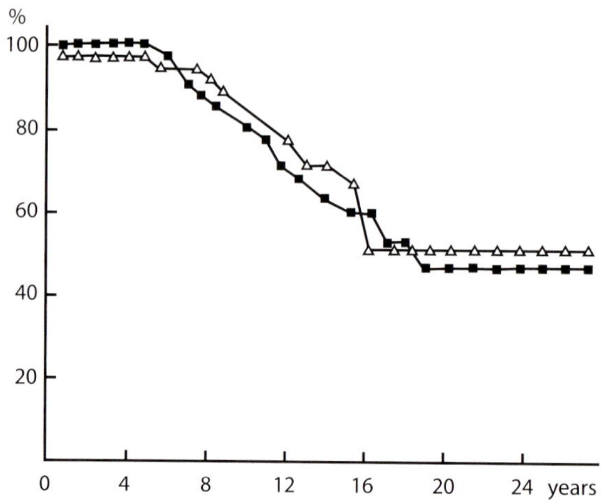

Figure 43.1

Cumulative survival rate (*x-axis*) of alcohol-induced chronic pancreatitis in operated (*black squares*) and nonoperated (*open triangles*) patients (modified from [8])

is higher for those who continue to drink [13]. The main causes of death for these patients are cardiovascular disease, hepatic cirrhosis, extrapancreatic or pancreatic cancer, postoperative complications, complications of chronic pancreatitis or of diabetes, and alcoholism [4,6–8,11–13]. In general, less than 20% of deaths are directly related to chronic pancreatitis.

What we do During the Follow-up

The treatment of this disease remains a challenging puzzle; pain is the main clinical manifestation of the disease and the main problem is its treatment. Although medical management of pain may be one of the therapeutic modalities [47,48], in the past as well as in the present, surgical management has been the main option, especially in the case of intractable pain [49]. In our experience, about 50% of all patients with chronic pancreatitis are treated medically, and about 50% by surgery. Pancreatic resection or drainage plays an important role in treating patients with pain, achieving a lasting resolution in about 70% of cases [50–52]. However, in recent years, other therapeutic options have been applied in clinical practice mainly for the relief of pain: endoscopic therapy [53], thoracoscopic splanchnicectomy [54,55], and extracorporeal shock-wave lithotripsy [56].

For many years, the success of these therapeutic modalities has been seen only from a medical point of view [22], but successful medical therapy reflects only one aspect of the multidimensional approach to these patients, which is also composed of the sensitive and functional aspects of day-to-day life. Furthermore, the evolution of chronic pancreatitis is not easy to study due to its relative rarity, delay in diagnosis, and finally, because of its long course many experiences of generations of researchers in a specific referral period are effectively lost.

Studies of the evaluation of the outcome of chronic pancreatitis recognize three main phases. In the first phase the studies on the description of morbidity and mortality regarded the surgical procedures performed [57–59] and were very limited in their ability to evaluate the evolution of the disease, being able to give information only on surgical morbidity and mortality, and were not able to give information on the middle- and long-term evaluation on pancreatic function (diabetes, malnutrition), recurrent pain, and loss in working days.

In the second phase, many papers have explored the evolution of chronic pancreatitis from a clinical point of view, describing the nutritional status of the patients, the appearance of complications, the frequency of hospitalizations, and the occurrence of diabetes mellitus. The limit of this approach lies in the strict medical evaluation, without taking into account the perspective of the patients.

The third phase consists of studies describing the history of chronic pancreatitis using an approach based both on the medical and on the patient's point of view. These studies utilize appropriate questionnaires administered to the patients and containing questions regarding their daily lives. Health-related quality of life, subjectively perceived by the patient, is becoming a major issue in the evaluation of any therapeutic intervention, mainly in patients with chronic or hard to cure diseases, where the aim of the intervention is to keep patients either symptom free and able to live in the community for a long time, or to reduce the discomfort caused by the disease. In chronic pancreatitis patients this approach was carried out for the first time by surgeons and endoscopists who have explored the quality of life in relation to their interventional approaches, but only a few of them have used structured and validated questionnaires [60–67]; furthermore, the time interval between the intervention and the assessment of the health-related quality of life was quite low in these studies, ranging from 3 to 74 months.

Quality of Life

Studies evaluating the quality of life in chronic pancreatitis involving mixed medical-surgical patients have been published only in the last few years [5,68–70]. Three of these studies utilized a questionnaire called Medical Outcome Study 36-Item Short-Form Health Survey (SF-36) [5,68,69] and in the most recent study, a questionnaire constituting two different modules, the European Organization for Research and Treatment of Cancer Quality of Life Questionnaire-C30 (EORTC QLQ-C30) and the Quality of Life Questionnaire pancreatic cancer module (QLQ-PAN26), which had previously been tested in pancreatic cancer patients [70]. All four studies demonstrat ed that patients with chronic pancreatitis have a substantially impaired quality of life and, most importantly, the impairment of the quality of life in younger patients is higher than in older ones, with obvious economic consequences for society.

Regarding gender, in the Italian study [5], the impairment of various domains was more pronounced in females: this finding differs from the German studies [68,69]. This may be explained, at least in part, by the fact that Italian females affected by chronic pancreatitis have a poor acceptance of the disease. These different findings reflect the importance of the studies on the quality of life because they show the cultural differences among the various countries.

Among the various clinical variables examined as possible factors related to chronic pancreatitis, only pain was able to significantly impair all eight domains of the SF-36, thus confirming that pain control is the main therapeutic option to be taken into account in order to improve the quality of life in patients with chronic pancreatitis, and suggesting that much effort should be made in order to identify more efficacious therapies capable of controlling this symptom.

Surprisingly, in the Italian study [5], neither the pancreatic surgery nor endoscopic therapy were able to substantially modify the various physical and mental domains investigated by the SF-36; this is in contrast to previous studies regarding the various surgical and endoscopic options [60,61–66,71–73]. This difference may be due to the fact that these studies enrolled a highly selected group of patients with a short time interval between the intervention and the assessment of the health-related quality of life (3–74 months). Another possible bias present in these surgical/endoscopic studies is that their data were not adjusted for sex and age.

It is worth noting that diabetes and major alterations of the Wirsung duct (which are expressions of long-standing chronic pancreatitis), as well as a decreased body mass index (which is an expression of maldigestion) are able to impair physical and mental domains [5,68,69].

Comorbidities were not significantly related to the quality of life of these patients [5,68]. A possible explanation of this phenomenon is the fact that chronic pancreatitis per se determines a high impairment of the quality of life, and comorbidities add truly little, since these patients already had low values of most of the SF-36 domains.

An important point is that a percentage varying from 4 to 10% [5,70] missed responses or refused to complete the questionnaires. In the Italian study [5], this group was better characterized; the patients who refused to complete the questionnaire were male patients, actual smokers with a long duration of alcohol consumption, with a long duration of the disease, and free of pain at the time of the study. Patients with the aforementioned characteristics are probably candidates for an intensive psychological approach in order to counterbalance their unwillingness to improve their relationship with the disease.

The main differences between the four studies exploring the quality of life in chronic pancreatitis patients [5,68–70] are:

1. The studies utilizing the SF-36 questionnaire had a control group that consisted of the general population [5,68,69], whereas the study utilizing the EORTC QLQ-C30 and the QLQ-PAN26 did not [70].
2. The studies utilizing the SF-36 had a high number of chronic pancreatitis patients coming from the country where the studies were carried out, whereas the study utilizing the EORTC QLQ-C30 and the QLQ-PAN26 enrolled 66 patients from four different countries (Germany, Italy, South Africa, and the United Kingdom).
3. Finally, all of the patients utilizing the SF-36 questionnaire were fluent in the native language [5,68,69], whereas Afrikaans-speaking patients in South Africa completed the English version of the EORTC QLQ-C30 and the QLQ-PAN26 [70].

What conclusions can we draw from the studies that have assessed the quality of life in chronic pancreatitis patients? First of all, it is necessary to choose a widely accepted questionnaire on the quality of life in order to render the various studies in different populations of chronic pancreatitis patients comparable. We need further studies comparing the various questionnaires in order to identify the questionnaire that is the most useful in routinely evaluating our patients in the office. In this respect, one of the characteristics of the questionnaire that should be taken into consideration is time to complete it. For example, SF-36 and EORTC QLQ-C30 are time-consuming because they require more than 5 min to complete, whereas SF-12 is quite fast, requiring no more than 2 min to answer and it gives the same information as SF-36 [74]. Finally, all future studies on the management of chronic pancreatitis should include a proven effective questionnaire in order to evaluate the point of view of the patient on the various treatments employed: we need to know not only the objective results of new treatment modalities, but also how the patients feel about them [75].

Conclusion

In the advanced stages of chronic pancreatitis, severe exocrine pancreatic insufficiency appears as well as diabetes mellitus in both operated and nonoperated patients. These two conditions have a very negative impact on the quality of life of our patients. Cancer degeneration, often associated with smoking, also seems to occur in the advanced period. Finally, the assessment of the quality of life in chronic pancreatitis may modify our approach to the treatment of these patients also in the late stage of the disease.

References

1. Gullo L, Barbara L, Labò G (1988) Effect of cessation of alcohol use on the course of pancreatic dysfunction in alcoholic pancreatitis. Gastroenterology 95:1063–1068
2. Ammann RW, Heitz PU, Kloppel G (1996) Course of alcoholic chronic pancreatitis: a prospective clinicomorphological long-term study. Gastroenterology 111:224–231
3. Etemad B, Whitcomb DC (2001) Chronic pancreatitis: diagnosis, classification, and new genetic developments. Gastroenterology 120:682–707
4. Gullo L, Costa PL, Labò G (1977) Chronic pancreatitis in Italy. Aetiological, clinical and histological observations. Rendic Gastroenterol 9:97–104
5. Pezzilli R, Morselli Labate AM, Ceciliato R, Frulloni L, Cavestro GM, Comparato G, Ferri B, Corinaldesi R, Gullo L (2005) Quality of life in patients with chronic pancreatitis. Dig Liver Dis 37:181–189
6. Sarles H, Sarles JC, Camatte R, Muratore R, Gaini M, Guien C, Pastor J, Le Roy F (1965) Observations on 205 confirmed cases of acute pancreatitis, recurring pancreatitis, and chronic pancreatitis. Gut 6:545–559
7. Bernades P, Belghiti J, Athouel M, Maliardo N, Breil P, Fekete F (1983) Histoire naturelle de la pancreatite chronique: etude de 120 cas. Gastroenterol Clin Biol 7:8–13
8. Ammann RW, Akovbiantz A, Largiader F, Schueler G (1984) Course and outcome of chronic pancreatitis. Longitudinal study of a mixed medical-surgical series of 245 patients. Gastroenterology 86:820–828
9. Dani R, Mott CB, Guarita DR, Nogueira CE (1990) Epidemiology and etiology of chronic pancreatitis in Brazil: a tale of two cities. Pancreas 5:474–478
10. Lankisch PG, Lohr-Happe A, Otto J, Creutzfeldt W (1993) Natural course in chronic pancreatitis. Pain, exocrine and endocrine pancreatic insufficiency and prognosis of the disease. Digestion 54:148–155
11. Layer P, Yamamoto H, Kalthoff L, Clain JE, Bakken LJ, DiMagno EP (1994) The different courses of early and late onset idiopathic and alcoholic chronic pancreatitis. Gastroenterology 107:1481–1487
12. Miyake H, Harada H, Kunichik K, Ochi K, Kimura I (1987) Clinical course and prognosis of chronic pancreatitis. Pancreas 2:378–385
13. Hayakawa T, Kondo T, Shibata T, Sugimoto Y, Kitagawa M (1989) Chronic alcoholism and evolution of pain and prognosis in chronic pancreatitis. Dig Dis Sci 34:33–38
14. Gullo L, Costa PL, Fontana G, Labò G (1976) Investigation of exocrine pancreatic function by continuous infusion of caerulein and secretin in normal subjects and in chronic pancreatitis. Digestion 14:97–107
15. Gullo L, Ventrucci M, Tomassetti P, Migliori M, Pezzilli R (1999) Fecal elastase 1 determination in chronic pancreatitis. Dig Dis Sci 44:210–213

16. Isaksson G, Ihse I (1983) Pain reduction by oral pancreatic enzyme preparation in chronic pancreatitis. Dig Dis Sci 28:97–102
17. Slaff J, Jacobson D, Tillmann CR, Curngton C, Toskes P (1984) Protease-specific suppression of pancreatic exocrine secretion. Gastroenterology 87:44–52
18. Halgreen H, Thorsgaard Pedersen N, Worning H (1986) Symptomatic effect of pancreatic enzyme therapy in patients with chronic pancreatitis. Scand J Gastroenterol 21:104–108
19. Mossner J, Secknus R, Meyer J, Niederau C, Adler G (1992) Treatment of pain with pancreatic extracts in chronic pancreatitis: results of a prospective placebo-controlled multicenter trial. Digestion 53:54–66
20. Malesci A, Gaia E, Fioretta A, Bocchia P, Ciravegna G, Cantor P, Vantini I (1995) No effect of long-term treatment with pancreatic extract on recurrent abdominal pain in patients with chronic pancreatitis. Scand J Gastroenterol 30:392–398
21. Gullo L, Parenti M, Monti L, Pezzilli R (1990) Diabetic retinopathy in chronic pancreatitis. Gastroenterology 98:1577–1581
22. Gullo L, Barbara L (1991) Treatment of pancreatic pseudocysts with octreotide. Lancet 338:540–541
23. Gullo L, Pezzilli R, De Giorgio R (1996) Effect of octreotide on pain in patients with chronic pancreatitis. Dig Surg 13:465–468
24. Lowenfels AB, Maisonneuve P, Cavallini G, Ammann RW, Lankisch PG, Andersen JR, Dimagno EP, Andren-Sandberg A, Domellof L (1993) Pancreatitis and the risk of pancreatic cancer. International Pancreatitis Study Group. N Engl J Med 328:1433–1437
25. Pradeep B, Sonnenberg A (1995) Pancreatitis is a risk factor for pancreatic cancer. Gastroenterology 109:247–251
26. Ekbom A, McLaughlin JK, Karlsson BM, Nyren O, Gridley G, Adami HO, Fraumeni JF Jr (1994) Pancreatitis and pancreatic cancer: a population-based study. J Natl Cancer Inst 86:625–627
27. Karlson BM, Ekbom A, Josefsson S, McLaughlin JK, Fraumeni JF Jr, Nyren O (1997) The risk of pancreatic cancer following pancreatitis: an association due to confounding? Gastroenterology 113:587–592
28. Gullo L, Tomassetti P, Migliori M, Casadei R, Marrano D (2001) Do early symptoms of pancreatic cancer exist that can allow an earlier diagnosis? Pancreas 22: 210–213
29. Lowenfels AB, Maisonneuve P, DiMagno EP, Elitsur Y, Gates LK Jr, Perrault J, Whitcomb DC (1997) Hereditary pancreatitis and the risk of pancreatic cancer. International Hereditary Pancreatitis Study Group. J Natl Cancer Inst 89:442–446
30. Hansen TH, Laursen M, Christensen E, Worning H (1995) Chronic pancreatitis and extrapancreatic cancer: a retrospective study among 181 patients with chronic pancreatitis. Int J Pancreatol 18:235–239
31. Bradley EL III (1987) The natural history of splenic vein thrombosis due to chronic pancreatitis: Indications for surgery. Int J Pancreatol 2:87–92
32. Woods MS, Traverso LW, Kozarek RA, Brandabur J, Hauptmann E (1995) Successful treatment of bleeding pseudoaneurysms of chronic pancreatitis. Pancreas 10:22–30
33. Bender JS, Bouwman DL, Levison MA, Weaver DW (1995) Pseudocysts and pseudoaneurysms: surgical strategy. Pancreas 10:143–147
34. Segal I, Parekh D, Lipschitz J, Gecelter G, Myburgh JA (1993) Treatment of pancreatic ascites and external pancreatic fistulas with a long-acting somatostatin analogue (Sandostatin). Digestion 54 (Suppl 1):53–58
35. Saed ZA, Ramirez FC, Hepps KS (1993) Endoscopic stent placement for internal and external pancreatic fistulas. Gastroenterology 105:1213–1217
36. Gullo L, Casadei R, Campione O, Grigioni W, Marrano D (1995) Alcoholic liver disease in alcoholic chronic pancreatitis: a prospective study. Ital J Gastroenterol 27:69–72
37. Grant BR, Dufour MC, Harford TC (1988) Epidemiology of alcoholic liver disease. Semin Liver Dis 8:12–25
38. Fitzgerald O, Fitzgerald P, Fennelly J, McMullin JP, Boland SJ (1963) A clinical study of chronic pancreatitis. Gut 4:193–216
39. Sarles H, Crousillat B (1978) Frequence des arteriopathies dans les pancreatites chroniques. Gastroenterol Clin Biol 2:791–796
40. Sambin P, Levrat R, Girard M (1971) Les angiopathies de la pancreatite chronique. J Med Lyon 52:425–438
41. Tuzhilin SA, Dreiling DA (1975) Cardiovascular lesions in pancreatitis. Am J Gastroenterol 63:381–388
42. Gullo L, Stella A, Labriola E, Costa PL, Descovich G, Labo G (1982) Cardiovascular lesions in chronic pancreatitis: a prospective study. Dig Dis Sci 27:716–722
43. Gullo L, Tassoni U, Mazzoni G, Stefanini F (1996) Increased prevalence of aortic calcification in chronic pancreatitis. Am J Gastroenterol 91:759–761
44. Witteman JCM, Kok FJ, Van Saase JLCM, Valkenburg HA (1986) Aortic calcification as a predictor of cardiovascular mortality. Lancet 2:1120–1122
45. Levy P, Milan C, Pignon JP, Baetz A, Bernades P (1989) Mortality factors associated with chronic pancreatitis. Unidimensional and multidimensional analysis of a medical-surgical series of 240 patients. Gastroenterology 96:1165–1172
46. Frey CF, Mayer KL (2003) Comparison of local resection of the head of the pancreas combined with longitudinal pancreaticojejunostomy (Frey procedure) and duodenum-preserving resection of the pancreatic head (Beger procedure). World J Surg 27:1217–1230
47. Singh VV, Toskes PP (2003) Medical therapy for chronic pancreatitis pain. Curr Gastroenterol Rep 5:110–116
48. Czako L, Takacs T, Hegyi P, Pronai L, Tulassay Z, Lakner L, Dobronte Z, Boda K, Lonovics J (2003) Quality of life assessment after pancreatic enzyme replacement therapy in chronic pancreatitis. Can J Gastroenterol17:597–603
49. Liao Q, Zhao YP, Wu WW, Li BL, Li JY (2003) Diagnosis and treatment of chronic pancreatitis. Hepatobiliary Pancreat Dis Int 2:445–448
50. Beger HG, Schlosser W, Friess HM, Buchler MW (1999) Duodenum-preserving head resection in chronic pancreatitis changes the natural course of the disease: a single-center 26-year experience. Ann Surg 230:512–519
51. Ihse I, Borch K, Larsson J (1990) Chronic pancreatitis: results of operations for relief of pain. World J Surg 14:53–58
52. Evans JD, Wilson PG, Carver C, Bramhall SR, Buckels JA, Mayer AD, McMaster P, Neoptolemos JP (1997) Outcome of surgery for chronic pancreatitis. Br J Surg 84:624–629
53. Gabbrielli A, Mutignani M, Pandolfi M, Perri V, Costamagna G (2002) Endotherapy of early onset idiopathic chronic pancreatitis: results with long-term follow-up. Gastrointest Endosc 55:488–493

54. Howard TJ, Swofford JB, Wagner DL, Sherman S, Lehman GA (2002) Quality of life after bilateral thoracoscopic splanchnicectomy: long-term evaluation in patients with chronic pancreatitis. J Gastrointest Surg 6:845–852
55. Leksowski K. Thoracoscopic splanchnicectomy for the relief of pain due to chronic pancreatitis. Surg Endosc 15:592–596
56. Holm M, Matzen P (2003) Stenting and extracorporeal shock wave lithotripsy in chronic pancreatitis. Scand J Gastroenterol 38:328–331
57. Warren KW (1969) Surgical management of chronic relapsing pancreatitis. Am J Surg 117:24–32
58. Leger L, Lenriot JP, Lemaigre G (1974) Five to twenty year followup after surgery for chronic pancreatitis in 148 patients. Ann Surg 180:185–191
59. Frey CF, Child CG, Fry W (1976) Pancreatectomy for chronic pancreatitis. Ann Surg 184:403–413
60. Howard TJ, Swofford JB, Wagner DL, Sherman S, Lehman GA (2002) Quality of life after bilateral thoracoscopic splanchnicectomy: long-term evaluation in patients with chronic pancreatitis. J Gastrointest Surg 6:845–852
61. Bloechle C, Izbicki JR, Knoefel WT, Kuechler T, Broelsch CE (1995) Quality of life in chronic pancreatitis – results after duodenum-preserving resection of the head of the pancreas. Pancreas 11:77–85
62. Broome AH, Eisen GM, Harland RC, Collins BH, Meyers WC, Pappas TN (1996) Quality of life after treatment for pancreatitis. Ann Surg 223:665–670
63. Sohn TA, Campbell KA, Pitt HA, Sauter PK, Coleman JA, Lillemo KD, Yeo CJ, Cameron JL (2000) Quality of life and long-term survival after surgery for chronic pancreatitis. J Gastrointest Surg 4:355–364
64. Huang JJ, Yeo CJ, Sohn TA, Lillemoe KD, Sauter PK, Coleman J, Hruban RH, Cameron JL (2000) Quality of life and outcomes after pancreaticoduodenectomy. Ann Surg 231:890–898
65. Witzigmann H, Max D, Uhlmann D, Geissler F, Ludwig S, Schwarz R, Krauss O, Lohmann T, Keim V, Hauss J (2002) Quality of life in chronic pancreatitis: a prospective trial comparing classical Whipple procedure and duodenum-preserving pancreatic head resection. J Gastrointest Surg 6:173–179
66. Brand B, Kahl M, Sidhu S, Nam VC, Sriram PV, Jaeckle S, Thonke F, Soehendra N (2000) Prospective evaluation of morphology, function, and quality of life after extracorporeal shockwave lithotripsy and endoscopic treatment of chronic calcific pancreatitis. Am J Gastroenterol 95:3428–3438
67. Strate T, Taherpour Z, Bloechle C, Mann O, Bruhn JP, Schneider C, Kuechler T, Yekebas E, Izbicki JR (2005) Long-term follow-up of a randomized trial comparing the Beger and Frey procedures for patients suffering from chronic pancreatitis. Ann Surg 241:591–598
68. Wehler M, Nichterlein R, Fischer B, Farnbacher M, Reulbach U, Hahn EG, Schneider T (2004) Factors associated with health-related quality of life in chronic pancreatitis. Am J Gastroenterol 99:138–146
69. Wehler M, Reulbach U, Nichterlein R, Lange K, Fischer B, Farnbacher M, Hahn EG, Schneider T (2003) Health-related quality of life in chronic pancreatitis: a psychometric assessment. Scand J Gastroenterol 38:1083–1089
70. Fitzsimmons D, Kahl S, Butturini G, van Wyk M, Bornman P, Bassi C, Malfertheiner P, George SL, Johnson CD (2005) Symptoms and quality of life in chronic pancreatitis assessed by structured interview and the EORTC QLQ-C30 and QLQ-PAN26. Am J Gastroenterol 100:918–926
71. Izbicki JR, Bloechle C, Broering DC, Kuechler T, Broelsch CE (1998) Longitudinal V-shaped excision of the ventral pancreas for small duct disease in severe chronic pancreatitis: prospective evaluation of a new surgical procedure. Ann Surg 227:213–219
72. Witzigmann H, Max D, Uhlmann D, Geissler F, Schwarz R, Ludwig S, Lohmann T, Caca K, Keim V, Tannapfel A, Hauss J (2003) Outcome after duodenum-preserving pancreatic head resection is improved compared with classic Whipple procedure in the treatment of chronic pancreatitis. Surgery 134:53–62
73. Rios GA, Adams DB (2001) Outcome of surgical treatment of chronic pancreatitis associated with sphincter of Oddi dysfunction. Am Surg 67:462–466
74. Pezzilli R, Morselli-Labate AM, Frulloni L, Cavestro GM, Ferri B, Comparato G, Gullo L, Corinaldesi R (2006) The quality of life in patients with chronic pancreatitis evaluated using the SF-12 questionnaire: a comparative study with the SF-36 questionnaire. Dig Liver Dis 38:109–115
75. Pezzilli R, Fantini L (2005) Chronic pancreatitis: assessing the quality of life. JOP 6:406–409

Pancreatic Cancer

Chapter 44 Epidemiology of Pancreatic Cancer *489*
A. B. Lowenfels, P. Maisonneuve

Chapter 45 Pathology of Pancreatic Cancer *497*
R. H. Hruban, A. Maitra, N. Fukushima

Chapter 46 Genetic Pathways in Pancreatic Tumorigenesis *513*
E. Gallmeier, S. E. Kern

Chapter 47 The Clinical Assessment of Pancreatic Cancer *527*
E. J. Shin, M. I. Canto

Chapter 48 The Staging of Pancreatic Cancer *541*
J. R. Rodríguez, C. Fernandez-del Castillo

Chapter 49 Oncological Management of Pancreatic Cancer in Advanced Stages *549*
D. Laheru

Chapter 50 Indications for Resection of Pancreatic Cancer *559*
O. J. Hines, H. A. Reber

Chapter 51 The Kausch-Whipple Pancreatectomy *567*
C. R. Ferrone, M. F. Brennan

Chapter 52 Pylorus-Preserving Pancreatico-duodenectomy *581*
R. D. Schulick, J. L. Cameron

Chapter 53 Management of Tumor Invasion/Adhesion to the Superior Mesenteric-Portal Vein During Pancreatectomy *593*
F. Mosca, U. Boggi, M. Del Chiaro

Chapter 54 Margin Status Following Pancreaticoduodenectomy for Pancreatic Adenocarcinoma: Implications of R Status *611*
C. P. Raut, G. Varadhachary, H. Wang, E. P. Tamm, J. B. Fleming, D. B. Evans

Chapter 55 Subtotal Left Resection for Pancreatic Cancer *625*
A. Nakeeb, B. Safar

Chapter 56 Total Pancreatectomy for Pancreatic Cancer *639*
J. Y. Tracey, M. Bouvet, A. R. Moossa

Chapter 57 Laparoscopic Management of Pancreatic Neoplasms *653*
C. G. S. Hüscher, C. Ponzano, M. Di Paola

Chapter 58 Bypass Procedures in the Treatment of Nonresectable Carcinoma of the Head of the Pancreas *665*
M. G. House, K. D. Lillemoe

Chapter 59 Resected Pancreatic Cancer *675*
G. R. Varadhachary, J. L. Abbruzzese

Chapter 60 Management of Locally Advanced and Recurrent Pancreas Cancer *689*
A. Jimeno, M. Hidalgo

Chapter 61 Survival After Medical and Surgical Treatment of Pancreatic Adenocarcinoma *695*
J. F. Tseng, C. Fernandez-del Castillo, A. L. Warshaw

Chapter 44

A. B. Lowenfels · P. Maisonneuve

Epidemiology of Pancreatic Cancer

With an overall mortality approaching 100%, pancreatic cancer remains a significant challenge for both surgeons and their patients. Because of its location deep within the abdomen, diagnosis of this cancer is still much more difficult than for other gastrointestinal tumors. At the time of detection, many of these tumors are already inoperable, suitable for only palliative therapy. There is a final problem: unlike tumors arising in other parts of the digestive tract, there are no widely accepted screening tools such as endoscopy for tumors of the esophagus, stomach, and colon.

Even though these tumors are rare, ranking 13th in a worldwide list of cancer incidence, for the reasons cited above, pancreas cancer ranks 4th as a cause of death in the USA, and 8th as a global cause of cancer death [1]. In this chapter we will review the epidemiology of pancreatic cancer, emphasizing the occurrence of this tumor in various countries, time-trends, risk factors, inherited disorders leading to pancreatic cancer, screening, and preventive aspects.

Descriptive Epidemiology

Because of its high mortality rates, incidence rates and mortality rates can be used nearly interchangeably to describe the frequency of this cancer. Table 44.1 compares the number of cases of digestive tract cancer in developed and less developed countries [2]. As can be seen, from a global viewpoint, the current burden of pancreatic cancer is greatest in developed countries, but by the end of the next decade, the number of cases in developed and less developed countries will be nearly the same. The large increase noted in less developed countries can be explained by anticipated aging of the population, decreasing death rates from competing causes such as infectious disease, and increasing prevalence of smoking.

A study of various world countries (Table 44.2) demonstrates clear differences in the age-adjusted incidence of this tumor in several different international populations. These wide differences are consistent with an important role for regional environmental factors.

Table 44.1. Estimated cases of digestive tract cancer in the years 2000and 2020 (with permission from [2])

Region	Organ	Estimated cases (2000)	Estimated Cases (2020)	Estimated Increase (%)
Developed	Large bowel	610,591	806,176	32%
	Stomach	334,011	439,842	32%
	Pancreas	127,416	168,453	32%
	Liver	106,950	142,836	34%
	Esophagus	71,163	94,251	33%
Less developed	Stomach	543,026	983,414	81%
	Liver	457,406	801,685	75%
	Esophagus	341,163	624,574	83%
	Large bowel	334,123	592,146	77%
	Pancreas	88,969	162,401	83%

Table 44.2. Male and female age-adjusted mortality rates per 100,000 for pancreatic cancer in various countries: 1981–2000 (with permission from [3]). *CI* Confidence interval, *AA* age-adjusted

	Male			Female		
Country	AA rate	Lower 95% CI of AA rate	Upper 95% CI of AA rate	Age-adjusted rate	Lower 95% CI of AA rate	Upper 95% CI of AA rate
Australia	6.6	6.4	6.7	4.5	4.4	4.6
Austria	8.9	8.8	9.1	6.0	5.9	6.1
Canada	7.7	7.6	7.8	5.4	5.3	5.4
France	7.3	7.3	7.4	3.8	3.8	3.9
Hungary	10.5	10.3	10.7	6.2	6.1	6.3
Ireland	8.4	8.1	8.6	5.5	5.3	5.7
Italy	7.2	7.2	7.3	4.4	4.4	4.5
Japan	8.4	8.3	8.4	4.7	4.7	4.7
New Zealand	6.6	6.3	6.8	4.4	4.2	4.6
Singapore	4.7	4.4	5.0	3.2	3.0	3.4
Spain	5.6	5.5	5.6	3.2	3.2	3.2
UK, England and Wales	7.0	7.0	7.1	4.9	4.9	5.0
UK, Northern Ireland	6.8	6.4	7.2	4.9	4.7	5.2
UK, Scotland	7.2	7.0	7.4	5.3	5.1	5.4
USA	7.5	7.5	7.5	5.3	5.3	5.3

Gender Differences

Throughout the world, male rates for pancreatic cancer exceed female rates by 40–50%. This excess is most likely caused by male/female smoking differences. As female smoking rates increase, as is currently occurring in the USA, we can predict a rise in the incidence of pancreatic cancer in females.

Racial Factors

As with many other cancer sites, there are racial differences in the incidence of pancreatic cancer. For example, age-specific and age-adjusted pancreatic cancer rates are approximately 50% higher in the American black population than in comparable white populations [4]. The explanation is unclear, but may be related to differences in smoking habits, or perhaps to racial differences in the rate of degradation of tobacco-derived carcinogens [5].

Maoris, an aboriginal group, comprise 10–13% of the total population of New Zealand and a smaller percentage of the Australian population. This racial group has a high risk of pancreatic cancer, with female rates being unexpectedly higher than male rates [6].

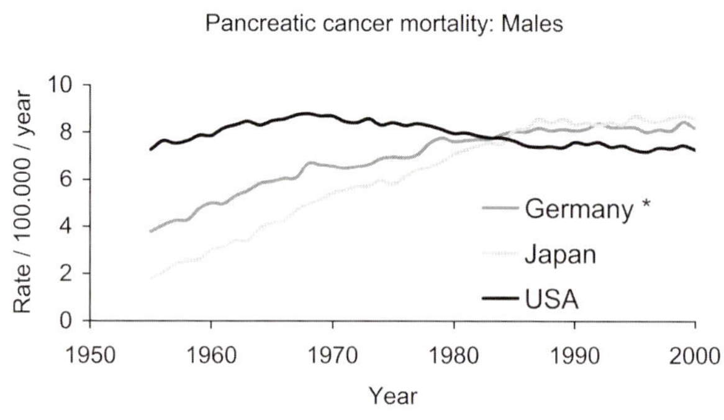

Figure 44.1

Time trends in male mortality from pancreatic cancer. Data from [2]

Time Trends

In many countries there has been an apparent increase in pancreatic cancer over the past several decades [7]. Part of this increase can be traced to more accurate diagnosis: with the availability of newer scanning techniques including computed tomography, magnetic resonance imaging, and endoscopic ultrasound scans, along with the increased use of fine-needle aspiration, the diagnosis of pancreatic cancer has become much more reliable.

In addition to more accurate diagnosis, part of the increase in pancreatic cancer can be traced to an increase in smoking – the strongest known risk factor for pancreatic cancer. Figure 44.1 examines the male pancreatic cancer mortality rate per 100,000 per year in three developed countries: Germany, Japan, and the USA. In all three countries mortality rates have increased since the 1960s, but in the USA there has been a recent modest decline, attributable to a reduction in smoking.

Risk Factors

Smoking

Smoking is the most thoroughly studied factor that increases the risk of contracting pancreatic cancer. There is almost uniform agreement in published studies that smoking doubles the risk of pancreatic cancer [8–10]. Based on a relative risk of two, and a smoking prevalence of, say, 30% in the general population, then smoking can be calculated to cause about one-quarter of the total burden of pancreatic cancer. The risk of pancreatic cancer is proportional to both the duration and the intensity of smoking, and it takes several years for the risk to diminish after the cessation of smoking.

Only about 1 or 2% of all smokers will ever contract pancreatic cancer compared to about 10% of smokers who will develop lung cancer. Clearly, smokers who do or do not develop a tobacco-related cancer must differ with respect to susceptibility to tobacco carcinogens [11].

Diet and Pancreatic Cancer

It is tempting to assume that the country and region-specific difference in the frequency of pancreatic cancer are related to dietary differences. It seems intuitive that a diet rich in nutrient-providing fruits and vegetables would lower the risk of various cancers, including pancreatic cancer. Unfortunately this appealing hypothesis has been difficult to substantiate. For example, a recent cohort study based on nearly 125,000 persons found that consuming a "prudent" diet (high in fruits and vegetables, low in meats and fats) did not reduce the risk of pancreatic cancer [12]. Many dietary studies have depended upon data from case-control studies where dietary intake from patients with pancreatic cancer is compared to dietary data from control subjects without pancreatic cancer. This popular study design can lead to spurious conclusions because information about diet is difficult to ascertain with a high degree of accuracy.

There is a possible link between obesity resulting from increased caloric consumption or a sedentary life style and pancreatic cancer [13–15]. Measures to avoid obesity will have other benefits in addition to helping to reduce the frequency of pancreatic cancer.

Preexisting Diseases and the Risk of Pancreatic Cancer

Chronic Pancreatitis

Chronic pancreatitis can be an idiopathic disease, an inherited genetic disorder, but is most frequently caused by heavy consumption of alcohol. All types of chronic pancreatitis, including tropical pancreatitis found in southern Indian and parts of Africa, can increase the risk of pancreatic cancer [16]. The exact mechanism is unknown, but is presumably related to increased cell turnover, which increases the likelihood of defective repair of damaged cells, leading to disturbed cellular architecture (pancreatic intraepithelial neoplasias) and eventually to pancreatic cancer [17]. Various studies have looked at the relationship between chronic pancreatitis and pancreatic cancer: all demonstrate a severalfold increased risk. In one large retrospective cohort study, there was a 10- to 20-fold increased risk of pancreatic cancer, even for patients with chronic pancreatitis for at least 5 years prior to the onset of pancreatic cancer [18].

About 1% of patients with chronic pancreatitis suffer from hereditary pancreatitis, an autosomal dominant inherited genetic disorder with an onset in childhood or in teenage. The cumulative risk of pancreatic cancer to age 70 years in these patients has been estimated to be almost 40% [19,20]. The high risk is presumably caused by the long duration of chronic pancreatitis.

Diabetes

This is a much more common disorder than pancreatitis, and has been established as a predisposing cause of pancreatic cancer. A recent meta-analysis of 36 studies (9,220 pancreatic cancer patients) suggests that the overall risk of pancreatic cancer is about 60% greater than in the background population of patients without diabetes (Fig. 44.2) [21]. The authors found an excess risk associated with diabetes even in the group of patients where diabetes had been present for 10 or more years. The risk is limited to patients with

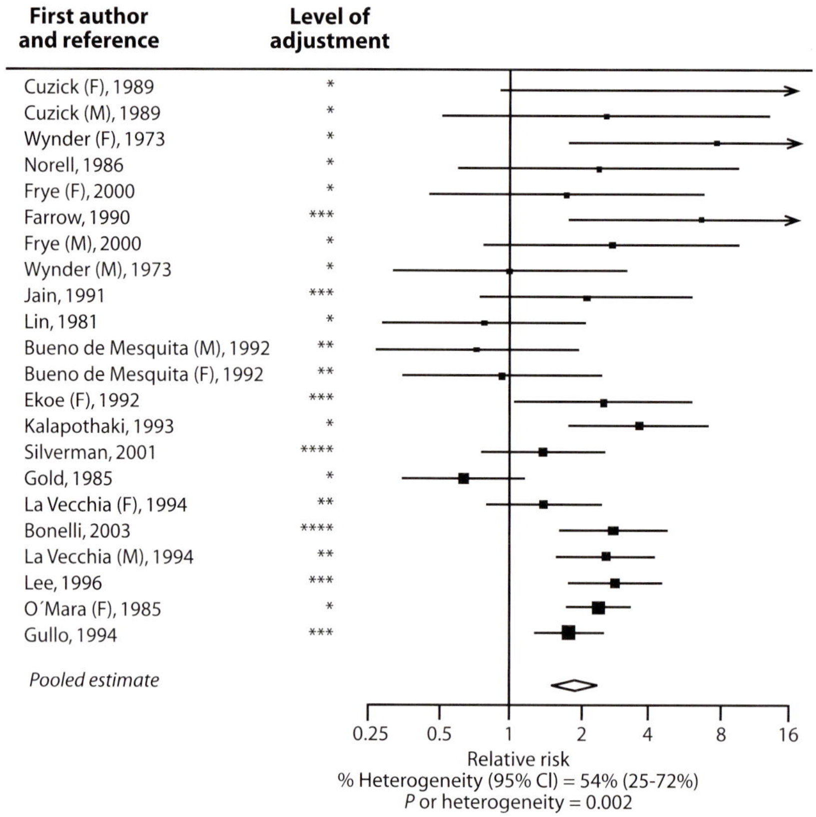

Figure 44.2

Diabetes and the risk of pancreatic cancer (with permission from [21]). *CI* Confidence interval. *Adjustment for age and sex; **adjustment for age, sex, and smoking or a marker of social class; ***adjustment for age, sex, smoking, and social class; ****adjustment for age, sex, smoking, social class, and dietary variables

type II diabetes; the rarer type I diabetes does not appear to be associated with pancreatic cancer.

Surgeons are aware that the onset of symptoms or signs suggestive of either pancreatitis or diabetes can also be an early indication of pancreatic cancer. Approximately 1% of recent-onset diabetics older than age 50 years will eventually be found to have an underlying pancreatic cancer [22]. At present there are no recommendations to screen patients with recent-onset diabetes for either pancreatitis or pancreatic cancer.

Infectious Diseases

Infectious diseases are a proven cause of liver and stomach cancer – two of the world's commonest tumors. Is there any evidence that either bacterial or viral infection can cause pancreatic cancer? Several studies have suggested a possible link between *Helicobacter pylori* infection and the subsequent development of pancreatic cancer [23–25]. However, the risk of pancreatic cancer is not especially elevated in those areas where *H. pylori* infection is common (i.e., developing and/or tropical countries). The possible relationship between *H. pylori* infection and pancreatic cancer merits further investigation.

Genetic Epidemiology

Several inherited germ-line cancer disorders have been linked with pancreatic cancer and some of these inherited diseases lead to early onset pancreatic cancer [26–36]. Of these, BRCA2 is the commonest, found in approximately 7–10% of patients with sporadic pancreatic cancer and in 10–20% of patients where there is a family history of pancreatic cancer. Most of these germ-line diseases are inherited in an autosomal dominant fashion except for three autosomal recessive disorders: ataxia-telangiectasia, cystic fibrosis, and Fanconi anemia. The probable genetic mutation is known for many inherited diseases where there is an increased risk of pancreatic cancer. Familial pancreatic cancer is an exception, but several groups are actively searching for the underlying genetic mutation. For surgeons, it is important to ask patients with pancreatic cancer about a family history of either pancreatic or other types of cancer to determine whether there is an underlying germ-line disorder.

Epidemiology of Pancreatic Surgery: Outcome Studies

Is the outcome following surgery for pancreatic cancer related to either hospital volume or to surgical experience? Several reports have studied this issue with similar findings: both the volume of surgery performed at a center and the experience of the operating surgeon have an impact on hospital mortality (Table 44.3)

As pointed out by Birkmeyer et al., even at a high-volume center, selecting an experienced surgeon will reduce operative mortality [41]. Furthermore, patients who receive therapy at centers with increased hospital volume or by more experienced surgeons have better survival statistics compared to other patients.

These findings suggest that operations for pancreatic cancer have a better short- and long-term outcome if performed at high-volume centers by experienced surgeons. In the USA, regionalization will increase travel time for these patients by an estimated 30 min [43]. Moreover, regionalization of patient care for pancreatic cancer will increase the opportunity for participation in much-needed randomized trials.

Preventive Aspects and Screening

Are there any drugs that effectively reduce the risk of pancreatic cancer? Certain anti-inflammatory agents have been shown to reduce the risk of some cancers and in this category of drugs, aspirin has been the most widely studied [44–48]. These studies are contradictory, so as yet there is no firm evidence that aspirin or other anti-inflammatory drugs protect patients against pancreatic cancer. But since aspirin is widely used as a preventive agent to reduce the risk of heart disease and possibly large bowel cancer, it may eventually prove to be helpful in preventing pancreatic cancer.

In some studies a reduced risk of cancer has been noted in persons with allergies, presumably caused by an alteration in the immune system. A recent meta-analysis of 13 population-based studies found that individuals with various types of allergies but especially in persons with atopic allergy, had a significant reduction in the risk of pancreatic cancer (Fig. 44.3) [49]. The realization of the importance of the immune system in pancreatic cancer has been the basis for current research on vaccine therapy for the treatment of pancreatic cancer [50]

Are there any special populations where the risk of pancreatic cancer is high enough to justify screening? At present, the only patients where the risk might be

Table 44.3. Impact of surgical and hospital volume on outcome after pancreatic surgery. *SEER* Surveillance Epidemiology and End Results

Author [reference]	Year	Population	Findings
Begg [37]	1998	USA SEER Medicare	12.9% operative mortality in low-volume centers compared to 5.8% in high volume centers
Gordon [38]	1999	State of Maryland	Adjusted mortality rate 12.5 times higher (95% CI = 6–25.8) in low- versus high-volume centers
Finlayson [39]	2003	USA nationwide sample	13.1% operative mortality in low-volume centers compared to 5.8% in high-volume centers
Backman [40]	2003	England, Wales	Longer survival for patients treated in high-volume centers (hazard ratio = 0.88, 95% CI = 0.83–0.93)
Birkmeyer [41]	2003	USA Medicare	Both surgical volume and hospital volume predict operative mortality. For surgeons performing <2-yearly operations mortality was 14.7%, compared to 4.6% mortality for surgeons with >4-yearly operations
Parks [42]	2004	Scotland 1993–1997	8% overall 30-day mortality unaffected by hospital or surgical volume. Risk of death at 3 years higher in patients treated by nonpancreatic specialists

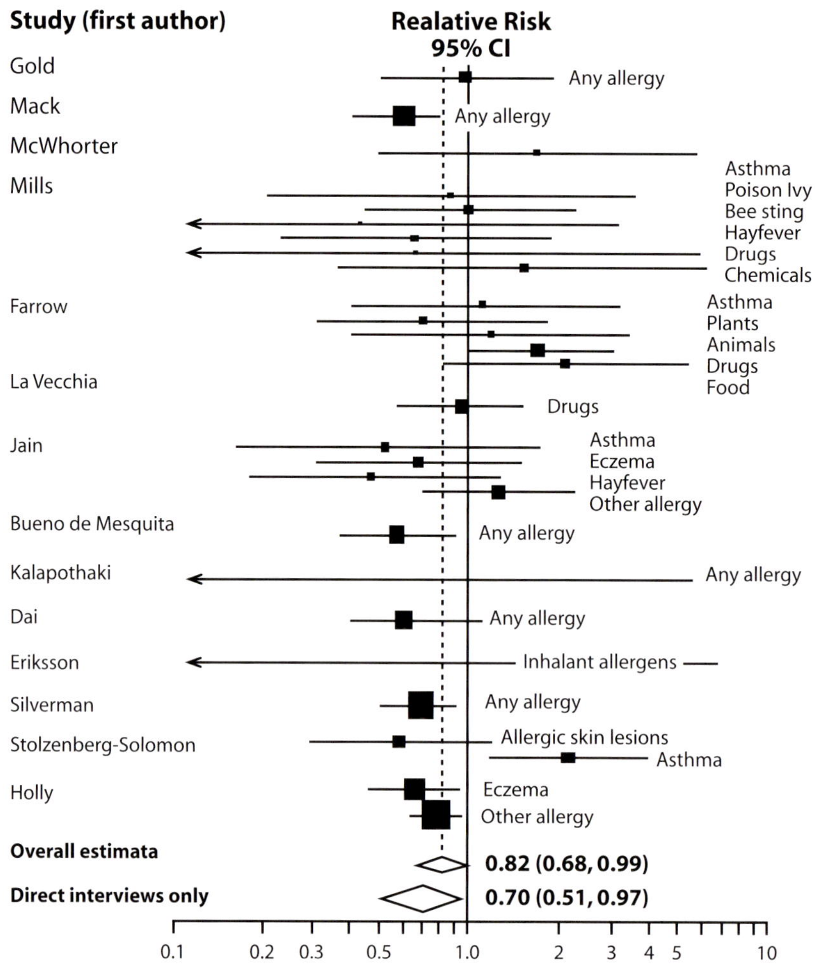

Figure 44.3

Relationship between allergy and pancreatic cancer (with permission from [49])

sufficiently high to make screening worthwhile are those rare individuals with the hereditary form of pancreatitis and perhaps patients with a strong family history of pancreatic cancer [51]. If screening is offered to these patients it should be performed as part of a research protocol in selected referral centers.

Summary

Within developed countries the burden of pancreatic cancer is remarkably similar, with an overall male and female cumulative incidence of about 1 and 0.65%. In most developed countries pancreatic cancer ranks high in the list of cancer mortality, being fourth in the USA and fifth in Japan and the UK.

The causes of pancreatic cancer remain obscure, with smoking, which doubles the risk of pancreatic cancer, the most clearly defined risk factor. Two antecedent diseases, diabetes and chronic pancreatitis, increase the likelihood of developing pancreatic cancer, but symptoms of both conditions can sometimes be the first manifestation of pancreatic cancer.

Since about 25–30% of pancreatic cancer is caused by smoking, efforts to control this important risk factor will substantially reduce the impact of pancreatic cancer. Only a few small groups of patients such as those with hereditary pancreatitis or familial pancreatic cancer are suitable for screening, which at present, should be performed as part of a research protocol.

Acknowledgments

Supported in part by grants from the C.D. Smithers Foundation, and Solvay Pharmaceuticals (ABL) and the Italian Association for Cancer Research (PM)

References

1. Parkin DM, Bray F, Ferlay J, Pisani P (2005) Global cancer statistics, 2002. CA Cancer J Clin 55:74–108
2. Globocan (2002) http://www-dep.iarc.fr/globocan/database.htm. 9-13-2005
3. Canques http://canques.seer.cancer.gov. 9-29-2005
4. Coughlin SS, Calle EE, Patel AV, Thun MJ (2000) Predictors of pancreatic cancer mortality among a large cohort of United States adults. Cancer Causes Control 11:915–923
5. Richie JP, Carmella SG, Muscat JE, Scott DG, Akerkar SA, Hecht SS (1997) Differences in the urinary metabolites of the tobacco-specific lung carcinogen 4-(methynitrosamino)-1-(3-pyridyl)-1-butanone in black and white smokers. Cancer Epidemiol Biomarkers Prev 6:783–790
6. Phillips AR, Lawes CM, Cooper GJ, Windsor JA (2002) Ethnic disparity of pancreatic cancer in New Zealand. Int J Gastrointest Cancer 31:137–145
7. Imamura Y, Mizuno S (2005) Comparison of pancreatic cancer mortality in five countries: France, Italy, Japan, UK and USA from WHO mortality database (1960–2000). Jpn J Clin Oncol 35:283–286
8. Silverman DT, Dunn JA, Hoover RN, Schiffman M, Lillemoe KD, Schoenberg JB, et al (1994) Cigarette smoking and pancreas cancer: a case-control study based on direct interviews. J Natl Cancer Inst 86:1510–1516
9. Doll R, Peto R, Wheatley K, Gray R, Sutherland I (1994) Mortality in relation to smoking: 40 years' observations on male British doctors [see comments]. BMJ 309:901–911
10. Lin Y, Tamakoshi A, Kawamura T, Inaba Y, Kikuchi S, Motohashi Y, et al (2002) A prospective cohort study of cigarette smoking and pancreatic cancer in Japan. Cancer Causes Control 13:249–254
11. Li D, Jiao L, Li Y, Doll MA, Hein DW, Bondy ML, et al (2006) Polymorphisms of cytochrome P4501A2 and N-acetyltransferase genes, smoking, and risk of pancreatic cancer1. Carcinogenesis 27:103–111
12. Michaud DS, Skinner HG, Wu K, Hu F, Giovannucci E, Willett WC, et al (2005) Dietary patterns and pancreatic cancer risk in men and women. J Natl Cancer Inst 97:518–524
13. Calle EE, Rodriguez C, Walker-Thurmond K, Thun MJ (2003) Overweight, obesity, and mortality from cancer in a prospectively studied cohort of U.S. adults. N Engl J Med 348:1625–1638
14. Ji BT, Chow WH, Gridley G, McLaughlin JK, Dai Q, Wacholder S, et al (1995) Dietary factors and the risk of pancreatic cancer: a case-control study in Shanghai China. Cancer Epidemiol Biomarkers Prev 4:885–893
15. Michaud DS, Giovannucci E, Willett WC, Colditz GA, Stampfer MJ, Fuchs CS (2001) Physical activity, obesity, height, and the risk of pancreatic cancer. JAMA 286:921–929
16. Lowenfels AB, Maisonneuve P, Lankisch PG (1999) Chronic pancreatitis and other risk factors for pancreatic cancer. Gastroenterol Clin North Am 28:673–85, x
17. Maitra A, Fukushima N, Takaori K, Hruban RH (2005) Precursors to invasive pancreatic cancer. Adv Anat Pathol 12:81–91
18. Lowenfels AB, Maisonneuve P, Cavallini G, Ammann RW, Lankisch PG, Andersen JR, et al (1993) Pancreatitis and the risk of pancreatic cancer. International Pancreatitis Study Group. N Engl J Med 328:1433–1437
19. Lowenfels AB, Maisonneuve P, DiMagno EP, Elitsur Y, Gates-LK J, Perrault J, et al (1997) Hereditary pancreatitis and the risk of pancreatic cancer. International Hereditary Pancreatitis Study Group. J Natl Cancer Inst 89:442–446
20. Howes N, Lerch MM, Greenhalf W, Stocken DD, Ellis I, Simon P, et al (2004) Clinical and genetic characteristics of hereditary pancreatitis in Europe. Clin Gastroenterol Hepatol 2:252–261
21. Huxley R, Ansary-Moghaddam A, Berrington DG, Barzi F, Woodward M (2005) Type-II diabetes and pancreatic cancer: a meta-analysis of 36 studies. Br J Cancer 92:2076–2083
22. Chari ST, Leibson CL, Rabe KG, Ransom J, de Andrade M, Petersen GM (2005) Probability of pancreatic cancer following diabetes: a population-based study. Gastroenterology 129:504–511
23. Stolzenberg-Solomon RZ, Blaser MJ, Limburg PJ, Perez-Perez G, Taylor PR, Virtamo J, et al (2001) Helicobacter pylori seropositivity as a risk factor for pancreatic cancer. J Natl Cancer Inst 93:937–941
24. Raderer M, Wrba F, Kornek G, Maca T, Koller DY, Weinlaender G, et al (1998) Association between Helicobacter pylori infection and pancreatic cancer. Oncology 55:16–19
25. Nilsson HO, Stenram U, Ihse I, Wadstrom T (2002) Re: Helicobacter pylori seropositivity as a risk factor for pancreatic cancer. J Natl Cancer Inst 94:632–633
26. Efthimiou E, Crnogorac-Jurcevic T, Lemoine NR, Brentnall TA (2001) Inherited predisposition to pancreatic cancer. Gut 48:143–147
27. Real FX, Malats N, Lesca G, Porta M, Chopin S, Lenoir GM, et al (2002) Family history of cancer and germline BRCA2 mutations in sporadic exocrine pancreatic cancer. Gut 50:653–657
28. Schmid RM (2002) Genetic basis of pancreatic cancer. Best Pract Res Clin Gastroenterol 16:421–433
29. Petersen GM, Hruban RH (2003) Familial pancreatic cancer: where are we in 2003? J Natl Cancer Inst 95:180–181
30. Hahn SA, Greenhalf B, Ellis I, Sina-Frey M, Rieder H, Korte B, et al (2003) BRCA2 germline mutations in familial pancreatic carcinoma. J Natl Cancer Inst 95:214–221
31. Ghiorzo P, Pastorino L, Bonelli L, Cusano R, Nicora A, Zupo S, et al (2004) INK4/ARF germline alterations in pancreatic cancer patients. Ann Oncol 15:70–78
32. Rogers CD, van der Heijden MS, Brune K, Yeo CJ, Hruban RH, Kern SE, et al (2004) The genetics of FANCC and FANCG in familial pancreatic cancer. Cancer Biol Ther 3:167–169
33. Goldstein AM (2004) Familial melanoma, pancreatic cancer and germline CDKN2A mutations. Hum Mutat 23:630
34. Koopmann J, Goggins M, Hruban RH (2004) Case 7-2004: hereditary melanoma and pancreatic cancer. N Engl J Med 350:2623–2624
35. Lynch HT, Deters CA, Lynch JF, Brand RE (2004) Familial pancreatic carcinoma in Jews. Fam Cancer 3:233–240
36. Couch FJ, Johnson MR, Rabe K, Boardman L, McWilliams R, de Andrade M, et al (2005) Germ line Fanconi anemia complementation group C mutations and pancreatic cancer. Cancer Res 65:383–386
37. Begg CB, Cramer LD, Hoskins WJ, Brennan MF (1998) Impact of hospital volume on operative mortality for major cancer surgery. JAMA 280:1747–1751
38. Gordon TA, Bowman HM, Bass EB, Lillemoe KD, Yeo CJ, Heitmiller RF, et al (1999) Complex gastrointestinal surgery: impact of provider experience on clinical and economic outcomes. J Am Coll Surg 189:46–56
39. Finlayson EV, Goodney PP, Birkmeyer JD (2003) Hospital volume and operative mortality in cancer surgery: a national study. Arch Surg 138:721–725

40. Bachmann MO, Alderson D, Peters TJ, Bedford C, Edwards D, Wotton S, et al (2003) Influence of specialization on the management and outcome of patients with pancreatic cancer. Br J Surg 90:171–177
41. Birkmeyer JD, Stukel TA, Siewers AE, Goodney PP, Wennberg DE, Lucas FL (2003) Surgeon volume and operative mortality in the United States. N Engl J Med 349:2117–2127
42. Parks RW, Bettschart V, Frame S, Stockton DL, Brewster DH, Garden OJ (2004) Benefits of specialisation in the management of pancreatic cancer: results of a Scottish population–based study. Br J Cancer 91:459–465
43. Birkmeyer JD, Siewers AE, Marth NJ, Goodman DC (2003) Regionalization of high-risk surgery and implications for patient travel times. JAMA 290:2703–2708
44. Anderson KE, Johnson TW, Lazovich D, Folsom AR (2002) Association between nonsteroidal anti-inflammatory drug use and the incidence of pancreatic cancer. J Natl Cancer Inst 94:1168–1171
45. Jacobs EJ, Connell CJ, Rodriguez C, Patel AV, Calle EE, Thun MJ (2004) Aspirin use and pancreatic cancer mortality in a large United States cohort. J Natl Cancer Inst 96:524–528
46. Menezes RJ, Huber KR, Mahoney MC, Moysich KB (2002) Regular use of aspirin and pancreatic cancer risk. BMC Public Health 2:18
47. Schernhammer ES, Kang JH, Chan AT, Michaud DS, Skinner HG, Giovannucci E, et al (2004) A prospective study of aspirin use and the risk of pancreatic cancer in women. J Natl Cancer Inst 96:22–28
48. Coogan PF, Rosenberg L, Palmer JR, Strom BL, Zauber AG, Stolley PD, et al (2000) Nonsteroidal ant-inflammatory drugs and risk of digestive cancers at sites other than the large bowel. Cancer Epidemiol Biomarkers Prev 9:119–123
49. Gandini S, Lowenfels AB, Jaffee EM, Armstrong TD, Maisonneuve P (2005) Allergies and the risk of pancreatic cancer: a meta-analysis with review of epidemiology and biological mechanisms. Cancer Epidemiol Biomarkers Prev 14:1908–1916
50. Laheru D, Jaffee EM (2005) Immunotherapy for pancreatic cancer – science driving clinical progress. Nat Rev Cancer 5:459–467
51. Durie P, Lerch MM, Lowenfels, AB, Maisonneuve P, Ulrich CD, Whitcomb DC (eds) (2002) Genetic Disorders of the Exocrine Pancreas. An Overview and Update. Karger, Basel

Chapter 45

R. H. Hruban · A. Maitra · N. Fukushima

Pathology of Pancreatic Cancer

A thorough understanding of the pathology of the pancreas is critical to the proper surgical management of patients with pancreatic disease. Some neoplasms of the pancreas are entirely benign and can be managed conservatively, while others are highly lethal malignancies that are best treated by aggressive surgical resection. This chapter provides a broad overview of the pathology of pancreatic neoplasia with emphasis on features important for the surgical management of patients with pancreatic disease.

Recent developments in our understanding of pancreatic neoplasia will also be discussed, particularly the growing recognition that a variety of noninvasive precursor lesions can give rise to invasive pancreatic cancer. These noninvasive precursor lesions create an opportunity to cure pancreatic neoplasia before an invasive cancer develops. At the same time they present a significant clinical management problem because there is precious little evidence-based medicine on which to judge when the benefit of removing a precursor lesion outweighs the risks of surgery.

In this chapter we will broadly divide our discussion of neoplasms of the pancreas into a description of those with predominantly exocrine differentiation and those with predominantly endocrine differentiation. The discussion of exocrine neoplasms will be further subdivided into those that are cystic and those that are solid.

Neoplasms of the Exocrine Pancreas

Cystic Neoplasms

Some of the characteristics of cystic neoplasms of the pancreas are compared in Table 45.1.

Serous Cystadenomas

These are benign epithelial neoplasms that are composed of uniform cuboidal glycogen-rich cells that form numerous small cysts containing serous fluid [8,32]. The mean age at diagnosis is 65 years (range 18–91 years), and most (70%) arise in women [16]. Presenting signs and symptoms are usually related to the presence of a large mass lesion in the abdomen. Most serous cystadenomas have a characteristic gross appearance (Fig. 45.1). They are well-demarcated masses composed of innumerable small cysts filled with straw-colored fluid [8,16,32]. Serous cystic neo-

Table 45.1. Cystic neoplasms of the pancreas

	Serous cystic neoplasm	Mucinous cystic neoplasm	Intraductal papillary mucinous neoplasm	Solid-pseudopapillary neoplasm
Mean age (years)	65	45	63	28
Gender (male:female)	30:70	10:90	60:40	10:90
Location within the pancreas	Evenly distributed	Body and tail	Head	Evenly distributed
Cyst contents	Watery straw colored fluid	Thick tenacious mucin	Thick tenacious mucin	Hemorrhagic
Connectivity to larger pancreatic ducts	No	No	Yes	No
Epithelial lining	Cuboidal, glycogen rich	Columnar, mucinous	Columnar, mucinous	Noncohesive uniform cells
Stroma	Nonspecific	Ovarian-type	Nonspecific	Delicate capillaries

plasms typically have a large central stellate scar that may calcify and they usually do not communicate with the pancreatic duct system. The calcified central scar is often appreciable on computerized tomography scans, and the lack of communication of the cysts with the duct system can be demonstrated by endoscopic retrograde cholangiopancreatography [56]. Gross variants include the macrocystic or oligocystic serous cystadenoma, the solid serous adenoma, and the combined well-differentiated endocrine neoplasm/serous cystadenoma. Because they form large unilocular masses, oligocystic serous cystadenomas can clinically mimic pseudocysts and mucinous cystic neoplasms [11,14,17,19,36,61]. Solid serous adenomas can grossly mimic pancreatic endocrine neoplasms (PENs) [55], and the combined well-differentiated endocrine neoplasm/serous cystadenoma is associated with the von Hippel-Lindau (VHL) syndrome [23,50,51].

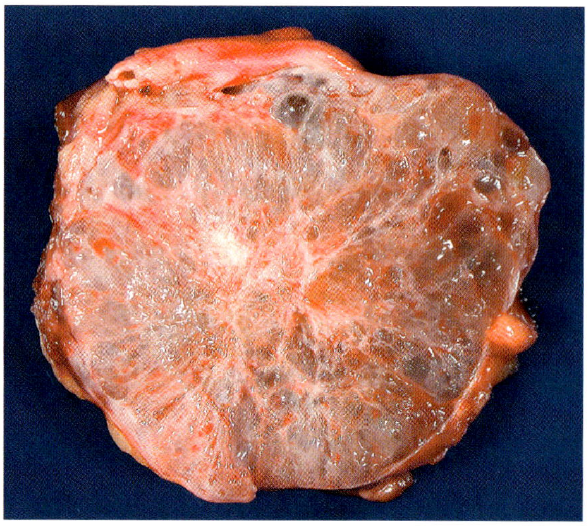

Figure 45.1

Serous cystadenoma. Gross cross-section revealing a well-demarcated mass composed of innumerable small cysts

Microscopically, serous cystadenomas are composed of cuboidal clear cells with uniform, centrally placed round nuclei (Fig. 45.2) [8,16,32]. The cells are optically clear because they contain abundant glycogen, and this glycogen can be highlighted by the periodic acid Schiff (PAS) stain.

At the genetic level, biallelic inactivation of the *VHL* gene has been reported both in serous cystadenomas in patients with the VHL syndrome and in adenomas in patients without VHL (nonsyndromic or sporadic adenomas) [45,66].

The vast majority of serous cystic neoplasms are entirely benign [8,16,32]. Only a handful of case reports of aggressive behavior have been reported. Serous cystic neoplasms that have metastasized are designated serous cystadenocarcinomas [18,54,69,75].

Mucinous Cystic Neoplasms

These are cystic epithelial neoplasms that are composed of mucin-producing epithelial cells associated with an ovarian type of stroma [32,70,71]. The vast majority arise in women (95%), although well-documented cases, including cases with ovarian stroma, have been reported in men [32,42,70,71]. The mean age at diagnosis is 45 years, and like serous cystade-

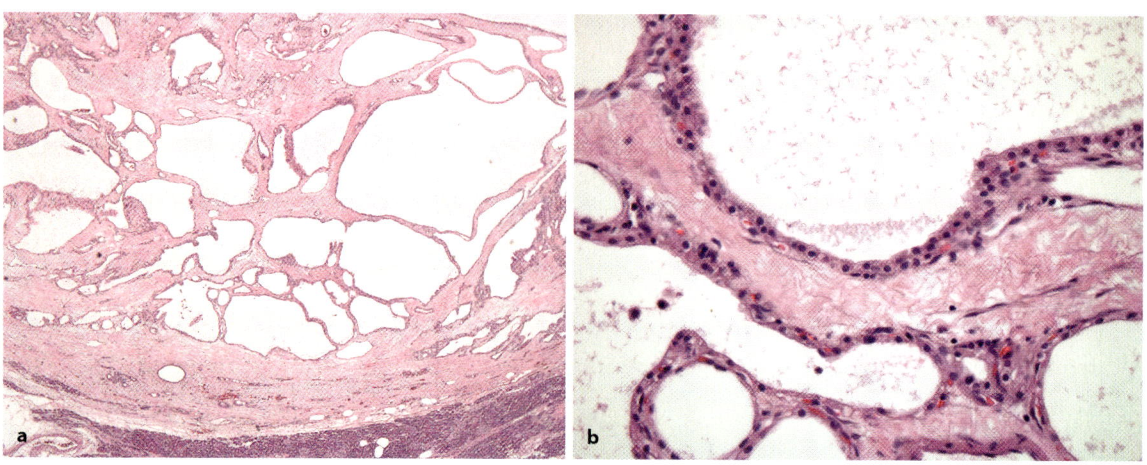

Figure 45.2

Serous cystadenoma. Low (a) and high-power (b) views demonstrating numerous small cysts lined by cuboidal epithelium with clear cytoplasm nomas, most patients present with signs and symptoms related to a large intra-abdominal mass lesion. Most arise in the body or tail of the pancreas and most mucinous cystic neoplasms do not communicate with the larger pancreatic ducts [32,70,71].

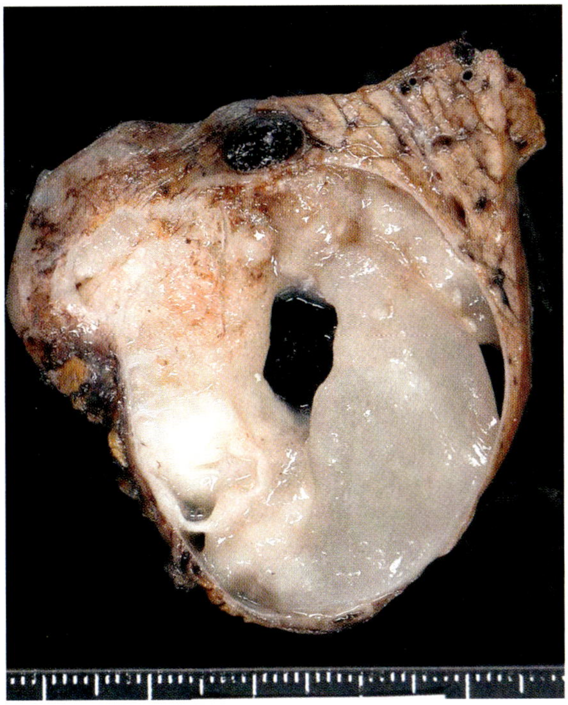

Figure 45.3

Mucinous cystic neoplasm. Gross cross-section revealing a large cystic neoplasm. The cyst is filled with thick tenacious mucin. Note the solid component on the left

Mucinous cystic neoplasms are usually solitary and large (mean 7–10 cm) [32,70,71]. They typically are well-demarcated and have a thick pseudocapsule. On sectioning they can be seen to be composed of multiple large (typically between 1 and 3 cm) cysts filled with thick tenacious mucin (Fig. 45.3). Some of the cysts may contain hemorrhagic fluid. The lining of the cysts is usually smooth in mucinous cystadenomas, while nodules and papillary excrescences can be seen in malignant examples.

Two features characterize mucinous cystic neoplasms at the light microscopic level (Fig. 45.4) [32,70,71]. First, the cysts are lined by columnar, mucin-containing epithelium. Second, the stroma has the appearance of ovarian stroma [20]. As noted grossly, the cysts typically do not communicate with the pancreatic ducts.

Noninvasive mucinous neoplasms can be categorized into mucinous cystic neoplasm with low-grade dysplasia (adenoma), mucinous cystic neoplasm with moderate dysplasia, and mucinous cystic neoplasm with high-grade dysplasia (carcinoma in situ) based on the degree of architectural and cytological atypia of the epithelial cells [32,70,71]. Remarkably, there is often significant heterogeneity in the degree of dysplasia in a single mucinous cystic neoplasm [15]. Parts of the lesion may be lined by completely bland epithelium, while elsewhere in the same tumor there may be high-grade dysplasia or even an invasive cancer [15]. It is therefore critically important to understand that biopsy or partial sampling cannot be used to evaluate the degree of dysplasia in a mucinous cystic neoplasm.

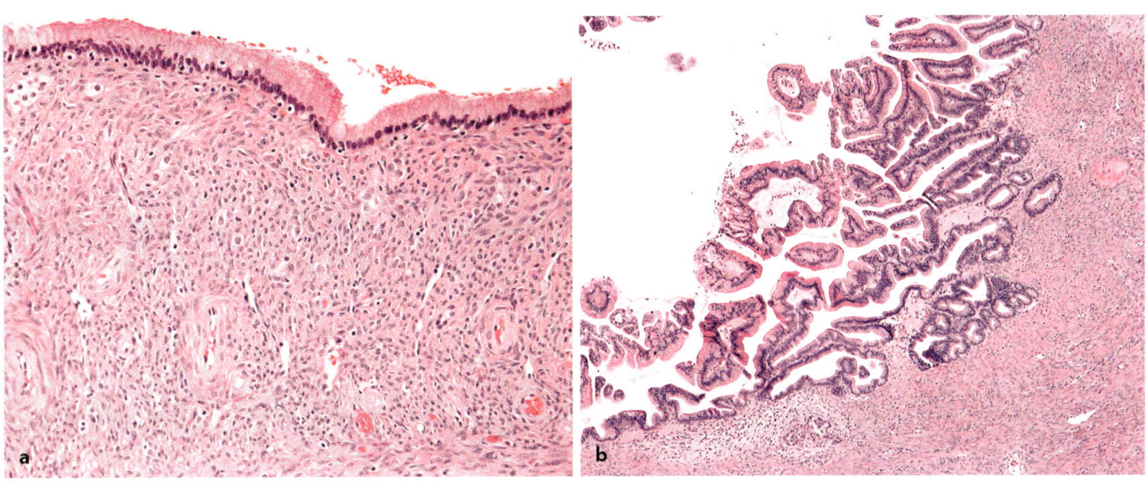

Figure 45.4

Mucinous cystic neoplasm. Microscopic images with mild dysplasia (a) and higher-grade dysplasia bordering on carcinoma in situ (b). Note the ovarian type of stroma

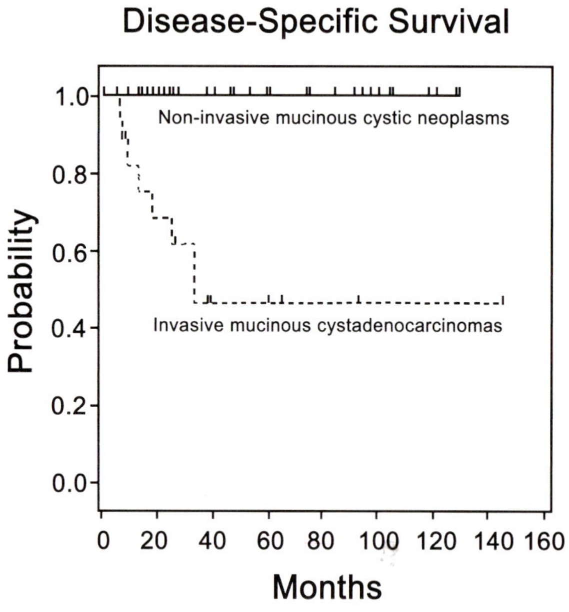

Figure 45.5

Mucinous cystic neoplasm survival curve comparing surgically resected patients with and without an associated invasive component (reprinted with permission [71])

One-third of all mucinous cystic neoplasms are associated with an invasive carcinoma, and this carcinoma is usually an invasive ductal adenocarcinoma or one of its variants. These neoplasms, not surprisingly, are designated a mucinous cystic neoplasm with an associated invasive adenocarcinoma. We try to avoid the less specific term "mucinous cystadenocarcinoma," because it can be applied to both lesions with in situ carcinoma and lesions with an invasive carcinoma. The identification of an invasive component has critical prognostic significance (Fig. 45.5). Patients with surgically resected mucinous cystic neoplasms that have been completely resected, thoroughly examined microscopically, and found not to have an associated invasive carcinoma have a close to 100% disease-specific survival rate [32,70,71]. By contrast, the 2-year survival rate for patients with a mucinous cystic neoplasm with an associated invasive carcinoma is approximately 67% and the 5-year survival rate is approximately 50% [32,70,71]. Confusion arises when mucinous cystic neoplasms are biopsied or inadequately sampled for microscopic examination. In these instances partial sampling may give the erroneous impression that a carcinoma is benign [15]. Simply put, the only way to determine whether a mucinous cystic neoplasm is benign is to completely resect the neoplasm and completely examine it microscopically.

Other adverse prognostic factors include the extent of invasion, patient age >50 years, and lymph node and distant metastases [32]. It should be noted that the survival rate for patients with a mucinous cystic neoplasm with an associated invasive adenocarcinoma is significantly better than that for patients with an invasive adenocarcinoma not associated with a mucinous cystic neoplasm.

Intraductal Papillary Mucinous Neoplasms

Intraductal papillary mucinous neoplasms (IPMNs) are grossly visible mucin-producing epithelial neoplasms that grow predominantly within the main pancreatic duct or one of its branches, and usually have papillary architecture [22,32,33,46]. IPMNs are slightly more common in men than in women (male to female ratio of 60:40), and the mean age at diagnosis is 63 years (range of 25–94 years) [60]. Interestingly, patients with an IPMN with an associated invasive carcinoma tend to be 3–5 years older than patients with noninvasive IPMNs [60].

IPMNs typically produce large quantities of mucin, and this mucin usually significantly dilates the pancreatic ducts, and often can be seen extruding from the ampulla of Vater, a finding virtually diagnostic of an IPMN [32,33,46]. Patients often present with signs and symptoms related to duct obstruction including abdominal pain, anorexia, weight loss, and recurrent episodes of pancreatitis.

Most IPMNs arise in the head of the pancreas (70%), although some involve the body and tail, and some diffusely involve the entire gland [32,33,46]. In contrast to mucinous cystic neoplasms, IPMNs can be multifocal. By definition, IPMNs involve the larger pancreatic ducts. Those that involve the main pancreatic duct are designated "main duct type," those that involve the secondary branches of the main pancreatic duct are designated "branch duct type," and those that involve both the main and branch ducts are called "combined type."

At the gross level, most IPMNs are intraductal, papillary, and clearly mucin-producing (Fig. 45.6) [32,33,46]. Noninvasive IPMNs tend to be smaller than IPMNs with an associated invasive carcinoma. An associated solid or gelatinous nodule should suggest the possibility of an associated invasive carcinoma. The microscopic findings parallel the gross findings. IPMNs are composed of intraductal mucin-secreting columnar epithelial cells with varying degrees of atypia (Fig. 45.7). Noninvasive IPMNs can be classified into three groups: IPMN with low-grade dysplasia (adenoma), IPMN with moderate dys-

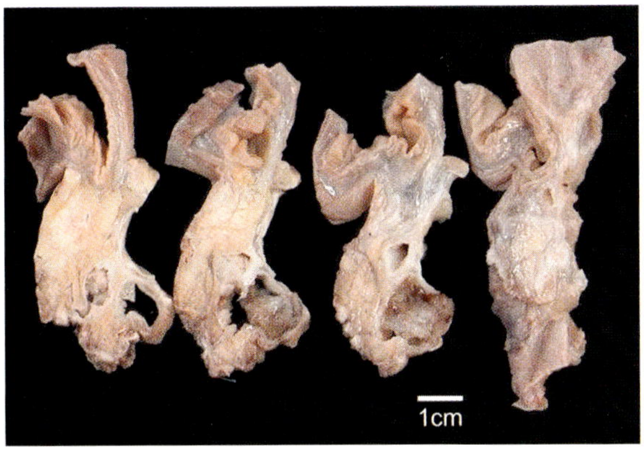

Figure 45.6

Intraductal papillary mucinous neoplasm (IPMN). Serial sections of the pancreas revealing an intraductal papillary mass (lower portion of the specimen). The duodenum is towards the top

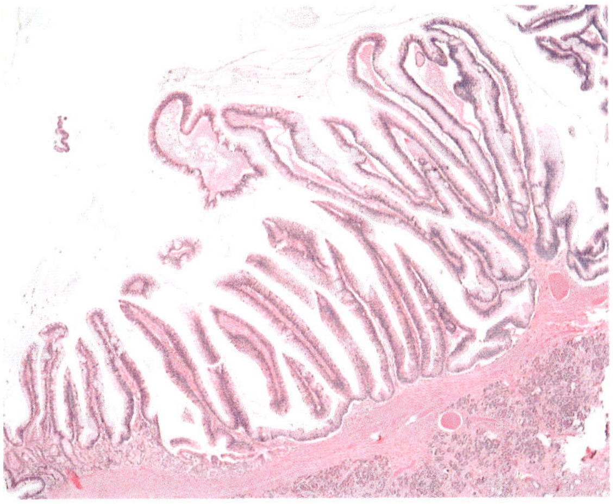

Figure 45.7

IPMN. This example is composed of long finger-like papillae lined by columnar mucin-producing epithelium. Not the prominent luminal mucin

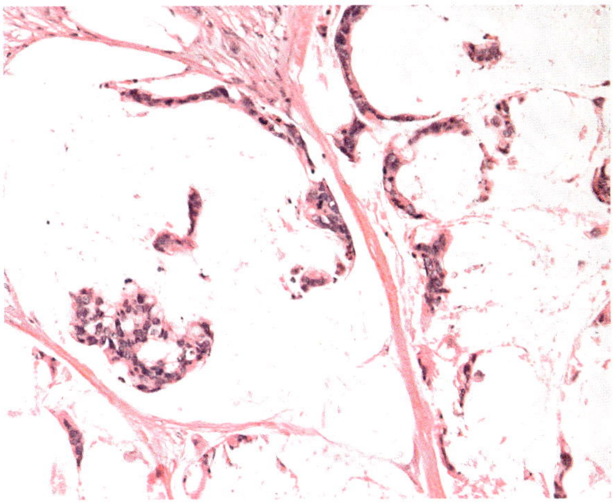

Figure 45.8

Colloid carcinoma. This neoplasm is composed of gland-forming mucin-producing epithelial cells embedded in extracellular pools of mucin

plasia, and IPMN with high-grade dysplasia (carcinoma in situ) based on the greatest degree of cytoarchitectural atypia present. In most cases immunohistochemical labeling will reveal the expression of the mucins MUC2 and MUC5AC [4]. In contrast to most ductal adenocarcinomas, most IPMNs are MUC1 negative.

In contrast to mucinous cystic neoplasms, the stroma associated with IPMNs is composed of relatively acellular collagen. Thus, IPMNs differ from mucinous cystic neoplasms in three important respects [21]. First, IPMNs are intraductal neoplasms while mucinous cystic neoplasms do not usually connect with the duct system. Second, IPMNs have an acellular stroma while mucinous cystic neoplasms have a distinctive ovarian-type stroma, and third, IPMNs can be multifocal, while mucinous cystic neoplasms are almost always solitary.

One-third of IPMNs have an associated invasive carcinoma [32,33,46]. This invasive carcinoma can be a typical ductal adenocarcinoma, or, in half the cases, it is a colloid (mucinous noncystic) adenocarcinoma [59]. Colloid carcinomas are characterized by abundant extracellular mucin production (Fig. 45.8). It is important to classify the type of invasive carcinoma because patients with IPMNs with an associated invasive colloid carcinoma appear to have a better prognosis than do patients with an IPMN with an associated invasive ductal adenocarcinoma [5].

The presence or absence of an associated invasive carcinoma is the single most important factor in determining patient prognosis [10,32,33,46,60]. Surgically resected noninvasive IPMNs have a 90–100% 5-year survival rate, while the 5-year survival rate for patients with an IPMN associated with an invasive carcinoma is 40% [10,60]. Prognosticators in patients with an IPMN with an associated invasive carcinoma include size of the invasive carcinoma, lymph node status, and the presence or absence of distant metastases. As noted earlier, patients with an invasive colloid carcinoma tend to do better than patients with an invasive ductal adenocarcinoma.

Slow growth and a prominent noninvasive growth phase provide an opportunity to surgically resect these neoplasms while they are still curable. The management of a patient with noninvasive IPMNs is, however, not always clear. Although there have been several reports of patients with an IPMN who were followed for years without progression of their disease, some noninvasive IPMNs clearly do progress to invasive cancer over time. Furthermore, the inability preoperatively to determine with certainty whether an invasive carcinoma component is present in an IPMN suggests that the decision to observe a patient with a known IPMN should not be taken lightly. Some have suggested that the size of an IPMN and the presence or absence of an associated mural nodule can guide treatment.

The multifocality of disease suggests that after the surgical resection of a noninvasive IPMN, patients are still at risk for additional neoplasms in the unresected portion of their gland [10,60]. Careful follow-up of patients, even those with noninvasive disease, is therefore warranted.

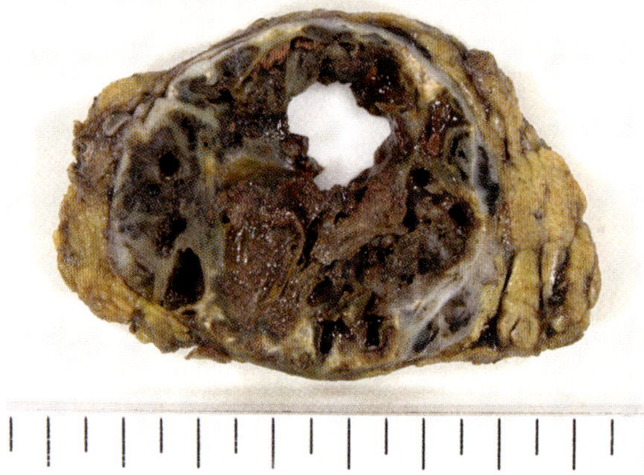

Figure 45.9

Solid-pseudopapillary neoplasm. The neoplasm appears relatively well-demarcated and contains solid areas as well as areas with prominent cystic degeneration and hemorrhage

Solid-Pseudopapillary Neoplasms

Solid-psuedopapillary neoplasms are low-grade malignant epithelial neoplasms composed of discohesive polygonal cells [1,32,43]. These cells surround delicate blood vessels and form solid masses with frequent cystic degeneration and intracystic hemorrhage. The majority of solid-pseudopapillary neoplasms occur in women (90%) in their 20s and 30s (mean age 28 years) [43]. Patients usually present with nonspecific symptoms related to an intra-abdominal mass, but some solid-pseudopapillary neoplasms rupture and cause hemoperitoneum.

Solid-pseudopapillary neoplasms can arise anywhere in the pancreas. They are often large (mean size 9–10 cm) and most appear grossly well-demarcated [42]. On cross-section most are solid and cystic (Fig. 45.9); the cystic areas are poorly defined and filled with necrotic debris and blood in various states of degeneration [43]. Rare solid-pseudopapillary neoplasms are completely solid, while other cases are almost completely cystic.

Solid-pseudopapillary neoplasms have a distinctive histologic appearance, but, remarkably, the direction of differentiation ("cell of origin") of these neoplasms is not well defined. The solid areas are richly vascular with delicate capillary-sized blood vessels and are composed of sheets of uniform cells with oval nuclei (Fig. 45.10). The nuclei often have a prominent nuclear groove. The cystic areas of the tumor are the product of degenerative changes within the neoplasm. The neoplastic cells are noncohesive and spaces between the cells are filled with necrotic debris and blood. Hyaline globules, foam cells, and cholesterol

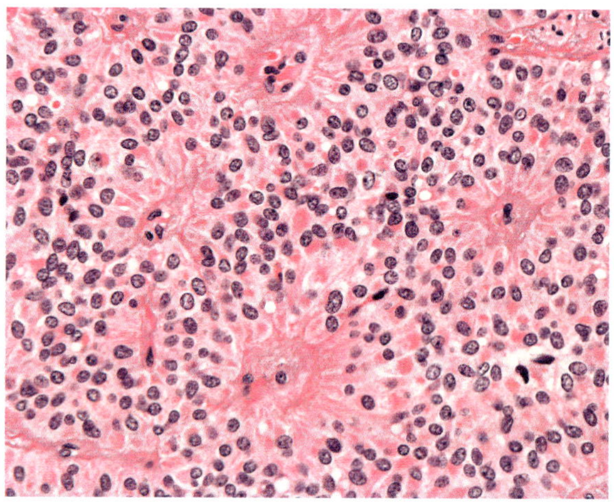

Figure 45.10

Solid-pseudopapillary neoplasm. The neoplastic cells are relatively uniform and surround delicate capillaries

crystals are typically present. The hyaline globules stain with the PAS stain.

Immunohistochemical labeling reveals the expression of vimentin, α-1 antitrypsin, and CD10 by the neoplastic cells [43,47,52]. In addition, >90% of solid-pseudopapillary neoplasms harbor genetic mutations in exon 3 of the *β-catenin* gene and these neoplasms show an abnormal nuclear pattern of labeling with antibodies to the β-catenin protein (Fig. 45.11) [1,63]. This latter feature is particularly useful in establishing the diagnosis.

Direct extension into adjacent organs can be seen, and a small minority (10%) of solid-pseudopapillary

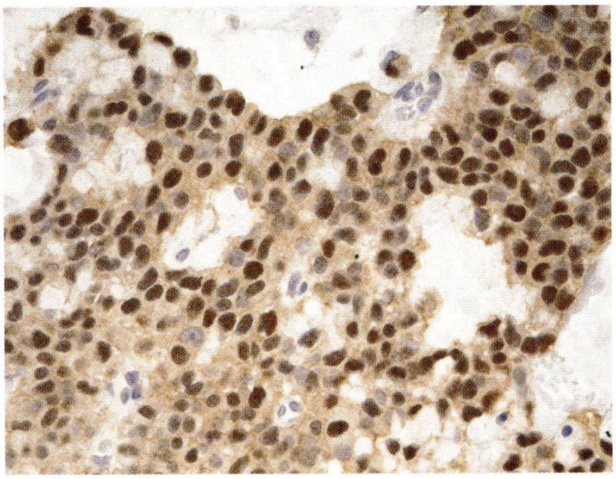

Figure 45.11

Solid-pseudopapillary neoplasm. Immunohistochemical labling for the β-catenin demonstrates the abnormal nuclear accumulation of the protein

neoplasms metastasize to distant organs including lymph nodes and the liver. Solid-pseudopapillary neoplasms often subtly infiltrate into the adjacent pancreatic parenchyma, a feature that does not have prognostic significance.

Surgical resection is the treatment of choice and long-term survival can even be achieved after the resection of metastases. It is rare for patients to die of their disease, but two patients with a particularly aggressive variant of solid-pseudopapillary neoplasm in which an undifferentiated component was present have recently been described [64].

Cystic Change in a Usually Solid Neoplasm

This can mimic a usually cystic neoplasm. Cystic change has been described in almost all usually solid neoplasms of the pancreas including ductal adenocarcinomas, pancreatic endocrine neoplasms, and even in intrapancreatic schwannomas.

Solid Exocrine Neoplasms

Some characteristics of solid exocrine neoplasms are compared in Table 45.2.

Infiltrating Ductal Adenocarcinoma

Infiltrating ductal adenocarcinoma is an invasive malignant epithelial neoplasm with glandular (ductal) differentiation [32,41]. It is the most common malignancy of the pancreas and it is also the most aggressive. This year it is estimated that 37,170 Americans will be diagnosed with pancreatic cancer and that 33,37 will die from the disease [34].

Common presenting signs and symptoms include epigastric pain that radiates to the back, weight loss, diabetes mellitus, jaundice, clay-colored stools, dark urine, pruritus, nausea, painless jaundice, and spontaneously appearing and disappearing thromboses (Trousseau's syndrome) [9,32,41].

Most infiltrating ductal adenocarcinomas arise in the head of the gland, but they may also arise in the body and tail [32,41]. The mean size of surgically resectable carcinomas of the head of the gland is 3 cm, and 5 cm for those arising in the tail of the gland. Ductal adenocarcinomas are usually poorly defined, firm, densely sclerotic masses (Fig. 45.12). The neoplastic cells often extend beyond the grossly identifiable tumor. Microscopically, these cancers are composed of gland-forming, mucin-producing epithelial cells admixed with a dense desmoplastic stroma (Fig. 45.13). In contrast to the normal pancreas, these neoplastic glands are haphazardly arranged. Perineural and lymphovascular invasion are common, and perineural invasion within the tumor is associated with perineural extension of the carcinoma into the retroperitoneum [28,74]. Ductal adenocarcinomas often obstruct the pancreatic duct. As a result, the nonneoplastic pancreatic parenchyma usually shows changes of chronic pancreatitis and, in some instanc-

Table 45.2. Solid neoplasms of the exocrine pancreas

	Ductal Adenocarcinoma	Acinar Cell Carcinoma	Pancreatoblastoma
Usual age at diagnosis (years)	60–80	Peak incidence in the 60s, a mean of 58	Mean 9.8 with a bimodal age distribution (newborn to 4, and 19–56)
Gender (male to female)	1.3:1	3.6:1	1.3–2:1
Presenting symptoms	Jaundice, pain, weight loss, cachexia	15% develop metastatic fat necrosis	Nonspecific, associated with Beckwith-Wiedemann syndrome
Direction of differentiation	Gland formation	Exocrine enzyme production (lipase, chymotrypsin, trypsin)	Acinar and squamoid nests

es, dilatation of the pancreatic duct (retention cyst formation).

A variety of systems have been established to grade the degree of differentiation in ductal adenocarcinomas [32,41]. Basically, the more closely the neoplastic glands resemble normal pancreatic ductal epithelium, the better differentiated the carcinoma. Well-differentiated ductal adenocarcinomas are composed of uniform well-formed glands with little or no architectural complexity or nuclear pleomorphism. Mitoses are rare and when present have a normal appearance. The neoplastic glands are less well formed in moderately differentiated ductal adenocarcinomas, and they are poorly formed in poorly differentiated ductal adenocarcinomas. In addition, there is a loss of polarity of the cells, greater nuclear pleomorphism, more mitoses, and more atypical mitotic figures as the degree of differentiation decreases.

Immunohistochemical labeling will reveal the expression of cytokeratin, particularly cytokeratins 7, 8, 13, 18, and 19 [32,41]. In addition, most ductal adenocarcinomas express epithelial membrane antigen (also known as MUC 1), carcinoembryonic antigen, carbohydrate antigen 19-9 (CA 19-9), B72.3 (TAG-72), CA 125, and DUPAN 2 [32,41]. Slightly more than a half of ductal adenocarcinomas show a complete loss of expression of Dpc4 (Fig. 45.14) [26,58,73].

Several genetic alterations in ductal adenocarcinomas have recently been defined. These include inactivation of tumor suppressor genes (*p16/CDKN2A*, *TP53*, *DPC4*) and activation of oncogenes (*KRAS2*, *AKT2*, *MYB*, *AIB1*) [32,41]. In addition, inactivation of one of the DNA mismatch repair genes (*MLH1* or *MSH2*) can be demonstrated in a small minority (4%) of ductal adenocarcinomas [24,72]. These latter carcinomas often have a distinct microscopic appearance called "medullary" histology (see below). In addition, the activation of the sonic hedgehog and notch signaling pathways appears to be common in ductal adenocarcinomas [7,48,65]. It is hoped that the identification of the genes altered in pancreatic cancer will lead to new methods for the early detection of pancreatic cancer and possibly mechanism-based therapies.

As noted earlier, the prognosis for patients diagnosed with pancreatic cancer is dismal [32,41]. The overall 5-year survival rate remains below 4%. Resectability is by far the most important prognostic factor. Prognosticators for surgically resected patients include stage, margin status, tumor size, major vessel involvement, degree of differentiation, and lymph node status.

Although these survival figures seem bleak, we believe that the recent recognition that infiltrating ductal adenocarcinomas arise from histologically well-defined, noninvasive precursor lesions provides an enormous opportunity to cure this disease. Just as infiltrating colorectal cancers arise from noninvasive adenomas, so too is it now clear that infiltrating ductal adenocarcinoma of the pancreas can arise from well-defined noninvasive precursor lesions called pancreatic intraepithelial neoplasias (PanINs) [30,31,62]. PanINs are noninvasive epithelial proliferations that are confined to the smaller ducts of the pancreas (Fig. 45.15). PanINs can show varying degrees of architectural and nuclear atypia. Those with minimal atypia are designated PanIN-1, those with moderate atypia PanIN-2, and those with significant atypia PanIN-3. A large body of clinical, morphological and molecular evidence makes it clear that some of these PanIN lesions progress to invasive ductal adenocarcinoma [30,31]. Simply put, lives will be saved if techniques can be developed to diagnose and treat PanINs before they progress to invasive cancer.

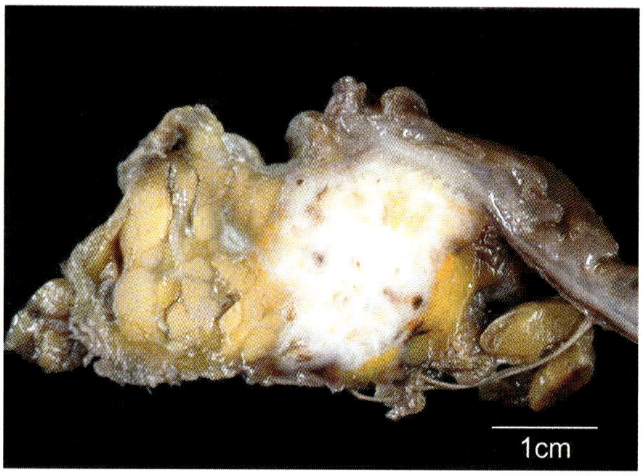

Figure 45.12

Ductal adenocarcinoma. Gross cross-section revealing a poorly defined sclerotic mass

The immediate question raised by the recognition of PanINs is what should be done when a PanIN is found at a surgical margin. Controlled studies to answer this question have not been performed. It is generally agreed that PanIN-1 and PanIN-2 are common in the population and that no additional therapy is needed if they are present at a margin. PanIN-3 is more difficult. While it is clear that some PanINs progress to invasive cancer, it is not known how frequently PanIN-3 progresses to invasive cancer, nor is it known how rapidly. That being said, additional pancreatic parenchyma should be resected for a PanIN-3 only when the patient can easily tolerate the procedure and when the patient's life expectancy is

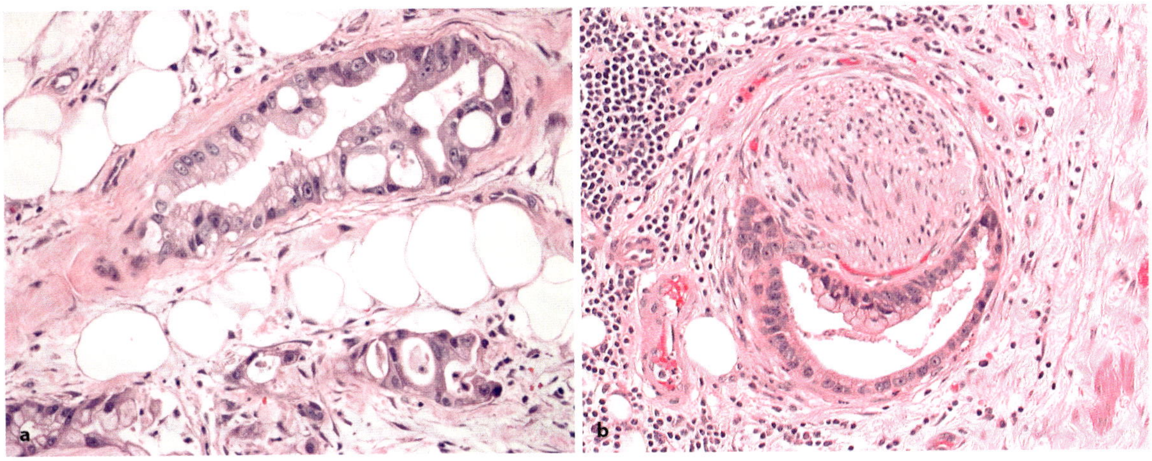

Figure 45.13

Ductal adenocarcinoma. Poorly formed glands composed of markedly atypical cells infiltrating into fat (a) and around a nerve (b)

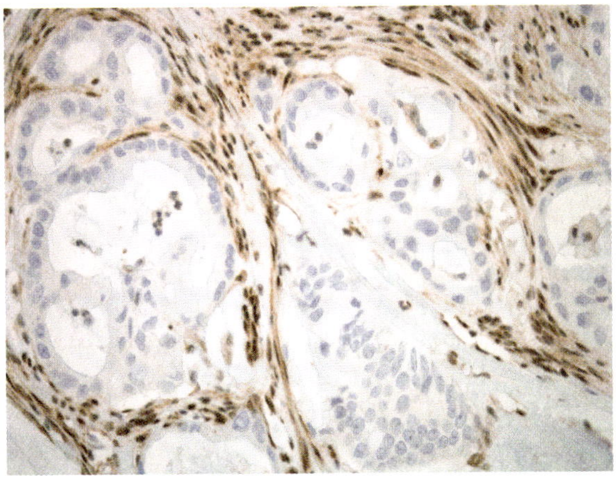

Figure 45.14

Ductal adenocarcinoma. Immunohistochemical labeling for Dpc4 revealing the complete loss of expression in the neoplastic glands. Note that the nonneoplastic stromal cells show a normal pattern of intact expression

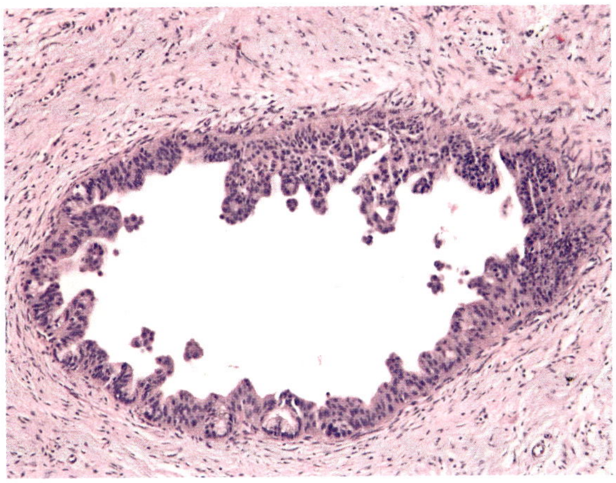

Figure 45.15

Pancreatic intraepithelial neoplasia (PanIN). This PanIN lesion shows marked atypia and would be classified as a PanIN-3 lesion

long enough that leaving a precursor behind would present a significant risk.

Variants of Adenocarcinoma

Several variants of ductal adenocarcinoma of the pancreas have been described. The most important include adenosquamous carcinoma, colloid carcinoma, hepatoid carcinoma, medullary carcinoma, signet ring cell carcinoma, undifferentiated carcinoma with osteoclast-like giant cells, and undifferentiated carcinoma. Adenosquamous carcinomas, as the name suggests, have significant components with both glandular and squamous differentiation [32]. They are a particularly aggressive variant of ductal carcinoma. Colloid carcinomas are characterized by abundant extracellular mucin production (Fig. 45.8) [5,59]. They are almost always associated with an intraductal papillary mucinous neoplasm and they appear to have a better prognosis than most ductal adenocarcinomas. Medullary carcinomas are characterized by poor differentiation, a syncytial growth pattern, and pushing borders [24,72]. They are interesting because, as noted earlier, they often show inactivation of one of

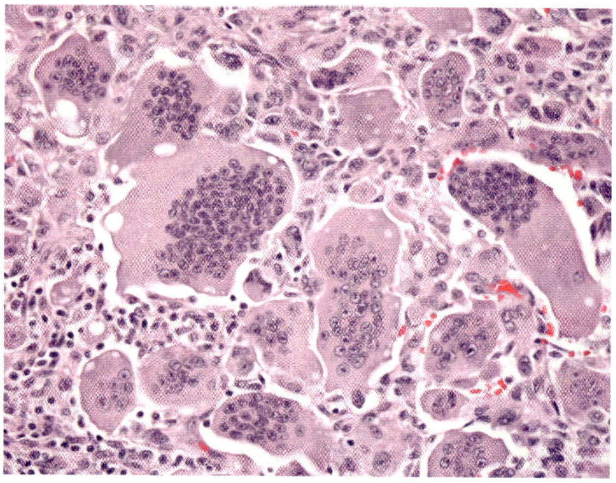

Figure 45.16

Undifferentiated carcinoma with osteoclast-like giant cells. Note the giant cells with numerous uniform nuclei scattered amongst atypical mononuclear cells

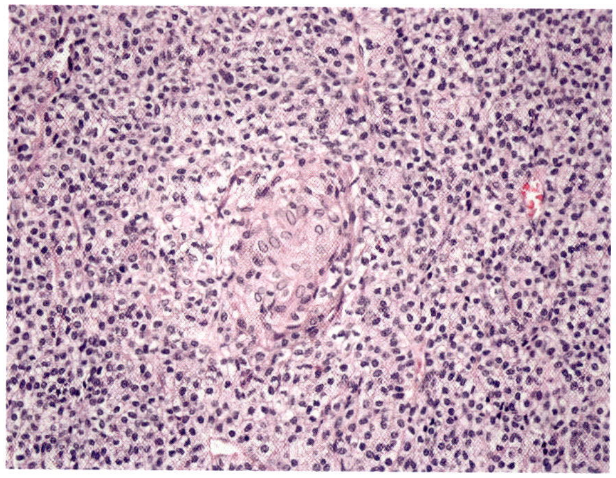

Figure 45.17

Acinar cell carcinoma. The neoplastic cells form small acini, they have abundant granular cytoplasm, and they frequently have single prominent nucleoli

the DNA mismatch repair genes. They may have a better prognosis and, based on experience in the treatment of medullary carcinomas of the colon, they may have a unique response to certain forms of chemotherapy. Signet ring cell carcinomas need to be distinguished from metastatic lobular carcinoma of the breast and signet ring cell gastric cancer metastatic to the pancreas. Undifferentiated carcinoma with osteoclast-like giant cells is a striking neoplasm composed of undifferentiated neoplastic mononuclear cells admixed with large benign-appearing multinucleated giant cells (Fig. 45.16) [68]. The direction of differentiation of these distinctive neoplasms was unknown for years, but it now appears that they are epithelial neoplasms with reactive multinucleated giant cells. Undifferentiated carcinomas are highly malignant neoplasms with little or no differentiation.

Acinar Cell Carcinoma

This is a malignant epithelial neoplasm with pancreatic exocrine (acinar) differentiation [2,32,38,39]. This differentiation can be established by the demonstration of exocrine enzyme production by the neoplasm (lipase, trypsin, chymotrypsin, etc.), or by the finding of zymogen granules at the ultrastructural level. Most patients are adults (mean 58 years), but acinar cell carcinomas can also occur in childhood [2,32,38,39]. The male to female ratio is as high as 3:1. Patients usually present with nonspecific symptoms related to a large mass lesion, but 15% of patients with acinar cell carcinomas present with the syndrome of metastatic fat necrosis. This dramatic syndrome is caused by the release of large quantities of lipase into the circulation, and is characterized by peripheral eosinophilia, polyarthralgias, and multiple foci of subcutaneous fat necrosis.

Grossly, most acinar cell carcinomas are large (mean 10 cm), well-demarcated, and soft and fleshy [2,32,38,39]. Microscopically, in contrast to ductal adenocarcinomas, most acinar cell carcinomas are cellular with little desmoplastic stroma. The neoplastic cells form small lumina, similar to nonneoplastic acini (Fig. 45.17). The nuclei contain single prominent nucleoli, and the cytoplasm has a granular appearance. Immunohistochemical labeling will reveal the expression of exocrine enzymes including lipase, chymotrypsin and trypsin. Electron microscopy, although rarely performed anymore, shows that the neoplastic cells contain numerous zymogen granules. Acinar cell carcinomas are very aggressive neoplasms, and the 5-year survival rate is only 5–10% [2, 32, 38, 39].

Pancreatoblastoma

Pancreatoblastoma is a distinctive malignant epithelial neoplasm with multiple lines of differentiation including acinar differentiation and squamoid nests [3,29,32,40]. Most pancreatoblastomas occur in children (mean age 9.8 years), but well-characterized cases have been reported in adults as well. Pancreatoblastomas are slightly more common in males than females, and many of the reported cases have been in Asians. Pancreatoblastomas have been reported in newborns with Beckwith-Wiedemann syndrome [35,44].

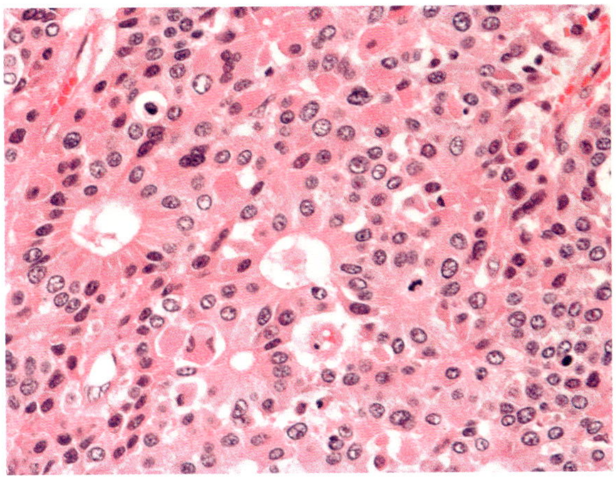

Figure 45.18

Pancreatoblastoma. A squamoid nest is present in the center of the field.

Grossly, pancreatoblastomas are usually large (mean 10 cm), well-demarcated, and on cut section they have a lobulated appearance. Microscopically, pancreatoblastomas, by definition, have at least two components an acinar cell component and squamoid nests (Fig. 45.18). Other components are also frequently present including cells with endocrine, ductal, and even mesenchymal differentiation. An immature component composed of small immature monotonous cells can also been seen.

The genetic changes of pancreatoblastomas are interesting. Like other neoplasms that arise in association with Beckwith-Wiedemann syndrome, pancreatoblastomas show loss of the maternal copy of the short arm of chromosome 11p near the *WT-2* locus (11p15.5) [3]. In addition, mutations in the *β-catenin* gene are seen in 50–80% of pancreatoblastomas [3].

Pancreatoblastomas are fully malignant neoplasms. One-third of patients have metastases at diagnosis and half will die from their disease. Not surprisingly, patients with unresectable disease and patients with metastases at presentation have a worse prognosis.

Neoplasms of the Endocrine Pancreas

Well-Differentiated PENs

Well-differentiated PENs are also known as islet cell tumors [12,32,37]. These neoplasms can be broadly grouped into nonsyndromic and syndromic PENs. Nonsyndromic PENs, as the name suggests, are tumors not associated with a clinical syndrome caused by excess hormone production. Syndromic PENs are neoplasms associated with both elevated serum hormone levels and clinical symptoms or findings associated with increased hormone levels (Table 45.3). Approximately 45% of syndromic PENs are insulinomas, 20% gastrinomas, 15% glucagonomas, 10% vasoactive intestinal polypeptide-secreting tumors, and 5% somatostatinomas [12,32,37].

Table 45.3. Pancreatic endocrine neoplasms (modified from Klimstra with permission [37]). *VIPoma*=Vasoactive-intestinal-polypeptide-secreting tumor

Type	Subtype	Size	Cell type	Syndrome	Clinical findings
Microadenoma		<0.5 cm	Any	None	None
Nonfunctional		Any	Any	None	Mass lesion
Functional	Insulinoma	Any	Beta cell	Insulinoma syndrome	Hypoglycemia
	Glucagonoma	Any	Alpha cell	Glucagonoma syndrome	Skin rash, stomatitis, diabetes
	Somatostatinoma	Any	Delta cell	Somatostatinoma syndrome	Diabetes, cholelithiasis
	VIPoma	Any	Unknown	Verner-Morrison syndrome	Watery diarrhea, hypokalemia, achlorhydria
	Gastrinoma	Any	G cell	Zollinger-Ellison Syndrome	Peptic ulcers
Poorly differentiated	Small-cell carcinoma	Any	Unknown		Aggressive metastatic carcinoma
	Large-cell endocrine carcinoma	Any	Unknown		Aggressive carcinoma

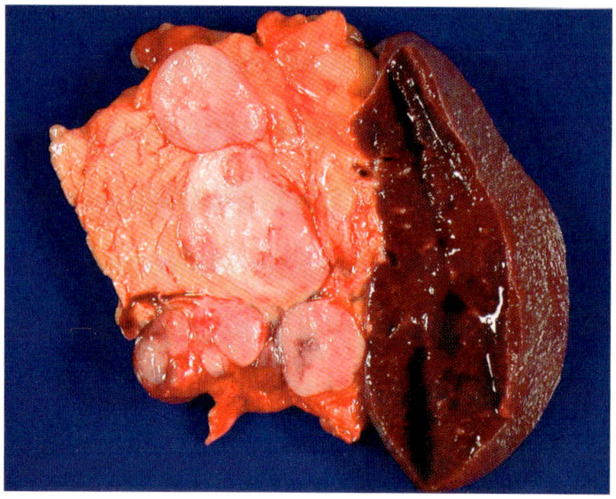

Figure 45.19

Pancreatic endocrine neoplasm (PEN). This example arose in the tail of the pancreas and has already spread to three adjacent lymph nodes

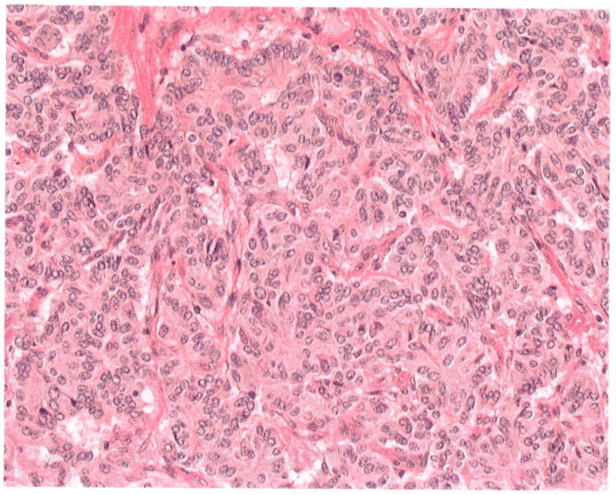

Figure 45.20

PEN. Microscopically these neoplasms are composed of uniform cells with a "salt and pepper" chromatin pattern

Most PENs form grossly well-demarcated uniform soft tan masses (Fig. 45.19). They are occasionally cystic, and cystic PENs can mimic other cystic neoplasms of the pancreas such as mucinous cystic neoplasms. Well-differentiated PENs less than 0.5 cm are designated microadenomas and are essentially always benign [12,32,37].

Microscopically, PENs are characterized by nests, ribbons or trabeculae of uniform cells (Fig. 45.20) [12,32,37]. These cells characteristically have "salt and pepper" nuclei and, by definition, a low mitotic rate. PENs immunohistochemically label with antibodies to the general endocrine markers chromogranin, synaptophysin, and CD56, and may also label with antibodies to specific endocrine peptides such as insulin, glucagon, and somatostatin (Table 45.3). It is important to note that immunohistochemical labeling for an endocrine peptide does not make a PEN syndromic. The designation of syndromic should only be applied to PENs associated with a clinical syndrome. Conversely, not all syndromic PENs label with antibodies to a specific endocrine hormone. In these latter instances it is believed that either the endocrine peptide is quickly released and therefore does not accumulate intracellularly, or that the antibody used to label the neoplasm was to an epitope not found on the peptide made by the tumor [12,32,37]. Electron microscopy will reveal dense core neurosecretory granules that measure 100–350 nm.

Some of the genetic alterations driving the development of PENs have recently been elucidated [27,49]. For example, patients with multiple endocrine neoplasia type 1 (MEN-1) have a germline mutation in the *menin* gene, and PENs in patients with MEN-1 show biallelic inactivation of the *menin* gene [6,25,67].

Well-differentiated PENs are significantly less aggressive than ductal adenocarcinomas. The 5-year survival for patients with a nonfunctioning PEN is 65% and the 10-year survival is 45% [12,32,37]. Unfortunately it is hard to predict the outcome of patients with well-differentiated PENs. As noted earlier, virtually all microadenomas (those less than 0.5 cm) are benign. PENs <2 cm with a low mitotic count and no large vessel invasion or metastases almost always follow a benign course. Prognosticators for larger PENs include size, mitotic rate, vascular invasion, extrapancreatic extension, necrosis, and lymph node or more distant metastases.

Small-Cell Carcinomas

Small-cell carcinomas of the pancreas are extremely rare [13,53,57]. Most small-cell carcinomas in the pancreas are actually metastases from a lung primary. Nonetheless, rare small-cell carcinomas primary to the pancreas do occur. These are highly malignant neoplasms and usually disseminated at diagnosis. Histologically, small-cell carcinomas are cellular neoplasms with an extremely high mitotic rate (>10 per 10 high-power fields), nuclear molding, and necrosis. Undifferentiated large-cell neuroendocrine carcinomas have also been described in the pancreas. Little is known about these rare neoplasms, but they are believed to behave similarly to large-cell neuroendocrine carcinomas of the lung.

Other Neoplasms in the Pancreas

Most of the neoplasms that occur outside of the pancreas can also occur within the pancreas. This includes mesenchymal neoplasms and lymphomas. The pathological findings for these neoplasms when they arise within the pancreas parallel those of similar neoplasms that arise outside of the gland.

Although rare, metastases to the pancreas have to be considered in the differential diagnosis of a pancreatic mass. We have seen examples of renal cell carcinoma, breast cancer, melanoma, and gastric carcinoma metastatic to the pancreas that have mimicked primary pancreatic neoplasms.

Conclusions

One of the more exciting developments in the last decade has been the demonstration that invasive ductal adenocarcinoma arises from histologically well-defined, noninvasive precursor lesions, including mucinous cystic neoplasms, IPMNs, and pancreatic intraepithelial neoplasia. These precursor lesions represent an opportunity to cure pancreatic neoplasia, but they also present a challenge to the surgeon, who must decide when to intervene in a given patient.

The pathologic diagnosis forms the cornerstone of good surgical management of a patient with pancreatic disease. Conversely, accurate pathologic diagnoses are dependent on an integration of clinical and pathologic findings (Tables 45.1–45.3). Excellent communication between surgeon and pathologist is therefore essential for good patient care.

References

1. Abraham SC, Klimstra DS, Wilentz RE, Wu T-T, Cameron JL, Yeo CJ, Hruban RH (2002) Solid-pseudopapillary tumors of the pancreas are genetically distinct from pancreatic ductal adenocarcinomas and almost always harbor beta-catenin mutations. Am J Pathol 160:1361–1369
2. Abraham SC, Wu TT, Hruban RH, Lee JH, Yeo CJ, Conlon K, Brennan MF, Cameron JL, Klimstra DS (2002) Genetic and immunohistochemical analysis of pancreatic acinar cell carcinoma: frequent allelic loss on chromosome 11p and alterations in the APC/beta-catenin pathway. Am J Pathol 160:953–962
3. Abraham SC, Wu TT, Klimstra DS, Finn L, Hruban RH (2001) Distinctive molecular genetic alterations in sporadic and familial adenomatous polyposis-associated pancreatoblastomas: frequent alterations in the APC/beta-catenin pathway and chromosome 11p. Am J Pathol 159:1619–1627
4. Adsay NV, Merati K, Basturk O, Iacobuzio-Donahue CA, Levi E, Cheng JD, Sarkar FH, Hruban RH, Klimstra DS (2004) Pathologically and biologically distinct types of epithelium in intraductal papillary mucinous neoplasms: delineation of an "intestinal" pathway of carcinogenesis in the pancreas. Am J Surg Pathol 28:839–848
5. Adsay NV, Pierson C, Sarkar F, Abrams J, Weaver D, Conlon K, Brennan MF, Klimstra DS (2001) Colloid (mucinous noncystic) carcinoma of the pancreas. Am J Surg Pathol 25:26–42
6. Bartsch D, Kopp I, Bergenfelz A, Rieder H, Munch K, Jager K, Deiss Y, Schudy A, Barth P, Arnold R, Rothmund M, Simon B (1998) MEN1 gene mutations in 12 MEN1 families and their associated tumors. Eur J Endocrinol 139:416–20
7. Berman DM, Karhadkar SS, Maitra A, Montes DO, Gerstenblith MR, Briggs K, Parker AR, Shimada Y, Eshleman JR, Watkins DN, Beachy PA (2003) Widespread requirement for Hedgehog ligand stimulation in growth of digestive tract tumours. Nature 425:846–851
8. Capella C, Solcia E, Klöppel G, Hruban RH (2000) Serous cystic neoplasms of the pancreas. In: Hamilton SR, Aaltonen LA (eds) World Health Organization Classification of Tumours. Pathology and Genetics of Tumours of the Digestive System. IARC Press, Lyon, pp 231–233
9. Chari ST, Leibson CL, Rabe KG, Ransom J, de Andrade M, Petersen GM (2005) Probability of pancreatic cancer following diabetes: a population-based study. Gastroenterology 129:504–511
10. Chari ST, Yadav D, Smyrk TC, DiMagno EP, Miller LJ, Raimondo M, Clain JE, Norton IA, Pearson RK, Petersen BT, Wiersema MJ, Farnell MB, Sarr MG (2002) Study of recurrence after surgical resection of intraductal papillary mucinous neoplasm of the pancreas. Gastroenterology 123:1500–1507
11. Chatelain D, Hammel P, O'Toole D, Terris B, Vilgrain V, Palazzo L, Belghiti J, Levy P, Ruszniewski P, Flejou JF (2002) Macrocystic form of serous pancreatic cystadenoma. Am J Gastroenterol 97:2566–2571
12. Chetty R, Asa SL (2004) Pancreatic endocrine tumors: an update. Adv Anat Pathol 11:202–210
13. Chetty R, Clark SP, Pitson GA (1993) Primary small cell carcinoma of the pancreas. Pathology 25:240–242
14. Cohen-Scali F, Vilgrain V, Brancatelli G, Hammel P, Vullierme MP, Sauvanet A, Menu Y (2003) Discrimination of unilocular macrocystic serous cystadenoma from pancreatic pseudocyst and mucinous cystadenoma with CT: initial observations. Radiology 228:727–733
15. Compagno J, Oertel JE (1978) Mucinous cystic neoplasms of the pancreas with overt and latent malignancy (cystadenocarcinoma and cystadenoma). A clinicopathologic study of 41 cases. Am J Clin Pathol 69:573–580
16. Compton CC (2000) Serous cystic tumors of the pancreas. Semin Diagn Pathol 17:43–55
17. Egawa N, Maillet B, Schroder S, Mukai K, Klöppel G (1994) Serous oligocystic and ill-demarcated adenoma of the pancreas: a variant of serous cystic adenoma. Virchows Arch 424:13–17
18. Eriguchi N, Aoyagi S, Nakayama T, Hara M, Miyazaki T, Kutami R, Jimi A (1998) Serous cystadenocarcinoma of the pancreas with liver metastases. J Hepatobiliary Pancreat Surg 5:467–470
19. Fujiwara H, Ajiki T, Fukuoka K, Mitsutsuji M, Yamamoto M, Kuroda Y (2000) Macrocystic serous cystadenoma of the pancreas. J Hepatobiliary Pancreat Surg 7:92–96

20. Fukushima N, Mukai K (1997) 'Ovarian-type' stroma of pancreatic mucinous cystic tumor expresses smooth muscle phenotype. Pathol Int 47:806–808
21. Fukushima N, Mukai K (2000) Differential diagnosis between intraductal papillary-mucinous tumors and mucinous cystic tumors of the pancreas. Int J Surg Pathol 8:271–278
22. Fukushima N, Mukai K, Kanai Y, Hasebe T, Shimada K, Ozaki H, Kinoshita T, Kosuge T (1997) Intraductal papillary tumors and mucinous cystic tumors of the pancreas: clinicopathologic study of 38 cases. Hum Pathol 28:1010–1017
23. Girelli R, Bassi C, Falconi M, De Santis L, Bonora A, Caldiron E, Sartori N, Salvia R, Briani G, Pederzoli P (1997) Pancreatic cystic manifestations in von Hippe-Lindau disease. Int J Pancreatol 22:101–109
24. Goggins M, Offerhaus GJ, Hilgers W, Griffin CA, Shekher M, Tang D, Sohn TA, Yeo CJ, Kern SE, Hruban RH (1998) Pancreatic adenocarcinomas with DNA replication errors (RER+) are associated with wild-type K-ras and characteristic histopathology. Poor differentiation, a syncytial growth pattern, and pushing borders suggest RER+. Am J Pathol 152:1501–1507
25. Gortz B, Roth J, Krahenmann A, de Krijger RR, Muletta-Feurer S, Rutimann K, Saremaslani P, Speel EJ, Heitz PU, Komminoth P (1999) Mutations and allelic deletions of the MEN1 gene are associated with a subset of sporadic endocrine pancreatic and neuroendocrine tumors and not restricted to foregut neoplasms. Am J Pathol 154:429–36
26. Hahn SA, Schutte M, Hoque AT, Moskaluk CA, da Costa LT, Rozenblum E, Weinstein CL, Fischer A, Yeo CJ, Hruban RH, Kern SE (1996) DPC4, a candidate tumor suppressor gene at human chromosome 18q21.1. Science 271:350–353
27. Hessman O, Lindberg D, Einarsson A, Lillhager P, Carling T, Grimelius L, Eriksson B, Akerstrom G, Westin G, Skogseid B (1999) Genetic alterations on 3p, 11q13, and 18q in nonfamilial and MEN 1-associated pancreatic endocrine tumors. Genes Chromosomes Cancer 26:258–264
28. Hirai I, Kimura W, Ozawa K, Kudo S, Suto K, Kuzu H, Fuse A (2002) Perineural invasion in pancreatic cancer. Pancreas 24:15–25
29. Horie A, Yano Y, Kotoo Y, Miwa A (1977) Morphogenesis of pancreatoblastoma, infantile carcinoma of the pancreas; report of two cases. Cancer 39:247–254
30. Hruban RH, Adsay NV, Albores-Saavedra J, Compton C, Garrett E, Goodman SN, Kern SE, Klimstra DS, Klöppel G, Longnecker DS, Lüttges J, Offerhaus GJ (2001) Pancreatic intraepithelial neoplasia: a new nomenclature and classification system for pancreatic duct lesions. Am J Surg Pathol 25:579–586
31. Hruban RH, Goggins M, Parsons JL, Kern SE (2000) Progression model for pancreatic cancer. Clin Cancer Res 6:2969–2972
32. Hruban RH, Pitman MB, Klimstra DS (2006) Atlas of tumor pathology. Tumors of the pancreas. 4th series, Fascicle 6. Armed Forces Institute of Pathology, Washington, DC
33. Hruban RH, Takaori K, Klimstra DS, Adsay NV, Albores-Saavedra J, Biankin AV, Biankin SA, Compton C, Fukushima N, Furukawa T, Goggins M, Kato Y, Klöppel G, Longnecker DS, Lüttges J, Maitra A, Offerhaus GJ, Shimizu M, Yonezawa S (2004) An illustrated consensus on the classification of pancreatic intraepithelial neoplasia and intraductal papillary mucinous neoplasms. Am J Surg Pathol 28:977–987
34. Jemal A, Tiwari RC, Murray T, Ghafoor A, Samuels A, Ward E, Feuer EJ, Thun MJ (2004) Cancer statistics, 2004. CA Cancer J Clin 54:8–29
35. Kerr NJ, Fukuzawa R, Reeve AE, Sullivan MJ, Fukazawa R (2002) Beckwith-Wiedemann syndrome, pancreatoblastoma, and the wnt signaling pathway. Am J Pathol 160:1541–1542
36. Khurana B, Mortele KJ, Glickman J, Silverman SG, Ros PR (2003) Macrocystic serous adenoma of the pancreas: radiologic-pathologic correlation. AJR Am J Roentgenol 181:119–123
37. Klimstra DS (2005) Tumors of the endocrine system. In: Von Hoff DD, Evans DB, Hruban RH (eds) Pancreatic Cancer, Jones and Bartlett, Boston, pp 586–599
38. Klimstra DS, Heffess CS, Oertel JE, Rosai J (1992) Acinar cell carcinoma of the pancreas. A clinicopathologic study of 28 cases. Am J Surg Pathol 16:815–837
39. Klimstra DS, Longnecker DS (2000) Acinar cell carcinoma. In: Hamilton SR, Aaltonen LA (eds) World Health Organization Classification of Tumours. Pathology and Genetics of Tumours of the Digestive System. IARC Press, Lyon, pp 241–243
40. Klimstra DS, Wenig BM, Adair CF, Heffess CS (1995) Pancreatoblastoma. A clinicopathologic study and review of the literature. Am J Surg Pathol 19:1371–1389
41. Klöppel G, Hruban RH, Longnecker DS, Adler G, Kern SE, Partanen TJ (2000) Ductal adenocarcinoma of the pancreas. In: Hamilton SR, Aaltonen LA (eds) World Health Organization Classification of Tumours. Pathology and Genetics of Tumours of the Digestive System. IARC Press, Lyon, pp 221–230
42. Klöppel G, Kosmahl M (2001) Cystic lesions and neoplasms of the pancreas. The features are becoming clearer. Pancreatology. 1:648–655
43. Klöppel G, Lüttges J, Klimstra DS, Hruban RH, Kern SE, Adler G (2000) Solid-pseudopapillary neoplasm. In: Hamilton SR, Aaltonen LA (eds) World Health Organization Classification of Tumours. Pathology and Genetics of Tumours of the Digestive System. IARC Press, Lyon, pp 246–248
44. Koh TH, Cooper JE, Newman CL, Walker TM, Kiely EM, Hoffmann EB (1986) Pancreatoblastoma in a neonate with Wiedemann-Beckwith syndrome. Eur J Pediatr 145:435–438
45. Latif F, Tory K, Gnarra J, Yao M, Duh F-M, Orcutt ML, Stackhouse T, Kuzmin I, Modi W, Geil L, Schmidt L, Zhou F, Li H, Wei MH, Chen F, Glenn G, Choyke P, Walther MM, Weng Y, Duan D-SR, Dean M, Glavac D, Richards FM, Crossey PA, Ferguson-Smith MA, Le Paslier D, Chumakov I, Cohen DJ, Chinault AC, Maher ER, Linehan WM, Zbar B, Lerman MI (1993) Identification of the von Hippel-Lindau disease tumor suppressor gene. Science 260:1317–1320
46. Longnecker DS, Adler G, Hruban RH, Klöppel G (2000) Intraductal papillary-mucinous neoplasms of the pancreas. In: Hamilton SR, Aaltonen LA (eds) World Health Organization Classification of Tumours. Pathology and Genetics of Tumours of the Digestive System. IARC Press, Lyon, pp 237–240
47. Miettinen M, Partanen S, Fräki O, Kivilaakso E (1987) Papillary cystic tumor of the pancreas. An analysis of cellular differentiation by electron microscopy and immunohistochemistry. Am J Surg Pathol 11:855–865
48. Miyamoto Y, Maitra A, Ghosh B, Zechner U, Argani P, Iacobuzio-Donahue CA, Sriuranpong V, Iso T, Meszoely IM, Wolfe MS, Hruban RH, Ball DW, Schmid RM, Leach SD (2003) Notch mediates TGF alpha-induced changes in epithelial differentiation during pancreatic tumorigenesis. Cancer Cell 3:565–576

49. Moore PS, Missiaglia E, Antonello D, Zamo A, Zamboni G, Corleto V, Falconi M, Scarpa A (2001) Role of disease-causing genes in sporadic pancreatic endocrine tumors: MEN1 and VHL. Genes Chromosomes Cancer 32:177–81
50. Mukhopadhyay B, Sahdev A, Monson JP, Besser GM, Reznek RH, Chew SL (2002) Pancreatic lesions in von Hippel-Lindau disease. Clin Endocrinol (Oxf) 57:603–608
51. Neumann HP, Dinkel E, Brambs H, Wimmer B, Friedburg H, Volk B, Sigmund G, Riegler P, Haag K, Schollmeyer P (1991) Pancreatic lesions in the von Hippel-Lindau syndrome. Gastroenterology 101:465–471
52. Notohara K, Hamazaki S, Tsukayama C, Nakamoto S, Kawabata K, Mizobuchi K, Sakamoto K, Okada S (2000) Solid-pseudopapillary tumor of the pancreas: immunohistochemical localization of neuroendocrine markers and CD10. Am J Surg Pathol 24:1361–1371
53. O'Connor TP, Wade TP, Sunwoo YC, Reimers H, Palmer DC, Silverberg AB, Johnson FE (1992) Small cell undifferentiated carcinoma of the pancreas. Report of a patient with tumor marker studies. Cancer 70:1514–1519
54. Okata T, Nonami T, Miwa T, Yamada F, Ando K, Tathmatsu T, Sugie S, Kondo T (1991) Hepatic metastasis of serous cystadenocarcinoma resected 4 years after operation – a case report. Nippon Shokakibyo Gakkai Zasshi 88:2719–2723
55. Perez-Ordonez B, Naseem A, Lieberman PH, Klimstra DS (1996) Solid serous adenoma of the pancreas. The solid variant of serous cystadenoma? Am J Surg Pathol 20:1401–1405
56. Procacci C, Graziani R, Bicego E, Bergamo-Andreis IA, Guarise A, Valdo M, Bogina G, Solarino U, Pistolesi GF (1997) Serous cystadenoma of the pancreas: report of 30 cases with emphasis on the imaging findings. J Comput Assist Tomogr 21:373–382
57. Reyes CV, Wang T (1981) Undifferentiated small cell carcinoma of the pancreas: a report of five cases. Cancer 47:2500–2502
58. Schutte M, Hruban RH, Hedrick L, Cho KR, Nadasdy GM, Weinstein CL, Bova GS, Isaacs WB, Cairns P, Nawroz H, Sidransky D, Casero RA, Meltzer PS, Hahn SA, Kern SE (1996) DPC4 gene in various tumor types. Cancer Res 56:2527–2530
59. Seidel G, Zahurak M, Iacobuzio-Donahue CA, Sohn TA, Adsay NV, Yeo CJ, Lillemoe KD, Cameron JL, Hruban RH, Wilentz RE (2002) Almost all infiltrating colloid carcinomas of the pancreas and periampullary region arise from in situ papillary neoplasms: a study of 39 cases. Am J Surg Pathol 26:56–63
60. Sohn TA, Yeo CJ, Cameron JL, Hruban RH, Fukushima N, Campbell KA, Lillemoe KD (2004) Intraductal papillary mucinous neoplasms of the pancreas: an updated experience. Ann Surg 239:788–797
61. Sperti C, Pasquali C, Perasole A, Liessi G, Pedrazzoli S (2000) Macrocystic serous cystadenoma of the pancreas: clinicopathologic features in seven cases. Int J Pancreatol 28:1–7
62. Takaori K, Hruban RH, Maitra A, Tanigawa N (2004) Pancreatic intraepithelial neoplasia. Pancreas 28:257–262
63. Tanaka Y, Kato K, Notohara K, Hojo H, Ijiri R, Miyake T, Nagahara N, Sasaki F, Kitagawa N, Nakatani Y, Kobayashi Y (2001) Frequent beta-catenin mutation and cytoplasmic/nuclear accumulation in pancreatic solid-pseudopapillary neoplasm. Cancer Res 61:8401–8404
64. Tang LH, Aydin H, Brennan MF, Klimstra DS (2005) Clinically aggressive solid-pseudopapillary tumors of the pancreas. Am J Surg Pathol 29:512–519
65. Thayer SP, di Magliano MP, Heiser PW, Nielsen CM, Roberts DJ, Lauwers GY, Qi YP, Gysin S, Fernandez-del Castillo C, Yajnik V, Antoniu B, McMahon M, Warshaw AL, Hebrok M (2003) Hedgehog is an early and late mediator of pancreatic cancer tumorigenesis. Nature 425:851–856
66. Vortmeyer AO, Lubensky IA, Fogt F, Linehan WM, Khettry U, Zhuang Z (1997) Allelic deletion and mutation of the von Hippel-Lindau (VHL) tumor suppressor gene in pancreatic microcystic adenomas. Am J Pathol 151:951–956
67. Weinhaeusel A, Vierhapper H, Schlegl R, Wagner T, Muhr D, Scheuba C, Niederle B, Haas OA (2000) A novel mutation E179K of the MEN1 gene predisposes for multiple endocrine neoplasia-type 1 (MEN1). Hum Mutat 16:533
68. Westra WH, Sturm PJ, Drillenburg P, Choti MA, Klimstra DS, Abores-Saavedra J, Montag A, Offerhaus GJ, Hruban RH (1998) K-ras oncogene mutations in osteoclast-like giant cell tumors of the pancreas and liver: genetic evidence to support origin from the duct epithelium. Am J Surg Pathol 22:1247–1254
69. Widmaier U, Mattfeldt T, Siech M, Beger HG (1996) Serous cystadenocarcinoma of the pancreas. Int J Pancreatol 20:135–139
70. Wilentz RE, Albores-Saavedra J, Hruban RH (2000) Mucinous cystic neoplasms of the pancreas. Semin Diagn Pathol 17:31–42
71. Wilentz RE, Albores-Saavedra J, Zahurak M, Talamini MA, Yeo CJ, Cameron JL, Hruban RH (1999) Pathologic examination accurately predicts prognosis in mucinous cystic neoplasms of the pancreas. Am J Surg Pathol 23:1320–1327
72. Wilentz RE, Goggins M, Redston M, Marcus VA, Adsay NV, Sohn TA, Kadkol SS, Yeo CJ, Choti MA, Zahurak M, Johnson KA, Tascilar M, Offerhaus GJ, Hruban RH, Kern SE (2000) Genetic, immunohistochemical, and clinical features of medullary carcinoma of the pancreas: a newly described and characterized entity. Am J Pathol 156:1641–1651
73. Wilentz RE, Su GH, Dai JL, Sparks AB, Argani P, Sohn TA, Yeo CJ, Kern SE, Hruban RH (2000) Immunohistochemical labeling for Dpc4 mirrors genetic status in pancreatic adenocarcinomas: a new marker of DPC4 inactivation. Am J Pathol 156:37–43
74. Yi SQ, Miwa K, Ohta T, Kayahara M, Kitagawa H, Tanaka A, Shimokawa T, Akita K, Tanaka S (2003) Innervation of the pancreas from the perspective of perineural invasion of pancreatic cancer. Pancreas 27:225–229
75. Yoshimi N, Sugie S, Tanaka T, Aijin W, Bunai Y, Tatematsu A, Okada T, Mori H (1992) A rare case of serous cystadenocarcinoma of the pancreas. Cancer 69:2449–2453

Chapter 46

E. Gallmeier · S. E. Kern

Genetic Pathways in Pancreatic Tumorigenesis

Tumorigenesis is a multistep process. The accumulation of newly acquired capabilities promotes cell autonomy, eventually transforming normal cells into malignant cells [1]. The predominant mechanism may be the accumulation of genetic alterations, providing certain selective advantages, in a select subset of genes [2]. Our understanding of the development of pancreatic cancer is hence based upon the identification and characterization of the genes that are mutated in this tumor type.

Although the term "pancreatic cancer" comprises several histopathologically distinguishable tumor entities, including acinar cell carcinomas, pancreatoblastomas, solid-pseudopapillary tumors, mucinous cystic tumors, and intraductal papillary mucinous neoplasms, it commonly refers to pancreatic ductal adenocarcinomas, which represent the most common form of pancreatic neoplasms [3]. We focus here on a comprehensive summary of the genetic alterations identified in pancreatic ductal adenocarcinomas and their functional implications for pancreatic cancer tumorigenesis.

Genetic Alterations in Pancreatic Cancer

The mutated genes in pancreatic ductal adenocarcinoma are summarized in Table 46.1. They are divided into three distinct functional groups: oncogenes, tumor-suppressor genes and genome-maintenance genes. The mutations can further be distinguished by their mutation origin (somatic or germline) and by their predominant mutagenic mechanism (chromosomal or microsatellite instability).

Mutations originate either somatically (acquired) or in the germline (inherited). As germline mutations are present in each cell of an affected individual, some germline mutations can confer an increased cancer susceptibility, implicating the respective genes in causing familial cancer syndromes. Familial pancreatic cancer syndromes, as it turns out, involve genes that can also be somatically mutated in sporadic pancreatic cancer (e.g., *CDKN2A*, *TP53*, *STK11*, see below). On the other hand, although the familial cancer syndrome juvenile polyposis is caused by germline mutations of *SMAD4*, a gene that is frequently somatically mutated in pancreatic cancer, this syndrome is thus far not linked to an increased risk of pancreatic cancer.

As in colorectal cancer, two distinct tumor categories exist in pancreatic cancer, distinguishable by the predominant mutagenic mechanism. Most pancreatic cancers exhibit chromosomal instability (CIN), which causes gross numeric chromosomal changes that result in aneuploidy [4–6]. A second category is characterized by microsatellite instability (MSI) [7, 8], which causes a drastically decreased fidelity of DNA replication and repair due to defects in DNA mismatch-repair. MSI tumors thus exhibit frequent errors in copying of DNA sequences, which occur particularly pronounced at repetitive sequences termed microsatellites. MSI occurs rather infrequently in pancreatic cancer. It is found in a tumor subset distinguishable from the majority of tumors in its histopathological features as well as its genetic alterations. Pancreatic carcinomas having MSI have a medullary histologic pattern [9] and very frequently harbor mutations in the *TGFBR2* or *ACVR2* genes. Also, unlike most pancreatic CIN tumors, they usually lack mutations in the *KRAS* gene [9–11].

Epigenetic Alterations in Pancreatic Cancer

In addition to genetic alterations, changes in gene function can be caused by epigenetic mechanisms, such as the transcriptional gene silencing through hypermethylation of gene promoters or, vice versa, gene activation through promoter hypomethylation, as well as loss of imprinting and certain chromatin modifications (for a review, see [12]). Some of these epigenetic mechanisms could also play a role during pancreatic cancer development and appear to be complementary to the genetic alterations (e.g., [13–15]). In contrast to the latter, however, the significance of epi-

Table 46.1. Genetic alterations in pancreatic cancer.

Gene name	Frequency	Pathway	Mutation origin	References
Oncogenes				
KRAS	90%	Ras	somatic	[16, 17]
BRAF (in KRAS wt tumors)	4%	Ras	somatic	[19]
AKT2 (amplification)	10–20%	mTor	somatic	[20, 21]
CCNE (amplification)	6%	Fbxw7-CyclinE	somatic	[19]
MYB (amplification)	10%	-	somatic	[22]
NCOA3/AIB1 (amplification)	30%	-	somatic	[23, 24]
Tumor-suppressor genes				
CDKN2A	85%	Rb	somatic > germline	[26, 29]
TP53	50–75%	p53	somatic > germline	[33, 35]
SMAD4	55%	TGF-β superfamily	somatic	[37]
TGFBR1	1%	TGF-β superfamily	somatic	[10]
TGFBR2	5% (mainly MSI)	TGF-β superfamily	somatic	[10]
ACVR1B	2%	TGF-β superfamily	somatic	[39]
ACVR2	5% (mainly MSI)	TGF-β superfamily	somatic	[11]
STK11	5%	mTor	somatic > germline	[40, 43]
MAP2K4	4%	SAPK	somatic	[44, 45]
RB1	rare	Rb	?	[65]
FBXW7	?	Fbxw7-cyclin E	somatic	[19]
Genome maintenance genes				
BRCA2	7% (sporadic) 17% (familial)	Fanconi anemia	germline > somatic	[47-50]
FANCC	3%	Fanconi anemia	somatic > germline	[51-53]
FANCG	1%	Fanconi anemia	germline	[51]
(MLH1)[a]	(4%)	(mismatch-repair)	-	[18]

[a] MLH1 appears not to be genetically, but rather epigenetically inactivated in pancreatic cancer

genetic changes during tumorigenesis cannot be determined unambiguously. Genetic changes that occur in tumors at a rate higher than expected by chance obviously must play a causal role, as there is statistical evidence for their selective advantage. In contrast, the relevance of epigenetic inactivation of a gene cannot be proven as readily because it is a potentially reversible event and because the "chance rate" at which it occurs in tumors is not known.

Oncogenes

Mutated (proto-)oncogenes contribute to cancer development by conferring an increased state of activation, often resulting in constitutive activation instead of the usual conditional, regulated activation of the encoded protein. Activating mutations comprise subtle, intragenic (point) mutations, gene amplification, and possibly, although not yet demonstrated in pancreatic cancer, specific chromosomal translocations.

The most commonly mutated oncogene in pancreatic cancer is *KRAS*, having a mutation rate of at least 90% [16, 17]. The few remaining tumors lacking mutations in *KRAS* often have a medullary histologic pattern [9, 18]. In addition, *BRAF* mutations have been found in *KRAS* wildtype, but not in a panel of *KRAS* mutant, pancreatic cancers [19].

Gene amplification, accompanied by overexpression of the respective protein, has been reported for a number of genes in pancreatic cancer, including the *CCNE* (cyclin E) gene in a few cases [19], the *AKT2* gene in 10–20% of tumors [20, 21], the *MYB* gene in 10% [22], and the *NCOA3* (*AIB1*) gene in at least 30%

[23, 24]. Although gene amplification and resultant protein overexpression render these genes potential oncogenes, there are at least two caveats to consider. First, the amplicons involved in the amplification process typically represent large DNA sequences, including more than one gene, and thus complicate or preclude the unambiguous determination of the culprit oncogene contained therein. Second, and even more importantly, the rate at which random amplifications occur by chance in tumors is unknown, posing a similar problem as explained above for epigenetic phenomena: Whether the amplifications were "selected for" by the tumor or rather accumulate simply by structural reasons and genetic drift, is difficult to prove. Thus, the significance of gene amplifications for pancreatic cancer development remains unclear.

Tumor-Suppressor Genes

Unlike oncogenes, mutations in tumor-suppressor genes contribute to cancer development by inactivation rather than activation of the affected gene. The underlying genetic mechanisms include point mutations, deletions, and (potentially) insertions. Tumor-suppressor genes are recessive, and thus inactivation of both alleles is usually necessary to confer a cellular change. An exception is provided by dominant-negative mutations, which can inactivate gene function upon mutation of only one allele [25]. Biallelic inactivation is frequently achieved by the combination of a subtle mutation (e.g., point mutation) accompanied by the gross deletion of the second allele (e.g., loss of a chromosomal arm or a whole chromosome), termed loss of heterozygosity (LOH) or allelic loss. In addition, the inactivation of tumor-suppressor genes can be achieved by epigenetic mechanisms [12]. The tumor-suppressor genes identified in pancreatic cancer will be classified here by their mutation frequencies. Tumor-suppressor genes that are mutated at a high frequency include *CDKN2A* (p16), *TP53*, and *SMAD4* (*DPC4*, deleted in pancreatic cancer). Those mutated at low frequency include *STK11* (*LKB1*), *MAP2K4* (*MKK4*), *TGFBR1*, *TGFBR2*, *ACVR1B*, *ACVR2*, *RB1*, and *FBXW7* (*CDC4*).

The most commonly mutated tumor-suppressor gene is *CDKN2A*, encoding the p16 protein [26]. This gene is somatically inactivated, either by intragenic mutation or by homozygous deletion, in nearly 85% of pancreatic cancers. In addition, *CDKN2A* is epigenetically inactivated by transcriptional silencing in most of the remaining tumors [27]. Germline mutations of *CDKN2A* are also found in the familial atypical multiple mole melanoma (FAMMM) syndrome [28], which predisposes to pancreatic cancer [29].

TP53 (behind *CDKN2A*) represents the second most commonly mutated gene in human cancer. *TP53* encodes the p53 protein and is somatically mutated in 50–75% of pancreatic cancers [30–33].In addition, germline mutations of *TP53* are found in the Li-Fraumeni syndrome [34], another familial cancer syndrome that predisposes to pancreatic cancer [35].

SMAD4 is somatically mutated in 55% of pancreatic cancers [36, 37] and *SMAD4* germline mutations cause the otherwise unrelated familial cancer syndrome juvenile polyposis [38]. In addition to the frequent inactivation of *SMAD4*, mutations occurring at lower frequencies have been identified in several functionally related genes (see below). These include the genes encoding the transforming growth factor β (TGF-β) receptors type I (*TGFBR1*, 1%) and II (*TGFBR2*, 5%) [10] as well as the genes encoding the activin receptors type I (*ACVR1B*, 2%) and II (*ACVR2*, 5%) [11, 39]. *TGFBR2* and *ACVR2* mutations occur at mononucleotide tracts in most MSI pancreatic cancers and are rarely found in non-MSI pancreatic cancers.

STK11 is somatically mutated in 5% of pancreatic cancers [40], and germline mutations are found in the familial cancer syndrome Peutz-Jeghers [41, 42], which predisposes to pancreatic cancer [43]. Mutations in *MAP2K4* have been reported in a variety of tumor types, including pancreatic cancer, and occur at a similar low rate (3–6%) [44–46]. *FBXW7* is another putative tumor-suppressor gene in pancreatic cancer, but only one somatic mutation has been reported yet. Although the frequency and significance of *FBXW7* mutations is hence unknown, functional evidence suggests that *FBXW7* mutations could contribute to pancreatic cancer development by causing the overexpression of *CCNE* [19] (see below).

Genome-Maintenance Genes

In contrast to the activation of oncogenes and the inactivation of tumor-suppressor genes, the inactivation of genome-maintenance genes should not provide a direct selective advantage to a cell. Instead, the impairment of genome-maintenance genes can lead to an increased mutation rate, driving tumorigenesis by enabling a cell to experience a greater number of potentially advantageous mutations. The mechanisms by which genome-maintenance genes are inactivated are similar to those described for tumor-suppressor genes. Due to our incomplete understanding of their functions, a clear-cut distinction between tumor-suppressor and genome-maintenance genes is often not possible.

Mutations of genome-maintenance genes in pancreatic cancer include the Fanconi anemia genes *FANCD1/BRCA2*, *FANCC*, and *FANCG*. *FANCD1/BRCA2* is mutated in 7–10% of sporadic pancreatic cancers, depending on the population studied. Although the first mutation is usually inherited, these *FANCD1/BRCA2* germline mutations do not appear to convey a high penetrance for pancreatic cancer in general [47, 48]. *FANCD1/BRCA2* mutations also occur in 12–17% of familial pancreatic cancers [49, 50], rendering this gene the most frequently mutated gene identified to date in cases of familial pancreatic cancer. The *FANCC* and *FANCG* genes are mutated in 3% and 1%, respectively, of pancreatic cancers [51–53].

Biallelic germline mutations in any of the Fanconi anemia genes, including *FANCC*, *FANCG*, and *FANCD1/BRCA2*, cause the familial cancer syndrome Fanconi anemia, and heterozygous germline mutations in some of these genes might increase the risk of pancreatic cancer [51, 53]. As pancreatic cancer is a very late-onset disease, a potential predisposition of Fanconi anemia patients to this malignancy might be masked by the early onset of other malignancies, especially the development of acute myeloid leukemia during childhood and the development of a variety of solid tumors mainly during adulthood [54–56].

A subset of pancreatic cancers exhibit the MSI phenotype, indicating the impairment of DNA mismatch-repair genes such as *MLH1* or *MSH2*. The absence of Mlh1 protein expression in 4% of pancreatic cancers [18] is probably caused by epigenetic inactivation of the *MLH1* gene, accompanied by promoter hypermethylation [57–59]. Separately, germline mutations of *MLH1* are found in the hereditary nonpolyposis colorectal carcinoma syndrome (HNPCC) [60], a familial cancer syndrome in which pancreatic cancers occasionally occur [61].

Functional Implications

The functional implications of the gene alterations summarized above are revealed by the known roles of their encoded proteins in molecular signaling pathways. Whereas oncogenes and tumor-suppressor genes are involved predominantly in growth-controlling pathways, genome-maintenance genes are implicated in DNA repair. Several of the pathways altered in human carcinogenesis have been reviewed [62]. Of these, the following are related to pancreatic cancer.

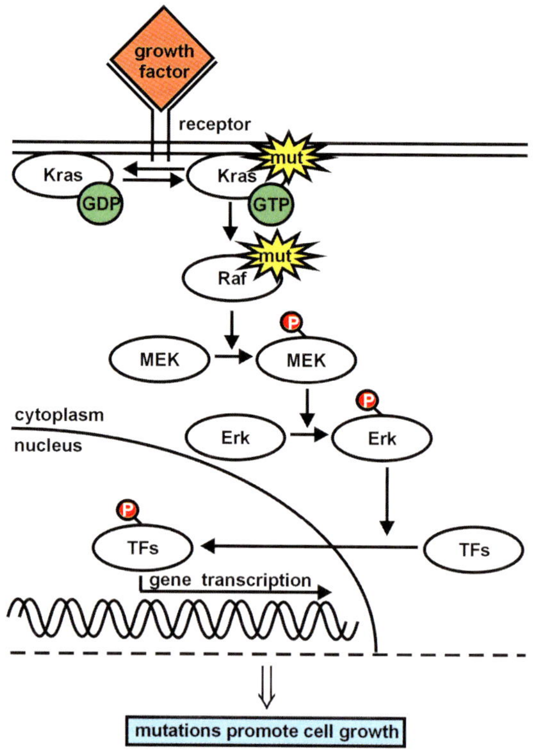

Figure 46.1

The Ras pathway. *P* Phosphorylation, *mut* mutation, *TFs* transcription factors

The Ras Pathway

The Ras pathway represents a growth-promoting pathway and is linked to pancreatic cancer by mutations in the *KRAS* and *BRAF* genes. Taken together, the high mutation rate of *KRAS* and the additional *BRAF* mutations in *KRAS* wildtype tumors indicate this pathway to be dysregulated in virtually all pancreatic cancers.

The *KRAS* gene encodes a guanine nucleotide-binding protein, Kras, which is located at the inner surface of the plasma membrane. Kras, in its active state, is bound to GTP, whereas in its inactive state, it is bound to GDP. Kras possesses an intrinsic GTPase activity that hydrolyzes GTP to GDP. The oncogenic mutations in *KRAS*, which exclusively occur at codons 12, 13, and 61, impair the GTP hydrolysis and thus the downregulation of Kras activity. Constitutively active Kras putatively results in the continuous transmission of growth-promoting signals or an exaggerated response to signals initiated by growth-factor receptors. One of the best-characterized effector pathways of Kras mediates the activation of certain

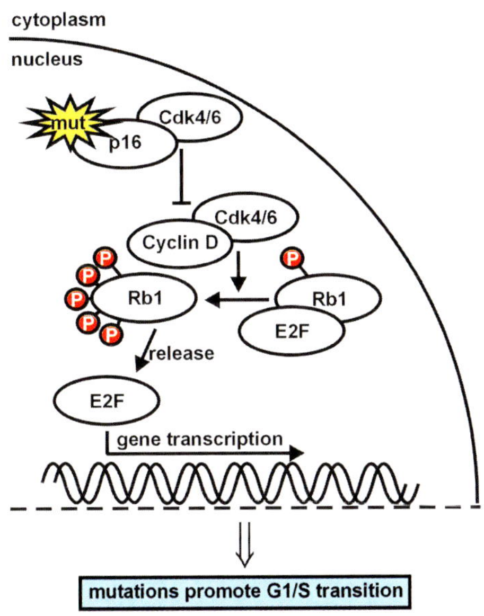

Figure 46.2

The Rb pathway

transcription factors (e.g., Elk1) via activation of the serine/threonine kinase Raf, which, in turn, triggers the mitogen-activating protein (MAP) kinase kinase (MEK)/Erk phosphorylation cascade (Fig. 46.1; for a review, see [63]). As the Ras pathway mediates growth signals, mutations in *KRAS* or *BRAF*, which cause its constitutive activation in tumors, are thought to promote cell growth.

The Rb Pathway

The Rb pathway represents a key regulator of the G1/S transition in the cell cycle and is linked to pancreatic cancer by mutations in the *CDKN2A* gene, encoding the p16 protein. Inactivation of *CDKN2A*, either by homozygous deletion, intragenic mutation, or epigenetic silencing, accounts for dysregulation of the Rb pathway in approximately 98% of pancreatic cancers [27]. Consequently, inactivation of the *RB1* gene itself, which is frequently found in a variety of other tumor types, appears to only play a minor role in pancreatic cancer tumorigenesis, mutations of *RB1* being rare [64, 65].

The Rb protein, in its active state, binds the transcription factor E2F and thereby inhibits E2F-induced gene transcription. Cdk4 and the closely related Cdk6, when bound to cyclin D, hyperphosphorylate Rb, which causes the dissociation of Rb from E2F. E2F release leads to the transcription of S-phase-promoting genes, causing or aiding cell entry into S-phase, where DNA synthesis commits the cell to another round of cell division. Binding of p16 to Cdk4 inactivates Cdk4. Thus, p16 blocks the progression of the cell from the G1- to S-phase by preventing Cdk4/Cyclin D-induced Rb-hyperphosphorylation (Fig. 46.2; for a review, see [66]). Mutations in p16 interfere with p16/Cdk4-binding, which ultimately results in the promotion of the G1/S-transition.

The p53 Pathway

The p53 pathway is linked to pancreatic cancer by mutations in the *TP53* gene. This gene encodes a transcription factor, p53, which regulates several cellular processes, among which the two best characterized are cell cycle control and programmed cell death, particularly in the cellular response to experimental DNA damage or oncogenic stress.

In normal cells, p53 is usually expressed at low levels due to its fast protein turnover. Nascent p53 can either be stabilized and activated or, instead, inactivated by proteolysis. p53 inactivation is mediated by Mdm2, which regulates the ubiquitin-mediated degradation of p53, but can also directly bind to p53 and thereby interfere with its transcriptional activity. Phosphorylation of p53, as by Chek2 and other protein kinases, may be the means to stabilize p53. Activated p53 binds to specific DNA sequences [67] and induces gene expression of a large variety of target genes, including genes involved in cell cycle regulation, for example *CDKN1A* (p21), *SFN* (14-3-3-σ), and *GADD45*, and genes involved in the regulation of apoptosis, for example *BAX*, *BBC3* (*PUMA*), and *PMAIP1* (*NOXA*). p53 also induces the transcription of *MDM2*, which establishes a negative feedback loop, controlling p53 protein levels. Mutations in *TP53* usually cause p53 inactivation by impairing its DNA-binding capability [68], thus interfering with p53-specific gene transcription [31].

As p53 appears as a central regulator of cell cycle checkpoints and controlled cell death, *TP53* mutations should result in the dysregulation of these cell growth-controlling mechanisms (Fig. 46.3; for a review, see [69]).

The TGF-β Superfamily Pathway

The pathway involving the TGF-β superfamily of cell surface receptors is linked to pancreatic cancer by mutations in the *SMAD4*, *TGFBR1*, *TGFBR2*, *ACVR1B*, and *ACVR2* genes.

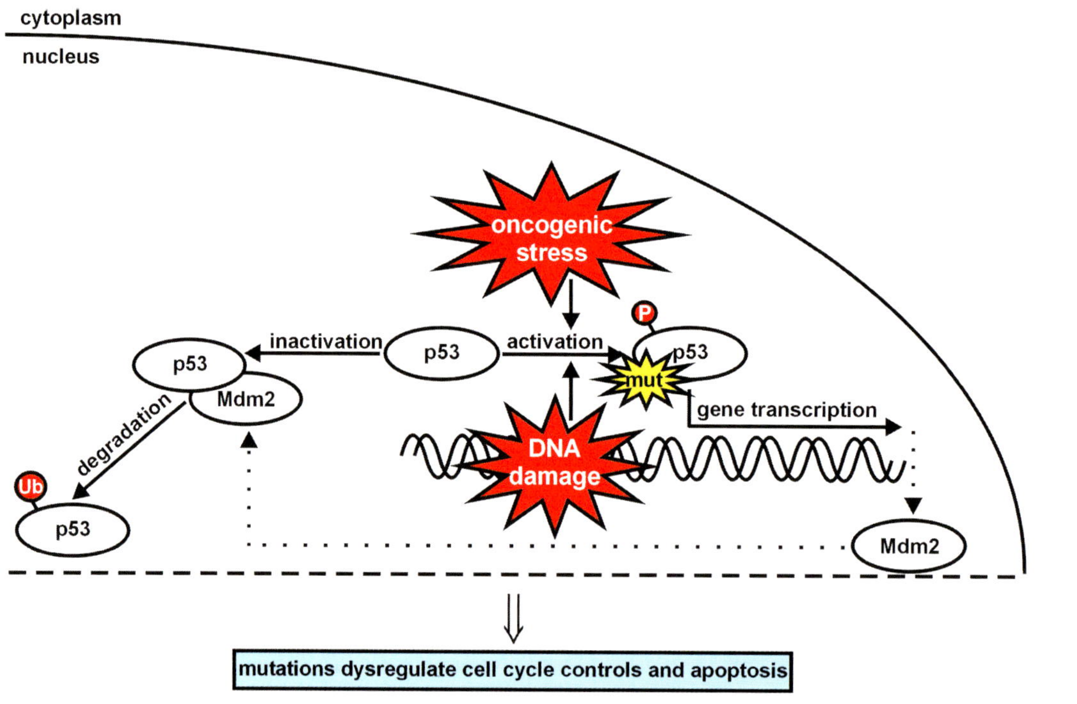

Figure 46.3

The p53 pathway. *Ub* Ubiquitin

Upstream signals initiated from ligands bound to the TGF-β superfamily receptors are mediated via a group of Smad proteins. These Smad proteins can be divided into three distinct groups, receptor-regulated Smads (R-Smads), inhibitory Smads (I-Smads), and the common-partner Smad (Co-Smad) [70]. Upon ligand binding, receptors of the TGF-β superfamily cause the phosphorylation of R-Smads, which can be inhibited by I-Smads, such as Smad7. Consecutively, the R-Smads heterodimerize with Smad4, associated with the nuclear translocation of the Smad complex. This complex binds to sequence-specific enhancers as a transcription factor, initiating the gene expression of target genes that are presumably involved in tumor suppression. Mutations in *SMAD4* can interfere with the above signaling pathway via at least four distinct mechanisms. First, homozygous *SMAD4* deletions as well as certain *SMAD4* missense mutations that cause protein instability result in loss of protein expression [71], which represents the most common mechanism responsible for *SMAD4* inactivation in pancreatic cancer [72]. *SMAD4* mutations can also impair DNA-binding of the Smad complex or impede its transcriptional activity, even when its DNA-binding functions are retained. Finally, *SMAD4* mutations can prevent the nuclear translocation of the Smad complex, per-

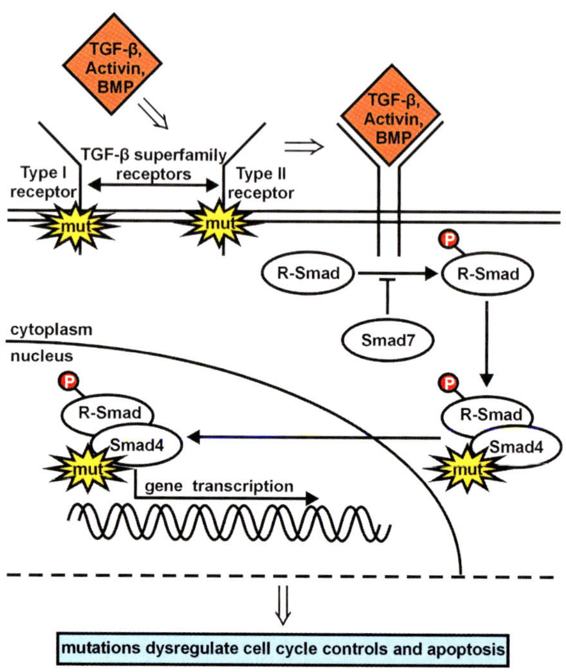

Figure 46.4

The transforming growth factor β (*TGF-β*) superfamily pathway

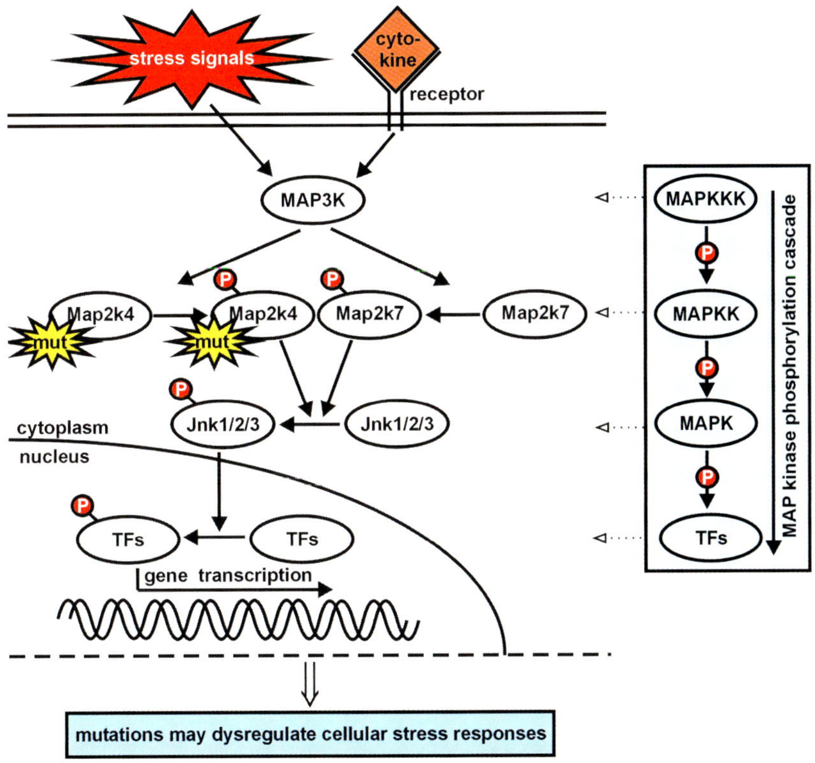

Figure 46.5

The stress-activated protein kinase pathway

haps by disrupting the binding capability of Smad4 to the other Smad proteins. As nuclear *SMAD4* is implicated in the negative control of cell growth via the regulation of cell cycle arrest and apoptosis [73], its inactivation caused by any of the above mechanisms could be oncogenic (Fig. 46.4; for a review, see [74])

Less frequently than mutations in *SMAD4*, mutations in the upstream receptor genes *TGFB1*, *TGFB2*, *ACVR1B*, and *ACVR2* can cause inactivation of the TGF-β superfamily signaling pathway in pancreatic cancer (for a review on TGF-β receptors, see [75]). Intriguingly, Smad4 does not appear to be uniformly indispensable in every cell type for mediating the growth-inhibitory effects of TGF-β, as some cells, in contrast to others, do not become resistant to the TGF-β-initiated effects upon *SMAD4* gene disruption [76–79]. Accordingly, mutations of genes in the TGF-β superfamily signaling pathway are not mutually exclusive, as would be presumed in a strictly linear pathway [33], and mutations of *SMAD4*, along with mutations of some other genes in this pathway, have been reported [10, 80].

The MAP Kinase Pathways

Signaling in the MAP kinase (MAPK) pathways is achieved by similar phosphorylation cascades, consisting of groups of serine/threonine kinases. A variety of upstream signals activate a MAPK kinase kinase (MAP3K), which phosphorylates a MAPK kinase (MAP2K), in turn phosphorylating a MAPK. The biological effects of the downstream MAPK are mediated via phosphorylation and activation of a variety of transcription factors that eventually initiate the transcription of genes involved in cell growth, development, apoptosis, and inflammation. Three MAPK pathways have been defined by their major downstream target at the MAPK level, namely Erk, p38, and Jnk.

There are at least two lines of evidence that link the development of pancreatic cancer to these MAPK pathways. First, the Ras pathway (Fig. 46.1) constitutes a MAPK pathway, with Raf representing the MAP3K, MEK representing the MAP2K and Erk representing the MAPK. Furthermore, the stress-activated protein kinase (SAPK) pathway, representing

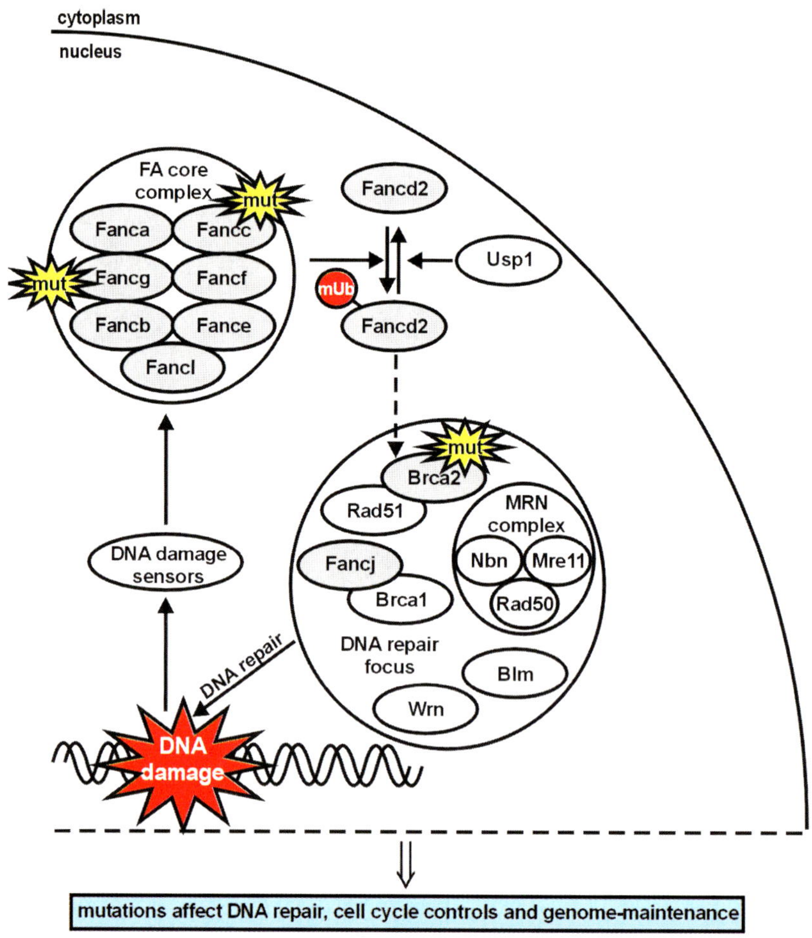

Figure 46.6

The Fanconi anemia pathway mUb Monoubiquitination

the Jnk/MAPK pathway, can be linked to pancreatic cancer by mutations in the *MAP2K4* gene. The upstream MAP3K in this pathway can be activated by proinflammatory cytokines via cell-surface receptors or various environmental stress signals. This leads to the phosphorylation of Map2k4 and Map2k7, which both are necessary for the efficient phosphorylation and activation of Jnk. Jnk then phosphorylates and activates certain transcription factors, including Jun and Atf2 (Fig. 46.5; for a review, see [81]). Mutations in *MAP2K4* impair, but do not completely abrogate, the downstream signaling to Jnk. As the SAPK pathway is not clearly tied to the cell-growth-regulatory functions of classical tumor-suppressor pathways, the mechanism by which *MAP2K4* could act as a tumor-suppressor gene remains poorly understood.

The Fanconi Anemia/Brca2 Pathway

The Fanconi anemia/Brca2 pathway is implicated in DNA repair and cell-cycle control and can be linked to pancreatic cancer by mutations in the *FANCC*, *FANCG*, and *FANCD1/BRCA2* genes. The proteins encoded by these genes appear to act in a common DNA damage response pathway, especially during the repair of DNA interstrand crosslinks and double-strand breaks. DNA damage leads to the activation of a nuclear multisubunit complex, comprising the Fanca, Fancb, Fancc, Fance, Fancf, Fancg, Fancl, and at least two other, as yet unknown, proteins. This complex activation, presumably coordinated by DNA-damage sensor proteins, causes the monoubiquitination of Fancd2, which, in turn, interacts via a yet incompletely understood mechanism with several DNA-repair proteins. These DNA-repair proteins co localize in DNA-repair foci and include Fancd1/Brca2

(Fig. 46.6). As Fancd1/Brca2 interacts directly with Rad51 and is required for proper Rad51 function, the Fanconi anemia/Brca2 pathway is thought to be involved in DNA-repair by homologous recombination (for a review, see [82]). The recent discoveries that *FANCJ* is synonymous with the DNA-helicase *BRIP1* (BRCA1-interacting protein) [83–85], and that *FANCM* represents the human ortholog of the bacterial DNA-repair protein Hef [86, 87], further support a direct function of the Fanconi anemia pathway in DNA-repair. The Fanconi anemia genes are therefore considered to represent genome-maintenance genes. In addition, they might have tumor-suppressive functions either related to or independent from the Fanconi anemia/Brca2 pathway.

The Fanconi anemia/Brca2 pathway serves as a good example to illustrate how genetic knowledge could directly translate into clinical applications. DNA interstrand-crosslinking agents are among the most commonly used chemotherapeutic drugs for anticancer therapy. *FANCC* and *FANCG* mutations confer an increased sensitivity to these drugs, an effect robustly observed in any *FANCC* and *FANCG* pathway-deficient cell line and depending only on the disruption of the respective gene [52, 82, 88]. Therefore, treatment regimens using DNA interstrand-crosslinking agents could be selectively or particularly beneficial for patients having pancreatic cancers harboring *FANCC* or *FANCG* mutations.

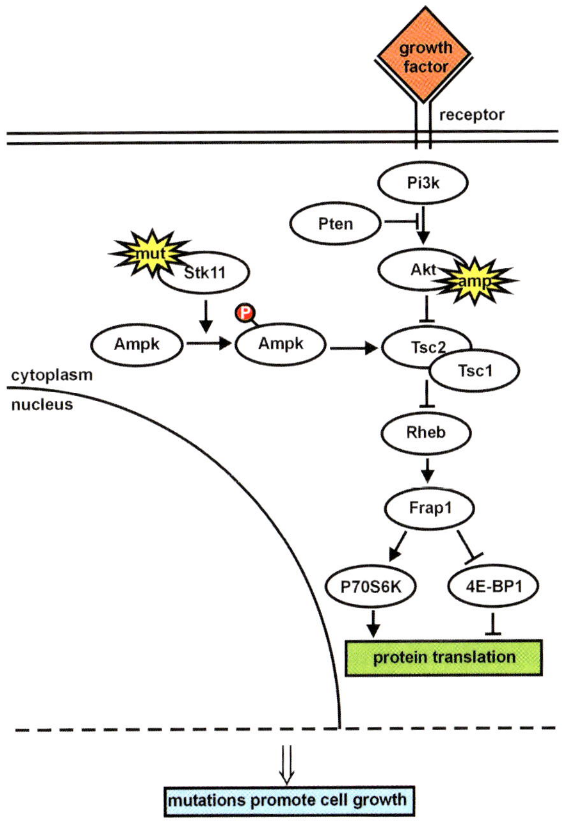

Figure 46.7

The mTor (Frap1) pathway. *amp* Amplification

The Mammalian Target of Rapamycin (mTor) Pathway

The mTor (Frap1) pathway has recently drawn considerable attention, especially as it can be pharmacologically modulated by rapamycin and its derivatives, and thus represents a potential molecular target for anticancer therapy. This pathway is implicated in the regulation of cell growth, probably due to the control of key regulators of protein translation, and can be linked to pancreatic cancer via two distinct mechanisms, mutations in the *STK11* (*LKB1*) gene and amplification of the *AKT2* gene.

The Tsc1/Tsc2 proteins play a central role in this pathway by inhibiting Frap1, which promotes protein translation via P70S6K and 4E-BP1. The upstream phosphoinositide 3-kinase activates Akt, which, in turn, activates Frap1 by suppressing Tsc1/Tsc2 [89]. *AKT2 a*mplification and concomitant Akt2 overexpression thus promote Frap1 signaling. In contrast, Stk11 suppresses Frap1 signaling via AMPK-mediated Tsc1/Tsc2 activation [90]. Thus, inactivating *STK11* mutations as well as (activating) *AKT2* amplification could result in the impaired suppression of growth-promoting effects of Frap1 signaling and could therefore both be oncogenic (Fig. 46.7; for a review, see [91]).

Interestingly, this pathway is linked to a large variety of human tumors by frequent alterations in other genes, including activating mutations in *PIK3CA* [92–96] and inactivating mutations in *PTEN* [97]. However, no mutations in these latter genes have been found in pancreatic cancer [98–100].

The Fbxw7-Cyclin E Pathway

The functional connection between Fbxw7 and cyclin E is illustrated by mutations in the putative tumor-suppressor gene *FBXW7* (*CDC4*) and amplification of the putative oncogene *CCNE* (cyclin E) in pancreatic cancer.

Cyclin E is a key regulator of the cell cycle, controlling the transition from G1-phase to S-phase. High levels of cyclin E promote G1/S progression and can be achieved in pancreatic cancer by at least two mechanisms: first, gene amplification of *CCNE* leads to cyclin E overexpression, and second, Fbxw7 negatively regulates cyclin E expression and thus, mutations in *FBXW7* increase cyclin E levels, an effect observed in pancreatic and other cancers [19, 101] (for a review, see [102]).

The Hedgehog Pathway

The Hedgehog pathway is implicated in the development of a variety of cancers including pancreatic cancer [103, 104]. Although no evidence has been found for genetic alterations in this pathway [105–107], there are examples supporting a role for epigenetic mechanisms to modulate the activity of this pathway in pancreatic cancer [108].

Future Directions and Clinical Applications

As illustrated in this chapter, considerable progress has been made during the last 15 years concerning the identification of genes associated with pancreatic cancer tumorigenesis. The recent completion of the Human Genome Project as well as significant technical advances will further aid to reduce cost and effort in this direction of research. Despite the considerable insight gained into tumorigenesis by these descriptive genomics, a thorough understanding of the precise function of the identified genes is lacking. Unfortunately, there is as yet no perfect system to study gene functions in human cancer, particularly in pancreatic cancer. Commonly used in vitro models, employing either exogenous gene overexpression to mimic physiologic gene function or short-interfering RNA (siRNA) technology to decrease the levels of the protein encoded by the gene under investigation, are prone to certain artifacts, and even gene-knockout models have limitations in terms of generalizability or clonal variability. Thus, the establishment of novel, better models to functionally characterize the identified genes will be the next major scientific challenge upon the completion of a comprehensive analysis of gene mutations in pancreatic cancer.

It appears that the genes that are mutated at a high frequency have naturally drawn more attention than those mutated at low frequency, and thus much more effort has been devoted to study the functional roles of the former. There is probably a plethora of genes that are mutated at low frequency in pancreatic cancer, which could nevertheless be equally important for its development. The recognition of a function of these genes in common pathways would not only strengthen the relevance of certain pathways in pancreatic cancer tumorigenesis, but could additionally unravel mutations in other genes implicated or related to the respective pathway. A good example, illustrating the significance of low-frequency mutations in pancreatic cancer involves the *TGFBR1*, *TGFBR2*, *ACVR1B*, *ACVR2* receptor genes. These genes are functionally related within the TGF-β superfamily signaling pathway, which has commanded high attention since the finding of the more common *SMAD4* mutations. Another example is the Fanconi anemia/Brca2 pathway. The Fanconi anemia genes *FANCC* and *FANCG* are mutated at a low rate in pancreatic cancer. However, upon the summing of all the known mutations including *FANCD1/BRCA2*, this pathway is recognized to be impaired in a significant fraction of pancreatic cancers.

The comprehensive identification and functional characterization of genes mutated at high and low frequency in pancreatic cancer is important not only to understand the biology of the malignancy, but also to develop clinical applications that directly benefit the patients. For example, the identification of germline mutations that confer an increased susceptibility to pancreatic cancer offers a screening test for subpopulations at risk. The establishment of a panel of genetic or other reliable alterations specific for pancreatic cancer (or, ideally, even the precursor lesions) could lead to applications that allow an earlier detection of the disease in the future. Finally, a better mechanistic understanding of the function of the genes mutated in pancreatic cancer could eventually yield targets for rational, genotype-based therapeutic strategies for individual patients.

References

1. Hanahan D, Weinberg RA (2000) The hallmarks of cancer. Cell 100:57–70
2. Vogelstein B, Kinzler KW (1993) The multistep nature of cancer. Trends Genet 9:138–141
3. Wilentz RE, Hruban RH (1998) Pathology of cancer of the pancreas. Surg Oncol Clin N Am 7:43–65
4. Griffin CA, Hruban RH, Morsberger LA, Ellingham T, Long PP, Jaffee EM, Hauda KM, Bohlander SK, Yeo CJ (1995) Consistent chromosome abnormalities in adenocarcinoma of the pancreas. Cancer Res 55:2394–2399
5. Johansson B, Bardi G, Heim S, Mandahl N, Mertens F, Bak-Jensen E, Andren-Sandberg A, Mitelman F (1992) Nonrandom chromosomal rearrangements in pancreatic carcinomas. Cancer 69:1674–1681
6. Lengauer C, Kinzler K.W, Vogelstein B (1998) Genetic instabilities in human cancers. Nature 396:643–649

7. Thibodeau SN, Bren G, Schaid D (1993) Microsatellite instability in cancer of the proximal colon. Science 260:816–819
8. Ionov Y, Peinado MA, Malkhosyan S, Shibata D, Perucho M (1993) Ubiquitous somatic mutations in simple repeated sequences reveal a new mechanism for colonic carcinogenesis. Nature 363:558–561
9. Goggins M, Offerhaus GJ, Hilgers W, Griffin CA, Shekher M, Tang D, Sohn TA, Yeo CJ, Kern SE, Hruban RH (1998) Pancreatic adenocarcinomas with DNA replication errors (RER+) are associated with wild-type K-ras and characteristic histopathology. Poor differentiation, a syncytial growth pattern, pushing borders suggest RER+. Am J Pathol 152:1501–1507
10. Goggins M, Shekher M, Turnacioglu K, Yeo CJ, Hruban RH, Kern SE (1998) Genetic alterations of the transforming growth factor beta receptor genes in pancreatic and biliary adenocarcinomas. Cancer Res 58:5329–5332
11. Hempen PM, Zhang L, Bansal RK, Iacobuzio-Donahue CA, Murphy KM, Maitra A, Vogelstein B, Whitehead RH, Markowitz SD, Willson JK, Yeo CJ, Hruban RH, Kern SE (2003) Evidence of selection for clones having genetic inactivation of the activin A type II receptor (ACVR2) gene in gastrointestinal cancers. Cancer Res 63:994–999
12. Feinberg AP, Tycko B (2004) The history of cancer epigenetics. Nat Rev Cancer 4:143–153
13. Sato N, Maitra A, Fukushima N, van Heek NT, Matsubayashi H, Iacobuzio-Donahue CA, Rosty C, Goggins M (2003) Frequent hypomethylation of multiple genes overexpressed in pancreatic ductal adenocarcinoma. Cancer Res 63:4158–4166
14. Ueki T, Toyota M, Sohn T, Yeo CJ, Issa JP, Hruban RH, Goggins M (2000) Hypermethylation of multiple genes in pancreatic adenocarcinoma. Cancer Res 60:1835–1839
15 Ueki T, Toyota M, Skinner H, Walter KM, Yeo CJ, Issa JP, Hruban RH, Goggins M (2001) Identification and characterization of differentially methylated CpG islands in pancreatic carcinoma. Cancer Res 61:8540–8546
16 Almoguera C, Shibata D, Forrester K, Martin J, Arnheim N, Perucho M (1988) Most human carcinomas of the exocrine pancreas contain mutant c-K-ras genes. Cell 53:549–554
17 Caldas C, Kern SE (1995) K-ras mutation and pancreatic adenocarcinoma. Int J Pancreatol 18:1–6
18 Wilentz RE, Goggins M, Redston M, Marcus VA, Adsay NV, Sohn TA, Kadkol SS, Yeo CJ, Choti M, Zahurak M, Johnson K, Tascilar M, Offerhaus GJ, Hruban RH, Kern SE (2000) Genetic immunohistochemical clinical features of medullary carcinoma of the pancreas: a newly described and characterized entity. Am J Pathol 156:1641–1651
19 Calhoun ES, Jones JB, Ashfaq R, Adsay V, Baker SJ, Valentine V, Hempen PM, Hilgers W, Yeo CJ, Hruban RH, Kern SE (2003) BRAF and FBXW7 (CDC4 FBW7 AGO SEL10) mutations in distinct subsets of pancreatic cancer: potential therapeutic targets. Am J Pathol 163:1255–1260
20 Cheng JQ, Ruggeri B, Klein WM, Sonoda G, Altomare DA, Watson DK, Testa JR (1996) Amplification of AKT2 in human pancreatic cells and inhibition of AKT2 expression and tumorigenicity by antisense RNA. Proc Natl Acad Sci U S A 93:3636–3641
21 Miwa W, Yasuda J, Murakami Y, Yashima K, Sugano K, Sekine T, Kono A, Egawa S, Yamaguchi K, Hayashizaki Y, Sekiya T (1996) Isolation of DNA sequences amplified at chromosome 19q131-q132 including the AKT2 locus in human pancreatic cancer. Biochem Biophys Res Commun 225:968–974
22 Wallrapp C, Muller-Pillasch F, Solinas-Toldo S, Lichter P, Friess H, Buchler M, Fink T, Adler G, Gress TM (1997) Characterization of a high copy number amplification at 6q24 in pancreatic cancer identifies c-myb as a candidate oncogene. Cancer Res 57:3135–3139
23 Henke RT, Haddad BR, Kim SE, Rone JD, Mani A, Jessup JM, Wellstein A, Maitra A, Riegel AT (2004) Overexpression of the nuclear receptor coactivator AIB1 (SRC-3) during progression of pancreatic adenocarcinoma. Clin Cancer Res 10:6134–6142
24 Ghadimi BM, Schrock E, Walker RL, Wangsa D, Jauho A, Meltzer PS, Ried T, (1999) Specific chromosomal aberrations and amplification of the AIB1 nuclear receptor coactivator gene in pancreatic carcinomas. Am J Pathol 154:525–536
25 Herskowitz I (1987) Functional inactivation of genes by dominant negative mutations. Nature 329:219–222
26 Caldas C, Hahn SA, da Costa LT, Redston MS, Schutte M, Seymour AB, Weinstein CL, Hruban RH, Yeo CJ, Kern SE (1994) Frequent somatic mutations and homozygous deletions of the p16 (MTS1) gene in pancreatic adenocarcinoma. Nat Genet 8:27–32
27. Schutte M, Hruban RH, Geradts J, Maynard R, Hilgers W, Rabindran SK, Moskaluk CA, Hahn SA, Schwarte-Waldhoff I, Schmiegel W, Baylin SB, Kern SE, Herman JG (1997) Abrogation of the Rb/p16 tumor-suppressive pathway in virtually all pancreatic carcinomas. Cancer Res 57:3126–3130
28 Gruis NA, van der Velden PA, Sandkuijl LA, Prins DE, Weaver-Feldhaus J, Kamb A, Bergman W, Frants RR (1995) Homozygotes for CDKN2 (p16) germline mutation in Dutch familial melanoma kindreds. Nat Genet 10:351–353
29 Lynch HT, Fusaro RM (1991) Pancreatic cancer and the familial atypical multiple mole melanoma (FAMMM) syndrome. Pancreas 6:127–131
30 Redston MS, Caldas C, Seymour AB, Hruban RH, da Costa L, Yeo CJ, Kern SE (1994) p53 mutations in pancreatic carcinoma and evidence of common involvement of homocopolymer tracts in DNA microdeletions. Cancer Res 54:3025–3033
31 Kern SE, Pietenpol JA, Thiagalingam S, Seymour A, Kinzler KW ,Vogelstein B (1992) Oncogenic forms of p53 inhibit p53-regulated gene expression. Science 256:827–830
32 Pellegata NS, Sessa F, Renault B, Bonato M, Leone BE, Solcia E, Ranzani GN (1994) K-ras and p53 gene mutations in pancreatic cancer: ductal and nonductal tumors progress through different genetic lesions. Cancer Res 54:1556–1560
33 Rozenblum E, Schutte M, Goggins M, Hahn SA, Panzer S, Zahurak M, Goodman SN, Sohn TA, Hruban RH, Yeo CJ, Kern SE (1997) Tumor-suppressive pathways in pancreatic carcinoma. Cancer Res 57:1731–1734
34 Srivastava S, Zou ZQ, Pirollo K, Blattner W, Chang EH (1990) Germ-line transmission of a mutated p53 gene in a cancer-prone family with Li-Fraumeni syndrome. Nature 348:747–749
35 Varley JM (2003) Germline TP53 mutations and Li-Fraumeni syndrome. Hum Mutat 21:313–320
36 Schutte M, Hruban RH, Hedrick L, Cho KR, Nadasdy GM, Weinstein CL, Bova GS, Isaacs WB, Cairns P, Nawroz H, Sidransky D, Casero RA Jr, Meltzer PS, Hahn SA, Kern SE (1996) DPC4 gene in various tumor types. Cancer Res 56:2527–2530
37. Hahn SA, Schutte M, Hoque AT, Moskaluk CA, da Costa LT, Rozenblum E, Weinstein CL, Fischer A, Yeo CJ, Hruban RH, Kern SE (1996) DPC4 a candidate tumor suppressor gene at human chromosome 18q211. Science 271:350–353

38 Howe JR, Roth S, Ringold JC, Summers RW, Jarvinen HJ, Sistonen P, Tomlinson IP, Houlston RS, Bevan S, Mitros FA, Stone EM, Aaltonen LA (1998) Mutations in the SMAD4/DPC4 gene in juvenile polyposis. Science 280:1086–1088
39 Su GH, Bansal R, Murphy KM, Montgomery E, Yeo CJ, Hruban RH, Kern SE (2001) ACVR1B (ALK4 activin receptor type 1B) gene mutations in pancreatic carcinoma. Proc Natl Acad Sci U S A 98:3254–3257
40 Su GH, Hruban RH, Bansal RK, Bova GS, Tang DJ, Shekher MC, Westerman AM, Entius MM, Goggins M, Yeo CJ, Kern SE (1999) Germline and somatic mutations of the STK11/LKB1 Peutz-Jeghers gene in pancreatic and biliary cancers Am J Pathol 154:1835–1840
41 Jenne DE, Reimann H, Nezu J, Friedel W, Loff S, Jeschke R, Muller O, Back W, Zimmer M (1998) Peutz-Jeghers syndrome is caused by mutations in a novel serine threonine kinase. Nat Genet:18 38–43
42. Hemminki A, Markie D, Tomlinson I, Avizienyte E, Roth S, Loukola A, Bignell G, Warren W, Aminoff M, Hoglund P, Jarvinen H, Kristo P, Pelin K, Ridanpaa M, Salovaara R, Toro T, Bodmer W, Olschwang S, Olsen AS, Stratton MR de la Chapelle A, Aaltonen LA (1998) A serine/threonine kinase gene defective in Peutz-Jeghers syndrome. Nature 391:184–187
43 Giardiello FM, Welsh SB, Hamilton SR, Offerhaus GJ, Gittelsohn AM, Booker SV, Krush AJ, Yardley JH, Luk GD (1987) Increased risk of cancer in the Peutz-Jeghers syndrome. N Engl J Med 316:1511–1514
44 Teng DH, Perry WL III, Hogan JK, Baumgard M, Bell R, Berry S, Davis T, Frank D, Frye C, Hattier T, Hu R, Jammulapati S, Janecki T, Leavitt A, Mitchell JT, Pero R, Sexton D, Schroeder M, Su PH, Swedlund B, Kyriakis JM, Avruch J, Bartel P, Wong AK, Tavtigian SV, et al (1997) Human mitogen-activated protein kinase kinase 4 as a candidate tumor suppressor. Cancer Res 57:4177–4182
45 Su GH, Hilgers W, Shekher MC, Tang DJ, Yeo CJ, Hruban RH, Kern SE (1998) Alterations in pancreatic biliary breast carcinomas support MKK4 as a genetically targeted tumor suppressor gene. Cancer Res 58:2339–2342
46 Su GH, Song JJ, Repasky EA, Schutte M, Kern SE (2002) Mutation rate of MAP2K4/MKK4 in breast carcinoma. Hum Mutat 19:81
47. Goggins M, Schutte M, Lu J, Moskaluk CA, Weinstein CL, Petersen GM, Yeo CJ, Jackson CE, Lynch HT, Hruban RH, Kern SE (1996) Germline BRCA2 gene mutations in patients with apparently sporadic pancreatic carcinomas Cancer Res 56:5360–5364
48 Ozcelik H, Schmocker B, Di Nicola N, Shi XH, Langer B, Moore M, Taylor BR, Narod SA, Darlington G, Andrulis IL, Gallinger S, Redston M (1997) Germline BRCA2 6174delT mutations in Ashkenazi Jewish pancreatic cancer patients. Nat Genet 16:17–18
49 Murphy KM, Brune KA, Griffin C, Sollenberger JE, Petersen GM, Bansal R, Hruban RH, Kern SE (2002) Evaluation of candidate genes MAP2K4 MADH4 ACVR1B BRCA2 in familial pancreatic cancer: deleterious BRCA2 mutations in 17%. Cancer Res 62:3789–3793
50 Hahn SA, Greenhalf B, Ellis I, Sina-Frey M, Rieder H, Korte B, Gerdes B, Kress R, Ziegler A, Raeburn JA, Campra D, Grutzmann R, Rehder H, Rothmund M, Schmiegel W, Neoptolemos JP, Bartsch DK (2003) BRCA2 germline mutations in familial pancreatic carcinoma. J Natl Cancer Inst 95:214–221
51 van der Heijden MS, Yeo CJ, Hruban RH, Kern SE (2003) Fanconi anemia gene mutations in young-onset pancreatic cancer. Cancer Res 63:2585–2588
52 van der Heijden MS, Brody JR, Gallmeier E, Cunningham SC, Dezentje DA, Shen D, Hruban RH, Kern SE (2004) Functional defects in the Fanconi anemia pathway in pancreatic cancer cells. Am J Pathol 165:651–657
53 Couch FJ, Johnson MR, Rabe K, Boardman L, McWilliams R, de Andrade M, Petersen G (2005) Germ line Fanconi anemia complementation group C mutations and pancreatic cancer. Cancer Res 65:383–386
54 Kutler DI, Singh B, Satagopan J, Batish SD, Berwick M, Giampietro PF, Hanenberg H, Auerbach AD (2003) A 20-year perspective on the International Fanconi Anemia Registry (IFAR). Blood 101:1249–1256
55. Alter BP (2003) Cancer in Fanconi anemia, 1927–2001. Cancer 97:425–440
56. Rosenberg PS, Greene MH, Alter BP (2003) Cancer incidence in persons with Fanconi anemia. Blood 101:822–826
57. Kane MF, Loda M, Gaida GM, Lipman J, Mishra R, Goldman H, Jessup JM, Kolodner R (1997) Methylation of the hMLH1 promoter correlates with lack of expression of hMLH1 in sporadic colon tumors and mismatch repair-defective human tumor cell lines. Cancer Res 57:808–811
58. Herman JG, Umar A, Polyak K, Graff JR, Ahuja N, Issa JP, Markowitz S, Willson JK, Hamilton SR, Kinzler KW, Kane MF, Kolodner RD, Vogelstein B, Kunkel TA, Baylin SB (1998) Incidence and functional consequences of hMLH1 promoter hypermethylation in colorectal carcinoma. Proc Natl Acad Sci U S A 95:6870–6875
59. Veigl ML, Kasturi L, Olechnowicz J, Ma AH, Lutterbaugh JD, Periyasamy S, Li GM, Drummond J, Modrich PL, Sedwick WD, Markowitz SD (1998) Biallelic inactivation of hMLH1 by epigenetic gene silencing, a novel mechanism causing human MSI cancers. Proc Natl Acad Sci U S A 95:8698–8702
60. Lynch HT, Lynch JF (2000) Hereditary nonpolyposis colorectal cancer. Semin Surg Oncol 18:305–313
61. Lynch HT, Voorhees GJ, Lanspa SJ, McGreevy PS, Lynch JF (1985) Pancreatic carcinoma and hereditary nonpolyposis colorectal cancer: a family study. Br J Cancer 52:271–273
62. Vogelstein B, Kinzler KW (2004) Cancer genes and the pathways they control. Nat Med 10:789–799
63. Shields JM, Pruitt K, McFall A, Shaub A, Der CJ (2000) Understanding Ras: 'it ain't over 'til it's over'. Trends Cell Biol 10:147–154
64. Barton CM, McKie AB, Hogg A, Bia B, Elia G, Phillips SM, Ding SF, Lemoine NR (1995) Abnormalities of the RB1 and DCC tumor suppressor genes: uncommon in human pancreatic adenocarcinoma. Mol Carcinog 13:61–69
65. Huang L, Lang D, Geradts J, Obara T, Klein-Szanto AJ, Lynch HT, Ruggeri BA (1996) Molecular and immunochemical analyses of RB1 and cyclin D1 in human ductal pancreatic carcinomas and cell lines. Mol Carcinog 15:85–95
66. Classon M, Harlow E (2002) The retinoblastoma tumour suppressor in development and cancer. Nat Rev Cancer 2:910–917
67. Kern SE, Kinzler KW, Bruskin A, Jarosz D, Friedman P, Prives C, Vogelstein B (1991) Identification of p53 as a sequence-specific DNA-binding protein. Science 252:1708–1711
68. Kern SE, Kinzler KW, Baker SJ, Nigro JM, Rotter V, Levine AJ, Friedman P, Prives C, Vogelstein B (1991) Mutant p53 proteins bind DNA abnormally in vitro. Oncogene 6:131–136

69. Oren M (2003) Decision making by p53: life, death and cancer. Cell Death Differ 10:431–442
70. Massague J, Wotton D (2000) Transcriptional control by the TGF-beta/Smad signaling system. EMBO J 19:1745–1754
71. Maurice D, Pierreux CE, Howell M, Wilentz RE, Owen MJ, Hill CS (2001) Loss of Smad4 function in pancreatic tumors: C-terminal truncation leads to decreased stability. J Biol Chem 276:43175–43181
72. Iacobuzio-Donahue CA, Song J, Parmiagiani G, Yeo CJ, Hruban RH, Kern SE (2004) Missense mutations of MADH4: characterization of the mutational hot spot and functional consequences in human tumors. Clin Cancer Res 10:1597–1604
73. Dai JL, Bansal RK, Kern SE (1999) G1 cell cycle arrest and apoptosis induction by nuclear Smad4/Dpc4: phenotypes reversed by a tumorigenic mutation. Proc Natl Acad Sci U S A 96:1427–1432
74. Elliott RL, Blobe GC (2005) Role of transforming growth factor Beta in human cancer. J Clin Oncol 23:2078–2093
75. Shi Y, Massague J (2003) Mechanisms of TGF-beta signaling from cell membrane to the nucleus. Cell 113:685–700
76. Hocevar BA, Brown TL, Howe PH (1999) TGF-beta induces fibronectin synthesis through a c-Jun N-terminal kinase-dependent, Smad4-independent pathway. EMBO J 18:1345–1356
77. Zhou S, Buckhaults P, Zawel L, Bunz F, Riggins G, Dai JL, Kern SE, Kinzler KW, Vogelstein B (1998) Targeted deletion of Smad4 shows it is required for transforming growth factor beta and activin signaling in colorectal cancer cells. Proc Natl Acad Sci U S A 95:2412–2416
78. Dai JL, Schutte M, Bansal RK, Wilentz RE, Sugar AY, Kern SE (1999) Transforming growth factor-beta responsiveness in DPC4/SMAD4-null cancer cells. Mol Carcinog 26:37–43
79. de Winter JP, Roelen BA, ten Dijke P, van der Burg B, van den Eijnden-van Raaij AJ (1997) DPC4 (SMAD4) mediates transforming growth factor-beta1 (TGF-beta1) induced growth inhibition and transcriptional response in breast tumour cells. Oncogene 14:1891–1899
80. Grady WM, Myeroff LL, Swinler SE, Rajput A, Thiagalingam S, Lutterbaugh JD, Neumann A, Brattain MG, Chang J, Kim SJ, Kinzler KW, Vogelstein B, Willson JK, Markowitz S (1999) Mutational inactivation of transforming growth factor beta receptor type II in microsatellite stable colon cancers. Cancer Res 59:320–324
81. Kyriakis JM, Avruch J (2001) Mammalian mitogen-activated protein kinase signal transduction pathways activated by stress and inflammation. Physiol Rev 81:807–869
82. D'Andrea AD, Grompe M (2003) The Fanconi anaemia/BRCA pathway. Nat Rev Cancer 3:23–34
83. Levran O, Attwooll C, Henry RT, Milton KL, Neveling K, Rio P, Batish SD, Kalb R, Velleuer E, Barral S, Ott J, Petrini J, Schindler D, Hanenberg H, Auerbach A.D (2005) The BRCA1-interacting helicase BRIP1 is deficient in Fanconi anemia. Nat Genet 37:931–933
84. Levitus M, Waisfisz Q, Godthelp BC, Vries YD, Hussain S, Wiegant WW, Elghalbzouri-Maghrani E, Steltenpool J, Rooimans MA, Pals G, Arwer, F, Mathew CG, Zdzienicka MZ, Hiom K, De Winter JP, Joenje H (2005) The DNA helicase BRIP1 is defective in Fanconi anemia complementation group J. Nat Genet 37:934–945
85. Bridge WL, Vandenberg CJ, Franklin RJ, Hiom K (2005) The BRIP1 helicase functions independently of BRCA1 in the Fanconi anemia pathway for DNA crosslink repair. Nat Genet 37:953–957
86. Mosedale G, Niedzwiedz W, Alpi A, Perrina F, Pereira-Leal JB, Johnson M, Langevin F, Pace P, Patel KJ (2005) The vertebrate Hef ortholog is a component of the Fanconi anemia tumor-suppressor pathway. Nat Struct Mol Biol 12:763–771
87. Meetei AR, Medhurst AL, Ling C, Xue Y, Singh TR, Bier P, Steltenpool J, Stone S, Dokal I, Mathew CG, Hoatlin M, Joenje H, de Winter JP, Wang W (2005) A human ortholog of archaeal DNA repair protein Hef is defective in Fanconi anemia complementation group M. Nat Genet 37:958–963
88. Gallmeier E, Calhoun ES, Rago C, Brody JR, Cunningham SC, Hucl T, Gorospe M, Kohli M, Lengauer C, Kern SE (2006) Targeted disruption of FANCC and FANCG in human cancer provides a preclinical model for specific therapeutic options. Gastroenterology 130:2145–2154
89. Inoki K, Li Y, Zhu T, Wu J, Guan K.L (2002) TSC2 is phosphorylated and inhibited by Akt and suppresses mTOR signalling. Nat Cell Biol 4:648–657
90. Shaw RJ, Bardeesy N, Manning BD, Lopez L, Kosmatka M, DePinho RA, Cantley LC (2004) The LKB1 tumor suppressor negatively regulates mTOR signaling. Cancer Cell 6:91–99
91. Inoki K, Corradetti MN, Guan KL (2005) Dysregulation of the TSC-mTOR pathway in human disease. Nat Genet 37:19–24
92. Campbell IG, Russell SE, Choong DY, Montgomery KG, Ciavarella ML, Hooi CS, Cristiano BE, Pearson RB, Phillips WA (2004) Mutation of the PIK3CA gene in ovarian and breast cancer. Cancer Res 64:7678–7681
93. Lee JW, Soung YH, Kim SY, Lee HW, Park WS, Nam SW, Kim SH, Lee JY, Yoo NJ, Lee SH (2005) PIK3CA gene is frequently mutated in breast carcinomas and hepatocellular carcinomas. Oncogene 24:1477–1480
94. Bachman KE, Argani P, Samuels Y, Silliman N, Ptak J, Szabo S, Konishi H, Karakas B, Blair BG, Lin C, Peters BA, Velculescu VE, Park BH (2004) The PIK3CA gene is mutated with high frequency in human breast cancers. Cancer Biol Ther 3:772–775
95. Broderick DK, Di C, Parrett TJ, Samuels YR, Cummins JM, McLendon RE, Fults DW, Velculescu VE, Bigner DD, Yan H (2004) Mutations of PIK3CA in anaplastic oligodendrogliomas, high-grade astrocytomas, medulloblastomas. Cancer Res 64:5048–5050
96. Samuels Y, Wang Z, Bardelli A, Silliman N, Ptak J, Szabo S, Yan H, Gazdar A, Powell SM, Riggins GJ, Willson JK, Markowitz S, Kinzler KW, Vogelstein B, Velculescu VE (2004) High frequency of mutations of the PIK3CA gene in human cancers. Science 304:554
97. Sansal I, Sellers WR (2004) The biology and clinical relevance of the PTEN tumor suppressor pathway. J Clin Oncol 22:2954–2963
98. Gallmeier E, Calhoun ES, Kern SE (2004) No mutations in PIK3CA identified in pancreatic carcinoma. J Neg Observ Genet Oncol 8:2
99. Okami K, Wu L, Riggins G, Cairns P, Goggins M, Evron E, Halachmi N, Ahrendt SA, Reed AL, Hilgers W, Kern SE, Koch WM, Sidransky D, Jen J (1998) Analysis of PTEN/MMAC1 alterations in aerodigestive tract tumors. Cancer Res 58:509–511
100. Goggins M, Hilgers W, Kern SE (1998) Normal PTEN gene in pancreatic cancer. J Neg Observ Genet Oncol 2:2

101. Rajagopalan H, Jallepalli PV, Rago C, Velculescu VE, Kinzler KW, Vogelstein B, Lengauer C (2004) Inactivation of hCDC4 can cause chromosomal instability. Nature 428:77–81
102. Reed SI (2003) Ratchets and clocks: the cell cycle, ubiquitylation and protein turnover. Nat Rev Mol Cell Biol 4:855–864
103. Thayer SP, di Magliano MP, Heiser PW, Nielsen CM, Roberts DJ, Lauwers, GY, Qi YP, Gysin S, Fernandez-del Castillo C, Yajnik V, Antoniu B, McMahon M, Warshaw AL, Hebrok M (2003) Hedgehog is an early and late mediator of pancreatic cancer tumorigenesis. Nature 425:851–856
104. Berman DM, Karhadkar SS, Maitra A, Montes De Oca R, Gerstenblith MR, Briggs K, Parker AR, Shimada Y, Eshleman JR, Watkins DN, Beachy PA (2003) Widespread requirement for Hedgehog ligand stimulation in growth of digestive tract tumours. Nature 425:846–851
105. Gallmeier E, Kern SE (2003) No homozygous deletions of PTC1 in pancreatic adenocarcinoma. J Neg Observ Genet Oncol 7: 8
106. Gallmeier E, Kern SE (2003) No activating mutations of Smoothened in pancreatic adenocarcinoma. J Neg Observ Genet Oncol 7:9
107. Gallmeier E, Kern S. (2004) No mutations in SUFU identified in pancreatic adenocarcinoma. J Neg Observ Genet Oncol 8:1
108. Martin ST, Sato N, Dhara S, Chang R, Hustinx SR, Abe T, Maitra A, Goggins M (2005) Aberrant methylation of the human hedgehog interacting protein (HHIP) gene in pancreatic neoplasms. Cancer Biol Ther 4:728–733

Chapter 47

E. J. Shin · M. I. Canto

The Clinical Assessment of Pancreatic Cancer

Despite many scientific advances in the past 50 years, pancreatic cancer remains one of the most deadly cancers in the United States, with a 5-year survival rate of less than 5% [1]. Pancreatic adenocarcinoma is the fourth leading cause of cancer-related death, and is second only to colorectal cancer as a cause of gastrointestinal-related cancer death [2]. The American Cancer Society predicted that 32,180 people in the United States (16,100 men and 16,080 women) would be diagnosed with, and about 31,800 would die of pancreatic cancer in 2005 [1]. The World Health Organization estimated a worldwide incidence of 216,400 cases and 213,500 deaths as a result of pancreatic cancer in 2000 [3].

Multiple factors have contributed to the poor prognosis of patients diagnosed with pancreatic cancer.

1. Due to the nonspecific nature of the symptoms and signs of pancreatic adenocarcinoma, patients are often diagnosed at a relatively advanced stage.
2. Pancreatic cancer tends to disseminate early in its natural history, and commonly during the preclinical phase of the disease [4, 5].
3. The only definitive therapy is surgical resection since pancreatic adenocarcinoma is resistant to most medical therapy [4]; however, most are deemed unresectable at the time of diagnosis. Between 1985 and 1995, only 9% of more than 100,000 pancreatic cancer patients in the National Cancer Data Base were eligible for surgical resection [6].

Symptoms and Signs

Given the high mortality rate of pancreatic cancer, it is imperative to make an early diagnosis. However, it is extraordinarily difficult to diagnose early pancreatic adenocarcinoma based on signs and clinical symptoms alone. Due to the nonspecific characteristics of the early symptoms and its insidious nature, pancreatic cancer is often mistaken for other illnesses [7, 8]. Moreover, the pancreas is a relatively inaccessible organ for physical examination [8].

Although the traditional teaching has touted painless jaundice as the classic presenting symptom for pancreatic adenocarcinoma, patients will often present with epigastric pain characterized by dull ache in the midepigastrum radiating to the back [9, 10]. Pain is usually improved with leaning forward and may be worse at night and in the supine position. The epigastric pain radiating to the back is believed to be due to perineural and splanchnic neuronal compression or invasion and from organ compression [10, 11]. Abdominal pain is a common symptom regardless of the location of the pancreatic tumor [12]. However, pain is reported more often by patients with a mass in the body and tail of the pancreas (90%) compared to those with mass in the head of the pancreas (70%) [13].

For pancreatic adenocarcinoma located in the head of the pancreas, clinical symptoms are often related to direct biliary or pancreatic duct invasion, or biliary duct compression. Symptoms are often nonspecific and include jaundice with pruritus, abdominal pain or dyspepsia, nausea and vomiting (secondary to partial or complete small-bowel obstruction from compression or invasion of the second portion of the duodenum), diarrhea or steatorrhea (secondary to pancreatic or bile duct obstruction), anorexia, generalized malaise, and insomnia [9, 10, 14–17]. Patients with tumors in the pancreatic body or tail often present with weight loss and abdominal pain.

An association has been found between jaundice as the presenting symptom and the location of the pancreatic lesion. Jaundice was found in 65–90% of the patients with mass in the head of the pancreas and in <20% of the patients with mass in the body or the tail of the pancreas [18, 19]. Jaundice as an initial presenting symptom has also been associated with improved prognosis, as supported by data that patients with jaundice are more likely to have resectable lesions at the time of diagnosis when compared to patients without jaundice [8, 18, 20].

A population-based case-control study was conducted to determine the signs and symptoms that may help in making an earlier diagnosis of pancreatic cancer [8]. When compared to the control population, patients with pancreatic adenocarcinoma were more likely to report appetite loss, abdominal pain of at least 6 weeks in duration, weight loss, jaundice, pale stool, dark urine, and usual bloating and belching (odds ratio >10) [8].

A less common presentation of pancreatic adenocarcinoma is pancreatitis, thought to be secondary to significant obstruction of the pancreatic duct from the tumor. Consequently, for patients with no obvious risk factors for pancreatitis, a pancreatic malignancy must be considered, especially in the older population [4, 21]. Another uncommon presentation of pancreatic cancer is new-onset diabetes mellitus, which can be observed in 6–68% of patients [22, 23].

Physical Examination

On physical examination, the most common finding is jaundice and excoriations from pruritus. Sometimes hepatomegaly from liver congestion or metastatic disease, splenomegaly from portal vein thrombosis, nontender palpable gallbladder (Courvoisier's sign), and a palpable pancreatic mass can be appreciated [14]. Invasion of the splenic artery or vein can lead to a left upper quadrant bruit in approximately 25% of the patients with tumors in the pancreatic body and tail [24]. With progression of disease, a nodular liver, ascites, and evidence of cachexia can also be identified. Other signs of metastatic disease include enlargement of the left supraclavicular lymph node (Virchow's node), periumbilical lymphadenopathy (Sister Mary Joseph's node), and pelvic metastatic tumor in the rectouterine/rectovesical space felt on rectal examination (Blumer's shelf) [14, 25]. Heme-occult-positive stool or evidence of frank gastrointestinal hemorrhage and physical findings associated with gastric outlet obstruction can be seen with invasion of the pancreatic cancer into the duodenum. Migratory superficial thrombophlebitis (Trousseau's sign) is classically associated with pancreatic malignancy and can occur in up to 10% of patients [26].

Laboratory Tests

Routine laboratory tests may reveal elevated liver function tests, especially serum bilirubin, alkaline phosphatase, and gamma-glutamyl transpeptidase. A mild elevation of transaminases can be seen, as well as mild anemia and coagulopathy from the malabsorption of fat-soluble vitamins and decreased production of vitamin K-dependent clotting factors by the liver. However, patients may also have a completely normal laboratory panel, especially in cases of mass in the tail of the pancreas. Thus, the diagnosis of pancreatic cancer is usually made by imaging studies and analysis of tissue biopsy samples.

Tumor Markers

Currently, there is no tumor-specific marker for pancreatic cancer. Multiple tumor-associated markers have been studied for the purpose of diagnosis and follow-up of pancreatic adenocarcinoma. The most extensively used tumor-associated marker is cancer-associated antigen 19-9 (CA19-9), a carbohydrate antigen related to the Lewis blood group antigen associated with circulating mucins, with a reported sensitivity of 79–91% and specificity of 93% [27]. However, the level of CA19-9 is closely related to the tumor burden. It is not uncommon for patients with small tumors to have normal CA19-9 values. It has been estimated that CA19-9 is elevated in only half of patients with tumors of 2 cm or less in size [28]. One study found that at a cutoff value of 37 U/ml, sensitivity and specificity were 76.7% and 87.1%, respectively [29]. If the level is greater than 120 μ/ml, however, the positive predictive value is 100% for malignancy [30].

An ideal screening test would be sensitive, specific, and cost-effective. Unfortunately, CA19-9 is not adequately sensitive or specific for use as a screening test for patients with low clinical suspicion due to the low incidence of pancreatic adenocarcinoma in the general population [15]. Interestingly, in patients who are Lewis a-b negative (7–10% of the population), serum levels of CA19-9 are low or absent [31, 32]. Furthermore, there are many nonmalignant conditions that can be associated with elevated levels of CA19-9, including biliary tract obstruction with cholangitis, pancreatitis, cirrhosis, cholecystitis, inflammatory diseases of the bowel, and autoimmune conditions including rheumatoid arthritis, systemic lupus erythematosus, and scleroderma.

Currently, the best use of CA19-9 is in evaluating effectiveness of cancer treatments, both surgical resection and chemotherapy, by following the patient's levels over time. A general rule is the higher the CA 19-9 level prior to surgery, the higher the tumor burden and the less likely that the tumor is resectable. In fact, patients with very high levels of CA19-9 (greater than 1000 μ/ml) are often noted to have advanced disease with low probability of surgically unresectability [33]. For patients who undergo surgical resection, decreasing or stable CA19-9 levels postoperatively are associated with longer survival, whereas increasing levels suggest recurrence or progression of disease [15, 34].

More accurate tumor markers are being tested to improve the early detection and prognosis of pancreatic cancer. By comparing patients with resectable pancreatic adenocarcinoma, chronic pancreatitis, and healthy controls, macrophage inhibitory cytokine 1 (MIC-1) appears to perform better than CA19-9 in differentiating between patients with pancreatic cancer from healthy controls, but not from chronic pancreatitis [35]. However, more research is needed to determine its applicability in clinical setting.

Abdominal Imaging

There are many imaging modalities available for patients undergoing evaluation for suspected pancreatic adenocarcinoma. Typically, diagnosis of pancreatic cancer is usually made by one or a combination of the following imaging studies: transabdominal ultrasound (US), contrast-enhanced, multiphase, multidetector, helical computed tomography (CT), magnetic resonance imaging (MRI), magnetic resonance cholangiopancreatography (MRCP), endoscopic retrograde cholangiopancreatography (ERCP), and endoscopic ultrasound (EUS).

Transabdominal US

Traditionally, transabdominal US has been used as the initial study in patients presenting with jaundice because of its availability, low cost, and low patient risk. However, the quality of this imaging, in particular, is highly dependent upon the skill of the operator. Furthermore, the quality of the study can be hindered by the body habitus of the patient, and presence or absence of overlying bowel loops [36]. The entire pancreas can be visualized only 25% of the time [37–39]. When visualized, pancreatic cancer appears as a solid hypoechoic, hypovascular mass with irregular margins [22, 36, 38–40]. Dilatation of the main pancreatic duct from the tumor mass as well as biliary system can be seen when the tumor is located in the head of the pancreas [36]. The sensitivity of transabdominal US has been reported from as low as 44% [41] to as high as 94% [36, 42, 43], and its specificity ranges from 90 to 99% [43, 44].

Contrast-Enhanced Helical CT

With the recent technological advances in CT, it has become possible to achieve a better visualization of pancreatic masses. Thin-section, multiphase, multidetector (usually 4–64), contrast-enhanced helical CT scanning leads to the continuous acquisition of large volume of information in a single breath, making it possible for a retrospective three-dimensional reconstruction of images [36, 45]. Thus, helical CT has good diagnostic accuracy, with a sensitivity of 85–95% and specificity of 95% for the detection of pancreatic cancer. Of note, the sensitivity of helical CT is related directly to the size of the tumor. For tumors <15 mm, the sensitivity of helical CT is cited as 67%, and for tumors greater than 15 mm, the sensitivity is 100% [46].

The most common finding at CT is a hypodense mass at the head of the pancreas (nearly 60%), in the body (15%), or in the tail (5%) [47–49]. Approximately 80% of small pancreatic tumors are isodense on delayed imaging [50]. A less common finding is enlargement of the entire pancreas [51].

Aside from detecting the mass lesion, CT is very useful for detecting vascular involvement (particularly, portal vein, celiac axis, and superior mesenteric artery and vein), which may determine surgical resectability, as well as metastatic lesions, peritoneal implants, and lymphadenopathy. Tumors seen to invade the superior mesenteric artery or the celiac axis are deemed unresectable, given that surgical resection with negative margins is not possible [4]. In contrast, visualization of occlusion of splenic vein with perigastric collaterals at CT does not always exclude surgical resection as an option [14]. When the helical CT determines the tumor to be resectable, up to 75% of tumors are confirmed to be resectable during surgery [15]. When the helical CT detects vascular involvement or other signs of unresectability, including periportal collaterals, dilated small peripancreatic veins (suggesting portal vein occlusion), distant metastatic lesions, or invasion of nearby organs, nearly all are confirmed to be unresectable during surgery [15, 52]. The most frequent reasons for aborted surgical resection are small peritoneal or metastatic liver implants and tumor involvement of the vasculature [53].

Magnetic Resonance Imaging

As a result of the recent advances in CT, there has been no significant advantage is found with routine MRI and magnetic resonance angiography for diagnosis and/or staging of pancreatic masses. The reported sensitivity and specificity ranged from 83–87% to 81–100%, respectively [54, 55]. Sheridan et al. found that there were no significant differences in detection of the mass lesion, but MRI was shown to be significantly better than helical CT in accurately determining surgical resectability (87% vs 76%, P=0.02) [56]. However, Nishiharu et al. found that helical CT was significantly superior to MRI in diagnosing peripancreatic tissue, portal vein, and/or peripancreatic artery (P<0.01) [57]. Thus, it appears that the choice of CT or MRI in the evaluation of patients with suspected pancreatic cancer depends upon the patient characteristics as well as the local expertise with the imaging techniques.

Pancreatic cancer tends to appear as a mass with lower signal intensity than that of the surrounding normal pancreatic parenchyma in T1-weighted images [50]. On T2-weighted images, the tumor tends to appear hyperintense or isointense when compared to the normal pancreatic parenchyma [57]. Vascular involvement was identified when perivascular fat planes were infiltrated by a tumor encircling of a vessel [50, 58].

Heavily-T2-weighted imaging sequences with prolonged echo times are utilized in MRCP to depict the biliary tree, the pancreatic duct, the liver, and the surrounding vascular structures. A study of 124 patients cited an 84% sensitivity and 97% specificity for MRCP in diagnosing pancreatic cancer [59]. MR images obtained through the MRCP protocol offer an excellent view of both the biliary tree and the pancreatic duct. With quality approaching that of the cholangiogram [14], it has, in many instances, replaced diagnostic ERCP in the evaluation algorithm for suspected pancreatic cancer, especially in light of the possibility of significant complications from ERCP, including bleeding, perforation, pancreatitis, and sedation-related adverse events [60]. Dilatation of the common bile duct, the pancreatic duct, or both may be an indication of underlying pancreatic malignancy [50]. However, a normal-caliber pancreatic duct can be see in up to 20% of the patients with documented pancreatic cancer [61]. One area that may be poorly visualized is the pancreatic tail if the patient is unable to hold his/her breath for the test [36].

One distinct disadvantage of MRI/MRCP is the claustrophobia and anxiety that some patients experience in closed systems, leading to either patient refusal or need for sedation. This may be less problematic with open MRI machines. In addition, it is not possible to image patients with a metallic prosthesis, artificial heart valves, or pacemakers.

Endoscopic Retrograde Cholangiopancreatography

With the advances in MRCP, the role of diagnostic ERCP has diminished, and it is increasingly reserved for therapeutic indications. Nonetheless, the diagnostic value of ERCP for diagnosing pancreatic cancer is high, with a sensitivity of 92% and a specificity of 96% (as cited by Nidederau and Grendell [62]). The most challenging diagnostic dilemma involves chronic pancreatitis leading to either false-positive or false-negative findings for pancreatic cancer on ERCP. A classic finding on ERCP is the "double-duct sign," which represents strictures or stenosis of both the common bile duct and the main pancreatic duct. Importantly, this finding can occasionally be seen in processes other than pancreatic cancer, including chronic pancreatitis [63, 64]. Even when the double-duct sign is not seen, there is usually an abnormality in the pancreatobiliary system, including pancreatic duct obstruction, pancreatic duct strictures greater than 1 cm in length, irregular pancreatic duct strictures, or stenoses, often in combination with loss of side branches [63]. A review of 530 ERCP examinations proved that it is a highly sensitive diagnostic tool, with only 15 (2.8%) normal pancreatograms seen in patients with pancreatic cancer [53, 65].

The role of preoperative biliary decompression is controversial. The initial driving force behind preoperative biliary stenting was early nonrandomized studies, which suggested a reduction in the mortality rate for jaundiced patients who underwent biliary decompression prior to surgical resection [66–72]. Despite the expected outcome of a decrease in bilirubin and alkaline phosphatase levels and increases in nutritional and performance status, subsequent studies have not yet proven that preoperative biliary drainage results in significant clinical benefit or reduction of postoperative morbidity and mortality rates [73–76]. In fact, several subsequent studies have reported higher morbidity and mortality rates when surgical resection is performed after preoperative biliary decompression [4, 73, 77–79]. Furthermore, in a meta-analysis, Sewnath et al. suggested that patients who had biliary stenting prior to surgery had a higher overall complication rate when compared to patients who did not undergo preoperative biliary stenting [80]. It also appeared that there was no benefit to preoperative biliary decompression. In addition, several studies have found no significant differences in complication rates except for slightly higher rate of wound infection for the group with preoperative biliary stenting [81–83].

Although no consensus has been achieved, most would concur that routine preoperative biliary drainage is not indicated in cases where prompt surgical resection is anticipated [78]. However, patients with significant metabolic or nutritional deficits, those developing cholangitis or sepsis, those entering into neoadjuvant therapeutic trials, or those in whom a delay in surgical intervention is necessary may benefit from preoperative biliary decompression [14, 78]. Generally, for patients with potentially resectable pancreatic cancer who require biliary decompression, a plastic stent, placed either endoscopically or percutaneously, is preferred [78].

Endoscopic Ultrasound

EUS is able to provide high-resolution imaging of the pancreas and nearby structures due to the close proximity of the high-frequency US probe (usually 7.5–12 MHz) in the stomach and duodenum to the pancreas during upper endoscopy, overcoming the extrinsic factor limiting transabdominal US. There are two types of EUS endoscopes available: radial scanning and linear array. The radial-scanning type produces images perpendicular to the axis of the scope, producing 360° images, with the transducer appearing as a "bulls eye" within the image [84]. The linear-array type, on the other hand, produces images parallel to the axis of the scope. When fine-needle aspiration (FNA) is performed during EUS, the linear-array echoendoscope is used because the needle can be visualized and manipulated in real time as it enters the target lesion [85].

Currently, EUS appears to be the most accurate imaging tool for the detection and local staging of pancreatic cancer. The sensitivity (91–99%) and the specificity (100%) of EUS-FNA are significantly better than those of conventional CT [86–89]. In a recent prospective comparison of EUS and dual-phase multidetector CT at a single academic center, the sensitivity of EUS for detection of a pancreatic mass was significantly greater than that of CT (98% versus 86%, respectively, P=0.012) [90]. EUS has been shown to be superior to CT and MRI, particularly for the detection of small pancreatic lesions <2 cm in diameter (Fig. 47.1) [54, 86, 91]. EUS may be superior to helical CT for the evaluation of patients with obstructive jaundice [92]. However, with the advances in CT technology, the multidetector helical CT with three-dimensional reconstruction of images appear to be as good as or superior to EUS in predicting the unresectability of pancreatic cancer [35, 85, 90, 93–96]. In other single-center studies, EUS was not very good for determining resectability [97].

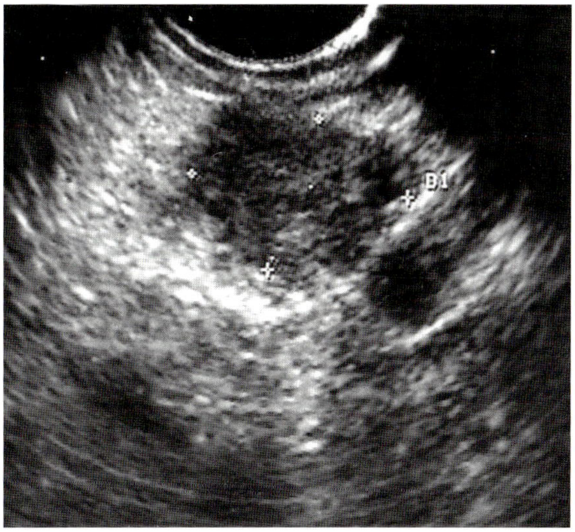

Figure 47.1

Endoscopic ultrasound (EUS) image (Pentax linear-array echoendoscope, 7.5 Mhz) of a small, resectable pancreatic mass (1.1 cm) in the pancreatic tail immediately adjacent to the splenic vein. EUS-guided fine needle aspiration showed adenocarcinoma, which was confirmed by surgical resection and pathology. A computed tomography (CT) scan and endoscopic retrograde cholangiopancreatography (ERCP) failed to make the diagnosis

In a prospective study examining the EUS features in 115 patients, pancreatic cancer was most often seen as a hypoechoic (98.3%; Fig. 47.1), nonhomogeneous (84.7%), solid mass (88.1%) with irregular borders (78%) (Fig. 47.2) [50, 98]. A second prospective study examined the EUS features in 45 patients with pancreatic cancer to assess the characteristics associated with vascular involvement. The most common features identified were irregular venous walls (87%), loss of interface (78%), and proximity of the mass to the vessel (73%) [99]. The most accurate sign was the visualization of irregular venous walls; however, it had a low sensitivity rate (47%) due to the relative inability of EUS to detect superior mesenteric vein invasion. Furthermore, vascular involvement can be suggested by the presence of a tumor within the vessel lumen, obliteration of a vessel, and/or the presence of collateral vessels on EUS [50].

EUS is helpful as a highly specific diagnostic test to follow an indeterminate clinical presentation consisting of laboratory finding (mildly elevated CA19-9) or radiologic pancreatic abnormality, such as "fullness," acute pancreatitis (Fig.47.2), focal enlargement of the pancreas, or dilated pancreatic or bile duct (Fig. 47.3).

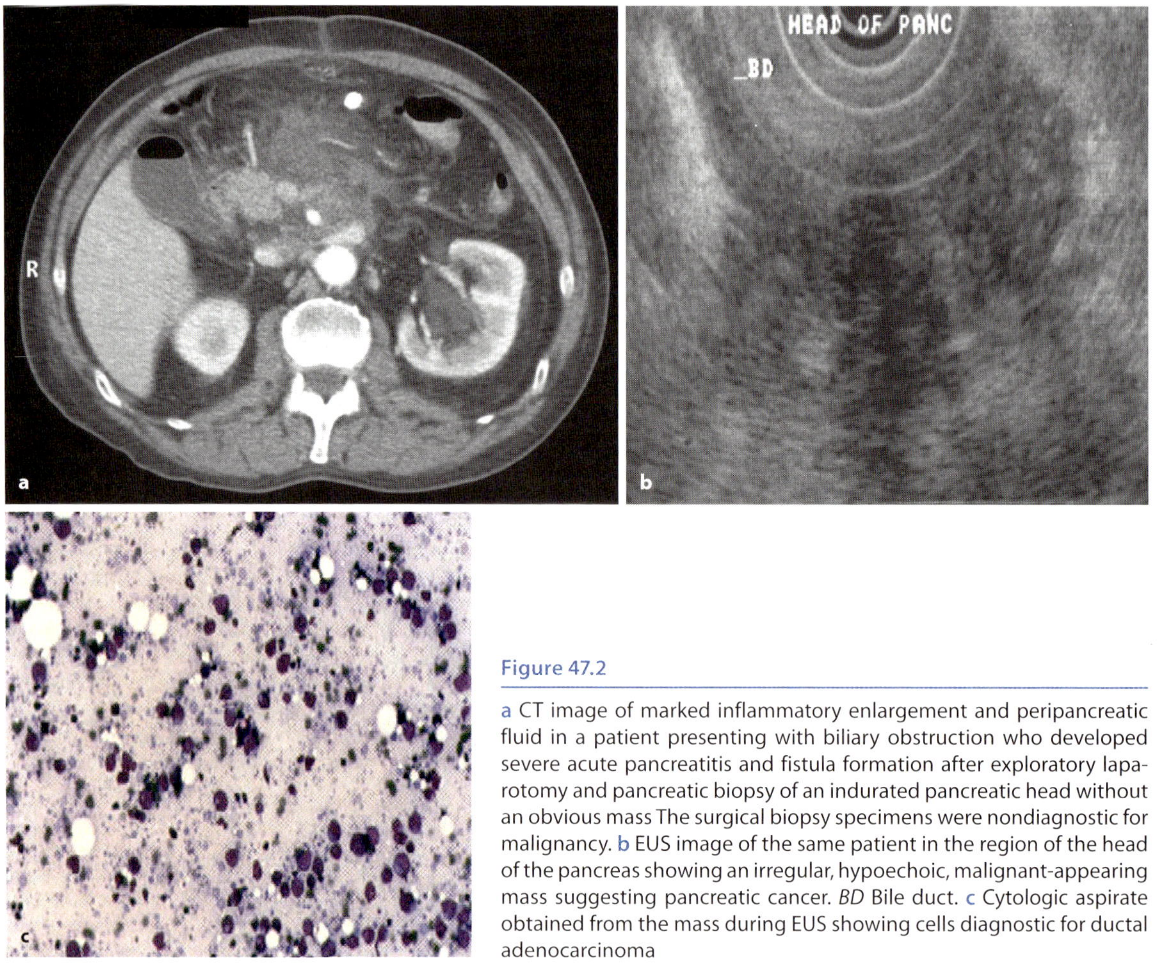

Figure 47.2

a CT image of marked inflammatory enlargement and peripancreatic fluid in a patient presenting with biliary obstruction who developed severe acute pancreatitis and fistula formation after exploratory laparotomy and pancreatic biopsy of an indurated pancreatic head without an obvious mass The surgical biopsy specimens were nondiagnostic for malignancy. b EUS image of the same patient in the region of the head of the pancreas showing an irregular, hypoechoic, malignant-appearing mass suggesting pancreatic cancer. *BD* Bile duct. c Cytologic aspirate obtained from the mass during EUS showing cells diagnostic for ductal adenocarcinoma

Indeed, the presence of a completely normal EUS examination performed by an experienced endosonographer has a very high likelihood of predicting the absence of pancreatic cancer [100]. Long-term follow-up (minimum 6 months, median follow-up 23.9 months) of 80 patients with clinically indeterminate suspicion of pancreatic cancer and a normal pancreas by EUS showed a negative predictive value of 100%.

The sensitivity of EUS for the detection of pancreatic cancer is high (91–98% [101, 90]), but is not 100%. A retrospective case series of 20 patients with missed pancreatic cancers from different centers in the United States showed that chronic pancreatitis (11/20 cases), diffusely infiltrating carcinoma, a prominent split between the dorsal/ventral pancreas, and a recent episode of acute pancreatitis were associated factors [102]. Importantly, when EUS was repeated 2–3 months following a negative exam, a pancreatic mass was found. Hence, if a patient does not undergo surgical exploration, EUS should be repeated within 3 months if there is a strong clinical suspicion of pancreatic cancer and all imaging tests, including EUS, are negative.

Pseudotumors from focal chronic pancreatitis can be quite difficult to differentiate from pancreatic cancer (Table 47.1; Fig. 47.3) [103]. The EUS diagnosis of pancreatic cancer in patients with underlying chronic pancreatitis may be more challenging as compared to those without chronic pancreatitis [104]. The use of power Doppler during EUS may increase the sensitivity to 93% for the diagnosis of pancreatic cancer; the absence of power Doppler signal (i.e., a hypovascular pattern) may help differentiate between cancer and pseudotumoral chronic pancreatitis [105].

EUS-Guided FNA

One distinct advantage of EUS over other radiologic imaging modalities is the ability to sample lesions and provide a tissue diagnosis. EUS-FNA is not routinely necessary in an operable patient with a resectable

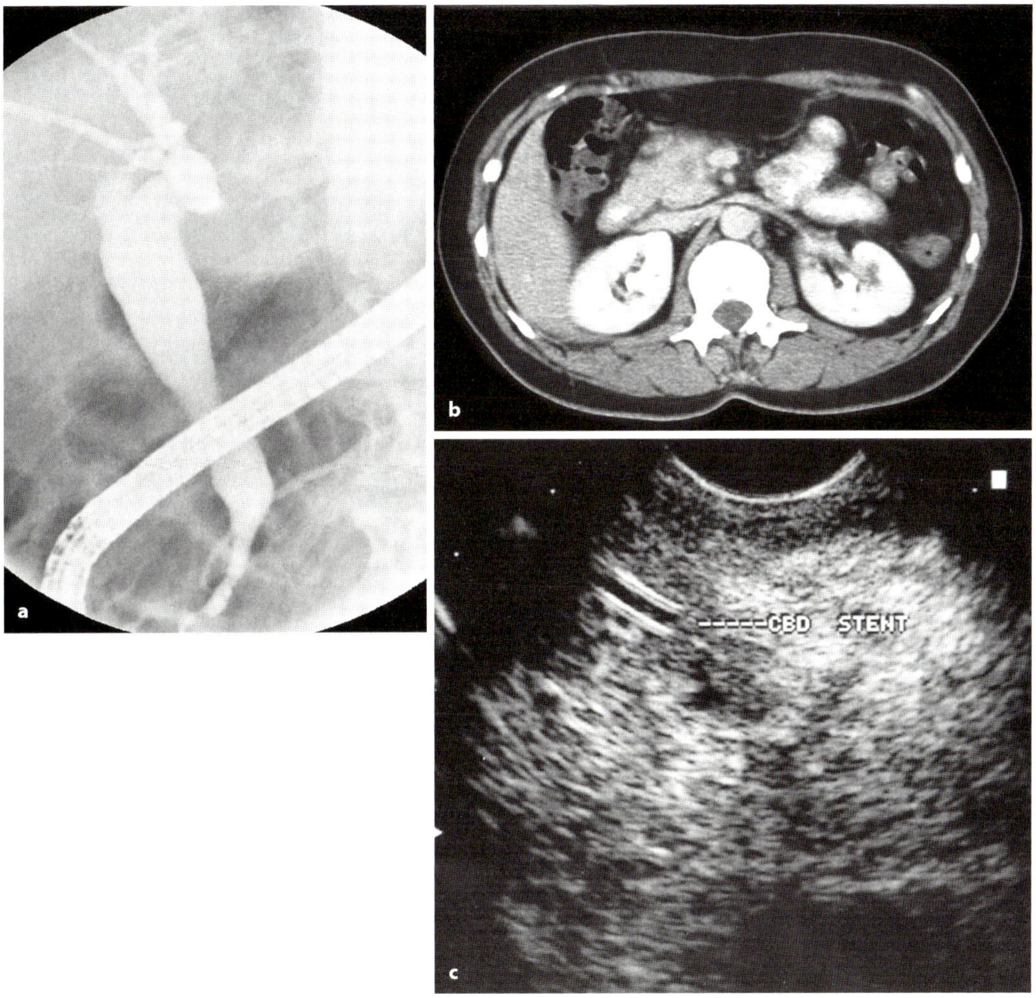

Figure 47.3

a ERCP image showing dilated extrahepatic and intrahepatic bile ducts and distal bile duct stricture in an elderly patient with history of abdominal pain, anorexia, weight loss, depression, and elevated serum cancer-associated antigen 19-9 (CA19-9). b Abdominal CT image showing an indeterminate mass in the pancreatic head. c EUS image showing an echogenic biliary stent (*CBD STENT*) within the bile duct stricture but no pancreatic mass. A Whipple procedure was performed and the final diagnosis was chronic pancreatitis with no evidence of malignancy

Table 47.1. Limitations of endoscopic ultrasound for the diagnosis of pancreatic malignancy

1. Operator dependency
2. Limited availability
3. Requires sedation
4. Altered anatomy or luminal obstruction results in unsuccessful or incomplete imaging
5. Limited penetration depth

pancreatic mass by CT and a clinical presentation consistent with malignancy. However, patients with indeterminate lesions (Figs. 47.2 and 47.4), patients with no symptoms and an incidentally detected pancreatic lesion, patients with evidence of biliary obstruction but no obvious mass (Fig. 47.3), those with locally invasive cancers or metastatic disease visualized at the time of EUS or prior to EUS imaging (by US, CT, or MRI) may benefit from an EUS-FNA. Transgastric or transduodenal EUS-guided FNA can be used to obtain tissue samples for cytology, instead of the traditional percutaneous biopsy technique, which carries with it a theoretical risk of tumor seeding [14]. Furthermore, there is theoretically less risk of

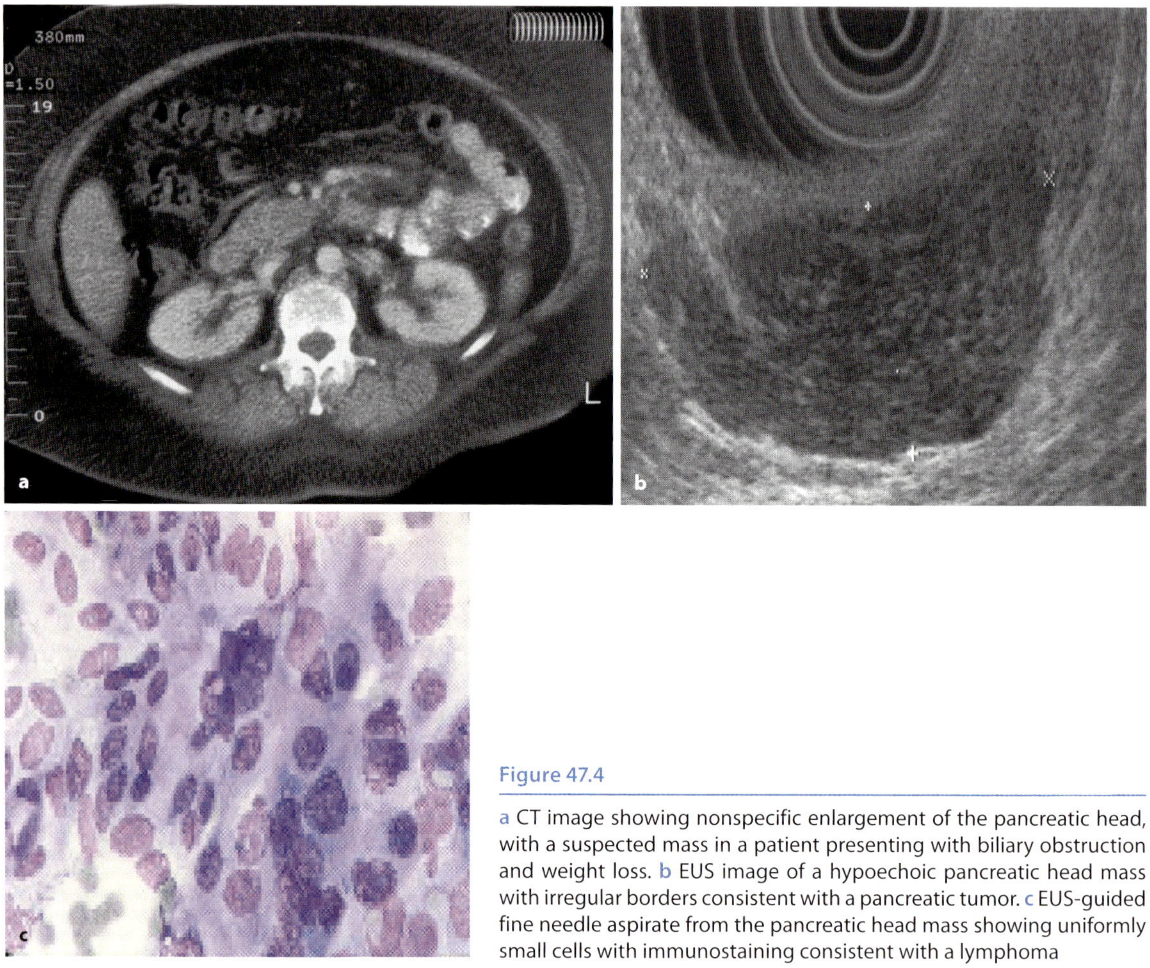

Figure 47.4

a CT image showing nonspecific enlargement of the pancreatic head, with a suspected mass in a patient presenting with biliary obstruction and weight loss. b EUS image of a hypoechoic pancreatic head mass with irregular borders consistent with a pancreatic tumor. c EUS-guided fine needle aspirate from the pancreatic head mass showing uniformly small cells with immunostaining consistent with a lymphoma

tumor seeding with EUS-FNA due to the transduodenal approach for head of pancreas masses, which results in puncture through tissue that would usually be removed during a Whipple procedure. In a retrospective study examining 489 patients, EUS-FNA had sensitivity of 79.9%, a specificity of 98.8%, a positive predictive value of 99.2%, a negative predictive value of 72.5%, and an accuracy of 86.5%. However, in a prospective series from medical centers with EUS expertise, the sensitivity of EUS-FNA of suspected pancreatic lesions has a sensitivity of 93%, a specificity of 100%, and a diagnostic accuracy of 95% for pancreatic lesions [106]. In a large series of 233 patients, the sensitivity, specificity, and accuracy of EUS-FNA for the diagnosis of pancreatic malignancy was 91%, 100%, and 92%, respectively [101]. Furthermore, recent studies suggest that the addition of tumor markers such as p53 immunostaining of EUS-FNA specimens [107] and analysis of mutant *K-RAS* in FNA specimens and pancreatic juice [108] may supplement the diagnosis of conventional cytology.

The main limitations of EUS for the diagnosis of pancreatic malignancy are shown in Table 47.1. EUS is highly operator dependent and pancreatic EUS is technically more difficult and requires greater experience and training than other nonpancreatic imaging sites. Secondly, EUS is less readily available than US, CT, or MRI, and third, EUS is more invasive than other standard radiologic tests, requiring intravenous sedation and its attendant small risk of adverse events. The overall complication rate of EUS-FNA for pancreatic lesion diagnosis is 1–2% and is attributable to perforation, pancreatitis (0.64% [109]), infection, and sedation-related side effects [101, 110]. Furthermore, although imaging of the pancreas can be technically completed in the vast majority of cases, altered anatomy and high-grade obstruction of the esophageal, gastric, or duodenal lumen may result in unsuccessful or incomplete imaging. Finally, EUS alone may not allow complete tumor staging because of limited penetration depth, and distant metastatic disease in the right liver lobe, peritoneum, and pelvis will not be detected.

CT- or US-Guided Percutaneous Biopsy

Percutaneous biopsy is of limited utility in patients in whom surgical intervention is planned for potentially resectable pancreatic lesion. The ranges calculated from previous studies for sensitivity, specificity, positive predictive value, and diagnostic accuracy are 64–98%, 80–100%, 98.4–100%, and 74.4–96%, respectively. In contrast, the negative predictive value has varied widely from 16 to 86%, with a recent retrospective study value of 47.1–48.6% [111]. Even with repeated sampling, a negative result cannot definitively exclude malignancy, since smaller tumors, which are more likely to be resectable, are also more likely to be missed by sampling error [14]. There is also a concern that tumor seeding will occur with percutaneous biopsy, either along the needle tract or via intraperitoneal spread [14, 112–114].

Percutaneous biopsy may be of use in unresectable pancreatic cancer to guide neoadjuvant or palliative chemoradiation therapy, or if there is a suspicion of pancreatic lymphoma [14]. Metastatic lesions in the right liver lobe or those that are peripheral and potentially beyond the reach of EUS-FNA are more favorably diagnosed by percutaneous FNA. However, currently, percutaneous biopsy sampling has largely been supplanted by EUS-FNA for primary pancreatic cancers due to the absence of pain (resulting from intravenous sedation), the ability to take multiple samples until diagnostic tissue is obtained (often requiring 5–6 passes or more with bedside cytology evaluation), and the short distance between the needle and the target (which enables increased force in very hard cancers). EUS-FNA produced greater accuracy when evaluating lesions <3 cm in size when compared to percutaneous biopsy under US or CT guidance (P=0.015) [111].

Cytologic diagnosis of pancreatic malignancy may be problematic for both percutaneous and EUS-guided FNA due to the relative paucity of malignant cells in highly sclerotic, hard tumors. Hence, the absence of malignant cells in fine-needle aspirates does not rule out a diagnosis of pancreatic cancer. In recent years, there has been increasing interest in improving the yield of EUS-FNA with tumor markers, such as immunohistochemical staining for *K-RAS* point mutations [103] and p53 protein overexpression [107]. In a prospective evaluation of pancreatic masses, investigators showed that p53 immunostaining increased the sensitivity (from 76% to 91%) and overall accuracy (from 79% to 92%) compared to conventional cytology without a change in specificity (91%) [107]. In a study of 62 patients with pancreatic cancer and 15 patients with chronic pancreatitis, the sensitivity of EUS-FNA was 82% (overall accuracy 86%); 74% of aspirates from malignant pancreatic masses and none of the aspirates from areas of focal chronic pancreatitis showed *K-RAS* mutations [103]. Another study showed improved accuracy of conventional cytologic analysis of aspirates (accuracy=61%) with the addition of quantitative analysis of *K-RAS* mutations in EUS FNA aspirates (accuracy =81%) and pancreatic juice (accuracy=88%).

Diagnostic Approach to the Patient with Suspected Pancreatic Cancer

Currently, there is no established consensus on a diagnostic algorithm for patients with suspected pancreatic cancer based on signs, symptoms, and laboratory findings. At our institution, we typically begin the evaluation with a multidetector, contrast-enhanced helical CT scan with a three-dimensional pancreas protocol. If the CT shows a discrete pancreatic mass without distant metastatic disease and/or local vascular invasion, then no other diagnostic or staging tests are needed prior to surgery. If there is nonspecific pancreatic enlargement but no mass, or if an indeterminate mass lesion is seen, EUS will be performed to confirm the presence and location of a malignant-appearing lesion and to obtain a FNA for tissue diagnosis. EUS-FNA will also be performed if there is clearly local vascular encasement or invasion or distant metastatic disease by CT. In the latter situation, medical and radiation oncology evaluation is obtained if the patient and family are interested in palliative therapy.

In patients with a potentially resectable pancreatic mass lesion and clinical presentation consistent with a tumor, there is usually no need to perform EUS-FNA. However, physicians must always have a high index of suspicion for other types of pancreatic and secondary tumors and pseudotumors that may be difficult to distinguish from pancreatic cancer (Table 47.2). If there are large, bulky abdominal lymph nodes, or a primary cancer at a different site (particularly breast, colon, or melanoma), EUS-FNA may be helpful in distinguishing between primary pancreatic ductal adenocarcinoma and pancreatic lymphoma (Fig. 47.4), or metastatic carcinoma to the pancreas. Patients with autoimmune sclerosing pancreatitis may present with a diffusely enlarged hypoechoic pancreas and/or a focal irregular hypoechoic mass lesion [115] and EUS-FNA can provide tissue that could confirm this diagnosis if there are chronic inflamma-

Table 47.2. Differential diagnosis of pancreatic cancer

Diagnosis	Pancreatic cancer-like clinical findings
Chronic pancreatitis	Weight loss (due to malabsorption), diabetes, abdominal pain, and dilatation of the pancreatic and/or bile duct
Autoimmune sclerosing pancreatitis	Jaundice, abdominal pain, weight loss, pancreatic mass
Cholangiocarcinoma	Biliary obstruction, jaundice, weight loss, abdominal pain
Ampullary adenocarcinoma	Biliary and/or pancreatic duct obstruction, jaundice, weight loss, abdominal pain
Ampullary adenomas	Biliary and/or pancreatic duct obstruction, abdominal pain
Metastatic cancer to the pancreas	Mass in pancreas, abdominal lymphadenopathy, liver metastasis
Pancreatic cysts	Mass in pancreas
Intraductal papillary mucinous neoplasms	Mass in pancreas, dilated pancreatic duct, pancreatitis, abdominal pain
Pancreatic neuroendocrine tumors	Mass in pancreas, liver metastasis
Pancreatic lymphoma	Mass in pancreas, abdominal lymphadenopathy
Sarcomas	Mass in pancreas
Choledocholithiasis	Biliary obstruction, jaundice, abdominal pain
Viral hepatitis	Jaundice, elevated liver function tests
Drug-induced jaundice	Jaundice, elevated liver function tests
Alcoholic liver disease	Jaundice, elevated liver function tests

tory cells and no malignant cells, when the clinical presentation is consistent (elevated immunoglobulin G). A trial of corticosteroids may be warranted in this setting. The distinction between inflammatory non-neoplastic masses, for example acute pancreatitis (Fig. 47.2), chronic pancreatitis (Fig. 47.3), and autoimmune sclerosing pancreatitis, pancreatic lymphoma, and metastatic carcinoma to the pancreas is critical, given the change in therapeutic approach and marked impact on patient management. For example, patients with pancreatic lymphoma could be given external beam radiation and chemotherapy, and patients with autoimmune pancreatitis respond well to systemic steroids.

If there is evidence of biliary obstruction with cholangitis, or if a delay to surgical intervention is anticipated, preoperative biliary decompression with a stent is often performed, either endoscopically or percutaneously. Barring any complications, patients with potentially resectable lesions should proceed to surgical intervention in a timely fashion. If the lesion is deemed unresectable, a metal expendable endoprosthesis may be placed for biliary obstruction for palliation.

References

1. Cancer Facts and Figures (2005). American Cancer Society 2005
2. Ahlgren JD (1996) Epidemiology and risk factors in pancreatic cancer. Semin Oncol 23:241–250
3. Parkin DM, Bray F, Ferlay J, Pisani P (2001) Estimating the world cancer burden: Globocan 2000. Int J Cancer 94:153–156
4. Li D, Xie K, Wolff R, Abbruzzese JL (2004) Pancreatic cancer. Lancet 363:1049–1057
5. Ettinghausen SE, Schwartzentruber DJ, Sindelar WF (1995) Evolving strategies for the treatment of adenocarcinoma of the pancreas. A review. J Clin Gastroenterol 21:48–60
6. Schneider G, Siveke JT, Eckel F, Schmid RM (2005) Pancreatic cancer: basic and clinical aspects. Gastroenterology 128:1606–1625
7. Hermann RE, Cooperman AM (1979) Current concepts in cancer: cancer of the pancreas. N Engl J Med 301:482–485
8. Holly EA, Chaliha I, Bracci PM, Gautam M (2004) Signs and symptoms of pancreatic cancer: a population-based case-control study in the San Francisco Bay area. Clin Gastroenterol Hepatol 2:510–517
9. Brand R (2004) Pancreatic cancer. Dis Mon 50:545–555
10. Barkin JS, Goldstein JA (1999) Diagnostic approach to pancreatic cancer. Gastroenterol Clin North Am 28:709–722
11. Raijman I, Levin B (1995) Exocrine tumors of the pancreas. In: Cohen S, Pounder RE, Kalser MH (eds) Bockus Gastroenterology, 5th edn. WB Saunders, Philadelphia pp 2984–3001
12. Braganza JM, Howat HT (1972) Cancer of the pancreas. Clin Gastroenterol 1:219–237

13. Furukawa H, Okada S, Saisho H, Ariyama J, Karasawa E, Nakaizumi A, Nakazawa S, Murakami K, Kakizoe T (1996) Clinicopathologic features of small pancreatic adenocarcinoma. A collective study. Cancer 78:986–990
14. Lillemoe KD, Yeo CJ, Cameron JL (2000) Pancreatic cancer: state-of-the-art care. CA Cancer J Clin 50:241–268
15. Barkin JS, Goldstein JA (2000) Diagnostic and therapeutic approach to pancreatic cancer. Biomed Pharmacother 54:400–409
16. DiMagno EP (1999) Pancreatic cancer: clinical presentation, pitfalls and early clues. Ann Oncol 10:140–142
17. Parks RW, Garden OJ (2000) Ensuring early diagnosis in pancreatic cancer. Practitioner 244:336–338, 340–341, 343
18. Moossa AR (1982) Pancreatic cancer: approach to diagnosis, selection for surgery and choice of operation. Cancer 50:2689–2698
19. Gullick HD (1959) Carcinoma of the pancreas; a review and critical study of 100 cases. Medicine (Baltimore) 38:47–84
20. Kalser MH, Barkin J, MacIntyre JM (1985) Pancreatic cancer. Assessment of prognosis by clinical presentation. Cancer 56:397–402
21. Lin A, Feller ER (1990) Pancreatic carcinoma as a cause of unexplained pancreatitis: report of ten cases. Ann Intern Med 113:166–167
22. Warshaw AL, Fernandez-del Castillo C (1992) Pancreatic carcinoma. N Engl J Med 326:455–465
23. Rosa JA, Van Linda BM, Abourizk NN (1989) New-onset diabetes mellitus as a harbinger of pancreatic carcinoma. A case report and literature review. J Clin Gastroenterol 11:211–215
24. Greenberger NJ (2001) Pancreatic Disease. In: Noble J (ed) Textbook of Primary Care Medicine, 3rd edn. Mosby, St. Louis, pp 974–975
25. Sohn TA, Yeo CJ (2002) Pancreatic and periampullary carcinoma (nonendocrine). In: Shackelford RT, Zuidema GD, Yeo CJ (eds) Shackelford's Surgery of the Alimentary Tract, 5th edn. WB Saunders, Philadelphia, pp III63–III85
26. Hruban RH, Wilentz RE (2005) The Pancreas. In: Kumar V, Abbas AK, Fausto N, Robbins SL, Cotran RS (eds) Robbins and Cotran Pathologic Basis of Disease, 7th edn. Elsevier Saunders, Philadelphia, p 951
27. Scholmerich J (1993) Diagnosis of pancreatic cancer. In: Beger HG, Buchler M, Malfertheiner P (eds) Standards in Pancreatic Surgery. Springer-Verlag, Berlin, p 578
28. Lynch HT, Smyrk T, Kern SE, Hruban RH, Lightdale CJ, Lemon SJ, Lynch JF, Fusaro LR, Fusaro RM, Ghadirian P (1996) Familial pancreatic cancer: a review. Semin Oncol 23:251–275
29. Kim HJ, Kim MH, Myung SJ, Lim BC, Park ET, Yoo KS, Seo DW, Lee SK, Min YI (1999) A new strategy for the application of CA19-9 in the differentiation of pancreaticobiliary cancer: analysis using a receiver operating characteristic curve. Am J Gastroenterol 94:1941–1946
30. Hyoty M, Hyoty H, Aaran RK, Airo I, Nordback I (1992) Tumour antigens CA 195 and CA 19-9 in pancreatic juice and serum for the diagnosis of pancreatic carcinoma. Eur J Surg 158:173–179
31. Ritts RE, Pitt HA (1998) CA 19-9 in pancreatic cancer. Surg Oncol Clin N Am 7:93–101
32. Lamerz R (1999) Role of tumour markers, cytogenetics. Ann Oncol 10:145–149
33. Glenn J, Steinberg WM, Kurtzman SH, Steinberg SM, Sindelar WF (1988) Evaluation of the utility of a radioimmunoassay for serum CA 19-9 levels in patients before and after treatment of carcinoma of the pancreas. J Clin Oncol 6:462–468
34. Montgomery RC, Hoffman JP, Riley LB, Rogatko A, Ridge JA, Eisenberg BL (1997) Prediction of recurrence and survival by post-resection CA 19-9 values in patients with adenocarcinoma of the pancreas. Ann Surg Oncol 4:551–556
35. Koopmann J, Rosenzweig CN, Zhang Z, Canto MI, Brown DA, Hunter M, Yeo C, Chan DW, Breit SN, Goggins M (2006) Serum markers in patients with resectable pancreatic adenocarcinoma: macrophage inhibitory cytokine 1 versus CA19-9. Clin Cancer Res 12:442–446
36. Brand R (2001) The diagnosis of pancreatic cancer. Cancer J 7:287–297
37. Friedman AC, Krudy AG Jr, Shawker TH (1987) Pancreatic neoplasms. In: Friedman AC (ed) Radiology of the Liver, Biliary Tract, Pancreas, and Spleen. Williams and Wilkins, Baltimore, p 1110 p, [1] p. of plates
38. Ormson MJ, Charboneau JW, Stephens DH (1987) Sonography in patients with a possible pancreatic mass shown on CT. AJR Am J Roentgenol 148:551–555
39. Campbell JP, Wilson SR (1988) Pancreatic neoplasms: how useful is evaluation with US? Radiology 167:341–344
40. Del Maschio A, Vanzulli A, Sironi S, Castrucci M, Mellone R, Staudacher C, Carlucci M, Zerbi A, Parolini D, Faravelli A, Cantaboni A, Garancini P, Di Carlo V (1991) Pancreatic cancer versus chronic pancreatitis: diagnosis with CA 19-9 assessment, US, CT, and CT-guided fine-needle biopsy. Radiology 178:95–99
41. Forsmark CE, Albert CA, Lambiase L, Vogel SB, Torres GM, Summerlin BJ, Toskes PP (1993) Diagnostic tests for pancreatic cancer [abstract]. Gastrointest Endosc 39:314
42. Pollock D, Taylor KJ (1981) Ultrasound scanning in patients with clinical suspicion of pancreatic cancer: a retrospective study. Cancer 47:1662–1665
43. Karlson BM, Ekbom A, Lindgren PG, Kallskog V, Rastad J (1999) Abdominal US for diagnosis of pancreatic tumor: prospective cohort analysis. Radiology 213:107–111
44. Maringhini A, Ciambra M, Raimondo M, Baccelliere P, Grasso R, Dardanoni G, Lanzarone F, Cottone M, Sciarrino E, Pagliaro L (1993) Clinical presentation and ultrasonography in the diagnosis of pancreatic cancer. Pancreas 8:146–150
45. Ferrucci JT (1999) Biliopancreatic malignancy current diagnostic possibilities: an overview. Ann Oncol 10:143–144
46. Legmann P, Vignaux O, Dousset B, Baraza AJ, Palazzo L, Dumontier I, Coste J, Louvel A, Roseau G, Couturier D, Bonnin A (1998) Pancreatic tumors: comparison of dual-phase helical CT and endoscopic sonography. AJR Am J Roentgenol 170:1315–1322
47. Freeny PC (1989) Radiology of the pancreas. Curr Opin Radiol 1:81–93
48. Freeny PC, Marks WM, Ryan JA, Traverso LW (1988) Pancreatic ductal adenocarcinoma: diagnosis and staging with dynamic CT. Radiology 166:125–133
49. Clark LR, Jaffe MH, Choyke PL, Grant EG, Zeman RK (1985) Pancreatic imaging. Radiol Clin North Am 23:489–501
50. Tamm E, Charnsangavej C (2001) Pancreatic cancer: current concepts in imaging for diagnosis and staging. Cancer J 7:298–311

51. Wittenberg J, Simeone JF, Ferrucci JT Jr, Mueller PR, vanSonnenberg E, Neff CC (1982) Non-focal enlargement in pancreatic carcinoma. Radiology 144:131–135
52. Vedantham S, Lu DS, Reber HA, Kadell B (1998) Small peripancreatic veins: improved assessment in pancreatic cancer patients using thin-section pancreatic phase helical CT. AJR Am J Roentgenol 170:377–383
53. Fernandez-del Castillo C, Jimenez RE (2002) Pancreatic cancer, cystic pancreatic neoplasms, and other nonendocrine pancreatic tumors. In: Feldman M, Friedman LS, Sleisenger MH (eds) Sleisenger Fordtran's Gastrointestinal and Liver Disease: Pathophysiology, Diagnosis, Management, 7th edn. Saunders, Philadelphia, pp 970–987
54. Muller MF, Meyenberger C, Bertschinger P, Schaer R, Marincek B (1994) Pancreatic tumors: evaluation with endoscopic US, CT, and MR imaging. Radiology 190:745–751
55. Vellet AD, Romano W, Bach DB, Passi RB, Taves DH, Munk PL (1992) Adenocarcinoma of the pancreatic ducts: comparative evaluation with CT and MR imaging at 1.5 T. Radiology 183:87–95
56. Sheridan MB, Ward J, Guthrie JA, Spencer JA, Craven CM, Wilson D, Guillou PJ, Robinson PJ (1999) Dynamic contrast-enhanced MR imaging and dual-phase helical CT in the preoperative assessment of suspected pancreatic cancer: a comparative study with receiver operating characteristic analysis. AJR Am J Roentgenol 173:583–590
57. Nishiharu T, Yamashita Y, Abe Y, Mitsuzaki K, Tsuchigame T, Nakayama Y, Takahashi M (1999) Local extension of pancreatic carcinoma: assessment with thin-section helical CT versus with breath-hold fast MR imaging – ROC analysis. Radiology 212:445–452
58. Sironi S, De Cobelli F, Zerbi A, Angeli E, Balzano G, Taccagni G, Di Carlo V, Del Maschio A (1996) Pancreatic adenocarcinoma: assessment of vascular invasion with high-field MR imaging and a phased-array coil. AJR Am J Roentgenol 167:997–1001
59. Adamek HE, Albert J, Breer H, Weitz M, Schilling D, Riemann JF (2000) Pancreatic cancer detection with magnetic resonance cholangiopancreatography and endoscopic retrograde cholangiopancreatography: a prospective controlled study. Lancet 356:190–193
60. Aliperti G (1996) Complications related to diagnostic and therapeutic endoscopic retrograde cholangiopancreatography. Gastrointest Endosc Clin N Am 6:379–407
61. Vitellas KM, Keogan MT, Spritzer CE, Nelson RC (2000) MR cholangiopancreatography of bile and pancreatic duct abnormalities with emphasis on the single-shot fast spin-echo technique. Radiographics 20:939–957; quiz 1107–1108, 1112
62. Niederau C, Grendell JH (1992) Diagnosis of pancreatic carcinoma. Imaging techniques and tumor markers. Pancreas 7:66–86
63. Menges M, Lerch MM, Zeitz M (2000) The double duct sign in patients with malignant and benign pancreatic lesions. Gastrointest Endosc 52:74–77
64. Schlauch D, Kohler B, Riemann JF (1993) Double-duct-sign – is it always cancer? Endoscopy 25:489–490
65. Freeny PC (1989) Radiologic diagnosis and staging of pancreatic ductal adenocarcinoma. Radiol Clin North Am 7:121–12
66. Denning DA, Ellison EC, Carey LC (1981) Preoperative percutaneous transhepatic biliary decompression lowers operative morbidity in patients with obstructive jaundice. Am J Surg 141:61–65
67. Gobien RP, Stanley JH, Soucek CD, Anderson MC, Vujic I, Gobien BS (1984) Routine preoperative biliary drainage: effect on management of obstructive jaundice. Radiology 152:353–356
68. Gundry SR, Strodel WE, Knol JA, Eckhauser FE, Thompson NW (1984) Efficacy of preoperative biliary tract decompression in patients with obstructive jaundice. Arch Surg 119:703–708
69. Hatfield AR, Tobias R, Terblanche J, Girdwood AH, Fataar S, Harries-Jones R, Kernoff L, Marks IN (1982) Preoperative external biliary drainage in obstructive jaundice. A prospective controlled clinical trial. Lancet 2:896–869
70. Nakayama T, Ikeda A, Okuda K (1978) Percutaneous transhepatic drainage of the biliary tract: technique and results in 104 cases. Gastroenterology 74:554–559
71. Norlander A, Kalin B, Sundblad R (1982) Effect of percutaneous transhepatic drainage upon liver function and postoperative mortality. Surg Gynecol Obstet 155:161–166
72. Lygidakis NJ, van der Heyde MN, Lubbers MJ (1987) Evaluation of preoperative biliary drainage in the surgical management of pancreatic head carcinoma. Acta Chir Scand 153:665–668
73. Heslin MJ, Brooks AD, Hochwald SN, Harrison LE, Blumgart LH, Brennan MF (1998) A preoperative biliary stent is associated with increased complications after pancreatoduodenectomy. Arch Surg 133:149–154
74. Gouma DJ, Moody FG (1984) Preoperative percutaneous transhepatic drainage: use or abuse. A clinical review. Surg Gastroenterol 3:74–80
75. Karsten TM, Allema JH, Reinders M, van Gulik TM, de Wit LT, Verbeek PC, Huibregtse K, Tytgat GN, Gouma DJ (1996) Preoperative biliary drainage, colonisation of bile and postoperative complications in patients with tumours of the pancreatic head: a retrospective analysis of 241 consecutive patients. Eur J Surg 162:881–888
76. Lai EC, Mok FP, Fan ST, Lo CM, Chu KM, Liu CL, Wong J (1994) Preoperative endoscopic drainage for malignant obstructive jaundice. Br J Surg 81:1195–1198
77. Povoski SP, Karpeh MS Jr, Conlon KC, Blumgart LH, Brennan MF (1999) Association of preoperative biliary drainage with postoperative outcome following pancreaticoduodenectomy. Ann Surg 230:131–142
78. Ujiki MB, Talamonti MS (2005) Surgical management of pancreatic cancer. Semin Radiat Oncol 15:218–225
79. Povoski SP, Karpch MS, Conlon KL, et al (1998) Positive intraoperative bile cultures at the time of pancreaticoduodenectomy are associated with preoperative biliary drainage and subsequent development of postoperative infectious complications and mortality. Gastroenterology 114:A537
80. Sewnath ME, Karsten TM, Prins MH, Rauws EJ, Obertop H, Gouma DJ (2002) A meta-analysis on the efficacy of preoperative biliary drainage for tumors causing obstructive jaundice. Ann Surg 236:17–27
81. Sewnath ME, Birjmohun RS, Rauws EA, Huibregtse K, Obertop H, Gouma DJ (2001) The effect of preoperative biliary drainage on postoperative complications after pancreaticoduodenectomy. J Am Coll Surg 192:726–734
82. Pisters PW, Hudec WA, Hess KR, Lee JE, Vauthey JN, Lahoti S, Raijman I, Evans DB (2001) Effect of preoperative biliary decompression on pancreaticoduodenectomy-associated morbidity in 300 consecutive patients. Ann Surg 234:47–55
83. Sohn TA, Yeo CJ, Cameron JL, Pitt HA, Lillemoe KD (2000) Do preoperative biliary stents increase postpancreaticoduodenectomy complications? J Gastrointest Surg 4:258–267; discussion 267–268

84. Kalloo AN, Norwitz L, Yeo CJ (2006) Chronic Pancreatitis. Digestive Disease Library: The Johns Hopkins Medical Institutions Gastroenterology Hepatology Resource Center
85. Buscail L, Faure P, Bournet B, Selves J, Escourrou J (2005) Interventional endoscopic ultrasound in pancreatic diseases. Pancreatology 6:7–16
86. Rosch T, Braig C, Gain T, Feuerbach S, Siewert JR, Schusdziarra V, Classen M (1992) Staging of pancreatic and ampullary carcinoma by endoscopic ultrasonography. Comparison with conventional sonography, computed tomography, and angiography. Gastroenterology 102:188–199
87. Rosch T, Lorenz R, Braig C, Feuerbach S, Siewert JR, Schusdziarra V, Classen M (1991) Endoscopic ultrasound in pancreatic tumor diagnosis. Gastrointest Endosc 37:347–352
88. Rosch T, Lightdale CJ, Botet JF, Boyce GA, Sivak MV Jr, Yasuda K, Heyder N, Palazzo L, Dancygier H, Schusdziarra V, et al (1992) Localization of pancreatic endocrine tumors by endoscopic ultrasonography. N Engl J Med 326:1721–1726
89. Rosch T, Lorenz R, Braig C, Classen M (1992) Endoscopic ultrasonography in diagnosis and staging of pancreatic and biliary tumors. Endoscopy 24:304–308
90. DeWitt J, Devereaux B, Chriswell M, McGreevy K, Howard T, Imperiale TF, Ciaccia D, Lane KA, Maglinte D, Kopecky K, LeBlanc J, McHenry L, Madura J, Aisen A, Cramer H, Cummings O, Sherman S (2004) Comparison of endoscopic ultrasonography and multidetector computed tomography for detecting and staging pancreatic cancer. Ann Intern Med 141:753–763
91. Nakaizumi A, Uehara H, Iishi H, Tatsuta M, Kitamura T, Kuroda C, Ohigashi H, Ishikawa O, Okuda S (1995) Endoscopic ultrasonography in diagnosis and staging of pancreatic cancer. Dig Dis Sci 40:696–700
92. Maluf-Filho F, Sakai P, Cunha JE, Garrido T, Rocha M, Machado MC, Ishioka S (2004) Radial endoscopic ultrasound and spiral computed tomography in the diagnosis and staging of periampullary tumors. Pancreatology 4:122–128
93. Gress F, Gottlieb K, Sherman S, Lehman G (2001) Endoscopic ultrasonography-guided fine-needle aspiration biopsy of suspected pancreatic cancer. Ann Intern Med 134:459–464
94. Soriano A, Castells A, Ayuso C, Ayuso JR, de Caralt MT, Gines MA, Real MI, Gilabert R, Quinto L, Trilla A, Feu F, Montanya X, Fernandez-Cruz L, Navarro S (2004) Preoperative staging and tumor resectability assessment of pancreatic cancer: prospective study comparing endoscopic ultrasonography, helical computed tomography, magnetic resonance imaging, and angiography. Am J Gastroenterol 99:492–501
95. Clarke DL, Thomson SR, Madiba TE, Sanyika C (2003) Preoperative imaging of pancreatic cancer: a management-oriented approach. J Am Coll Surg 196:119–129
96. Roche CJ, Hughes ML, Garvey CJ, Campbell F, White DA, Jones L, Neoptolemos JP (2003) CT and pathologic assessment of prospective nodal staging in patients with ductal adenocarcinoma of the head of the pancreas. AJR Am J Roentgenol 180:475–480
97. Ahmad NA, Lewis JD, Siegelman ES, Rosato EF, Ginsberg GG, Kochman ML (2000) Role of endoscopic ultrasound and magnetic resonance imaging in the preoperative staging of pancreatic adenocarcinoma. Am J Gastroenterol 95:1926–1931
98. Brand B, Pfaff T, Binmoeller KF, Sriram PV, Fritscher-Ravens A, Knofel WT, Jackle S, Soehendra N (2000) Endoscopic ultrasound for differential diagnosis of focal pancreatic lesions, confirmed by surgery. Scand J Gastroenterol 35:1221–1228
99. Brugge WR, Lee MJ, Kelsey PB, Schapiro RH, Warshaw AL (1996) The use of EUS to diagnose malignant portal venous system invasion by pancreatic cancer. Gastrointest Endosc 43:561–567
100. Catanzaro A, Richardson S, Veloso H, Isenberg GA, Wong RC, Sivak MV Jr, Chak A (2003) Long-term follow-up of patients with clinically indeterminate suspicion of pancreatic cancer and normal EUS. Gastrointest Endosc 58:836–840
101. Raut CP, Grau AM, Staerkel GA, Kaw M, Tamm EP, Wolff RA, Vauthey JN, Lee JE, Pisters PW, Evans DB (2003) Diagnostic accuracy of endoscopic ultrasound-guided fine-needle aspiration in patients with presumed pancreatic cancer. J Gastrointest Surg 7:118–128
102. Bhutani MS, Gress FG, Giovannini M, Erickson RA, Catalano MF, Chak A, Deprez PH, Faigel DO, Nguyen CC (2004) The No Endosonographic Detection of Tumor (NEST) Study: a case series of pancreatic cancers missed on endoscopic ultrasonography. Endoscopy 36:385–389
103. Takahashi K, Yamao K, Okubo K, Sawaki A, Mizuno N, Ashida R, Koshikawa T, Ueyama Y, Kasugai K, Hase S, Kakumu S (2005) Differential diagnosis of pancreatic cancer and focal pancreatitis by using EUS-guided FNA. Gastrointest Endosc 61:76–79
104. Barthet M, Portal I, Boujaoude J, Bernard JP, Sahel J (1996) Endoscopic ultrasonographic diagnosis of pancreatic cancer complicating chronic pancreatitis. Endoscopy 28:487–491
105. Saftoiu A, Popescu C, Cazacu S, Dumitrescu D, Georgescu CV, Popescu M, Ciurea T, Gorunescu F (2006) Power Doppler endoscopic ultrasonography for the differential diagnosis between pancreatic cancer and pseudotumoral chronic pancreatitis. J Ultrasound Med 25:363–372
106. Chang KJ, Nguyen P, Erickson RA, Durbin TE, Katz KD (1997) The clinical utility of endoscopic ultrasound-guided fine-needle aspiration in the diagnosis and staging of pancreatic carcinoma. Gastrointest Endosc 45:387–393
107. Itoi T, Takei K, Sofuni A, Itokawa F, Tsuchiya T, Kurihara T, Nakamura K, Moriyasu F, Tsuchida A, Kasuya K (2005) Immunohistochemical analysis of p53 and MIB-1 in tissue specimens obtained from endoscopic ultrasonography-guided fine needle aspiration biopsy for the diagnosis of solid pancreatic masses. Oncol Rep 13:229–234
108. Tada M, Komatsu Y, Kawabe T, Sasahira N, Isayama H, Toda N, Shiratori Y, Omata M (2002) Quantitative analysis of K-ras gene mutation in pancreatic tissue obtained by endoscopic ultrasonography-guided fine needle aspiration: clinical utility for diagnosis of pancreatic tumor. Am J Gastroenterol 97:2263–2270
109. Eloubeidi MA, Gress FG, Savides TJ, Wiersema MJ, Kochman ML, Ahmad NA, Ginsberg GG, Erickson RA, Dewitt J, Van Dam J, Nickl NJ, Levy MJ, Clain JE, Chak A, Sivak MV, Jr, Wong R, Isenberg G, Scheiman JM, Bounds B, Kimmey MB, Saunders MD, Chang KJ, Sharma A, Nguyen P, Lee JG, Edmundowicz SA, Early D, Azar R, Etemad B, Chen YK, Waxman I, Shami V, Catalano MF, Wilcox CM (2004) Acute pancreatitis after EUS-guided FNA of solid pancreatic masses: a pooled analysis from EUS centers in the United States. Gastrointest Endosc 60:385–389
110. Bhutani MS, Hawes RH, Baron PL, Sanders-Cliette A, van Velse A, Osborne JF, Hoffman BJ (1997) Endoscopic ultrasound guided fine needle aspiration of malignant pancreatic lesions. Endoscopy 29:854–858

111. Volmar KE, Vollmer RT, Jowell PS, Nelson RC, Xie HB (2005) Pancreatic FNA in 1000 cases: a comparison of imaging modalities. Gastrointest Endosc 61:854–861
112. Ferrucci JT, Wittenberg J, Margolies MN, Carey RW (1979) Malignant seeding of the tract after thin-needle aspiration biopsy. Radiology 130:345–346
113. Weiss SM, Skibber JM, Mohiuddin M, Rosato FE (1985) Rapid intra-abdominal spread of pancreatic cancer. Influence of multiple operative biopsy procedures. Arch Surg 120:415–416
114. Warshaw AL (1991) Implications of peritoneal cytology for staging of early pancreatic cancer. Am J Surg 161:26–29; discussion 29–30
115. Farrell JJ, Garber J, Sahani D, Brugge WR (2004) EUS findings in patients with autoimmune pancreatitis. Gastrointest Endosc 60:927–936

Chapter 48

J. R. Rodríguez · C. Fernandez-del Castillo

The Staging of Pancreatic Cancer

Advances in imaging technology have delivered profound improvements in our ability to evaluate the pancreas and surrounding structures and stage a malignancy if detected. The result has been a decrease in the number of patients having to undergo multiple invasive procedures and unnecessary laparotomies. The degree to which these advances have impacted survival and health-related quality of life in the current treatment of pancreatic cancer remains to be shown.

Resectability and Staging

In 2005 there will be an estimated 32,180 new cases of pancreatic cancer in the USA along with 31,800 new deaths [1]. Unfortunately, only about 20% of these new diagnoses are determined to be surgically resectable [2–4]. These are the only patients with any possibility of cure. For the rest, the prognosis is extremely poor. We will attempt to provide a succinct, pragmatic approach to the clinical staging of pancreatic cancer.

Patients who are diagnosed with pancreatic cancer are placed into three categories once staging is completed: (1) patients with distant metastases (liver, peritoneum, distant lymph nodes, and occasionally other organs), (2) patients with locally advanced disease precluding curative resection, and (3) patients with no metastasis and tumors that are resectable for possible cure. The treating physician's goal during clinical staging of pancreatic cancer should be to provide a minimally invasive, safe, and cost-effective method that will enable healthcare providers to formulate the optimum treatment strategy for an individual patient. This is accomplished through a history and physical examination, laboratory and radiographic studies, and if appropriate, diagnostic laparoscopy. Staging also provides a standardized method to compare outcomes between similar groups of patients, to appropriately categorize patients into novel clinical trials and perhaps most importantly, provides patients, families and physicians with useful prognostic information.

Clinical Contributions to Staging

Jaundice and pain are the most common presenting symptoms of pancreatic adenocarcinomas. Since the majority of these lesions are located in the head of the gland in proximity to the bile duct and ampulla, they may become symptomatic earlier in the course of illness relative to lesions in the body and tail. Pain may or may not be present in early disease and should not be considered a sign of unresectability. Physical findings conspicuous for advanced disease include marked weight loss, abdominal ascites, left supraclavicular adenopathy, palpable abdominal mass, and migrating thrombophlebitis. The carbohydrate antigen CA 19-9 is the only readily available tumor marker that has been shown to contribute to preoperative staging. High levels (>600 U/ml) have been correlated with a high likelihood of unresectability [5]. However, this finding should not preclude complete radiologic evaluation of the suspected tumor. Conversely, very low CA 19-9 levels (<100 U/ml) may obviate the need for staging laparoscopy (SL). A recent study from the Fox-Chase Cancer Center found a low diagnostic yield from SL in 63 patients with CA 19-9 levels of <100 U/ml. In their study, none of these patients were identified as having metastatic disease [6].

Computed Tomography

Arterial and venous phase-contrast enhanced, multidetector, pancreatic protocol computed tomography (MDCT) is the cornerstone in the evaluation of the patient with suspected pancreatic cancer [7]. It provides a wealth of information and becomes the principal branching point in the imaging algorithm. Detailed images delineate the size and extent of spread of the tumor and provide information pertaining to the extent of vascular involvement and enlarged lymph nodes (Figs. 48.1 and 48.2). Dual-phase scanning is especially useful for evaluating suspected pancreatic neoplasms. Arterial phase imaging is indicated for de-

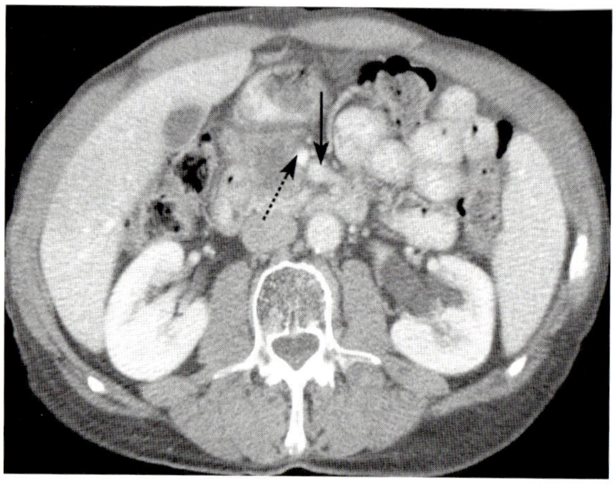

Figure 48.1

Borderline resectable low-attenuation mass in the head of the pancreas that extends along the anterior margin of the superior mesenteric vein (SMV; *dashed arrow*), with an intact fat plane between the SMV and superior mesenteric artery (SMA; *solid arrow*)

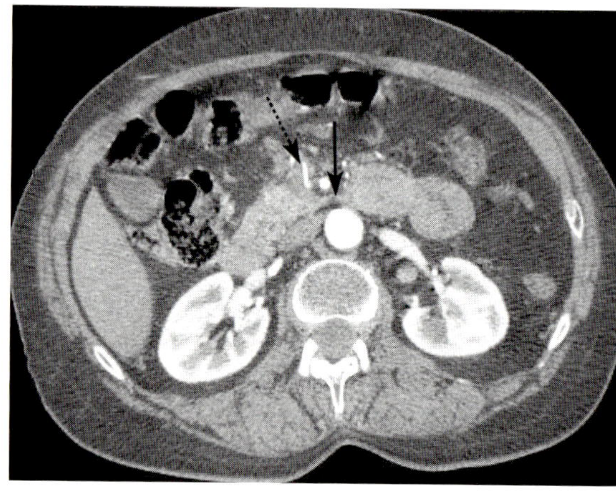

Figure 48.2

Dual-phase multidetector computed tomography (MDCT) image of a locally advanced, unresectable pancreatic cancer involving the SMA (*solid arrow*) and its branches (*dashed arrow*)

tection of small hypervascular lesions such as islet cell tumors, which are frequently inconspicuous on portal venous phase images. Three-dimensional reconstructions provide comprehensive additional information about the anatomy of the vessels, the relationship and possible involvement of vascular structures in the vicinity of focal pancreatic lesions, and the degree and level of dilatation of obstructed pancreatic and biliary ducts. Reduced image acquisition times and increasing data processing speeds have rendered the classical visceral artery angiogram virtually obsolete in the staging of pancreatic cancer. Computed tomography (CT) does, however, have its weaknesses. Ionizing radiation, intravenous contrast allergy and contrast-induced nephropathy are well known risks. MDCT also has poor sensitivity for lesions less than 1 cm in size such as peritoneal implants, which may occur early in the natural history of pancreatic adenocarcinoma [8]. Peripancreatic inflammation when one or more secondary signs are seen can render potential malignancies difficult to characterize and may result in indeterminate CT findings.

Endoscopic Ultrasound

In those patients who have nonspecific MDCT scan findings such as "fullness" in the head of the pancreas, especially in the setting of known pancreatitis, endoscopic ultrasound (EUS) offers an excellent test with which to diagnose and stage a patient with potential pancreatic cancer. It also allows for the acquisition of tissue for pathologic diagnosis via fine-needle aspiration (FNA) because of the proximity of the high-frequency probe on the end of the flexible endoscope to the tumor (Fig. 48.3). Vascular evaluation is complemented by color flow Doppler sonography. However, EUS does not replace MDCT images for assessing resectability [9, 10]. It is by its nature a limited evaluation that is invasive, and has demonstrated significant user dependence. It also relies on the active involvement of a cytopathologist [11]. At the Massachusetts General Hospital (MGH), EUS is a useful adjunct for further characterizing small tumors or in cases where tissue diagnosis is required for the purposes of determining adjuvant or neoadjuvant therapy [12]. When clinical or radiographic characteristics suggest the possibility of a diagnosis different than adenocarcinoma, EUS and FNA is recommended.

Laparoscopy

Diagnostic laparoscopy or SL provides valuable complementary data to that of MDCT in many cases. The principal candidates are those who are found to have no evidence of distant metastasis on MDCT. Its main utility lies in the ability to detect and biopsy liver or peritoneal implants that are not visible radiologically (Figs. 48.4 and 48.5) or in a few cases even macroscopically, since peritoneal washings can be positive in the absence of visible metastasis [13, 14]. In a series reported by MGH, notably shorter survival times were observed in patients with positive cytology for

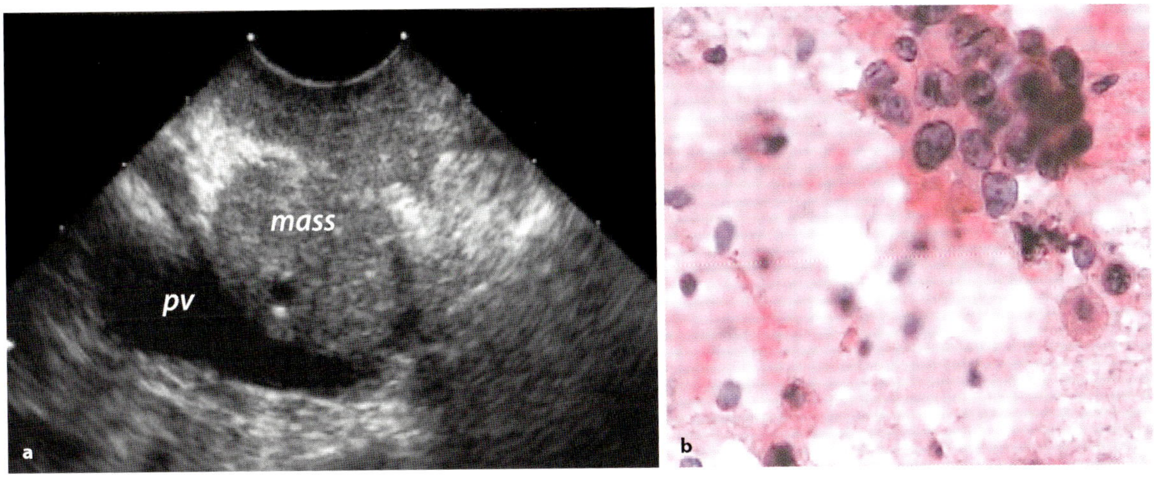

Figure 48.3

a Endoscopic ultrasound (EUS) examination demonstrating a pancreatic head mass with portal vein invasion. b Fine-needle aspiration (FNA) of the pancreatic head mass demonstrating well-differentiated adenocarcinoma

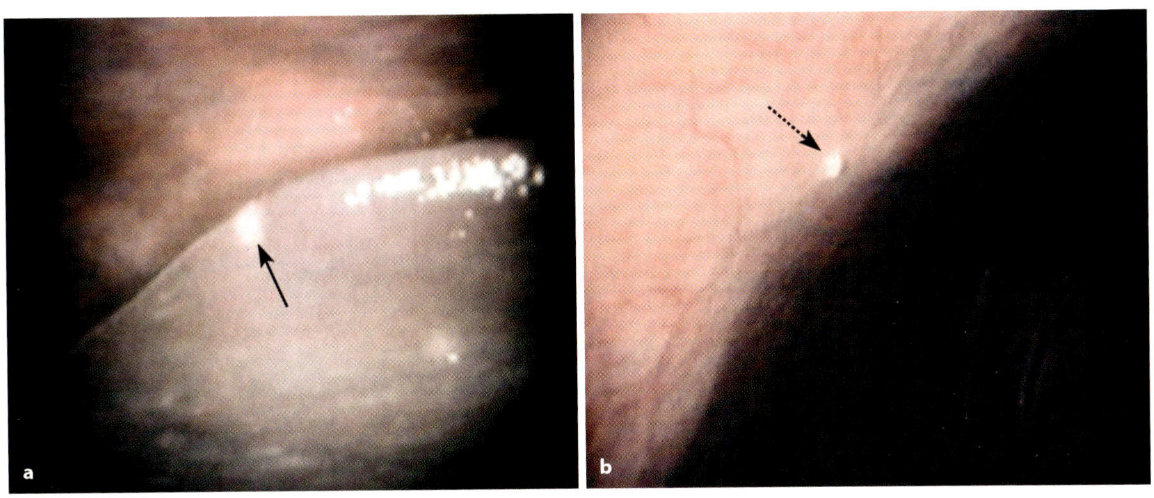

Figure 48.4

Unsuspected liver (a, *solid arrow*) and peritoneal implants (b, *dashed arrow*) in a patient with pancreatic cancer believed to be resectable preoperatively

malignant cells during SL compared to those with negative results (Fig. 48.6) [15]. Several series have demonstrated the utility of SL in upstaging a tumor that was initially believed to be resectable [13, 16–21]. Metastatic implants are more likely to be seen in cancers involving the body and tail of the gland [22]. Patients with large tumors in the head (>2 cm) also benefit from SL. In rare instances, patients discovered to have tumors smaller than this can avoid laparoscopy since these patients are less likely to have metastasis. Finally, laparoscopy is also useful for patients with locally advanced, unresectable disease to properly determine their candidacy for novel protocols, radiotherapy, or neoadjuvant treatment that may potentially downstage their tumors to resectability. Some authors have advocated advanced techniques incorporating extensive dissection and laparoscopic ultrasonography [16, 21, 23–26]. We favor an expeditious examination, peritoneal washings and biopsy of suspicious areas on peritoneal surfaces. In our opinion, the "simple" SL is more appealing because the expertise required lies within the scope of most general surgeons, allowing triage prior to transferring a patient to a high-volume center.

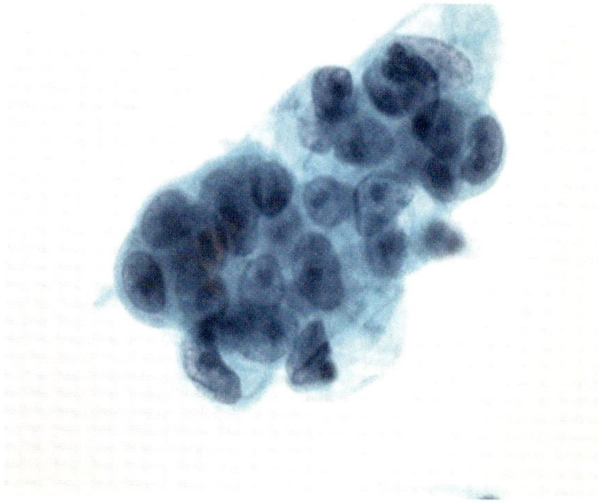

Figure 48.5

Peritoneal wash with positive results for malignancy showing a cluster of adenocarcinoma cells with nuclear overlapping and cytomorphologic features of malignancy, including an increased nuclear to cytoplasmic ratio and nuclear membrane irregularities

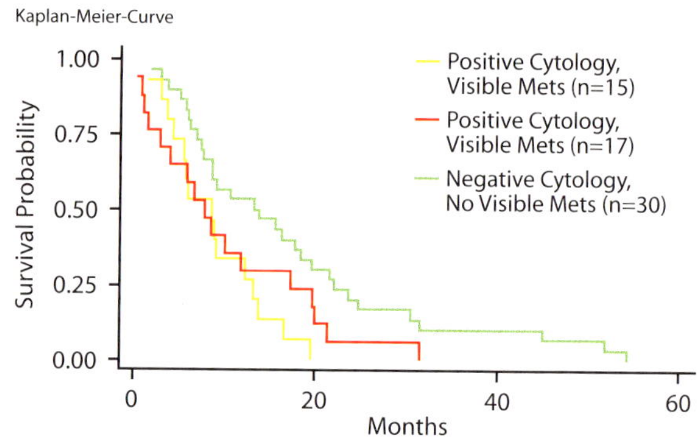

Figure 48.6

Survival time of patients with pancreatic cancer, comparing patients ($n = 15$) with positive test results for malignant cells (*Positive Cytology*) from peritoneal-fluid cytology and no metastases (*Mets*; *yellow line*), patients ($n = 17$) with positive results and visible metastases (*red line*), and patients ($n = 30$) with negative test results (*Negative Cytology*) for malignant cells

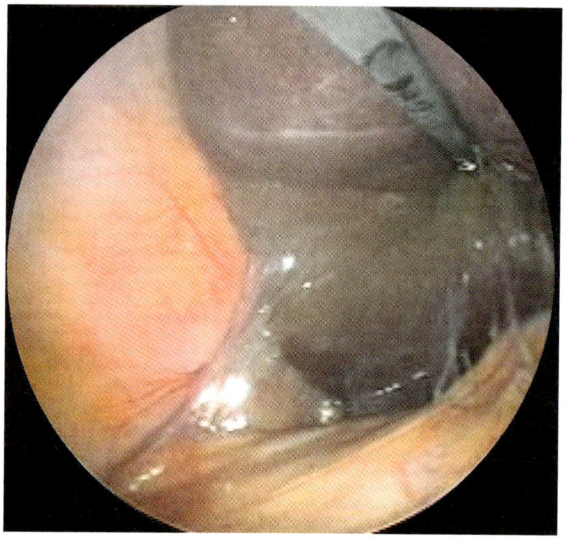

Figure 48.7

Inspection of the undersurface of the liver is performed utilizing a rod inserted through the second trocar

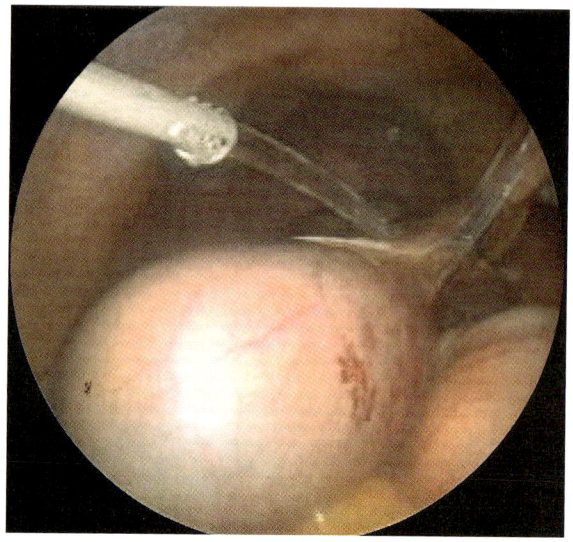

Figure 48.8

Peritoneal washings are obtained by instilling 500 ml of 0.9% normal saline into the abdomen and tilting the operating table

Surgical Technique

SL using two trocars (both 5 mm) can be performed in either the inpatient or outpatient setting under general anesthesia as long as provisions are made for postlaparoscopy admission in the event that a complication occurs. The steps are outlined below:

1. The patient is positioned supine on the operating table and the entire abdomen is prepped. Access can be achieved with a Veress needle through a 5-mm infraumbilical incision.
2. Adequate pneumoperitoneum is obtained to a pressure of 15 mmHg.
3. A 5-mm scope is inserted and visual inspection of the lower and upper abdomen is completed, paying particular attention to the liver surfaces.

4. A second trocar (5 mm) is inserted in the right upper quadrant, through which a rod is inserted that can be used to lift areas of the liver so that the undersurface can be inspected, or to manipulate other viscera (Fig. 48.7).
5. Any existing free fluid is aspirated, and peritoneal washings are obtained by instilling 500 ml of 0.9% normal saline into the abdomen and tilting the operating table (Fig. 48.8). This will occasionally (9.6%) yield an unexpected diagnosis of disseminated cancer in the peritoneal cavity [13].
6. A complete visual inspection of the entire abdominal and pelvic cavities is completed, including the diaphragm omentum, transverse mesocolon, ligament of Treitz, hilum of the liver, and hepatoduodenal ligament.
7. Specimens of peritoneal, liver, omental nodules, or enlarged nodes are taken with the biopsy forceps inserted through the second trocar.
8. After hemostasis is confirmed the instruments are withdrawn, the CO_2 is allowed to escape, and skin incisions are closed.

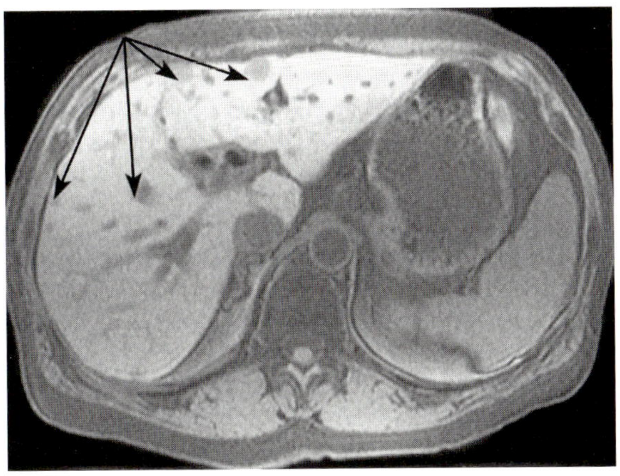

Figure 48.9

Magnetic resonance image with gadolinium demonstrating multiple hepatic lesions consistent with metastatic disease (*solid arrows*)

Magnetic Resonance Imaging

The image utility of MRI is comparable to that supplied by CT in the staging of pancreatic cancer [27]. New advances include fast breath-hold pulse sequences that increase detail by decreasing respiratory variation, gadolinium-enhanced MRI to evaluate arterial and venous patency, magnetic resonance cholangiopancreatography reconstructions, which may diminish the role of ERCP, and manganese administration to help delineate pancreatic neoplasms since pancreatic adenocarcinomas do not take up manganese [28–30]. MRI is more sensitive than helical CT for detecting small liver metastases (Fig. 48.9). At present, MRI has not replaced MDCT as the initial imaging tool in the staging algorithm of suspected pancreatic cancer, although it may eventually do so. It is more expensive

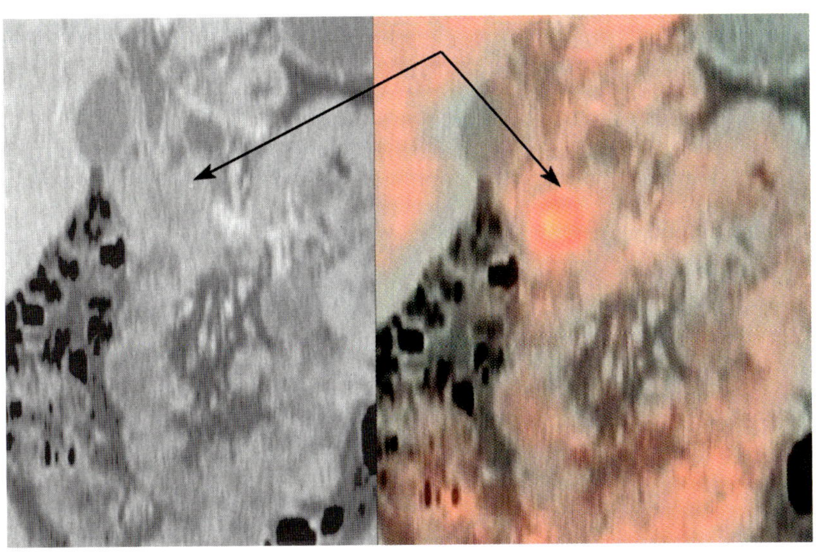

Figure 48.10

Coronal reconstruction positron emission tomography/computed tomography demonstrating a large tumor in the head of the pancreas (*solid arrows*)

and the acquisition and interpretation of data is more time consuming. There are specific instances that might favor this more costly evaluation, including patient allergies to iodine-based contrast medium or patients at high risk for contrast-induced nephropathy.

Positron Emission Tomography

Positron emission tomography (PET) is being used increasingly in oncology, as it provides images of physiologic function. It is based on tumor ability to take up radiolabeled tracer (18-fluorodeoxyglucose). In pancreatic cancer, it may have utility in revealing unsuspected metastatic disease that are as small as 1 cm in diameter, and to follow or monitor patients for recurrence following various treatments, in whom the normal anatomic planes are disrupted or modified [31]. Furthermore, it may be more sensitive than CT for detecting cancers less than 2 cm. However, false-positive results may be encountered in patients with enlarged bile ducts and granulomas [32]. Simultaneous examination by PET and CT has been developed with the aim of improving the limited anatomic information offered by PET alone (Fig. 48.10) [33, 34]. At present there is no evidence to support its routine use in the staging of pancreatic cancer. Further evaluation using a prospective study considering cost-effectiveness is necessary to clarify the appropriate role of PET in the staging of pancreatic cancer.

Intraoperative Staging

Ultimately, the final decision regarding resectability is made in the operating room by the surgeon. The entire peritoneal cavity is inspected, including the liver surfaces, and suspicious nodules are sent for frozen section. A wide Kocher maneuver allows for examination of the head of the pancreas and excludes invasion into the retroperitoneum, in the region of the vena cava. Technical resectability is assessed through the evaluation of the tumor relationship to the major surrounding vessels. If the surgeon determines tumor resectability after mobilization of the gland and inspection of the superior mesenteric vein and portal vein junction, a Whipple resection ensues. In some instances portal vein resection with reconstruction can be performed. If the tumor is determined to be unresectable, a confirming tissue diagnosis should be obtained.

Postoperative Staging

The final consideration in the staging process is pathologic examination of the resected specimen. The most recent staging classification published by the American Joint Committee on Cancer (AJCC) for pancreatic adenocarcinoma is presented in Table 48.1 [35]. This table demonstrates that tumor stage and prognosis are affected by tumor size, the degree of tumor extension into adjacent tissues, and regional lymph node metastasis. This information is important to the surgeon in formulating a concept of the patient's prognosis and in considering adjuvant strategies such as chemotherapy and radiation.

Table 48.1. American Joint Committee on Cancer staging classification for pancreatic adenocarcinoma

Definitions			
Primary Tumor (T)			
TX	Primary tumor cannot be assessed		
T0	No evidence of primary tumor		
Tis	Carcinoma in situ		
T1	Tumor limited to the pancreas 2 cm or less in greatest dimension		
T2	Tumor limited to the pancreas more than 2 cm in greatest dimension		
T3	Tumor extends beyond the pancreas but without involvement of the celiac axis or the superior mesenteric artery (unresectable primary tumor)		
Regional Lymph Nodes (N)			
NX	Regional lymph nodes cannot be assessed		
N0	No regional lymph node metastasis		
N1	Regional lymph node metastasis		
Distant Metastasis (M)			
MX	Distant metastasis cannot be assessed		
M0	No distant metastasis		
M1	Distant metastasis		
Stage Grouping			
0	Tis	N0	M0
IA	T1	N0	M0
IB	T2	N0	M0
IIA	T3	N0	M0
IIB	T1	N1	M0
	T2	N1	M0
	T3	N1	M0
III	T4	Any N	M0
IV	Any T	Any N	M1

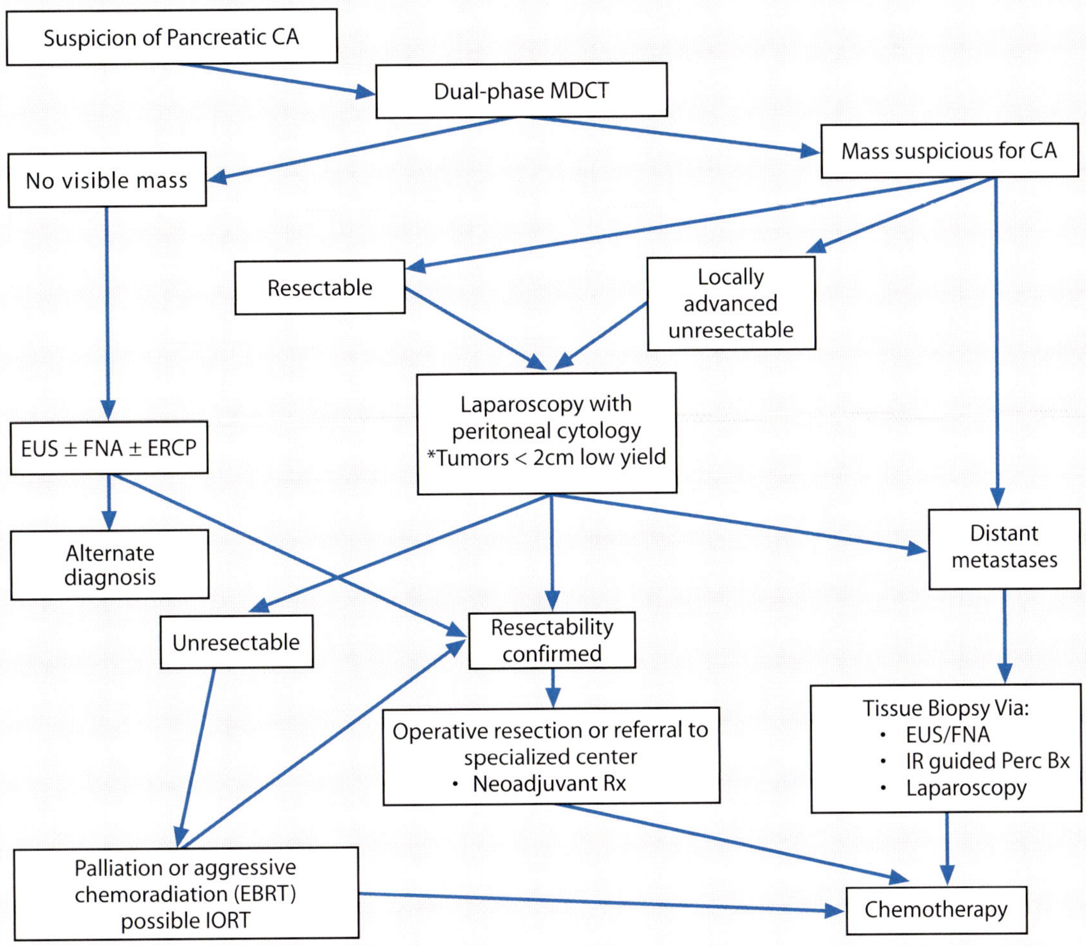

Figure 48.11

Massachusetts General Hospital preoperative staging algorithm for patients with suspected pancreatic cancer. *CA* Cancer, *ERCP* endoscopic retrograde cholangiopancreaticography, *EBRT* external beam radiotherapy, *IORT* intraoperative radiotherapy, *Rx* radiation therapy, *IR* Interventional Radiology, *Perc Bx* percutaneous biopsy

Approach to Preoperative Staging

An algorithm detailing the preoperative staging strategy for pancreatic carcinoma at MGH is presented in Fig. 48.11. It emphasizes the central role of MDCT scanning as the initial step in the evaluation of a patient with suspected pancreatic cancer as well as the importance of staging laparoscopy with peritoneal cytology in the staging algorithm. SL is most useful for patients considered resectable (especially those with tumors ≥2 cm and those located in the body and tail of the gland) as well as those considered to have locally advanced unresectable tumors.

References

1. Cancer Facts and Figures (2005) American Cancer Society, Atlanta
2. Beger HG, Rau B, Gansauge F, Poch B, Link KH (2003) Treatment of pancreatic cancer: challenge of the facts. World J Surg 27:1075–1084
3. Li D, Xie K, Wolff R, Abbruzzese JL (2004) Pancreatic cancer. Lancet 363:1049–1057
4. Lockhart AC, Rothenberg ML, Berlin JD (2005) Treatment for pancreatic cancer: current therapy and continued progress. Gastroenterology 128:1642–1654
5. Steinberg WM, Gelfand R, Anderson KK, et al (1986) Comparison of the sensitivity and specificity of the CA19-9 and carcinoembryonic antigen assays in detecting cancer of the pancreas. Gastroenterology 90:343–349

6. Karachristos A, Scarmeas N, Hoffman JP (2005) CA 19-9 levels predict results of staging laparoscopy in pancreatic cancer. J Gastrointest Surg 9:1286–1292
7. Horton KM, Fishman EK (2002) Adenocarcinoma of the pancreas: CT imaging. Radiol Clin North Am 40:1263–1272
8. Ott DJ (1999) Pancreatic tumors: efficacy of newer CT techniques matches that of endoscopic sonography. Am J Gastroenterol 94:1414–146
9. Wren SM, Ralls PW, Stain SC, Kasiraman A, Carpenter CL, Parekh D (1996) Assessment of resectability of pancreatic head and periampullary tumors by color flow Doppler sonography. Arch Surg 131:812–817; discussion 7–8
10. Aslanian H, Salem R, Lee J, Andersen D, Robert M, Topazian M (2005) EUS diagnosis of vascular invasion in pancreatic cancer: surgical and histologic correlates. Am J Gastroenterol 100:1381–1385
11. Klapman JB, Logrono R, Dye CE, Waxman I (2003) Clinical impact of on-site cytopathology interpretation on endoscopic ultrasound-guided fine needle aspiration. Am J Gastroenterol 98:1289–1294
12. Midwinter MJ, Beveridge CJ, Wilsdon JB, Bennett MK, Baudouin CJ, Charnley RM (1999) Correlation between spiral computed tomography, endoscopic ultrasonography and findings at operation in pancreatic and ampullary tumours. Br J Surg 86:189–193
13. Jimenez RE, Warshaw AL, Rattner DW, Willett CG, McGrath D, Fernandez-del Castillo C (2000) Impact of laparoscopic staging in the treatment of pancreatic cancer. Arch Surg 135:409–414; discussion 414–415
14. Ellsmere J, Mortele K, Sahani D, et al (2005) Does multidetector-row CT eliminate the role of diagnostic laparoscopy in assessing the resectability of pancreatic head adenocarcinoma? Surg Endosc 19:369–373
15. Makary MA, Warshaw AL, Centeno BA, Willet CG, Rattner DW, Fernandez-del Castillo C (1998) Implications of peritoneal cytology for pancreatic cancer management. Arch Surg 133:361–365
16. Conlon KC, Dougherty E, Klimstra DS, Coit DG, Turnbull AD, Brennan MF (1996) The value of minimal access surgery in the staging of patients with potentially resectable peripancreatic malignancy. Ann Surg 223:134–140
17. Gloor B, Todd KE, Reber HA (1997) Diagnostic workup of patients with suspected pancreatic carcinoma: the University of California-Los Angeles approach. Cancer 7:1780–1786
18. Holzman MD, Reintgen KL, Tyler DS, Pappas TN (1997) The role of laparoscopy in the management of suspected pancreatic and periampullary malignancies. J Gastrointest Surg 1:236–244
19. Friess H, Kleeff J, Silva JC, Sadowski C, Baer HU, Buchler MW (1998) The role of diagnostic laparoscopy in pancreatic and periampullary malignancies. J Am Coll Surg 186:675–682
20. Saldinger PF, Reilly M, Reynolds K, et al (2000) Is CT angiography sufficient for prediction of resectability of periampullary neoplasms? J Gastrointest Surg 4:233–237; discussion 8–9
21. Pisters PW, Lee JE, Vauthey JN, Charnsangavej C, Evans DB (2001) Laparoscopy in the staging of pancreatic cancer. Br J Surg 88:325–337
22. Fernandez-del Castillo C, Rattner DW, Warshaw AL. Standards for pancreatic resection in the 1990s. Arch Surg 1995;130(3):295-9; discussion 9-300
23. John TG, Greig JD, Carter DC, Garden OJ (1995) Carcinoma of the pancreatic head and periampullary region. Tumor staging with laparoscopy and laparoscopic ultrasonography. Ann Surg 221:156–164
24. Minnard EA, Conlon KC, Hoos A, Dougherty EC, Hann LE, Brennan MF (1998) Laparoscopic ultrasound enhances standard laparoscopy in the staging of pancreatic cancer. Ann Surg 228:182–187
25. Kwon AH, Inui H, Kamiyama Y (2002) Preoperative laparoscopic examination using surgical manipulation and ultrasonography for pancreatic lesions. Endoscopy 34:464–468
26. Shoup M, Brennan MF, McWhite K, Leung DH, Klimstra D, Conlon KC (2002) The value of splenic preservation with distal pancreatectomy. Arch Surg 137:164–168
27. Trede M, Rumstadt B, Wendl K, et al (1997) Ultrafast magnetic resonance imaging improves the staging of pancreatic tumors. Ann Surg 226:393–405
28. Diehl SJ, Lehmann KJ, Gaa J, McGill S, Hoffmann V, Georgi M (1999) MR imaging of pancreatic lesions. Comparison of manganese-DPDP and gadolinium chelate. Invest Radiol 34:589–595
29. Adamek HE, Albert J, Breer H, Weitz M, Schilling D, Riemann JF (2000) Pancreatic cancer detection with magnetic resonance cholangiopancreatography and endoscopic retrograde cholangiopancreatography: a prospective controlled study. Lancet 356:190–193
30. Ly JN, Miller FH (2002) MR imaging of the pancreas: a practical approach. Radiol Clin North Am 40:1289–1306
31. Annovazzi A, Peeters M, Maenhout A, Signore A, Dierckx R, Van De Wiele C (2003) 18-fluorodeoxyglucose positron emission tomography in nonendocrine neoplastic disorders of the gastrointestinal tract. Gastroenterology 125:1235–1245
32. Frohlich A, Diederichs CG, Staib L, Vogel J, Beger HG, Reske SN (1999) Detection of liver metastases from pancreatic cancer using FDG PET. J Nucl Med 40:250–255
33. Beyer T, Townsend DW, Brun T, et al (2000) A combined PET/CT scanner for clinical oncology. J Nucl Med 41:1369–1379
34. Heinrich S, Goerres GW, Schafer M, et al (2005) Positron emission tomography/computed tomography influences on the management of resectable pancreatic cancer and its cost-effectiveness. Ann Surg 242:235–243
35. American Joint Committee on Cancer staging classification for pancreatic adenocarcinoma Cancer Staging Manual, 6th edn (2002) Springer-Verlag, New York

Chapter 49

D. Laheru

Oncological Management of Pancreatic Cancer in Advanced Stages

Historically, 5-fluorouracil (5-FU)-based chemotherapy has been the most widely studied chemotherapeutic agent for all stages of pancreatic cancer. Despite more recent attempts to modify the delivery of 5-FU, response rates have remained unchanged in the 10–20% range with median survival of 4–5 months for patients with stage IV disease [1–5].

The Role of Gemcitabine in Metastatic Pancreatic Cancer

Gemcitabine is a prodrug deoxycytidine (2'-deoxy-2',2'-difluorocytidine monohydrochloride) analogue that is metabolized by deoxycytidine kinase to active diphosphate and triphosphate (dFdCTP) nucleosides. These metabolites inhibit ribonucleotide reductase with the effect of decreasing intracellular levels of required deoxynucleotide triphosphates for continued DNA synthesis. In addition, gemcitabine triphosphate directly competes with dCTP for incorporation into DNA. Recently, gemcitabine has demonstrated promise as an active agent in treating pancreatic cancer. Casper and colleagues reported the results of a phase II trial using weekly gemcitabine at 800–1250 mg/m^2 in 44 patients with unresectable pancreatic cancer. The response rate was noted to be 11% but with a median survival of 5.6 months and a 1-year actuarial survival of 23% [6]. Subsequently, Burris and colleagues randomized 126 patients with unresectable pancreatic cancer to either gemcitabine (1000 mg/m^2 weekly over a 30-min infusion × 7 followed by 1 week of rest then weekly × 3 every 4 weeks) or 5-FU (600 mg/m^2 weekly). Although the primary endpoints were issues related to quality of life, median survival was 5.7 months in the gemcitabine arm compared to 4.4 months in the 5-FU arm. In addition, 1-year survival was 18% in the gemcitabine arm compared to 2% in the 5-FU arm (p=0.0025) with median time to progression also favoring gemcitabine (9 weeks compared to 4 weeks in the 5-FU arm, p=0.0002). Gemcitabine was well tolerated with the majority of side effects related to grade 3 or 4 neutropenia (26%) without associated infections, low-grade fevers (30%), and nausea and vomiting (9.5% and 3.2%). The Food and Drug Administration (FDA) has since approved gemcitabine (1996) as a first-line therapy in metastatic pancreatic cancer [7]. In addition, Rothenberg and colleagues evaluated gemcitabine (1000 mg/m^2 weekly × 7 with 1 week off then weekly × 3 with 1 week off) in 63 patients with unresectable disease who had been previously treated with 5-FU. The overall salvage response was 10.5%, with median time to progression at 2.5 months and median survival at 3.85 months, with a toxicity profile similar to first-line therapy [8]. Recent strategies include identifying alternative dosing schedules of gemcitabine that might both enhance drug delivery to tumor cells and identify synergistic combinations with other chemotherapeutic agents. Tempero and colleagues randomized 93 patients to either gemcitabine (2200 mg/m^2) over the standard 30-minute infusion or gemcitabine (1500 mg/m^2) at a rate of 10 mg/m^2/min. With analysis completed on 67 patients, the response rate was 17% vs. 3% in favor of the longer infusion rate. In addition, median survival (6.1 months vs. 4.7 months) and 1-year survival (23% vs. 0%) favored the longer infusion rate [9].

Combination Chemotherapy

Recent efforts have focused on developing strategies that would enhance the efficacy of gemcitabine and ultimately improve on median survival. Table 49.1 summarizes the most recent studies.

Gemcitabine with 5-FU

Preclinical data have also demonstrated a synergistic and noncrossresistant effect of 5-FU when given with gemcitabine [4]. However, the combination of 5-FU and gemcitabine has not consistently resulted in significant improvement over gemcitabine alone. Early

Table 49.1. Selected phase II and recent phase III chemotherapy studies in advanced pancreatic cancer. *PR* Partial response, *CR* complete response, *5-FU* 5-fluorouracil, *Gem* gemcitabine, *FDR* fixed dose rate, *NR* not recorded, *NS* not significant

Study	Patients (*n*)	Chemotherapy	PR/CR rate	Median survival (months)		1-year survival
Burris (1997) [7]	63	5-FU bolus	0 (0%)	4.4		2%
	63	Gemcitabine	3 (5.4%)	5.7	p=0.0025	18%
Heinemann (2006) [19]	96	Gem	NR	6		NR
	99	Gem+cisplatin	NR	7.5	p=0.15	NR
Rocha Lima (2004) [25]	173	Gem	8 (4.4%)	6.6		21%
	169	Gem+irinotecan	27 (16%)	6.3	p=NS	22%
Ko (2007) [20]	49	Gem	2/22 (9%)	5		9%
	43	Fixed-dose Gem	1/17 (5%)	8	(p=0.013)	29%
O'Reilly (2004) [26]	174	Gem	11 (6.3%)	6.3		21%
	175	Gem + exatecan	14 (8.2%)	6.7	(p=NS)	23%
Richards (2004) [16]	283	Gem	26 (9.1%)	6.3		21%
	282	Gem + pemetrexed	52 (18.3%)	6.2	(p=0.85)	20%
Louvet (2005) [23]	156	Gem	27 (17.3%)	7.1		28%
	157	Gem (FDR) + oxaliplatin	42 (26.8%)	9	(p=NS)	35%
Cunningham (2005) [14]	266	Gem +/– capecitabine	19 (7%)	6		19%
	267	Gem + capecitabine	37 (14%)	7.4	(p=NS)	26%

studies had designed the use of gemcitabine with bolus infusion 5-FU with no significant improvement when compared to single-agent gemcitabine [10]. However, subsequent studies focusing on infusional schedules of 5-FU with gemcitabine suggested a clinical parallel to the data using infusional 5-FU in the therapy of metastatic colorectal cancer. Hidalgo et al. examined the combination of 5-FU administered as a continuous infusion (200 mg/m^2 throughout study) with gemcitabine 700–900 mg/m^2 weekly × 3 repeated every 4 weeks. The reported median survival was 10.3 months [11]. In addition, Louvet reported a phase II study of infusional 5-FU and leukovorin (leukovorin 400 mg/m^2 in a 2-h infusion followed by a 5-FU 400 mg/m^2 bolus followed by 2–3 g/m^2 continuous infusion 5-FU in a schedule known as LV5FU2) with gemcitabine 1000 mg/m^2 on day 3, repeat cycle every 2 weeks. The reported median survival was 9 months [12]. However, a study by Hess using gemcitabine (1000 mg/m^2 days 1 and 8) and capecitabine (starting 500 mg/m^2 divided bid × 14 days) in 36 patients with advanced pancreas cancer repeated every 21 days. The median survival was 6.4 months [13]. Most recently, a phase III study of gemcitabine + capecitabine (gemcitabine 1000 mg/m^2 weekly × 3 weeks, repeat every 4 weeks + capecitabine 1660 mg/m^2/day × 3 weeks repeated every 4 weeks) versus gemcitabine alone (gemcitabine 1000 mg/m^2 weekly × 7 with 1 week off for cycle 1 followed by weekly × 3 weeks repeat every 4 weeks) was completed in 533 patients with advanced pancreatic cancer. The response rate was 14% versus 7% in favor of the combination. More importantly, the median survival was 7.4 months with a 1-year survival of 26%, versus 6 months (p<.05) with a 1-year survival of 19% also in favor of the combination therapy [14]. Several modulators of 5-FU have been examined previously, including interferon-alpha and N-(phosphonoacteyl)-L-aspartate disodium, none of which have been any additional benefit. There has been interest in examining other 5-FU formulations either alone or with gemcitabine, including the multitargeted folate inhibitor pemetrexed that has activity against thymidylate synthase, dihyrofolate reductase, and glyncinamide ribonucleotide formyltransferase [15]. A phase III study of gemcitabine alone (1000 mg/m^2 weekly × 3 every 4 weeks) versus gemcitabine + pemetrexed (gemcitabine 1250 mg/m^2 on days 1 and 8, and pemetrexed 500 mg/m^2 on day 8 all repeated every 3 weeks) in patients with advanced pancreatic cancer demonstrated an improvement in response rate (18% versus 9%) but no improvement in median survival (6.3 months versus 6.2 months) [16].

Gemcitabine with Platinum Chemotherapy

Another potentially synergistic agent that has been used with gemcitabine is cisplatin. This combination is thought to be synergistic either by enhancing dFdCTP incorporation into DNA or via increasing DNA adduct formation [17,18]. Early studies identified median survival from 5.6 to 8.2 months. This combination has recently been examined in two phase III studies. Colucci and colleagues treated 107 patients with advanced pancreas cancer with either gemcitabine alone at standard dose and schedule or gemcitabine and cisplatin (25 mg/m^2 weekly × 3 every 4 weeks). The combination of gemcitabine and cisplatin improved median time to disease progression (2.7 months for GEMCITABINE alone versus 5 months for combination gemcitabine/cisplatin, p=0.048) with no significant differences in toxicities. However, while the median survival for gemcitabine group was 5 months compared to 7.5 months for the combination chemotherapy, the p value of 0.43 was not statistically significant [18]. More recently, Heinemann presented the phase III data of 195 patients randomized to either gemcitabine alone, standard dose and schedule, versus gemcitabine and cisplatin (50 mg/m^2 weekly × 3 repeated every 4 weeks) [19]. While a difference in median survival was noted (6 months for gemcitabine alone versus 8.3 months for the combination), this was not statistically significant. Ko and colleagues have completed a phase II study of 51 metastatic pancreas cancer patients with gemcitabine (1000 mg/m^2 at the fixed dose infusion of 10 mg/m^2/min) with cisplatin (20 mg/m^2) on days 1 and 15, a schedule repeated every 28 days. Toxicities were primarily grade 3/4 hematologic toxicities. The median time to progression was 3.9 months, with a median survival of 7.1 months [20].

Gemcitabine with Oxaliplatin

Oxaliplatin is a diaminocyclohexane-platinum compound that received FDA approval in August 2002 for use in combination with infusional 5-FU and leukovorin for the treatment of patients with colorectal cancer whose disease has recurred or become worse following initial therapy with a combination of irinotecan with bolus 5-FU and leukovorin. Based on preclinical data that identified synergistic antitumor activity, oxaliplatin has since also been evaluated in combination with gemcitabine in patients with advanced pancreatic cancer. The French Cooperative group GERCOR examined gemcitabine 1000 mg/m^2 as a 10-mg/m^2/min prolonged infusion administered on day 1 in combination with oxaliplatin 100 mg/m^2 as a 2-h infusion administered on day 2 repeated every 2 weeks in 64 patients with chemonaïve metastatic pancreas cancer. The response rate was noted to be 30.6%, with a clinical benefit response of 40%. Median progression-free survival and overall survival were 5.3 months and 9.2 months, respectively, with a 36% 1-year survival. The combination was safe, with reported side effects including grade 3 or 4 neutropenia/thrombocytopenia of 11%, nausea and vomiting of 14%, diarrhea of 6.2%, and peripheral neuropathy of 11% [21].

The North Central Cancer Treatment Group completed a phase I study of gemcitabine and oxaliplatin in 18 patients with metastatic pancreas cancer. Dose-limiting toxicities of neutropenia and severe infection were identified at the maximum tolerated dose of gemcitabine 1250 mg/m^2 (day 1 and day 8 every 21 days) and oxaliplatin 130 mg/m^2 (day 1 every 21 days) [22].

Recently, Louvet presented a phase III study of 326 patients randomized to gemcitabine with oxaliplatin (gemcitabine 1000 mg/m^2 as a 10-mg/m^2/min prolonged infusion administered on day 1 in combination with oxaliplatin 100 mg/m^2 as a 2-h infusion administered on day 2 repeated every 2 weeks) versus gemcitabine (1000 mg/m^2 standard 30-min infusion) alone. While there was a difference in response rate (27% versus 17%) and progression-free survival (5.8 months versus 3.7 months), there was no difference with respect to median survival (9 months versus 7.1 months, p=0.13) [23]. Even had an improvement in median survival been identified, it would have been difficult to interpret unequivocally as the study design included two variables with respect to the standard gemcitabine (gemcitabine versus gemcitabine and oxaliplatin as well as the variable of standard 30-min gemcitabine infusion versus the fixed dose infusion at 10 mg/m^2/min). Recently, the Eastern Cooperative Oncology Group completed a phase III study of gemcitabine alone at standard 30-min infusion, gemcitabine at a standard dose but at the 10 mg/m^2/min infusion rate, and gemcitabine at the 10-mg/m^2/min infusion rate with oxaliplatin. The results are expected to be presented in 2006.

Gemcitabine with Topoisomerase I Inhibitors

Rocha Lima completed a phase II study of 45 patients treated with gemcitabine 1000 mg/m^2 over 30 min and irinotecan 100 mg/m^2 both weekly × 2 repeated every 3 weeks. Median survival was 5.7 months [24].

Rocha Lima presented the follow-up phase III study recently of 353 patients randomized to either gemcitabine alone or gemcitabine + irinotecan. While there was a higher response rate for combination gemcitabine and irinotecan (16% vs. 4%), the median survival was no different (6.6 months for gemcitabine alone versus 6.3 months for the combination) [25]. O'Reilly and colleagues have tested a more contemporary topoisomerase inhibitor, exatecan (2 mg/m^2 every 3 weeks) with gemcitabine (1000 mg/m^2 days 1 and 8 repeated every 3 weeks) versus gemcitabine alone in 349 patients with advanced pancreatic cancer. The median survival was 6.7 months for gemcitabine + exatecan versus 6.2 months for gemcitabine alone (p=0.52) [26].

Gemcitabine with Taxanes

The combination of gemcitabine and docetaxel was developed based on early reports suggesting that docetaxel was very active as single agent in patients with pancreatic cancer [27]. Cascinu et al. from the Italian Group for the Study of Digestive Tract Cancer reported a phase I/II study of docetaxel 70–80 mg/m^2 on day 8 and gemcitabine 1000 mg/m^2 on days 1 and 8 every 21 days. The maximum tolerated dose of the regimen was 70 mg/m^2 of docetaxel, with higher doses resulting in dose-limiting hematological toxicity. Eighteen patients were treated in the phase II portion of the study with only 1 partial response (5.5%) and a median survival of 5.4 months, which resulted in early termination of the study since gemcitabine as a single agent would achieve similar clinical efficacy [28]. Jacobs et al. conducted a phase II study of docetaxel 75 mg/m^2 on day 1 and standard gemcitabine 1000 mg/m^2 on days 1, 8, and 15 every 28 days in 34 patients with advanced disease. The regimen had to be modified to a weekly docetaxel schedule of 40 mg/m^2 on days 1 and 8 with gemcitabine 1000 mg/m^2 administered on the same days every 21 days after 13 of the first 18 patients developed grade 2–3 hematological toxicity. Overall, 10 patients achieved a partial response (30%) for a median time to progression of 6 months and a median survival of 10.5 months [29]. The combination of gemcitabine-docetaxel (gemcitabine 800 mg/m^2 days 1 and 8 and docetaxel 85 mg/m^2 every 3 weeks) has been compared to cispl atin-docetaxel (cisplatin 75 mg/m^2 on day 1 and docetaxel 75 mg/m^2 on day 1 every 21 days) in a randomized phase II study conducted by the European Organization for Research and Treatment of Cancer. Preliminary data from this study indicates that both regimens are equally effective, with a response rate of 16% and median survival of 7.6 and 7.1 months, respectively [30]. In addition, Ryan and colleagues reported a phase II trial of gemcitabine (600 mg/m^2 on days 1, 8, and 15 repeated every 28 days) and taxotere (60 mg/m^2 every 28 days) in 34 patients with advanced disease. The response rate was noted to be 18%, with a median survival of 8.9 months [31].

The combination of docetaxel-gemcitabine is currently one of the experimental arms of the CALGB 89904, phase III randomized clinical trial in which patients with advanced pancreatic cancer are randomized to treatment with fixed-dose rate gemcitabine (10 mg/m^2/minute × 150 min on day 1,8, and 15 every 28 days), gemcitabine-cisplatin (gemcitabine 1000 mg/m^2 on days 1, 8, and 15 and cisplatin 50 mg/m^2 on days 1 and 15), gemcitabine-docetaxel (gemcitabine 1000 mg/m^2 on days 1 and 8, and docetaxel 40 mg/m^2 on days 1 and 8 every 21 days), and gemcitabine-irinotecan (gemcitabine 1000 mg/m^2 days 1 and 8, and irinotecan 100 mg/m^2 on days 1 and 8).

Gemcitabine with Other Chemotherapy Combinations

There has been additional interest based on preclinical data in synergistically combining multiple chemotherapy agents with gemcitabine. Early data would suggest that such combinations have similar safety profiles with some of the gemcitabine combinations and are active schedules. Fine and colleagues have published preliminary data with a schedule known as GTX (gemcitabine 750 mg/m^2 at 10 mg/m^2/min fixed-dose infusion on days 4 and 11, taxotere 30 mg/m^2 over 30 min on days 4 and 11, xeloda 1500 mg/m^2 p.o. divided doses bid days on days 1–14 repeated every 21 days) in 44 patients with locally advanced (12 patients) and metastatic disease (32 patients). Of note, approximately 23% of patients had received prior first-line chemotherapy. Toxicities included grade 3 diarrhea and hand-foot syndrome (20%), grade 3 neutropenia (25%), and grade 2 asthenia (20%). Partial responses were identified in 47% of patients. The median survival for both groups has not been reported [32].

Kozuch and colleagues treated 34 patients who had been previously treated with gemcitabine either alone or in combination with a schedule known as G-FLIP (day 1: gemcitabine 500 mg/m^2 over 50 min, leukovorin 300 mg over 30 min, irinotecan 80 mg/m^2 over 80 min, 5-FU bolus 400 mg/m^2 over 10 min then 600 mg/m^2 over 8 h. Day 2: leukovorin 300 mg over

30 min, 5-FU bolus 400 mg/m^2 over 10 min, cisplatin 50-75 mg/m^2 with mannitol over 45 minutes, and 5-FU 600 mg/m^2 over 8 h). Toxicities were largely hematologic. Median survival for this pretreated group was 10.3 months [33]. The schedule has since been modified to gemcitabine (500 mg/m^2), irinotecan (120 mg/m^2), bolus 5-FU 400 mg/m^2, and leukovorin (300 mg/m^2) all on day 1, followed by a 24-h infusion of 5-FU (1500 mg/m^2) and cisplatin (35 mg/m^2) on day 2, with the schedule repeating every 2 weeks, in a 23 patient follow-up study (including 11 patients with pancreatic cancer). Grade 3/4 toxicities included thrombocytopenia (3%), anemia (6%), neutropenia (16%) with fever (10%), and thrombosis (23%). Of the 11 pancreas cancer patients, 1 experienced a complete response and 2 a partial responses [34].

New Drugs in Pancreatic Cancer

The identification of overexpressed/underexpressed genes and tumor-dependant growth pathways, and the search for tumor-specific proteins or antigens have been the focus of much cancer research. The rationale to develop these drugs in pancreatic cancer comes from the better understanding of the biological basis of the disease that has made possible the identification and validation of some of these targets in pancreatic cancer [35]. In addition, as evidenced by the previous studies using gemcitabine in combination with other chemotherapy agents, the continued poor prognosis of patients with this disease suggests that conventional chemotherapy has reached a plateau with regard to improving outcome. Table 49.2 summarizes key selected studies conducted with novel drugs in pancreatic cancer.

Matrix Metalloproteinase Inhibitors

The matrix metalloproteinases (MMPs) are a group of closely related proteases that are dysregulated in the majority of human neoplasms including pancreatic cancer. The increased activity of these enzymes has been related to tumor growth, progression, invasion, generation of blood vessels, and metastasis. Several inhibitors of the MMPs have been developed as anticancer agents and two of then, marimastat and BAY12-9566 have been more extensively studied in pancreatic cancer [36].

Marimastat is a hydroxamate peptidomimetic broad-spectrum inhibitor of the MMP family, including MMPs 1, 2, and 9. In phase I studies in pancreatic cancer, doses from 10 to 25 mg orally twice a day were well tolerated. Evans and colleague reported a phase II study that enrolled 113 patients with advanced pancreas cancer. Of the patients who were treated with a 25 mg once a day dose, 90% reported a 30% decline or stabilization in the tumor marker CA-19-9 and a median survival of 3.8 months. The median survival overall was 3.8 months. Twenty-nine percent of the patients developed arthralgias, the most common toxicity encountered with marimastat [37]. The efficacy and toxicity of marimastat 10 mg twice a day with gemcitabine (standard dose and infusion time) was compared to gemcitabine + placebo in a phase III study of 239 patients with advanced disease. There was no improvement in any parameter of outcome in the combined treatment group. The 1-year survival was 18% for the combination versus 17% for gemcitabine alone, with a median survival of 165 days (combination) versus 164 days (gemcitabine alone) [38]. The second MMP inhibitor extensively studied in pancreatic cancer is BAY12-9566, a peptidomimetic inhibitor specific

Table 49.2. Selected phase II and recent phase III studies of chemotherapy and molecular targeted agents for advanced pancreatic cancer

Study	Patients (*n*)	Molecular-targeted agent	Chemotherapy	PR/CR rate	Median survival (months)		1-year survival
Bramhall (2002) [38]	119	Placebo	Gen	11%	5.5		17%
	120	Marimastat	Gem	16%	5.5	(p=0.95)	18%
Moore (2003) [39]	139	None	Gem	5%	6.6		25%
	138	BAY12-9566	none	1%	3.7	(p <0.001)	10%
Xiong (2004) [52]	41	Cetuximab	Gem	12%	7.6		32%
Kindler (2004) [43]	40	Bevacizumab	Gem	27%	12.4		54%
Van Cutsem (2004) [47]	347	Placebo	Gem	8%	6.4		27%
	341	Tipifarnib	Gem	6%	6.1	(p=0.75)	24%
Moore (2005) [53]	260	Placebo	Gem	8%	6.4		17%
	261	Erlotinib	Gem	8%	6	(p=0.05)	24%

for MMP-2 and MMP-9. The drug (800 mg bid every day) was compared in a phase III study to single-agent gemcitabine (standard dose and infusion). Of a planned sample of 350 patients, 277 were enrolled after an interim analysis demonstrated that patients treated with gemcitabine had a significantly better time to tumor progression (3.5 versus 1.7 months, $p<0.001$) and overall survival (6.6 versus 3.7 months, $p<0.001$) [39]. In summary, these studies suggest that current MMP inhibitors do not have relevant antitumor activity in patients with advanced metastatic pancreatic cancer. Whether or not these drugs or newer-generation analogs would be effective in earlier stages of pancreatic cancer remains to be determined.

Angiogenesis Inhibitors

It is now generally accepted that tumors require the generation of blood vessels to grow, invade, and metastasize [40–42]. The drug of this class that appears more promising is pancreatic cancer is bevacizumab; a recombinant humanized monoclonal antibody against vascular endothelial growth factor (VEGF), a growth factor that has been implicated in pancreatic cancer progression in several preclinical studies. Bevacizumab has been studied in combination with gemcitabine in a phase II study in patients with pancreatic cancer [43]. Forty patients with advanced or locally advanced pancreatic cancer received gemcitabine 1000 mg/m^2 on days 1, 8, and 15 every 28 days and bevacizumab, 10 mg/kg intravenously on days 1 and 15. Results from the first 26 evaluable patients have been reported with a response rate of 27%, median time to tumor progression of 5.3 months, median survival of 12.4 months, and an estimated 1-year survival of 54%. Grade 3/4 toxicities included neutropenia (25%), anemia (3%), thrombocytopenia (5%), thrombosis (10%), hypertension (3%), and proteinuria (3%), In addition, there were two grade 5 toxicities (gastrointestinal bleed and bowel perforation) Correlative studies suggest that patients with higher baseline levels of VEGF (>82.5 pg/dl) tend to fare slightly worse. There is currently a phase III clinical trial through Cancer and Leukemia Group B of gemcitabine + bevacizumab versus gemcitabine + placebo. The study will reach study accrual by 2006.

Inhibitors of the Oncogene Ras

Mutations in the oncogene Ras is the most frequent genetic abnormality in pancreatic cancer. Because Ras requires farnesylation in order to be active, a posttranslational modification mediated by the enzyme farnesyltransferase, inhibitors of this enzyme have been developed as potential Ras inhibitors [44,45]. Two of these agents, tipifarnib and lonafarnib have been studied in disease-oriented studies in pancreatic cancer. Tipifarnib was tested in a single-agent phase II study in patients with advanced pancreatic cancer; it was administered at a dose of 300 mg orally twice a day for 21 of 28 days. Twenty patients were treated with no objective responses and a median survival of 19.7 weeks. Correlative studies conducted in peripheral blood mononuclear cells demonstrated partial inhibition of the target farnesyltransferase enzyme [46]. Van Cutsem and colleagues subsequently reported a randomized phase III study comparing the combination of R115777 (200 mg bid every day) with gemcitabine (standard dose and infusion) against gemcitabine plus placebo in 688 patients with advanced pancreatic cancer. The median overall survival was 193 days for the experimental arm versus 182 days for the control arm ($p=0.75$) [47]. Lonafarnib was evaluated in a randomized phase II study in comparison to gemcitabine. The 3-month progression-free survival rate for patients treated with lonafarnib was 23% and 31% for gemcitabine, and the median overall survival was 3.3 months and 4.4 months, respectively. There were two partial responses in patients treated with lonafarnib and one partial response observed in one patient treated with gemcitabine. Overall, lonafarnib was better tolerated than gemcitabine in that study [48].

Inhibitors of the Epidermal Growth Factor Receptor Family of Receptors

The epidermal growth factor receptor (EGFR) family of receptors includes four related transmembrane receptors, each of which are composed of an external ligand binding domain, a transmembrane domain, and an intracellular domain with tyrosine kinase (TK) activity. These receptors are frequently dysregulated in cancer and have been associated with the process of tumor growth, invasion, and metastasis, stimulating considerable interest in developing these drugs for cancer treatment. Pharmacologically, the inhibitors of the EGFR belong to two broad classes of drugs including monoclonal antibodies against the extracellular domain of the receptor and small molecules inhibitors of the intracellular TK domain [49,50]. Studies conducted in pancreatic cancer have tested mainly the combination of these drugs with gemcitabine.

Safran and collaborators reported a phase II study of trastuzumab (4 mg/kg loading followed by 2 mg/kg/week), a monoclonal antibody that targets the Her-2 receptor, in combination with gemcitabine (standard dose and infusion) in 34 patients with pancreatic cancer who were Her-2/neu positive. Thirty patients were 2+ positive and 4 patients were 3+ positive. Confirmed partial responses were observed in 2 of 32 patients (6%). The median survival and 1-year survival were 7 months and 19%, respectively [51]. Abbruzzese and collaborators conducted a phase II study of gemcitabine and cetuximab, a monoclonal antibody against the EGFR in EGFR-positive pancreatic cancer patients; 41 patients were treated in the study. The overall response rate was 12.5%, with a median survival of 6.7 months and 1-year survival of 33% [52]. There is currently a phase III clinical trial through the Southwest Oncology Group of gemcitabine + bevacizumab versus gemcitabine + placebo. The study will reach study accrual by 2006. The second clinically relevant classes of agents that inhibit the EGFR are small-molecule inhibitors of the receptor TK. There are several of these agents currently in clinical development. Erlotinib has been developed the most extensively for pancreatic cancer. More recently, the results of a phase III study that compared the survival of patients with pancreatic cancer treated with gemcitabine alone or in combination with erlotinib have been reported. A total of 569 patients with locally advanced or advanced pancreatic cancer were randomized to either gemcitabine (standard dose and infusion) plus placebo or gemcitabine plus erlotinib 100–150 mg daily (the majority of patients received 100 mg). The combined regimen was well tolerated. Patients treated with erlotinib had a statistically better median survival of 6.37 months versus 5.91 months (p=0.025) [53]. On the basis of this trial, in November 2005 the FDA approved erlotinib for use in combination with gemcitabine for the first-line treatment of advanced pancreatic cancer.

Summary

In summary, 5-FU, gemcitabine, and erlotinib are the only FDA-approved chemotherapeutic/molecular targeted agents in advanced pancreatic cancer. Although the efficacy of gemcitabine may be augmented by innovative dosing schedules or by the use of synergistic drug combinations, much work remains to be completed. There are several molecular targeted agents that are being tested in early clinical trials or, in the case of bevacizumab and erlotinib, in phase III trials.

References

1. Ahlgren JD (1996) Chemotherapy for pancreatic carcinoma. Cancer 78:653–663
2. DeCaprio JA, Mayer RJ, Gonin R, et al (1991) Fluorouracil and high dose leukovorin in previously untreated patients with advanced pancreatic adenocarcinoma: results of a phase II trial. J Clin Oncol 9:2128–2133
3. Crown J, Casper ES, Botet J, et al (1991) Lack of efficacy of high dose leukovorin and fluorouracil in patients with advanced pancreatic adenocarcinoma. J Clin Oncol 9:1682–1686
4. Peters GJ, van der Wilt CL, van Moorsel CJ, et al (2000) Basis for effective combination cancer chemotherapy with antimetabolites. Pharmacol Ther 87:227–253
5. DiMagno E, Reber HA, Tempero MA (1999) AGA technical review on the epidemiology, diagnosis, and treatment of pancreatic ductal adenocarcinoma. Gastroenterology 117:1463–1484
6. Casper E, Green MR, Kelson DP, et al (1994) Phase II trial of gemcitabine (2,2'-difluorodeoxycytidine) in patients with adenocarcinoma of the pancreas. Invest New Drugs 12:29–34
7. Burris HA III, Moore MJ, Cripps MC, et al (1997) Improvements in survival and clinical benefit with gemcitabine as first-line therapy for patients with advanced pancreatic cancer : a randomized trial. J Clin Oncol 15:2403–2413
8. Rothenberg ML, Moore MJ, Cripps MC, et al (1996) a phase II trial of Gemcitabine in patients with 5-FU refractory pancreas cancer. Ann Oncol 7:347–353
9. Tempero M, Plunkett W, van Haperen V, et al (1999) Randomized phase II trial of dose intense gemcitabine by standard infusion vs. fixed dose rate in metastatic pancreatic adenocarcinoma. Proc Am Soc Clin Oncol 18:273a (abstract 1048)
10. Berlin JD, Adak S, Vaughn DJ, et al (2000) a phase II study of gemcitabine and 5-fluorouracil in metastatic pancreatic cancer: an Eastern Cooperative Oncology Group Study. Oncology 58:215–218
11. Hidalgo M, Castellano D, Paz-Ares, L, et al (1999) Phase I–II study of gemcitabine and fluorouracil as a continuous infusion in patients with pancreatic cancer. J Clin Oncol 17:585–592
12. Louvet C, Andre T, Hammel P, et al (2001) Phase II trial of bimonthly leukovorin, 5-fluorouracil and gemcitabine for advanced pancreatic adenocarcinoma (FOLFUGEM). Ann Oncol 12:675–679
13. Hess V, Salzberg M, Borner M, et al (2003) Combining capecitabine and gemcitabine in patients with advanced pancreatic carcinoma: a phase I/II trial. J Clin Oncol 21:66–68
14. Cunningham D, Chau I, Stocken D, et al (2005) GemCAP – phase III randomized comparison of gemcitabine versus gemcitabine plus capecitabine in patients with advanced pancreatic cancer. Eur J Cancer 3:12 (abstract PS11)
15. Miller KD, Picus J, Blanke C, et al (2000) Phase II study of the multi-targeted anti-folate LY231514 (ALIMTA, MTA, pemetrexed disodium) in patients with advanced pancreatic cancer. Ann Oncol 11:101–103
16. Richards DA, Kindler HL, Oettle H, et al (2004) A randomized phase III study comparing gemcitabine + pemetrexed versus gemcitabine in patients with locally advanced and metastatic pancreas cancer. J Clin Oncol 22:14S (abstract 4007)

17. Philip PA, Zalupski MM, Vaitkevicius VK, et al (2001) Phase II study of Gemcitabine and cisplatin in the treatment of patients with advanced pancreatic cancer. Cancer 92:569–577
18. Colucci G, Giuliani F, Gebbia V, et al (2002) Gemcitabine alone or with cisplatin for the treatment of patients with locally advanced and/or metastatic pancreatic carcinoma. Cancer 94:902–910
19. Heinemann V, Quietzsch D, Gieseler F, et al (2006) Randomized phase III trial of gemcitabine plus cisplatin compared with gemcitabine alone in advanced pancreatic cancer. J Clin Oncol 24:3946–3952
20. Ko A, Dito E, Schillinger B, et al (2006) Phase II trial of fixed dose rate gemcitabine with cisplatin for metastatic adenocarcinoma of the pancreas. J Clin Oncol 24:379–385
21. Louvet C, Andre T, Lledo G, et al (2002) Gemcitabine combined with oxaliplatin in advanced pancreatic adenocarcinoma: final results of a GERCOR multi-center phase II study. J Clin Oncol 20:1512–1518
22. Alberts SR, Townley PM, Goldberg RM, et al (2003) Gemcitabine and oxaliplatin for metastatic pancreatic adenocarcinoma: a North Central Cancer Treatment Group phase II study. Ann Oncol 14:580–585
23. Louvet C, Labainca R, Hammel P, et al (2005) Gemcitabine in combination with oxaliplatin compared with gemcitabine alone in locally advanced or metastatic pancreatic cancer: results of a GERCOR and GISCAD phase III trial. J Clin Oncol 23:3509–3516
24. Rocha Lima C, Savarese D, Bruckner H, et al (2002) Irinotecan plus gemcitabine induces both radiographic and CA19-9 tumor marker responses in patients with previously untreated advanced pancreatic cancer. J Clin Oncol 20:1182–1191
25. Rocha Lima C, Green M, Rotche R, et al (2004) Irinotecan plus gemcitabine results in no survival advantage compared with gemcitabine monotherapy in patients with locally advanced or metastatic pancreatic cancer despite increased tumor response rate. J Clin Oncol 22:3776–3783
26. O'Reilly EM, Abou-Alfa G, Letourneau R, et al (2004) A randomized phase III trial of DX-8951f (exatecan mesylate; DX) and gemcitabine (GEM) versus gemcitabine alone in advanced pancreatic cancer (APC). J Clin Oncol 22:14S (abstract 4006)
27. Rougier P, Adenis A, Ducreux M, et al (2000) A phase II study: docetaxel as first-line chemotherapy for advanced pancreatic adenocarcinoma. Eur J Cancer 36:1016–1025
28. Cascinu S, Gasparini G, Catalano V, et al (1999) A phase I/II study of gemcitabine and docetaxel in advanced pancreatic cancer: a report from the Italian Group for the Study of Digestive Tract Cancer (GISCAD). Ann Oncol 10:1377–1379
29. Jacobs AD, Otero H, Picozzi VJ, et al (2004) Gemcitabine combined with docetaxel for the treatment of unresectable pancreatic adenocarcinoma. Cancer Invest 22:505–514
30. Heinemann V (2002) Gemcitabine in the treatment of advanced pancreatic cancer: a comparative analysis of randomized trials. Semin Oncol 29:9–16
31. Ryan DP, Kulke MH, Fuchs CS, et al (2002) a phase II study of gemcitabine and docetaxel in patients with metastatic pancreatic cancer. Cancer 94:97–103
32. Fine RL, Fogelman D Sherman W, et al (2003) The GTX regimen: a biochemically synergistic combination for advanced pancreatic cancer. Proc Am Soc Clin Oncol 22:281 (abstract 1129)
33. Kozuch P, Grossbard ML, Barzdins A, et al (2001) Irinotecan combined with gemcitabine, 5-fluorouracil, leukovorin and cisplatin (G-FLIP) is an effective and non-cross resistant treatment for chemotherapy refractory metastatic pancreatic cancer. Oncologist 6:488–495
34. Rachamalla R, Malamud S, Grossbard M, et al (2004) Phase I dose-finding study of biweekly irinotecan in combination with fixed doses of 5-Fluorouracil/lekovorin, gemcitabine and cisplatin (G-FLIP) in patients with advanced pancreatic cancer or other solid tumors. Anticancer Drugs 15:211–217
35. Adjei A, Hidalgo M (2005) Intracellular signal transduction pathway proteins as targets for cancer therapy. J Clin Oncol 23:5386–5403
36. Purcell WT, Rudek M, Hidalgo M (2002) Development of matrix metalloproteinase inhibitors in cancer therapy. Hematol Oncol Clin North Am 16:1189–1227
37. Evans J, Stark A, Johnson C, et al (2001) a phase II trial of marimastat in advanced pancreatic cancer. Br J Cancer 85:1865–1870
38. Bramhall S, Schulz J, Nemunaitis, J et al (2002) a double blind placebo-controlled randomized study comparing gemcitabine and marimastat with gemcitabine alone and placebo as first line therapy in patients with advanced pancreatic cancer. Br J Cancer 87:161–167
39. Moore MJ, Hamm J, Dancey J, et al (2003) Comparison of gemcitabine versus the matrix metalloproteinase inhibitor BAY 12-9566 in patients with advanced or metastatic adenocarcinoma of the pancreas: a phase III trial of the National Cancer Institute of Canada Clinical Trials Group. J Clin Oncol 21:3296–3302
40. Wey J, Fan F, Gray M, et al (2005) Vascular endothelial growth factor receptor-1 promotes migration and invasion in pancreatic cancer cell lines. Cancer 104:427–438
41. Korc M (2003) Pathways for aberrant angiogenesis in pancreatic cancer. Mol Cancer 2:8–15
42. Wolff RA (2002) Exploiting molecular targets in pancreatic cancer. Hematol Oncol Clin North Am 16:139–157
43. Kindler H, Friberg G, Stadler W, et al (2004) Bevacizumab plus gemcitabine is an active combination in patients with advanced pancreatic cancer: interim results of an ongoing Phase II trial from the University of Chicago Phase II Consortium. Paper presented at American Society of Clinical Oncology Gastrointestinal Symposium. San Francisco, CA, Jan 22–24, 2004 (abstract 86)
44. Li D, Xie K, Wolff R, et al (2004) Pancreatic cancer. Lancet 363:1049–1057
45. Dempke W (2003) Farnesyltransferase inhibitors – a novel approach in the treatment of advanced pancreatic carcinomas. Anticancer Res 23:813–818
46. Cohen S, Ho L, Ranganathan S, et al (2003) Phase II and pharmacodynamic study of the farnesyltransferase inhibitor R115777 as initial therapy in patients with metastatic pancreatic adenocarcinoma. J Clin Oncol 21:1301–1306
47. Van Cutsem E, van de Velde H, Karasek P, et al (2004) Phase III trial of gemcitabine plus tipifarnib compared with gemcitabine plus placebo in advanced pancreatic cancer. J Clin Oncol 22:1430–1438
48. Lersch C, Van Cutsem E, Amado R, et al (2001) Randomized phase II study of SCH 66336 and gemcitabine in the treatment of metastatic adenocarcinoma of the pancreas. Proc Am Soc Clin Oncol 20:(abstract 608)

49. Ueda S, Ogata S, Tsuda H, et al (2004) The correlation between cytoplasmic over-expression of epidermal growth factor receptor and tumor aggressiveness: poor prognosis in patients with pancreatic ductal adenocarcinoma. Pancreas 29:e1–8
50. Xiong HQ, Abbruzzese J (2002) Epidermal growth factor receptor-targeted therapy for pancreatic cancer. Semin Oncol 5:31–37
51. Safran H, Iannitti D, Ramanathan R, et al (2004) Herceptin and gemcitabine for metastatic pancreatic cancers that over-express HER-2-neu. Cancer Invest 22:706–712
52. Xiong HQ, Rosenberg A, LoBuglio A, et al (2004) Cetuximab, a monoclonal antibody targeting the epidermal growth factor receptor, in combination with gemcitabine for advanced pancreatic cancer: a multi-center phase II trial. J Clin Oncol 22:2610–2616
53. Moore M, Goldstein D, Hamm J, et al (2005) Erlotinib improves survival when added to gemcitabine in patients with advanced pancreatic cancer. A phase III trial of the National Cancer Institute of Canada Clinical Trials Group [NCIC–CTG]. Proceedings of the 2005 Gastrointestinal Cancers Symposium, Orlando, FL, January 27–29 (abstract 77)

Chapter 50

O. J. Hines · H. A. Reber

Indications for Resection of Pancreatic Cancer

Of the options currently available for patients with pancreatic cancer, surgical resection offers the only potential for cure, and probably provides the best palliation as well. Thus, in the absence of certain clear contraindications (which will be discussed), most patients with this disease deserve to be explored. The decision to actually resect a pancreatic cancer is complex and based on sophisticated imaging, assessment of operative risk, an understanding of tumor biology and current clinical data, and the experience that only a focused clinical practice can bring. In this chapter, we will discuss this decision-making process to the point of resection, including the assessment made in the operating room. Because much of the approach is based on personal experience, which obviously varies among so-called experts, we will try to offer a balanced perspective where controversy may exist. The pancreas can be the site of several different types of cancer, but our comments refer to the most common form, the so-called ductal adenocarcinoma of the pancreas.

The Initial Encounter

Most patients who are thought to have pancreatic cancer have undergone an initial evaluation by a primary care physician or gastroenterologist, and they are referred to a surgeon only if there is no obvious evidence of unresectability. Clear evidence of unresectability on a CT scan would include liver metastasis or peritoneal disease. While there is general agreement that tumor resection is contraindicated in the presence of such advanced disease, there are certain misconceptions that also influence referral patterns and even affect surgical decision-making.

Many physicians feel that tumors that exceed a certain size are unresectable, and they may even fail to refer the patient to a surgeon for an opinion. It is true that small pancreatic tumors (<2 cm diameter) are more likely to be resectable than larger ones. Nevertheless, the majority of pancreatic cancers located in the head of the gland are larger than that by the time the diagnosis is made and an operation is performed. For example, at the University of Erlangen in Germany, of all resections of tumors in the head of the gland, 15% were 1–2 cm in diameter, 33.4% were 2–3 cm, 23.3% were 3–4 cm, and 27.8% were >4 cm [1]. At the University of California, Lost Angeles Medical Center over the period 1989–1994, 26% of the resections were for tumors 1–2 cm in diameter, 17% were 2–3 cm, 22% were 3–4 cm, 26% were 4–5 cm, and 9% were >5 cm in diameter. Thus, it should be apparent that no patient should be denied the chance for a resection because of a tumor that is considered too large.

As part of an evaluation for pancreatic cancer, the physician may test serum tumor markers including CA19-9 and CEA. CA19-9 is a monosialoganglioside/glycolipid that is present in the serum of healthy individuals (<40 U/ml). CA19-9 levels are elevated in pancreatic, hepatocellular, gastric, colorectal, and ovarian cancer. CA19-9 can also rise in benign conditions of extrahepatic biliary obstruction such as pancreatitis and choledocholithiasis. High levels of CA19-9 (>300 U/ml) correlate with advanced disease [2]. Because the serum level of CA19-9 is related to the tumor burden, values above 1,000 U/ml have been considered to signal the presence of widespread and unresectable disease [3, 4]. Although it is uncommon to find a localized tumor with such high CA19-9 levels, we have resected the tumor in some patients whose levels were elevated to that degree. Thus, CA19-9 levels by themselves should not be a reason to consider a patient unresectable. CEA levels are less reliable than CA19-9 for the diagnosis and management of pancreatic cancer, but are often utilized in combination with CA19-9 [5].

Finally, no patient should be considered too old to undergo a Whipple operation for pancreatic cancer. Each patient should undergo the usual preoperative assessment for major abdominal surgery, and decisions about operability based on those results rather than chronological age. Several studies have documented the safety of pancreatic resection in the older population [6–8].

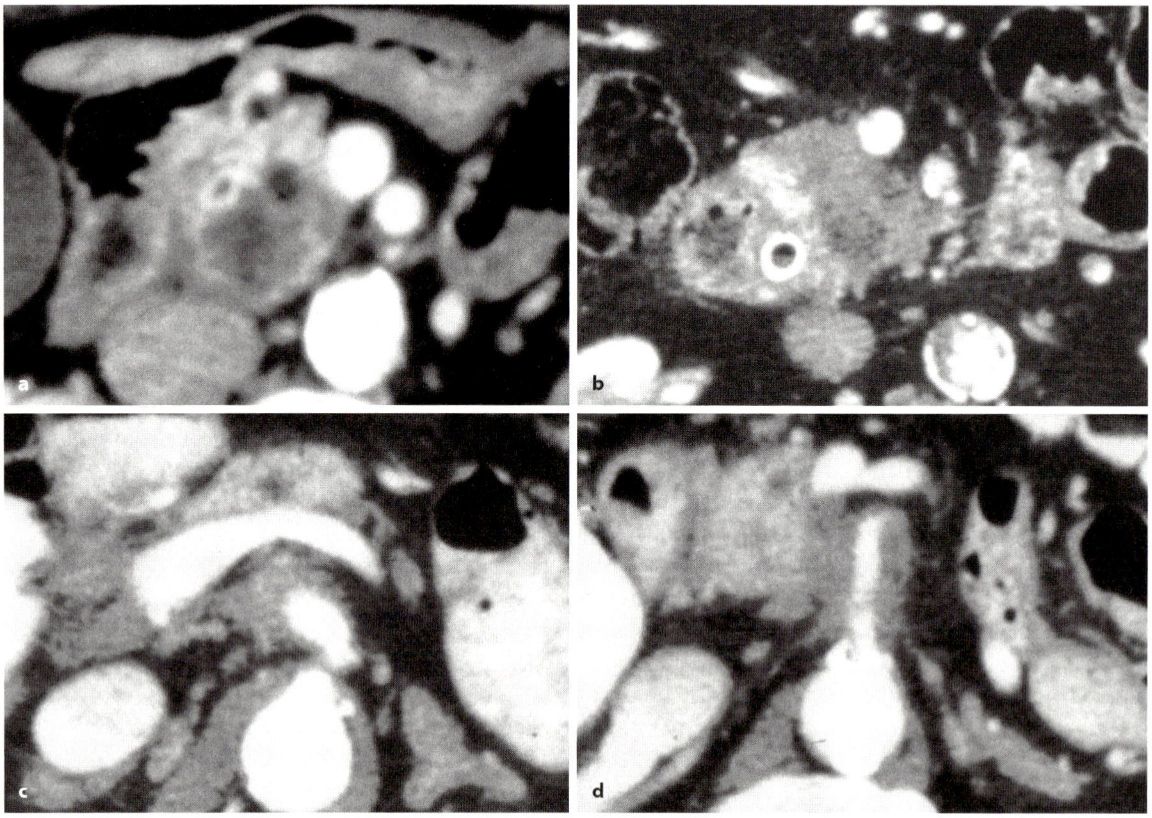

Figure 50.1

Computed tomography (CT) scan of the pancreas and progressive involvement of the superior mesenteric vein (SMV). The likelihood of being able to resect a pancreatic head lesion can be based on the degree to which (i.e., percentage) the SMV is in contact with the tumor. Involvement of the vein: a 25%, b 25–50%, c 50-75%, d 75–100%

Determination of Resectability

In most centers, the single most valuable study to stage patients with pancreatic cancer is the helical computed tomography (CT) scan done according to a specific "pancreatic protocol". This requires 2- to 3-mm collimation through the pancreas itself, intravenous contrast, and separate scans for both the pancreas and liver during the arterial and venous phases. Appropriate software permits the recreation of images that provide extraordinary detail about the tumor and its relationship to important adjacent structures. Nevertheless, for a variety of reasons, some patients still cannot be categorized with certainty into a resectable or unresectable group.

In the absence of distant metastatic disease, most unresectable patients have locally extensive disease that involves adjacent large blood vessels (e.g., hepatic or superior mesenteric arteries, superior mesenteric or portal veins), or has spread to adjacent regional lymph nodes not removed as part of the usual Whipple specimen (e.g., celiac nodes, retroduodenal nodes between the vena cava and aorta). Enlarged lymph nodes can be seen on CT, but inflammatory nodes cannot be distinguished from neoplastic ones. Thus, the mere presence of large nodes should not be the reason that a CT scan is interpreted as showing an unresectable tumor.

In our experience, the ability of CT to predict resectability is about 85% [9]. Errors are usually due to small liver or peritoneal metastases that were undetected or cancer that invades the superior mesenteric or portal vein. The ability of the CT scan to predict that a tumor will be unresectable has been reported to be as high as 95% [10]. In fact, the accuracy of such a prediction is related to the expertise of the radiologist, the nature of the CT finding on which the prediction is based, and to the experience and philosophy of the surgeon. Thus, if the apparent presence of liver metastases is the basis for the prediction of unresectability, the level of reliability is high. If the radiologist finds evidence for tumor invasion of the supe-

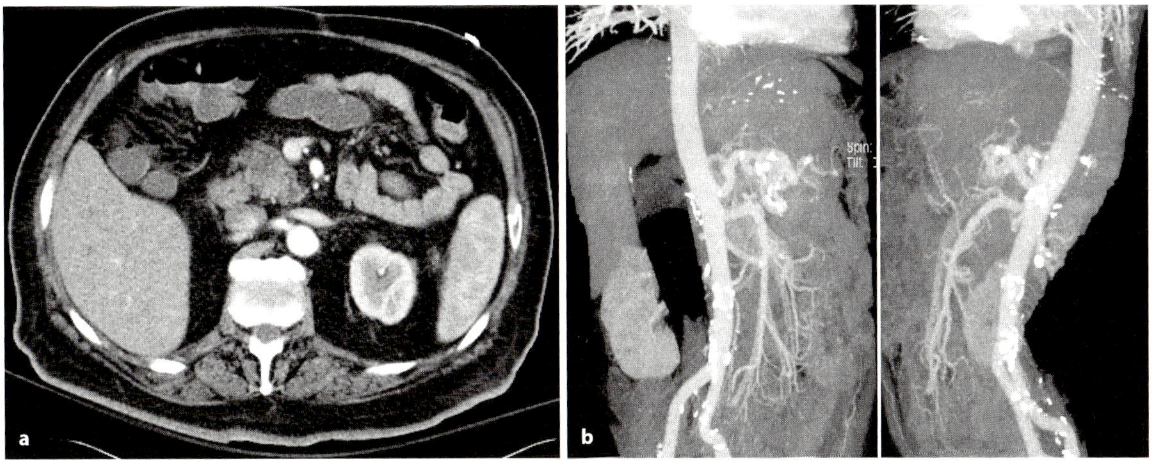

Figure 50.2

CT scan (a) and CT angiography (b) of the same patient with a pancreatic head mass. The angiography demonstrates the arterial vasculature from a right lateral and complete left lateral position

rior mesenteric vein, the implications of such a finding may be less clear (Fig. 50.1). For example, there may be loss of the normal fat plane between the vein and the tumor, for a variable distance around the circumference of the vessel. This raises the question of unresectability because of vascular invasion, but the tumor may merely be contiguous with or adherent to the vein. In many cases when the tumor is in contact with as much as 50% of the vein circumference, we have been able to peel the vein off of the adherent tumor. Degrees of contact of more than 50% are more likely to represent true invasion and unresectability. So too is narrowing or distortion of the vein. Even when the tumor invades the vein, we will occasionally resect the tumor and a part of the vessel wall, in an effort to palliate a patient who seems to be a reasonable candidate. While we do not believe that such patients are cured by the resection, some are undoubtedly palliated.

Endoscopic ultrasound (EUS) also has the potential to provide information about resectability, but the quality of the information is highly operator dependent. We will often refer patients for EUS when the CT findings suggest vascular invasion, but the findings are equivocal. When the EUS interpretation is that of complete vascular occlusion by the tumor, this reliably indicates unresectability. But we have been less impressed by predictions of resectability with lesser degrees of involvement, even by experienced operators [11]. We have resected tumors when the EUS report indicated an unresectable lesion and have also found that the tumor was unresectable because it did involve major vessels, even though the EUS reported no evidence of vascular involvement. The reliability of EUS predictions increases not only with the experience of the endoscopist, but also with the increasing collaboration between the endoscopist and surgeon. We prefer that the EUS (and CT) interpretation be given as a specific description of the findings (e.g., the tumor is in contact with 30% of the circumference of the wall of the portal vein, but does not appear to invade or distort it), rather than a statement as to whether the tumor is resectable.

Using EUS technology, the physician can also safely and reliably obtain fine-needle aspirates of primary tumors and lymph nodes for cytologic examination. The sensitivity is 85% and specificity is almost 100% [12]. As indicated earlier, metastatic disease in lymph node basins outside of the area of resection (e.g., celiac nodes) precludes resection.

The use of preoperative angiography of the abdominal vasculature has largely been replaced by CT. If the surgeon feels an angiographic image is required to assess resection, the radiologist can supply reformatted images demonstrating striking detail of the superior mesenteric vein, portal vein, superior mesenteric artery, celiac axis, and hepatic arteries (Fig. 50.2).

Staging and Resectablity

The tumor, nodal involvement, and metastasis (TNM) definitions and 6th edition of the American Joint Committee on Cancer staging for pancreatic cancer is presented in Table 50.1 [13]. Patients with stage 0, I, or

Table 50.1. The American Joint Committee on Cancer (AJCC) has designated staging by tumor, nodal involvement, and metastases (TNM) classification

TNM definitions	
Primary tumor (T)	
TX:	Primary tumor cannot be assessed
T0:	No evidence of primary tumor
Tis:	Carcinoma in situ
T1:	Tumor limited to the pancreas, ≤2 cm in greatest dimension
T2:	Tumor limited to the pancreas, >2 cm in greatest dimension
T3:	Tumor extends beyond the pancreas but without involvement of the celiac axis or the superior mesenteric artery
T4:	Tumor involves the celiac axis or the superior mesenteric artery (unresectable primary tumor)
Regional lymph nodes (N)	
NX:	Regional lymph nodes cannot be assessed
N0:	No regional lymph node metastasis
N1:	Regional lymph node metastasis
Distant metastasis (M)	
MX:	Distant metastasis cannot be assessed
M0:	No distant metastasis
M1:	Distant metastasis
AJCC stage groupings	
Stage 0	Tis, N0, M0
Stage IA	T1, N0, M0
Stage IB	T2, N0, M0
Stage IIA	T3, N0, M0
Stage IIB	T1, N1, M0
	T2, N1, M0
	T3, N1, M0
Stage III	T4, any N, M0
Stage IV	Any T, any N, M1

II disease are generally considered resectable. Some surgeons also will resect tumors in patients with stage III disease (tumor invasion of the celiac or superior mesenteric arteries; see below); we will not. Patients whose tumors are confined to the pancreas, and even with involved lymph nodes in areas that are usually removed with the standard pancreaticoduodenectomy, are candidates for resection. Some patients with invasion of the superior mesenteric or portal veins also may be.

Intraoperative Assessment

Laparoscopy is commonly used to operatively stage patients with pancreatic cancer. Some surgeons have used it, in the majority of cases, as a separate procedure in the outpatient setting, and the findings guide the subsequent workup. More often, laparoscopy is performed immediately before laparotomy under the same anesthetic; if evidence of unresectability is found, the operation is concluded or a palliative bypass may be performed. We perform it selectively. We have not used laparoscopy in patients who appear to have resectable lesions on helical CT, and who are good candidates for resection. In a recent review of our own data, resection was possible in 85% of our patients who were judged to have resectable cancers of the head of the pancreas after CT scan. Of the remaining 15% of the total who did not have resectable cancers, small liver or peritoneal metastases, which might have been seen laparoscopically, were the reason in only half. Thus, if all of our patients had undergone laparoscopy as a routine, at best less than 10% might have been spared subsequent laparotomy. We do use laparoscopy in certain circumstances. Examples include some patients with pancreatic cancer and CT evidence of liver or other metastases not proven preoperatively, patients with a very high serum level of CA19-9, and some patients with ascites who probably have peritoneal metastases. We will often also use it in patients with cancers of the body or tail of the pancreas.

We usually explore patients through a bilateral subcostal incision. After a general exploration of the abdominal contents for evidence of distant metastatic disease (e.g., liver or peritoneal seeding), the transverse colon is elevated and the base of the transverse mesocolon overlying the duodenum and head of the pancreas is examined. While tumor invasion here does not preclude resection, it does require removal of a portion of the mesocolon in order to excise all grossly apparent cancer. However, because invasion of the mesocolon is also usually accompanied by tumor involvement of the superior mesenteric vein, this finding generally signifies unresectability.

Although we usually follow a routine in the mobilization of the various structures for a pancreaticoduodenectomy (e.g., Kocher maneuver first, entrance into the lesser sac, and mobilization of the greater curve of the stomach next, skeletonization of the superior mesenteric vein), we depart from this routine when there is a specific area of concern that was raised in the preoperative evaluation. For example, if large celiac nodes were known to be present, we would expose and biopsy them first. If there were a question of hepatic artery involvement by tumor, we would begin the dissection in the hepatoduodenal ligament. In the absence of such concerns, the final determination of resectability usually depends upon whether the superior mesenteric and/or portal veins are free of the tumor. This requires exposure of the vessels above and below the neck of the pancreas, usually with ligation and division of the tributaries of the superior mesenteric vein, and elevation of the pancreatic neck from the underlying vessels. It is usually easy to determine whether the vein is free anteriorly, but adherence laterally or posteriorly, which would preclude resection, may be harder to ascertain. Some clue may come from a combined visual and tactile assessment of the tumor mass in relation to the course of the exposed superior mesenteric – portal vein. Still we will occasionally decide to resect the tumor only to find that the vessels are adherent to it in these areas. Then we would resect the involved portion of the vein. If the vein is suspected of being involved by tumor, and we decided against resection, we would biopsy some of the adherent tissue to confirm that tumor was present. Sometimes this assessment is confounded by the presence of pancreatitis, caused by preoperative manipulations (e.g., endoscopic retrograde cholangiopancreatography, stent placement, fine-needle aspiration). Then the adherence may be inflammatory rather than because of tumor invasion, and the biopsy specimens would not show cancer. In any case, if histologic proof of cancer was not obtained preoperatively and a decision is made against resection, the diagnosis should be confirmed during the operation so that chemotherapy can be given later. This is done most easily and safely by obtaining a fine-needle aspirate of the mass in the head of the pancreas.

In patients with pancreatitis and adherence of the pancreas to the vein, it may not be possible to tell whether the adherence is from tumor invasion or inflammation. Then we usually will not resect, but will conclude the procedure and recommend that the patient undergo neoadjuvant therapy for 2–3 months. This allows the inflammatory component to resolve, and provides for treatment of the cancer until a reevaluation and a consideration for reexploration can be made. If the tumor is deemed unresectable because of confirmed neoplastic invasion of the vessels, then we follow a similar protocol. In this latter group, the neoadjuvant treatment has been given for about 6 months, with the hope that downstaging may occur [14]. Although this is not common (about 10% of such patients), we have several long-term survivors in this highly select group.

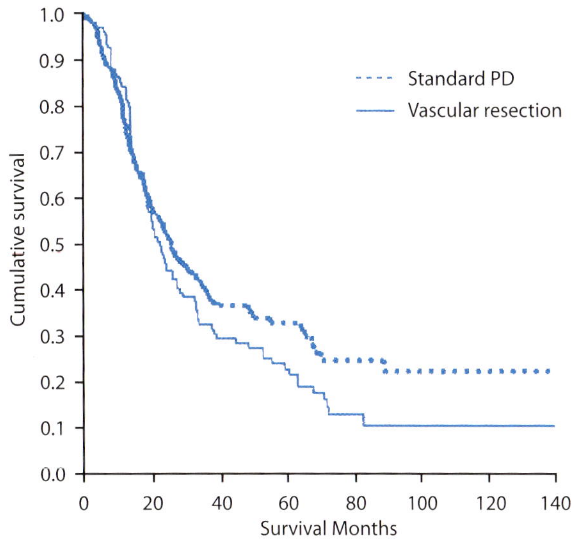

Figure 50.3

Kaplan-Meier survival curves in patients with pancreatic adenocarcinoma who underwent standard pancreaticoduodenectomy (*PD*) or PD with vascular resection and reconstruction. The median survival for standard PD was 26.5 months. The median survival for PD with vascular resection was 23.4 months [15]

Some surgeons are more willing to resect tumors along with segments of vein when there is evidence of superior mesenteric or portal venous involvement, and have shown that the operation can be done safely [15, 16]. Reported survival statistics (operative mortality rate and long term survival) are similar to those for patients who undergo resection where there was no vessel involvement and vessels were not resected (Fig. 50.3). However, because patients with vessel involvement are not cured by resection, we agree with the majority of surgeons who do not routinely resect in this situation.

Body and Tail Pancreatic Cancer

In general, patients with adenocarcinoma of the body and tail of the pancreas present with more advanced disease than patients with tumors in the head of the pancreas. The majority of these patients remain asymptomatic until they have developed advanced local or systemic disease. Of course, the tumors in the latter patients are not resected. Traverso recently reported that two times as many patients with left-sided tumors (53%) as right-sided tumors have unrecognized distant disease [17]. On the other hand, even patients with locally extensive disease may be candidates for resection [18–20].

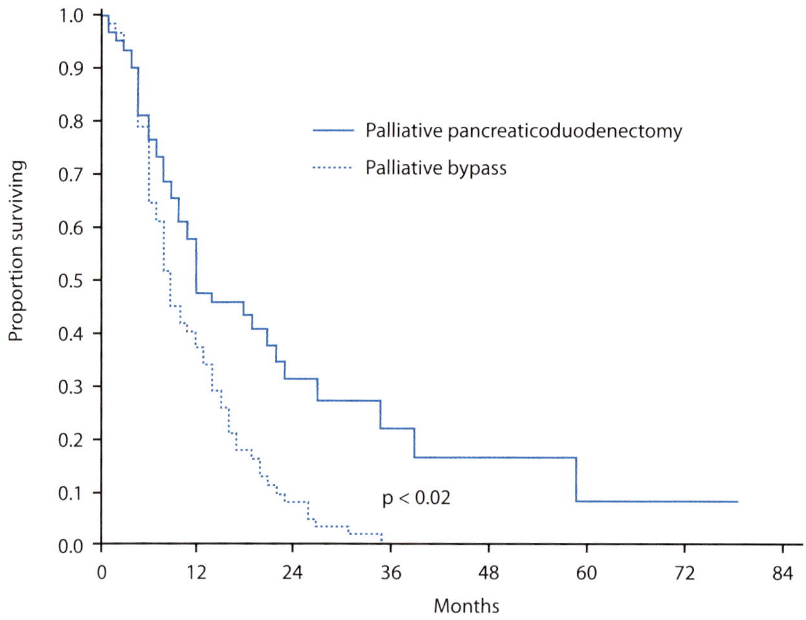

Figure 50.4

Actuarial survival curves (Kaplan-Meier) for patients undergoing palliative PD ($N = 64$) and palliative bypass ($N = 62$) [21]

Patients are evaluated with CT scan to determine whether there is any evidence of liver or peritoneal disease. If this is not apparent we usually perform laparoscopy to start the operation. If there is no evidence of distant spread of the tumor, we proceed with open resection. Involvement of the splenic artery or vein does not contraindicate resection, but extension of the tumor into either the celiac or superior mesenteric artery does. We routinely resect celiac and superior mesenteric artery lymph nodes and the surrounding soft tissue, so obvious involvement of nodes in these areas does not preclude resection of the tumor.

Local extension of the tumor into the spleen is not necessarily a contraindication to resection since the spleen should routinely be removed as part of the specimen. In addition, local extension into the mesocolon or colon may also be resected en bloc in selected cases. While this is unlikely to cure the patient, we think that it may provide palliation if it can be done safely. Recently, there have been several case series describing the safety of laparoscopic distal pancreatectomy for benign pancreatic tumors. It is our opinion that this procedure has yet to be shown efficacious in the case of adenocarcinoma, and we would not recommend it in that situation.

Palliative Resection of Pancreatic Cancer

Although the intent of resection in the case of pancreatic cancer is cure, in most cases this is not the result, and the patient eventually succumbs to the disease. So in most cases of resection, the procedure is palliative. Resection clearly improves survival in patients who are properly selected as outlined earlier. The operative mortality rate of pancreaticoduodenectomy is low and the morbidity manageable.

If a tumor is found to be unresectable at the time of surgery, a bypass of the stomach and/or biliary tree is often performed. In the event that the tumor eventually obstructs either the stomach or the bile duct, the patient will have another route for drainage and further intervention is not likely to be required. A pancreaticoduodenectomy would accomplish the same and, some would argue, may be better than bypass alone. Some investigators have reported a survival advantage of several months (Fig. 50.4) over those undergoing bypass alone [21, 22]. Others have reported equal survival to patients who were undergoing curative resection; however, this may simply reflect the overall poor prognosis for both groups. It is also unclear whether the patients who underwent palliative resection were appropriately matched with those who had a so-called curative operation. Some also suggest that there is the potential for better pain control for resected patients, since the tumor has been removed. Indeed, although it seems intuitively apparent that certain patients with limited local or even distant disease may benefit from resection, there are insufficient data available to routinely recommend it.

Summary

When assessing a patient with pancreatic cancer for resection, a pancreas protocol CT scan may be the only test required. If it shows a mass in the pancreas without evidence of metastatic disease or vascular involvement, surgery may be undertaken without further diagnostic studies. If the CT shows distant metastases, this should be confirmed histologically, and the patient triaged to a nonsurgical treatment protocol. The same is true with unequivocal involvement of the hepatic, celiac, or superior mesenteric artery, or superior mesenteric or portal vein. If there are suspicious lymph nodes or possible involvement of one of the aforementioned blood vessels by tumor, EUS may be helpful. At the time of EUS, confirmation by fine-needle aspiration of node involvement outside of the pancreaticoduodenectomy resection field precludes resection. So too does an unequivocal finding of vascular invasion. However, we usually operate on any patient who remains with an equivocal assessment. Laparoscopy is performed first when metastatic disease is suspected. If none is found, laparotomy is performed and the tumor is resected as long as intraoperative maneuvers suggest the absence of vascular invasion by the cancer.

References

1. Becker V, Stommer P (1993) Pathology and classification of tumours of the pancreas. In: Trede M, Carter DC (eds) Surgery of the Pancreas. Churchill Livingston, New York, pp 399-421
2. Tian F, Appert HE, Myles J, Howard JM (1992) Prognostic value of serum CA 19-9 levels in pancreatic adenocarcinoma. Ann Surg 215:350–355
3. Forsmark CE, Lambiase L, Vogel SB (1994) Diagnosis of pancreatic cancer and prediction of unresectability using the tumor-associated antigen CA19-9. Pancreas 9:731–734
4. Schlieman MG, Ho HS, Bold RJ (2003) Utility of tumor markers in determining resectability of pancreatic cancer. *Arch Surg* 138:951–956
5. Yasue M, Sakamoto J, Teramukai S, et al (1994) Prognostic values of preoperative and postoperative CEA and CA19.9 levels in pancreatic cancer. Pancreas 9:735–740
6. Richter A, Niedergethmann M, Lorenz D, Sturm JW, Trede M, Post S (2002) Resection for cancers of the pancreatic head in patients aged 70 years or over. Eur J Surg 168:339–344
7. Fong Y, Blumgart LH, Fortner JG, et al (1995) Pancreatic or liver resection for malignancy is safe and effective for the elderly. Ann Surg 222:426–434
8. Sohn TA, Yeo CJ, Cameron JL, Lillemoe KD, Talamini MA, Hruban RH, Sauter PK, Coleman J, Ord SE, Grochow LB, Abrams RA, Pitt HA (1998) Should pancreaticoduodenectomy be performed in octogenarians? J Gastrointest Surg 2:207–216
9. Lu DS, Reber HA, Krasny RM, Kadell BM, Sayre J (1997) Local staging of pancreatic cancer: criteria for unresectability of major vessels as revealed by pancreatic-phase, thin-section helical CT. Am J Roentgenol 168:1439–1443
10. House MG, Yeo CJ, Cameron JL, Campbell KA, Schulick RD, Leach SD, Hruban RH, Horton KM, Fishman EK, Lillemoe KD (2004) Predicting resectability of periampullary cancer with three-dimensional computed tomography. J Gastrointest Surg 8:280–288
11. Aslanian H, Salem R, Lee J, Andersen D, Robert M, Topazian M (2005) EUS diagnosis of vascular invasion in pancreatic cancer: surgical and histologic correlates. Am J Gastroenterol 100:1381–1385
12. Volmar KE, Vollmer RT, Jowell PS, Nelson RC, Xie HB (2005) Pancreatic FNA in 1000 cases: a comparison of imaging modalities. Gastrointest Endosc 61:854–861
13. Green FL, Page DL, Fleming ID, et al (eds) (2002) AJCC Cancer Staging Manual (6th edn). Springer, New York
14. Todd KE, Gloor B, Lane JS, Isacoff WH, Reber HA (1998) Resection of locally advanced pancreatic cancer after downstaging with continuous-infusion 5-fluorouracil, mitomycin-C, leucovorin, and dipyridamole. J Gastrointest Surg 2:159–566
15. Tseng JF, Raut CP, Lee JE, Pisters PW, Vauthey JN, Abdalla EK, Gomez HF, Sun CC, Crane CH, Wolff RA, Evans DB (2004) Pancreaticoduodenectomy with vascular resection: margin status and survival duration. J Gastrointest Surg 8:935–949
16. Hartel M, Niedergethmann M, Farag-Soliman M, Sturm JW, Richter A, Trede M, Post S (2002) Benefit of venous resection for ductal adenocarcinoma of the pancreatic head. Eur J Surg 168:707–712
17. Liu RC, Traverso LW (2005) Diagnostic laparoscopy improves staging of pancreatic cancer deemed locally unresectable by computed tomography. Surg Endosc 19:638–642
18. Johnson CD, Schwall G, Flechtenmacher J, Trede M (1993) Resection for adenocarcinoma of the body and tail of the pancreas. Br J Surg 80:1177–1179
19. Dalton RR, Sarr MG, van Heerden JA, et al (1992) Carcinoma of the body and tail of the pancreas: is curative resection justified? Surgery 111:489–494
20. Brennan MF, Moccia RD, Klimstra D (1996) Management of adenocarcinoma of the body and tail of the pancreas. Ann Surg 223:506–511
21. Lillemoe KD, Cameron JL, Yeo CJ, Sohn TA, Nakeeb A, Sauter PK, Hruban RH, Abrams RA, Pitt HA (1996) Pancreaticoduodenectomy. Does it have a role in the palliation of pancreatic cancer? Ann Surg 223:718–725
22. Wagner M, Redaelli C, Lietz M, Seiler CA, Friess H, Buchler MW (2004) Curative resection is the single most important factor determining outcome in patients with pancreatic adenocarcinoma. Br J Surg 91:586–594

Chapter 51

C.R. Ferrone · M.F. Brennan

The Kausch-Whipple Pancreatectomy

Allen Oldfather Whipple, a Clinical Director of Memorial Sloan-Kettering Cancer Center (MSKCC), is often credited with developing the operation of pancreaticoduodenectomy in 1935 while at the Presbyterian Hospital in New York City [1,2]. However, Professor Codivilla of Bologna performed a pancreaticoduodenectomy for a distal gastric cancer involving the duodenum in 1898 [3] and Professor W. Kausch performed a pancreaticoduodenectomy in 1909 for a small carcinoma of the ampulla of Vater [4]. The operation has evolved over the twentieth century from a two-stage procedure with significant morbidity and mortality to a one-stage procedure that can be performed expeditiously and safely.

Preoperative Investigation and Preparation

Metastatic disease needs to be excluded through a combination of preoperative imaging and diagnostic laparoscopy. Once metastatic disease has been excluded, vascular invasion determines resectability. Arterial encroachment or encasement, in our opinion, precludes resection for cure, since extended radical procedures have not translated into overall survival benefit [5,6]. Venous encroachment of the superior mesenteric vein (SMV) or portal vein (PV) in the absence of varices does not preclude resection. However, venous encroachment is often an indicator of more advanced disease, which has a high likelihood of extension to the celiac artery or superior mesenteric artery (SMA). At MSKCC, 58 (17%) of 332 patients underwent pancreatic resection with PV resection for isolated PV involvement. The overall mortality was slightly higher for those patients undergoing PV resection (3% vs. 5%), however, the median survival (13 months) was equivalent [7]. At MD Anderson, similar results were obtained when isolated resection of the SMV, PV, or SMV-PV confluence was performed in 141 patients; a higher complication rate (21%), higher rate of R1 resections (22% vs. 12%), but a similar overall survival compared to those patients who did not undergo vascular resection (median survival of 23.4 vs. 26.5 months) [8].

Imaging

Thin-cut pancreatic protocol computed tomography (CT) scans with contrast are able to rule out gross invasion or encroachment. More subtle degrees of involvement, which can be suspected when clear fat planes cannot be identified surrounding the celiac axis or the SMA, can be more difficult to discern. With improved CT scans and dedicated protocol-driven vascular phase imaging, angiography no longer has a role in the evaluation of pancreatic adenocarcinoma or endocrine tumors. Three-dimensional reconstruction of the vasculature can add definition in select cases.

Endoscopic Ultrasound

Endoscopic ultrasound (EUS), although operator dependent, can provide important additional information regarding resectability. In a series of 81 patients, overall EUS correlation with surgical pathology was 85% for T stage and 72% for N stage. More specifically, correlation was as follows: T1 92%, T2 85%, T3 93%, N0 72%, and N1 72% [9]. CT failed to detect a mass in 26% of patients and had a lower correlation than EUS for T (30%) and N (55%) staging; T1 65%, T2 67%, T3 38%, N0 52%, and N1 100% [9]. EUS was also more effective than thin-cut CT scans at detecting the involvement of the portal-mesenteric axis by the tumor (87–93% vs. 62–67%, $p = 0.04$) [9,10]. The utility of EUS does decrease if the patient has chronic pancreatitis, a recent episode of acute pancreatitis (<4 weeks), a diffusely infiltrating carcinoma, or a prominent ventral/dorsal split [11].

Positron Emission Tomography

The role of 18-flurodeoxyglucose positron emission tomography (FDG-PET) has not been established. Multiple studies report that FDG-PET changed the management of 40% of patients thought to be resectable by identifying metastatic disease. Higashi et al. found that FDG PET detected distant metastases or unexpected lesions not seen on CT scans in 35 of 93 (38%) patients; 3 distant lymph node metastases, 10 liver metastases, 9 peritoneal disseminations, 9 bone and multiple metastases, and 4 other malignancies [12–15]. We have found PET to be of limited value and have not incorporated it into our routine preoperative work-up.

Laparoscopy

Once gross metastatic disease and vascular encroachment have been excluded, laparoscopy is able to save up to 35% of patients a laparotomy [16,17]. Retrospective reviews at MSKCC and Massachusetts General Hospital (MGH) demonstrated that 10–34% of patients deemed resectable by preoperative evaluation were found to have occult advanced disease on laparoscopy [18,19].

Preoperative Preparation

The majority of patients with pancreatic head adenocarcinoma will present with jaundice and weight loss. Metabolic derangements need to be corrected. Preoperative nutritional support is of limited value despite the inanition seen in these patients. We do not routinely preoperatively biopsy pancreatic lesions. However, both CT-guided or EUS-guided biopsy procedures can be performed if a preoperative diagnosis is necessary and would change management. Patients are given a limited bowel preparation and a single dose of preoperative intravenous antibiotics. A second-generation cephalosporin such as cefotetan, or newer combinations such as piperacillin/tazobactam provide appropriate coverage for the most common organisms contaminating bile, which are the primary source of intra-abdominal and wound infections [20].

Preoperative Biliary Drainage

Approximately 70% of patients present with jaundice. Preoperative biliary drainage should be avoided in potentially resectable patients if their operation is imminent, due to the significant increase in complications following stent placement. Preoperative biliary drainage has been shown to significantly increase the rate of infectious complications, intra-abdominal abscesses, and postoperative deaths [21–23]. Biliary drainage, however, does play an important role in patients who are unresectable and in symptomatic patients whose resection must be delayed.

Rationale for Surgical Treatment

Surgical resection provides the only potential cure for patients with pancreatic adenocarcinoma. The primary goal is an R0 resection. On multivariate analyses from numerous high-volume institutions, a negative margin is consistently a significant predictor of overall survival [24]. However, for the resected patient the current American Joint Committee on Cancer (AJCC)/TNM staging system is relatively nondiscriminatory in its attempt to predict patient survival. Therefore, we have created a pancreatic adenocarcinoma nomogram using the MSKCC prospective database [25]. The nomogram, which combines individual clinicopathological and operative data to predict survival at 1, 2, and 3 years from initial resection, is able to provide more accurate survival predictions than the AJCC staging system. This nomogram has recently been validated using another institutional-based series [26].

Indications and Contraindications

Any symptomatic or suspicious pancreatic lesion should be resected. As discussed previously, metastatic disease and arterial encroachment are contraindications to surgical resection and need to be ruled out prior to taking the patient to the operating room. As a significant proportion of patients with pancreatic adenocarcinoma are elderly, medical comorbidities need to be considered. We have shown, however, that pancreatic resections in 138 selected patients over the age of 70 years did not have a significantly increased morbidity or mortality rate when compared to younger patients [27].

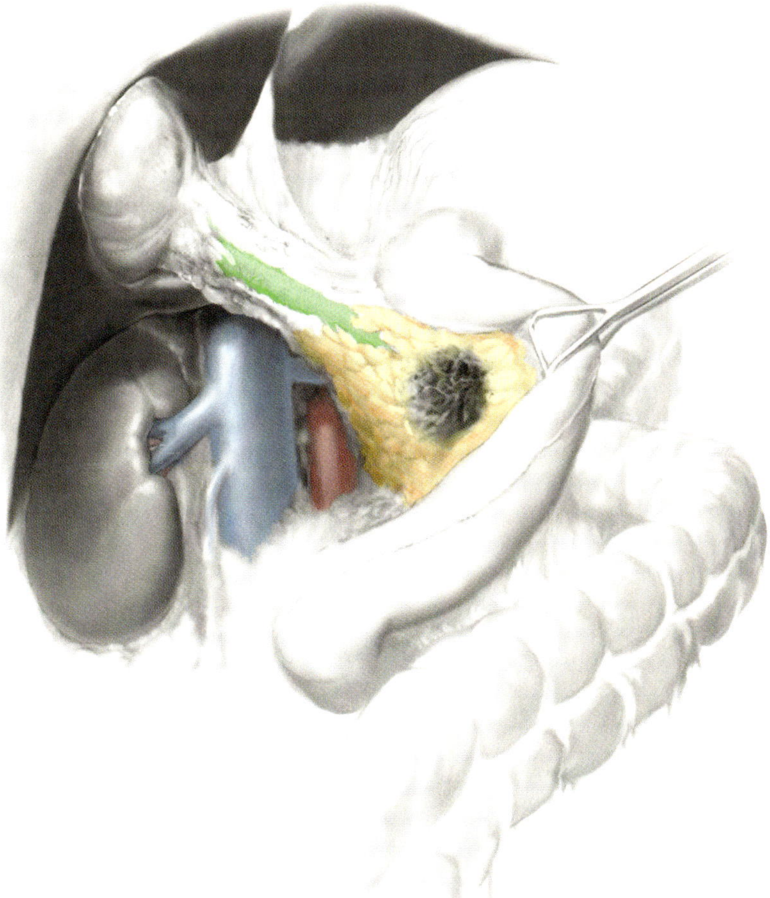

Figure 51.1
The colon is mobilized from the right upper quadrant and the pancreas is elevated. The duodenum can be retracted by the hand of the assistant or using a soft noncrushing clamp

Operative Approach

Diagnostic laparoscopy is performed by placing a supraumbilical 10-mm camera port via a vertical incision. Washings can be performed via a 5-mm port placed subcostally in the right upper quadrant. Once metastatic disease and transverse mesocolon invasion has been ruled out, a vertical upper-midline incision or a bilateral subcostal incision can be performed. A recent meta-analysis comparing vertical incisions with transverse incisions demonstrated that patients have less postoperative pain and fewer pulmonary complications with transverse incisions. A vertical incision, however, is associated with a shorter operative time, less muscular division, and better possibilities for extension of the incision [28]. The abdomen is carefully entered, the liver is palpated, and absence of invasion of the transverse mesocolon is confirmed. Our approach to determine resectability begins by mobilizing the right colon from the right upper quadrant (Fig. 51.1). The retroperitoneal tissues are then incised and the right renal vein is identified at its confluence with the inferior vena cava (IVC; Fig. 51.2). The IVC is then dissected free of all tissue preserving the gonadal vessels. The third and fourth part of the duodenum is reflected and the pancreas elevated so that a hand can be passed behind the pancreas to palpate the tumor mass. This maneuver can usually determine whether there is extension posteriorly to the side of the SMA. If extension of tumor from the head of the pancreas to the SMA is encountered, mesenteric vein or PV involvement is likely. Certainly, gross invasion or adherence by palpation of the SMA would result in termination of the procedure; however, this is rarely found given adequate preoperative imaging.

Once the artery is deemed to be free of tumor, the omentum is elevated and the lesser sac is entered. The omentum is detached from the colon and the inferior border of the pancreas is identified. The anterior surface of the SMV is identified, the right gastroepiploic

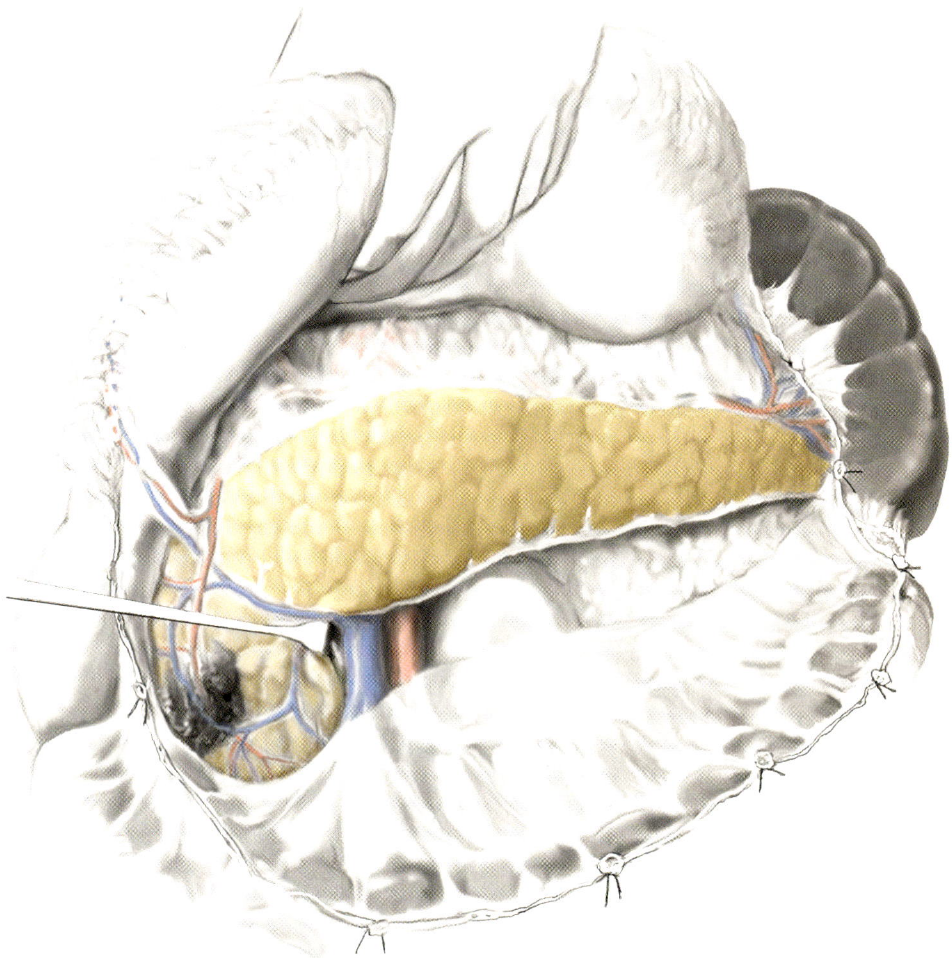

Figure 51.2

The greater omentum is detached from the colon in an avascular plane with the use of the cautery. The base of the mesocolon, at the inferior border of the pancreas, is incised to identify the anterior and right border of the superior mesenteric vein (SMV), displacing the uncinate upwards and to the right

vein is divided, and the anterior branch of the inferior pancreaticoduodenal vein is ligated just below the pancreas (Fig. 51.2). The latter vessel should be ligated, as tension on this vessel can result in bothersome bleeding. The middle colic vessels draining into the SMV should be carefully preserved unless tethered or involved with a low-lying tumor. However, the middle colic vein can usually be divided with impunity. The presence of any significant varices in the omentum or colonic varices should raise concern as to PV or SMV obstruction.

The pancreas is now elevated off of the anterior surface of the SMV to determine whether or not there is adherence. Since this is essentially an avascular plane, bleeding presupposes firm tethering by the tumor to the posterior or right side of the SMV-splenic vein confluence. If this dissection is free, attention is turned to the superior border of the pancreas. Careful dissection of the pancreas off of the PV is performed and the superior and inferior openings are connected with a large Kelley clamp.

Attention is now turned to the hepatic artery (HA), where there are commonly enlarged, often inflammatory nodes that need to be carefully dissected free to avoid bothersome hemorrhage. The magnitude of the common HA pulse is carefully examined to avoid missing a median arcuate ligament syndrome or aberrant/accessory hepatic arterial supply. The gastroduodenal artery (GDA) is now identified and if there is no adherence or encasement of the common HA, it is doubly ligated and divided. Prior to formal division and ligation of the GDA, temporary occlusion and pal-

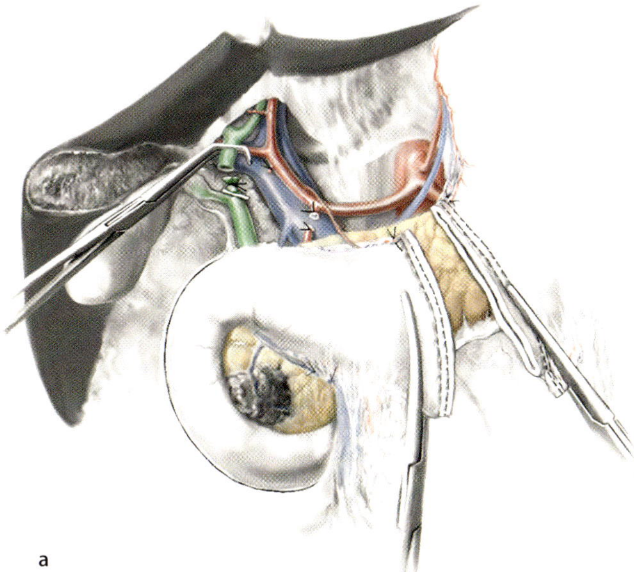

a

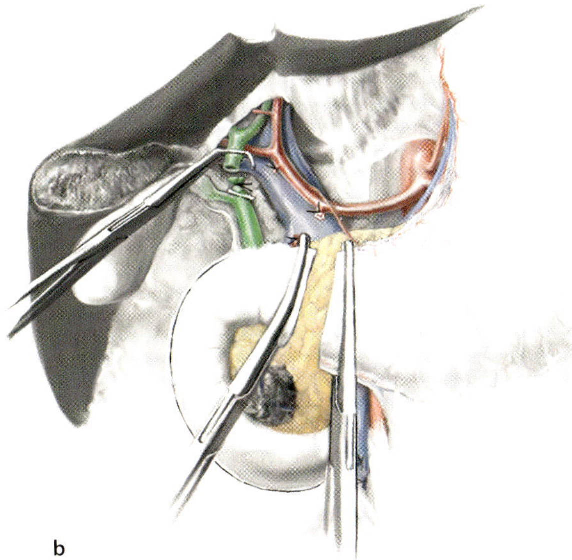

b

Figure 51.3

The bile duct is divided below a pediatric Satinsky clamp. The distal bile duct is suture ligated or closed with a hemostatic clip. The stomach is divided with Kocher clamps and a stapler leaving the proximal clamp for the site of anastomosis. a Standard Whipple. b Pylorus preservation

pation of the distal common HA ensures no retrograde flow from the SMA to the HA. The PV at the superior aspect of the pancreas can now be dissected free.

We now turn our attention to the ligament of Treitz, but it is also perfectly acceptable to mobilize the gallbladder at this point. We prefer to do this later in the procedure because ligation of the cystic artery has the theoretical prospect of devascularizing the gallbladder and allowing the potential for infected bile to leak through the ischemic gallbladder wall. Mobilization of the ligament of Treitz is performed as far behind the mesenteric vessels as possible, while identifying the inferior mesenteric vein. Small branches of the jejunal vascular arcade of the most proximal part of the jejunum are then ligated and divided using hemoclips, or alternatively the Ligasure can be used. The bowel is transected with a gastrointestinal (GI) stapler. The free duodenum and very proximal jejunum are then carefully passed behind the mesenteric vessels.

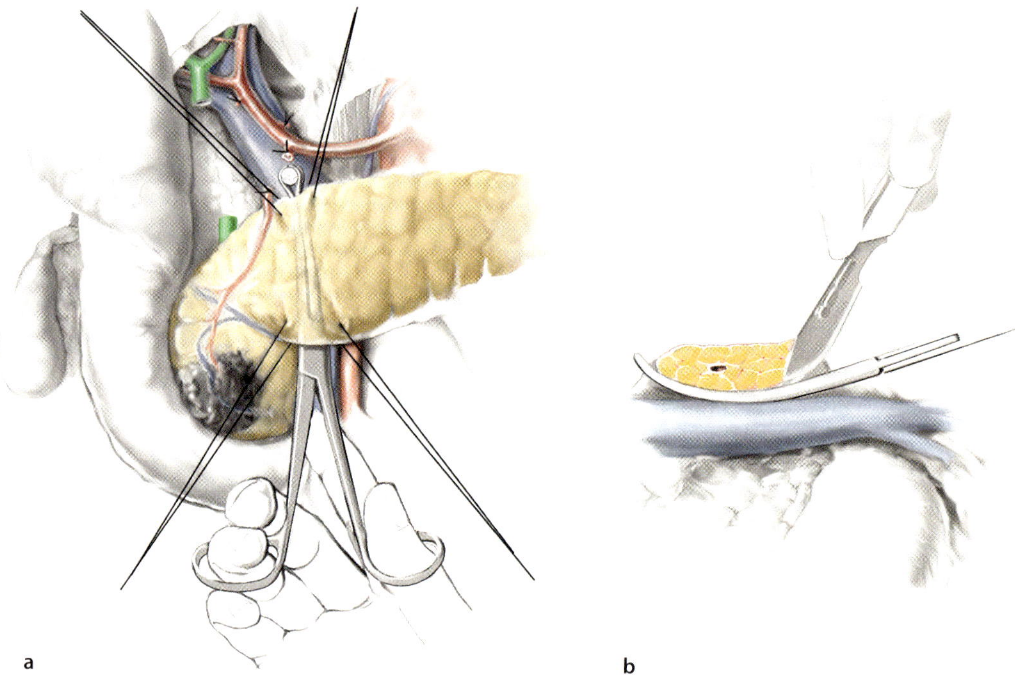

Figure 51.4

a Stay sutures in the inferior and superior border of the pancreas prevent hemorrhage when dividing the pancreas sharply. b We prefer to use a knife to divide the pancreas so as to have a clearly divided pancreatic mucosal division for subsequent anastomosis. A Kocher grooved director prevents injury to the portal vein

Attention is now directed to the stomach. The decision of whether to perform a pylorus-sparing operation needs to be made. Tran et al. prospectively randomized 170 patients to pylorus-preserving pancreaticoduodenectomy versus standard Whipple and found no significant difference in delayed gastric emptying, weight loss, operative time, or overall survival [29]. If the standard pancreaticoduodenectomy is performed, the greater omentum is completely divided to the border of the stomach. The stomach is then isolated, curved and straight Kocher clamps are placed at the site of the future gastrojejunal anastomosis, with the remaining stomach being divided by a GI stapler. The exposed staple line, which will not be utilized for the anastomosis, can be oversewn. The divided stomach is now reflected to the patient's right and the common hepatic duct is divided just above the entrance of the cystic duct (Fig. 51.3a, b). The common hepatic duct should be divided in the upper third where the blood supply from the right or common HA is better than in the middle third of the bile duct, which is a watershed area. A bile culture should be performed at the time of transection, especially if the patient has had a biliary stent in place. A frozen section of the duct margin is performed if patients are suspected of having a distal bile duct carcinoma. Prior to dividing the common bile duct, the most common arterial anomaly, a replaced right HA, needs to be ruled out. The lateral border of the common hepatic duct is now dissected free, with removal of the adjacent tissue and lymph nodes en bloc with the specimen.

Four stay sutures are placed at the inferior and superior border of the pancreatic neck to minimize hemorrhage (Fig. 51.4a). A Kocher grooved director is placed below the neck of the pancreas and a knife is used to divide the pancreas between the two sets of stay sutures (Fig. 51.4b). A suture is placed in the divided pancreatic duct on the specimen side, due to the theoretical possibility of contamination of the peritoneum with malignant cells.

The uncinate process remains as the only attachment. It is reflected from behind the SMV and is carefully dissected off of the right side and posterior aspect of the PV. This dissection is often easier if it is commenced from above, with careful attention to the origin of the SMA. The dissection plane along the right side of the SMA clears the artery and gives good exposure of the posterior PV. If the tumor is adherent to the PV, a resection may need to be performed. The specimen is now removed.

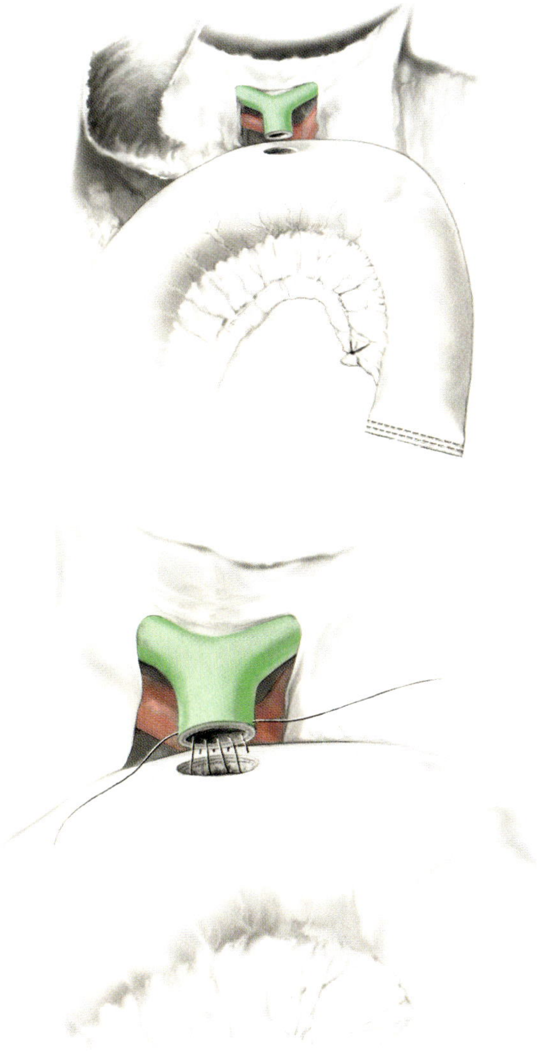

Figure 51.5

An end-to-side choledochojejunal anastomosis is performed first using a running 4-0 monofilament absorbable suture. We prefer a small mucosal incision and a larger serosal incision. If the bile duct is not dilated, interrupted sutures may be easier and more appropriate

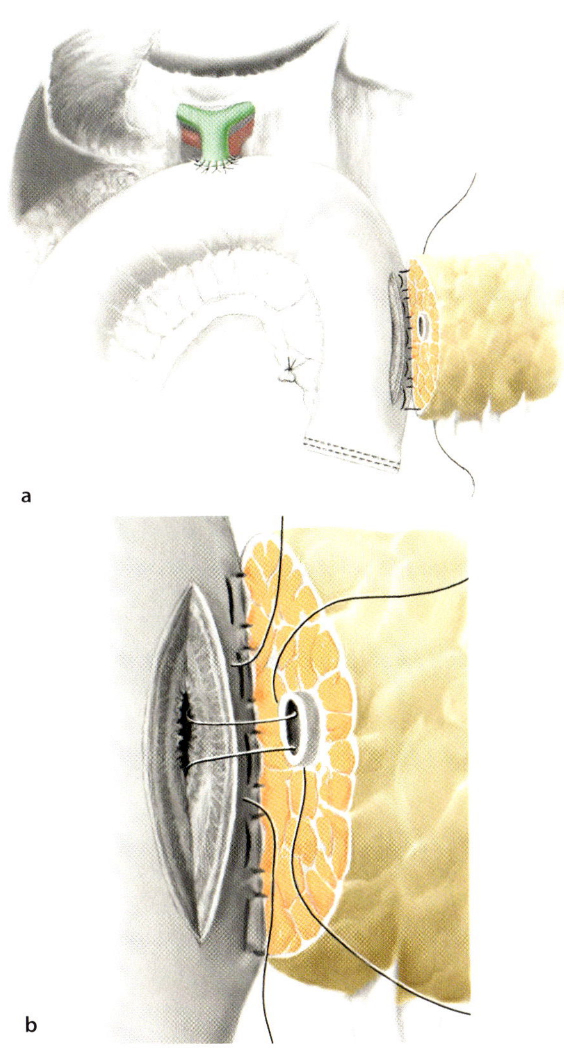

Figure 51.6

a The pancreatic anastomosis involves an anterior and posterior running 4-0 polydiaxonone suture (b), and even the smallest duct can usually accommodate four interrupted sutures at 12, 3, 6, and 9 o'clock

Reconstruction

For the standard pancreaticoduodenectomy the reconstruction begins with an end-to-side choledochojejunal anastomosis (Fig. 51.5). This is performed with a running 4-0 absorbable monofilament such as polydiaxonone suture (PDS). Using a pediatric Satinsky clamp the duct is held as an affixation stitch is placed in the left corner. An incision is made in the serosa, and a smaller one in the mucosa of the small bowel. A running posterior layer is designed to prolapse the mucosa of the bowel into the bile duct. For this, a greater "bite" is taken on the serosa of the bowel and the bile duct wall, than the mucosa of the bowel. The anterior layer is performed in a similar or direct over and over fashion, ensuring a patent noncicatricial anastomosis. The knots must approximate the tissue, but not so tight as to cut through the bile duct and produce a leak. In very small bile duct anastomoses, it is easier to place four or five interrupted sutures under direct vision, tying them after the posterior stitches have been placed.

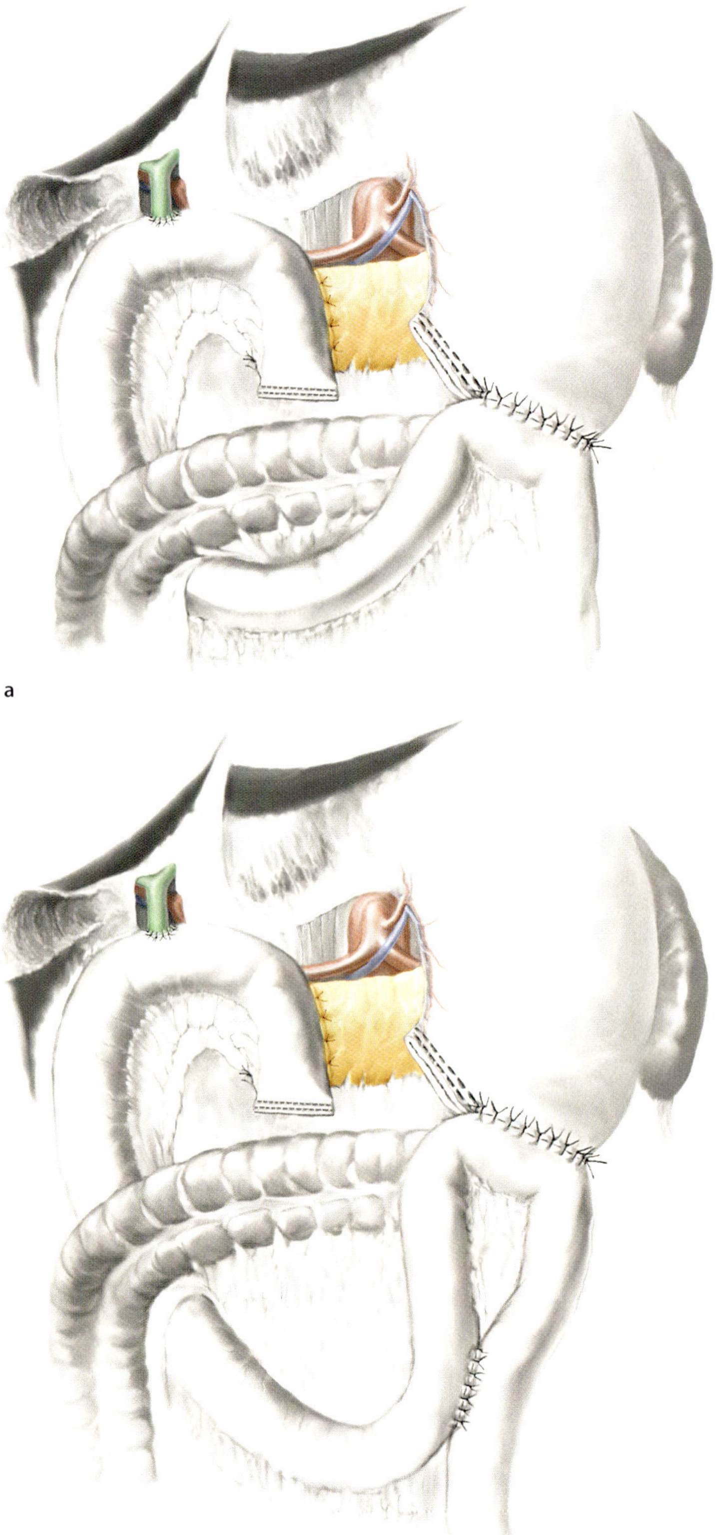

a

b

Figure 51.7

a The completed reconstruction. b Additionally side-to-side anastomosis (Braun´s) of the jejunum

A direct mucosa-to-mucosa anastomosis of the pancreatic duct to the sidewall of the jejunum is similarly made (Fig. 51.6). A posterior layer of running or interrupted 4-0 PDS sutures is placed to invaginate part of the posterior aspect of the pancreas into the sidewall of the jejunum. The serosa is then scored on the jejunum and a single posterior duct to mucosa stitch with 5-0 monofilament suture is placed. A small incision is then made in the mucosa and an interrupted 5-0 duct-to-mucosa anastomosis is completed. Similarly, anterior running or interrupted 4-0 PDS sutures are placed to invaginate the anterior pancreatic capsule into the sidewall of the jejunum. We rarely employ stents.

A standard antecolic gastrojejunostomy or duodenojejunostomy is created using a running 3-0 PDS suture. This anastomosis should be placed approximately 40 cm from the choledochojejunostomy to prevent reflux of food and acid into the liver (Fig. 51.7). The abdominal wall is now closed using two no. 1 PDS sutures and staples are applied to the skin.

Variations in Procedure

Dissection of the Mesenteric Vein from the Right

In mobilizing the third part of the duodenum, it may be easier to continue mobilizing the inferior border of the duodenum to the sidewall of the SMV, and mobilizing the uncinate process early in the procedure.

Early Division of the Common Bile Duct

Many surgeons will perform a biliary bypass regardless of whether the lesion is resectable. This allows for early division of the common bile duct, with excellent access to the suprapancreatic portion of the PV. This approach should also be considered in cases where there is concern for tumor adherence to the PV above the splenic vein confluence, or in cases where the dissection of the PV is difficult.

Frozen Section Biopsy Sampling of the Pancreas

Some surgeons advocate intraoperative biopsy sampling, in the absence of a preoperative diagnosis. We do not advocate this, since the decision for resection should be based predominantly on the preoperative and intraoperative clinical findings. However, it is important to emphasize to the patient and their family preoperatively that there is a possibility of the final diagnosis being benign.

Frozen section of the transected pancreatic margin should only be performed if the surgeon plans to act on the information. If the caliber or appearance of the duct of the transected pancreas is of concern, and a positive biopsy specimen would result in a further 1- to 3-cm resection of the pancreas with a similar reconstruction, then it should be considered. However, if there is concern for multifocal disease and total pancreatectomy would not be considered, frozen section becomes redundant. In addition, a positive posterior pancreatic margin is more common than a positive dissection margin.

Variations in Reconstruction

The Choledochojejunal Anastomosis

Significant debate revolves around suture material and technique: running continuous or interrupted sutures, use of stents, and the need for Roux-en-Y diversion. The authors are comfortable with a continuous running monofilament 4-0 PDS suture, and prefer not to use a stent. If an interrupted technique is used, we recommend starting with a posterior (12 o'clock) stitch then sutures at the 3 o'clock and 9 o'clock position to splay open the bile duct. Interrupted stitches are then placed through the wall of the bile duct and the full thickness of the jejunum, again taking care to incorporate the mucosa. The sutures are held on tags until the entire posterior row is complete and then tied down sequentially. The posterior sutures can be placed so that the knots are tied outside the biliary-jejunal lumen. The anterior row of sutures is now placed in the same fashion and tied down sequentially.

The Pancreatic Anastomosis

The pancreas can be directly invaginated into the jejunum. An end-to-end pancreaticojejunal invagination is usually performed by tailoring the pancreatic remnant to the sides of the small intestine (Fig. 51.8a). An interrupted posterior layer of absorbable or nonabsorbable sutures is placed between the posterior pancreas and the seromuscular layer of the jejunum. These sutures are placed circumferentially so that the end of the jejunum is sewn to the transected pancreas. An anterior outer layer is then placed to further insert the pancreas into the jejunum. Pancreaticogastrostomy can be performed in place of a pancreaticojejunostomy with no significant difference in outcome in terms of morbidity and mortality (Fig. 51.8b).

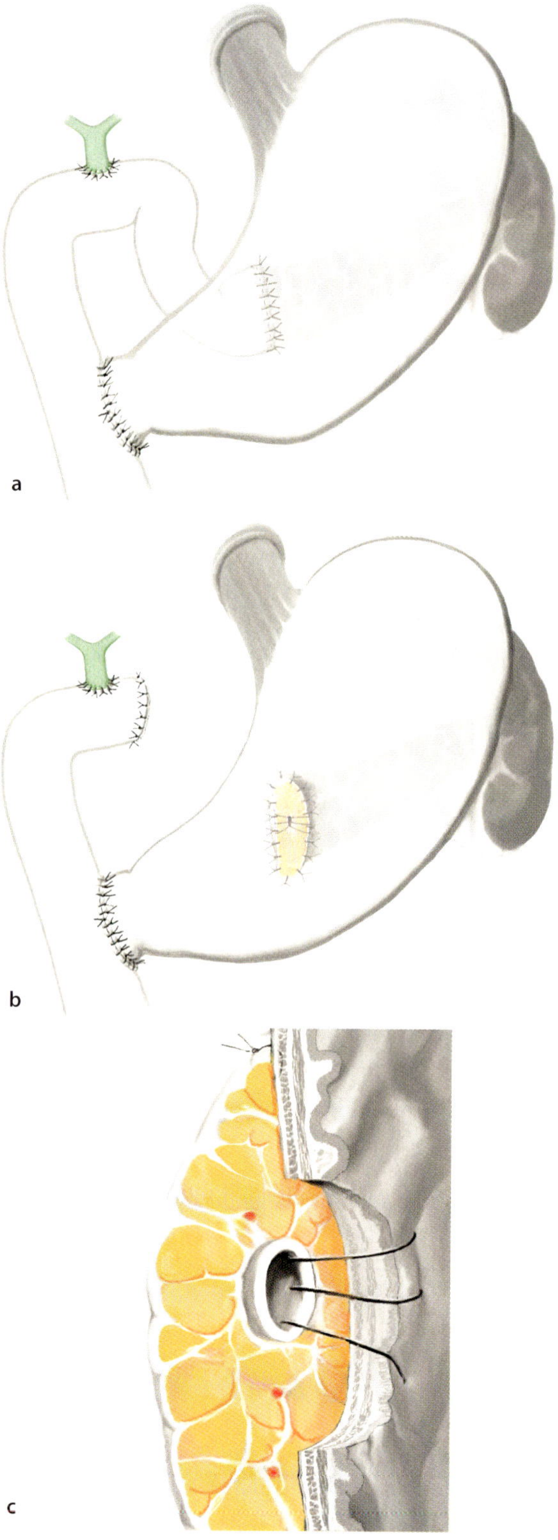

Figure 51.8

a End-to-end pancreaticojejunostomy. b Pancreaticogastrostomy. c Inner layer pancreatico-gastrostomosis

Reconstruction of Gastrointestinal Continuity

An important alternative to the approach outlined above is a Roux-en-Y reconstruction separating the gastric from the pancreatic and biliary anastomosis. Although some authors believe a pancreatic fistula would be easier to manage with a Roux-en-Y reconstruction, there is no good data to support this.

PV Resection

Major PV involvement usually indicates arterial encroachment and an unresectable tumor. However, all surgeons should be familiar with the technique for resecting the PV for those situations in which unanticipated adherence makes dissection of the right side of the PV difficult and unsafe. At least 2 cm and occasionally 3 cm of PV/SMV can be resected and an end-to-end anastomosis can be performed (Fig. 51.9a, b). If the site of attachment is below the splenic vein, a wedge resection can be performed with an end-to-end SMV reconstruction (Fig. 51.9c). With extension or invasion beyond the first jejunal branch, it is rarely, if ever, possible to safely resect the SMV. Ligation of the splenic vein and elevation of the small bowel is often required in order to obtain enough mobilization for a tension-free anastomosis. The vessels are clamped with pediatric vascular clamps and a running anastomosis with 4-0 Prolene suture is performed, with the final knot being tied over a nerve hook to allow for adequate expansion.

Postoperative Course

The median length of stay at MSKCC for the 472 patients resected between 1983 and 2000 was 14 days. However, in 2004 it was 10 days. The standard patient will be transferred to the floor after 4 h in the recovery room. The nasogastric tube is removed on the morning of postoperative day 1. If the patient appears to be clinically stable, clears can be started on postoperative day 3, followed by slow advancement to regular small meal feedings. In two randomized controlled studies performed at MSKCC, neither early postoperative total parenteral nutrition (TPN) nor enteral feeding was of any benefit [30,31]. The patients who received TPN actually had a higher incidence of complications, mainly related to infection.

The patients' blood glucose should be checked routinely to ensure there is no surgically induced diabetes. We do not routinely treat patients with antibiotics postoperatively; however, if the patient does develop a fever, thus necessitating antibiotics, we treat with an-

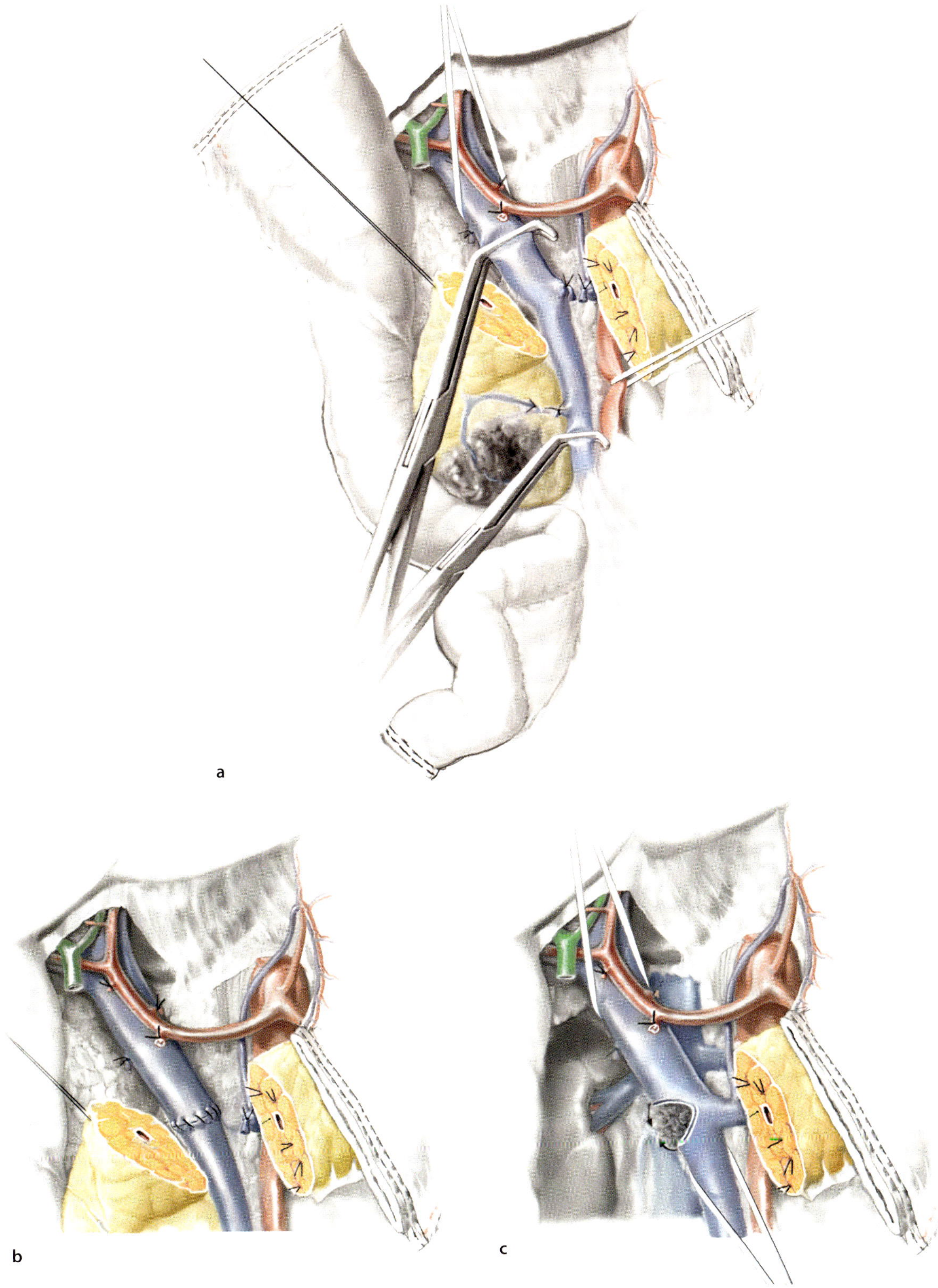

Figure 51.9

Portal vein reconstruction. If tumor involves 2–3 cm of the SMV, the portal vein, SMV, and splenoportal junction are dissected. a The splenic vein is ligated and divided at the splenoportal junction. Vascular clamps are placed proximally and distally. b Primary anastomosis of the veins using a running 4-0 or 5-0 Prolene suture is performed. c If the site of attachment is limited, a wedge resection with transverse closure ensures an adequate lumen tibiotics that are appropriate for the organisms in the bile culture that was obtained intraoperatively. The patient should also be maintained on ulcer prophylaxis to prevent the development of a marginal ulcer at the gastrojejunostomy site.

We do not routinely place intraoperative drains. In a randomized controlled trial at MSKCC, intraoperative drains did not demonstrate a decrease in morbidity and mortality [32]. However, if closed suction drains were placed intraoperatively, they can be removed once the drainage has significantly decreased to <30 ml/day and is not bilious. If drain output remains high and is not bilious, but the fluid amylase is low, the drain can be removed since the fluid is most likely serous and not a biliary or pancreatic leak.

Postoperative Complications and Short-Term Outcome

The patient, and where appropriate their family, need to have an understanding of the operation and its associated morbidity and mortality. Morbidity rates in the literature range from 21 to 44%, with the most prevalent complications including delayed gastric emptying, pancreatic fistulas/wound infections, and bleeding. The majority of intra-abdominal infections are due to an anastomotic leak or a contamination at the time of operation from a previously instrumented bile duct [8,33–35]. The majority of intra-abdominal collections can be drained percutaneously. However, if percutaneous drainage does not rapidly resolve the systemic effects of infection, reoperation must be considered. Older patients (>75 years) did not have a significantly increased mortality, but were more likely to require a stay in an intensive care unit, suffer a cardiac complication, and experience a compromised nutritional and functional status after major pancreatic resection [36]. At MSKCC the 30-day mortality of the 472 patients who underwent pancreaticoduodenectomy for pancreatic head adenocarcinoma between October 1983 and April 2000 was 2.8%.

Long-Term Outcome

The long-term outcome is determined largely by the pathology within the resected specimen. The 5-year survival for patients with a resected pancreatic adenocarcinoma ranges from 10 to 25% [35,37,38]. The actual 5-year survival for those resected at MSKCC is 11%, with 50% of them succumbing to pancreatic adenocarcinoma after 5 years [37].

References

1. Whipple AO, Parson WB, Mullins CR (1935) Treatment of carcinoma of the ampulla of Vater. Ann Surg 102:763–779
2. Whipple AO (1963) A reminiscence: pancreaticoduodenectomy. Rev Surg 20:221–225
3. Auve L (1908) Des pancreatectomies et specialement de la pancréatectomie céphalique. Rev Chir 37:335–385
4. Kausch W (1912) Das carcinom der papilla duodeni und seine radikale Entfernung. Beitr Z Clin Chir 78:439–486
5. Fortner JG (1973) Regional resection and pancreatic carcinoma. Surgery 73:799–800
6. Pedrazzoli S, DiCarlo V, Dionigi R, Mosca F, Pederzoli P, Pasquali C, Kloppel G, Dhaene K, Michelassi F (1998) Standard versus extended lymphadenectomy associated with pancreatoduodenectomy in the surgical treatment of adenocarcinoma of the head of the pancreas: a multicenter, prospective, randomized study. Lymphadenectomy Study Group. Ann Surg 228:508–517
7. Harrison LE, Klimstra DS, Brennan MF (1996) Isolated portal vein involvement in pancreatic adenocarcinoma. A contraindication for resection? Ann Surg 224:342–347; discussion 347–349
8. Tseng JF, Raut CP, Lee JE, Pisters PWT, Vauthey J, Abdalla EK, Gomez HF, Sun CC, Crane CH, Wolff RA, Evans DB (2004) Pancreaticoduodenectomy with vascular resection: margin status and survival duration. J Gastrointest Surg 8:935–950
9. Gress FG, Hawes RH, Savides TJ, Ikenberry SO, Cummings O, Kopecky K, Sherman S, Wierseman M, Lehman GA (1999) Role of EUS in the preoperative staging of pancreatic cancer: a large single-center experience. Gastrointest Endosc 50:786–791
10. Maluf-Filho F, Sakai P, Cunha JE, Garrido T, Rocha M, Machado MC, Ishioka S (2004) Radial endoscopic ultrasound and spiral computed tomography in the diagnosis and staging of periampullary tumors. Pancreatology 4:122–128
11. Bhutani MS, Gress FG, Giovannini M, Erikson RA, Catalano MF, Chak A, Deprez PH, Faigel DO, Nguyen CC (2004) The No Endosonographic Detection of Tumor (NEST) Study: a case series of pancreatic cancers missed on endoscopic ultrasonography. Endoscopy 36:385–389
12. Higashi T, Saga T, Nakamoto Y, Ishimori T, Fujimoto K, Doi R, Imamura M, Konishi J (2003) Diagnosis of pancreatic cancer using fluorine-18 fluorodeoxyglucose positron emission tomography (FDG PET) – usefulness and limitations in "clinical reality". Ann Nucl Med 17:261–279
13. Delbeke D, Rose DM, Chapman WC, et al (1999) Optimal interpretation of FDG-PET in the diagnosis, staging, and management of pancreatic carcinoma. J Nucl Med 40:1784–1791
14. Koyama K, Okamura T, Kawabe J, Nakata B, Chung KH, Ochi H, et al (2001) Diagnostic usefulness of FDG PET for pancreatic mass lesions. Ann Nucl Med 15:217–224
15. Mertz HR, Sechopoulos P, Delbeke D, Leach SD (2000) EUS, PET, and CT scanning for evaluation of pancreatic adenocarcinoma. Gastrointest Endosc 52:367–371
16. Mire F, Sauvanet A, Trivin F, Hammel P, O'Toole D, Palazzo L, Vilgrain V, Belghiti J, Ruszniewski P, Levy P (2004) Staging of pancreatic head adenocarcinoma with spiral CT and endoscopic ultrasonography: an indirect evaluation of the usefulness of laparoscopy. Pancreatology 4:436–440

17. Warshaw AL, Gu ZY, Wittenberg J, Waltman AC (1990) Preoperative staging and assessment of resectability of pancreatic cancer. Arch Surg 125:230–233
18. Merchant NB, Conlon KC (1998) Laparoscopic evaluation in pancreatic cancer. Semin Surg Oncol 15:155–165
19. Jimenez RE, Warshaw AL, Fernandez-Del Castillo C (2000) Laparoscopy and peritoneal cytology in the staging of pancreatic cancer. J Hepatobiliary Pancreat Surg 7:15–20
20. Povoski SP, Karpeh MS Jr, Conlon KC, Blumgart LH, Brennan MF (1999) Preoperative biliary drainage: impact on intraoperative bile cultures and infectious morbidity and mortality after pancreaticoduodenectomy. J Gastrointest Surg 3:496–505
21. Povoski SP, Karpeh MS, Conlon KC, Blumgart LH, Brennan MF (1999) Association of preoperative biliary drainage with postoperative outcome following pancreaticoduodenectomy. Ann Surg 230:131–142
22. Heslin MJ, Brooks AD, Hochwald SN, Harrison LE, Blumgart LH, Brennan MF (1998) A preoperative biliary stent is associated with increased complications after pancreatoduodenectomy. Arch Surg 133:149–154
23. Pisters PW, Hudec WA, Hess KR, Lee JE, Vauthey JN, Lahoti S, Raijman I, Evans DB (2001) Effect of preoperative biliary decompression on pancreaticoduodenectomy-associated morbidity in 300 consecutive patients. Ann Surg 234:47–55
24. Wagner M, Redaelli C, Lietz M, Seiler A, Friess H, Buechler MW (2004) Curative resection is the single most important factor determining outcome in patients with pancreatic adenocarcinoma. Br J Surg 91:586–594
25. Brennan MF, Kattan MW, Klimstra D, Conlon K (2004) Prognostic Nomogram for patients undergoing resection for adenocarcinoma of the pancreas. Ann Surg 240:293–298
26. Ferrone CR, Kattan MW, Thayer SP, Brennan MF, Warshaw AL (2005) Validation of post-resection pancreatic adenocarcinoma nomogram, for survival. J Clin Oncol 23:7529–7535
27. Fong Y, Blumgart LH, Fortner JG, Brennan MF (1995) Pancreatic or liver resection for malignancy is safe and effective for the elderly. Ann Surg 222:426–434; discussion 434–437
28. Grantcharov TP, Rosenberg J (2001) Vertical compared with transverse incisions in abdominal surgery. Eur J Surg 167:260–267
29. Tran KTC, Smeenk HG, van Eijck CHJ, Kazemier G, Hop WC, Greeve JWC, Terpstra OT, Zijlstra JA, Klinkert P, Jeekel H (2004) Pylorus preserving pancreaticoduodenectomy versus standard Whipple procedure. Ann Surg 240:738–745
30. Brennan MF, Pisters PW, Posner M, Quesada O, Shike M (1994) A prospective randomized trial of total parenteral nutrition after major pancreatic resection for malignancy. Ann Surg 220(4):436–441; discussion 441–444
31. Heslin MJ, Latkany L, Leung D, Brooks AD, Hochwald SN, Pisters PW, Shike M, Brennan MF (1997) A prospective, randomized trial of early enteral feeding after resection of upper gastrointestinal malignancy. Ann Surg 226:567–577; discussion 577–580
32. Conlon KC, Labow D, Leung D, Smith A, Jarnagin W, Coit DG, Merchant N, Brennan MF (2001) Prospective randomized clinical trial of the value of intraperitoneal drainage after pancreatic resection. Ann Surg 234;487–494
33. Yeo CJ, Cameron JL, Sohn TA, Lillemoe KD, Pitt HA, Talamini MA, Hruban RH, Ord SE, Sauter PK, Coleman J, Zahurak ML, Grochow LB, Abrams RA (1997) Six hundred fifty consecutive pancreaticoduodenectomies in the 1990s: pathology, complications, and outcomes. Ann Surg 226:248–260
34. Wagner M, Redaelli C, Lietz M, Seiler CA, Friess H, Buechler MW (2004) Curative resection is the single most important factor determining outcome in patients with pancreatic adenocarcinoma. Br J Surg 91:586–594
35. Richter A, Niedergethmann M, Sturm JW, Lorenz D, Post S, Trede M (2003) Long-term results of partial pancreaticoduodenectomy for ductal adenocarcinoma of the pancreatic head: 25 year experience. World J Surg 27:324–329
36. Lightner AM, Glasgow RE, Jordan TH, Krassner AD, Way LW, Mulvihill SJ, Kirkwood KS (2004) Pancreatic resection in the elderly. J Am Coll Surg 198:697–706
37. Conlon KC, Klimstra DS, Brennan MF (1996) Long-term survival after curative resection for pancreatic adenocarcinoma. Clinicopathologic analysis of 5-year survivors. Ann Surg 223:273–279
38. Fong Y, Blumgart LH, Fortner JG, et al (1995) Pancreatic or liver resection is safe and effective for the elderly. Ann Surg 222:426–434

Chapter 52

R. D. Schulick · J. L. Cameron

Pylorus-Preserving Pancreaticoduodenectomy

Surgical procedures to resect periampullary malignancies and benign processes have evolved over the last 100 years since Halsted from the Johns Hopkins Hospital reported the first successful resection of a periampullary cancer in 1899 [1]. He described a local ampullary resection with reanastomosis of the pancreatic and bile ducts into the duodenum for a woman who presented with obstructive jaundice. Codivilla is often credited with performing the first en bloc resection of the head of the pancreas along with the duodenum for periampullary carcinoma, but unfortunately, the patient did not survive the postoperative period [2]. The first successful two-stage pancreaticoduodenectomy (PD) was performed by Kausch in 1909 [3]. In 1914, Hirschel reported the first successful one-stage PD [4]. In the first third of the 20th century, most periampullary cancers that were operated on were managed by a transduodenal approach similar to that reported by Halsted. PD was not often considered as a viable option until 1935, with the report of Whipple and colleagues of three, two-stage, en bloc resections of the head of the pancreas and duodenum [5]. Over the next decade, several modifications and technical refinements were made in the operation. The procedure was rarely performed until the 1980s because of the high operative morbidity, mortality, and poor prognosis associated with periampullary malignancies. During the last three decades there have been significant advances in terms of our ability to diagnose and care for the family of diseases treated with PD, as well as an increased understanding of their pathogeneses.

Historical Rationale for Pylorus Preservation

For many years, the standard or classic PD (CPD) described by Kausch and Whipple, in which the antrum of the stomach is resected in addition to the head of the pancreas, duodenum, distal bile duct, and gallbladder, was the most commonly employed procedure. In an attempt to decrease the side effects related to antrectomy, which were thought to include postoperative weight loss, dumping, and marginal ulceration, Watson reported the first pylorus-preserving PD (PPPD) in 1944 [6]. The procedure was later championed and popularized by Traverso and Longmire [7]. The issues regarding the superiority of either CPD or PPPD can be grouped into differences in their oncologic scope (i.e., survival results), the difference in time and resources required to perform each (i.e., operative time and transfusion requirements), and the differences in postoperative complications (i.e., delayed gastric emptying, weight loss, marginal ulceration, and dumping).

Indications and Contraindications for PPPD

The indications for PD in general include the need to remove the head of the pancreas, duodenum, distal bile duct, and gallbladder (if present) for:

1. A mass in the head of the pancreas, distal bile duct, ampulla, or periampullary duodenum that is symptomatic or has the potential to be neoplastic and/or malignant.
2. A cystic process in the head of the pancreas that is symptomatic or has the potential to be or become malignant.
3. An inflammatory mass in the head of the pancreas that is symptomatic and refractory to medical management.
4. Severe trauma to the head of the pancreas or periampullary region.

In many cases, a precise preoperative diagnosis is not made and patients are taken to the operating room without biopsy, as this will not alter the decision to operate. The decision to perform either a CPD or PPPD is finalized in the operating room depending on the operative findings.

Contraindications to PPPD include:

1. Encroachment of a neoplastic process onto the duodenum, pylorus, or antrum.
2. Surgical absence of the pylorus or antrum.
3. Involvement of the duodenal bulb, pylorus, or antrum by ulcer disease or inflammatory process.
4. Ischemia of the remnant duodenum after resection of the PPPD specimen.

Surgical Technique of PPPD

The use of staging laparoscopy for lesions that are potentially malignant is controversial. In some centers, staging laparoscopy is always performed with the belief that it will save a significant number of patients the morbidity and mortality of exploratory laparotomy only to find metastatic or locally unresectable disease [8]. In general, the surgeons in these centers believe that if a patient is not resected for potential cure, they are best palliated by nonoperative means. In other centers, staging laparoscopy is not routinely used because of the belief that current cross-sectional imaging studies are so sensitive and specific and that it does not make sense to subject all patients to laparoscopy to pick up the few who have unresectable disease. In addition, some surgeons argue that as many as 20% of the unresectable patients with malignancy will eventually develop gastric outlet obstruction requiring surgical intervention, and the ability to perform a hepaticojejunostomy will more durably relieve obstructive jaundice [9]. Furthermore, an operative chemical splanchnicectomy can be performed at the same time to alleviate the pain caused by celiac involvement. In some centers, surgeons selectively use staging laparoscopy focusing on the subgroups of patients at highest risk of being unresectable [10]. For example, patients with adenocarcinoma involving the body or tail of the pancreas are more likely to have unresectable disease at the time of presentation because these lesions do not cause obstructive jaundice and are usually larger and more advanced at the time of diagnosis. Patients with periampullary duodenal, ampullary, and distal common bile duct adenocarcinoma are much more likely to be resectable because they often present with obstructive jaundice earlier in the course of their disease.

Exposure for a PD is obtained with either a vertical midline incision from the xiphoid process to just below the umbilicus, or a bilateral subcostal incision (Fig. 52.1). Exposure is greatly enhanced with the use of a mechanical retracting device.

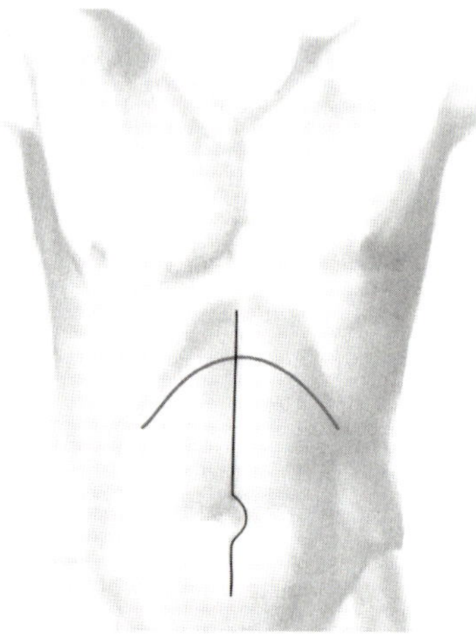

Figure 52.1

Upper midline or bilateral subcostal incisions for pancreaticoduodenectomy

The first portion of a PD is devoted to assessing the extent of disease as well as resectability. At open exploration, the entire liver is assessed for the presence of metastases not seen by preoperative imaging studies both by inspection and palpation. Intraoperative ultrasound is not routinely used unless preoperative imaging suggests the possibility of intraparenchymal metastatic disease in the liver. The celiac axis is carefully palpated and inspected for lymph node involvement. Tumor-bearing nodes within the resection zone do not contraindicate resection because long-term survival is sometimes achieved with peripancreatic nodal involvement. The parietal and visceral peritoneal surfaces, the omentum, the ligament of Treitz, the entire small and intra-abdominal large intestine, and the transverse mesocolon are carefully inspected for the presence of metastatic disease. An extensive Kocher maneuver is performed by elevating the duodenum and head of the pancreas out of the retroperitoneum and into the midline, allowing the visualization of the superior mesenteric artery at its origin from the aorta (Fig. 52.2). If the gallbladder is present, it is mobilized out of the gallbladder fossa, the cystic artery divided, and the cystic duct mobilized to the junction with the common bile duct. The common hepatic artery and proper hepatic artery should also be assessed to determine that they are free of tumor involvement.

If the intraoperative assessment reveals localized disease without tumor encroachment upon resection margins, the resection is usually relatively straightforward. If assessment reveals evidence of local tumor extension, giving the early impression of possible un-

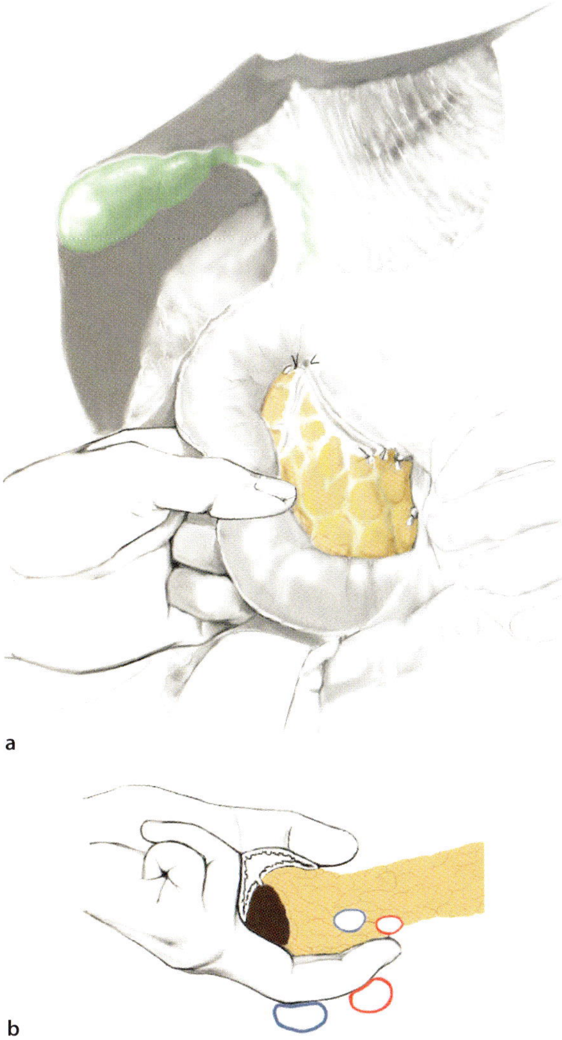

Figure 52.2

A Kocher maneuver will allow a periampullary mass to be fully palpated and will allow assessment of the location of the mass to the superior mesenteric artery and vein as well as the portal vein. *v.* Vein, *a.* artery

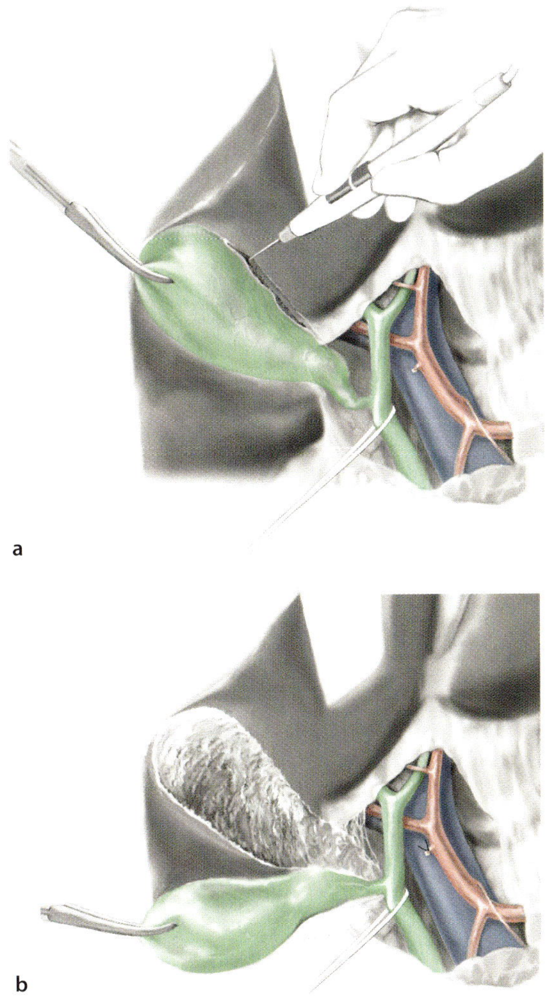

Figure 52.3

The gallbladder is mobilized off of the gallbladder fossa, the cystic artery is divided, and the common hepatic duct is divided

resectability, the sequence for performing the PD should be adjusted accordingly. The easiest and safest portions of the resection should be performed first, and the more difficult portions later. Tumors that initially appear unresectable are often successfully resected by patiently working where it is easiest first and finishing the more difficult portions later.

The distal common hepatic duct is divided close to the level of the cystic duct entry site early during the operation (Fig. 52.3). For distal common bile duct cancers or pancreatic cancers near this area, more margin on the bile duct into the hilus of the liver may be required. The bile duct is retracted caudally and a dissection plane is opened on the anterior surface of the portal vein. During these maneuvers, the portal structures should be assessed for a replaced right hepatic artery originating from the superior mesenteric artery. If found, this vessel should be dissected and protected from injury. If the patient appears to have an accessory right hepatic artery and a significant native right hepatic artery, the accessory vessel can often be taken without consequence. The gastroduodenal artery is next identified and clamped atraumatically. This maneuver confirms that the hepatic artery is not being supplied solely retrogradely through the superior mesenteric artery collaterals (in the setting of ce-

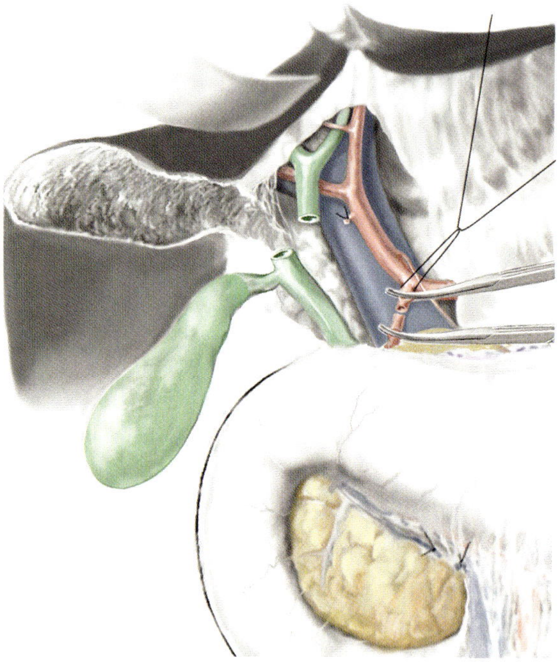

Figure 52.4

The gastroduodenal artery is divided after a confirmatory test clamp. *r.* Right

liac artery stenosis or occlusion). It also confirms that the structure is indeed the gastroduodenal artery and not the common hepatic artery coursing downwards. Once confirmed, the gastroduodenal artery is ligated (Fig. 52.4).

The superior mesenteric vein caudal to the neck of the pancreas can be identified by performing an extensive Kocher maneuver (Fig. 52.5). The superior mesenteric vein is identified running anterior to the third portion of the duodenum and is frequently surrounded by adipose tissue as it receives tributaries from the uncinate process and neck of the pancreas, the greater curve of the stomach, and from the transverse mesocolon. In this location, the superior mesenteric vein is identified by dissecting the fatty tissue of the transverse mesocolon away from the uncinate process of the pancreas. Division of the branches emptying into the anterior surface of the superior mesenteric vein allows continued cephalad dissection. Often a vein retractor lifting the inferior edge of the neck of the pancreas is useful for visualization. The plane anterior to the superior mesenteric vein is developed under direct vision, avoiding branches and tumor involvement. Care should be taken to avoid in-

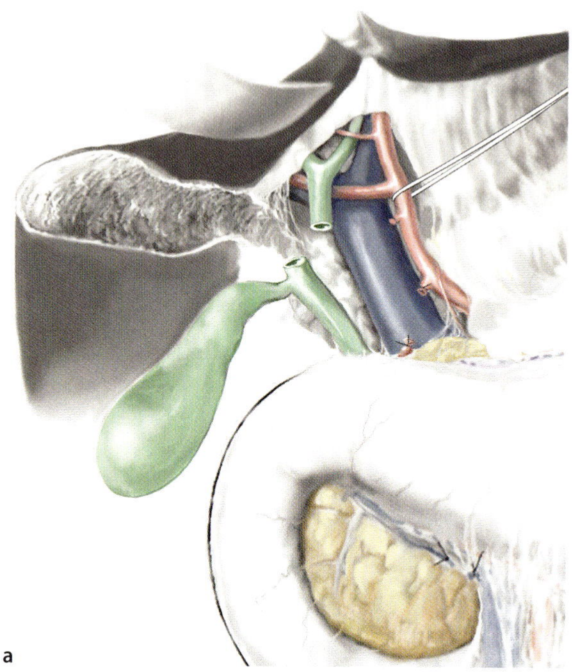

a

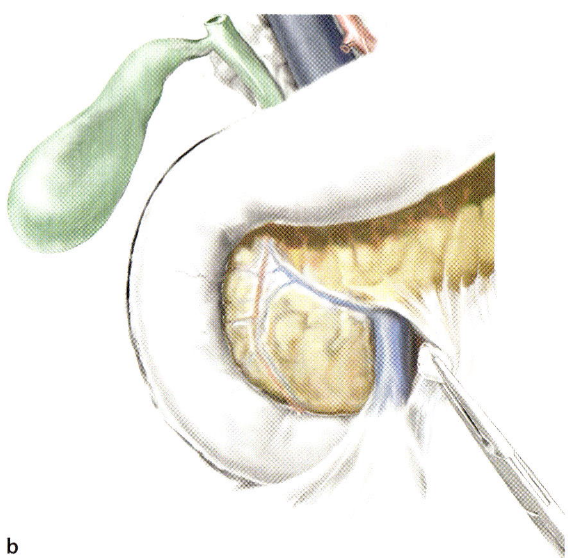

b

Figure 52.5

The plane between the portal vein and cephalad neck of the pancreas is begun from above (*left*). The plane between the superior mesenteric vein and caudal neck of the pancreas is begun from below (*right*)

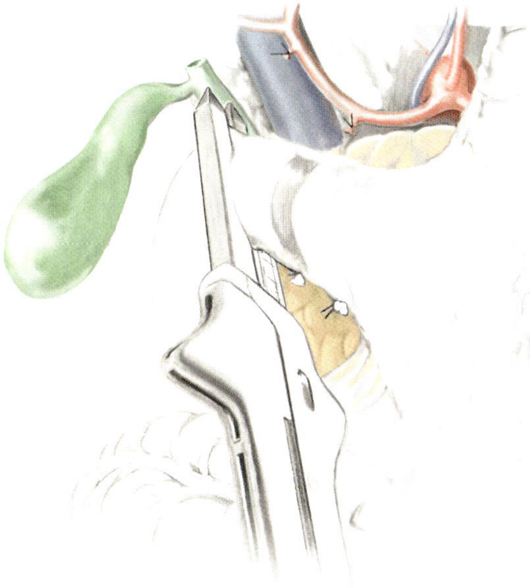

Figure 52.6

The duodenum is divided with a linear stapling device approximately 2–3 cm from the pylorus

advertent damage to the splenic vein as it joins the superior mesenteric vein posterior to the neck of the pancreas. After the plane anterior to the portal vein and superior mesenteric vein is complete, a Penrose drain is looped under the neck of the pancreas.

For a PPPD, the first and second portions of the duodenum are circumferentially dissected to free them from the tissues connecting them to the hepatoduodenal ligament and the pancreas. The duodenum is divided 2–3 cm distal to the pylorus with a linear stapling device (Fig. 52.6). The right gastric artery can often be spared, but may be taken if it allows better mobilization of the duodenum for reconstruction.

Stay sutures are place superiorly and inferiorly on the pancreatic remnant to reduce bleeding from the segmental pancreatic arteries running in those locations. The pancreatic neck is then divided after confirming a free plane anterior to the portal and superior mesenteric veins (Figs. 52.7 and 52.8). The Penrose drain previously placed behind the neck of the pancreas is used to elevate the pancreatic tissue to be divided and protect the underlying major veins. Some attention has been paid to the blood supply of the resection margin of the pancreatic remnant such that electrocautery should not be used to divide the pancreas [11]. The site of the main pancreatic duct should be noted so it can be incorporated into the subsequent reconstruction.

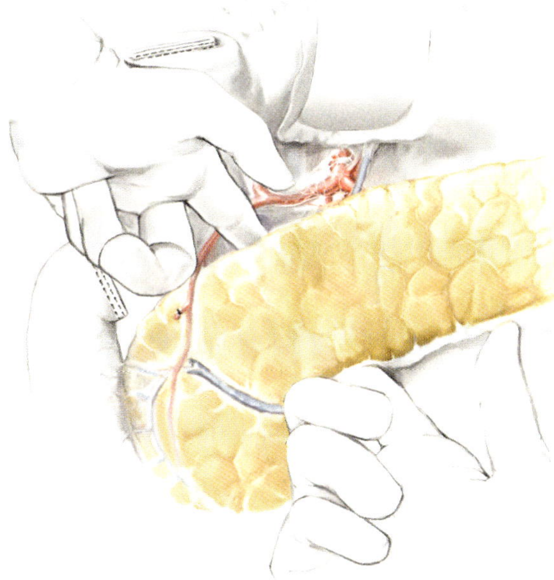

a

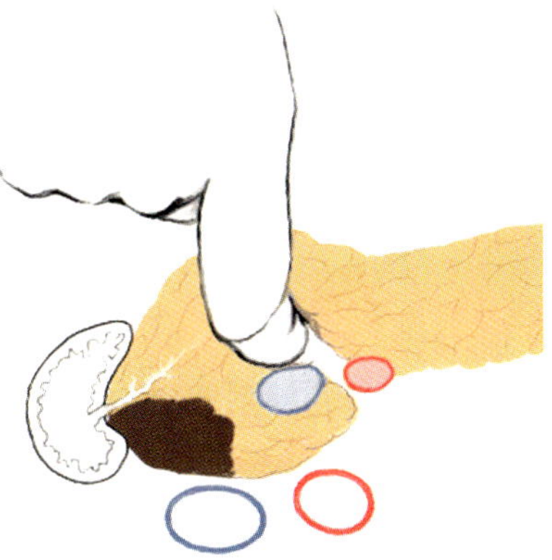

b

Figure 52.7

A complete tunnel is formed under the neck of the pancreas and over the portal and superior mesenteric veins.

The gastrointestinal tract is divided distally at a point of mobile jejunum, typically 20 cm distal to the ligament of Treitz (Fig. 52.9). The mesenteric vessels to this initial portion of the jejunum are carefully divided over clamps and tied to avoid bleeding. Once the proximal jejunum is separated from its mesentery, it can be delivered dorsal to the superior mesenteric vessels from the left to the right side (Fig. 52.10).

The specimen now remains connected by the uncinate process of the pancreas. This structure is separated from the portal vein, superior mesenteric vein, and superior mesenteric artery. This is performed by serially clamping, dividing, and tying the smaller branches off the portal and superior mesenteric ves-

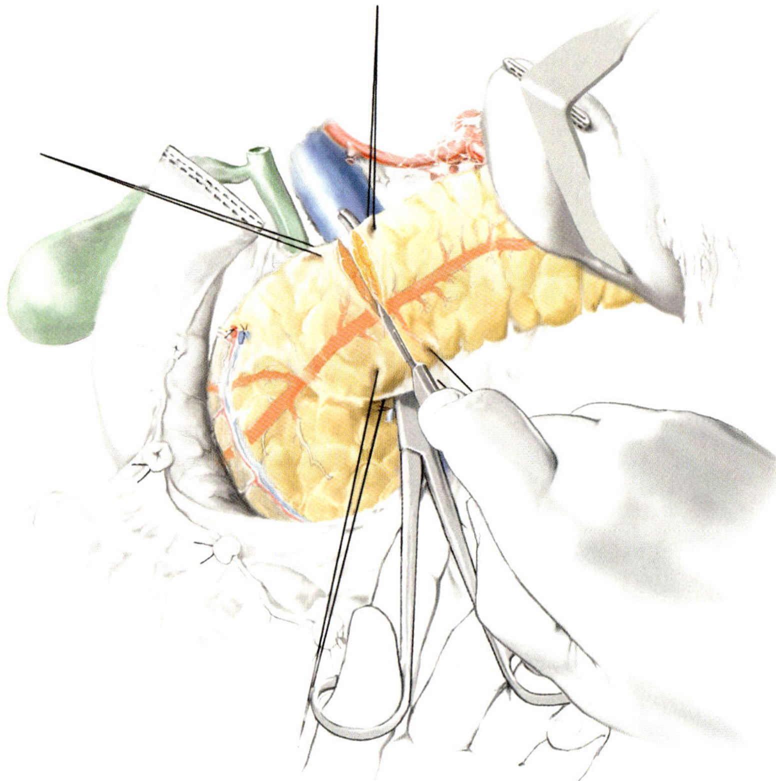

Figure 52.8

The neck of the pancreas is divided

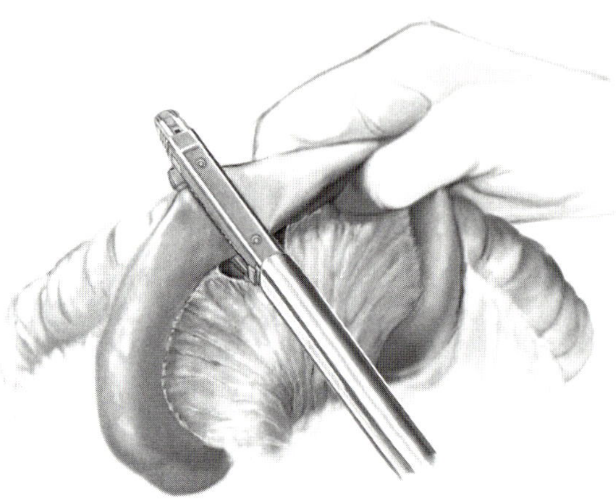

Figure 52.9

The proximal jejunum is divided and mobilized

sels (Fig. 52.11). Dissection should be performed flush with these structures to remove all pancreatic and nodal tissue in these areas. Great care is taken not to injure the superior mesenteric artery and vein at this level, but to remove completely the pancreatic tissue and lymph nodes near the vascular structures. With these areas dissected, the specimen is removed and the pancreatic neck margin, uncinate margin, and common hepatic duct margins are marked for the pathologists. To speed up analysis of these frozen section margins, the common hepatic duct margin and the pancreatic neck margin may be sampled earlier and sent to pathology while the main specimen is still being removed.

There are multiple options for reconstruction after PD. Most commonly, the reconstruction first involves the pancreas, followed by the bile duct, and then the duodenum. The issues and controversies surrounding the pancreatic and biliary reconstructions are outlined by multiple papers in the literature specifically addressing these issues.

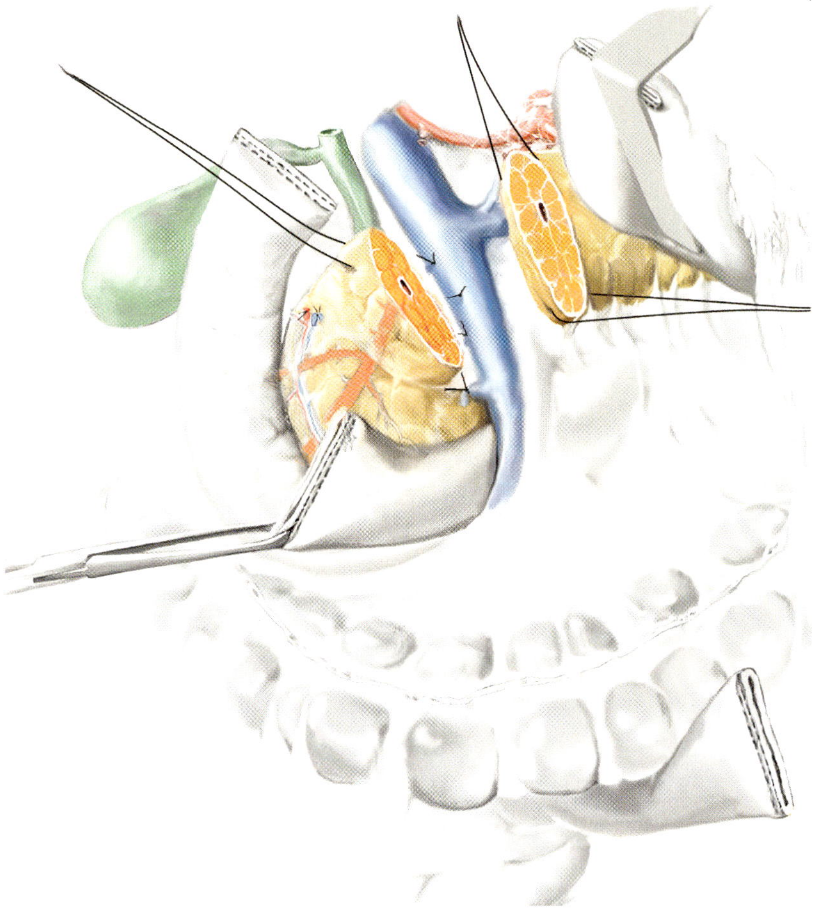

Figure 52.10

The proximal jejunal stump with third and fourth portions of the duodenum are mobilized under the ligament of Treitz

The most common reconstruction includes a retrocolic pancreaticojejunostomy, followed by a hepaticojejunostomy, and then a duodenojejunostomy. The pancreatic reconnection is the most problematic anastomosis out of the three and is responsible for much of the morbidity and mortality associated with the procedure.

Some groups favor a separate Roux-en-Y reconstruction for the pancreas. Controversy continues regarding the best type of pancreaticojejunostomy, the importance of duct-to-mucosa sutures, and the use of pancreatic duct stents. The pancreatic reconstruction is typically performed with either a duct-to-mucosal anastomosis or with an invagination technique. With either technique the proximal jejunum is brought through a defect in the mesocolon to the right of the middle colic artery. The duct-to-mucosal anastomosis is constructed in an end-to-side fashion whereby the outer back row consists of interrupted 3-0 silk sutures incorporating the capsule and parenchyma of the transected pancreas and submucosal bites of the jejunum. A small defect is then made in the jejunum, to which a duct-to-mucosa anastomosis is performed incorporating the pancreatic duct and the full thickness of the jejunum using interrupted 5-0 or 4-0 synthetic absorbable sutures (Fig. 52.12). Some surgeons prefer to stent this anastomosis with a 6-cm stent cut from a 5- or 8-French pediatric feeding tube. One half (3 cm) of the stent is placed into the pancreatic duct and the other half is placed into the jejunum. The stent is held in place with one of the absorbable sutures placed in the ductal anastomosis. This stent usually passes through the rest of the intestinal tract within a couple of weeks.

The invagination technique is typically performed with an end-to-end or end-to-side pancreaticojejunostomy. The pancreatic remnant should be circumferentially cleared and mobilized for 2–3 cm, to allow for an optimal anastomosis. The pancreaticojejunostomy is typically performed in two layers. The outer

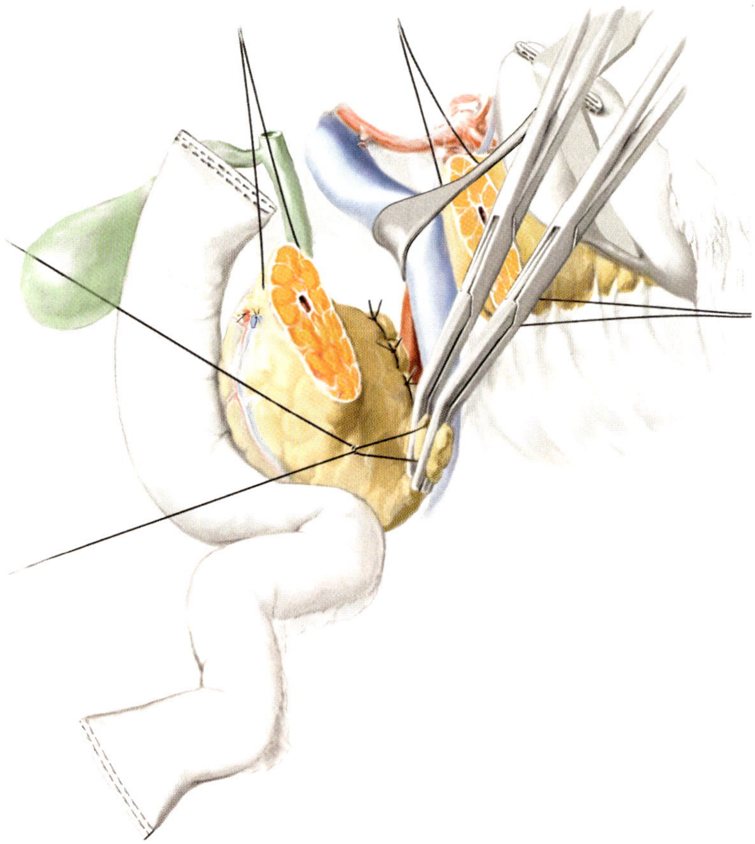

Figure 52.11

The uncinate portion of the pancreas is mobilized off of the portal and superior mesenteric veins, as well as, the superior mesenteric artery

layer consists of interrupted silk sutures that incorporate the capsule and parenchyma of the pancreas and the submucosal layer of the jejunum. The inner layer consists of a running 3-0 absorbable suture (or interrupted absorbable sutures) that incorporates the capsule and a portion of the parenchyma of the pancreas and the full thickness of the jejunum. The inner layer should incorporate the pancreatic duct for several bites, to splay it open. When completed, this anastomosis nicely invaginates the cut surface of the pancreatic neck into the jejunal lumen.

If the stomach is used to reconnect the pancreas, it is invaginated into the back wall of the stomach, as described previously for the jejunum. In a prospective randomized trial comparing pancreaticogastrostomy to pancreaticojejunostomy, there was no difference in the leak or fistula rate between the two types of anastomoses [12].

The biliary anastomosis is typically performed with an end-to-side hepaticojejunostomy approximately 5–10 cm distal on the jejunal limb from the pancreaticojejunostomy. This anastomosis is performed with a single layer of interrupted absorbable sutures (Fig. 52.13). If the patient has a percutaneous biliary stent, this is left in place, traversing the anastomosis. Preoperative biliary stenting remains controversial. Current data indicate that routine preoperative biliary stenting is of no benefit and carries potential risks, including an increased risk of wound or infectious complications, as well as an increased risk of pancreatic fistula formation [13–15]. Stenting should be used selectively in patients with obstructive jaundice who will have a substantial delay between initial presentation and definitive surgery, in patients who have undergone previous biliary-bypass surgery, and in rare patients with primary suppurative cholangitis. The method of stenting, endoscopic versus percutaneous, should be chosen based on local expertise.

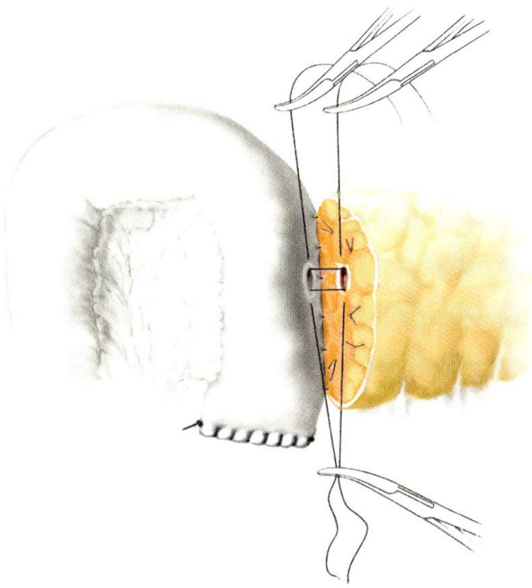

Figure 52.12

An end-to-side, duct-to-mucosa pancreaticojejunostomy. The outer layer consists of interrupted 3-0 silk sutures placed through the seromuscular layer of the intestines and through the capsule of the pancreas into the cut edge. The inner layer consists of interrupted 5-0 Maxon sutures through the duct and full thickness through a defect in the intestines incorporating the mucosa

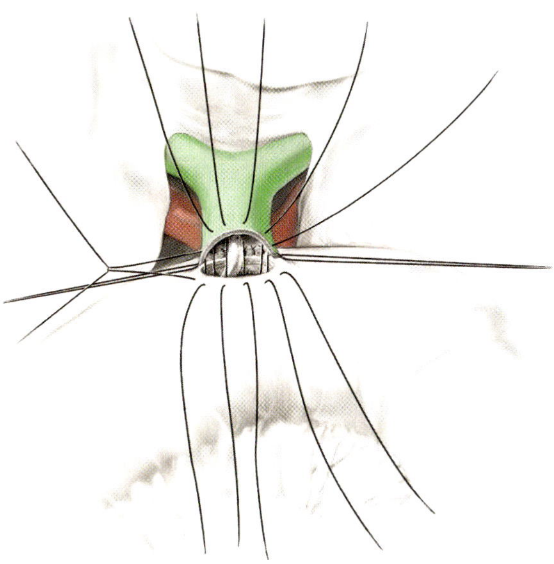

Figure 52.13

An end-to-side hepaticojejunostomy. The anastomosis is fashioned with interrupted 4-0 Maxon sutures

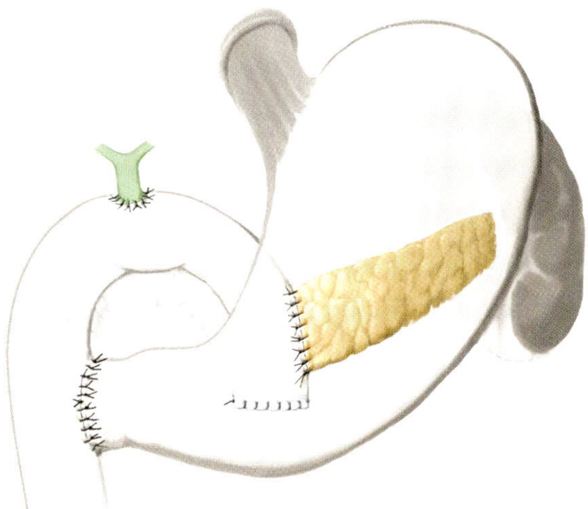

Figure 52.14

Reconstruction after pylorus-preserving pancreaticoduodenectomy. This drawing depicts a retrocolic duodenojejunostomy

The third anastomosis performed is the duodenojejunostomy in cases of pylorus preservation. This anastomosis is typically performed 10–15 cm downstream from the hepaticojejunostomy, proximal to the jejunum traversing the defect in the mesocolon (Fig. 52.14). Alternatively, this anastomosis can be performed in antecolic fashion with the jejunum distal to where it traverses the defect in the transverse mesocolon.

After the reconstruction is completed, closed suction drains are left in place to drain the biliary and pancreatic anastomoses. The defects at the ligament of Treitz, as well as around the jejunal limb through the transverse mesocolon should be closed. Some groups prefer not to place closed suction drains, accepting that if a fluid collection becomes clinically evident postoperatively, percutaneous drainage by interventional radiology may be required.

Table 52.1. Two large, recently published, randomized controlled clinical trials comparing classic pancreaticoduodenectomy (CPD) and pylorus-preserving pancreaticoduodenectomy (PPPD). *NS* Not significant

Year	Author		*n*	Operative time	Estimated blood loss	Pancreatic fistula	Delayed gastric emptying	Days in hospital	Operative mortality	Margin positive resection rate	Pancreas cancer median survival
2004	Tran et al. [16]	CPD	83	300 min	2000 ml	14%	23%	20	7%	17%	11 months
		PPPD	87	300 min	2000 ml	13%	22%	18	3%	26%	12 months
		P value		NS	NS	NS	NS	NS	NS	NS	NS
2005	Seiler et al. [17]	CPD	109	449 min	1500 ml	2%	45%	20	3%	21%	18 months
		PPPD	105	382 min	1198 ml	3%	31%	21	2%	9%	19 months
		P value		0.001	0.041	NS	NS	NS	NS	NS	NS

Early Postoperative Management

The postoperative management following PD consists of keeping the patient with nothing by mouth for 1 or 2 days, and then advancing the diet with liquids, and then solids as tolerated. The stomach is decompressed overnight after surgery with a nasogastric tube, which is usually removed the next morning unless there is an extraordinarily high output. The drains around the pancreatic anastomosis are removed once the patient has been on a regular diet. Drain amylase is checked prior to pulling the drains to check for leak or fistula.

Randomized Clinical Trials

Two large randomized clinical trials have been recently reported (Table 52.1). The first was a multicenter trial by Tran et al. [16], who reported on the randomization of 170 consecutive patients to either CPD or PPPD. There were no differences in median blood loss and duration of operation between the two groups. Delayed gastric emptying was observed at equivalent rates in the two groups. There was only a marginal difference in postoperative weight loss in favor of the CPD group. The rate of tumor-positive resection margins was not statistically significant. Long-term survival was not statistically significant between the two groups. They concluded that the CPD and PPPD groups were associated with comparable operative time, blood loss, hospital stay, mortality, morbidity, and incidence of delayed gastric emptying. The overall long-term and disease-free survival rates were comparable in both groups. They also concluded that both surgical procedures are equally effective for the treatment of pancreatic and periampullary carcinoma.

The second trial was a single-institution study in which 130 resectable patients were randomized to receive either a CPD or a PPPD [17]. There were significant differences in operative time and estimated blood loss favoring the PPPD group. There was no difference in perioperative morbidity including pancreatic fistula rate or delayed gastric emptying rate. Long-term survival, quality of life, and weight gain were identical in both groups. At 6 months postprocedure, capacity to work was better after PPPD. They concluded that both procedures were equally effective for the treatment of pancreatic and periampullary cancers. They also concluded that PPPD resection offers some minor advantages in the early postoperative period, but not in the long term.

References

1. Halsted WS (1899) Contributions to the surgery of the bile passages, especially of the common bile duct. Boston Med Surg J 141:645–654
2. Sauve L (1908) Des pancreatectomies et specialement de la pancreatectomie cephalique. Rev Chir 37:335–385
3. Kausch W (1912) Das carcinoma der papilla duodeni und seine radikale entfeinung. Beitr Z Clinc Chir 78:439–486
4. Hirschel G (1914) Die resection des duodenums mit der papille wegen karzinoims. Munchen Med Wochenschr 61:1728–1730
5. Whipple AO, Parsons WB, Mullins CR (1935) Treatment of carcinoma of the ampulla of Vater. Ann Surg 102:763–779
6. Watson K (1944) Carcinoma of the ampulla of Vater. Successful radical resection. Br J Surg 31:368–373
7. Traverso LW, Longmire WP Jr (1978) Preservation of the pylorus in pancreaticoduodenectomy. Surg Gynecol Obstet 146:959–962
8. Conlon KC, Dougherty E, Klimstra DS, Coit DG, Turnbull AD, Brennan MF (1996) The value of minimal access surgery in the staging of patients with potentially resectable peripancreatic malignancy. Ann Surg 223:134–140
9. Lillemoe KD (1998) Palliative therapy for pancreatic cancer. Surg. Oncol. Clin. North Am 7:199–216
10. Vollmer CM, Drebin JA, Middleton WD, Teefey SA, Linehan DC, Soper NJ, Eagon CJ, Strasberg SM (2002) Utility of staging laparoscopy in subsets of peripancreatic and biliary malignancies. Ann Surg 235:1–7
11. Strasberg SM, Drebin JA, Mokadam NA, Green DW, Jones KL, Ehlers JP, Linehan D (2002) Prospective trial of a blood supply-based technique of pancreaticojejunostomy: effect on anastomotic failure in the Whipple procedure. J Am Coll Surg 194:746–758
12. Yeo CJ, Cameron JL, Maher MM, Sauter PK, Zahurak ML, Talamini MA, Lillemoe KD, Pitt HA (1995) A prospective randomized trial of pancreaticogastrostomy versus pancreaticojejunostomy after pancreaticoduodenectomy. Ann Surg 222:580–588
13. Heslin MJ, Brooks AD, Hochwald SN, Harrison LE, Blumgart LH, Brennan MF (1998) A preoperative biliary stent is associated with increased complications after pancreaticoduodenectomy. Arch Surg 133:149–154
14. Povoski SP, Karpeh MS, Conlon KC, Blumgart LH, Brennan MF (1999) Association of preoperative biliary drainage with postoperative outcome following pancreaticoduodenectomy. Ann Surg 230:131–142
15. Sohn TA, Yeo CJ, Cameron JL, Pitt HA, Lillemoe KD (2000) Preoperative biliary stents in patients undergoing pancreaticoduodenectomy: increased risk of postoperative complications? J. Gastrointest Surg 4:258–267
16. Tran KT, Smeenk HG, van Eijck CH, Kazemier G, Hop WC, Greve JW, Terstra OT, Zijlstra JA, Klinkert P, Jeekel H (2004) Pylorus preserving pancreaticoduodenectomy versus standard Whipple procedure. Ann Surg 240:738–745
17. Seiler CA, Wagner M, Bachmann T, Redaelli CA, Schmied B, Uhl W, Friess H, Buchler MW (2005) Randomized clinical trial of pylorus-preserving duodenopancreatectomy versus classical Whipple resection – long term results. Br J Surg 92:547–556

Chapter 53

F. Mosca · U. Boggi · M. Del Chiaro

Management of Tumor Invasion/Adhesion to the Superior Mesenteric-Portal Vein During Pancreatectomy

A small percentage of patients diagnosed with pancreatic cancer have localized, "early", neoplasms that can be resected with wide, tumor-free, margins and hopefully cured by surgery alone [1]. Indeed, pancreas cancer typically pursues a high-grade biologic course that is characterized by early spread into retroperitoneal tissues, lymphatic nodes, perineural spaces, and peripancreatic vessels. Moreover, when first diagnosed, it is already associated with peritoneal and/or liver metastases [2], and circulating tumor cells have been detected in the blood and in the bone marrow of 28% and 24% of patients, respectively [3]. These observations demonstrate that complete tumor removal is rarely possible in patients diagnosed with duct cell adenocarcinoma of the pancreas, and that nearly all pancreatectomies done with curative intention are actually palliative procedures.

Between 30 and 35% of pancreatic cancers are deemed unresectable due to isolated involvement of the peripancreatic veins. Historically, the main reasons for not doing a resection were technical complexity of the operation, increased risk of postoperative complications, and lack of demonstrated survival benefit. Currently, it is clear that adding a venous resection to a pancreatectomy does not increase the postoperative risk (Table 53.1) [4–13], but there is still no sound evidence that it improves survival [14]. However, most reported series refer mainly to patients either scheduled for rescue procedures of extensively invasive tumors with no actual hope of cure [15], or in whom the decision to resect a venous segment was made intraoperatively, when tumor invasion of the peripancreatic veins was discovered too late to abort pancreatectomy and when dissection had already been carried out around or within tumor margins [16]. Accordingly, the majority of available data is not suitable for meaningful comparison with "standard" pancreatectomy and may not reflect the actual prognostic implications of a planned approach to tumor adhesion/invasion to the superior mesenteric/portal vein.

We describe herein the methods developed to achieve a "no-touch pancreatectomy" with en bloc resection of venous segments thought to be involved by pancreatic tumors. Long-term results, including comparisons with neoplasms undergoing bypass without resection, show that survival can be improved in carefully selected patients.

Table 53.1. Postoperative morbidity and mortality in recent series of pancreatectomy with associated resection of vascular segments. *NA* Not avail

First author	Reference	Year	Patients	Morbidity	Mortality
Harrison	[12]	1996	58	NA	5%
Leach	[13]	1998	31	30%	0%
Bachellier	[4]	2001	21	38.1%	4.7%
Shibata	[5]	2001	28	32%	4%
Van Greenen	[10]	2001	34	41%	0
Hartel	[7]	2002	68	27%	4%
Sasson	[9]	2002	37	35%	2.7%
Nakagohri	[6]	2003	33	NA	6.1%
Capussotti	[8]	2003	22	33.3%	0
Howard	[11]	2003	13	54%	NA
TOTAL			**345**	**34% (86/254)**	**3.7% (11/291)**

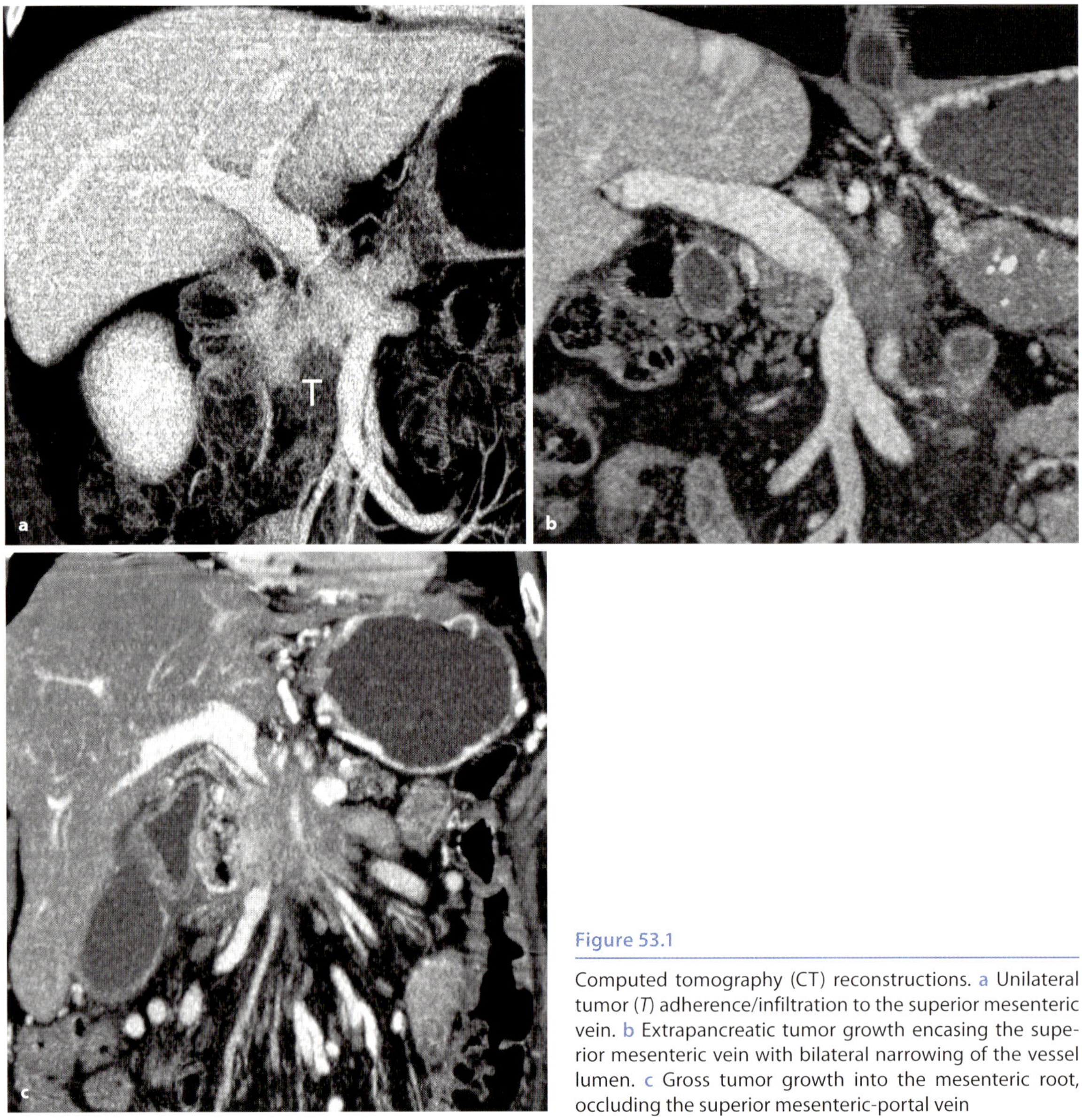

Figure 53.1

Computed tomography (CT) reconstructions. a Unilateral tumor (*T*) adherence/infiltration to the superior mesenteric vein. b Extrapancreatic tumor growth encasing the superior mesenteric vein with bilateral narrowing of the vessel lumen. c Gross tumor growth into the mesenteric root, occluding the superior mesenteric-portal vein

Rationale for Pancreatectomy with Associated Venous Resection

Long-term follow-up analyses show that between 95 and 97% of patients undergoing curative Whipple procedures for duct cell adenocarcinoma of the pancreas actually have occult tumor spread beyond the reach of the knife [2]. Consequently, one half of these patients die within 20 months after resection [17], 5-year survival usually does not exceed 10%, and deaths due to cancer recurrence continue to occur for up to 10 years after diagnosis [18]. It is not completely clear yet if these discouraging figures are caused by the high grade biology of pancreas cancer, the often delayed diagnosis, the lack of effective medical treatments, or by a combination thereof. However, despite the predictably low cure rate, patients with localized pancreas cancer are currently considered surgical candidates even when the tumor invades the surrounding organs or structures, such as the duodenum or the distal common bile duct, or is associated with lymph node metastases [19]. On the contrary, involvement of the superior mesenteric-portal vein is usually deemed a contraindication [20], despite there being no substantial proof that isolated vessel invasion implies enhanced cancer aggressiveness. It could actually reflect the perivenous origin of the tumor (Fig. 53.1a). This "localized vascular involvement," however, should be clearly separated from vessel encasement and extrapancreatic tumor growth (i.e., peripancreatic carcinomatosis; Fig. 53.1b) and/or full-thickness infiltration with intraluminal tumor propagation (Fig. 53.1c). While surgery cannot be of any significant benefit in either of the latter conditions, it could still be suitable in the former instance provided that no attempt is made at separating the tumor from the vessel. Indeed, breaching the thin margin between the tumor and the vessel could convert a potentially margin-negative (R_0) resection into a certain margin-positive (at least R_1) resection, thus laying the foundation for subsequent local tumor recurrence.

Selection Criteria

The importance of candidate selection cannot be overemphasized. Tumor type plays a fundamental role and indications vary widely between ductal adenocarcinoma of the pancreas and other pancreatic or periampullary malignancies (i.e., acinar cell carcinoma, neuroendocrine carcinoma, cystic neoplasms, ampullary carcinoma, and distal common bile duct carcinoma).

Preoperative Diagnostic Work-up

Preoperative evaluation includes physical examination, routine laboratory testing, chest radiography, ultrasonography, and contrast-enhanced multislice computed tomography in all patients. Laparoscopic staging [21, 22] is used to address specific issues (e.g., rule out the presence of peritoneal carcinomatosis suspected, but not demonstrated, with other diagnostic modalities), while angiography and endoscopic retrograde cholangiopancreatography are not employed.

Assessment of Resectability

Current preoperative imaging methods, above all computed tomography, usually anticipate the need for venous resection during pancreatectomy. At the time of initial surgical exploration, however, local tumor extension should be further defined before attempting any dissection around the tumor. In detail, after checking the liver and peritoneum for distant metastases, the head of the pancreas is inspected and palpated so as to further define the relationships between the tumor and the superior mesenteric vein. Contact ultrasonography is performed next using high-frequency probes (Fig. 53.2).

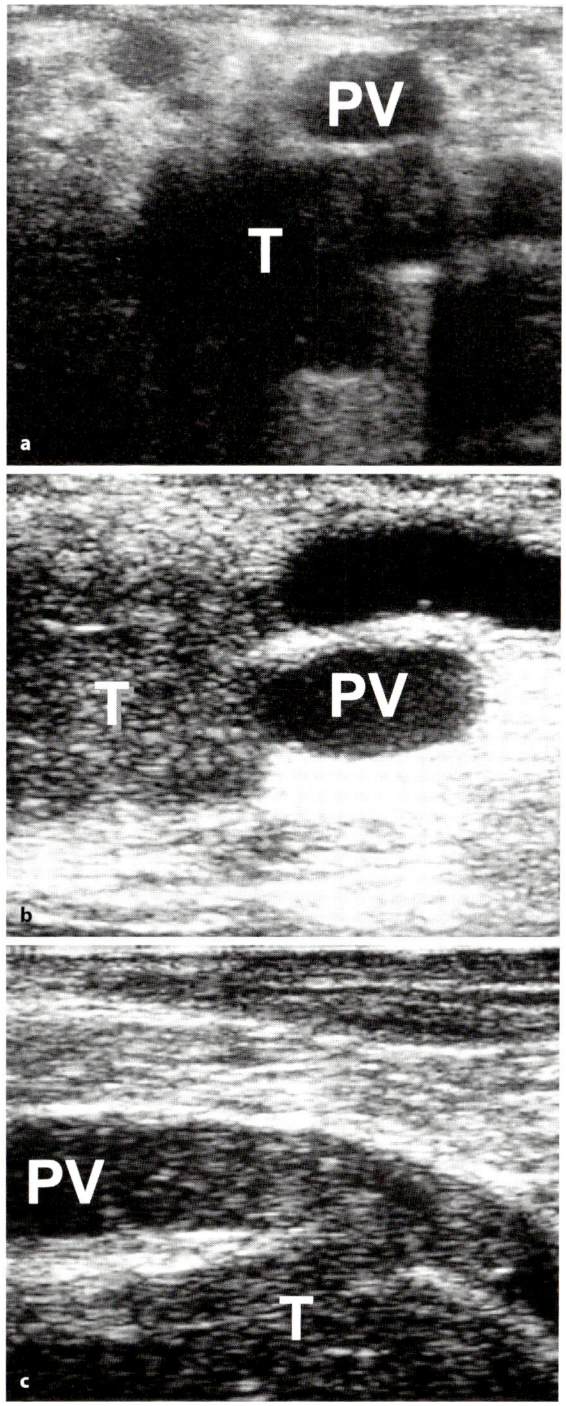

Figure 53.2

Contact ultrasonography. a A well-defined hyperechoic non-tumoral plane clearly separates a pancreatic tumor (*T*) from the portal vein (*PV*). b Tumor adherence/invasion to the portal vein. c Tumor growth into the portal vein causing thrombotic occlusion of the vessel

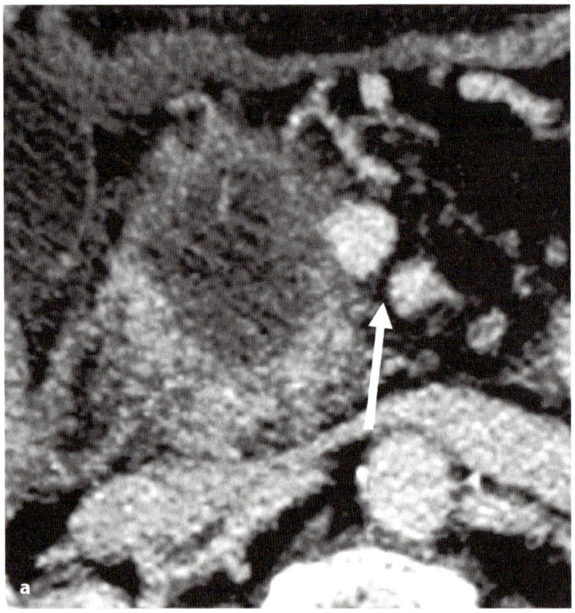

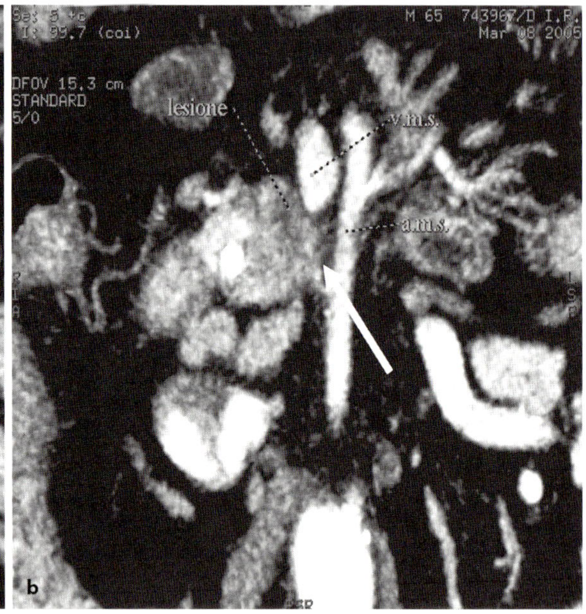

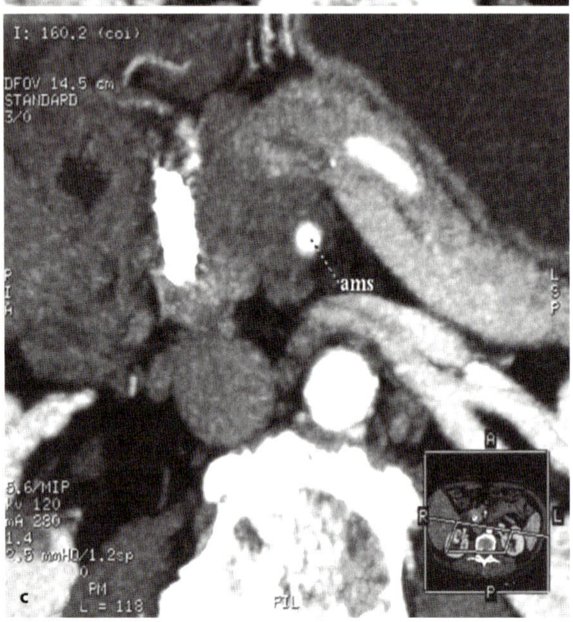

Figure 53.3

a CT scan showing an intact fat plane (*arrow*) between a pancreatic tumor (*T*) and the superior mesenteric artery. b CT reconstruction showing tumoral propagations (*arrow*) extending into the retroperitoneal margin and reaching the right lateral aspect of the superior mesenteric artery (*a.m.s.*). c CT scan showing gross tumor growth into the retroperitoneal margin, encasing the superior mesenteric artery (*ams*). *v.m.s.* Superior mesenteric vein

Indications and Contraindications

During the first period of our experience (November 1987 through July 1998) pancreatic tumors were considered resectable if confined to the pancreas and if vascular involvement permitted resection and reconstruction, irrespective of tumor type [23]. Afterwards, resection continued to be indicated when technically feasible only for tumors other than ductal adenocarcinoma of the pancreas. For pancreas cancer, mainly based on the experiences reported by Ishikawa et al. in 1992 [24] and Nakao et al. in 1995 [25], indications were restricted to unilateral (<180°) segmental vascular involvement. Special attention was also paid to exclude cases with deep tumor extension at the retroperitoneal margin [13, 16, 24, 26], defined by the absence of an intact fat plane between the tumor and the right lateral wall of the superior mesenteric artery (Fig. 53.3). Isolated arterial involvement was not considered an absolute contraindication. Tumors with concurrent involvement of multiple vessels or extending deeply in the retroperitoneum were considered eligible for resection only if responsive to neoadjuvant treatments.

Surgical Techniques

For right-sided resections and total pancreatectomies our procedure of choice is a modified pylorus-preserving pancreatectomy, as described previously [27]. For digestive reconstruction we prefer to use a single retrocolic, or occasionally antecolic, jejunal loop anastomosed sequentially to the pancreatic remnant, the hepatic duct, and the first duodenal portion. Soft pancreatic remnants, thought to be at high risk of pancreatic fistula, have also been duct injected with neoprene or other sclerosing agents [28], although in the last 8 years this technique has been employed only occasionally.

When tumor adherence/invasion to the superior mesenteric/portal vein is suspected, the vein is encircled above and below the involved segment; dissecting the tumor off the vessel wall is not attempted. Planning for a circumferential sleeve resection rather than for a tangential excision allows safer and easier dissection in nontumoral tissues (Figs. 53.4 and 53.5). Resected segments are usually reconstructed using autologous interposition grafts. The internal jugular vein seems to be particularly suitable for this purpose since its size usually matches that of the resected segment, including the slight increase of caliber that is observed from proximal to distal [26]. Other possible conduits are the iliac veins, the superficial femoral veins, and the left renal vein [24]. Occasionally, when a total pancreatectomy is necessary but the distal splenic vein is not involved by the tumor, clockwise rotation of the splenic vein can provide a further reconstruction option (Fig. 53.6). The ovarian vein or the greater saphenous vein can be used for patch closure of side-wall resections, but not as jump grafts [29]. Although a direct anastomosis without an interposing graft is facilitated by ligating and dividing the splenic vein, we have always preferred to preserve the splenic vein to avoid sinistral hypertension with its inherent complications [30]. When necessary, the splenic vein has been anastomosed end-to-side to the reconstructed superior mesenteric-portal vein (Fig. 53.7). When an interposition graft is necessary but no autologous segments are available or suitable, the last alternative to prosthetic conduits are cadaveric veins preserved between 0 and 4°C in Terasaki solution for less than 7 days. We do not advise the use of vascular prostheses of any type due to the well-known risk of intra-abdominal infection following pancreatectomy.

In most patients the venous segment involved is the superior mesenteric vein. After achieving proximal and distal venous control, above and below the tumor, the first jejunal loop is completely mobilized so that it need not be further mobilized to remove the specimen. Then, after dividing the neck of the pancreas, the retroperitoneal margin is approached from the left aspect of the superior mesenteric-portal vein, instead of from the right side. Starting at the mesenteric root and proceeding along the right lateral aspect of the superior mesenteric artery, the en bloc specimen, including the head of the pancreas and the superior mesenteric vein, is detached from its retroperitoneal attachments (Fig.53.4b). To facilitate this maneuver, the distal splenic vein is encircled and mobilized widely. With this approach, most locoregional nodes are resected en bloc with the head of the pancreas. During the dissection of the superior mesenteric artery, attention should be paid to spare the left sided portion of the nerve plexus, since circumferential stripping has been associated with troublesome diarrhea [31]. When this anterior approach is difficult, such as in male patients with omental obesity, an alternative approach is from the back: the small bowel and right colon, completely mobilized, are displaced onto the upper abdomen, thus exposing the posterior aspect of the pancreatic head-mesenteric root. From this route the superior mesenteric artery is promptly located and is more readily accessible (Fig. 53.8). In either instance, after completing the dissection of the retroperitoneal margin, the superior mesenteric-portal vein and the splenic vein are the only residual attachments that prevent specimen removal (Fig. 53.4c). Occasionally, when the superior mesenteric-portal vein is chronically suboccluded due to compression or infiltration, closure of collateral veins causes splanchnic stasis. The ensuing edema and swelling of the intestines as well as the scattered bleeding from venous hypertension make the above-described dissection difficult. In these patients we prefer to cross-clamp the superior mesenteric artery and vein, divide the superior mesenteric vein, quickly complete the dissection of the retroperitoneal margin en bloc with the head of the pancreas, remove the specimen, and immediately reconstruct the superior mesenteric-portal vein (Fig. 53.9). When the superior mesenteric vein is involved proximally in the mesenteric root, where three large veins usually merge to constitute the main trunk of the vein, it should be decided how many veins should be eventually reconstructed before the specimen has been completely mobilized. The importance of a timely decision is twofold. First, severe postoperative complications can result from vein ligation in the absence of appropriate collateral drainage. Secondly, if more than one vein needs to be reconstructed, the use of an interposition graft may become

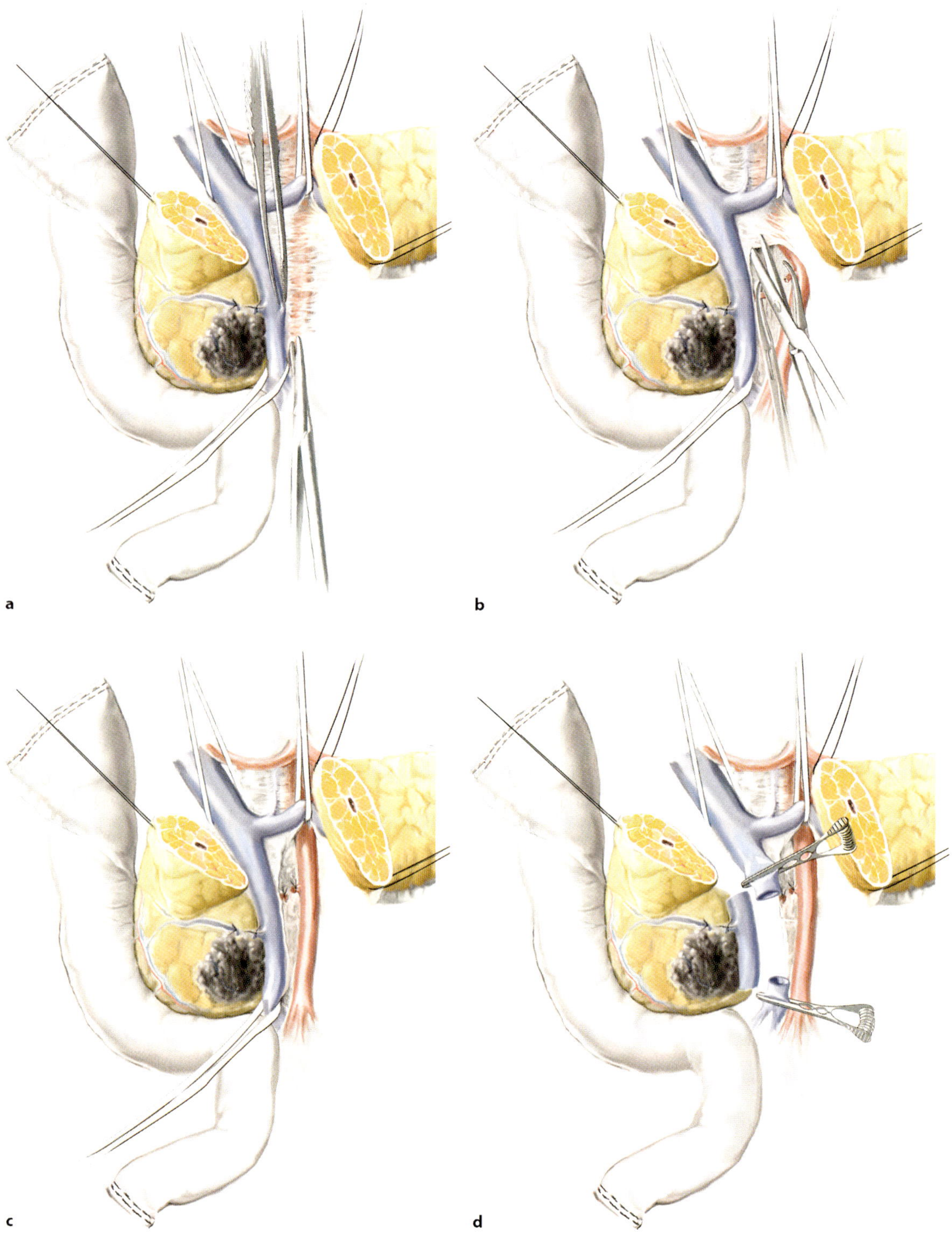

Figure 53.4

a The superior mesenteric vein is approached from its left side, starting distal to the tumor. b Dissection proceeds proximally along the right lateral margin of the superior mesenteric artery, until the entire retroperitoneal margin is divided. c The superior mesenteric/portal vein and the splenic vein are the only left structures that prevent specimen removal. d The specimen has been resected en bloc with a sleeve segment of the superior mesenteric vein

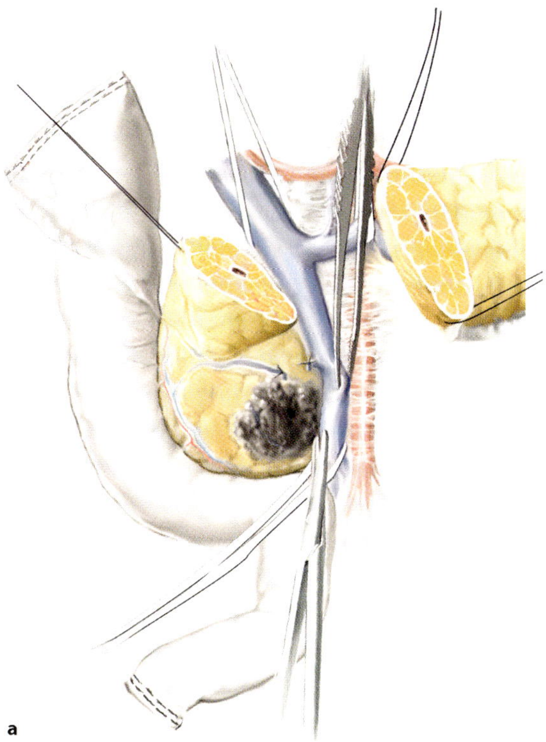

Figure 53.5

a The superior mesenteric vein is approached from its right side. Dissection is carried out around the tumor and the venous segment deemed to be involved so as to allow lateral clamping and side-wall resection. b The specimen has been resected en bloc with a small patch of the superior mesenteric vein

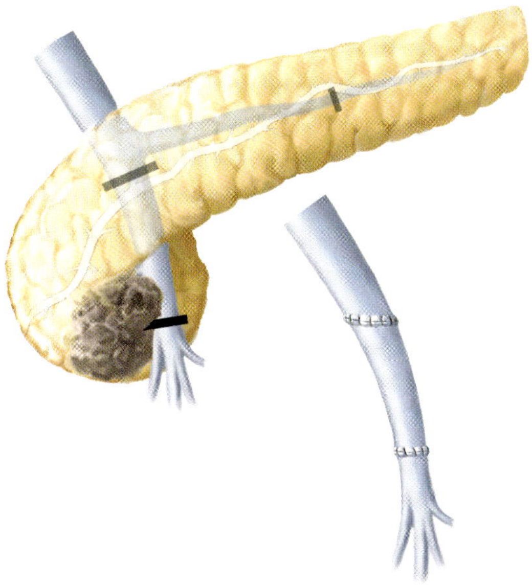

Figure 53.6

Reconstruction of the superior mesenteric vein by clockwise rotation of uninvolved splenic vein during total pancreatectomy

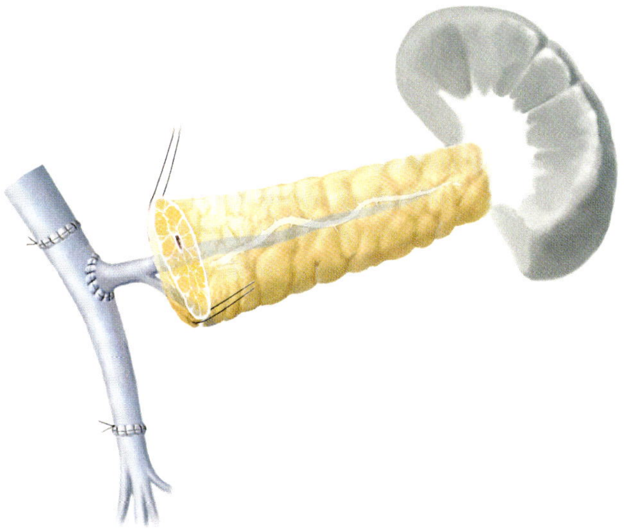

Figure 53.7

The splenic vein is anastomosed end-to-side to the interposition graft used to reconstruct the superior mesenteric/portal vein

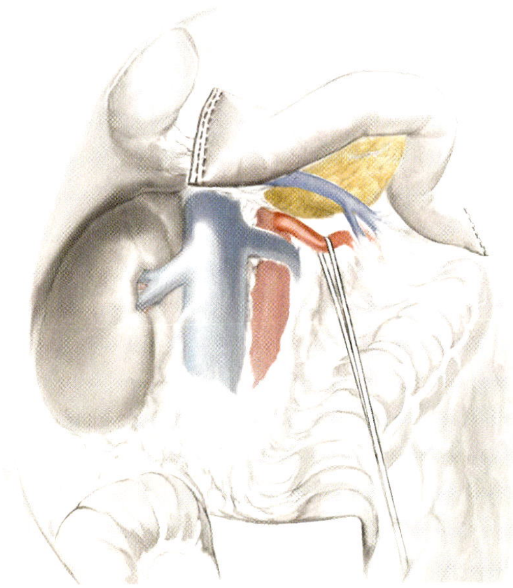

Figure 53.8

Complete mobilization and upper displacement of the intestines provides a further, posterolateral, way of approaching the superior mesenteric artery and dissecting the retroperitoneal margin en bloc with the vein segment that should be resected. *inf* Infiltration, *av* adventitia

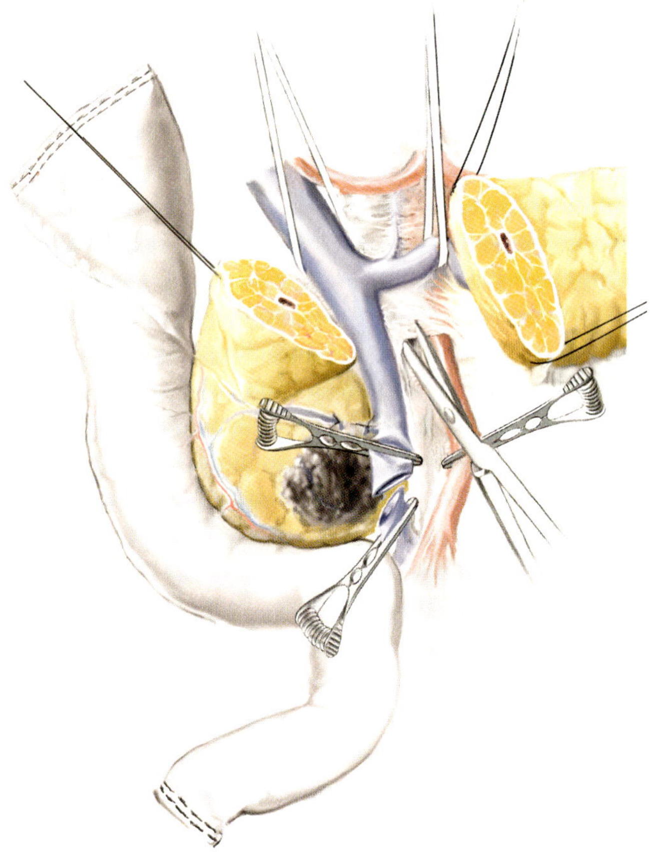

Figure 53.9

After crossclamping the superior mesenteric artery and vein, the dissection of the retroperitoneal margin is quickly completed so as to allow immediate reconstruction and solve the splanchnic stasis

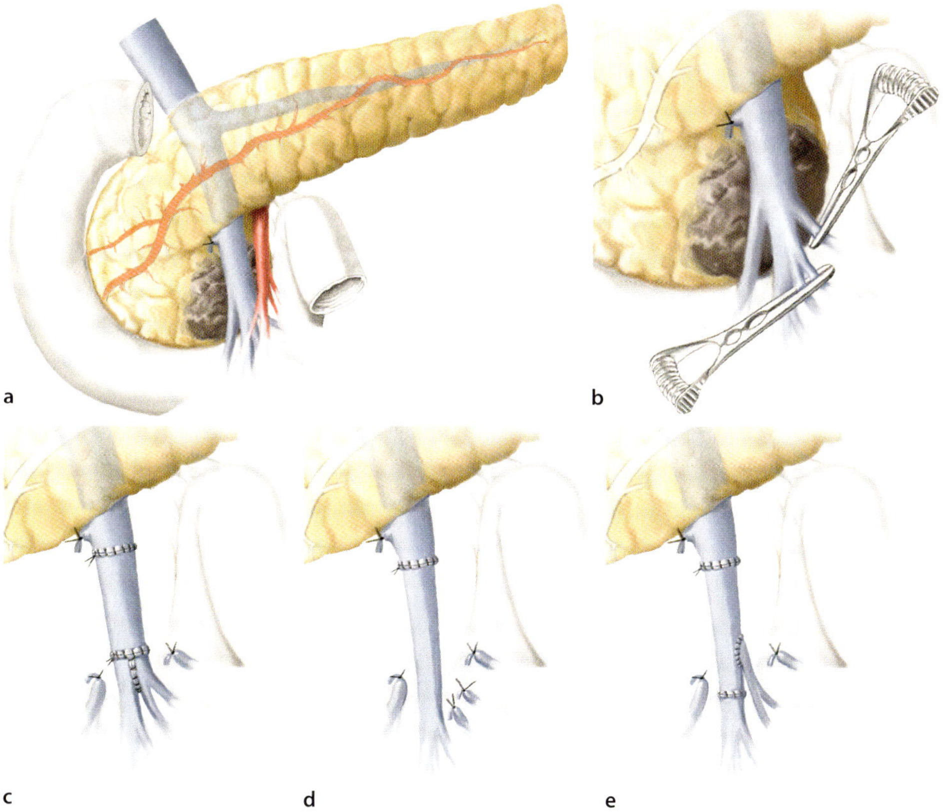

Figure 53.10

a Pancreas tumor adherent/invading the proximal segment of the superior mesenteric vein. b Tributary veins are individually crossclamped during dissection in order to verify the efficacy of collateral drainage. Intestine viability and splanchnic stasis are noted repeatedly. c Direct, end-to-end reconstruction of the superior mesenteric vein. Only the largest tributary has been anastomosed. d Reconstruction of the superior mesenteric vein using an interposition graft. The proximal anastomosis incorporates two tributaries. e Reconstruction of the superior mesenteric vein using an interposition graft. One tributary is anastomosed end-to-side to the jump graft

necessary so as to allow side implantation of collaterals, and it should be made available when the dissection has been completed. The first jejunal vein, a large vein that crosses the superior mesenteric artery posteriorly, can be ligated with no consequences. However, before deciding to ligate any of these large veins they should be individually crossclamped while dissection progresses so as to have time to verify the occurrence of intestinal stasis (Fig. 53.10).

Another important issue is avoiding blood pooling in the splanchnic circulation and reducing the time during which the often cholestatic liver is deprived of portal inflow. Direct reconstruction, by end-to-end anastomosis, requires quick suturing, although crossclamping the superior mesenteric artery can reduce intestinal edema. When an interposition graft is required, staged occlusion of venous pedicles, coupled with concurrent crossclamping of the superior mesenteric artery, seems to be preferable. Thus, in a case of isolated involvement of the superior mesenteric vein, the vessel is clamped below the tumor and divided, thus allowing the surgeon to perform the proximal anastomosis while portal flow is partially nourished by the splenic vein and some intestinal venous effluent is maintained, if the inferior mesenteric vein was not ligated. Then, after removal of the specimen, portal flow is abolished only during the construction of the proximal anastomosis. When the splenoportal junction is also resected, the splenic vein is anastomosed end-to-side to the interposition graft employed to replace the superior mesenteric-portal vein. This anastomosis does not usually require crossclamping of the jump graft, as lateral partial occlusion is usually sufficient. Avoiding splanchnic stasis is an important goal of pancreatectomy with associated vascular resection. Indeed, the ensuing intestinal and pancreatic stump edema not only complicate the completion of the procedure, but may also have negative consequences on the healing of digestive anastomoses.

Heparin is not usually given intraoperatively and postoperative antithrombotic prophylaxis is not enhanced as compared with our standard practice (calcium heparin 0.2 ml three times daily until the patient is fully ambulant). The patency of vascular reconstructions is checked daily during the early postoperative period by ultrasound-Doppler; equivocal findings are confirmed by computed tomography.

Postoperative Complications

The spectrum of complications occurring after pancreatectomy associated with resection of a vein segment does not differ from that observed after standard pancreatectomies. Perhaps the only specific complication is thrombosis of the reconstructed vessel. This is associated with quick accumulation of ascitic fluid and usually becomes evident as a rapid increase in abdominal girth. Intestinal edema and swelling contribute to abdominal distension and are also associated with failure to pass flatus, absence of intestinal sounds, and gaseous distension of bowel loops. Worsening jaundice may also be noted along with other signs of poor liver function such as cutaneous and/or mucous hemorrhage. Laboratory tests reveal hepatic function decompensation.

Data from the literature show that venous thrombosis develops in 1.7–3.7% of reconstructed vascular segments [4, 12]. In our own experience, nonocclusive venous thrombosis occurred in two patients (2%).

Treatment depends on the likelihood that collaterals can bypass the occluded vein. More specifically, one can anticipate the development of valid collateral circulation when the ileocolic and inferior mesenteric veins were not ligated (Fig. 53.11a). In these patients, treatment includes full intravenous heparinization for 1 week followed by oral warfarin sodium for 6 months. On the contrary, when the colic veins are sacrificed (Fig. 53.11b) or when the thrombosis occurs in the portal vein itself, there is little likelihood that effective collateral circulation can develop. In these patients, if the thrombosis is complete, rescue should be attempted by surgical thrombectomy. The underlying cause of thrombosis should be defined at relaparotomy and any technical faults corrected. Also, the viability of the intestine should be carefully evaluated, including the integrity of all enteric anastomoses. Postoperative management should include enhanced anticoagulation prophylaxis and daily ultrasound Doppler surveillance.

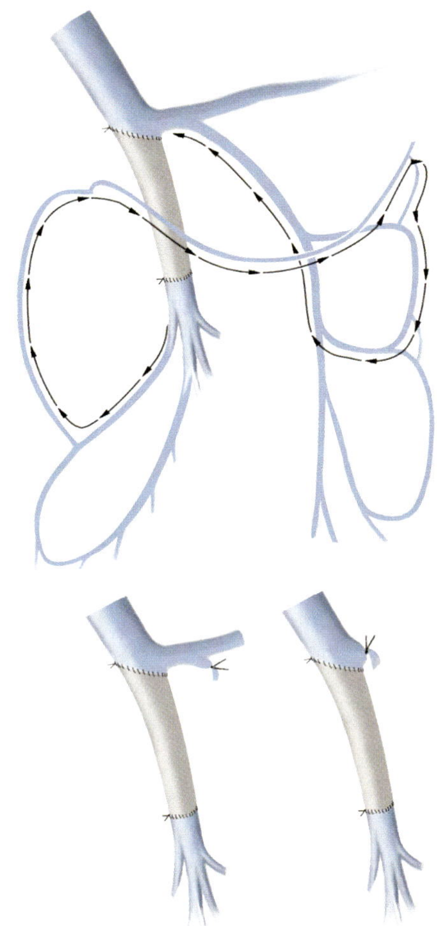

a

b

Figure 53.11

a Thrombosed superior mesenteric vein bypassed through colic veins. b Effective collateral splanchnic drainage is not expected to develop if thrombosis is occlusive and the inferior mesenteric vein (or the splenic vein) was ligated

Results

Literature Review

Recent data (Table 53.1) demonstrate that the morbidity and mortality associated with pancreatectomies with simultaneous portal-mesenteric vein resection usually do not exceed those recorded following conventional procedures. Increased morbidity or mortality should therefore no longer be felt as a major disincentive for vein resection at the time of pancreatectomy. In addition, if early pioneering experiences with regional pancreatectomy [32] are not considered, available survival data do not show a negative prognostic impact of vein resection. Bachellier et al., in their analysis of 31 pancreatoduodenectomies with resection of the portal-mesenteric vein, report a 2-

year survival rate of 22%, which basically overlaps the 24% recorded following conventional pancreatectomy [4]. Similarly, in the experience of Nakagohri et al., the median survival time of 33 patients undergoing portal-mesenteric vein resection was not worse than that recorded in 48 conventional pancreatectomies (15 vs 10 months; p = not significant) [6]. Similar results were reported by Leach et al. (median survival time 22 vs. 20 months) [13], Harrison et al. (median survival time 13 vs. 17 months) [12], Tseng et al. (median survival time 23.43 vs 26.5 months) [14], and Hartel et al. (5-year survival 22% vs 24%) [7]. Moreover, resection of venous segments thought to be surgically infiltrated seems to be associated with a survival advantage when pathology fails to demonstrated actual tumor invasion. This intriguing observation, reported by Nakagohri [6] and by Hartel [7], however, is not universally confirmed [14] and remains controversial.

Personal Series

Between November 1987 and December 2004, 1,641 patients diagnosed with pancreatic or periampullary tumors were admitted to our Department. Of these, 743 patients (45.3%) underwent pancreatectomy, including 138 patients (8.3%) who required associated resection of vascular segments. One hundred and three vein segments were resected in 102 patients (6.2%; one patient had segmental resections of the portal-mesenteric vein and the retropancreatic inferior vena cava). Side-wall resections (28/103; 27%) were usually repaired with wide patch grafts (Fig. 53.12), while sleeve resections (75/103; 73%) were reconstructed using interposition grafts (52/103; 50%: left internal jugular vein 42/103, 41%; cadaver donor iliac vein graft 8/103, 8%, gonadal vein 1/103, <1%; PTFE graft 1/103, <1%; Fig. 53.13) or direct anastomosis (23/103; 22%; Fig. 53.14).

Hospital stay averaged 21.9 days (range 10–74 days). Postoperative complications occurred in 36 patients (35.3%) and were fatal in 6 of them (5.9%; Table 53.2). All portal-mesenteric thromboses were nonocclusive and were treated conservatively.

Pathology demonstrated pancreatic duct cell adenocarcinoma in 84 out of 102 patients (Tables 53.3 and 53.4). Overall, 85 venous segments were resected and 77 (91%) were analyzed (Table 53.4).

For patients diagnosed with ductal adenocarcinoma, survival at 1, 3, and 5 years was 58.5%, 15%, and 10.5%, respectively (median survival time 15 months; Fig. 53.15). Tumor invasion of the tunica intima was

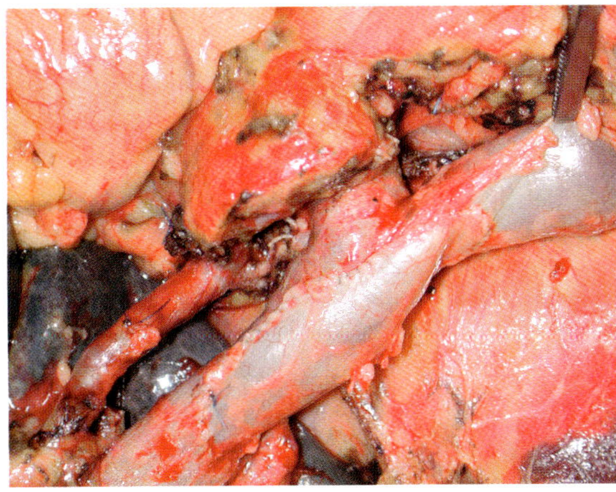

Figure 53.12

Intraoperative picture showing patch closure of large side-wall resection

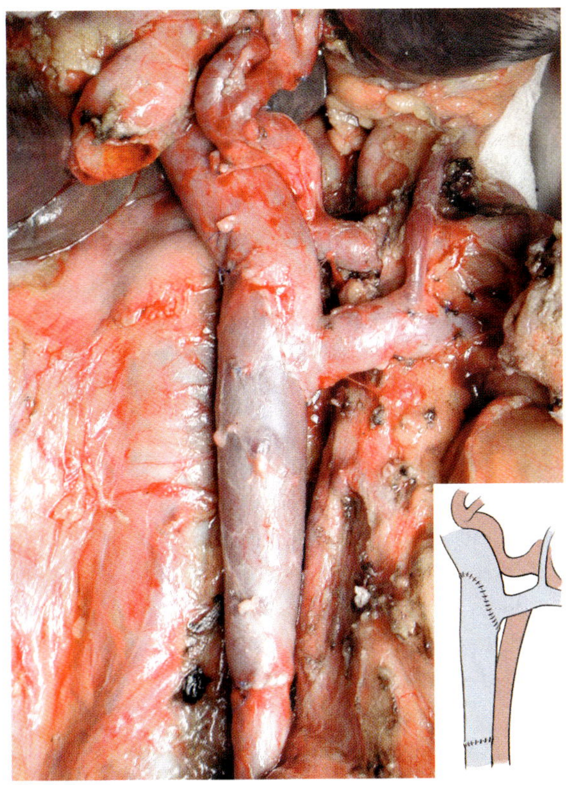

Figure 53.13

Intraoperative picture showing reconstruction of sleeve resection of the superior mesenteric vein using an autologous interposition graft (left internal jugular vein)

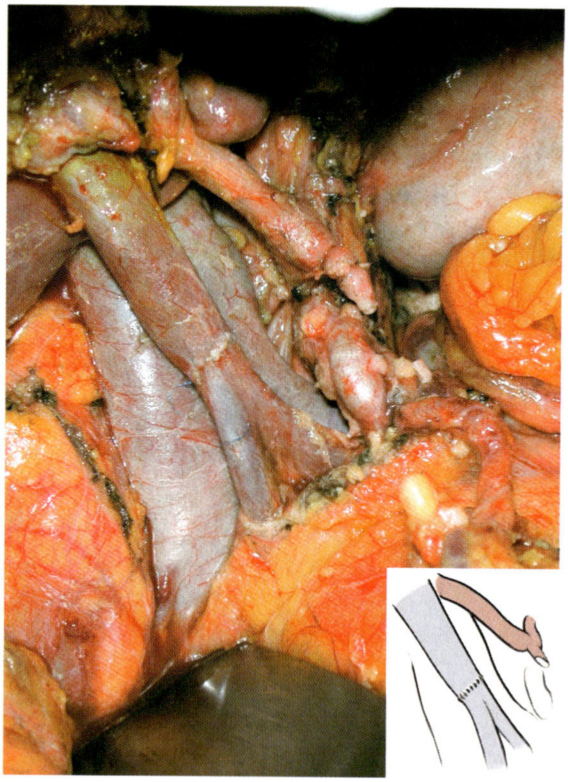

Figure 53.14

Intraoperative picture showing end-to-end reconstruction of sleeve resection of the superior mesenteric vein

associated with lower survival rates (46.4%, 7.7%, and 7.7% at 1, 3, and 5 years, respectively) as compared with tumor invasion limited to the tunica media, adventia, or no actual vein infiltration (62.6%, 19.3%, and 15.5% at 1, 3, and 5 years, respectively; $p = 0.04$; Fig. 53.16). Radical (R_0) resection improved survival as compared with resection with microscopic tumor residual (R_1; Fig. 53.17). Adjuvant chemotherapy also improved survival as compared to no postoperative

Table 53.2. Postoperative complications

Complication	Number	%
Pancreatic fistula	10	9.8
Hemorrhage	6*	5.8
Delayed gastric emptying	4	3.9
Multiple organ failure	3***	2.9
Peripancreatic fluid collection	3	2.9
Nonocclusive portal thrombosis	2	2
Heart attack	2*	2
Respiratory complications	2*	2
Stroke	1	1
Stump pancreatitis	1	1
Brittle diabetes	1	1
Gastric perforation	1	1
TOTAL	**36**	**35.3**

* Mortality

Table 53.3. Tumor histology

Tumor type	Number	%
Pancreatic ductal adenocarcinoma	84	82.3
Distal common bile duct cholangiocarcinoma	3	2.9
Pancreatic neuroendocrine carcinoma	2	1.9
Pancreatic adenosquamous carcinoma	1	0.9
Pancreatic squamous carcinoma	1	0.9
Pancreatic papillary carcinoma	1	0.9
Pancreatic mucinous carcinoma	1	0.9
Pancreatic mucinous cystadenoma	1	0.9
Pancreatic serous cystadenoma	1	0.9
Gall bladder carcinoma	1	0.9
Retroperitoneal sarcoma	1	0.9
Gastrointestinal stromal tumor	1	0.9
Pancreatic metastases from renal cell carcinoma	1	0.9
Pancreatic metastases from testicular seminoma	1	0.9
Gastric carcinoma	1	0.9
Chronic pancreatitis	1	0.9

Table 53.4. Pathology of ductal adenocarcinoma

Characteristic			Number or mean	% or range
Mean tumor diameter			4 cm	1.5–11 cm
Perineural invasion			62	73.8%
Residual tumor	R_0		66	78.6%
	R_1		18	21.4%
	R_2		0	-
Lymph node metastases	N_0		16	19.0%
	N_1		68	80.9%
Stage	I		0	-
	IIa		15	31.2%
	IIb		66	78.6%
	III		0	-
	IV		3	3.6%
Vein invasion[a]	None		29	37.6%
	Proven		48	62.4%
		to the adventitia	8	16.7%
		to the media	23	47.9%
		to the intima[b]	17	35.4%

[a] 77 vein segments examined out of 85 resected
[b] Including four cases with thrombosis

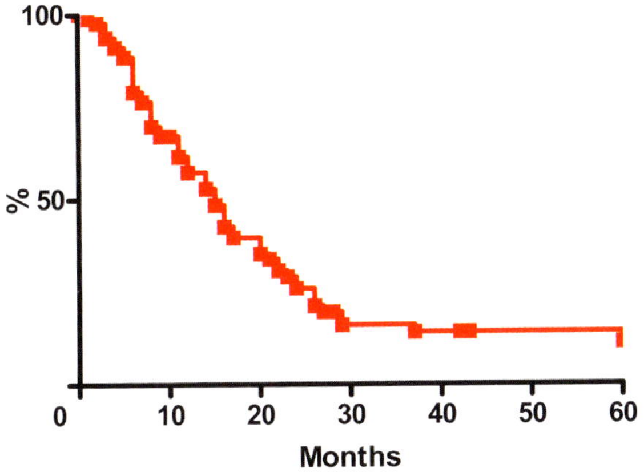

Figure 53.15

Survival curve of patients diagnosed with ductal pancreatic adenocarcinoma undergoing vein resection at the time of pancreatectomy

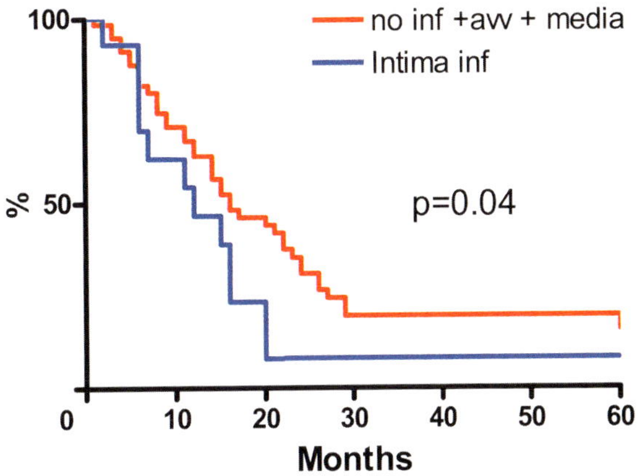

Figure 53.16

Survival curves of patients diagnosed with ductal pancreatic adenocarcinoma categorized on the basis of demonstration of actual tumor invasion and depth of tumor infiltration. *Inf* Infiltration, *aw* adventitia, *media* tunica media, *Intima* tunica intima

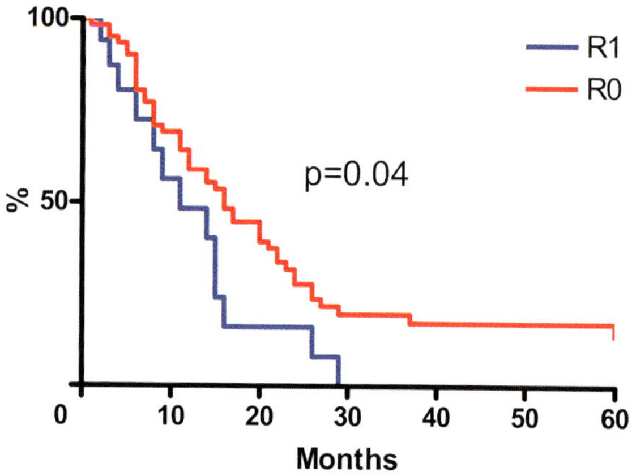

Figure 53.17

Survival curves of patients diagnosed with ductal pancreatic adenocarcinoma categorized on the basis of tumor residual. *R0* No residual tumor, *R1* microscopic residual tumor

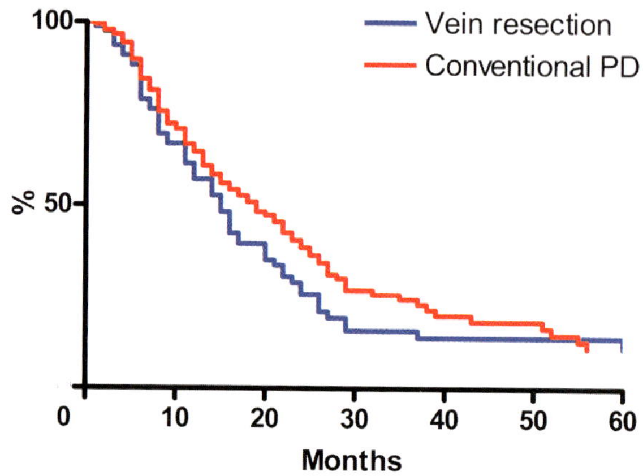

Figure 53.19

Survival curves of patients diagnosed with ductal pancreatic adenocarcinoma undergoing either pancreatectomy *(PD)* alone or pancreatectomy plus vein resection

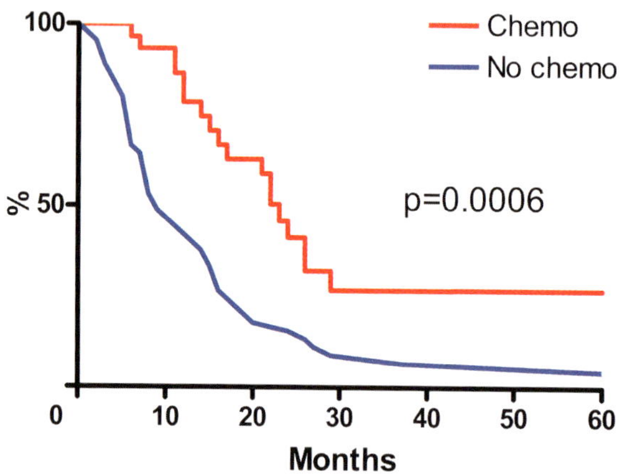

Figure 53.18

Survival curves of patients diagnosed with ductal pancreatic adenocarcinoma categorized on the basis of implementation of adjuvant medical treatment. *Chemo* Chemotherapy

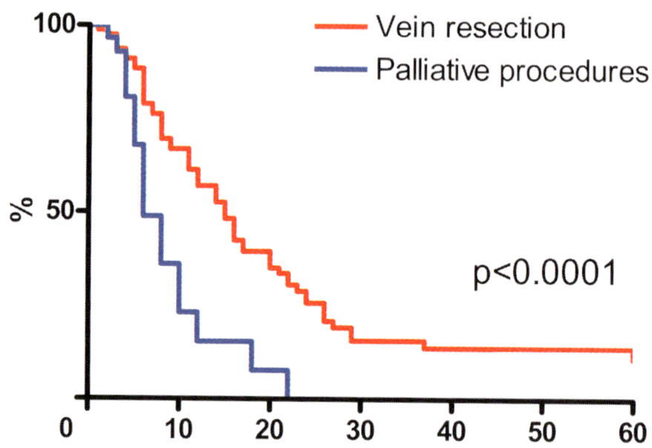

Figure 53.20

Survival curves of patients diagnosed with ductal pancreatic adenocarcinoma undergoing either pancreatectomy plus vein resection or palliation without tumor resection

treatment (Fig. 53.18). Overall, survival of patients requiring vein resection at the time of pancreatectomy was not different from that of contemporary patients undergoing pancreatectomy alone (Fig. 53.19), and was superior to that of patients with tumors of equivalent clinical and surgical stages undergoing bypass palliation or exploratory laparotomy (Fig. 53.20).

For patients diagnosed with tumor types other than ductal adenocarcinoma of the pancreas, survival at 1, 3, and 5 years was 81.9%, 67%, and 43.1%, respectively (median survival time 59 months; Fig. 53.21).

Conclusions

In pancreatic ductal adenocarcinoma the high mortality rate from cancer recurrence makes the distinction between curative and palliative resection inappropriate, even when dealing with small neoplasms thought to be "early" cancers. Nonetheless, most patients do benefit from resection, especially if margin negative (R_0), since tumor removal improves the quality of life [33], prolongs survival [34], and remains the only therapeutic venue that permits cure [35]. Pancreatectomy, however, should not be seen as the only

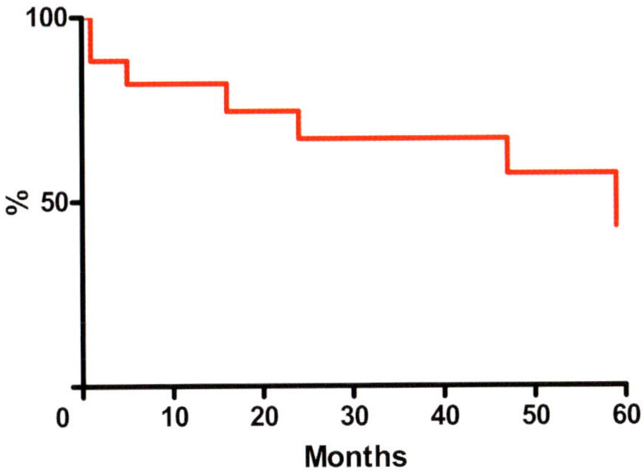

Figure 53.21

Survival curve of patients diagnosed with tumor types other than ductal pancreatic adenocarcinoma undergoing pancreatectomy plus vein resection

treatment of pancreatic cancer, but rather as one of the major steps in a complex treatment plan that includes, and strongly relies on, the implementation of effective adjuvant and/or neoadjuvant regimens. Without effective medical treatment, the difference between resection and palliation could indeed be so poorly defined that the nihilistic paradigm of Crile [36] could still find some advocates. On the contrary, the availability of effective neoadjuvant, adjuvant, and immunotherapy, could broaden current surgical perspectives, making pancreatectomy more beneficial even for patients with locally advanced pancreatic cancers.

While awaiting the availability of new oncologic treatments, however, pancreatic surgeons should continue to realize that the few hopes of cure for patients diagnosed with pancreas cancer begin with margin-negative pancreatectomy. Current data do not allow one to draw any firm conclusion regarding the actual prognostic implications of isolated venous involvement. Thus, resection should be pursued also when vein invasion is suspected, if there is reasonable hope that it can be margin negative. To make this difficult decision, pancreatic surgeons should be familiar with techniques for vascular resection and reconstruction, thus eliminating any interference from technical issues (i.e., practical difficulties in dealing with the large peripancreatic vessels) or fear of increasing the risk of postoperative complications. Moreover, when deciding between resection and palliation, pancreatic surgeons should remember that true vascular invasion is difficult to differentiate from inflammatory adhesions, even by the most sophisticated imaging methods and careful surgical exploration. In addition, in the absence of tissue diagnosis, even differentiating between duct cell adenocarcinoma and other tumor types may be difficult, if not impossible. Paradoxically, a few patients thought to have locally advanced pancreatic cancers may actually have benign pancreatic disease, and final diagnosis may require large, core biopsy specimens that may be difficult to obtain without resection. Misdiagnosing a benign pancreatic disease as an inoperable pancreatic cancer has obvious personal, social, and healthcare consequences that cannot be overemphasized. Our experience not only confirms that not all vascular segments thought to be radiologically and surgically infiltrated have actual tumor ingrowths, but also that not all pancreatic tumors thought to be invasive are malignant. Thus, when dealing with pancreatic malignancies, differentiating between inflammatory and tumoral adhesions, and even between benign and malignant pancreatic tumors, may not be easy or obvious. Despite the current multidisciplinary approach to pancreatic diseases, most of the weight of these decisions remains with the surgeon, since they largely depend on his/her intraoperative judgment. For instance, no final proof can be obtained, either pre- or intraoperatively, that adhesions between pancreatic tumors and the portal-mesenteric vein are neoplastic or inflammatory before trial dissection is carried out. However, especially in the case of adventitial infiltration, even this maneuver cannot accurately differentiate inflammation from superficial tumor invasion. Dissection close to, or within, tumor margins may leave behind an otherwise resectable microscopic tumor. Accordingly, Yeo et al. have reported that the portal margin of pancreatic specimens from patients without suspected vein invasion is microscopically infiltrated in 7% [37]. Ishikawa and co-workers also showed that intraoperative cytology on touch smears of exposed superior mesenteric-portal veins that appeared to be intact at the macroscopic level, demonstrated occult tumor invasion in 30%. Following vein resection, tumor invasion was confirmed in six out of seven patients, being limited to the tunica adventitia in five and extending into the tunica media in one [38]. The approach described herein was developed mostly to face the challenges posed by these borderline cases. Indeed, planned en bloc venous resection is not only technically easier, but also enhances the probability of achieving a R_0 resection as compared with intraoperative methods that are usually more oriented to solve accidental, and often unanticipated, technical problems than to assure margin-negative resection. Accordingly, our results show that pancreatectomy with en-bloc vein resection clearly improves survival when compared to bypass procedures, and it achieves the same results of standard pancreatic resections without vein resection in terms of postoperative complications and long-term survival. The sum of these comparisons demonstrates that en bloc vein resection during pancreatectomy is beneficial. Indeed, it prolongs survival when compared to palliation and it does not worsen the postoperative course when compared with conventional pancreatectomy. Demonstrating a survival benefit in comparison with the latter group of patients would not have been logical. On the contrary, achieving equivalent survival outcomes underscores that, at least in many patients, vein involvement actually reflects the perivascular tumor location and is not a marker of higher tumor grade. Our results, confirmed by other groups [14], do not fully contradict published experiences showing poor survival following vein resection [39]. Indeed, the scanty survival results recorded in several series can be mostly explained by selection bias due to inclusion of patients with overtly incurable cancers, such as those involving multiple vessels [13], or those in whom previously unsuspected venous involvement was managed on demand [40].

The lower grade of periampullary tumors and pancreatic neoplasms, other than ductal adenocarcinoma, makes the outlook of patients diagnosed with these tumor types, and undergoing pancreatectomy with venous resection, clearly valuable and worth pursuing.

References

1. Richter A, Niedergethmann M, Sturm JW, Lorenz D, Post S, Trede M (2003) Long-term results of partial pancreaticoduodenectomy for ductal adenocarcinoma of the pancreatic head: 25-year experience. World J Surg 27:324–329
2. Pawlik TM, Abdalla EK, Barnett CC, Ahmad SA, Cleary KR, Vauthey JN, Lee JE, Evans DB, Pisters PW (2005) Feasibility of a randomized trial of extended lymphadenectomy for pancreatic cancer. Arch Surg 140:584–589; discussion 589–591
3. Picozzi VJ, Kozarek RA, Traverso LW (2003) Interferon-based adjuvant chemoradiation therapy after pancreaticoduodenectomy for pancreatic adenocarcinoma. Am J Surg 185:476–480
4. Bachellier P, Nakano H, Oussoultzoglou E, et al (2001) Is panceaticoduodenectomy with mesentericoportal venous resection safe and worthwhile? Am J Surg 182:120–129
5. Shibata C, Kobari M, Tsuchiya T, et al (2001) Pancreatectomy combined with superior mesenteric portal vein resection for adenocarcinoma of the pancreas. World J Surg 25:1002–1005
6. Nakagohri T, Kinoshita T, Konishi M, et al (2003) Survival benefit of portal vein resection for pancreatic cancer. Am J Surg 186:149–153
7. Hartel M, Niedergethmann M, Farag-Soliman M, et al (2002) Benefit of venous resection for ductal adenocarcinoma of the pancreatic head. Eur J Surg 168:707–712
8. Capussotti L, Massucco P, Ribero D, et al (2003) Extended lymphadenectomy and vein resection for pancreatic head cancer: outcomes and implications for therapy. Arch Surg 138:1316–1322
9. Sasson AR, Hoffman JP, Ross EA, et al (2002) En bloc resection for locally advanced cancer of the pancreas: is it worthwhile? J Gastroint Surg 6:147–158
10. van Greenen RCI, ten Kate MFJW, de Wit LT, et al (2001) Segmental resection and wedge excision of the portal or superior mesenteric vein during pancreatoduodenectomy. Surgery 129:158–163
11. Howard TJ, Villanustre N, Moore SA, et al (2003) Efficacy of venous reconstruction in patients with adenocarcinoma of the pancreatic head. J Gastrointest Surg 7:1089–1095
12. Harrison LE, Klimstra DS, Brennan MF (1996) Isolated portal vein involvement in pancreatic adenocarcinoma. A contraindication for resection? Ann Surg 224:342–3347; discussion 347–349
13. Leach SD, Lee JE, Charnsangavej C, et al (1998) Survival following pancreaticoduodenectomy with resection of the superior mesenteric–portal vein confluence for adenocarcinoma of the pancreatic head. Br J Surg 85:611–617
14. Tseng JF, Raut CP, Lee JE, et al (2004) Pancreaticoduodenectomy with vascular resection: margin status and survival duration. J Gastrointest Surg 8:935–950
15. Lillemoe KD, Cameron JL, Yeo CJ, et al (1996) Pancreaticoduodenectomy: does it have a role in the palliation of pancreatic cancer? Ann Surg 223:718–728
16. Cusack JC, Fuhrman GM, Lee JE, et al (1994) Managing unsuspected tumor invasion of the superior mesenteric–portal venous confluence during pancreaticoduodenectomy. Am J Surg 168:352–354
17. Neoptolemus JP, Stocken DD, Dunn JA, et al (2001) Influence of resection margins on survival for patients with pancreatic cancer treated by adjuvant chemoradiation and/or chemotherapy in ESPAC-1 randomized controlled trial. Ann Surg 234:758–768
18. Pisters PW, Evans DB, Leung DH, et al (2001) Surgery for ductal adenocarcinoma of the pancreatic head. World J Surg 25:533–534
19. Yeo CJ, Cameron JL (2000) The treatment of pancreatic cancer. Ann Chir Gynaecol 89:225–233
20. Launois B, Stasik C, Bardaxoglou E, et al (1999) Who benefits from portal vein resection during pancreaticoduodenectomy for pancreatic cancer? World J Surg 23:926–929
21. Pietrabissa A, Di Candio G, Giulianotti PC, Carobbi A, Boggi U, Mosca F (1996) Operative technique for the laparoscopic staging of pancreatic malignancy. Min Invas Ther Allied Technol 5:274–280
22. Pietrabissa A, Caramella D, Di Candio G, Carobbi A, Boggi U, Rossi G, Mosca F (1999) Laparoscopy and laparoscopic ultrasonography of pancreatic cancer: a critical appraisal. World J Surg 23:998–1002; discussion 1003
23. Fortner JG (1984) Regional pancreatectomy for cancer of the pancreas, ampulla and other related sites. Tumor staging and results. Ann Surg 199:418–425

24. Ishikawa O, Ohigashi H, Imaoka S, et al (1992) Preoperative indications for extended pancreatectomy for locally advanced pancreas cancer involving the portal vein. Ann Surg 215:231–236
25. Nakao A, Harada A, Nonami T, et al (1995) Clinical significance of portal invasion by pancreatic head carcinoma. Surgery 117:50–55
26. Bold RJ, Charnsangavej C, Cleary KR, et al (1999) Major vascular resection as part of pancreaticoduodenectomy for cancer: radiologic, intraoperative, and pathologic analysis. J Gastrointest Surg 3:233–243
27. Mosca F, Giulianotti PC, Balestracci T, et al (1997) Long-term survival in pancreatic cancer: pylorus-preserving versus Whipple pancreatoduodenectomy. Surgery 122:553–566
28. Di Carlo V, Chiesa R, Pontiroli AE, et al (1989) Pancreatoduodenectomy with occlusion of the residual stump by Neoprene injection. World J Surg 13:105–110; discussion 110–111
29. Kubota K, Makuuchi M, Sugawara Y, et al (1998) Reconstruction of the hepatic and portal veins using a patch graft from the right ovarian vein. Am J Surg 176:295–297
30. Harada N, Imaizumi T, Hatori T, Fukuda A, Takasaki K (2000) Extended radical operation for pancreatic head cancer – the role of portal resection. In: Dervenis CG, Bassi C (eds) Pancreatic Tumors Achievements and Perspectives. Georg Thieme, Germany, pp 211–215
31. Kawabata A, Hamanaka Y, Suzuki T (1998) Potentiality of dissection of the lymph nodes with preservation of the nerve plexus around the superior mesenteric artery. Hepatogastroenterology 45:236–241
32. Fortner JG, Kim DK, Cubilla A, et al (1977) Regional pancreatectomy: en bloc pancreatic, portal vein and lymph node resection. Ann Surg 186:42–50
33. Nieveen van Dijkum EJM, Kuhlmann KFD, Terwee CB, et al (2005) Quality of life after curative or palliative surgical treatment of pancreatic and periampullary carcinoma. Br J Surg 92:471–477
34. Yeo CJ, Sohn TA, Cameron JL, et al (1998) Periampullary adenocarcinoma: analysis of 5-year survivors. Ann Surg 227:821–831
35. Conlon KC, Klimstra DS, Brennan MF (1996) Long-term survival after curative resection for pancreatic ductal adenocarcinoma. Clinicopathologic analysis of 5-year survivors. Ann Surg 223:273–279
36. Crile G (1970) The advantages of bypass operations over radical pancreatoduodenectomy in the treatment of pancreatic carcinoma. Surg Gynecol Obstet 130:1049–1053
37. Yeo CJ, Cameron JL, Lillemoe KD, et al (2002) Pancreaticoduodenectomy with or without distal gastrectomy and extended retroperitoneal lymphadenectomy for periampullary adenocarcinoma, part 2: randomized controlled trial evaluating survival, morbidity, and mortality. Ann Surg 236:355–366; discussion 366–368
38. Ishikawa O, Ohigashi H, Sasaki Y, et al (1998) Intraoperative cytodiagnosis for detecting a minute invasion of the portal vein during pancreatoduodenectomy for adenocarcinoma of the pancreatic head. Am J Surg 175:477–481
39. Allema JH, Reinders ME, van Gulik TM et al (1994) Portal vein resection in patients undergoing pancreatoduodenectomy for carcinoma of the pancreatic head. Br J Surg 81:1642–1646
40. Launois B, Franci J, Bardaxoglou E, et al (1993) Total pancreatectomy for ductal adenocarcinoma of the pancreas with special reference to resection of the portal vein and multicentric cancer. World J Surg 17:122–127

Chapter 54

C.P. Raut · G. Varadhachary · H. Wang · E.P. Tamm · J.B. Fleming · D.B. Evans

Margin Status Following Pancreaticoduodenectomy for Pancreatic Adenocarcinoma: Implications of R Status

Margin assessment is necessary to determine the adequacy of resection following pancreaticoduodenectomy. Numerous studies have reported that a positive margin of resection is an independent predictor of poor long-term survival following pancreaticoduodenectomy for pancreatic adenocarcinoma [1–10]. However, most of these studies did not describe the system or technique used for the pathologic evaluation of surgical specimens and, therefore, margin analysis, and did not distinguish margins that were grossly positive from those that were microscopically positive. For studies in which survival duration is an endpoint of analysis, and for all prospective clinical trials, the margin status of resected specimens must be determined. All pancreatic resections should be classified according to residual disease status (termed "R" factor): R0, no gross or microscopic residual disease; R1, microscopic residual disease (microscopically positive surgical margins with no gross residual disease); and R2, grossly evident residual disease [11].

The surgical margins for pancreaticoduodenectomy specimens routinely evaluated by histology include the pancreatic transection margin, the common bile duct (or hepatic duct) transection margin, the gastrointestinal transection margins, and the soft-tissue margin adjacent to the proximal superior mesenteric artery (SMA). We refer to the mesenteric soft tissue and perineural tissue to the right of the proximal 3–4 cm of the SMA as the SMA margin; some refer to this as the retroperitoneal, mesenteric, or uncinate margin (Fig. 54.1) [12]. While the pancreatic and bile duct margins may be re-resected if the intraoperative frozen section analysis suggests a positive margin, the SMA margin cannot be re-resected because in general, surgeons do not resect the SMA for adenocarcinoma. Therefore, the most common margin found to be positive after pancreaticoduodenectomy is the SMA margin [13, 14]. A microscopically positive SMA margin is usually due to perineural and lymphatic invasion along the autonomic plexus surrounding the SMA and celiac axis, and for that reason, R1 resections may occur (and be unavoidable) in up to 10–20% of patients following a grossly negative tumor resection. However, most R2 resections can be avoided by accurate interpretation of the preoperative computed tomography (CT) images.

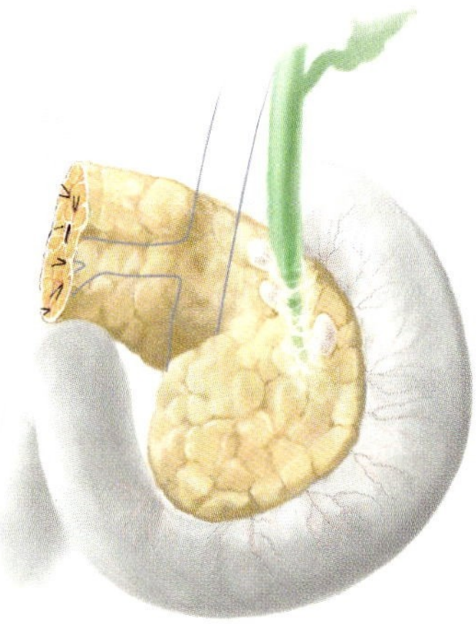

Figure 54.1

Illustration of a pancreaticoduodenectomy specimen demonstrating how the superior mesenteric artery (SMA) margin should be inked at the time of permanent section pathologic examination. This margin cannot be retrospectively evaluated if the margin was not inked for identification at the time of gross inspection. *SMPV* Superior mesenteric portal vein

The pathologist cannot usually differentiate an R1 (microscopically positive) from an R2 (grossly positive) SMA margin in the absence of information regarding the retroperitoneal dissection, which should be included in the operative dictation. The R designation should always be listed in the dictated operative report by having the surgeon wait to sign-off on the operative report until the pathology report is available for review and therefore the status of the SMA margin determined. For example, if the surgeon states that gross tumor was encountered when completing the SMA dissection, a positive histologic margin should result in the R2 designation in the operative report and the medical record. If the surgeon states (in the operative report) that there was no gross evidence of tumor extension to the SMA margin, then a positive histologic margin should result in the R1 designation in the operative report and the medical record.

The Importance of Preoperative Diagnostic Imaging

Preoperative evaluation of the patient with suspected or biopsy-proven pancreatic cancer includes physical examination, routine laboratory testing, chest radiography, and contrast-enhanced, thin-section, dual-phase (pancreatic parenchymal and portal venous phase) multislice CT of the abdomen with images of the pelvis to evaluate for peritoneal disease. The CT criteria utilized at our institution to define a potentially resectable pancreatic tumor include the absence of tumor extension to the SMA, celiac axis, and common hepatic artery (CHA), and a patent superior mesenteric portal vein (SMPV) confluence (Table 54.1) [15]. This implies a normal tissue plane between the tumor and adjacent arterial structures (Fig. 54.2), and the technical ability to resect and reconstruct the SMPV confluence if the tumor cannot be separated from the SMV or portal vein (PV) [16]. Locally advanced, surgically unresectable tumors are defined as those that encase the celiac axis and/or SMA or that occlude the superior mesenteric vein (SMV), PV, or SMPV confluence (Fig. 54.3). We have defined the term "encasement" to describe a vessel–tumor relationship in which a tumor is inseparable from the vessel for >180° of the circumference of the vessel. We use the term "abutment" to describe a vessel–tumor relationship in which a tumor is inseparable from the vessel for ≤180° of the circumference of the vessel.

With recent advances in pancreatic imaging, the distinction between resectable (stage I or II) and locally advanced (stage III) disease may be difficult or

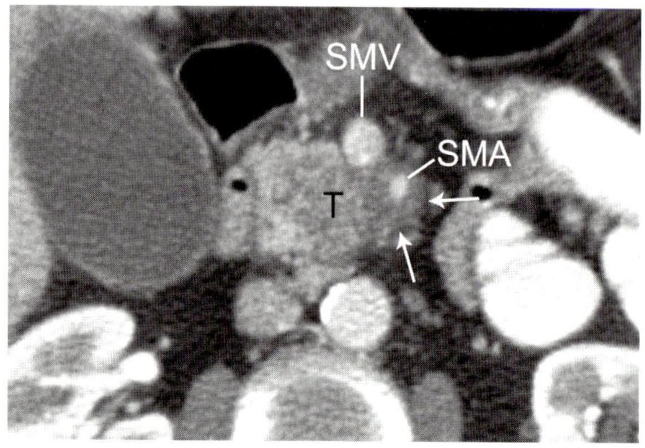

Figure 54.2

Axial contrast-enhanced computed tomography (CT) image from the pancreatic parenchymal phase of a resectable pancreatic cancer (*long white arrows*) that contacts (*short white arrow*) the superior mesenteric vein (SMV) but is separated from the SMA by an intact tissue plane (*white arrowhead*). Resection and reconstruction of a portion of the SMV may be necessary. A biliary stent (*ST*) is also present

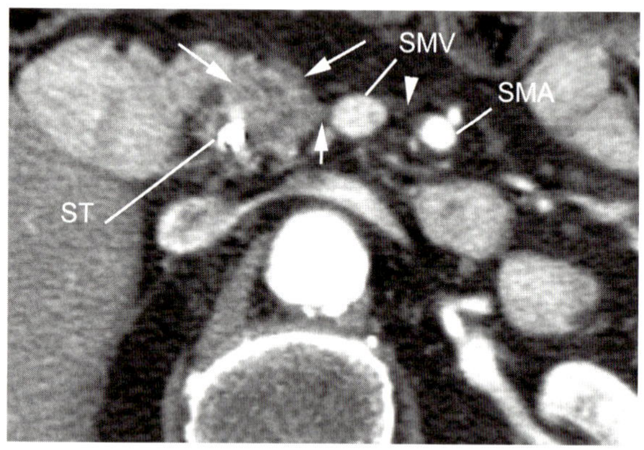

Figure 54.3

Axial contrast-enhanced CT image of a locally advanced pancreatic cancer (*black T*) due to encasement of the SMA. The medial extent of the tumor is identified by the *arrows*. The SMV is anterior and lateral to the SMA

Table 54.1. M.D. Anderson definitions for the preoperative staging of localized pancreatic cancer. *SMA* Superior mesenteric artery, *SMV/PV* superior mesenteric vein/portal vein

Vessel	Resectable	Borderline resectable	Locally advanced
SMA	Normal tissue plane between tumor and vessel	Tumor abutment ≤180° or ≤50% of the circumference of the artery	Tumor encasement (>180°)
Celiac axis/ common hepatic artery	Normal tissue plane between tumor and vessel	Short-segment encasement or abutment of the common hepatic artery (typically at the gastroduodenal origin)	Tumor encasement (>180°) of the celiac axis
SMV/PV	Patent SMV/PV confluence	Short-segment occlusion with suitable vessel above and below to allow for resection and reconstruction	Occlusion with no technical option for reconstruction

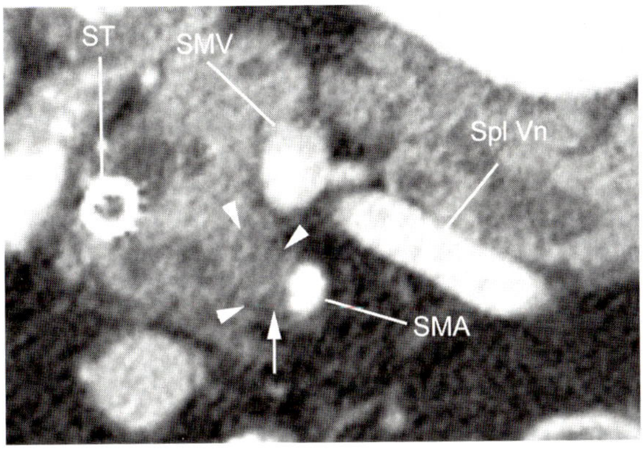

Figure 54.4

Axial contrast-enhanced CT image of a borderline resectable pancreatic cancer. The tumor (*white arrowheads*) abuts the SMA over approximately 135–180° of the circumference of the artery (see the area identified by the *arrow*). A metallic wall stent is present in the common bile duct. *Spl Vn* Splenic vein

blurred in selected cases, and the term "borderline resectable" is emerging to define these tumors. Our criteria for borderline resectable pancreatic cancer includes patients whose tumors exhibit "short segment" encasement of the hepatic artery, without celiac axis involvement (typically at the level of the gastroduodenal artery, GDA), that is amenable to resection and reconstruction; abutment of the SMA involving ≤180° of the circumference of the artery (Fig. 54.4); or short-segment occlusion of the SMV, PV, or SMPV confluence with a patent SMV below and patent PV above the area of tumor involvement to allow for vascular reconstruction if necessary. A patient with borderline resectable pancreatic head cancer is at especially high risk for a margin-positive resection with surgery alone. Therefore, we routinely utilize a multimodality approach to such patients involving chemotherapy or chemoradiation prior to surgery [17].

The development of multislice or multidetector CT (MDCT) allows imaging of the entire pancreas during peak contrast enhancement. In addition, scan data can be processed to display images in three-dimensional and multiplanar formats. Helical CT performed with contrast enhancement and a thin-section technique can accurately assess the relationship of the low-density tumor to the celiac axis, SMA, and SMPV confluence. For MDCT scanning at our institution, patients receive 1,000 ml of water or a 2% barium sulfate suspension (Readi-CAT; E-Z-EM, Westbury, NY, USA) to opacify the stomach and small bowel. Non-contrast-enhanced CT scans are then obtained through the liver and pancreas at a slice thickness of 5 mm to localize the pancreas. Intravenous (IV) contrast enhancement is achieved with nonionic contrast material (300–320 mg iodine/ml) administered by an automatic injector at a rate of 3–5 ml/s for a total of 150 ml. At least two phases of contrast-enhanced helical scanning are performed. On a 16-detector-row MDCT scanner, the first (pancreatic parenchymal) phase begins 36 s after contrast injection and is performed during a 10-s breathhold, with imaging obtained from the diaphragm through the horizontal portion of the duodenum at a slice thickness of 2.5 mm contiguous, reconstructed to 1.25-mm slice thickness every 0.625 mm for multiplanar reconstructions. Imaging during this first phase includes the pancreas at 40–46 s after contrast injection, which, at this rate of contrast injection, optimizes the difference in density between the pancreas and tumor (pancreatic parenchymal phase). The second (venous) phase, which is performed to look for metastases in the liver and abdomen, begins 60 s after the start of IV contrast injection and covers the entire liver and upper abdomen at a 2.5-mm slice thickness, which is then reconstructed to a 1.25-mm slice thickness every 0.625 mm.

The main limitation of multidetector CT is its low sensitivity for low-volume hepatic or peritoneal metastases. Studies suggest that up to 20% of patients who are thought to have resectable disease preoperatively actually have CT-occult metastatic disease found at laparoscopy or laparotomy. This number will vary depending on the quality of the CT images and the definitions used for local tumor resectability; high-quality images and precise, objective definitions of which tumors are resectable and which are locally advanced will minimize the potential for nontherapeutic laparotomies.

Surgical Considerations for Standard Pancreaticoduodenectomy and Extended Resections

The most important factors to consider prior to performing pancreaticoduodenectomy for adenocarcinoma are careful patient selection, apparent tumor biology, and relevant surgical anatomy and technique. The first of these factors, patient selection, comprises both patient- and tumor-related issues. Surgery should only be considered in patients with an Eastern Cooperative Oncology Group performance status of 0 or 1 and adequate end organ function to tolerate a major abdominal operation and potential complications. For example, it would be uncommon to con-

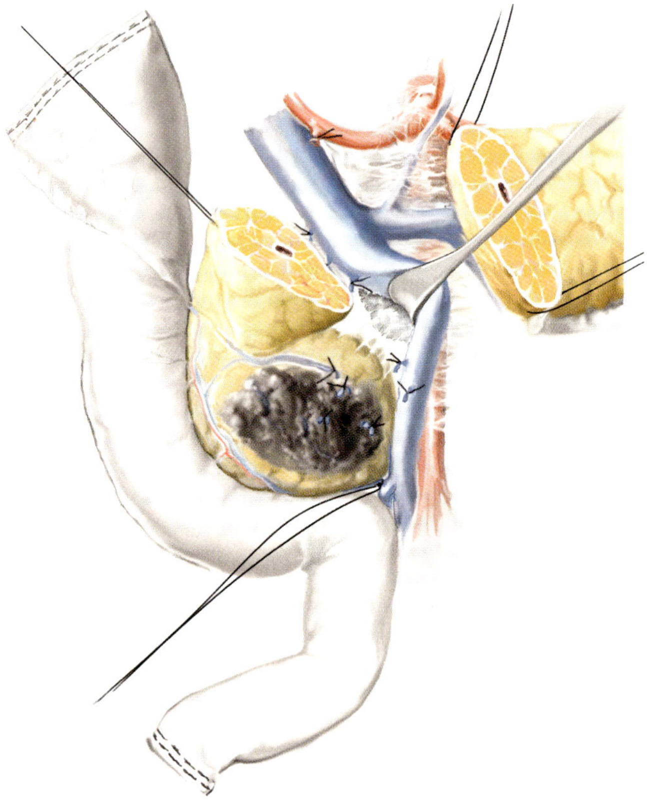

Figure 54.5

Illustration of the important surgical anatomy of the SMV at the level of the uncinate process. The SMV usually bifurcates into two main branches, one to the ileum and one to the jejunum. Adequate venous return from the small bowel requires that one or the other of these two main tributaries of the SMV is intact. The jejunal branch of the SMV (often referred to as the first jejunal branch) drains the proximal jejunum, travels posterior to the SMA, and enters the SMV along its posterolateral wall. The jejunal branch usually has a few venous tributaries that drain the uncinate process (*inset*). If necessary, the jejunal branch can be divided. Very rarely, the jejunal branch will travel anterior to the SMA

sider pancreaticoduodenectomy in a patient with significant cardiac, pulmonary, or renal comorbidities. Tumor-related factors are based on high-quality CT imaging, as discussed above. Importantly, if preoperative imaging suggests increased surgical complexity, one must ensure that the condition of the patient is suitable for increased operative time, blood loss, and potential hemodynamic fluctuations.

A second factor that must be considered is tumor biology. Outcomes may be affected by the size and local extent of the primary tumor, the presence or absence of suspicious regional lymph nodes, and the serum level of CA19-9. When the tumor biology is unfavorable (high CA19-9, tumor of borderline resectability), the delivery of systemic therapy with or without radiation therapy should be considered. One distinct advantage of a neoadjuvant treatment approach is to provide a sufficient time interval to assess the underlying tumor biology, thereby allowing for the selection of patients for surgery who have the highest likelihood of benefiting from pancreaticoduodenectomy. Neoadjuvant therapy also provides for potential downstaging (sterilizing the vessel/tumor interface) to maximize the chance for an R0/R1 resection. In addition, chemotherapy with or without radiation therapy, delivered before surgery, is often better tolerated, as surgical recovery does not complicate the delivery of treatment.

Finally, in considering surgical anatomy and technique, one must accurately analyze important tumor–vessel relationships prior to surgery, and have the technical ability to perform the maneuvers required to complete the planned operation. For example, if the tumor is inseparable from the posterolateral wall of the SMV on contrast-enhanced CT, it is a mistake to proceed with operation unless the surgeon has a strategy for vascular resection and the technical ability to remove part of the SMV and repair the vessel.

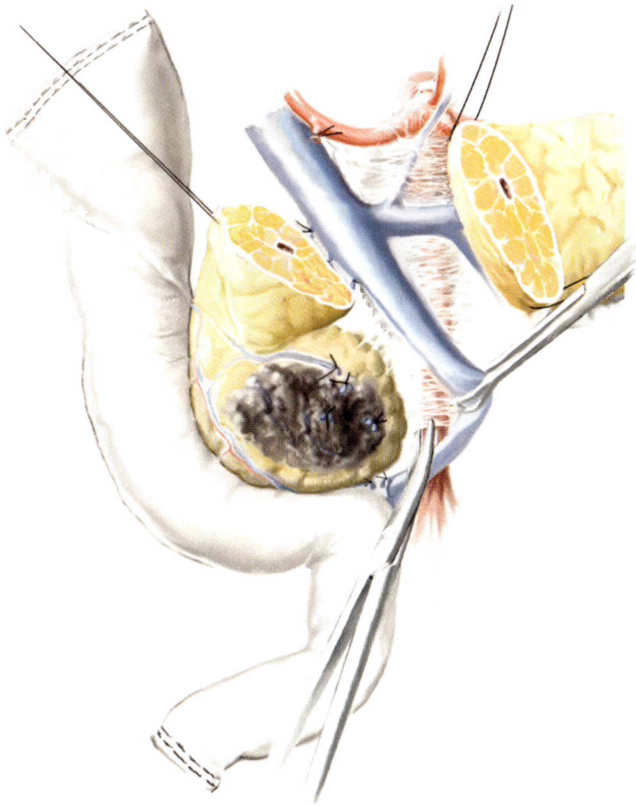

Figure 54.6

Illustration of the final step in resection of the specimen. Medial retraction of the SMPV confluence facilitates dissection of the soft tissues adjacent to the lateral wall of the proximal SMA; this site represents the SMA margin. The inferior pancreaticoduodenal artery (or arteries) is identified at its origin from the SMA, ligated, and divided

Contemporary CT images are extremely accurate in determining the extent of regional vascular involvement. The surgical plan can be precisely delineated prior to laparotomy, at which time the surgeon then needs to determine whether he or she has the technical ability to perform the operation required. Once the decision is made to proceed with the laparotomy and the abdomen is opened, there should be few instances when the primary tumor is determined to be unresectable for local reasons. In short, unresectability can be accurately determined by preoperative imaging.

The most important technical aspect of the pancreaticoduodenectomy operation is the final step in removal of the pancreatic head and uncinate process from the mesenteric vessels. Following pancreatic transection, proper mobilization of the SMV involves identification of the jejunal branch of the SMV (referred to by some as the first jejunal branch). This branch originates from the right posterolateral aspect of the SMV (at the level of the uncinate process), travels posterior to the SMA, and enters the medial (proximal) aspect of the jejunal mesentery [14]. Very rarely, the jejunal branch may course anterior to the SMA. The jejunal branch usually gives off one or two venous tributaries to the uncinate process; these tributaries should be divided (Fig. 54.5). Medial retraction of the SMPV confluence allows one to expose the SMA (Fig. 54.6). The specimen is then separated from the right lateral wall of the SMA, which is dissected to its origin at the aorta. Complete removal of the uncinate process from the SMV is required for full mobilization of the SMPV confluence and subsequent identification of the SMA. Failure to fully mobilize the SMPV confluence risks injury to the SMA and usually results in a positive margin of resection due to incomplete removal of the uncinate process and the mesenteric soft tissue adjacent to the SMA. Exposure of the SMA is necessary for direct ligation of the inferior pancreaticoduodenal arteries (usually two of them). Mass ligation of this vessel (or vessels) with mesenteric soft tissue is the major cause of postopera-

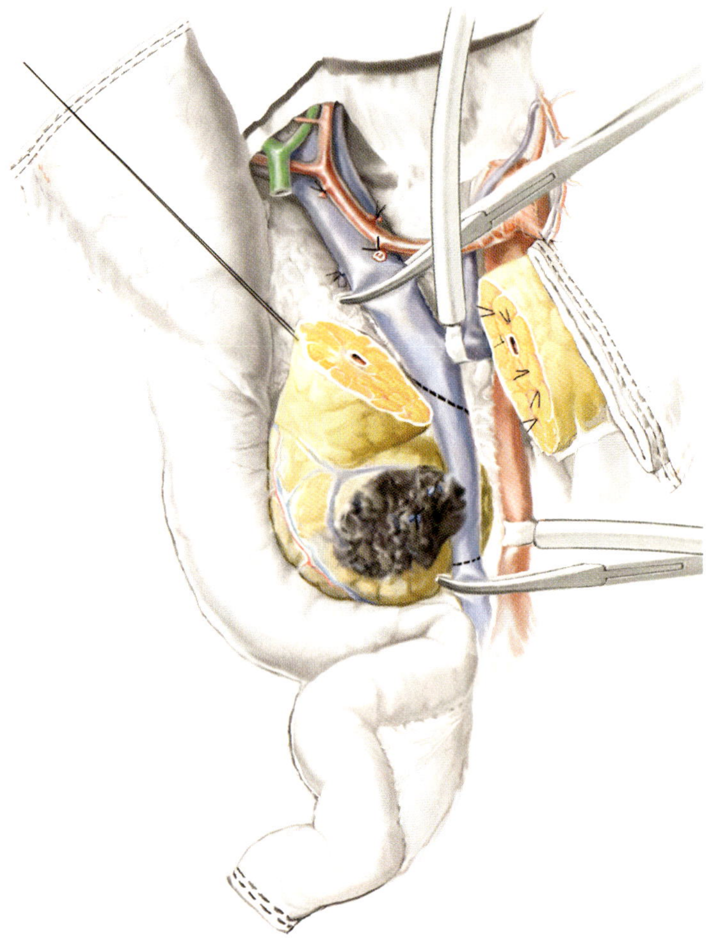

Figure 54.7.

Illustration of resection of the SMV with preservation of the splenic vein. The intact splenic vein tethers the portal vein, making a primary anastomosis impossible in most cases. With the splenic vein intact, one cannot complete the dissection of the specimen from the right lateral border of the SMA to the origin of this vessel in standard fashion. Therefore, options include either placing the graft prior to specimen removal, or separation of the pancreatic head first from the SMA by medial rotation of the specimen

tive retroperitoneal hemorrhage, as this vessel retracts from its poorly placed tie or ligature. The perineural and mesenteric tissue along the proximal SMA represents the SMA margin.

It is important to emphasize the distinction between regional pancreatectomy and pancreaticoduodenectomy with vascular resection and reconstruction as applied to patients with resectable and borderline resectable pancreatic cancer. We do not consider venous or arterial resection as an attempt to improve en-bloc lymphatic and soft-tissue clearance, as is performed in regional pancreatectomy [18]. It is unlikely that larger local-regional resections (to the left of the SMA and celiac axis) in poorly selected patients with advanced disease will impact survival. Vascular resection should be performed only in carefully selected patients who have resectable or borderline resectable disease as defined on high-quality CT and described above.

The need for venous resection should be anticipated whenever the tumor is inseparable from the SMPV confluence on preoperative CT imaging. Data from our institution have demonstrated that the need for venous resection at the time of pancreaticoduodenectomy does not influence survival duration [16]. However, this assumes that venous resection and reconstruction is performed only in patients with tumors that are otherwise resectable – meaning that there is no evidence of tumor extension to the celiac axis or SMA. The standard technique for segmental venous

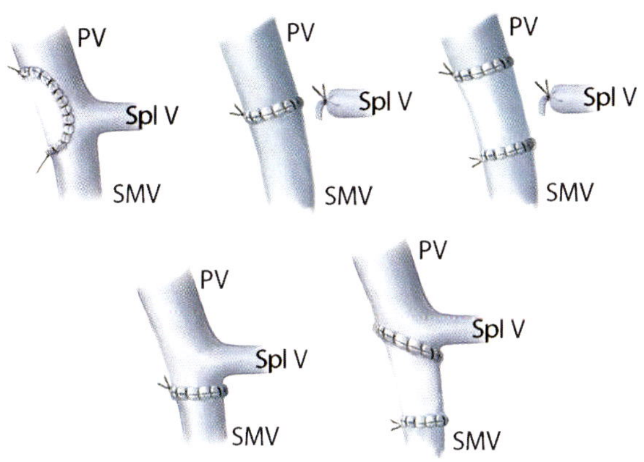

Figure 54.8

Illustration of the different types of venous reconstruction used at the time of pancreaticoduodenectomy. When a patch is needed we use the saphenous vein and when an interposition graft is needed we commonly use the left internal jugular vein (*IJ*). *PV* Portal vein. Modified from reference [16]

resection involves transection of the splenic vein. Division of the splenic vein allows complete exposure of the SMA medial to the SMV and provides increased SMV and PV length (as they are no longer tethered by the splenic vein) for a primary venous anastomosis following segmental vein resection. The retroperitoneal dissection is then completed by sharply dividing the soft tissues anterior to the aorta and to the right of the exposed SMA; the specimen is then attached only by the SMPV confluence. A generous 2- to 3-cm segment of SMPV confluence can be resected without the need for interposition grafting if the splenic vein is divided. Venous resection is always performed with inflow occlusion of the SMA, and systemic heparinization is usually employed prior to occluding the SMA. We have seen upper gastrointestinal hemorrhage due to sinistral portal hypertension following splenic vein ligation. This usually results when the splenic, inferior mesenteric, and left gastric veins are ligated. Mobilization of the pancreatic neck often results in ligation of the left gastric vein. If the inferior mesenteric vein enters the portion of SMV to be resected, then this vessel will also be divided. When the inferior mesenteric vein enters the splenic vein, it provides a route for collateral venous flow (when the splenic vein is divided) out of the splenic vein in a retrograde fashion; division of the splenic vein in this situation is usually well tolerated. We currently preserve the splenic vein–PV junction whenever possible (Fig. 54.7), especially if the inferior mesenteric vein needs to be ligated and divided. Splenic vein preservation is possible only when tumor invasion of the SMV or PV does not involve the splenic vein confluence. Preservation of the splenic vein–SMPV confluence significantly limits mobilization of the PV and prevents primary anastomosis of the SMV (following segmental SMV resection) unless segmental resection is limited to 2 cm or less. Therefore, in most patients who undergo SMV resection with splenic vein preservation, an interposition graft is required. Our preferred conduit for interposition grafting is the internal jugular vein (Fig. 54.8). Preservation of the splenic vein adds significant complexity to venous resection because it prevents direct access to the most proximal 3–4 cm of the SMA (medial to the SMV). Venous resection and reconstruction can be performed either before the specimen has been separated from the right lateral wall of the SMA or after complete mesenteric dissection by separating the specimen first from the SMA (currently our preferred approach). Both techniques require significant experience with pancreaticoduodenectomy and should only be performed by surgeons who are experienced in vascular resection and reconstruction at the time of pancreaticoduodenectomy.

In general, we limit arterial resection and reconstruction to the CHA, or resection (with or without reconstruction) of the right or left hepatic arteries in the setting of aberrant hepatic arterial anatomy. Segmental resection of the CHA may be considered when isolated arterial encasement is present usually occurring at the origin of GDA origin. The CHA-proper hepatic artery region is usually quite redundant and a primary anastomosis is often possible when the region of the GDA origin is resected. Occasionally, an interposition graft with reversed saphenous vein is required. Because the right and left hepatic arteries communicate within the liver, ligation of the right hepatic artery should be tolerated assuming a normal level of serum bilirubin and normal flow in the PV. However, because the proximal bile duct receives virtually all of its arterial supply from the right hepatic artery following interruption of cephalad flow from the GDA, we usually revascularize this vessel. The right hepatic artery may be encased by tumor when it arises from the celiac axis (with an early bifurcation and a low-lying right hepatic) or if it arises from the SMA. A replaced right hepatic artery arising from the SMA, unlike an accessory right hepatic artery, represents the only direct arterial inflow to the right hepatic lobe. While a right hepatic artery arising from the SMA is prone to tumor encasement at the posterosuperior border of the pancreatic head, pancreaticoduodenectomy in this situation often does not require removal of this vessel because the majority of resectable tumors are located more anteriorly in the pancreatic head or uncinate process. Rarely, the entire CHA may arise from the SMA (type IX); failure to recognize this anatomic variant and inadvertent ligation of the hepatic artery requires repair.

As multimodality therapy becomes more frequently applied to patients with more advanced (local) disease, such as those with borderline resectable pancreatic head cancer, the operative management will become more complicated from both a technical perspective and with regard to the impact of systemic therapies and radiation on the techniques of surgical resection and reconstruction. For example, if the radiation therapy is not done with careful attention to field size and technique, adjacent tissue effects may greatly complicate vascular dissection. In addition, the use of newer, targeted therapies may have implications for wound healing and the risk for intraoperative and postoperative hemorrhage. The recent advances in systemic therapy and radiation therapy techniques have major implications for the surgeon, making it even more important that complicated pancreatic cancer patients be treated by a multidisciplinary working group of experienced physicians.

Pathologic Assessment of the Pancreaticoduodenectomy Specimen

The template for the pathology reporting of pancreaticoduodenectomy specimens currently used at our institution appears in Table 54.2. Such templates are necessary to allow accurate transfer of pathologic data to prospective databases. The pathologic evaluation of the pancreaticoduodenectomy specimen begins with frozen-section analysis of the pancreatic

Table 54.2. Synoptic pathology template used at

M.D. Anderson Cancer Center for reporting of pancreaticoduodenectomy specimens
Specimen: Pancreaticoduodenectomy
Tumor Diagnosis: Histologic type of the tumor
Degree of Differentiation: well/moderate/poor
The tumor size: the maximal dimension in centimeters
Extrapancreatic extension: present/absent
Lymphovascular invasion: present/absent
Perineural invasion: present/absent
Retroperitoneal (SMA) margin status: positive/negative (if negative, the distance to inked margin in millimeters)
Bile duct margin status: positive/negative
Pancreatic transection margin status: positive/negative
Proximal stomach or duodenum margin status: positive/negative
Distal duodenum or jejunum margin status: positive/negative
Regional Lymph Nodes:
Total number of positive lymph nodes
Total number of lymph nodes examined
If vessel resection performed:
Name of the vessel removed
Presence or absence of vessel invasion and the layer of vessel wall involved:
perivascular connective tissue/vessel wall/into the lumen
Vascular resection margin status
Degree of treatment effect (if patient received preoperative therapy): reported as a
percentage of viable tumor cells, classified as <10%, 10–50%, 50–90%, >90%*
Final pTNM Staging (American Joint Committee on Cancer 6th edition):
pT: T1/T2/T3
pN: N0/N1
pMX: Distant metastasis

* Adapted from Evans et al. 1992 [23]

and common hepatic/bile duct transection margins, both of which are submitted en-face. Positive resection margins on the hepatic/bile duct or pancreas should be resected to a negative margin if possible. Complete permanent-section analysis of the pancreaticoduodenectomy specimen (Fig. 54.1) requires that it be oriented with the pathologist to accurately identify and assess the SMA margin of excision and other standard pathologic variables. Because we remove all tissue to the right of the SMA, further resection at the SMA/retroperitoneal margin is not possible. However, this margin must be identified and inked with the pathologist; it cannot be assessed retrospectively. The SMA margin of excision is then sectioned serially, perpendicular to the inked margin and entirely submitted for histologic examination after overnight fixation in 10% buffered formalin. If the SMA transection margin is negative, the closest distance from the inked SMA transection margin to tumor is then measured microscopically and reported in the final pathology report for all pancreaticoduodenectomy specimens.

Infiltrating ductal adenocarcinoma is the most common histologic type of pancreatic cancer. Grossly, ductal adenocarcinomas form firm, poorly defined masses with yellow to white cut surfaces, which obliterate the lobular architecture of the normal pancreas. The histology of well-differentiated ductal adenocarcinoma is characterized by well-formed large or medium-sized glands, often with a haphazard growth pattern. The glands are lined by cuboidal or columnar epithelial cells with basally located nuclei. Cytologic atypia and nuclear pleomorphism are often minimal. Distinguishing well-differentiated ductal adenocarcinoma from benign reactive glands can be extremely difficult. Close attention must be paid to the growth pattern and location of the glands and the cytologic details (nuclear pleomorphism within individual glands). Findings of vascular invasion, perineural invasion, or glands next to muscular arteries without intervening pancreatic parenchyma are diagnostic for carcinoma. Other helpful features in establishing the diagnosis of an adenocarcinoma include incomplete glandular formation, intraluminal necrotic debris, and loss of DPC4 protein expression, which is detected in about half of pancreatic ductal adenocarcinomas, but not in reactive benign ductal epithelium. Compared with well-differentiated ductal adenocarcinomas, incomplete glandular formation, greater variation in nuclear size, chromatin pattern, and prominence of nucleoli, and mitosis are more commonly seen in moderately differentiated ductal carcinomas. The neoplastic glands vary in size and shape and have abundant desmoplastic stroma. Poorly differentiated ductal carcinomas are composed of poorly formed glands, individual infiltrating tumor cells in desmoplastic stroma, and solid nests and sheets of tumor cells. The neoplastic cells often show marked pleomorphism, brisk mitotic activity, and little or no mucin production (Fig. 54.9).

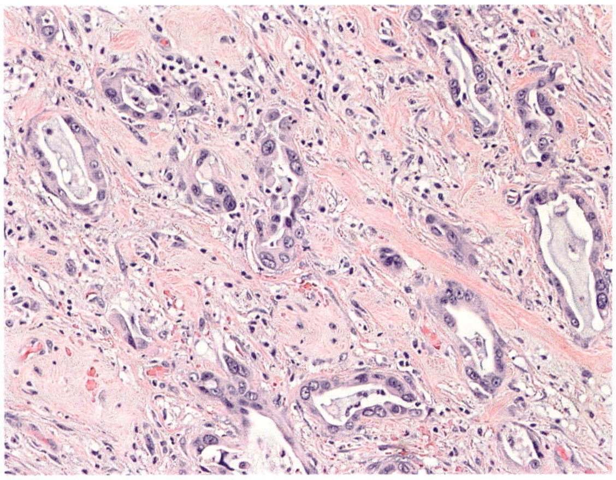

Figure 54.9

Moderately differentiated pancreatic ductal adenocarcinoma with intraluminal mucin and abundant dense desmoplastic stroma (hematoxylin and eosin, H&E, stain; original magnification ×100)

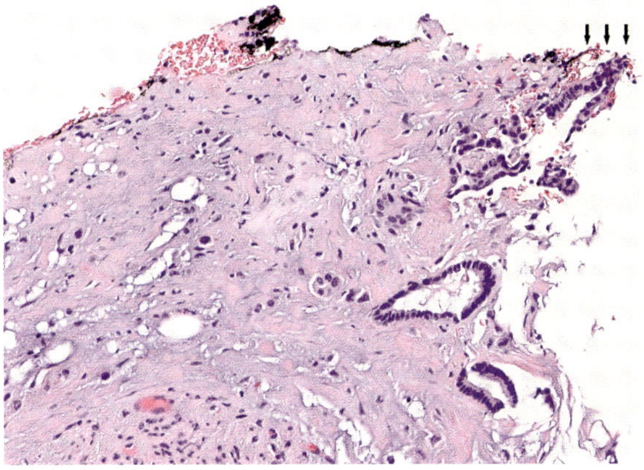

Figure 54.10

Positive SMA margin in a moderately-differentiated pancreatic ductal adenocarcinoma Black ink marks the SMA margin. The tumor cells are focally present at the inked SMA margin (marked with arrow) (H & E stain, original magnification 100x)

Tumor infiltration into perineural spaces is commonly seen in pancreatic adenocarcinoma. This is an important consideration because the SMA is surrounded by a neural plexus that provides visceral innervation to the small intestine. This neural plexus extends proximally to the celiac ganglion, which surrounds the aorta at and above the level of the celiac artery. Not surprisingly, therefore, infiltration of this mesenteric neural plexus is characteristic of pancreatic adenocarcinoma once it involves the SMA (Fig. 54.10).

Recent Results from the M.D. Anderson Cancer Center

We recently reported an analysis of 360 patients who underwent pancreaticoduodenectomy for adenocarcinoma of pancreatic origin in an effort to examine the impact of a microscopically positive resection margin (R1) on patterns of disease recurrence and survival [19]. Most patients received preoperative and/or postoperative chemotherapy and/or chemoradiation that included either protocol-based or off-protocol treatment. Concomitant chemotherapy included 5-fluorouracil, paclitaxel, gemcitabine, or capecitabine [20–22]. Chemotherapy given before or after chemoradiation consisted of gemcitabine alone or in combination. Patients were followed for a minimum of 12 months postoperatively or until death (if sooner). Follow-up consisted of physical examination, laboratory studies, and CT imaging at 3- to 4-month intervals for the first 2 years postoperatively, at 6-month intervals for years 3–5, and then at yearly intervals. The first site or sites of disease recurrence were classified as local, regional, or distant. Local recurrence was defined as recurrence in the region of the pancreatic bed and root of the mesentery. Regional recurrence was defined as recurrence in the soft tissues or lymph nodes beyond the pancreatic bed or within the peritoneal cavity (including ascites and/or wound implants). Distant recurrence was defined as recurrence in the liver, lungs, or other distant organs. Radiographic findings consistent with recurrent disease were considered adequate proof of recurrence; tissue confirmation was rarely obtained. Only first sites of recurrence were documented.

Resection margins were histologically positive (R1) in 60 (16.7%) and negative (R0) in 300 (83.3%) of the 360 patients. The SMA margin was positive in 53 (88.3%) of 60 patients with R1 resections; the remaining 7 patients (11.7%) had isolated positive pancreatic transection margins. Among the 53 patients with positive SMA margins, 5 also had other positive margins: 3 positive pancreatic transection margins, 1 positive bile duct transection margin, and 1 positive pancreatic and bile duct transection margins. Logistic regression was used to determine which covariates were significantly associated with an R1 resection. Operative blood loss (per 100 ml), the need for vascular resection, and tumor size were statistically significant by univariate analyses. When adjusting for these factors in a backward stepwise fashion, only operative blood loss (odds ratio, OR=1.03, 95% confidence interval, CI=1.01–1.06) and tumor size (OR=1.42, 95% CI=1.09–1.84) were associated with an R1 resection.

Table 54.3. Summary of studies evaluating the impact of margin status on survival. *R0* Margins grossly and microscopically negative, *R1* margins grossly negative but microscopically positive, *R2* margins grossly positive, *NA* not available

Author (year)	No. of patients (%)[a]	Resection status	Median R1/R2 survival (months)	Median R0 survival (months)
Raut (2006) [19]	60 (16.7)	R1	22	28
Neoptolemos (2001) [4]	101 (19)	R1	11	17
Benassai (2000) [1]	15 (20)	R1, R2	9	17
Sohn (2000) [7]	184 (30)	R1	12	19
Millikan (1999) [3]	22 (29)	R1	8	17
Nishimura (1997) [5]	70 (45)	R1, R2	6	12
Sperti (1996) [8]	19 (17)	R1, R2	7	14
Nitecki (1995) [6]	28 (16)	R2	9	NA
Yeo (1995) [10]	58 (29)	R1, R2	10	18
Willett (1993) [9]	37 (51)	R1	12	20
Gall (1991) [2]	47 (34)	R1, R2	7	11

[a] Number of patients (percentage) in study with R1 and/or R2 resections

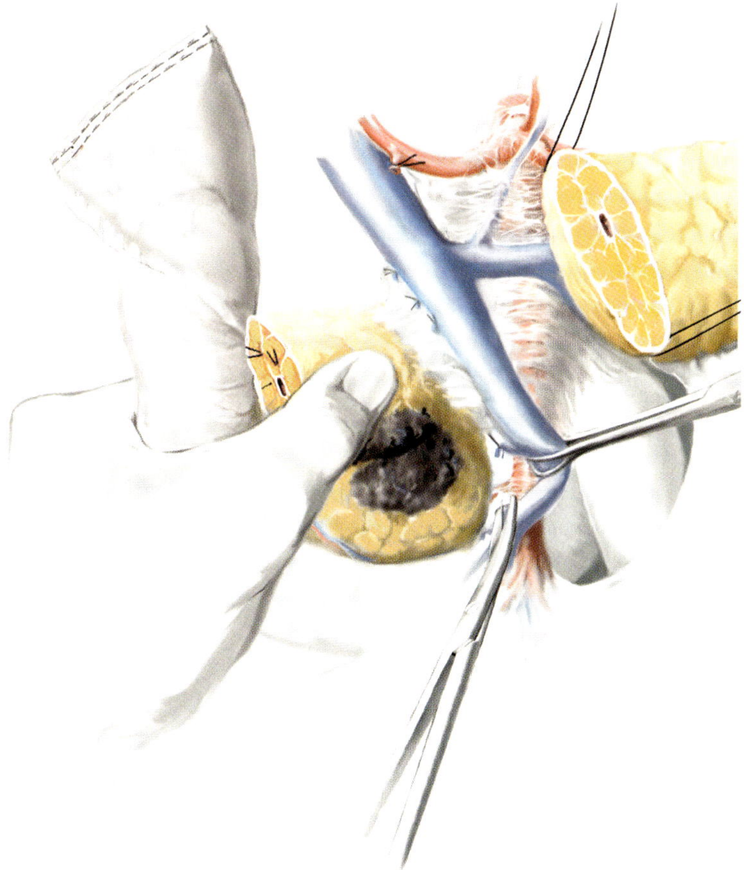

Figure 54.11

Illustration of attempted removal of the pancreaticoduodenectomy specimen from the mesenteric vessels without mobilization of the SMV and direct identification of the SMA. This technique may result is an SMA injury, and inadequate control of the inferior pancreaticoduodenal arteries due to their mass ligation with adjacent soft tissue. SMA injury and postoperative hemorrhage are avoidable complications if the SMA is routinely exposed for identification (rather than the surgeon relying on palpation). This technique also facilitates a complete retroperitoneal/mesenteric dissection, minimizing the potential for a margin-positive resection

The median survival for the 360 patients was 25.4 months. Log-rank tests were used to compare Kaplan-Meier survival curves for each prognostic factor of interest. On univariate analysis, lymph node metastases, R1 resection, and major perioperative complications were associated with decreased survival. Median survival was 21.5 months in 60 patients after an R1 resection, compared with 27.8 months in 300 patients after an R0 resection (p=0.027). Covariates that affected survival at the p<0.10 level of significance were included in a multivariate Cox proportional hazards model. After adjusting for these variables in a backwards stepwise fashion, only the presence of lymph node metastases (hazard ratio, HR=1.55), major perioperative complications (HR=1.40), and operative blood loss (HR=1.01) adversely affected overall survival. Although R status influenced survival on univariate analysis (HR=1.42, 95% CI=1.04–1.93), an R1 resection did not independently affect survival after controlling for all other variables.

Recurrent disease was identified in 41 (68.3%) of 60 patients who underwent an R1 resection and in 199 (66.3%) of 300 patients who underwent an R0 resection. Some patients developed first recurrence at more than one site. Resection margin status did not affect the pattern of first recurrence; the proportion of patients with local, regional, or distant sites of first recurrence was similar in the R0 and R1 resection groups.

This recently reported experience is in contrast to other reports in the literature (Table 54.3) that did not

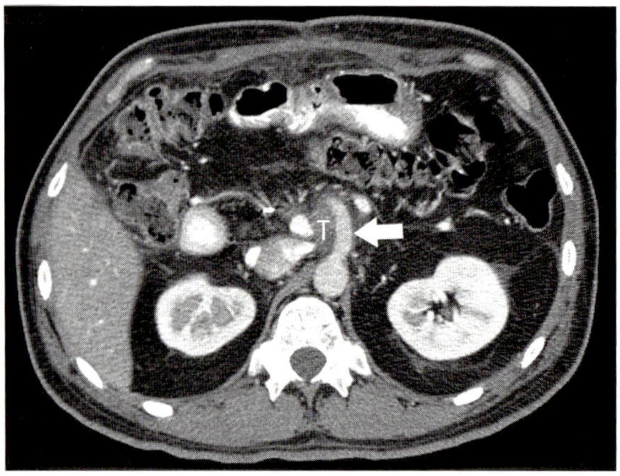

Figure 54.12

Axial contrast-enhanced CT image demonstrating residual low-density tumor (*T*) at the level of the SMA origin (*arrow*). The SMV can be seen to the right side of the residual tumor and just anterior to the inferior vena cava

utilize a standardized system for pathologic evaluation of the pancreaticoduodenectomy specimen. In the absence of accurate, real-time pathologic analysis of surgical specimens, assessment of margin status is impossible, as this information cannot be retrieved retrospectively. In our experience (and that of others), the majority of the R1 resections occur due to a positive SMA margin – a margin that probably receives less attention than it deserves given its major oncologic importance. This part of the operation is usually performed fairly quickly by placing a series of clamps along the right lateral border of the SMA, often without visible identification of the artery (Fig. 54.11). Such a technique is both dangerous (due to the possibility of SMA injury) and oncologically incorrect, frequently leaving gross tumor behind adjacent to the SMA (Fig. 54.12). Importantly, such incomplete resections usually go undocumented or are misclassified as an R1 resection.

<<Table 54.3 here>>

<<Figure 54.11 here>>

<<Figure 54.12 here>>

When a complete SMA dissection is performed, with no palpable or visible evidence of tumor, a microscopically positive margin of resection may still occur due to the infiltrative nature of pancreatic adenocarcinoma. The incidence of R1 resections in our experience was 17%; one would assume that the frequency of positive margins would increase when pancreaticoduodenectomy is performed in a multi-institutional setting where critical variables such as preoperative imaging, surgical technique, and pathologic assessment of the surgical specimen have not been standardized. This information is very important for the design of clinical trials involving surgery for patients with early-stage pancreatic cancer. In addition, all physicians, especially surgeons, need to emphasize the accurate reporting of margin status when pancreaticoduodenectomy is performed for cancer.

The impact of neoadjuvant therapy on surgical margin status remains an area of active investigation. In our experience, neoadjuvant therapy was not a statistically significant predictor of margin status; an R1 resection (positive SMA margin) occurred in 34 (13.4%) of 254 patients who received preoperative therapy and 20 (19.0%) of 105 patients who did not ($p=0.17$). However, these results were likely affected by significant selection bias. For example, patients who did not receive preoperative therapy may have had more favorable tumors (by multidisciplinary CT review) for immediate resection and been thought to be at lowest risk for an R1 resection. As systemic agents for pancreatic cancer become more effective, both alone and in combination with radiation therapy, the use of neoadjuvant therapy is likely to increase, especially in those patients most likely to undergo a positive margin resection.

Summary

The potential for a positive margin resection (R1, R2) can be minimized by careful attention to patient selection and operative technique. These variables are under the direct control of the surgeon and the multidisciplinary group of physicians caring for the patient with potentially resectable pancreatic cancer. A grossly positive resection (R2) should be avoided, as the survival duration following an R2 pancreaticoduodenectomy is no different than that of patients with stage III pancreatic cancer treated with nonsurgical therapies. However, an R1 resection appears to have a different implication for patient outcome. Our data suggest that the impact of a microscopically positive margin on survival duration may be less than was previously appreciated and is likely to occur in at least 15–20% of patients despite a gross complete pancreaticoduodenectomy. Such data are encouraging for those working on innovative multimodality solutions to the pancreatic cancer problem and emphasize the importance of surgical technique, especially with respect to the SMA dissection and contemporary methods of vascular resection and reconstruction in an effort to avoid R2 resections.

References

1. Benassai G, Mastrorilli M, Quarto G, et al (2000) Survival after pancreaticoduodenectomy for ductal adenocarcinoma of the head of the pancreas. Chir Ital 52:263–270
2. Gall FP, Kessler H, Hermanek P (1991) Surgical treatment of ductal pancreatic carcinoma. Eur J Surg Oncol 17:173–181
3. Millikan KW, Deziel DJ, Silverstein JC, et al (1999) Prognostic factors associated with resectable adenocarcinoma of the head of the pancreas. Am Surg 65:618–623; discussion 623–624
4. Neoptolemos JP, Stocken DD, Dunn JA, et al (2001) Influence of resection margins on survival for patients with pancreatic cancer treated by adjuvant chemoradiation and/or chemotherapy in the ESPAC-1 randomized controlled trial. Ann Surg 234:758–768
5. Nishimura Y, Hosotani R, Shibamoto Y, et al (1997) External and intraoperative radiotherapy for resectable and unresectable pancreatic cancer: analysis of survival rates and complications. Int J Radiat Oncol Biol Phys 39:39–49
6. Nitecki SS, Sarr MG, Colby TV, van Heerden JA (1995) Long-term survival after resection for ductal adenocarcinoma of the pancreas. Is it really improving? Ann Surg 221: 59–66
7. Sohn TA, Yeo CJ, Cameron JL, et al (2000) Resected adenocarcinoma of the pancreas – 616 patients: results, outcomes, and prognostic indicators. J Gastrointest Surg 4:567–579
8. Sperti C, Pasquali C, Piccoli A, Pedrazzoli S (1996) Survival after resection for ductal adenocarcinoma of the pancreas. Br J Surg 83:625–631
9. Willett CG, Lewandrowski K, Warshaw AL, et al (1993) Resection margins in carcinoma of the head of the pancreas. Implications for radiation therapy. Ann Surg 217:144–148
10. Yeo CJ, Cameron JL, Lillemoe KD, et al (1995) Pancreaticoduodenectomy for cancer of the head of the pancreas. 201 patients. Ann Surg 221:721–731
11. General Information on Cancer Staging and End-Results Reporting (2002) In: Greene FL, Page DL, Fleming ID, et al (eds) AJCC Cancer Staging Manual. Springer, New York, pp 1–16
12. Exocrine Pancreas (2002) In: Greene FL, Page DL, Fleming ID, et al (eds) AJCC Cancer Staging Manual. Springer, New York, pp 157–164
13. Scoggins CR, Lee JE, Evans DB (2005) Pancreaticoduodenectomy with en bloc vascular resection and reconstruction for localized carcinoma of the pancreas. In: VonHoff DD, Evans DB, Hruban RH, (eds) Pancreatic Cancer. Jones and Bartlett, Sudbury, MA, pp 321–334
14. Yen T, Abdalla E, Pisters PWT, Evans DB (2005) Pancreaticoduodenectomy. In: von Hoff DD, Evans DB, Hruban RH, (eds) Pancreatic Cancer. Jones and Bartlett, Sudbury, MA, pp 265–285
15. Tamm EP, Silverman PM, Charnsangavej C, Evans DB (2003) Diagnosis, staging, and surveillance of pancreatic cancer. Am J Roentgenol 180:1311–1323
16. Tseng JF, Raut CP, Lee JE, et al (2004) Pancreaticoduodenectomy with vascular resection: margin status and survival duration. J Gastrointest Surg 8:935–950
17. Varadhachary GR, Tamm EP, Crane C, et al (2005) Borderline resectable pancreatic cancer. Curr Treat Options Gastroenterol 8:377–384
18. Fortner JG (1973) Regional resection and pancreatic carcinoma. Surgery 73:799–800
19. Raut CP, Tseng JF, Sun CC, et al (2006) Impact of resection status on pattern of failure and survival after pancreaticoduodenectomy for pancreatic adenocarcinoma. In preparation 2006
20. Breslin TM, Hess KR, Harbison DB, et al (2001) Neoadjuvant chemoradiotherapy for adenocarcinoma of the pancreas: treatment variables and survival duration. Ann Surg Oncol 8:123–132
21. Pisters PWT, Wolff RA, Janjan NA, et al (2002) Preoperative paclitaxel and concurrent rapid-fractionation radiation for resectable pancreatic adenocarcinoma: toxicities, histologic response rates, event-free outcome. J Clin Oncol 20:2537–2544
22. Wolff RA, Evans DB, Crane C, et al (2002) Initial results of preoperative gemcitabine (GEM)-based chemoradiation for resectable pancreatic adenocarcinoma. Proc Am Soc Clin Oncol 21:130a
23. Evans DB, Rich TA, Byrd DR, et al (1992) Preoperative chemoradiation and pancreaticoduodenectomy for adenocarcinoma of the pancreas. Arch Surg 127:1335–1339

Chapter 55

Subtotal Left Resection for Pancreatic Cancer

A. Nakeeb · B. Safar

Over 200,000 people die each year of cancer of the pancreas. Pancreatic cancer is the fourth and the sixth leading cause of cancer deaths in the USA and Europe, respectively. In the USA it was estimated that nearly 33,000 new cases of pancreas cancer would be diagnosed in 2005, with almost 32,000 people dying of the disease in the same year [1]. The nonspecific symptoms associated with early pancreatic cancer, the inaccessibility of the pancreas to examination, the aggressiveness of the tumors, and the technical difficulties associated with pancreatic surgery make pancreatic cancer one of the most challenging diseases treated by surgeons. Surgical resection of pancreatic adenocarcinoma offers the only chance for long-term cure. Over the past two decades significant advances have been made in both the surgical techniques and the perioperative care of patients with pancreatic cancer. The perioperative mortality for pancreatic resections has been reduced to less than 3% in many high-volume centers.

Pathology

Approximately 65% of pancreatic cancers arise in the head, neck, or uncinate process of the pancreas; 15% originate in the body or the tail of the gland, and 20% diffusely involve the whole gland. Tumors of the pancreas are classified according to their cell of origin and can arise from either the exocrine or endocrine pancreas. Ductal adenocarcinomas account for more than 75% of all nonendocrine pancreatic cancers. Grossly, they are white–yellow, poorly defined, hard masses that often obstruct the distal common bile duct or main pancreatic duct. They are often associated with a desmoplastic reaction that causes fibrosis and chronic pancreatitis. Microscopically, they contain infiltrating glands of varying size and shape surrounded by dense, reactive fibrous tissue.

Ductal adenocarcinomas tend to infiltrate into vascular, lymphatic, and perineural spaces. At the time of resection, most ductal carcinomas have already metastasized to regional lymph nodes. In addition to the lymph nodes, pancreatic ductal adenocarcinoma frequently metastasizes to the liver (80%), peritoneum (60%), lungs, and pleurae (50–70%), and adrenal glands (25%). They can also directly invade the duodenum, stomach, transverse mesocolon, colon, spleen, and adrenal glands.

In a report of 235 elective distal pancreatectomies performed between 1984 and 1997 from The Johns Hopkins Hospital, 140 patients underwent resection for benign and malignant neoplasms of the pancreas [2]. The most common lesions found in the body and tail of the pancreas were benign cystadenomas (serous and mucinous) in 37%, ductal adenocarcinoma in 31%, neuroendocrine tumors in 24%, cyst adenocarcinoma in 4%, and other rare tumors including papillary and cystic tumors (Hamoudi tumor) in 3% and isolated solitary metastasis from renal cell carcinoma (1%).

Clinical Presentation

Many of the difficulties associated with the management of pancreatic cancer result from our inability to make the diagnosis at an early stage. The early symptoms of pancreatic cancer include anorexia, weight loss, abdominal discomfort, and nausea. Unfortunately, the nonspecific nature of these symptoms often leads to a delay in the diagnosis. Specific symptoms usually develop only after invasion or obstruction of nearby structures has occurred. In cases of advanced disease, cachexia, muscle wasting, or a nodular liver, consistent with metastatic disease, may be evident. Other physical findings in patients with disseminated cancer include left supraclavicular adenopathy (Virchow's node), periumbilical adenopathy (Sister Mary Joseph's node), and pelvic drop metastases (Blumer's shelf). Ascites can be present in 15% of patients.

Unlike tumors of the head of the pancreas which often present early with obstructive jaundice (85%), tumors of the body and tail present most commonly with vague symptoms including abdominal pain that often radiates to the back (84%), weight loss (42%), gastrointestinal symptoms (nausea, vomiting, early satiety, or anorexia; 35%), a palpable abdominal mass (14%), and new-onset diabetes mellitus (4%). As a result, patients with malignancies of the body and tail of the pancreas tend to present with larger tumors (3 cm vs. 5 cm) and at a more advanced stage than patients with cancers of the head of the pancreas [3].

In patients with localized cancer of the body and tail of the pancreas, laboratory values are frequently normal early in the course. Patients with pancreatic cancer may demonstrate a normochromic anemia and hypoalbuminemia secondary to the nutritional consequences of the disease. The serum concentration of many tumor markers may be increased in pancreatic cancer, but they all lack sensitivity and tumor specificity. The most extensively studied tumor marker for pancreatic cancer is CA19-9, a Lewis blood-group-related mucin glycoprotein. Approximately 5% of the population lacks the Lewis gene and therefore cannot produce CA19-9. When a normal upper limit of 37 U/ml is used, the accuracy of the CA19-9 level in identifying patients with pancreatic adenocarcinoma is only about 80%. When a higher cutoff value of more than 90 U/ml is used, the accuracy improves to 85%, and increasing the cutoff value to 200 U/ml increases the accuracy to 95% [4]. The combined use of CA19-9 and either ultrasonography, computed tomography (CT), or endoscopic retrograde cholangiopancreaticography can improve the accuracy of the individual tests, so that the combined accuracy approaches 100% for the diagnosis of pancreatic cancer. Levels of CA19-9 have also been correlated with prognosis and tumor recurrence. In general, higher CA19-9 values before surgery indicate an increased size of the primary tumor and increased rate of unresectability.

Pathologic Staging

Accurate pathologic staging of pancreatic cancer is important for providing prognostic information to patients and for comparing the results of various therapeutic trials. The American Joint Committee on

Table 55.1. American Joint Committee on Cancer Staging of Pancreatic Cancer (adapted from [5])

Stage grouping	T	N	M	5-year survival (%)
Stage IA	T1	N0	M0	20–30
Stage IB	T2	N0	M0	20–30
Stage IIA	T3	N0	M0	10–25
Stage IIB	T1,T2,T3	N1	M0	10–15
Stage III	T4	Any N	M0	0–5
Stage IV	Any T	Any N	M1	—

Tumor (T)

TX:	Primary tumor cannot be assessed
T0:	No evidence of primary tumor
Tis:	Carcinoma in situ
T1:	Tumor limited to the pancreas, 2 cm or less in greatest dimension
T2:	Tumor limited to the pancreas, more than 2 cm in greatest dimension
T3:	Tumor extends beyond the pancreas but without involvement of the celiac axis or the superior mesenteric artery
T4:	Tumor involves the celiac axis or the superior mesenteric artery (unresectable primary tumor)

Regional lymph nodes (N)

NX:	regional lymph nodes cannot be assessed
N0:	no regional lymph node metastasis
N1:	regional lymph node metastasis

Distant metastasis (M)

MX:	distant metastasis cannot be assessed
M0:	no distant metastasis
M1:	distant metastasis

Cancer (AJCC) staging for pancreatic cancer is shown in Table 55.1 [5]. This system, based on the TNM classification, takes into account the extent of the primary tumor (T), the presence of absence of regional lymph node involvement (N), and the presence or absence of distant metastatic disease (M).

Preoperative Staging

The goal of preoperative staging of pancreatic cancer is to determine the feasibility of surgery and the optimal treatment for each individual patient. At the time of diagnosis only 10% of patients have tumors confined to the pancreas, 40% have locally advanced disease, and more than 50% have distant spread. Unfortunately, only 10–20% of all patients are candidates for pancreatic resection. Therefore, accurate preoperative staging is important to determine which patients are candidates for curative resection and to avoid a nontherapeutic laparotomy in patients with unresectable disease. In many cases, either dynamic CT with intravenous contrast or magnetic resonance imaging (MRI) may provide all the information necessary. Using objective, specific, anatomy-based CT criteria that demonstrates: (1) the absence of extrapancreatic disease, (2) a patent superior mesenteric vein (SMV)-portal vein confluence, and (3) no evidence of direct tumor extension to the celiac axis, superior mesenteric artery or hepatic artery; the accuracy of high-quality helical CT scanning to identify potentially resectable pancreatic cancer approaches 85% [6]. For tumors of the body and tail of the pancreas, occlusion of the splenic vein with perigastric collaterals or involvement of the splenic artery does not always preclude resection and should not be considered a sign of unresectability.

Endoscopic ultrasonography (EUS) is a minimally invasive technique in which a high-frequency ultrasonographic probe is placed into the stomach and duodenum endoscopically and the pancreas is imaged. Tumors appear as hypoechoic areas in the pancreatic substance. The strengths of EUS techniques for pancreatic cancer are the clarification of small lesions (<2 cm) when CT findings are questionable or negative, detection of malignant lymphadenopathy, detection of vascular involvement, and the ability to perform EUS-guided fine-needle aspiration (FNA) for definitive diagnosis and staging. EUS is not effective in assessing metastatic disease to the liver. In patients for whom a tissue diagnosis is required (poor operative candidates or undergoing neoadjuvant therapy), EUS-guided FNA has been used to acquire tissue samples for cytologic analysis. This approach may avoid the risks of tumor seeding. The accuracy of EUS without FNA averages 85% for determining T-stage and 70% for determining N-stage disease. The combination of EUS and FNA has a sensitivity of 93% and a specificity of 100% for T stage and an accuracy of 88% for N stage [7].

Laparoscopy

The use of diagnostic laparoscopy in pancreatic cancer remains controversial. Proponents believe that laparoscopy can identify a substantial number of unresectable patients with advanced disease and, therefore, should be uniformly applied to all patients with potentially resectable tumors. On the other hand, opponents believe that the inherent cost of such a practice far outweighs the benefit to the small number of patients in whom diagnostic laparoscopy is useful. The liver and peritoneum are the most common sites of distant spread of pancreatic carcinoma. Once distant metastases have developed, survival is so limited that a conservative approach is usually indicated. Liver metastases larger than 1 cm in diameter can usually be detected by CT, but approximately 30% of these metastases are smaller and therefore may not be routinely detected. Moreover, peritoneal and omental metastases are usually only 1–2 mm in size and can frequently be detected only by direct visualization. With the recent improvements in CT imaging, the rate of positive peritoneal findings approaches 20–25% for all patients with pancreatic cancer and is significantly higher for patients with cancers of the body and tail. For example, patients presenting with obstructive jaundice secondary to tumors in the head of the pancreas typically have only a 15–20% incidence of unexpected intraperitoneal metastasis after routine staging studies. In contrast, unexpected peritoneal metastasis is found in up to 50% of patients with cancer of the body and tail of the pancreas [8]. Selective use of staging laparoscopy should be considered for patients at high risk of occult metastatic disease such as patients with: (1) large primary tumors, (2) lesions in the neck, body, or tail of the pancreas, (3) equivocal radiographic findings suggestive of occult distant metastatic disease, such as low-volume ascites, CT findings indicating possible carcinomatosis, and small hypodense regions in the hepatic parenchyma that suggest hepatic metastases that are not amenable to percutaneous biopsy, and (4) subtle clinical and laboratory findings suggesting more advanced disease (e.g., marked hypoalbuminemia and/or weight loss, significant increases in CA19-9 level, and relatively severe pain requiring narcotic analgesia).

The ultimate yield of staging laparoscopy for pancreatic cancer is dependant on the technique used. Simple laparoscopy with the examination and biopsy of the surface of the liver and the peritoneal surfaces will not identify patients with unresectable disease secondary to deep liver metastasis or locally advanced pancreatic cancer. Conlon and colleagues [9] describe a thorough multiport laparoscopic technique that mimics the staging and assessment of resectability of open surgery. Their technique involves the placement of a 10-mm trocar inserted in an infraumbilical position and the use of a 30° laparoscope. Operating ports are placed in the right (10 and 5 mm) and left (5 mm) upper quadrants. A systemic examination of the peritoneal cavity is performed. The primary tumor is assessed, and local extent, size, and fixation are noted. Extension to contiguous organs such as the colon, duodenum, liver, spleen, and stomach are identified. Cytological washings are taken from the right and left upper quadrants prior to manipulation of the primary or metastatic tumor. The patient is then placed in a 20° reverse Trendelenburg position to allow visualization of the liver. The hilus of the liver is visualized and the foramen of Winslow is examined; suspicious periportal lymph nodes are biopsied. The patient is then placed in a 10° Trendelenburg position, and the omentum is retracted cephalad to allow visualization of the ligament of Treitz. The mesocolon is inspected and then the gastrohepatic omentum is incised, exposing the caudate lobe of the liver, vena cava, and celiac axis. Celiac, portal, or perigastric nodes are sampled if necessary. During the examination, any suspicious lesions are biopsied and sent for frozen section. Unresectability is determined if one or more of the following are confirmed histologically: (1) hepatic, serosal, peritoneal, or omental metastases, (2) extrapancreatic extension of the tumor, (3) distant nodal metastasis, and (4) invasion or encasement of the celiac axis, hepatic artery, or superior mesenteric artery. Patients who are found to have portal or mesenteric vein encroachment by the tumor are considered potentially resectable and undergo exploratory laparotomy.

Preoperative Preparation

Every patient considered for a pancreatic resection needs a full evaluation of cardiac, pulmonary, and renal function. A full array of laboratory test must be obtained including a complete blood count, renal panel, and liver panel. A nutritional assessment needs to be made to make sure that the patient can undergo surgery safely; if the patient has severe weight loss or has an albumin of <3 g/dl, strong consideration for supplemental nutrition is indicated.

Since no attempt to save the spleen is made during distal pancreatic resection for carcinoma, the patient should receive vaccination against encapsulated organisms to prevent postsplenectomy sepsis. These include *Streptococcus pneumoniae*, *Neisseria meningitidis* and *Haemophilus influenzae* vaccines. The vaccines should be administered 1 or 2 weeks prior to the operation.

Resection of Carcinoma of the Body and Tail of the Pancreas

Distal pancreatic resection has been performed for a variety of conditions including inflammatory processes and benign and malignant tumors. The goals of surgical resection for carcinoma of the body and tail of the pancreas are to achieve complete excision of the tumor with a negative microscopic margin (R0) and resection of the draining regional lymph nodes. The lymphatic drainage of the body and tail of the pancreas are shown schematically in Fig. 55.1. The body and tail of the pancreas may be thought of as having four equally sized quadrants. Lymphatic vessels traveling from the four quadrants flow to lymphatics lying along the superior and inferior borders of the body and tail of the pancreas. Small lymph nodes lie along these lymphatics. The lymphatic vessels along the su-

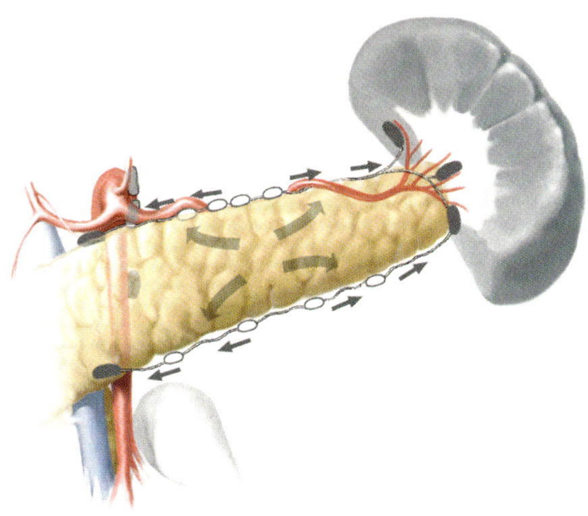

Figure 55.1

Schematic drawing of lymphatic drainage of body and tail of the pancreas (with permission from Strasberg et al. [10])

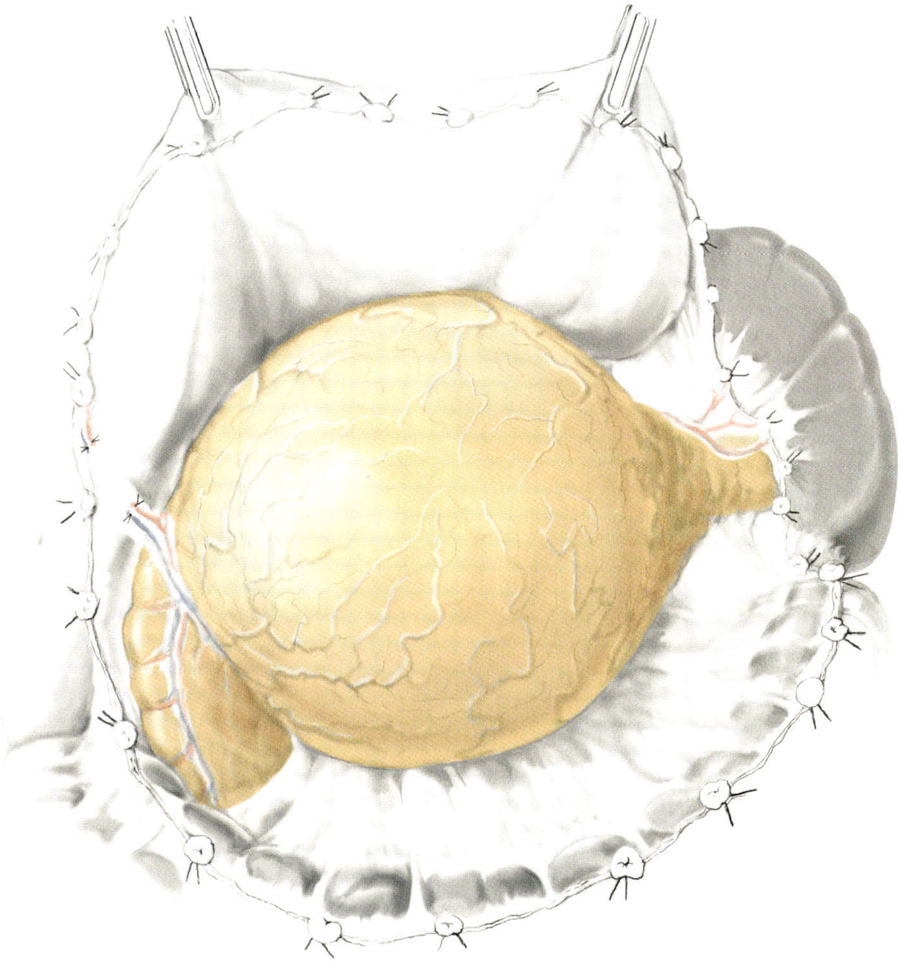

Figure 55.2

Exposure of the body and tail of the pancreas by dividing the gastrocolic ligament

perior and inferior borders of the left half of the body and tail drain to splenic nodes in the hilum of the spleen or gastrosplenic nodes in the gastrosplenic omentum. Lymphatic vessels coursing along the superior and inferior borders of the right half of the body drain to the gastroduodenal and infrapancreatic nodes. These four sets of nodes form a ring of nodes. The ring is one of the two nodal groups receiving lymph from the body and tail of the pancreas. The second major group of nodes lies anterior to the aorta in relation to the celiac and superior mesenteric arteries. This group receives lymph from the nodes of the ring, but is not exclusively an N2 node group. Pancreatic lymphatics may enter these nodes directly without first entering a node on the ring. Therefore, they should be considered as N1 and as N2 nodes [10].

Preoperative Preparation

Once the preoperative workup has been completed and the patient is cleared for surgery, a full bowel prep is used in case the transverse colon needs to be resected. Deep venous thrombosis prophylaxis with heparin or low-molecular-weight heparin is given preoperatively and sequential compression devices are placed on the lower extremities. Preoperative antibiotics (second- or third-generation cephalosporin) are given to cover for enteric pathogens. The patient is positioned supine on the operating table and several folded sheets are placed under the left flank to improve exposure.

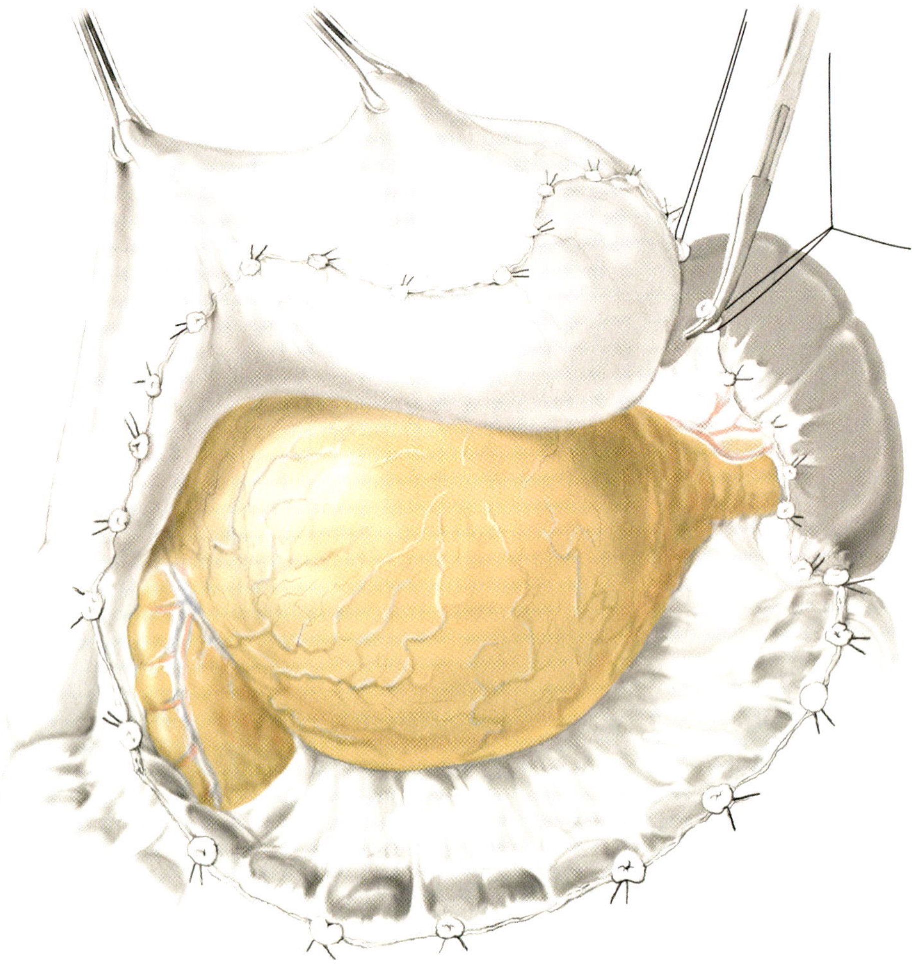

Figure 55.3

Division of the short gastric vessels and the splenocolic ligament

Operative Procedure

Incision

Once the staging laparoscopy is completed and distant metastatic disease to the liver and peritoneum has been ruled out, the peritoneal cavity is entered through a left subcostal incision that extends to the right of midline. An upper midline incision may also be used in thin patients. Once the abdomen is entered, a careful exploration is performed to confirm the absence of disseminated disease.

Exposure of the Pancreas

The lesser sac is entered by dividing the gastrocolic omentum (Fig. 55.2). This is achieved by lifting the greater omentum upwards and the transverse colon downwards. Alternatively, the greater omentum may be taken off the transverse colon and be left attached to the greater curve of the stomach. Once the lesser sac is entered, the posterior wall of the stomach is separated from the pancreas using sharp and blunt dissection to expose the body and tail of the pancreas. The duodenum is kocherized, and the head and the uncinate process of the pancreas are palpated and visualized. This allows for careful inspection and palpation of the entire gland. Intraoperative ultrasound may be used to further define the relationship between the tumor and the surrounding vascular structures.

Assessment of Resectability

Once the pancreas is exposed, the celiac axis and superior mesenteric vessels are identified and assessed to determine resectability. The splenic artery is iden-

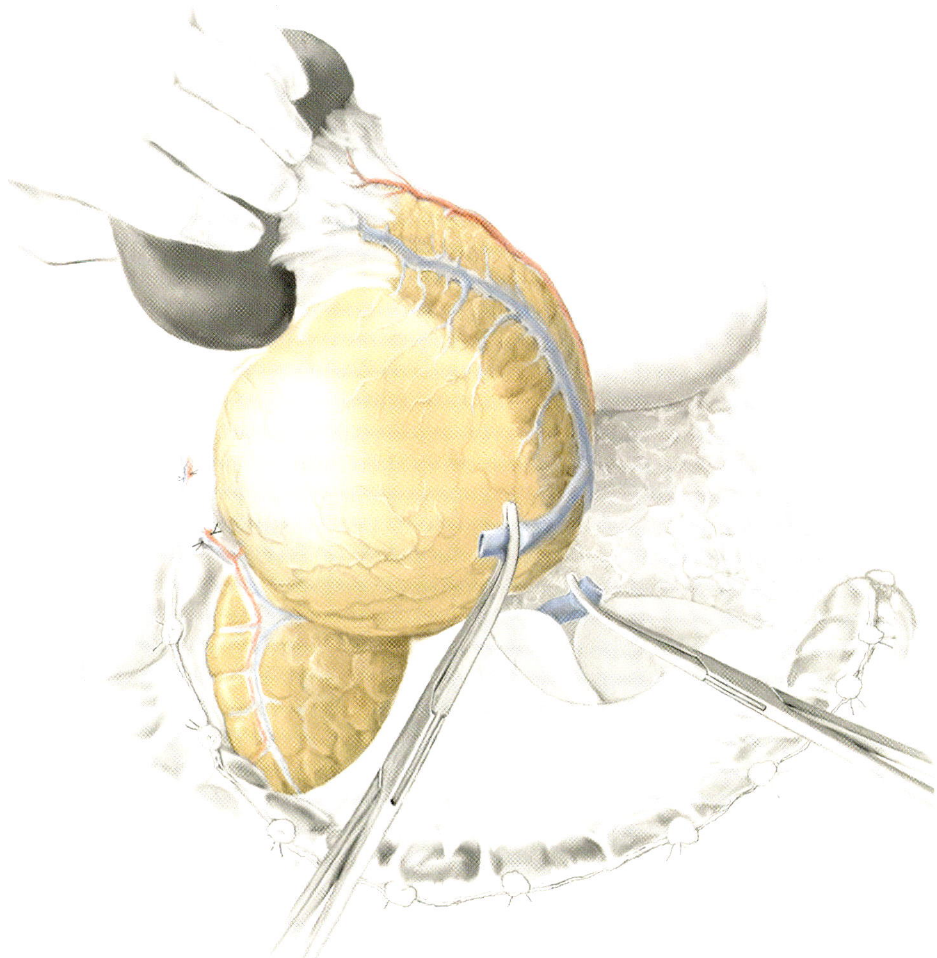

Figure 55.4

Mobilization of the spleen and body and tail of the pancreas with ligation of the inferior mesenteric vein (*v.*)

tified as it comes off the celiac axis and a vessel loop is placed around it. This step gives one control of the splenic artery and allows one to ligate it early in the procedure if bleeding should occur. Patients with a thrombosed splenic vein may have left-side portal hypertension and multiple collateral vessels leading from the spleen to the stomach via the short gastric vessels. In such circumstances, it is usually preferable to ligate and divide the splenic artery early in the procedure

Mobilization of the Spleen

The spleen is retracted toward the midline with the left hand (it should be compressed medially toward the spine rather than retracted anteriorly) and mobilized out of the retroperitoneum using electrocautery. The retroperitoneum usually consists of loose areolar tissue that is easily mobilized. The omental attachments anterior to the hilum of the spleen are divided between Kelly clamps and ligated with 2-0 silk (Fig. 55.3). The line of division is easily determined if the omentum has previously been completely taken off the transverse colon. As the division extends up toward and then along the greater curvature of the stomach, the vasa brevia are encountered and are doubly clamped, divided, and ligated. The splenic flexure of the colon is carefully dissected away from the inferior pole of the spleen, and the peritoneal attachments that make up the splenocolic ligament are divided.

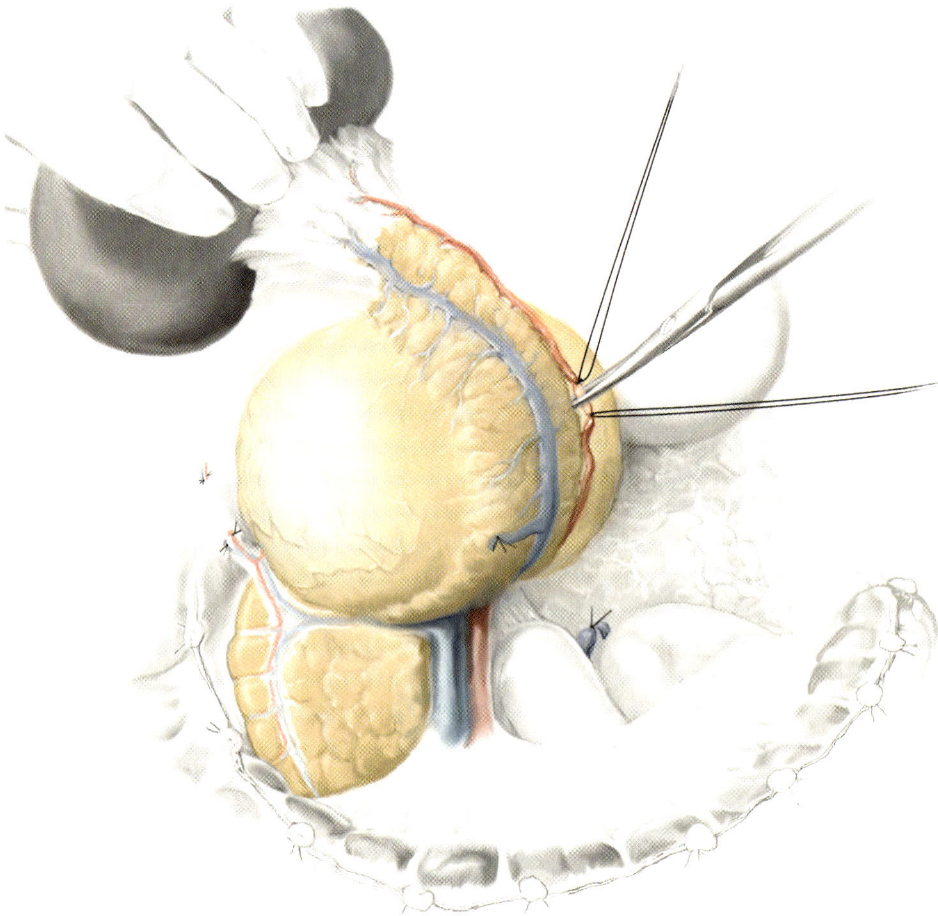

Figure 55.5

Ligation of the splenic artery (*a.*) at its origin from the celiac axis

Mobilization of the Pancreas

The tail and body of the pancreas are further mobilized out of the retroperitoneum by retracting the spleen and the tail of the pancreas medially. In the course of this mobilization, one must be careful not to injure the left adrenal gland, which often occupies a fairly superficial position in the retroperitoneum, anterior and medial to the superior pole of the left kidney. Care must also be taken not to carry the dissection too deep and risk injuring the kidney or renal vessels (Fig. 55.4). The splenic vein is easily identified in the middle portion of the posterior aspect of the pancreas. The inferior mesenteric vein, which joins the splenic vein at the middle of the body of the pancreas, is identified in the retroperitoneum just lateral to the ligament of Treitz and can be divided at this point.

Division of the Splenic Vessels

Further mobilization of the pancreas to the midline exposes the splenic artery origin at the celiac axis, which has been previously isolated with a vessel loop. Further mobilization of the pancreas to the midline exposes the point where the splenic artery comes off the celiac axis. The splenic artery is triply clamped, divided, and triply ligated with 2-0 silk and a 3-0 Prolene suture ligature near its point of origin (Fig. 55.5). At this point the SMV can be identified. The anterior plane of the SMV can be dissected between the vein and the neck of the gland. A Penrose drain can be looped under the neck to aid exposure. With larger pancreatic cancers, the splenic vein may be involved with tumor extension into the retroperitoneum, dividing the pancreatic neck at this point with the cautery can facilitate the dissection of the splenic and portal vein confluence under direct vision. The splenic vein is clamped, divided without

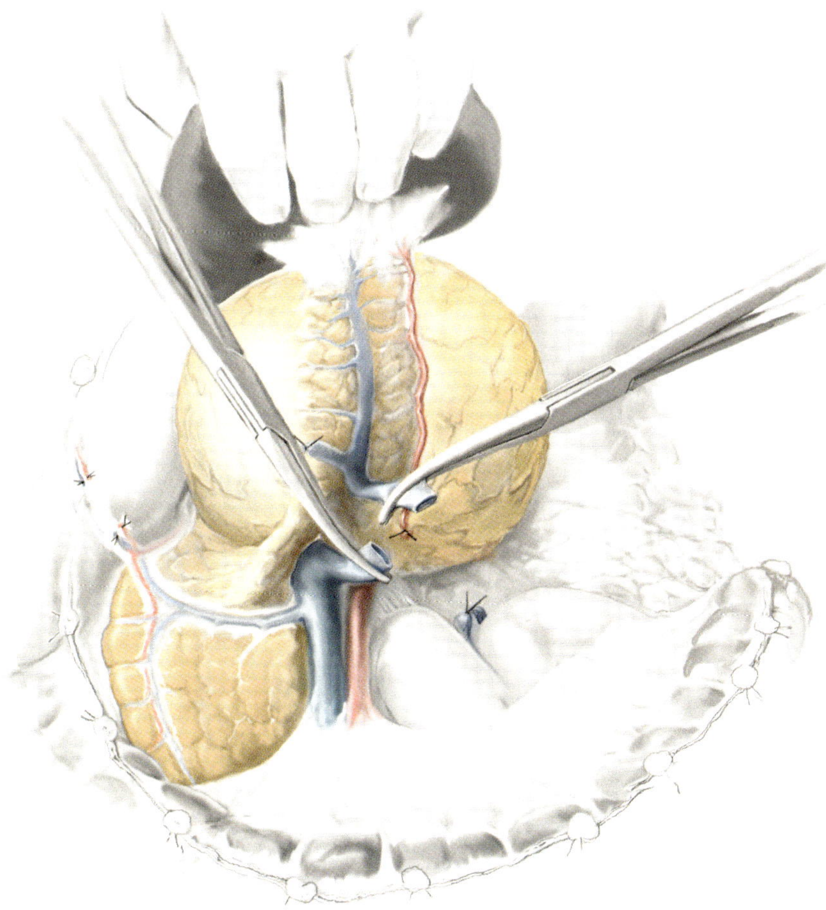

Figure 55.6

Division of the splenic vein at the superior mesenteric vein-portal vein confluence

compromising the portal vein/SMV, and ligated with 0 silk tie and 3-0 Prolene suture on the proximal stump (Fig. 55.6). If there is a pancreatic tumor arising from the proximal body of the gland, the splenic vein may be ligated flush with the SMV. At this location, it is best to oversew the vein with a continuous 3-0 Prolene suture so as not to compromise the SMV–portal vein complex.

Transection of the Neck of the Pancreas

The portal vein and the SMV are carefully dissected away from the undersurface of the neck of the pancreas. A row of overlapping horizontal mattress sutures of 3-0 absorbable synthetic material is placed in the neck of the pancreas just proximal to the point where it is to be divided (Fig. 55.7); using large needles that have been straightened makes this task simple even if the head–neck junction through which the needles are passed is thickened. The neck of the pancreas is then divided with the electrocautery (Fig. 55.8). The operative specimen should be sent to pathology for frozen section evaluation to ensure a negative microscopic margin. A row of figure-of-eight sutures of 3-0 absorbable synthetic suture material is placed over the end of the pancreas (Fig. 55.9). If the pancreatic duct can be identified, it should be separately oversewn with a figure-of-eight or mattress suture (again, of 3-0 absorbable synthetic suture material). The resection bed should be marked with titanium clips to guide postoperative radiation therapy if necessary.

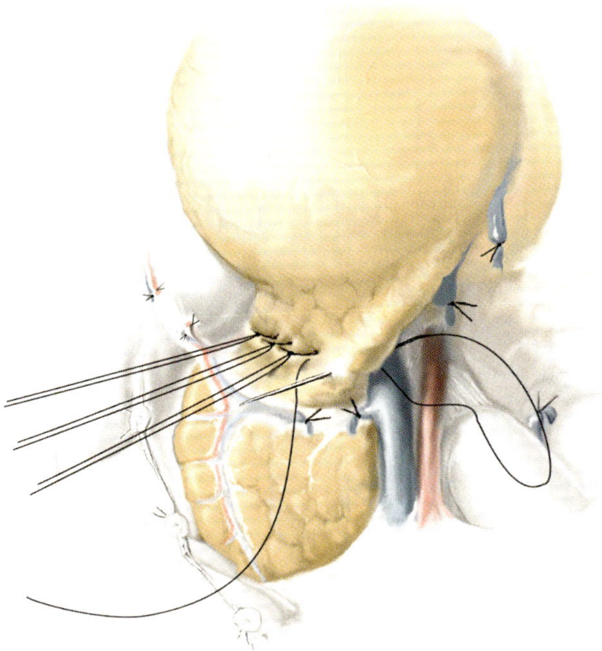

Figure 55.7

Placement of horizontal matress sutures in the neck of the pancreas prior to transection of the neck of the pancreas

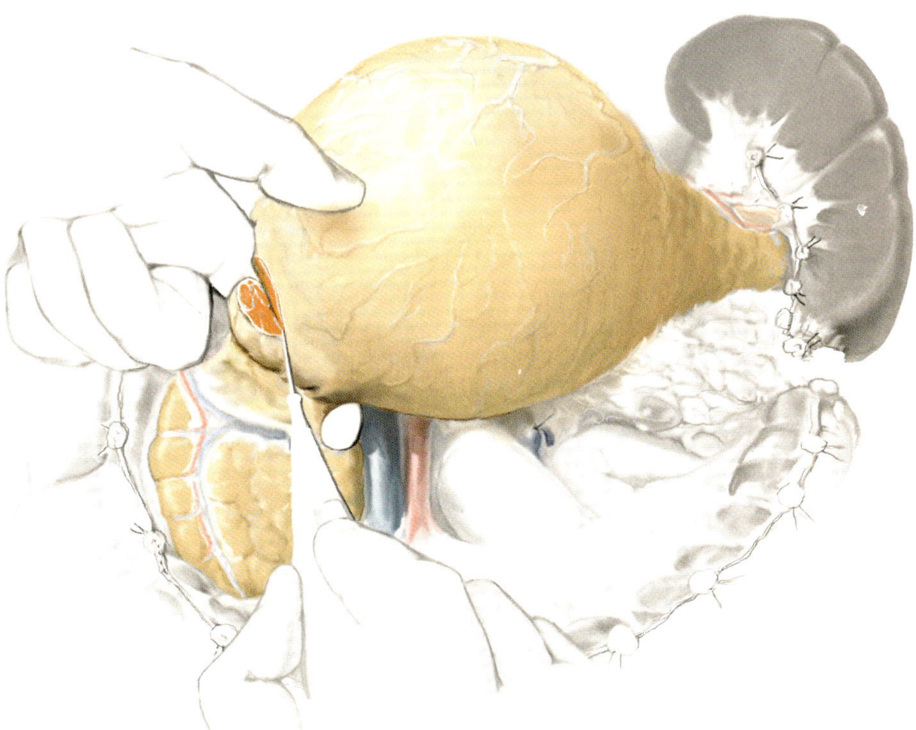

Figure 55.8

Transection of the pancreas with electrocautery

Closure

The abdomen is copiously irrigated with an antibiotic solution. The pancreatic remnant is drained with a closed-suction Silastic drain brought out through a stab wound in the left upper quadrant. There is no need to drain the splenic bed. The abdominal wall is closed with a single layer of continuous no. 1 absorbable synthetic monofilament sutures placed through and through all muscle and fascial layers. The subcutaneous tissues are irrigated with an antibiotic solution and the skin closed with either a continuous 4-0 absorbable synthetic suture or staples.

Antegrade Pancreatosplenectomy

One proposed strategy to improve outcome in patients with resectable pancreatic cancer is to increase the resection margin and perform more extensive lymph node clearance. Based on this ideology, a novel approach was recently advocated by Strasberg et al [10]. In this method, after dissection of the greater omentum off the colon and division of the short gastric vessels close to the stomach, the neck of the pancreas is elevated off the SMV and portal vein from below. The lesser omentum is opened, and the proper hepatic artery is followed proximally to the common hepatic and gastroduodenal arteries. The right gastric artery is divided to facilitate this dissection. The lymph nodes on the left border of the proper hepatic artery and portal vein and the lymph nodes anterior to the common hepatic artery are mobilized. The anterior surface of the portal vein is exposed by retracting the gastroduodenal artery to the right, and the tunnel behind the neck of the pancreas is completed. The neck of the pancreas is divided, and the pancreatic duct is oversewn with a figure-of-eight 5-0 synthetic absorbable suture. An extensive lymph node dissection is then carried out of the celiac lymph nodes; the splenic artery is identified at its origin from the celiac axis, ligated, and divided. Dissection from this point proceeds from right to left in one of two planes (i.e., anterior or behind the adrenal) in order to ensure negative posterior margins. Nodes along the front and left side of the superior mesenteric artery are removed. Based on the lymphatic drainage of the gland this procedure removes all N1 lymph nodes. In their report, 10 patients underwent the procedure with no postoperative mortality and acceptable morbidity. They concluded that this technique was safe and oncologically sound, however it took longer and was technically more challenging. Further studies are needed before this technique is widely adopted.

Postoperative Care

The implementation of case management and clinical pathway in surgical units has contributed to a decrease in the length of hospital stay. The patient is monitored postoperatively in an intensive care unit for the first 24 h. Laboratory tests should be checked in the recovery room as well as the morning of the first postoperative day; these include a complete blood count, electrolytes, liver function tests, and amylase. Mild pancreatitis can develop postoperatively and may explain the reason for an exaggerated inflammatory response. Frequent assessment of the blood glucose should be carried out and blood glucose should be kept under 150 in the postoperative period. Prophylactic antibiotics should not be continued for longer than 24 h. The nasogastric tube may be removed on day 1 postoperatively and the patient is allowed to have sips of liquids. As the diet is advanced over the next few days the peripancreatic drain is carefully checked for evidence of a pancreatic fistula. The drain can be removed once the patient is tolerating a regular diet and there is no evidence of a pancreatic leak. In the event of continued leak, the patient may be discharged with the drain and instructed to record daily output. Most fistulas close spontaneously without any further intervention.

Role of Prophylactic Somatostatin Analogues after Distal Pancreatic Resection

Pancreatic fistula and its potential sequelae (e.g., abscess, hemorrhage, sepsis) remain troublesome and at times life-threatening complications follow elective pancreatic resection. Pancreatic fistula has been reported to occur in more than 30% of patients undergoing elective pancreatic resections. Octreotide and vapreotide are synthetic analogues of native somatostatin that act by inhibiting pancreatic secretions. It has been proposed that the use of these agents may decrease the rate of fistula formation, accelerate fistula closure, and reduce postoperative complications.

Several prospective, randomized, double blinded, multicenter trials from Europe [11–14] have suggested a statistically significant decrease in overall postoperative complications after pancreatectomy with the use of perioperative octreotide (Table 55.2). The incidence of pancreas-specific complications was also reduced. These studies were not prospectively designed with the necessary power to study the specific question of complications related directly to the pancreatic anastomosis. In addition, these studies enrolled

Table 55.2. Prospective randomized controlled trials of prophylactic octreotide versus placebo for patients undergoing elective resection of the pancreas

First author	*N*	Pancreatic fistula Placebo (%)	 Octreotide Placebo (%)	Overall morbidity Octreotide Placebo (%)	 Octreotide (%)	Overall mortality (%)	 (%)
Buchler 1992 [11]	246	38	18	55	32	5.8	3.2
Pederzolli 1994 [12]	252	19	9	29	16	3.8	1.6
Montors 1995 [13]	218	20	9	36	22	5.6	8.1
Freiss 1995 [14]	247	22	10	30	16	0.8	1.6
Lowy 1997 [15]	110	6	12	25	30	0	2
Yeo 2000 [16]	211	11	9	34	40	0	1
Sarr[a] 2003 [17]	275	23	24	42	40	1.4	0

[a] Vapreotide was used instead of octreotide in this study

patients with chronic pancreatitis who would be expected to have a lower incidence of pancreatic leak.

In contrast, two large-center studies in the USA evaluating perioperative octreotide [15, 16] and one using vapreotide [17] failed to demonstrate any benefit of the somatostatin analogues after elective pancreatectomy for presumed pancreatic neoplasms. The most recent study by Sarr et al. [17] was a prospective, multicenter, randomized, double-blinded, placebo-controlled trial of vapreotide in 275 patients undergoing elective proximal, central, and distal pancreatectomy. There were no statistically significant differences between vapreotide- and placebo-treated patients in either pancreas-related complications (30.4% versus 26.4%, respectively) or in other complications not related to the pancreas (40% versus 42%, respectively). In the distal pancreatectomy subgroup (52 patients), no difference was found in the pancreas-specific complication rate (vapreotide 42% vs. placebo 27%). Soft pancreatic texture was the only statistically significant factor associated with pancreatic fistula ($P < 0.025$).

These studies demonstrate that prophylactic administration of octreotide does not uniformly reduce the incidence of pancreatic anastomotic leak, overall morbidity, or mortality after pancreatic resection. Routine use of octreotide for patients undergoing pancreatic resection cannot be supported on the basis of currently available data.

Postoperative Results

Despite the skepticism of surgeons earlier in the last century, pancreatic resection for pancreatic cancer can now be achieved safely at high-volume centers. Lillemoe et al. [2] reported their complication and mortality rate following distal pancreatectomy for a variety of diseases (Table 55.3). In their series they reported a 30-day mortality rate of 0.9% and an overall morbidity rate of 31%. They included new-onset diabetes mellitus in their complications, which was 8%, pancreatic fistula 5%, intra-abdominal abscess 4%, small-bowel obstruction 4%, and postoperative hemorrhage 4%. Fourteen patients required a second surgical procedure, most commonly for bleeding.

Prognosis

In the last two decades several institutions [3, 18–21] have reported their outcomes of distal pancreatectomy for the treatment of pancreas cancer (Table 55.4). Most suggest that the disease is less commonly found in the body and tail than in the head of the gland and that it is less likely to be resectable as it presents at a later stage. Nevertheless, if the tumor is resectable, the operation can be achieved with rare mortality and minimal morbidity at high-volume centers. In the largest series published for adenocarcinoma of the pancreas, Sohn et al. [3] examined the factors influencing long-term survival following resection. Of the 616 patients who underwent surgical resection, 52 (9%) were distal pancreatectomies for tumors in the body and tail of the gland. The overall survival for the

Table 55.3. Morbidity and mortality in 235 distal pancreatectomies

	N (235)	%
Mortality	2	0.9
Morbidity	71	31
New onset insulin dependent diabetes	19	8
Pancreatic fistula	12	5
Intra-abdominal abscess	10	4
Small bowel obstruction	10	4
Hemorrhage	9	4
Infection	8	3
Pulmonary	5	2
Miscellaneous	8	3
Reoperation	14	6
Length of stay (days)	15 (mean)	10 (median)

Table 55.4. Adenocarcinoma of the body and tail of the pancreas. *MSKCC* Memorial Sloan-Kettering Cancer Center

Institution	Year	*N*	Resected	Morbidity	Mortality	Median survival
John Hopkins [18]	1992	113	9 (8%)	4 (44%)	0	–
Heidelberg [19]	1993	105	13 (12%)	2 (15%)	0	13 months
Johns Hopkins [3]	2000	–	52	13 (25%)	1 (2%)	12 months
MSKCC [20]	2003	513	57 (11%)	–	0	12 months
Mayo Clinic [21]	2005	–	93a	43 (46%)	0	15.5 months

[a] Includes cystadenocarcinomas and invasive carcinoma associated with intraductal papillary mucinous neoplasm

entire cohort was 63% at 1 year and 17% at 5 years, with a median survival of 17 months. For left-sided tumors, the 1- and 5-year survival rates were 50% and 15%, respectively. Patients undergoing distal pancreatectomy for left-sided lesions had larger tumors (4.7 vs. 3.1 cm, $P < 0.0001$), but fewer node-positive resections (59% vs. 73%; $P = 0.03$) and fewer poorly differentiated tumors (29% vs. 36%; $P < 0.001$) as compared to those undergoing pancreaticoduodenectomy for right-sided tumors. Factors shown to have favorable independent prognostic significance by multivariate analysis were negative resection margins, tumor diameter <3 cm, estimated blood loss <750 ml, well/moderate tumor differentiation, and postoperative chemoradiation. In addition, tumor location in the head, neck, or uncinate process approached significance in the final multivariate model.

Summary

Pancreas cancer is deadly, with less than 5% of patients diagnosed with the disease surviving 5 years. Resection remains the only chance of cure for these patients. This calls for aggressive evaluation of patients with potential pancreatic cancer and improved screening methods in the future. A better understanding of tumor genetics and neoplastic progression models may lead to progress in early detection and perhaps chemoprevention. Improvements in abdominal imaging and the recognition of imageable precursor lesions may improve our ability to detect smaller, lower-staged neoplasms. At no time in the past has there been as much activity in the field of pancreatic adenocarcinoma. It is hoped that future developments in many areas currently under active study will improve the overall prognosis for patients with pancreatic or periampullary adenocarcinoma.

References

1. Surveillance, Epidemiology, and End Results (SEER) Program (www.seer.cancer.gov) SEER*Stat Database
2. Lillemoe KD, Kaushal S, Cameron JL, et al (1999) Distal pancreatectomy: indications and outcomes in 235 patients. Ann Surg 229:693–700
3. Sohn TA, Yeo CJ, Cameron JL, et al (2000) Resected adenocarcinoma of the pancreas 616 patients: results, outcomes, and prognostic indicators. J Gastrointest Surg 4:567–579
4. Ritts RE, Pitt HA (1998) CA 19-9 in pancreatic cancer. Surg Oncol Clin N Am 7:93–101
5. American Joint Committee on Cancer (2002) AJCC Cancer Staging Manual, 6th edn. Springer, New York, pp 157–164
6. Pisters PWT, Lee JE, Vauthey, et al (2001) Laparoscopy in the staging of pancreatic cancer. Br J Surg 88:325–337
7. Dye CE, Waxman I (2002) Endoscopic ultrasound. Gastroenterol Clin N Am 31:863–879
8. Barreiro CJ, Lillemoe KD, Koniaris LG, et al (2002) Diagnostic laparoscopy for periampullary and pancreatic cancer: What is the true benefit? J Gastrointest Surg 6:75–81
9. Conlon KC, Dougherty E, Klimstra DS, et al (1996) The value of minimal access surgery in the staging of patients with potentially resectable peripancreatic malignancy. Ann Surg 223:134–140
10. Strasberg SM, Drebin JA, Linehan D (2003) Radical antegrade modular pancreatosplenectomy. Surgery 133:521–527
11. Buchler M, Firess H, Klempa I, et al (1992) Role of octreotide in the prevention of postoperative complications following pancreatic resection. Am J Surg 163:125–131
12. Pederzolli P, Bassi C, Falconi M, Camboni MG (1994) Efficacy of octreotide in the prevention of complications of elective pancreatic surgery. Br J Surg 81:265–269
13. Montorsi M, Zago M, Mosca F, et al (1995) Efficacy of octreotide in the prevention of pancreatic fistula after elective pancreatic resections: a prospective controlled randomized trial. Surgery 117:26–31
14. Friess H, Beger HG, Sulkowsky U, et al (1995) Randomized controlled multicentre study of the prevention of complications by octreotide in patients undergoing surgery for chronic pancreatitis. Br J Surg 82:1270–1273
15. Lowy AM, Lee J, Pisters PWT, et al (1997) Prospective, randomized trial of octreotide to prevent pancreatic fistula after pancreaticoduodenectomy for malignant disease. Ann Surg 26:632–641
16. Yeo CJ, Cameron JL, Lillemoe KD, et al (2000) Does prophylactic octreotide decrease the rates of pancreatic fistula and other complications after pancreaticoduodenectomy? Results of a prospective randomized placebo-controlled trial. Ann Surg 232:419–429
17. Sarr MG, Pancreatic Surgery Group (2003) The potent somatostatin analogue vapreotide does not decrease pancreas-specific complications after elective pancreatectomy: a prospective, multicenter, double-blinded, randomized, placebo-controlled trial. J Am Coll Surg 196:556–564
18. Nordback IH, Hruban RH, Boitnott, et al (1992) Carcinoma of the body and tail of the pancreas. Am J Surg 164:26–31
19. Johnson CD, Schwall G, Flechtenmacher J, Trede M (1993) Resection for adenocarcinoma of the body and tail of the pancreas. Br J Surg 80:1177–1179
20. Shoup M, Conlon KC, Klimstra, Brennan MF (2003) Is extended resection for adenocarcinoma of the body or tail of the pancreas justified? J Gastrointest Surg 8:946–952
21. Christein JD, Kendrick ML, Iqbal CW, et al (2005) Distal pancreatectomy for resectable adenocarcinoma of the body and tail of the pancreas. J Gastrointest Surg 9:922–927

Chapter 56

J.Y. Tracey · M. Bouvet · A.R. Moossa

Total Pancreatectomy for Pancreatic Cancer

The historic evolution of total pancreatectomy parallels closely the earlier fate of total gastrectomy. At first, complete excision of either organ was thought to be incompatible with life. In the second quarter of the last century, however, major scientific and technical advances in surgery and other clinical disciplines led to their successful extirpation. Initially, total resection of either organ was reserved for very advanced tumors with resulting high morbidity and mortality. Then the operations were performed widely for various malignant and benign conditions, which coincided with a gradual decrease in the operative risk. In the 1970s and 1980s, our improved understanding of gastrointestinal physiology and resulting postoperative derangements in metabolic processes, combined with multiple advances in blood banking, anesthesia, and intensive care, gradually led to a more realistic, conservative, and selective approach to radical operations on either organ.

During the period 1950–1990, enthusiasm for total pancreatectomy for cancer in the head of the pancreas was fed by scientific findings, technical developments, and dissatisfaction with the outcomes of the Whipple procedure. At this time, the Whipple operation was still associated with high morbidity, mortality, and poor survival rates for this dismal disease, and this led to the search for a better operation.

The bulk of scientific evidence favoring total pancreatectomy suggested that all the ducts within the gland, regardless of location, were equally exposed to the same carcinogenic stimuli and potentially resulted in multicentric disease. Two important papers helped fuel this idea. In 1954, Ross reported two separate carcinomas 13 cm apart in the same gland and made a strong plea for total pancreatectomy for cancer in the head of the gland [1]. In addition, Sommers et al. [2] reported pancreatic duct hyperplasia, carcinoma-in-situ, and invasive carcinoma in the same resected specimen. It would be another 30 years before these beliefs were challenged by two important studies, which led to the eventual supplantation of the total pancreatectomy by the more pancreas-sparing Whipple operation.

Kloppel et al. [3] and Motojima et al. [4] showed that multiple lesions in a single gland were much less common than had previously been anticipated. In addition, the natural history and rate of progression of histological premalignant changes seen in the body and tail of the gland were totally unknown. Predicting the time frame from microscopic changes to frankly invasive cancer was impossible. Yet, there were still other arguments in favor of total pancreatectomy, including a more extensive lymphadenectomy, a decreased risk of tumor growth at the transected pancreatic margin, elimination of postoperative pancreatitis, and eradication of leakage at the pancreaticojejunal anastomosis.

By the 1990s the incidence of operative complications associated with the Whipple operation had decreased substantially due to the evolution of modern critical care, interventional drainage procedures, total parenteral nutrition, and antibiotic therapy. A sensible and rational compromise then occurred in the 1990s, when it became very clear from large institutional retrospective series that total pancreatectomy did not confer any survival benefit compared with the Whipple operation for cancer of the head of the pancreas. Thus, the Whipple operation once again became the first option for a cancer in the head of the gland and periampullary region, and total pancreatectomy is now reserved for specific instances only.

Indications

1. When there is definite multicentricity of the tumor as seen on imaging techniques, and/or on abdominal exploration.
2. Rare giant tumors, such as cystadenomas, cystadenocarcinomas, and sarcomas occupying virtually the entire gland.
3. Intraductal papillary mucin-secreting tumors of the pancreas that are diffuse throughout the gland (IPMN´S).
4. When there is obvious cancer documented (by frozen section histology) at the pancreatic transection margin during a Whipple operation.
5. When the patient is a long-standing insulin-requiring diabetic.

Contraindications

Absolute Contraindications

1. Evidence of peritoneal seeding.
2. Evidence of liver metastases.
3. Involvement of the celiac trunk, the superior mesentric artery, or the hepatic artery.
4. Extension into the aortic lymph nodes or adjoining organs including the stomach, colon, kidney, or spleen, which precludes negative margins.
5. Absence of an experienced surgical team.
6. Patient lacking alertness, intelligence, or willingness to manage diabetes mellitus.

Relative Contraindications

1. Invasion of the superior mesenteric/portal vein axis. In selected cases where the major venous trunk is minimally invaded, the idea of an en bloc excision of a segment of the venous trunk together with the specimen can be entertained provided a tumor-free surgical margin can be achieved. The venous trunk can then be reconstructed.
2. Severe obesity, which poses additional technical difficulties and is associated with higher operative risks.

Preoperative Investigations

A full history and physical examination is mandatory. A helical (spiral) or, multidetector abdominal computed tomography (CT) scan using the pancreatic protocol (intravenous contrast and oral water with thin slices through the pancreas) is essential. On imaging studies, attention is paid to the size of the lesion, the presence or absence of extrapancreatic invasion, nodal enlargement, and involvement of major vessels. In those cases where there is doubt about major vessel invasion, endoscopic ultrasound (EUS) can be a useful adjunct. Magnetic resonance cholangiopancreatography is emerging as the imaging modality of choice and it has the potential to replace both CT scans and EUS in the future, but at this time it is not always readily available.

If the tumor is deemed resectable by any of the imaging techniques, there is no need to perform a biopsy procedure. In addition, diagnostic endoscopic retrograde cholangiopancreatography and/or percutaneous transhepatic cholangiogram with or without biliary decompression are both avoided. Preoperative biliary manipulation has been shown to be associated with increased morbidity [5].

Preoperative Preparation

The necessary preoperative laboratory tests including a hemogram, full chemistry panel, liver function tests, coagulation panel, and tumor markers (CEA and CA19-9) are completed. If the tumor markers are elevated, they may be helpful later on for monitoring the tumor's response to surgery and/or adjuvant therapy. The patient is immunized against encapsulated organisms including *Neisseria meningitidis, Haemophilus influenzae*, and *Streptococcus pneumoniae* several days prior to the eventual splenectomy, which is part of the proposed operation.

The patient is advised to take only clear liquids for the 2 days prior to the operation, together with some mild laxative to provide a good mechanical bowel preparation. Nonabsorbable antibiotics may be added depending on the surgeon's personal preference. Vitamin K should be given subcutaneously 2 days prior to the operation, and again the morning of surgery. It is also continued for 2–3 days postoperatively. Packed red blood cells and fresh frozen plasma must be made available during the perioperative period. In addition, the patient should be kept well hydrated, especially in the presence of jaundice.

Informed Consent

The surgeon must have at least one comprehensive discussion with the patient and relatives. The operation must be explained in simple terms. All questions must be answered and the risks and benefits outlined and documented in the chart.

Immediate Preoperative Preparation

On the morning of the operation, a second, brief, question-and-answer period is held with the patient and relatives. Prophylactic antibiotics are given along with vitamin K and a proton pump inhibitor in the preoperative area. A second, and at times a third, round of antibiotics is given during the case, especially if major intraoperative bleeding is encountered. It should be mentioned that preoperative and intraoperative communication with the anesthesiologist are paramount. Intraoperative glucose and blood loss must be thoroughly monitored and communicated between the surgeon and anesthesiologist.

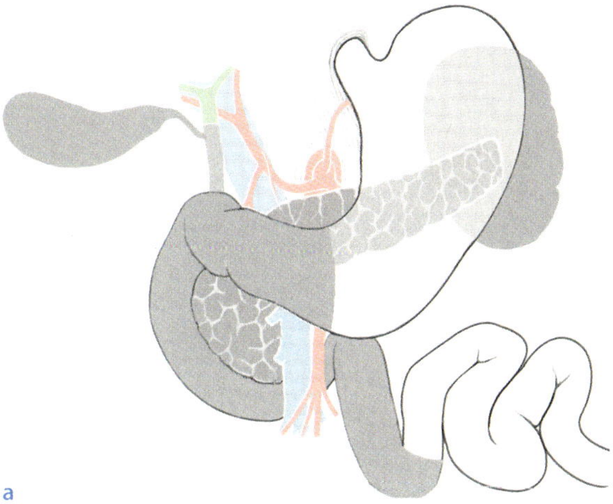

a

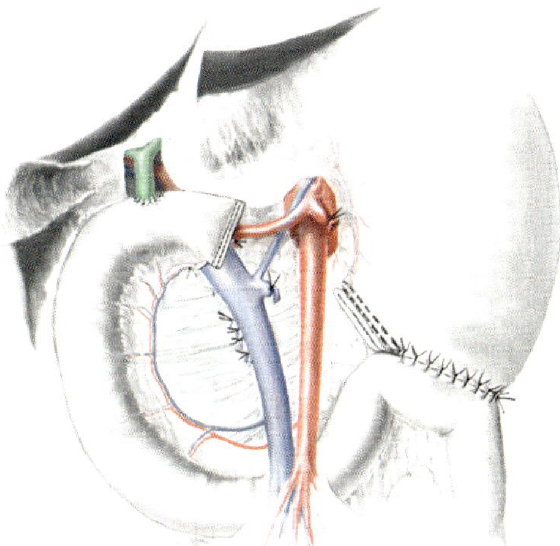

b

Figure 56.1

a Extent of resection (*shaded*) and b final reconstruction

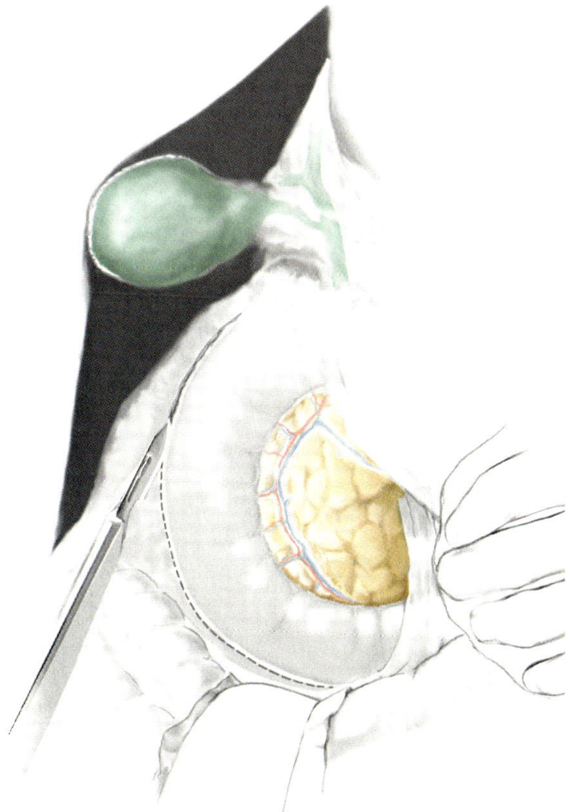

Figure 56.2

The *dotted line* indicates the peritoneal incision in front of the right kidney that is used to start the Kocher maneuver

The Operation

Preexploration laparoscopy to detect small, unsuspected peritoneal seeding or liver metastases is not routinely performed. It is only occasionally beneficial in cases where nonsurgical palliation is anticipated. The seven sacred principles of the operation can be summarized as follows: access, exposure, assistance, recognition and mobilization of anatomic structures, adherence to recognized tissue planes, and careful homeostasis. The anatomic extent of the operation and reconstruction are shown in Fig. 56.1.

The Incision

We usually adopt a bilateral subcostal incision approximately two finger-breadths below the costal margins. If the patient has a long, narrow subcostal angle, we advocate a long, vertical incision starting at the xiphisternum and continuing well below the umbilicus. Regardless of the incision chosen, the falsiform ligament is detached from the umbilicus, carefully mobilized, and preserved along its entire length into the liver for later use.

The liver and entire peritoneal cavity are carefully inspected for metastatic disease. In particular, the root of the mesentery in the regions of the transverse mesocolon and the ligament of Treitz are carefully inspected for tenting or puckering. If there is any question of tumor extension a biopsy sample is taken for frozen section histology. The presence of portal hypertension in association with these findings implies invasion of the root of the mesentery and occlusion of the superior mesenteric vein and virtually indicates unresectability.

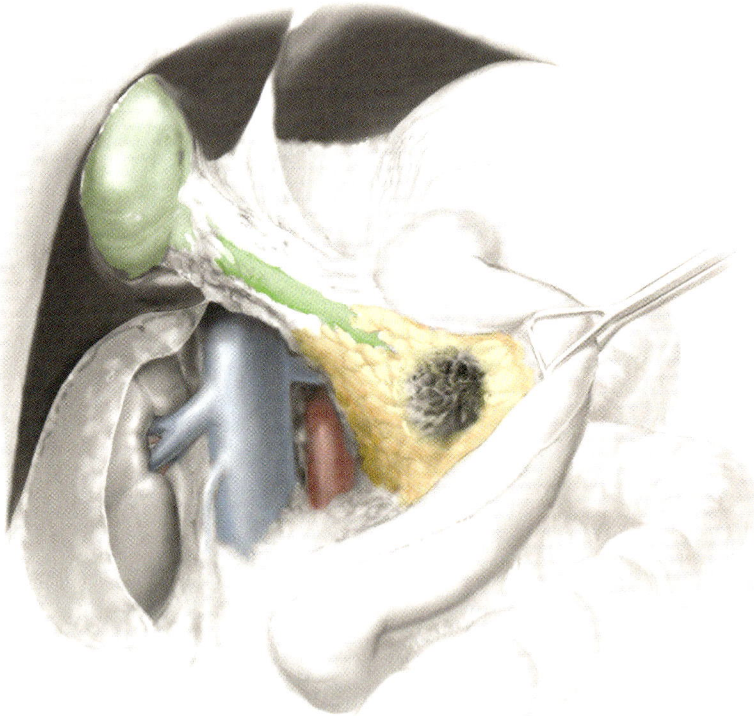

Figure 56.3

Full Kocher maneuver exposing the capsule of the right kidney, right renal vessels, inferior vena cava (*IVC*), right gonadal vein aorta, and left renal vein (*v.*)

Evaluation and Mobilization of the Pancreatoduodenal Region

Step 1: The Posterior Approach (an Extensive Kocher Maneuver)

The hepatic flexure of the colon is mobilized just enough to provide access to the duodenum and the head of the pancreas. The peritoneum lateral to the second part of the duodenum in front of the right kidney is incised, starting from the foramen of Winslow superiorly and continued down to the third part of the duodenum, where it is crossed by the transverse mesocolon and superior mesenteric vessels (Fig. 56.2). This maneuver should expose the retroperitoneal structures including the right kidney, the right renal vessels, the vena cava, the gonadal veins, and the left renal vein (Fig. 56.3).

As the third part of the duodenum is carefully mobilized from behind the superior mesenteric vessels, excessive traction should be avoided since small branches from the superior mesenteric vein can easily be torn, leading to troublesome bleeding. By palpating the posterior aspect of the uncinate process, the tumor and its lateral relationship to the superior mesenteric vessels can be appreciated (Fig. 56.4). With posterior palpation, attention should be paid to a po-

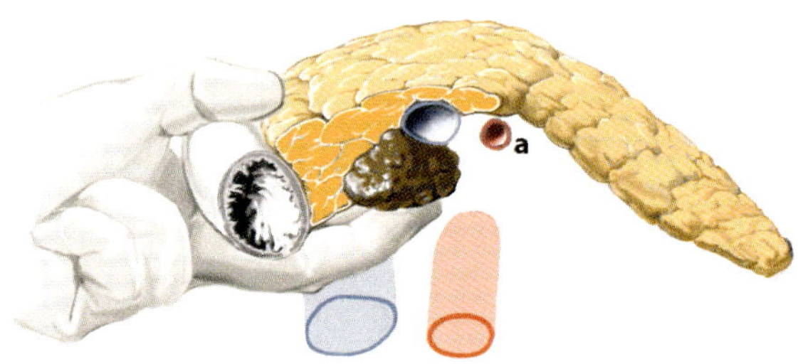

Figure 56.4

Palpation of mass in the head of pancreas to assess its relationship with the superior mesenteric vessels. *a.* Artery

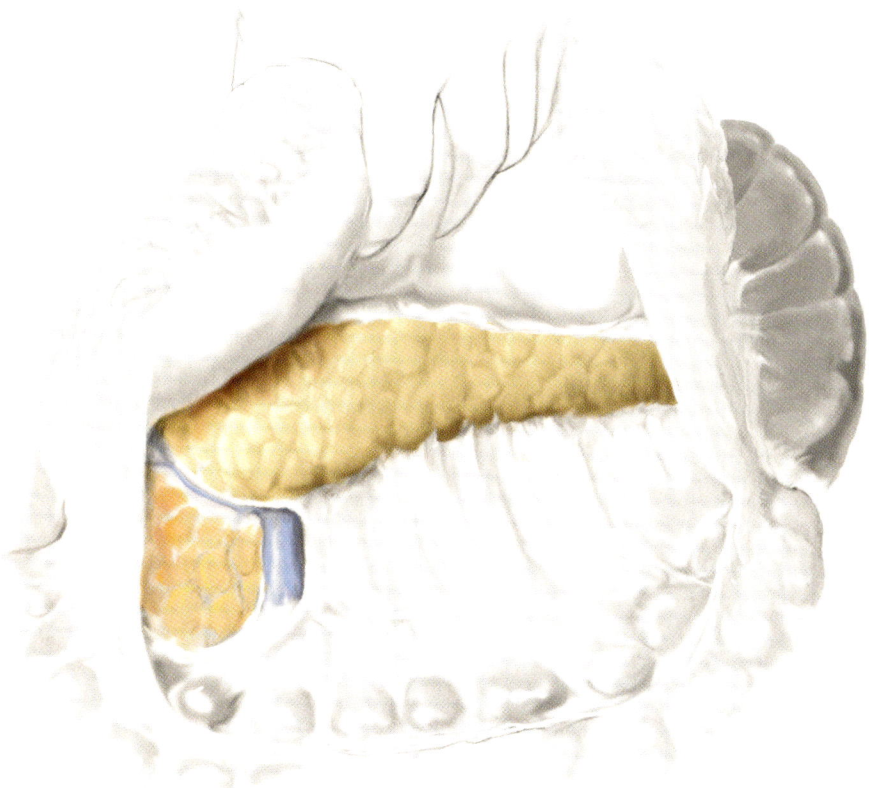

Figure 56.5

The transverse colon and mesocolon are retracted inferiorly to expose the inferior border of the pancreas. The middle colic vessels lead to the superior mesenteric vessels just behind the inferior border of the pancreatic neck

tential anatomic variant, the right hepatic artery (replaced right), or common hepatic artery (replaced common) originating from the superior mesenteric artery and coursing upward, behind the uncinate process and common bile duct. In about 20% of individuals, the right hepatic artery (replaced right), or the common hepatic artery (replaced common) arise from the superior mesenteric artery and run posterior to the uncinate process into the hepatoduodenal ligament. If the tumor is bulky, exposing the superior mesenteric vein laterally may be difficult. In such instances, the omentum is divided to expose the anterior aspect of the pancreas.

Step 2: The Anterior Approach

The omentum is detached from the transverse mesocolon along the relatively avascular plane to allow further entry into the lesser sac (Fig. 56.5). This is continued toward the left side of the abdomen and the spleen. Once the lesser sac is opened, the middle colic vein can be appreciated in the transverse mesocolon. The middle colic vein can be followed to its junction with the superior mesenteric vein just behind the inferior portion of the neck of the pancreas.

Step 3: The Superior Approach

The peritoneum overlying the portal triad is incised and all the soft tissue and lymphatics overlying the hepatic artery, common hepatic duct, and the portal vein are stripped inferiorly. At this juncture, the gallbladder is detached from the liver bed, starting with the fundus; the cystic artery is ligated and divided as usual.

The common hepatic duct can now be divided and used for traction in developing the plane anterior to the portal vein. The gastroduodenal artery is located as it leaves the hepatic artery, and is ligated and divided. This opens the superior aspect of the plane an-

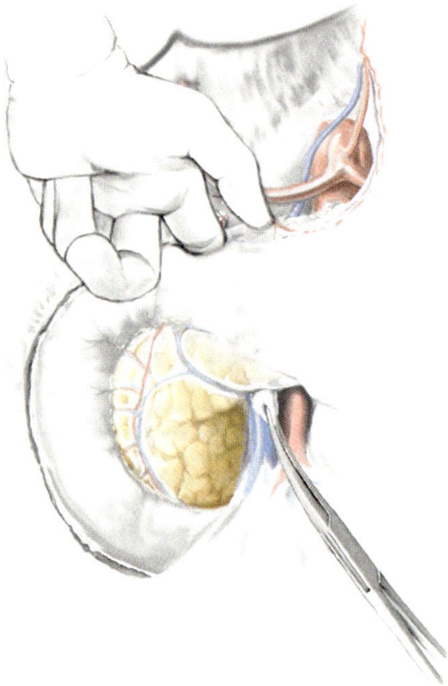

Figure 56.6

Using the index finger superiorly and a peanut sponge inferiorly, the neck of the pancreas (*P*) is bluntly elevated from the portal vein–superior mesenteric vein trunk (*T*)

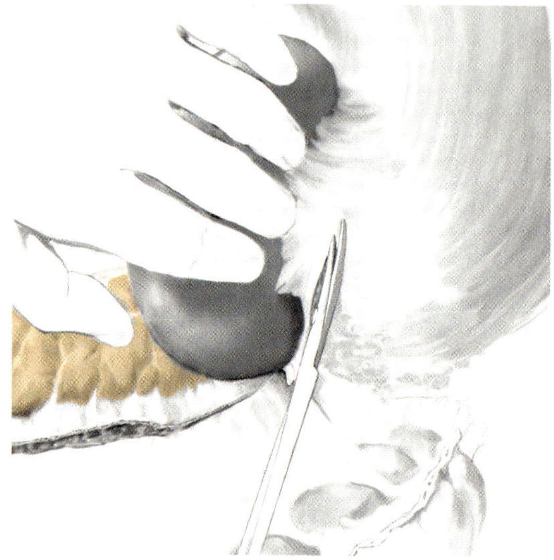

Figure 56.7

The dome of the spleen is retracted toward the right iliac fossa and the lienorenal ligament is divided to free the spleen and tail of the pancreas off the posterior parietal structures

terior to the portal vein behind the neck of the pancreas. If there is no invasion, this plane can be gently opened and an instrument may be passed behind the neck of the pancreas to elevate it. Alternatively, an index finger can be inserted from above, another one from below, anterior to the portal vein/superior mesenteric vein axis. If the plane is clear, resection can begin (Fig. 56.6).

<<Figure 56.6 here>>

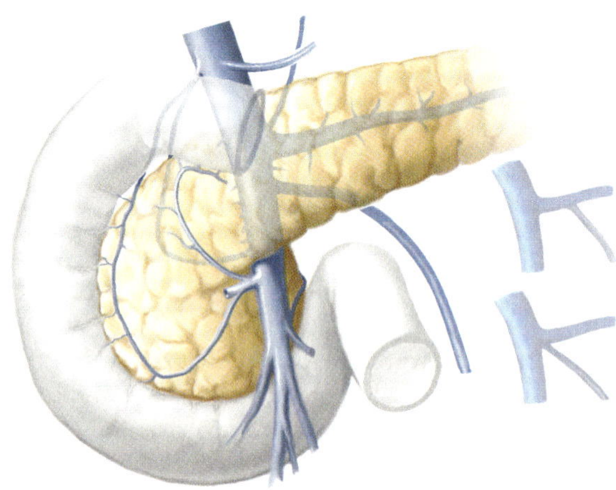

Figure 56.8

Anatomic relationship of the major veins to the neck and head of the pancreas

The Resection

Step 4: Mobilization and Transection of the Stomach

The omentum is serially detached from the greater curve of the stomach. The gastric branches of the gastroepiploic vessels are ligated and divided, going laterally along the fundus of the stomach. The lowest short gastric vessels may be ligated and divided now, or it may be easier once the spleen has been mobilized. The stomach is elevated anteriorly and a decision may then be made whether or not to preserve the entire stomach and first part of the duodenum. If "pylorus preservation" is desired, the first part of the duodenum is divided using a linear stapler. Alternatively, if an antrectomy is to be performed, the right gastric artery is ligated and divided at its origin from the hepatic or gastroduodenal artery. Termination of the left gastric vessels into the junction of the antrum and body of the stomach (crow's feet) are carefully ligated and divided. A linear stapler can be used at the junction of the antrum and the body of the stomach to transect the stomach. Care should be taken to preservc the left gastric artery and its esophageal branches.

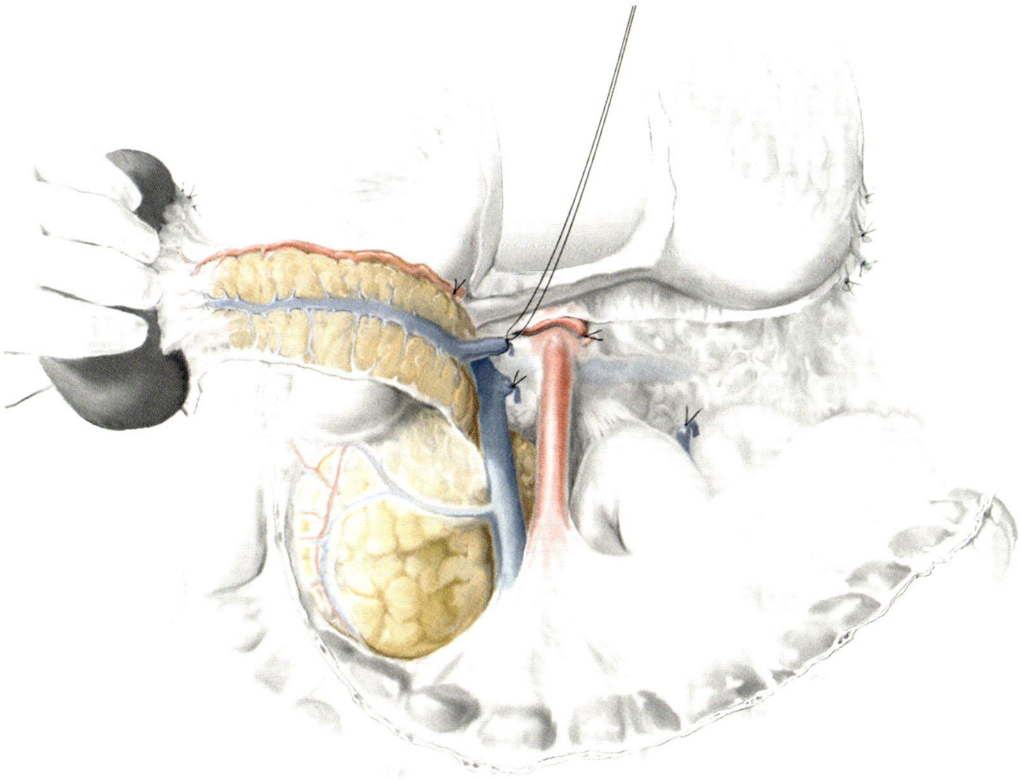

Figure 56.9

The spleen, tail, and body of the pancreas are retracted to the right. The splenic artery is ligated and divided at the celiac axis. The splenic vein is ligated and divided at its junction with the superior mesenteric vein (*SMV*). *SMA* Superior mesenteric artery

Step 5: Mobilization of the Spleen and Left Pancreas

Gentle traction is applied to the dome of the spleen in the direction of the right iliac fossa. This allows the division of the posterior leaf of the lienorenal ligament in front of the left kidney (Fig. 56.7). The splenocolic ligament is also divided to free the left colon inferiorly. The spleen and tail of the pancreas can then be mobilized anteriorly using blunt dissection. By elevating the tail of the gland and the spleen anteriorly and to the patient's right, the uppermost two or three short gastric vessels can be easily ligated and divided.

A vagotomy is not necessary as the risk of marginal ulceration is low following an antrectomy and the liberal use of proton pump inhibitors or H2 receptor antagonists virtually eliminates this complication.

Gentle blunt mobilization of the pancreatic tail continues from left to right and the spleen and pancreas, with the attached splenic vein on the posterior surface of the gland, are elevated. The inferior mesenteric vein is dealt with according to the anatomic variation of its termination (Fig. 56.8). If it enters the splenic vein it is ligated and divided close to the entry. If it enters the superior mesenteric vein, it is not disturbed [6].

The splenic artery is followed to its point of origin at the celiac axis, where it is doubly ligated and divided. The splenic vein is carefully dissected from its groove in the posterior aspect of the pancreas close to its junction with the portal vein, where it is doubly ligated and divided. This allows the neck of the pancreas to be elevated from the anterior aspect of the portal and superior mesenteric veins (Fig. 56.9). The specimen now remains attached by three areas only: the uncinate process and its fibro-fatty adherence to the superior mesenteric vessels, the upper small bowel with its midgut vascular attachments, and the peritoneum around the ligament of Treitz.

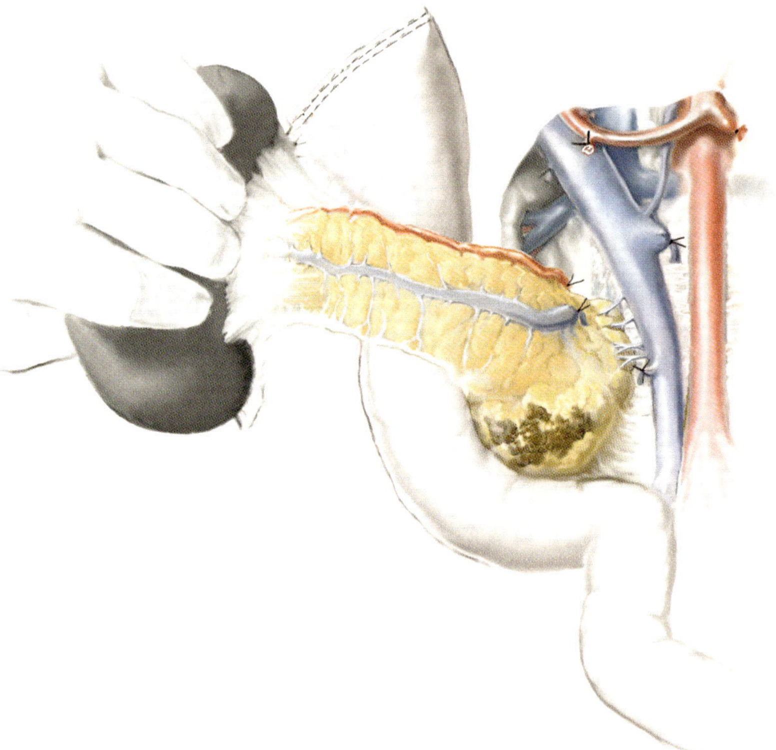

Figure 56.10

Ligation and division of the small veins draining into the superior mesenteric vein

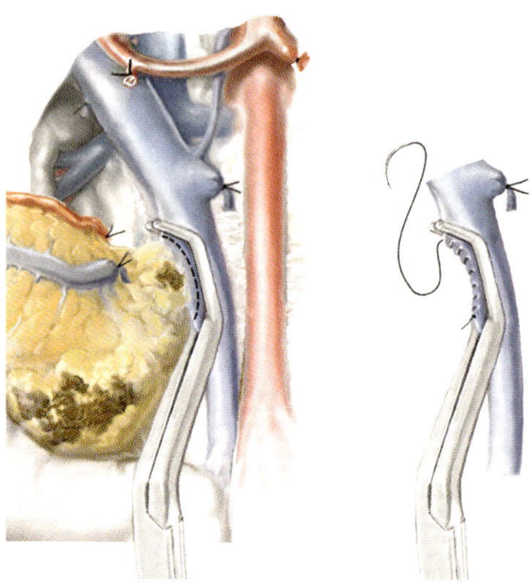

Figure 56.11

The use of a Statinsky clamp to excise a small portion of the portal vein (*1*) and superior mesenteric vein (*3*) due to tumor (*4*) invasion

Step 6: Freeing the Uncinate Process

With the retraction of the spleen, tail, and body and of the pancreas, along with the uncinate process to the right of the patient, the individual tributaries from the portal vein and superior mesenteric vein are made visible by gentle blunt dissection (Fig. 56.10). These vessels are individually controlled by ligatures and divided. In this way, the entire uncinate process can be gently detached from the anterior aspect of the root of the mesentery.

At this point, with all bridges burned, the posterior-lateral segment of the portal vein/superior mesenteric vein may be found to be invaded by tumor. If the invasion is minimal, a Statinsky clamp is used to obtain control of the venous trunk and the lateral edge of the vein can be excised along with the specimen (Fig. 56.11). In some instances, it may be necessary to excise a short segment of the vein with the specimen. In these cases an end-to-end anastomosis is performed with or without the use of an interposition vein graft comprised of a segment of iliac vein.

Once the trunk of the superior mesenteric/portal vein confluence is retracted medially using a vein retractor, the dissection continues one step posteriorly,

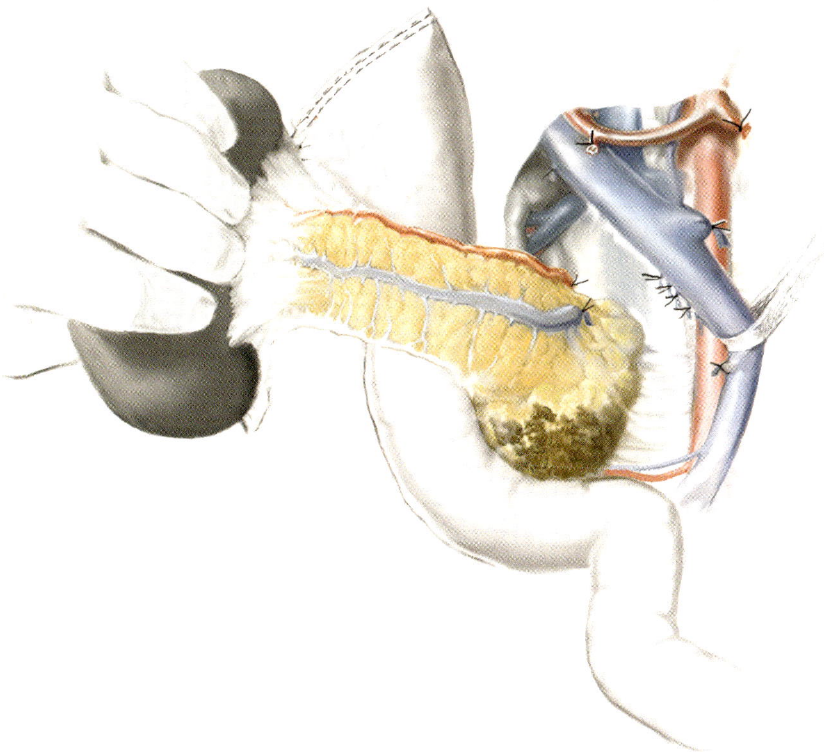

Figure 56.12

Freeing the uncinate process and the small arterial tributaries from the superior mesenteric artery after retracting the superior mesenteric vein to the left

to the bridge of tissue between the superior mesenteric artery and the uncinate process. Before dividing this attachment, it is important to carefully palpate once more the uncinate process posteriorly in order to check that there is no anatomic variation in the hepatic arterial blood supply (i.e., a common or replaced right hepatic artery). Occasionally, the preoperative imaging studies may identify such anatomic variation.

The multiple small arterial branches from the superior mesenteric artery to the uncinate process are not easily demonstrated. In practice, it is easier to stay on the adventitia of the superior mesenteric artery and to sequentially separate the tissue using a right-angle clamp or hemoclip to ligate and divide the fibro-fatty tissue joining the superior mesenteric artery to the uncinate process (Fig. 56.12).

Step 7: Division of the Ligament of Treitz and the Proximal Jejunum

The ligament of Treitz is exposed under the transverse mesocolon and the peritoneal attachment divided so that the duodenojejunal junction is free except for its vascular attachments. The upper jejunum is freed by ligating and dividing the inferior pancreaticoduodenal artery and the upper jejunal branches of the superior mesenteric vessels (Fig. 56.12). The uppermost two or three vessels of the jejunal mesentery are serially ligated and divided. This frees the upper small bowel, which then is mobilized and herniated beneath the root of the mesentery into the right upper quadrant. It should slide easily into the right subhepatic space where it can be divided using a linear gastrointestinal anastomosis stapler to free the entire specimen.

The Reconstruction

Prior to reconstruction, the entire operative field is irrigated with warm saline and inspected for small bleeding vessels, which can be controlled by ligature, hemoclips, or electrocautery (Fig.56.13). Once hemostasis has been achieved, the sequence of anastomoses is decided and is largely dependent on the surgeon's personal preference. We routinely oversew the staple

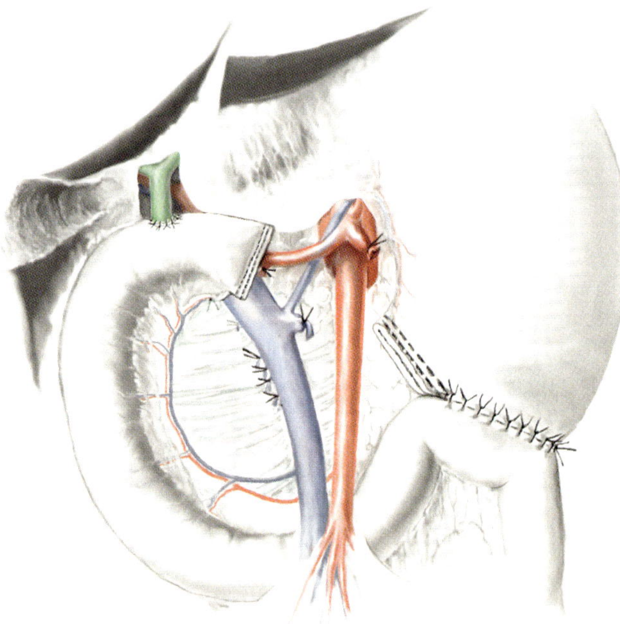

Figure 56.13

Gastrointestinal and biliary reconstruction following total pancreatoduodenectomy

lines of the upper proximal jejunum and the distal stomach with interrupted seromuscular sutures of 3.0 silk (Fig. 56.13).

The terminal end of the upper jejunum is pulled up behind the root of the mesentery into the right upper quadrant. The common hepatic duct is implanted into the side of the jejunum in an end-to-side manner using a single layer of full-thickness interrupted absorbable 3.0 vicryl sutures, care being taken to achieve mucosa-to-mucosa apposition. Once the posterior layer has been completed, a small piece of rolled gelfoam can be inserted across the anastomotic line in order to protect the back wall while the anterior layer is sewn. The gelfoam is left in place and disintegrates shortly after completion of the anastomosis. The falciform ligament is used as a buttressing patch to hold the upper jejunum behind and around the biliary–enteric anastomosis, helping to relieve tension on the anastomosis. The jejunum distal to the choledochojejunal anastomosis is arranged to create a new "C-loop" of jejunum, which is tacked to the residual lateral peritoneal lining in front of the right renal capsule (Fig. 56.13). The upper jejunum to the left of the superior mesenteric vessels is tacked to the surrounding cut peritoneal edges at the "old" ligament of Treitz and the transverse mesocolon to recreate a "new" ligament of Treitz. The stomach is brought through a gap created in the transverse mesocolon to the left of the middle colic vessels and a side-to-side posterior retrocolic gastrojejunostomy is created using a linear stapler; the staple line is reinforced with interrupted 3.0 seromuscular sutures (Fig. 56.13). The entire abdomen is again irrigated with copious amounts of warm saline and hemostasis assured. Two Jackson-Pratt or similar suction drains are used to drain the right subhepatic space posterior to the biliary–enteric anastomosis, and the left posterior subdiaphragmatic space. A nasogastric tube is left in place lying in the newly recreated "C-loop" of jejunum. The abdomen is closed with no. 1 Maxon sutures in two layers and the skin is closed with staples. If there is a generous layer of subcutaneous tissue, vertical mattress nylon sutures are used to occlude the subcutaneous dead space.

Postoperative Management

The patient is transferred to the intensive care unit and carefully monitored. All medications are given intravenously. Blood glucose is maintained between 70 and 140 mg/dl, by giving regular intravenous boluses of insulin. Alternatively, a continuous infusion of insulin may be employed. It is important to avoid subcutaneous injections of all medications since the patient's body fluids are in a state of flux and absorption is unpredictable. The patient is typically kept intubated on a respirator overnight. If the patient is stable, he/she is extubated the following morning and transferred from the intensive care unit to the ward or intermediate care unit, if appropriate. Nasogastric suction is continued for the next 4–5 days. Antibiotics are used perioperatively only. In general, the Jackson-Pratt drains are removed on the fourth or fifth prospective day, depending on the amount of drainage. The nasogastric tube is removed soon afterwards and oral intake is instituted. A suppository may be given to stimulate the restoration of gastrointestinal function and a bowel movement, which generally occurs at around post-operative day 7. When eating, the patient is instructed to take small, frequent, low-fat, high-carbohydrate and protein meals together with pancreatic enzyme supplements and a proton pump inhibitor. He/she is instructed about controlling the level of blood glucose and also how to administer injections of appropriate amounts of regular and long-acting insulin.

Complications of Total Pancreatectomy

Intraoperative Complications

Hemorrhage is the most frequent complication of total pancreatectomy and is best avoided by a thorough knowledge and appreciation of standard anatomy along with its variants. It is further controlled by meticulous dissection and ligation of all vessels along with replacement of blood and clotting factors as deemed appropriate.

Immediate Postoperative Complications

Bleeding

Hemorrhage is the commonest early postoperative complication of the operation. Thorough preoperative preparation, adequate transfusion of blood and clotting factors during the operation, and careful ligation of all vessels are essential. It is vital to double check all vascular areas for hemostasis before the abdomen is closed. In spite of these precautions, bleeding from the operative site through the drains may be alarming during the first 24 h. Reoperation is mandatory when there is reason to suspect a major bleeding site or when clot accumulation in the abdomen causes distention, tamponade, and/or when a consumption coagulopathy is recognized. However, in this type of situation one rarely, if ever, finds a discreet bleeding point at reoperation. Clots are gently evacuated and the whole abdomen irrigated prior to reclosure with drainage.

Hemobilia

Decompression of bile ducts that have been obstructed for several weeks often produces oozing from the walls of the bile passages. When this occurs in the postoperative period the jaundice may fail to improve or may even deepen temporarily. The hemobilia is occasionally very severe and the fluid coming out of the biliary tract as seen in the nasogastric tube appears to contain more blood than bile. This complication, in our experience, has always stopped spontaneously with the replacement of blood and blood-clotting factors. During this period it is essential to maintain a euvolemic state and to avoid acute tubular necrosis and potential hepatorenal failure.

Early fatal postoperative complications include generalized sepsis, mesenteric arterial and venous thrombosis, renal failure, hepatic failure, myocardial infarction, congestive heart failure, cerebrovascular accident, and pulmonary embolism.

Intermediate Complications

Delayed gastric emptying occurs in roughly 20–30% of patients with pylorus preservation and is usually self limiting. Other nonfatal complications may include pneumonitis, small-bowel obstructions, wound dehiscence, and atrial fibrillation. Bile leaks and bilomas may also occasionally occur. Intra-abdominal abscesses and wound infections may be significant, especially if the patient's biliary tree was stented preoperatively. Fecal fistulas and gastrojejunocolic fistulas are exceptionally rare but may occur.

Upper gastrointestinal bleeding due to stress ulceration or marginal ulceration is no longer a problem with the advent of adequate pharmacologic suppression of gastric acid secretion.

Late Complications

Recurrent cancer leading to other complications such as recurrent jaundice, cholangitis, gastric outlet obstruction, and a small bowel obstruction may occur. Other complications may occasionally develop due to adhesions and gastric intestinal reflux into the biliary tree and gastroesophageal reflux disease.

Long-Term Follow Up

The patient should be educated about, and monitored for, both endocrine and exocrine insufficiency since each may be fraught with problems that can shorten the patient's life.

Exocrine Insufficiency

Steatorrhea as defined by multiple loose, fatty, foul-smelling, stools and leads to dehydration, malabsorption, and weight loss. The patient must be taught to eat frequent low-fat meals and to take pancreatic enzyme supplements at the beginning of each meal. In addition, the patient is advised to take multivitamins and oral supplements up to three times a week.

Endocrine Insufficiency

The resulting diabetic state following total pancreatectomy necessitates comprehensive education for the patient and relatives. Once oral feeding is resumed, regular and long-acting (neutral protamine Hagedorn or lente) insulin is given in the morning, and usually a smaller dose given in the evening. It is important to start teaching the patient to monitor his own blood sugar regularly at least two times a day and to administer his own insulin in order to maintain a blood glucose level between 70 and 140 mg/dl. If the patient becomes hyperglycemic, exceeding the renal threshold for glucose, the patient will lose calories in the urine as well as fluid and electrolytes as a result of the osmotic diuresis. On the other hand, the patient and the relatives must be reminded that this form of diabetes is different from most in that hypoglycemia is a relatively common occurrence, probably due to the absence of pancreatic glucagon. These episodes can be avoided by increasing the intake of food or by decreasing the insulin dose, especially when physical activity is increased, and to carry glucose at all times. The occasional patient may die during a hypoglycemic attack and it is mandatory for the physician to reiterate this danger to the patient at each clinic visit. The patient should carry sugar with him/her at all times, including at the bedside. The patient must not miss any evening meals since this is the time that severe hypoglycemia most often develops. It may even be beneficial for all patients to experience an early hypoglycemic attack (i.e., tachycardia, sweating, undue nervousness) while he/she is still in hospital to see that these symptoms can easily be relieved by taking sugar.

Short-Term Outcome

The operative mortality is the same as that of the Whipple operation and should not exceed 1–2%. However, with both operations, the operative morbidity, if one were to include all categories of minor complications like superficial wound infection, atelectasis, urinary tract infections, and superficial vein phlebitis, is around 40%.

Long-Term Results

The patient is reviewed at regular intervals looking for metabolic disturbance as well as cancer recurrence. Full hematological and chemistry panels, as well as levels of CA19-9 and CEA are monitored every 2–3 months in the 1st year. The patient should have a periodic CT scan every 6 months for the first 2 years.

The vast majority of late deaths result from recurrent cancer. Our experience as well as that of others dictates that there are five poor prognostic factors following total pancreatectomy for cancer in the head of the pancreas. These are: (1) size of tumor greater than 2 cm, (2) extrapancreatic invasion, (3) presence of lymph node metastasis, (4) presence of perineural invasion, and (5) the presence of lymphatic and vascular invasion in the main tumor mass. Patients belonging to any of these groups are advised to have radiotherapy with 5-fluorouracil as a radio sensitizer, starting 5–6 weeks after the operation. The patient should also receive full cycles of gemcitabine chemotherapy empirically for at least the following year. The 5-year survival following total pancreatectomy is around 20–25%, but this may increase to 70–80% percent if the tumor is an intraductal mucin-producing neoplasm.

References

1. Ross DE (1954) Cancer of the pancreas; a plea for total pancreatectomy. Am J Surg 87:20–33
2. Sommers SC, Murphy SA, Warren S (1954) Pancreatic duct hyperplasia and cancer. Gastroenterology 27:629–640
3. Kloppel G, et al (1982) Classification of exocrine pancreatic tumors. Histological studies of 167 autopsy and 97 biopsy cases. Pathologe 3:319–38
4. Motojima K, et al (1993) Detection of point mutations in the Kirsten-ras oncogene provides evidence for the multicentricity of pancreatic carcinoma. Ann Surg 217:138–143
5. Povoski SP, et al (1999) Association of preoperative biliary drainage with postoperative outcome following pancreaticoduodenectomy. Ann Surg 230:131–242
6. Moossa AR (1980) Tumors of the Pancreas. Williams & Wilkins, Baltimore
7. Maingot R (1980) Abdominal Operations, 7th edn. Appleton-Century-Crofts, New York
8. Scott-Conner CEH (2002) Chassin's Operative Strategy in General Surgery: an Expositive Atlas, 3rd edn. Springer, New York
9. Trede M, Carter DC (1997) Surgery of the Pancreas, 2nd edn. Churchill Livingstone, New York
10. Moossa AR, Scott MH, M Lavelle-Jones (1984) The place of total and extended total pancreatectomy in pancreatic cancer. World J Surg 8: 895–899

Chapter 57

C. G. S. Hüscher · C. Ponzano · M. Di Paola

Laparoscopic Management of Pancreatic Neoplasms

Introduction

Pancreatico-duodenectomy (PD) still produces minimal survival benefits for cancer patients although it remains the only curative chance. Laparoscopy has been proven to reduce immune suppression and postoperative pain and discomfort, while providing enhanced vision and magnification of anatomic structures. The laparoscopic approach could add to the effectiveness of standard surgical treatments the less invasive endoscopic approach. Long term results of laparoscopic surgery have been shown to be at least equal (if not superior) to those of open surgery in the randomized trials [1-5]. So, beside the technical difficulties there is no reason to think that with laparoscopic PD we should aspect different results. From an oncologic point of view the quality of the dissection during a laparoscopic PD is without any doubt extremely accurate. A perfect visualisation is essential during such a difficult procedure that otherwise could not be completed without dramatic intra-operative complications.

Nevertheless, the history of laparoscopic pancreatico-duodenectomy is a brief one. In 1994 Gagner and Pomp reported, first in the literature, a laparoscopic PD, and in 1997 they published 10 more cases of laparoscopic PD [6-8]. In this experience the conversion rate was 40%, the average operative time was 8,5 hours and the hospital stay was 22.3 days.

Despite an accurate search on the Medline, we were able to find only another "large" series of laparoscopic PD which includes 25 patients, with excellent results in term of mortality and morbidity rate [9]. Such limited diffusion of laparoscopic PD is multifactorial; it is a technically demanding procedure, it requires a long operating time, and moreover the surgeon must be very experienced both in pancreatic and laparoscopic procedures. Furthermore, we could consider this operation like a two step highly demanding procedure: after a long, difficult and tiring demolition phase the surgeon is faced with an equally demanding reconstruction. We believe that the best option is to have a second "fresh" team to take over and complete the procedure. That means that two experienced teams should be available to perform a laparoscopic PD. Such an expertise is probably available only in selected centres. We present in this chapter the technique and the results of laparoscopic PD of what, to our knowledge, is the largest number of laparoscopic pancreatico-duodenectomy performed in a single centre.
Surgical technique of left and total pancreatectomy is also described.

Preoperative Investigation and Preparation for the Procedure

An accurate preoperative staging is essential to identify patients likely to benefit from radical surgery, as there is a general consensus that distant metastasis represent an absolute contraindication to surgery. Thus preoperative work-up must be extensive, including thin-section, multislice computed tomography scanning of the thorax and abdomen. The patient's general status is assessed by blood tests, plain chest

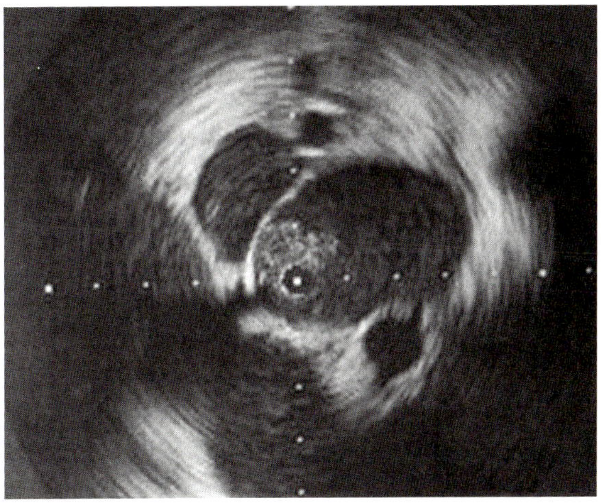

Figure 57.1

Intravascular ultrasonography: intraluminal vegetation (hyperechoic area in the center of the image) inside the portal vein. A lymph node is visible on the left upper part of the image, close to the hepatic artery. The common bile duct is visible in the inferior right part of the image, under the portal vein x-ray, spirometry, blood gas analysis, electrocardiogram, and echocardiography with systolic ejection fraction evaluation.

In case of a tumor located in the proximity of the portal vein, percutaneous intravascular ultrasonography is carried out to rule out portal vein invasion, which represents an absolute contraindication for the laparoscopic approach (Fig. 57.1).

For periampullary tumors, if jaundice is present, we try to avoid any drainage of the biliary tree whenever possible. If such a procedure is necessary, the positioning of a percutaneous drain under ultrasound guidance is preferred.

Rationale for Surgical Treatment

Surgeons willing to embark in laparoscopic pancreatic surgery should be aware that this is a new approach to a well-established procedure. The aim of this new approach is to decrease the surgical trauma for a poor-prognosis disease, providing a better quality of life for the patient. The immune response could also be better.

It must be underlined that despite the explosion of minimally invasive surgery in the treatment of gastrointestinal malignancies, very limited experience has been gained in laparoscopic pancreatic surgery, and few relevant studies are reported in the medical literature [6–8]. At present, the status of the knowledge to all of the potential advantages of the laparoscopic approach is theoretical, but absolutely far from being proven.

Indication and Contraindications

In our experience, all of the periampullary tumors, and tumors of the pancreatic head without portal vein invasion are suitable for a laparoscopic approach, as well as all left-sided tumors. Benign lesions of the pancreas, such as adenomas and cystoadenomas, ampullary and duodenal adenomas, insulinomas, and chronic pancreatitis mimicking a solid lesion, represent good indications for a laparoscopic approach. Portal hypertension secondary to hepatic cirrhosis is considered a contraindication.

Equipment

The following instruments and materials are required:

1. 30-degree angle view scope
2. Two coaxial needle-holders
3. Vascular laparoscopic forceps
4. Absorbable clip applicator (Lapro-clip, Tyco Health System)
5. Large- and small-size absorbable endoclip cartridges (Tyco Health System)
6. Argon beam coagulator
7. Argon beam probe
8. Generator for ultrasonically activated dissection (Ultracision, Ethicon Endosurgery, Cincinnati, Ohio, USA)
9. Ultrasonically activated 15 mm scissors (Ultracision, Ethicon Endosurgery, Cincinnati, Ohio, USA)
10. High-frequency monopolar and bipolar generators
11. Ultrasound cart with ultrasound laparoscopic probe
12. Endolinear stapler with vascular and parenchymal cartridges 45 mm in length
13. Vicryl (Ethicon, Sommeville, NJ, USA) Endoloops
14. Large-size titanium clip applier
15. Large-size Endobag
16. Air-tight abdominal wall protection/retrieval device (Lap-Disc; Ethicon)
17. Vessel loops in red, blue, and yellow colors

Although a minimally invasive procedure has been planned, a full set of traditional instruments should be available and ready in the operating room in case conversion to an open procedure becomes necessary.

Operating Room Setup and Patient Position

The patient is placed in a supine position, legs separated, with a 20-degree reverse-Trendelenburg tilt. The surgeon stands between the patient's legs with the camera assistant on his left side and a second assistant on his right side holding a liver retractor. The scrub nurse stays on the surgeon's right side. The rack with endoscopic equipment is on the patient's left. The use of two monitors is recommended. The high-frequency generator is on the left and slightly behind the surgeon (Fig. 57.2).

Port Placement

The procedure is accomplished with the aid of four 10- to 12-mm trocars. The first is inserted at the navel. Carbon dioxide pneumoperitoneum is then induced and the peritoneal cavity is carefully inspected to rule out peritoneal seeding. Two other trocars are

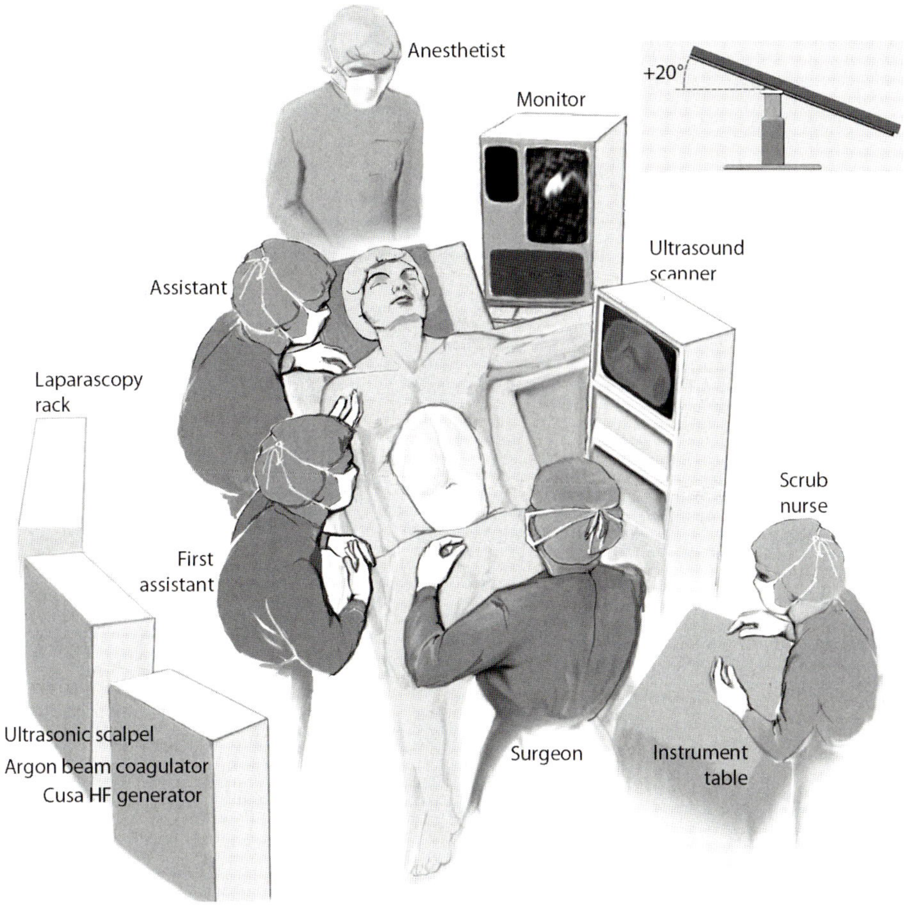

Figure 57.2

Theatre setup. *HF* High frequency

inserted through the abdominal wall in the left and right upper quadrants just below the costal margin at the level of the anterior axillary lines. A fourth cannula is placed in the midline, just below the xyphoid process (Fig. 57.3).

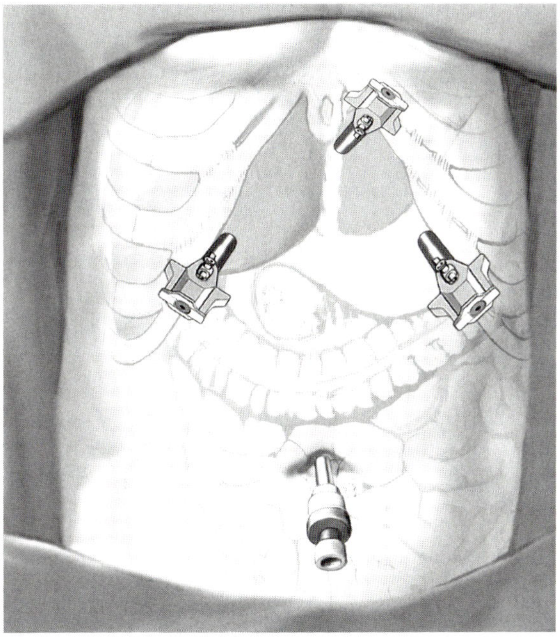

Figure 57.3

Trocar sites

Details of Laparoscopic Anatomy for Radical Extrafascial Duodenopancreatectomy

Perfect knowledge of the anatomy of the region is mandatory for a laparoscopic procedure. If areolar, avascular planes are important in open surgery, they are the very essence of laparoscopic surgery. Those planes came from the embryological development, and arise from the process of rotation that take place during the embryological life.

The key to understanding the final position of the pancreas and the fusion processes in the posterior abdominal wall, is the rotation of the stomach and midgut, and the formation of the mesogastric bursa.

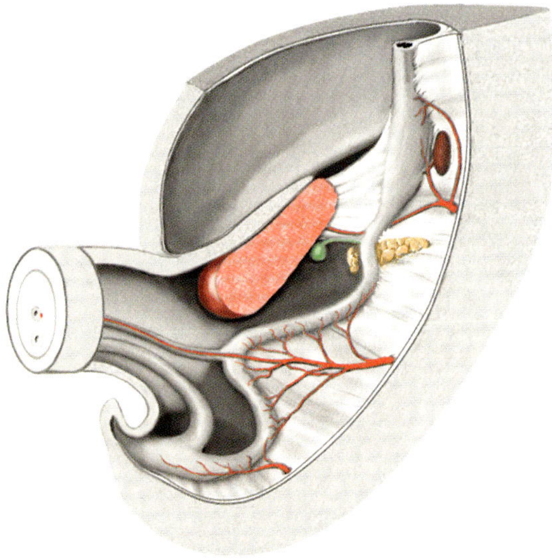

Figure 57.4

The initial disposition of the primitive intestinal loop. Note the position of the main vessels in the dorsal mesentery (celiac axis, superior and inferior mesenteric artery), which are named directive vessels of the peritoneum because they are the pivot around which the rotation of the umbilical loop takes place

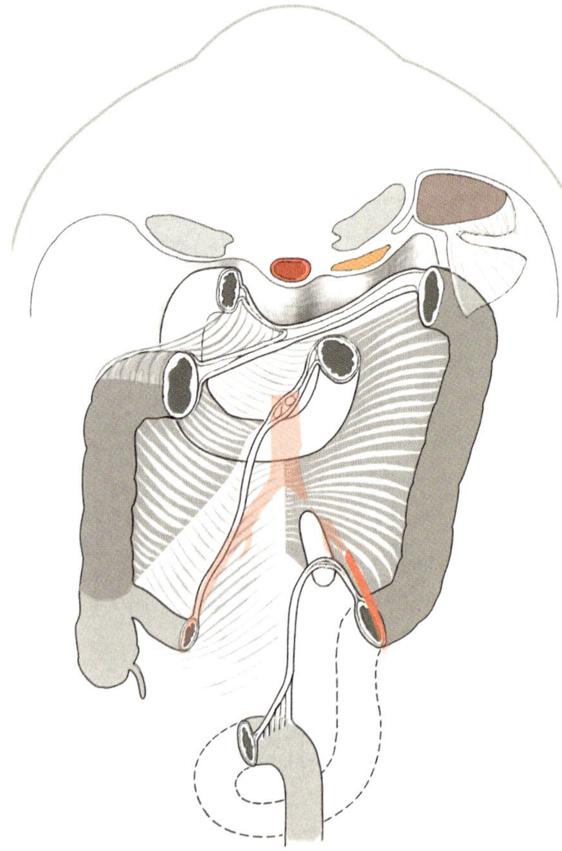

Figure 57.5

The disposition after the rotation is completed. The root of the transverse mesocolon goes from right to left and from down upwards, dividing the anterior aspect of the pancreatic head into two regions: supra- and inframesocolic. Toldt's fascia is showed in *grey* on both sides

The pancreas originated from two buds that appear toward the end of the 4th week of embryonic development: a dorsal bud located in the dorsal mesogastrium and a ventral bud located in the ventral mesentery (Fig. 57.4). At around the 5th week, the duodenum rotates to the right and posteriorly, and in so doing draws dorsally the common bile duct (CBD) and the ventral pancreas. As a result, the ventral pancreas comes to lie immediately below and behind the dorsal pancreas. The next phase results in fusion of the two pancreatic buds. While this structural development takes place, a spatial development also occurs as torsion of the intestinal loop takes place during its growth and differentiation. The primitive pancreas is initially located in a median sagittal plane within the dorsal mesentery. As a results of the rotation of the stomach, the body-tail of the pancreas and the splenic artery contained in the dorsal mesogastrium come to lie in a frontal plane, while the torsion of the duodenal loop and mesoduodenum brings the pancreatic head to the right. When the bowel comes back into the abdominal cavity, the final part of the rotation takes place. The cecum returns to the abdominal cavity in the left upper quadrant and makes a further rotation going right and downward to its definitive position. As a result of this rotation, the root of the transverse colon goes from right to left and from down upwards, thus dividing the head of the pancreas into two regions: supra- and submesocolic. The superior two-

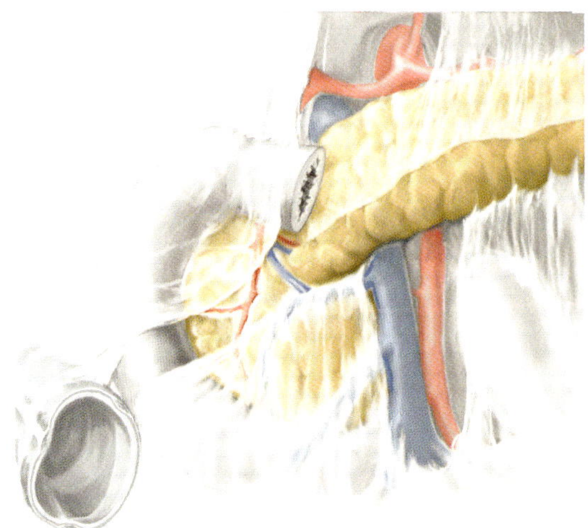

Figure 57.6

The anterior aspect of the head of the pancreas: Fredet's area and root of the transverse mesocolon thirds of the anterior aspect of the pancreas are adherent to the full thickness of the greater omentum and to the upper lining of transverse mesocolon, thus creating the so-called supramesocolic prepancreatic fascia or supramesocolic omental fascia. (Fig. 57.5). The inferior one-third of the anterior aspect of the pancreas is covered by the inferior lining of the transverse mesocolon, which is in contact with the peritoneum that overlies the duodenum. This contact creates a coalescent structure that extends from upside down and is known as the submesocolic preduodenopancreatic fascia of Fredet (Fig. 57.6) [10]. Lateral to the duodenum, both fasciae merge into the posterior duodenopancreatic fascia of Treitz, which, going downward, becomes Toldt's fascia of the right side. Fredet's fascia is left intact during the dissection, as we try to perform an "en bloc" removal of the pancreatic head covered anteriorly by Fredet's fascia and posteriorly by Treitz's fascia. The only opening in Fredet's fascia is right before the superior mesenteric vein (SMV), at the level where the Henlé (grastroomental) trunk merges into the vein.

Operative Technique

Laparoscopic Pylorus-Preserving Pancreaticoduodenectomy

The procedure starts by dividing the right side of the gastrocolic ligament. The lesser sac is entered, and the right gastroepiploic vessels are dissected and divided between absorbable clips. The stomach is lifted up to accomplish the dissection of the first part of the duodenum, which is divided with a linear endostapler, 2 cm distal to the pylorus. Before firing the stapler, the gastroduodenal artery must be identified as well as the gastro-omental trunk. The middle colic vein must be preserved, while the inferior pancreaticoduodenal vein can be ligated.

The hepatoduodenal ligament is dissected free (Fig. 57.7). The CBD is isolated and divided. A bulldog clamp can be positioned on the proximal stump of the CBD in order to avoid the bile dripping in the operative field. The common hepatic artery is dissected free and the gastroduodenal artery is identified and divided between absorbable clips (Fig. 57.8).

The peritoneum overlying the inferior aspect of the pancreas is opened. The SMV is dissected anteriorly from below, and a retropancreatic tunnel is created under direct visual control and with the help of magnification provided by the laparoscope (Fig. 57.9). The neck of the pancreas is then encircled with a loop lifted up and transected on the left side of the SMV with the Harmonic scalpel (HS). During the transection of the upper part of the gland, care must be taken to identify the main pancreatic duct.

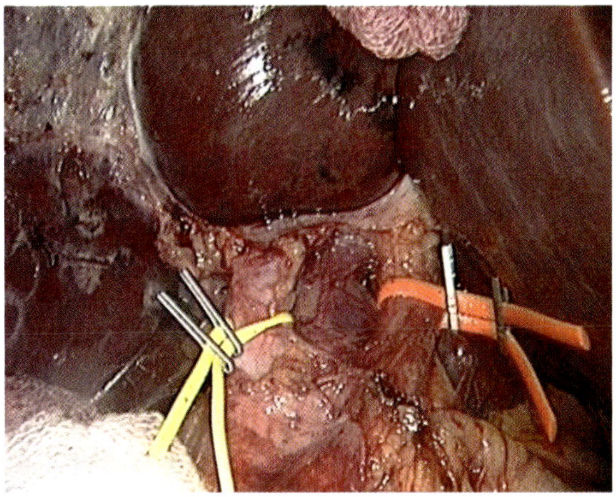

Figure 57.7

The elements of the hepatic pedicle are encircled with vessel loops of different colors. This preliminary step makes the vascular preparation safer and control of bleeding easier in case of vascular lesion, and facilitates the subsequent maneuvers

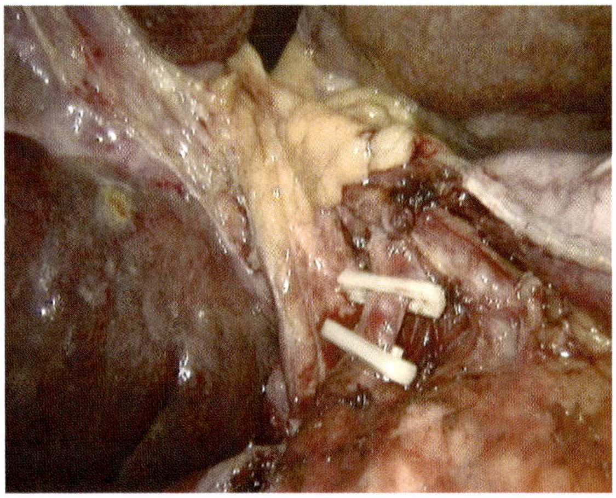

Figure 57.8

The gastroduodenal artery has been clipped with two absorbable clips. The proximal stump of the duodenum, which has been sectioned by an endogastrointestinal anastomosis device, is visible in the field

Kocher's maneuver can now be accomplished. This maneuver can be facilitated by the second assistant pulling leftward the first part of the duodenum with a Babcock clamp. Maximum attention is paid not to open Treitz's fascia behind the head of the pancreas. The hepatic flexure of the colon is mobilized and the front of the dissection can move to the inframesocolic space. The transverse colon is lifted up and the first jejunal loop dissected free and transected with an

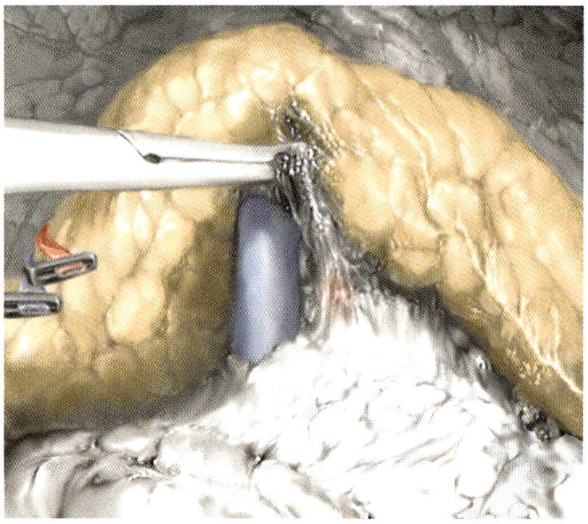

Figure 57.9

The retroisthmic tunnel is created under direct visual control. The portal vein is clearly visible in the field. The right gastroepiploic vessels, which had been clipped and divided are visible in the field

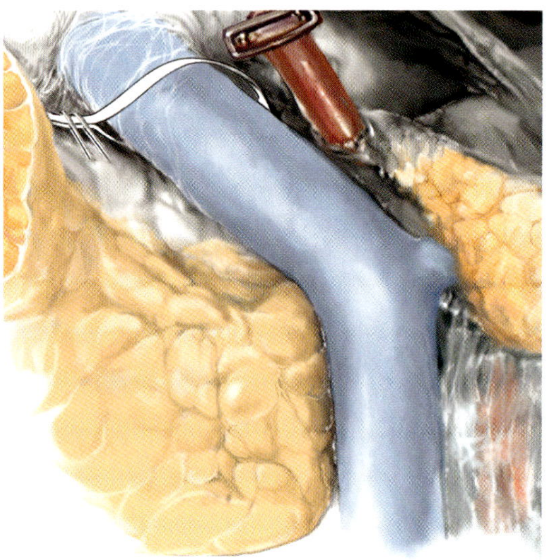

Figure 57.10

After the transection of the pancreas, its only remaining attachment is represented by the uncinate process. This shelf of pancreatic parenchyma is located posteriorly to the superior mesenteric vein and is deeply connected to the superior mesenteric artery. The superior mesenteric vein and the portal trunk are completely dissected free

endostapler loaded with a white cartridge. The ligament of Treitz is divided and from below the stapled proximal end of jejunum is transposed to the supramesocolic space by passing it behind the superior mesenteric artery (SMA) and SMV to emerge on the right side with the bulk of the specimen. At this stage the only remaining attachment of the pancreas is represented by the uncinate process. This shelf of pancreatic parenchyma is located posteriorly to the SMV and is deeply connected to the SMA (Fig. 57.10). While retracting the transected pancreas to the right, the uncinate process is detached using the harmonic scalpel and bipolar forceps. One must be aware that the uncinate process is extremely rich in vessels, notably the anastomotic branch to the pancreatic head from the dorsal pancreatic artery, the inferior-posterior pancreaticoduodenal artery (which can originate from a common trunk together with the first jejunal artery), and the inferior pancreatic vein. Therefore, the dissection must be extremely careful and hemostasis meticulous because hemorrhage arising from the uncinate may itself require conversion to open surgery and can be life-threatening in the postoperative period.

Reconstruction

The anastomoses are created in a retrocolic fashion in the following order: pancreaticojejunostomy, hepaticojejunostomy, and duodenojejunostomy. An end-to-side pancreaticojejunostomy is performed by placing the jejunal loop near the pancreatic stump. A running 3-0 polypropylene suture is used to approximate the posterior half of the gland to the jejunal wall. A small opening in the jejunal wall is made and a very short disposable stent (3–4 cm) inserted halfway into the pancreatic duct and halfway into the jejunum. Its purpose is to protect the posterior wall of the Wirsung jejunostomy, which is fashioned using two or three stitches of 3-/4-0 silk tightened with intracorporeal knots (Fig. 57.11). The anastomosis is completed by an anterior, running 3-0 polypropylene suture tied to the tail of the posterior running suture and further secured by absorbable clips.

The hepaticojejunal anastomosis is placed 10–12 cm from the pancreaticojejunal anastomosis, while the duodenojejunostomy is constructed a further 15 cm downstream. The bilioenteric anastomosis is performed by running a 4-0 absorbable monofilament suture, secured at the beginning and at the end by absorbable clips (Fig. 57.12). The tails of the stitches are tied together and further secured with an absorbable clip.

The last anastomosis performed ist the duodenojejunal one: jejunal loop is opened along the antimesenteric border. A posterior running suture is fashioned with a 3-0 absorbable monofilament including all layers of the bowel. The anastomosis is completed by an anterior extramucosal running stitch. The tails of the two running sutures are tightened together and further secured by absorbable clips.

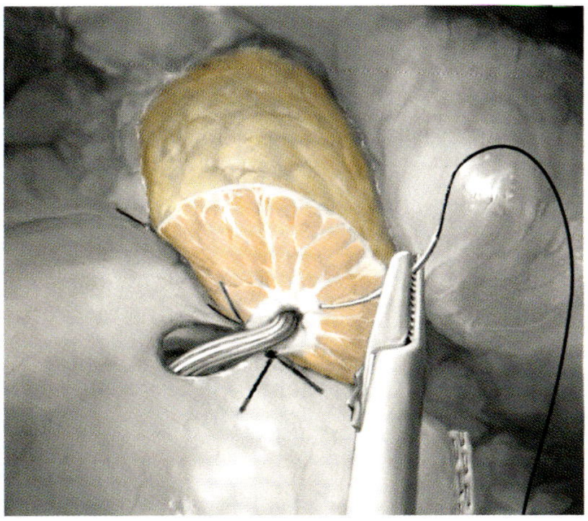

Figure 57.11

Pancreaticojejunal anastomosis: the posterior running suture is completed. A disposable stent is inserted into Wirsung's duct. The anastomosis between the pancreatic duct and jejunum is made with two or three stitches of silk tightened with intracorporeal knots

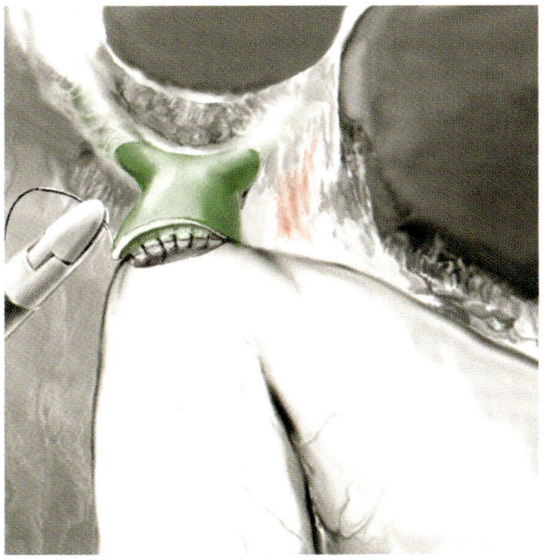

Figure 57.12

The bilioenteric anastomosis is made with the aid of two running, full-thickness sutures with an absorbable monofilament. The posterior layer is completed

Specimen Retrieval and Drain Placement

The specimen is introduced in a large Endobag inserted through the umbilical port, having first transferred the laparoscope to one of the lateral ports. The umbilical incision is enlarged to about 5 cm and, using the bag as a wall protector, the specimen is carefully delivered to the outside. The incision is partially closed, the pneumoperitoneum reestablished, and the laparoscope reintroduced. Hemostasis is checked and two suction drains are inserted. The first one is positioned between the pancreatic anastomosis posteriorly and the duodenojejunal anastomosis anteriorly, and brought outside through the incision made for the trocar on the left side. The second is left underneath the hepaticojejunostomy and brought out through the incision made for the trocar on the right side.

Laparoscopic Classic Whipple Procedure Without Pancreaticojejunal Anastomosis

This approach to the pancreatic remnant was firstly described in 1989 by Di Carlo et al. [11] and this first report of the technique seemed to give good results in term of incidence of lethal complications. In fact, we have abandoned this technique since the rate of pancreatic fistula was very high, at about 60%, while the mortality rate was not lowered. We therefore recommend a pancreaticojejunal anastomosis whenever possible.

Operative Technique

The gastrocolic ligament is opened and the lesser sac is entered. The greater curvature is mobilized. The hepatogastric ligament is opened and the stomach transected with several applications of a linear endostapler, as for a distal gastrectomy, preserving the left coronary vein and the left gastric artery. The stapler is loaded with a blue (normal tissue) or green (thick tissue) cartridge as required. The gastrohepatic ligament is dissected free and the common hepatic artery, the proper hepatic artery and the gastroduodenal artery are dissected free. The gastroduodenal artery is divided between absorbable clips. Once the cholecystectomy is accomplished, the dissection of the hepatic pedicle proceeds by dissecting the CBD and the portal trunk. This maneuver is made easier by the reduction of portal flow induced by the pneumoperitoneum. The CBD is transected with laparoscopic scissors above the cystic duct. The technique further proceeds as described above for the pylorus-preserving pancreaticoduodenectomy.

Reconstruction

The hepaticojejunostomy is performed as described above. The pancreatic stump is not anastomised. The pancreatic duct is catheterized and injected with cyanoacrylate. After the tissue-sealant injection, the opening is secured with one or two 3-0 polypropylene stitches.

A side-to-side gastro-jejunal anastomosis with the posterior wall of the stomach is then performed using a linear stapler loaded with a blue cartridge. The aperture remaining after removal of the stapler is closed with interrupted 3-0 polypropylene stitches, tightened with extracorporeal slipknots.

Specimen Retrieval and Drain Placement

Specimen retrieval is performed as described previously. Two suction drains are inserted. The first is positioned close to the pancreatic stump and passed through the subxyphoid incision, with the aim of achieving the shortest possible path in case a pancreatic fistula develops. The second is left beneath the hepaticojejunostomy.

Results

The preliminary results of laparoscopic pancreaticoduodenectomy have been reported elsewhere [12]. From November 1999 to December 2004, 47 patients underwent laparoscopic pancreaticoduodenectomy: 36 for malignant and 11 for benign disease. There were 28 (59.5%) males and 19 (40.5%) females, whose average age was 62±12 years (range from 38 to 84 years). In 11 cases (23.4%) the operation was converted to open surgery. In three cases conversion occurred during the creation of the pancreatic tunnel, because of adhesions between the tumor and the portal vein (two patients had T3 cancer with positive nodes, and one patient had portal vein infiltration who subsequently required portal vein resection). In four cases the procedure was converted during the final phase of the detachment of the uncinate process for tumor extension (all were T3 cancer with positive nodes). In two benign cases, the operation was converted for sclerosis due to pancreatitis. In one further patient the procedure was converted for diffuse bleeding due to a prolonged prothrombin time and International Normalized Ratio. The remaining patient was the only "emergency conversion" due to the rupture of the portal vein; this patient had severe chronic pancreatitis.

In 23 cases a laparoscopic pylorus-preserving pancreaticoduodenectomy was performed, and in 24 patients a Whipple procedure. In 22 patients a pancreaticojejunal anastomosis was not performed and the main pancreatic duct was occluded with cyanoacrylate glue.

The mean operative time was 384.5±76.9 min (range from 240 to 560 min) and the overall morbidity rate was 61.7% (29/47). In 12 patients a pancreatic leak was the only complication recorded, and in two further patients the only complication was delayed gastric empting and lymphorrhea, respectively. The overall pancreatic fistula rate was 38.3%, the incidence being greater among patients without pancreaticojejunal anastomosis (59%) than in those with pancreaticojejunal anastomosis (28%).

Postoperative complications requiring reoperation occurred in 13 patients: 6 bile leaks, 6 bleeds, 1 bowel occlusion. Three reoperations (27.2%) were necessary in the converted group, and 11 (30.5%) in the laparoscopic group. In those patients, the second operation was accomplished laparoscopically in six cases, thus only five patients in whom the procedure had been primarily completed laparoscopically were subsequently submitted to open surgery.

The mean number of dissected lymph nodes was 18±9 (range 2–40). Regional lymph node metastases were detected in 25 (69.5%) out of 36 patients with malignant disease. The medium length of postoperative stay was 19 ±11 days (range 8–51 days, median 14 days), and the 60-day postoperative mortality was 6.4% (3/47).

Left Pancreatectomy and Splenectomy

The equipment, operating room setup, patient position, and port placement do not differ from those for the previously described procedures (Figs. 57.1 and 57.2).

Operative Technique

The procedure starts with the mobilization of the splenic flexure of the colon. The lesser sac is entered by dividing the gastrocolic ligament. The greater curvature of the stomach is then mobilized by dividing the gastrosplenic ligament and coagulating the short gastric vessels with the HS. The splenic artery is identified and dissected free at the upper border of the pancreas. This maneuver is accomplished while the second assistant lifts up the stomach. Once the artery is completely dissected free, a right-angle clamp encircles the artery with a silicon loop secured with a nonabsorbable clip. This allows a rapid control of the splenic artery in case of bleeding during the dissection. The artery may now be divided between absorbable clips. It is recommended that the artery be divided proximally to the pancreatic artery of Arnold, which supplies the body and the tail of the pancreas (Fig. 57.13).

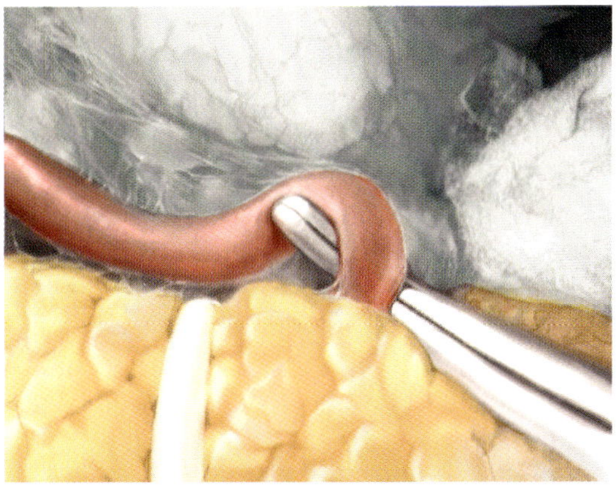

Figure 57.13

The artery is visible in the field above right-angled clamps. The splenic artery which supply the body and tail of the pancreas must be ligated to the befurcation.

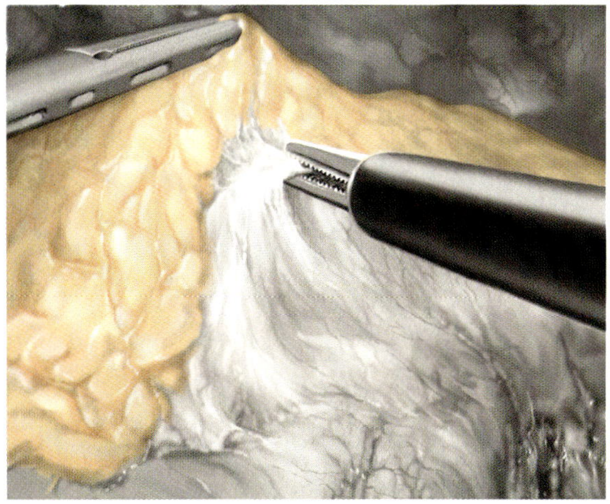

Figure 57.14

The retropancreatic tunnel is created: the peritoneum is divided along the inferior margin of the body and tail of the pancreas

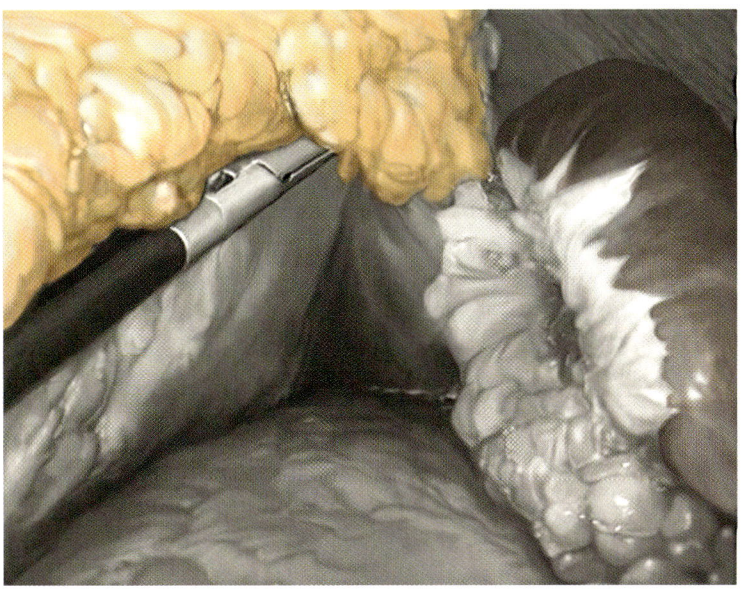

Figure 57.15

Left pancreatectomy with splenectomy: the plane of dissection is the avascular plane between mesogastric and Gerota's fasciae

At this stage, the retropancreatic tunnel can be performed. The peritoneum is divided along the inferior margin of the body and tail of the pancreas, corresponding to the insertion of the root of the transverse mesocolon on the posterior abdominal wall (Fig. 57.14). This dissection starts at the left border of the SMV or further to its left depending on the location of the tumor in the gland, and does not differ from the technique described for right-sided resections. The pancreas can be lifted up with a loop and divided. The mobilization of the body-tail of the gland is accomplished along the inferior border of the pancreas in the avascular plane between mesogastric and Gerota's fasciae (Fig. 57.15). The splenic vein is

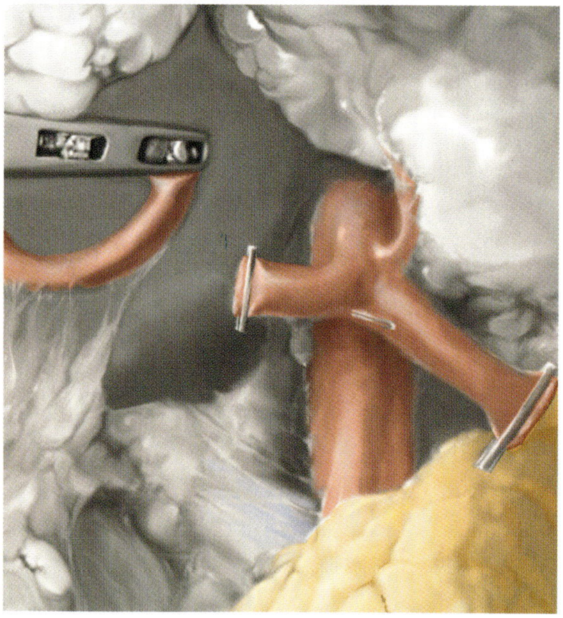

Figure 57.16

The celiac trunk is dissected completely free. The splenic artery is clipped as well as the hepatic artery. The distal stump of the hepatic artery is visible, lifted up by the forceps. The hepatic flow is controlled by visual examination of the color and tension of the liver. If there is any doubt, intraoperative Doppler ultrasound measurement can be used before the celiac trunk is resected

now dissected free and sectioned between absorbable clips or with an endostapler.

When the tumor is located in the body of the pancreas or at the neck, encasement of the celiac axis can be found. In this case, the celiac trunk can be resected with a vascular endostapler (Fig. 57.16). Care must be taken to preserve the gastroduodenal artery with its branches, namely the superior anterior and the superior posterior, which represent the only remaining hepatic arterial supply (Appleby procedure) [5].

Specimen Retrieval and Drain Placement

Specimen removal does not differ from previously described techniques. Usually only one suction drain is positioned in the left subphrenic space.

Total Pancreatectomy and Splenectomy

The equipment, operating room setup, patient position, and port placement are the same as for laparoscopic pancreaticoduodenectomy (Figs. 57.1 and 57.2).

Operative Technique

We have performed a laparoscopic total pancreatectomy in only two cases, so we still do not consider this procedure fully standardized. The first step of the operation involves mobilization of the right colonic flexure and of the duodenopancreatic bloc by means of a Kocher maneuver. The head of the pancreas and duodenum are mobilized from the posterior plane of the inferior vena cava (IVC) and the dissection is extended to the left to fully expose the IVC, the renal veins, the aorta, and the SMA (supramesocolic access according to Borelly; Fig. 57.17).

The left flexure of the colon is mobilized, the gastrocolic ligament is opened from right to left, and the greater curvature is mobilized. By retracting the stomach upward, the gastropancreatic fold is clearly visualized. This runs from the omental tuberosity of the pancreas to the lesser curvature of the stomach and it contains the left gastric vessels; these have to be preserved to assure an adequate blood supply to the gastric stump. The splenic artery is identified at the upper edge of the pancreas. It is dissected free, encircled with a silicon loop, and divided between absorbable clips or by an endostapler. The dissection proceeds leftward by dividing the superior leaflet of the transverse mesocolon along its insertion at the inferior margin of body and tail of the pancreas. This maneuver leads to the complete mobilization of body and tail of the pancreas along the avascular plane between the mesogastric and left Gerota's fasciae. The pancreas is encircled with silicon tape and lifted up. The splenopancreatic mobilization (Jinnai's maneuver) continues along the posterior margin of the spleen, from the lower to the upper pole, sectioning the splenorenal ligament, the lateral attachments to the abdominal wall, and the phrenosplenic ligament.

At this stage the vestibule of the lesser sac is entered, dissecting the lesser curvature of the stomach sufficiently for a gastric resection. Any left accessory hepatic artery within the lesser omentum should be carefully preserved. The line of transection should run from the point of van Goethen on the greater curvature (watershed between the right and left gastroepiploic vessels) to the lesser curvature: the nasogastric tube is withdrawn and the stomach is divided with multiple firings (usually three) of a 45-mm linear endostapler introduced through the left port. The stapler is loaded with a blue (normal tissue) or green (thick tissue) cartridge as required.

The elements of the hepatoduodenal ligament are dissected; the common hepatic artery is dissected free and encircled with a silicon loop. The gastroduodenal

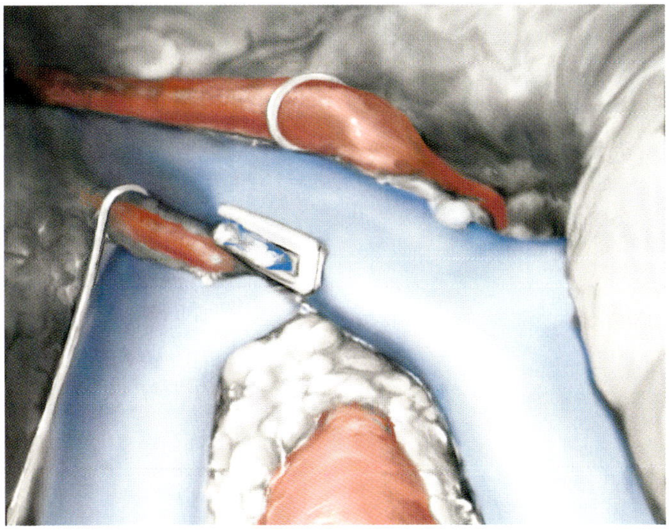

Figure 57.17

The portal trunk is visible in the field after the Kocher maneuver is accomplished: the inferior vena cava, the left renal vein, and the aorta are fully dissected. An accessory roght hepatic artery arising from the superior mesenteric artery is visible in the field encircled with a vessel loop

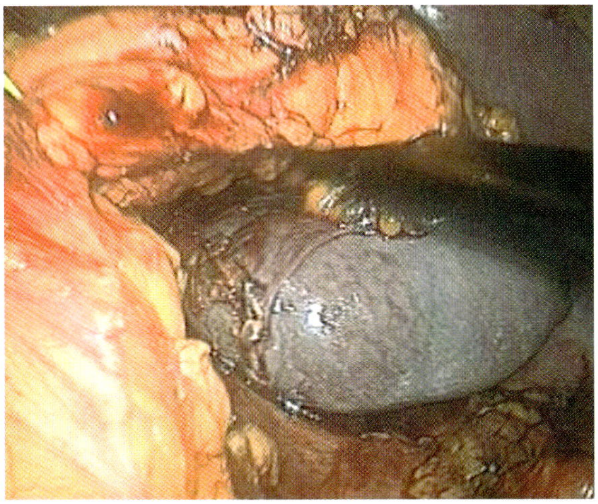

Figure 57.18

Total pancreatectomy: once the left pancreas and the spleen have been completely dissected, they are lifted and positioned in the right quadrant of the abdomen

artery is identified and sectioned between absorbable clips. After cholecystectomy is accomplished, the CBD is dissected free and divided. Dissecting the portal vein completes the dissection of the hepatic pedicle.

The peritoneum overlying the inferior aspect of the head of the pancreas is opened. A tunnel behind the pancreas is created by exposing the splenic vein until it reaches the confluence with the SMV. The splenic vein is then dissected and divided with a vascular endogastrointestinal anastomosis (white cartridge).

Moving to the inframesocolic compartment, the duodenojejunal flexure is identified and the jejunum is divided at a distance of at least 10 cm from the ligament of Treitz. The duodenum and the proximal jejunum are displaced to the right side of the inframesocolic compartment, passing underneath the superior mesenteric vessels. The splenopancreatic block is retracted to the right (Fig. 57.18), exposing the residual connections of the pancreas. The uncinate process behind the SMV is detached from the SMA by means of the HS and bipolar forceps.

Reconstruction Phase

The end-to-side hepaticojejunostomy and the side-to-side gastrojejunal anastomosis on the posterior wall of the stomach are fashioned as described earlier.

Specimen Retrieval and Drain Placement

Specimen removal does not differ from previously described techniques. Two suction drains are positioned. The first is left beneath the hepaticojejunostomy and passed through the right lateral incision. The second is positioned in the left subphrenic space.

References

1. COST Study Group: A comparison of laparoscopically assisted and open colectomy for colon cancer. N Engl J Med 2004; 350: 2050-9
2. Lacy AM, Garcia-Valdecasas JC, Delgado S, et al. Laparoscopy-assisted colectomy versus open colectomy for treatment of non-metastatic colon cancer: a randomised trial. Lancet 2002; 359:2224-9
3. JC Weeks, H. Nelson, S. Gelber, D. Sargent, G. Schroeder: Short-term quality of life outcomes following laparoscopic-assisted colectomy vs open colectomy for colon cancer. JAMA 2002; 287 (3): 321-8
4. PJ Guillou, P Quirke, H Thorpe et al: Short term endpoints of conventional versus laparoscopic-assisted surgery in patients with colorectal cancer (MRC CLASSIC trial): multicentre, randomised controlled trial. Lancet 2005; 365: 1718-26
5. The colon cancer laparoscopic and open resection study group (COLOR): Laparoscopic surgery versus open surgery for colon cancer: short-term outcomes of a randomised trial. Lancet Oncol 2005; 6: 477-84
6. Milone L., Turner P., Gagner M.: Laparoscopic surgery for pancreatic tumours, an update. Min Chir 59:165-73, 2004
7. Gagner M., Pomp A.: Laparoscopic pylorus-preserving pancreatico-duodenectomy. Surg Endosc. 1994; 8: 408-410
8. Gagner M., Pomp A.: Laparoscopic pancreatic resection: is it worthwhile?. J Gastrointest Surg. 1997; 1: 20-26
9. Dulucq J.L., Wintringer P., Mahajna A: Laparoscopic pancreaticoduodenectomy for benign and malignant disease. Surg Endosc. 2006; 20: 1045-1050

10 Fredet P.: Le péritoine. In Poirer and Charpy, editors: Traité d'anatomie humaine, Paris, 1905, Masson Publishing Co.

11 Di Carlo V., Chiesa R., Pontiroli A.E., et al. Pancreatico-duodenectomy with occlusion of the residual stump by neoprene injection. World J Surg, 13(1): 105-10, 1989

12 Hüscher C (2004) Laparoscopic Whipple Procedure. In: Cameron JL (ed) Current Surgical Therapy, 8th edn. Elsevier Mosby, Philadelphia 1266-74

13 Hirai I, Kimura W, Kamiga M, Mizutani M, Takeshida A, Watanabe T, Fuse A (2005) The significance of intraoperative Doppler ultrasonography inn evaluating hepatic arterial flow when assessing the indications for Appleby procedure for pancreatic body cancer. J Hepatobiliary Pancreat Surg 12: 55-60

Chapter 58

M. G. House · K. D. Lillemoe

Bypass Procedures in the Treatment of Nonresectable Carcinoma of the Head of the Pancreas

Adenocarcinoma of the pancreas, with an annual incidence of approximately 28,000, is the fourth leading cause of cancer-related mortality in men and women in the United States [1]. While complete surgical extirpation can improve the outlook for some patients, the 5-year survival for all patients with pancreatic adenocarcinoma ranges from 0.4 to 4% [2]. Patients who undergo complete surgical resection for localized adenocarcinoma of the head of the pancreas in addition to adjunctive chemotherapy experience a 5-year survival of only 20%, with a median survival of 18 months [3, 4]. Unfortunately, at the time of initial diagnosis, only 50% of patients with pancreatic cancer will be free of distant metastases, and less than 20% of these patients will have localized disease amenable to curative resection [3, 4]. Among patients who are felt to be candidates for curative resection on preoperative imaging, approximately 15–25% will be found to have occult metastases or locoregional vascular invasion at the time of exploration [5].

Even though the majority of patients with pancreatic cancer are not candidates for curative resection due to early metastatic spread or extensive locoregional tumor involvement, palliation of obstruction of the biliary tree and/or duodenum remains a key consideration in the surgical management of this disease. During the course of their disease, approximately 80% of patients with cancer involving the head of the pancreas will experience obstructive jaundice, and 20% will develop symptoms related to duodenal obstruction [6–10]. Depending on performance status and medical comorbidities, survival for patients with metastatic disease is approximately 3–6 months, while patients with nonmetastatic, locally advanced pancreatic cancer experience a median survival of approximately 6–12 months [6–8, 10]. Adequate palliation of biliary and duodenal obstruction has been shown to improve quality of life; therefore, every attempt, whether nonoperative or operative, should be made to palliate obstruction in virtually all patients with unresectable pancreatic cancer [9–12].

Surgical treatment has served as the traditional modality for palliating the symptoms associated with locally advanced pancreatic cancer; however, improved nonoperative strategies have proved to be reliable and durable in select patients with either biliary or duodenal obstruction [10, 13]. For patients with unequivocal evidence of unresectable disease during preoperative evaluation, or those at prohibitive operative risk, endoluminal methods for biliary and duodenal stenting should be attempted first, and open surgical bypass procedures should be reserved for treatment failures of nonsurgical (i.e., endoscopic or percutaneous) methods. Despite improvements in nonsurgical methods, open palliative bypass procedures for biliary and duodenal obstruction continue to be more durable long-term and require less reintervention [14]. For patients undergoing open exploration for equivocal radiographic signs of unresectable pancreatic cancer, surgical palliation is often indicated for those found to have nonmetastatic (or low-volume metastatic), unresectable disease intraoperatively.

Preoperative Investigation

Despite advances in computed tomography (CT) that have improved the preoperative assessment of tumor unresectability for patients with pancreatic cancer, approximately 20% of patients who are explored with curative intent will be found to have either occult metastases or locoregional vascular invasion (Table 58.1) [5]. Three-dimensional technology has enhanced the radiographic assessment of mesenteric vascular invasion by neoplasms arising from the head of the pancreas (Fig. 58.1); however, open surgical exploration continues to serve as the standard for determining tumor resectability. Endoscopic ultrasound (EUS) and diagnostic laparoscopy can be used selectively as adjuncts to CT in determining locoregional vascular invasion and occult metastatic disease, respectively.

Table 58.1. Resectability of periampullary tumors among patients undergoing three-dimensional computed tomography. From House et al. 2004 [5]

	Periampullary neoplasms[b]	Pancreatic adenocarcinomas
Resectability	95 (83%)	67 (79%)
Margin-negative resectability[a]	71 (75%)	49 (73%)
Total explorations	115	85

[a] Among resectable cases only
[b] Periampullary neoplasms include primary tumors of the pancreas, CBD, ampulla, and duodenum

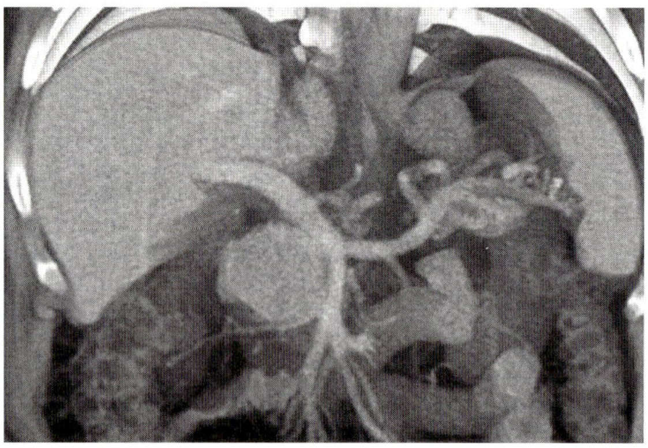

Figure 58.1

Three-dimensional axial-oblique reconstruction shows a low-density mass within the head of the pancreas that abuts, but does not encase the superior mesenteric vein (SMV) or portal vein (PV). The vessels appear patent with no evidence of displacement. This pancreatic adenocarcinoma was resected without the need for partial SMV or PV resection. (From House et al. 2004 [5])

Indications for Surgical Palliation

The majority of pancreatic adenocarcinomas arise in the head of the pancreas and possess a desmoplastic biology. Not surprisingly, 80% of patients with pancreatic adenocarcinoma will seek medical attention for symptoms related to jaundice secondary to mechanical obstruction of the intrapancreatic portion of the distal common bile duct [6–8, 11]. Another 20% of patients will develop mechanical obstruction of the duodenum, either at the time of diagnosis or during disease progression [15]. Obstructive jaundice can also be accompanied by refractory pruritus, anorexia, malabsorptive diarrhea, and liver failure. The development of gastric outlet obstruction only adds to the progressive malnutrition potentiated by the jaundiced state. Each of these conditions, particularly when combined, can lead to rapid generalized wasting. For these reasons, decompression of biliary obstruction and reestablishment of gastric emptying lead to a dramatic improvement in the overall medical condition, which contributes to a prolongation of comfortable survival.

For jaundiced patients with pancreatic cancer deemed unresectable based on preoperative evaluation, nonsurgical palliation is generally indicated except for the most terminally ill patients. Since its clinical inception in 1980, the use of endoscopically placed biliary endoprostheses has continued to evolve and now serves as the predominant modality for palliating obstructive jaundice in patients who are not candidates for curative resection [13]. Endoscopic attempts at biliary drainage fail in less than 10% of patients, usually as a result of tumor infiltration into the duodenal wall that prevents access to the ampulla [12, 16]. In the uncommon event that endoscopic management is unsuccessful, percutaneous transhepatic access can be obtained to allow external biliary drainage. In most cases, internal biliary drainage can be achieved after the initial external drainage procedure.

Duodenal or gastric outlet obstruction has traditionally been managed by surgery, but there is growing experience with endoluminal approaches to relieving obstruction [10]. In the past, endoscopic options included tube gastrostomy with jejunal extension for nutritional access; however, the development of self-expanding enteral stents has provided a reliable measure for palliating duodenal obstruction in patients who do not require surgical exploration to determine resectability. Despite early success with enteral stents in small series, complications can arise and include mucosal ulceration, duodenal perforation, stent migration, and tumor ingrowth leading to recurrent obstruction. Patients with reasonable life expectancy who fail endoscopic attempts at palliation or develop complications related to endoluminal stenting, may require surgical gastrojejunostomy.

Since most symptomatic patients with preoperative radiologic studies demonstrating unresectable disease can be adequately palliated with nonoperative techniques, there is little role for surgical palliation

Table 58.2. Impact of gastrojejunostomy on immediate postoperative outcomes after surgical palliation for unresectable preampullary cancer

	Gastrojejunostomy (*n*=44)	No gastrojejunostomy (*n*=43)
Perioperative deaths	0 (0%)	0 (0%)
Any complications	14 (32%)	14 (33%)
Cholangitis	4 (9%)	2 (5%)
Biliary anastomotic leak	3 (7%)	2 (5%)
Delayed gastric emptying	1 (2%)	1 (2%)
Wound infection	2 (5%)	0 (0%)
Pneumonia	1 (2%)	2 (5%)
Gastric anastomotic leak	0 (0%)	–
Postoperative hospital length of stay (days)	8.5±0.5	8.0±0.5

for a large subgroup of patients with pancreatic cancer. However, there does remain an important role for surgical palliation in those patients undergoing operation to attempt resection.

Diagnostic laparoscopy has become an important part of the staging of many patients with pancreatic cancer. In most situations when unresectable disease is found at laparoscopy in the form of liver metastasis or peritoneal implants, operative palliation is not generally indicated. In a series of 155 patients from the Memorial Sloan-Kettering Cancer Center who were found to have unresectable pancreatic adenocarcinoma at the time of staging laparoscopy, only 3 (2%) required an open procedure to palliate biliary or gastric obstruction during their lifetime [17]. Over two-thirds of the patients in this retrospective study were found to have either liver or peritoneal metastases, and the median survival was 6.2 months. Obstructive symptoms developed in 19 patients (12%), but the majority were managed without an open procedure. Jaundiced patients without gastric outlet obstruction who are found to have metastatic disease at the time of staging laparoscopy can usually be palliated successfully with endoscopic biliary stenting alone. Patients with gastric outlet obstruction who are determined to have unresectable disease at the time of staging laparoscopy, should undergo laparoscopic gastrojejunostomy [18].

Patients found to be unresectable at the time of laparotomy should be considered for operative palliation at that time, even those who have been stented endoscopically for obstructive jaundice. Unless the porta hepatis is inaccessible, both a biliary-enteric bypass and a gastrojejunostomy should be performed regardless of existing symptoms. The latter concept has been debated for years among surgeons. A least three meta-analyses of surgical series have suggested that 15–25% of patients found to be unresectable at the time of laparotomy and not provided with a gastrojejunostomy will eventually develop symptomatic duodenal obstruction [6, 8, 19, 20]. Two prospective randomized trials have provided level I evidence that supports performing a biliary-enteric bypass and a gastrojejunostomy for all patients who are determined to have unresectable disease at the time of laparotomy [9, 21]. One of these trials, conducted at the Johns Hopkins Hospital, randomized asymptomatic patients who were found to be unresectable at the time of laparotomy to either a prophylactic gastrojejunostomy or none [9]. Approximately 50% of the patients randomized to no prophylactic gastrojejunostomy were deemed unresectable on the basis of liver or peritoneal metastases. In this group, 19% of patients, who were not treated with a gastrojejunostomy developed late gastric outlet obstruction requiring therapeutic intervention prior to death; no patient who underwent a prophylactic gastrojejunostomy developed such problems. The addition of a gastrojejunostomy did not add to the perioperative morbidity, mortality, or length of stay related to the laparotomy (Table 58.2). These results have been confirmed subsequently by a multi-institutional study conducted in The Netherlands [18]. It is our opinion that all patients who are determined to be unresectable during open exploration for pancreatic head cancer should be considered for biliary-enteric bypass and gastrojejunostomy.

Despite these prospective data supporting prophylactic gastrojejunostomy for patients found to be unresectable at the time of exploratory laparotomy, there are some groups who believe that the limited long-term survival in patients with unresectable pancreatic cancer eliminates the need for prophylactic gastrojejunostomy, especially in patients with gross evidence of distant metastases.

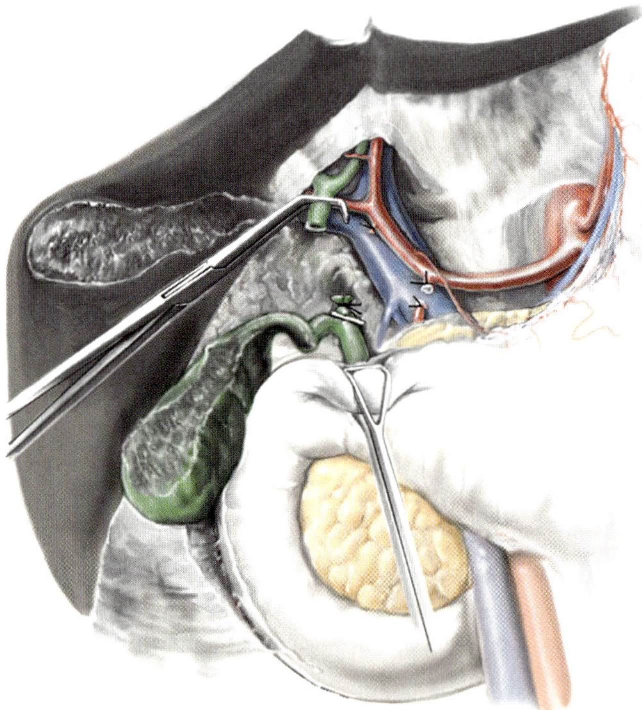

Figure 58.2

Division of the common hepatic duct permits easy identification of the PV above the proximal duodenum and neck of the pancreas. The bile duct can be clamped to prevent bile spillage during the subsequent dissection

Surgical Bypass Techniques for Biliary and Duodenal Obstruction

Despite advances in diagnostic radiography, many patients are not determined to be unresectable until the time of open surgical exploration. Thus, surgical palliation of existing or potential biliary and duodenal obstruction remains a major option in the management of unresectable pancreatic cancer. After entering the abdomen and assessing for metastatic disease, the duodenum is extensively mobilized out of the retroperitoneum to assess for involvement of the superior mesenteric artery (SMA) and to exclude the rare presence of aortic or caval invasion. If SMA invasion is determined, efforts are directed toward surgical palliation. Accurate assessment of tumor resectability in patients with equivocal radiographic findings usually necessitates a concomitant cholecystectomy and transection of the common bile or hepatic duct, which facilitates identification and dissection of the portal vein (Fig. 58.2). With extensive Kocherization of the third portion of the duodenum, the superior mesenteric vein (SMV) can be identified anteriorly and dissected along its anterior surface under the neck of the pancreas to its connection with the portal vein (Fig. 58.3). If tumor encasement of the SMV or portal vein is discovered, the chance for a margin-negative resection is unlikely, and a palliative double-bypass (biliary and gastric) procedure is begun. If tissue confirmation of pancreatic adenocarcinoma was not obtained preoperatively, a transduodenal core needle biopsy sample of the pancreatic head can be obtained.

Historically, most surgeons advocated an antecolic gastrojejunostomy due to concerns of placing the anastomosis in proximity to the tumor bed; however, there is now strong evidence that a retrocolic, isoperistaltic gastrojejunostomy is associated with a lower incidence of postoperative delayed gastric emptying and even late-occurring gastric outlet obstruction from locoregional tumor recurrence [6, 22]. The anastomosis should be fashioned with either a hand-sewn or stapled technique at the most dependent aspect of the greater curvature of the stomach, with a loop of jejunum approximately 20 cm from the ligament of Treitz (Fig. 58.4). The posterior gastrojejunostomy should be delivered below the transverse mesocolon and tacked in place (Fig. 58.5). Vagotomy is generally

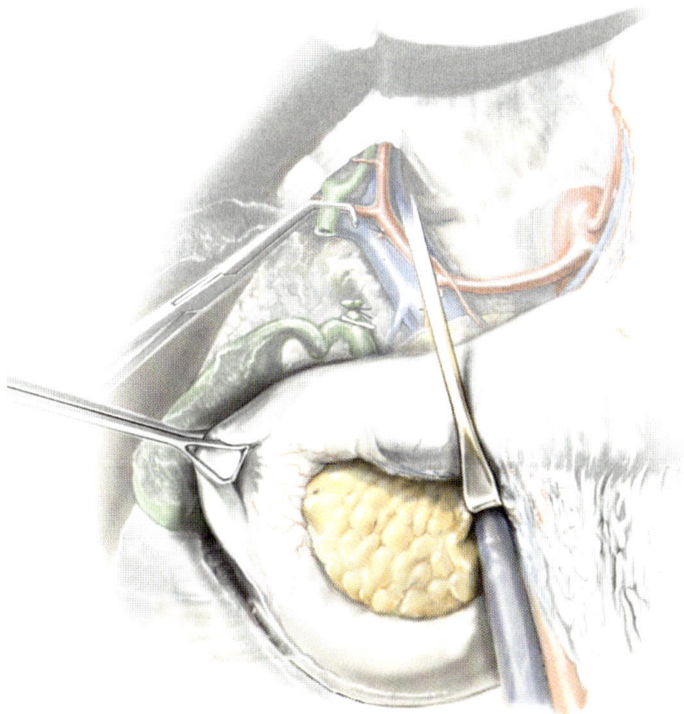

Figure 58.3

Once the second and third portions of the duodenum are Kocherized and the head of the pancreas is mobilized from the retroperitoneum, the anterior aspect of the SMV can be identified and traced along its course under the neck of the pancreas toward the PV. Tumor involvement of the lateral aspect of the SMV and PV can be assessed at this point

avoided during palliative gastrojejunostomy to prevent delayed gastric emptying.

Even though surgical biliary bypass can be accomplished with cholecystojejunostomy or choledochoduodenostomy, these two options are associated with overall inferior short- and long-term results and generally should be avoided. Most experienced pancreatic surgeons prefer using hepatico-(choledocho)-jejunostomy for internal drainage, especially since the bile duct must be transected to determine resectability in many patients. Biliary bypass can be accomplished with either a simple jejunal loop or a Roux-en-Y limb. Figure 58.6 shows diagrammatically a retrocolic loop hepaticojejunostomy approximately 50 cm downstream of the gastrojejunostomy. The hepaticojejunostomy should be constructed with a single interrupted layer of absorbable suture material in a tension-free, end-to-side manner (Fig. 58.7). A transanastomotic stent is not required; however, a percutaneous transhepatic stent, when present preoperatively, can be repositioned to decompress the anastomosis. A Braun jejunojejunostomy is performed between the efferent and afferent limbs leading to and away from the biliary-enteric anastomosis (Fig. 58.6). While a loop anastomosis requires slightly less operative time, the use of a defunctionalized Roux-en-Y jejunal limb seems to be associated with less anastomotic tension and can facilitate the management of potential biliary leaks. An operative drain can be positioned near the hepaticojejunostomy and brought out through the right abdominal wall.

The last step of surgical palliation for unresectable pancreatic cancer includes chemical splanchnicectomy. This procedure involves the injection of 20 ml of 50% alcohol on each side of the aorta at the level of the celiac axis (Fig. 58.8). The level of the celiac plexus is established by palpating the thrill of the common hepatic artery along its origin off the celiac axis.

In some surgeons' hands, laparoscopic palliation including gastrojejunostomy and biliary bypass is an alternative to open surgical palliation in patients with unresectable cancer. Several series involving limited numbers of patients have shown satisfactory short- and long-term results for both biliary bypass and gastrojejunostomy with laparoscopic procedures. Biliary bypass can be accomplished with either a cholecysto-

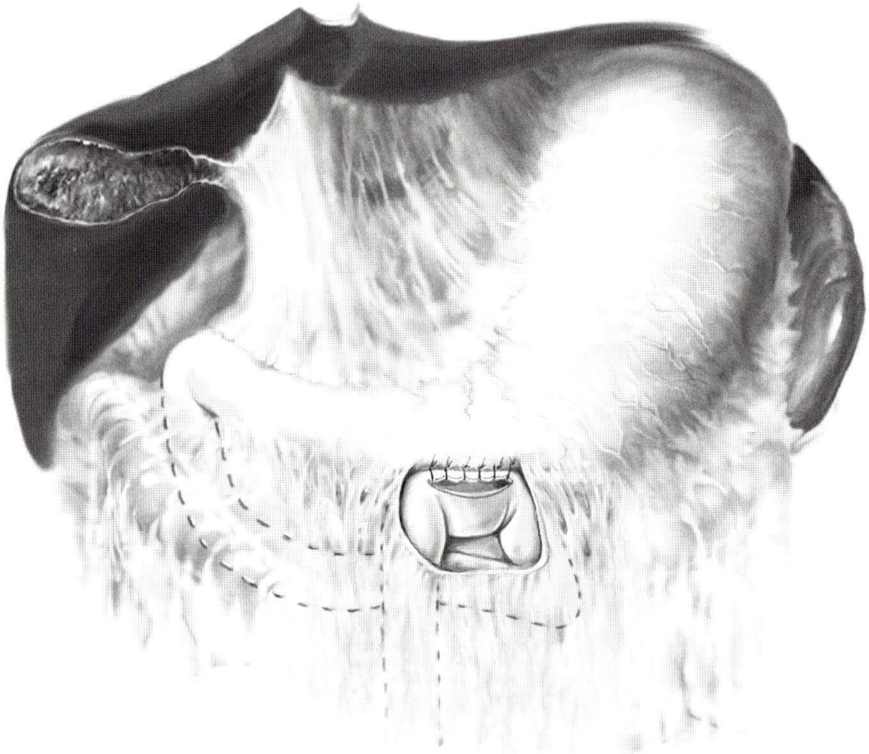

Figure 58.4

The most dependent portion of the greater curvature of the stomach is dissected free of its attachments to the greater omentum. A jejunal loop, approximately 30 cm downstream of the ligament of Treitz, is delivered through a rent in the transverse mesocolon, and a side-to-side, isoperistaltic gastrojejunostomy is performed

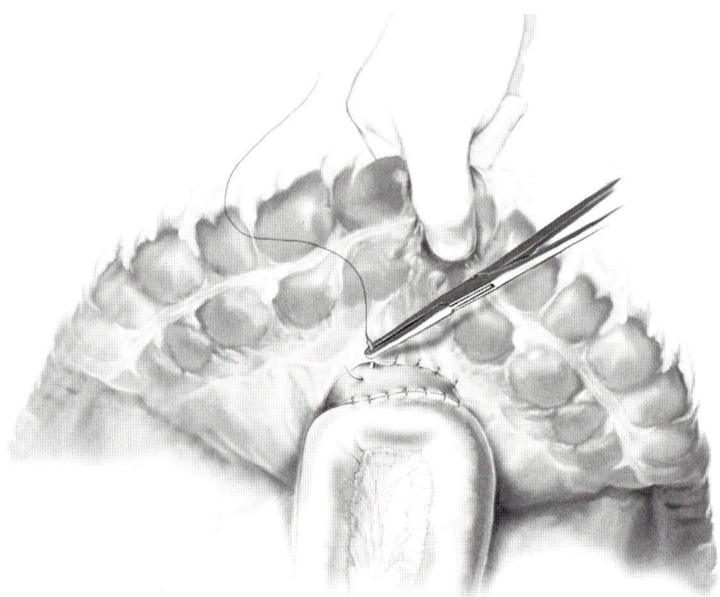

Figure 58.5

The retrocolic gastrojejunostomy is delivered below the rent in the transverse mesocolon, and the gastric side of the anastomosis is tacked to the inferior leaflet of the mesocolon

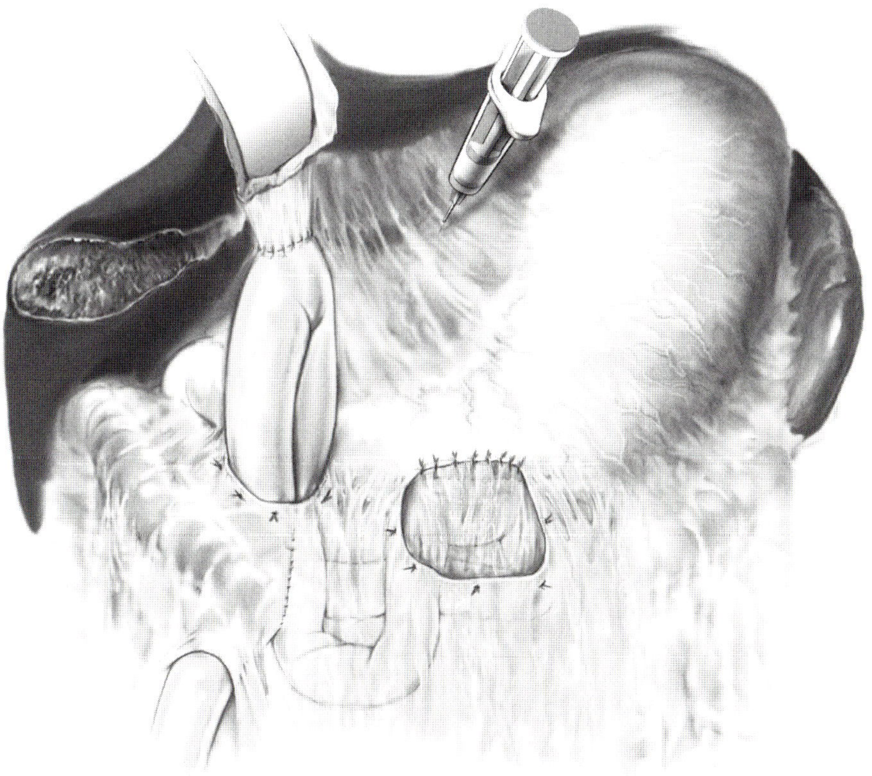

Figure 58.6

Approximately 50 cm downstream of the gastrojejunostomy, a jejunal loop is delivered through a second rent in the transverse mesocolon, and an end-to-side hepaticojejunostomy is performed. A side-to-side Braun jejunojejunostomy is performed at least 25 cm distal to the hepaticojejunostomy. The anastomosis between the jejunal loops is reduced below the transverse mesocolon and tacked in place to prevent herniation

Figure 58.7

The bile duct anastomosis to the jejunal loop can be performed at the level of the common hepatic duct (shown) or common bile duct in an end-to-side fashion using interrupted 4-0 or 5-0 absorbable sutures

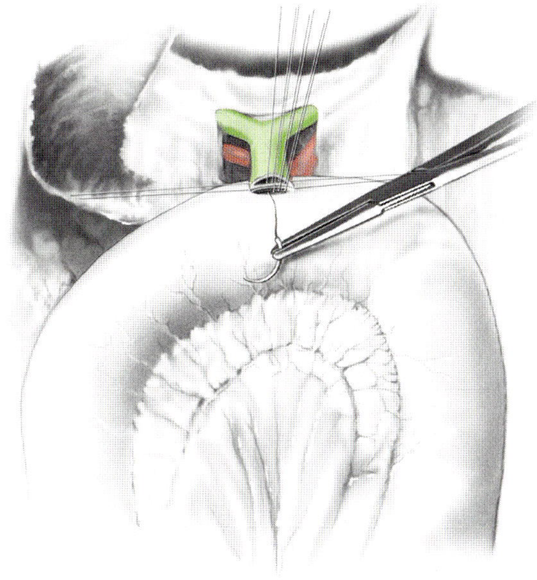

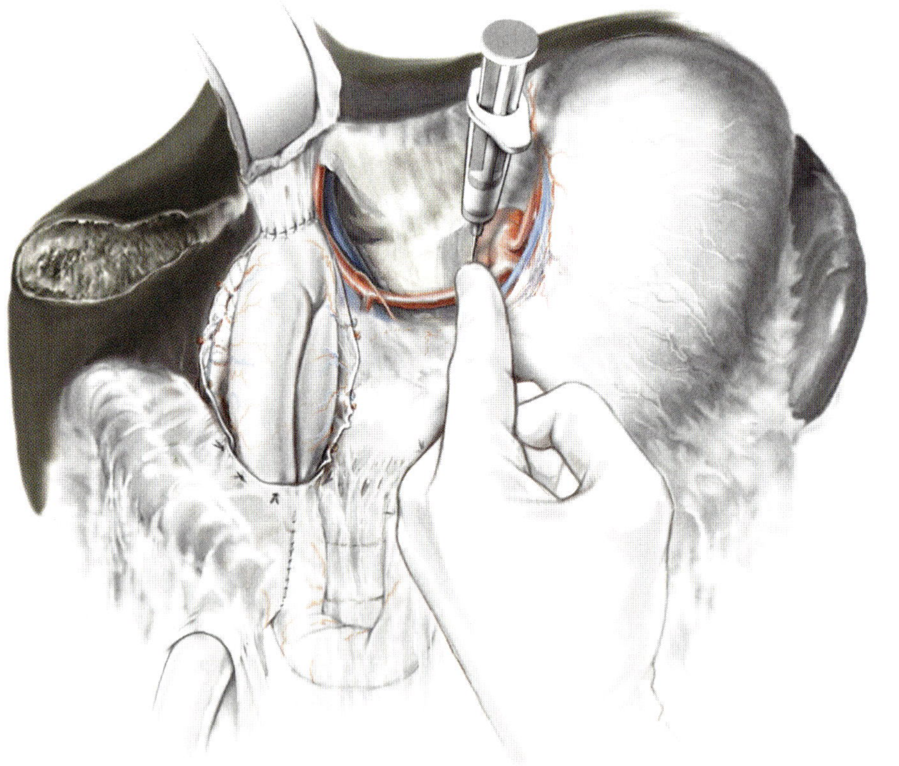

Figure 58.8

The chemical splanchnicectomy is carried out by injecting 20 ml of ethyl alcohol (50% solution) on each side of the aorta (*Ao*) at the level of the celiac axis. After opening the hepatoduodenal ligament, the common hepatic artery and splenic artery can be palpated as a thrill to determine the level of the celiac axis. *IVC* Inferior vena cava

jejunostomy or hepatico-(choledocho)-jejunostomy. Due to the limited long-term success associated with cholecystojejunostomy, the latter is the favored approach of surgeons with extensive laparoscopic experience. The hepaticojejunostomy can be constructed in either an end-to-side or side-to-side manner with either a Roux-en-Y jejunal limb or simple jejunal loop.

Postoperative Course after Surgical Palliation

Immediately after surgical double bypass, nasogastric decompression is used to prevent early postoperative nausea and emesis and can be removed within 24 h. Perioperative antibiotics should be discontinued within 24 h of operation, even for patients with deep jaundice unless they have recently experienced cholangitis. Patients are started on sips of liquids after removal of the nasogastric tube and are gradually advanced to a solid diet over the course of 2–3 days. Like all patients with advanced cancer, patients with unresectable pancreatic adenocarcinoma are at high risk for venous thrombosis and should receive appropriate antithrombotic therapy, including decompression devices of the lower extremities, early activity, and low-dose anticoagulation. All patients undergoing gastrojejunostomy should be maintained long-term on either histamine H_2-blockers or proton pump inhibitors to prevent marginal ulceration at the anastomosis. The operative drain can be removed safely after resumption of a diet and no evidence of leakage from the hepaticojejunostomy. The average length of hospital stay after a surgical double-bypass procedure is between 5 and 7 days. Percutaneous transhepatic biliary stents, when present, can be removed 4–6 weeks after the biliary bypass procedure. After recovery from a double-bypass procedure for unresectable pancreatic cancer, patients should be referred to medical and radiation oncology for consideration of appropriate therapy.

Table 58.3. Stent placement versus surgical biliary bypass for obstructive jaundice in patients with unresectable periampullary cancer. From Watanapa et al. (1992) [14]

	Percutaneous stent n=490		Endoscopic stent n=789		Surgical bypass n=180	
	Range	Mean	Range	Mean	Range	Mean
30-day mortality	6–33	9	0–20	14	0–31	12
Hospital stay (days)	13–18	14	3–26	7	9–30	17
Success rate (%)	76–100	92	82–100	90	75–100	93
Early complications (%)	4–67	16	8–34	21	6–56	31
Late complications (%)	7–38	28	13–45	28	5–47	16

Outcomes After Surgical Bypass Procedures

Survival after surgical palliation of obstructive jaundice secondary to pancreatic adenocarcinoma is on the order of 5–6 months, and in general does not depend on the type of procedure performed. Compared to nonoperative techniques, which carry a lower short-term morbidity, mortality, hospital stay, and cost, the major advantage of surgical biliary bypass is the lower incidence of late complications, namely recurrent jaundice and cholangitis (Table 58.3) [14]. Although open biliary and gastric bypass techniques carry a perioperative morbidity of 22% and a mortality of 3%, the long-term benefits associated with open palliation often outweigh these perioperative risks (Table 58.4) [6]. In contrast to the various forms of nonoperative palliation that require reintervention in over one-third of patients, operative biliary drainage procedures are associated with few late complications and require reintervention in less than 5% of patients [23].

Long-term pain related to pancreatic cancer is perhaps the most debilitating symptom associated with this disease and can quickly lead to the deterioration of the patient's quality of life. While only 30–40% of patients with pancreatic cancer report moderate to severe pain at the time of diagnosis, over 80% of patients with advanced cancer experience severe pain prior to death [24, 25]. Chemical splanchnicectomy can achieve acute pain relief in over 80% of patients and can prevent the subsequent onset of pain for up to 6 months postoperatively [24]. Furthermore, patients with severe preoperative pain who undergo a palliative chemical splanchnicectomy experience a significant improvement in overall survival [24].

Table 58.4. Postoperative complications after surgical palliation for unresectable preampullary cancer (n=180 patients)

Complication	% of patients
Mortality	3.1%
Overall morbidity	22%
Reoperation	1%
Delayed gastric emptying	9%
Pancreatic fistula	0%
Wound infection	4%
Bile leak	5%
Intra-abdominal abscess	4%
Cholangitis	2%
Pneumonia	0.3%
Postoperative length of stay (days)	10.1±0.3

Conclusions

Surgical palliative treatment for unresectable pancreatic cancer is directed at three major symptoms associated with disease progression: obstructive jaundice, cancer-related pain, and duodenal obstruction. Despite improvements in CT imaging, EUS, and laparoscopy to stage patients with pancreatic cancer, some patients are determined to be unresectable only at the time of open exploration. Surgical management can achieve successful and durable palliation of obstructive symptoms and cancer-related pain as a single procedure during laparotomy. To take advantage of the long-term advantages afforded by surgical palliation, operative procedures must be performed with acceptable morbidity. In patients with unresectable pancreatic cancer, quality of life should always be addressed.

References

1. Landis SH, Murray T, Bolden S, Wingo PA (1999) Cancer statistics, 1999. CA Cancer J Clin 49:8–31
2. Kalser MH, Barkin J, MacIntyre JM (1985) Pancreatic cancer. Assessment of prognosis by clinical presentation. Cancer 56:397–402
3. Ahrendt SA, Pitt HA (2002) Surgical management of pancreatic cancer. Oncology (Huntingt) 16:725–734; discussion 734, 736–78, 740, 743
4. Radiation therapy combined with Adriamycin or 5-fluorouracil for the treatment of locally unresectable pancreatic carcinoma. Gastrointestinal Tumor Study Group (1985) Cancer 56:2563–2568
5. House MG, Yeo CJ, Cameron JL, Campbell K, Schulick R, Leach S, Hruban R, Horton K, Fishman E, Lillemoe KD (2004) Predicting resectability of periampullary cancer using 3-dimensional computed tomography. J Gastrointest Surg 8:280–288
6. Sohn TA, Lillemoe KD, Cameron JL, Huang JJ, Pitt HA, Yeo CJ (1999) Surgical palliation of unresectable periampullary adenocarcinoma in the 1990s. J Am Coll Surg 188:658–666; discussion 666–669
7. Singh SM, Reber HA (1989) Surgical palliation for pancreatic cancer. Surg Clin North Am 69:599–611
8. Singh SM, Longmire WP Jr, Reber HA (1990) Surgical palliation for pancreatic cancer. The UCLA experience. Ann Surg 212:132–139
9. Lillemoe KD (1998) Palliative therapy for pancreatic cancer. Surg Oncol Clin N Am 7:199–216
10. Espinel J, Vivas S, Munoz F, Jorquera F, Olcoz JL (2001) Palliative treatment of malignant obstruction of gastric outlet using an endoscopically placed enteral Wallstent. Dig Dis Sci 46:2322–2324
11. Brandabur JJ, Kozarek RA, Ball TJ, Hofer BO, Ryan JA Jr, Traverso LW, Freeny PC, Lewis GP (1988) Nonoperative versus operative treatment of obstructive jaundice in pancreatic cancer: cost and survival analysis. Am J Gastroenterol 83:1132–1139
12. Arguedas MR, Heudebert GH, Stinnett AA, Wilcox CM (2002) Biliary stents in malignant obstructive jaundice due to pancreatic carcinoma: a cost-effectiveness analysis. Am J Gastroenterol 97:898–904
13. Soehendra N, Reynders-Frederix V (1980) Palliative bile duct drainage – a new endoscopic method of introducing a transpapillary drain. Endoscopy 12:8–11
14. Watanapa P, Williamson RC (1992) Surgical palliation for pancreatic cancer: developments during the past two decades. Br J Surg 79:8–20
15. Lillemoe KD, Cameron JL, Hardacre JM, Sohn TA, Sauter PK, Coleman J, Pitt HA, Yeo CJ (1999) Is prophylactic gastrojejunostomy indicated for unresectable periampullary cancer? A prospective randomized controlled trial. Ann Surg 230:322–328
16. Lichtenstein DR, Carr-Locke DL (1995) Endoscopic palliation for unresectable pancreatic carcinoma. Surg Clin North Am 75:969–988
17. Espat N, Brennan MF, Conlon K (1999) Patients with laparoscopically staged unresectable pancreatic adenocarcinoma do not require subsequent surgical biliary or gastric bypass. J Am Coll Surg 188:649–655
18. Nieveen van Dijkum EJ, Romijn MG, Terwee CB, de Wit LT, van der Meulen JH, Lameris HS, Rauws EA, Obertop H, van Eyck CH, Bossuyt PM, Gouma DJ. (2003) Laparoscopic staging and subsequent palliation in patients with peripancreatic carcinoma. Ann Surg 237:66–73
19. Warshaw AL, Gu ZY, Wittenberg J (1990) Preoperative staging and assessment of resectability of pancreatic cancer. Arch Surg 125:230–233
20. Trede M (1985) The surgical treatment of pancreatic carcinoma. Surgery 97:28–35
21. Van Heek NT, De Castro SM, van Eijck CH, van Geenen RC, Hesselink EJ, Breslau PJ, Tran TC, Kazemier G, Visser MR, Busch OR, Obertop H, Gouma DJ (2003) The need for a prophylactic gastrojejunostomy for unresectable periampullary cancer: a prospective randomized multicenter trial with special focus on assessment of quality of life. Ann Surg 238:894–902
22. Lillemoe KD, Sauter PK, Pitt HA, Yeo CJ, Cameron JL (1993) Current status of surgical palliation of periampullary carcinoma. Surg Gynecol Obstet 176: 1–10
23. Smith AC, Dowsett JF, Russell RC, Hatfield AR, Cotton PB (1994) Randomised trial of endoscopic stenting versus surgical bypass in malignant low bile duct obstruction. Lancet 344:1655–1660
24. Lillemoe KD, Cameron JL, Kaufman HS, Yeo CJ, Pitt HA, Sauter PK (1993) Chemical splanchnicectomy in patients with unresectable pancreatic cancer. A prospective randomized trial. Ann Surg 217:447–455; discussion 456–457
25. Gress F, Schmitt C, Sherman S, Ikenberry S, Lehman G (1999) A prospective randomized comparison of endoscopic ultrasound- and computed tomography-guided celiac plexus block for managing chronic pancreatitis pain. Am J Gastroenterol 94:900–905

Chapter 59

G.R. Varadhachary · J.L. Abbruzzese

Resected Pancreatic Cancer

Pancreatic cancer is a systemic disease for most patients, and two-thirds of patients have locally advanced or metastatic disease at the time of diagnosis. For the subset of patients (20%) who present with potentially resectable tumors, the 5-year survival rate for those whose tumors are successfully resected is approximately 15–20% and lower for those with positive nodes or margins [1]. Patients usually succumb to metastatic disease or locoregional failure.

As with other cancers, the rationale for postoperative therapy is to treat micrometastatic disease and improve survival in patients with resected cancer; unfortunately, despite more than two decades of research, there is no consensus on the best postoperative therapy for pancreatic adenocarcinoma. In a study reported in 1999, trends in disease stage, treatment patterns, and outcomes were analyzed for patients diagnosed with pancreatic adenocarcinoma between 1985 and 1995 [2]. Data were available for 100,313 patients. For the 9,044 patients who underwent pancreatectomy, the overall 5-year survival rate was 23.4%. Adjuvant treatment was used in 40% of cases and consisted of radiation therapy, chemotherapy, or both in 6.5%, 5.1%, and 28.3% of patients, respectively. The approach to adjuvant therapy also differs between high-volume centers in the USA and Europe.

Some of the barriers to determining the best postoperative therapy include poor surgical recovery that complicates the use of chemotherapy and chemoradiation therapy, poor patient selection and inadequate staging studies for patients in postoperative trials, lack of standardized criteria for evaluating resection margins, and lack of chemotherapy with significant activity in pancreatic adenocarcinoma. More recently, preoperative or neoadjuvant treatments have been explored as an alternative to adjuvant therapy. In this chapter, we review the data for adjuvant and neoadjuvant strategies for the treatment of pancreatic cancer.

Prognostic Indicators for Resected Pancreatic Cancer

Various prognostic factors for pancreatic cancer are discussed in the literature, including tumor size, margin resection status, nodal status, histologic differentiation, intraoperative blood transfusion, lymph-vascular invasion and adjuvant therapy. Of these, nodal status is the most important, with a 5-year overall survival rate of approximately 10% for node-positive patients and 25% for node-negative patients [3–5].

Lim and colleagues analyzed the prognostic factors influencing pancreatic cancer survival after curative resection using prospectively collected, population-based data [6]. They included 396 Medicare-eligible patients aged 65 years and older with localized pancreatic adenocarcinoma who had undergone surgical resection with curative intent while residing in one of the 11 Survival, Epidemiology, and End Results registries between 1991 and 1996. Linked Medicare data provided information on treatments and comorbidities, and linked census tract data provided sociodemographic information. The median overall survival duration for the study population was 17.6 months, with 1- and 3-year survival rates of 60.1% and 34.3%, respectively. Over time, survival duration appeared to gradually improve, and more patients underwent surgery in teaching centers. On univariate analysis, prognostic variables that reduced survival included African-American ethnicity, treatment outside of a teaching hospital, lack of adjuvant chemoradiation therapy, and histopathologic factors such as tumor size >2 cm in diameter, moderate-to-poor histologic tumor grade, and lymph node metastases. Higher socioeconomic status was associated with both an increased likelihood of receiving adjuvant therapy and improved overall survival. The strongest predictors of survival on multivariate analysis were adjuvant combined chemoradiation therapy, small tumors (<2 cm in diameter), negative lymph nodes, well-differentiated histologic features, having undergone surgery in a teaching hospital, and high socio-

Table 59.1. Margin status and survival data for resected pancreatic cancer

First author (Year)	Patients *n*	Patients with positive margin (R1 or R2) (%)	Median survival for margin-positive patients (months)	Median survival for margin-negative patients (months)
Yeo (1995) [7]	201	58 (29%)	10	18
Millikan (1999) [3]	75	22 (29)	8	17
Sohn (2000) [8]	616	184 (30)	12	19
Benassai (2000) [10]	75	15 (20)	9	26
Neoptolemos (2001) [11]	541	101 (19)	11	17
Takai (2003) [12]	94	64 (68)	8	23

economic status. The strongest survival determinant was postoperative adjuvant chemoradiation therapy.

Margin assessment is critical to determining the adequacy of resection and is an important prognostic feature of resected pancreatic cancer. The tissue to the right of the proximal 3–4 cm of the superior mesenteric artery (SMA) is called the retroperitoneal margin (some refer to this as the mesenteric or uncinate margin). The surgery is termed an "R0 resection" if no microscopic tumor is found at the margin. An "R1 resection" refers to a microscopically positive retroperitoneal margin after an otherwise complete resection, and a "R2 resection" refers to gross residual disease left behind after pancreaticoduodenectomy. Patients who have undergone R1 resections often have lower survival rates than those who have undergone R0 resections, independent of nodal status and other prognostic factors (Table 59.1) [3,7–12]. Benassai and colleagues reported single-institution survival data for 75 patients who underwent pancreaticoduodenectomy for pancreatic head adenocarcinomas between 1974 and 1995. The median overall survival duration after resection was 17 months, and the estimated 5-year survival rate was 18.7%. Forty-two percent of node-negative patients were alive at 5 years, compared with 8% of node-positive patients ($P < 0.001$). The 5-year survival rates for margin-negative resection and margin-positive resection were 23% vs. 0%, respectively ($P < 0.001$). Gender, age, and blood transfusion had no significant effect on survival. The authors concluded that the presence of positive resection margins was the strongest independent predictor of decreased survival. In a study by Millikan and colleagues, the only significant independent factors that improved survival were the absence of intraoperative blood transfusion ($P = 0.02$) and a negative resection margin ($P = 0.04$); patients who underwent R1 resections had a median survival of approximately 8 months.

In the more recent European Study Group for Pancreatic Cancer-1 (ESPAC-1) adjuvant study, 101 of 541 patients (19%) underwent R1 resections. The median overall survival duration of patients who underwent R1 resections was 11 months, compared with 17 months for patients who underwent R0 resections [11]. The benefit obtained with chemotherapy persisted in the presence of positive margins, but was lower than that found in patients with negative margins. In a separate paper on the benefit of adjuvant therapy in the context of margin positivity, the authors concluded that future trials of adjuvant treatments, as well as randomization and analysis, should be stratified by this important prognostic factor.

Radiation Alone as Adjuvant Therapy for Pancreatic Cancer

Locoregional failure is not uncommon in patients with resected pancreatic cancer. Pancreatic head and uncinate tumors (60–70% of all pancreatic adenocarcinomas) have several vital structures around them, including the superior mesenteric vein, portal vein, SMA, and celiac axis. Even after postoperative chemoradiation therapy, local recurrence rates can be as high as 50%, providing the rationale for the use of preoperative or postoperative radiation therapy [13]. As indicated above, an R1 resection complicates 10–30% of patients who have undergone pancreaticoduodenectomy. This is usually due to perineural and lymphatic invasion along the vessel wall. Rich neural networks envelop the pancreas and are connected to the local vascular structures. Invasion of the nerve sheaths surrounding the vessels increases the risk of a margin-positive resection. While an R2 resection can be avoided by interpreting the preoperative computerized tomography (CT) scans correctly, patients who undergo an R1 or R2 resection are at high risk for locoregional failure, similar to patients who have a positive radial margin, after rectal cancer surgery. In this setting postoperative radiation therapy can potentially decrease the risk of locoregional failure.

External-beam radiation therapy (EBRT) alone after potentially curative pancreatectomy has been shown to reduce local recurrence rates but does not improve overall survival. Therefore, intraoperative radiation therapy (IORT) has been studied in an attempt to improve local tumor control, thereby potentially affecting overall survival. IORT allows high doses of radiation to be delivered to tumors without increasing normal tissue toxicity because intraoperatively, normal tissues can be shielded or mobilized away from the radiation field. EBRT in combination with IORT has been studied in small single-institution phase II studies. Morganti and colleagues evaluated 17 patients with clinical stage T1-3, N0 or N1, M0 adenocarcinoma of the head of the pancreas who were treated with pancreatectomy and preoperative (5 Gy), intraoperative (10 Gy), and postoperative (50 Gy) radiation therapy [14]. All patients underwent intraoperative and postoperative radiation therapy and nine patients underwent preoperative radiation therapy. The median overall survival duration was 17.5 months and the 3- and 5-year overall survival rates were 41% and 18%, respectively. The local failure rate was 17.6% and the remaining patients died of metastatic disease.

Kokubo and colleagues retrospectively studied the survival of patients with pancreatic cancer treated with IORT, EBRT, or both after pancreatectomy [15]. Of 138 patients who had undergone potentially curative surgery between 1980 and 1997, 98 had an R0 margin, and the remaining 40 had a positive surgical margin. The usual EBRT dose was 45–55 Gy (1.5–2.0 Gy/day). The median IORT dose was 25 Gy in a single fraction. The 2-year survival rate for patients with R0 margins was 19%, and that for patients with R1 or R2 margins was 4% ($P < 0.005$). Disappointingly, although the median survival duration of patients with negative margins treated with IORT and EBRT was longer than that of those treated with surgery alone (17 vs. 11 months), there was no significant difference in long-term survival.

The only prospective randomized trial of IORT was conducted by the National Cancer Institute [16]. This study compared IORT with observation after pancreaticoduodenectomy. Twenty-four patients were randomly assigned to the two arms. Patients in the IORT arm who had extrapancreatic extension of their tumor also underwent EBRT (45–55 Gy). The mortality and morbidity rates did not significantly differ between the IORT and observation arms. The median survival duration was 18 months in the IORT arm and 12 months in the observation arm, but the difference was not statistically significant. Locoregional control was better in the IORT arm than in the observation arm (recurrences in 4 of the 12 patients versus all 12, respectively).

The results of these studies suggest that IORT can be given safely after pancreaticoduodenectomy and improves local control in selected patients. Because distant relapse limits survival in patients with pancreatic cancer, it is no surprise that neither IORT nor EBRT alone has any effect on overall survival. For now, IORT use should be restricted to clinical trials and selected patients.

Chemoradiation Therapy as Adjuvant Therapy for Pancreatic Cancer

The rationale for using chemotherapy alone or chemoradiation therapy is clear: pancreatic cancer metastasizes early, and despite early stage presentation and surgical intervention with curative intent, most patients die of disseminated disease. Therefore, most of the current preoperative and postoperative trials have a systemic therapy component to treat micrometastatic disease. There have been several randomized and nonrandomized trials of adjuvant chemoradiation therapy (selected trials are outlined in Table 59.2) [17–21]. The three trials most often cited are the Gastrointestinal Tumor Study Group (GITSG), the European Organization for Research and Treatment of Cancer (EORTC), and the European Study Group of Pancreatic Cancer (ESPAC-1) trials.

Moertel and colleagues of the GITSG were the first to study the role of adjuvant chemoradiation therapy in resected pancreatic cancer after finding encouraging survival data for radiation therapy and concurrent 5-fluorouracil (5-FU) chemotherapy in patients with locally advanced unresectable pancreatic cancer [22]. In the adjuvant treatment trial, patients were randomly assigned to either observation alone after pancreaticoduodenectomy or EBRT (40 Gy) given concurrently with a 500 mg/m^2/day bolus of 5-FU on the first 3 and last 3 days of radiation therapy [17,18]. This was followed by maintenance chemotherapy, 5-FU (500 mg/m^2/day) for 3 days, monthly for 2 years or until disease progression.

This study accrued poorly and after 8 years only 43 patients were available for analysis. Survival durations in the treatment versus surgery-alone arms were 20 months and 11 months, with 2-year survivals of

Table 59.2. Selected adjuvant therapy trials in resected pancreatic cancer. *GITSG* Gastrointestinal Tumor Study Group, *5-FU* 5-fluorouracil, *RT* radiation therapy, *EORTC* European Organization for Research and Treatment of Cancer, *JHH* Johns Hopkins Hospital, *ESPAC* European Study Group for Pancreatic Cancer, *IFN* interferon, *CDDP* cisplatin, *PVI* protracted venous infusion, *NA* not available

Trial, first author (year)	Primary (*n*)	Treatment	Patients (*n*) Adjuvant therapy vs. surgery alone	Median survivalmonths) Adjuvant therapy vs. surgery alone	*P* value
GITSG, Kalser (1985) [17]	Pancreas	5-FU + RT (40 Gy)	21	20	0.035
			22	11	
GITSG (1987) [18]	Pancreas	5-FU + RT (40 Gy)	30	18	-
Norway, Bakkevold (1993) [19]	Pancreas (47) Ampulla (14)	5-FU, doxorubicin, mitomycin-C	30	23	0.04
			31	11	
Milwaukee, Demeure (1998) [20]	Pancreas	5-FU + RT (50.4–54 Gy)	30	24.2	<0.05
			31	16.9	
EORTC, Klinkenbijl (1999) [21]	Pancreas (114) Periampullary (104)	5-FU + RT (40 Gy)	110	24.5	0.208
			108	19	
JHH, Abrams (1999) [54]	Pancreas (23) Periampullary (6)	5-FU + RT (50.4–57.6 Gy)	29	15.9	–
JHH, Sohn (2000) [8]	Pancreas	5-FU + RT (40–57.6 Gy)	333	19	<0.0001
			119	11	
ESPAC-1 Neoptolemos (2001) [23]	Pancreas	5-FU	146	17.4	0.19
			139	15.9	
Japan, Takada (2002) [55]	Pancreas (173)[a] Bile duct (139) Gallbladder (140) Ampulla (56)	5-FU, mitomycin-C	92a	17.8	0.45
				26.6	
Virginia Mason, Picozzi (2003) [26]	Pancreas	5-FU + IFN + CDDP + RT (45–54 Gy) followed by PVI 5-FU	43	NA	

[a] Of the eligible 158 patients with pancreatic carcinoma, 92 patients underwent curative resections

20% and 10%, respectively. Five of the 21 (24%) patients assigned to the chemoradiation therapy arm did not start treatment until more than 10 weeks after surgery because of prolonged postoperative recuperation. Given the encouraging results of this trial, another 32 patients were registered to the treatment arm after the study closed, and these results were confirmed. The GITSG trial made 5-FU-based EBRT the preferred postoperative treatment in the USA for pancreatic cancer. However, the study has been criticized for it's small sample size, low radiation dose of 40 Gy, and long accrual time.

Klinkenbijl and colleagues of the Gastrointestinal Tract Cancer Cooperative Group of the EORTC presented their adjuvant trial data in 1999 [21]. Between 1987 and 1995, 218 patients were randomized to receive either chemoradiation therapy (40 Gy in a split course and 5-FU as a continuous infusion at a dose of 25 mg/kg/day during EBRT) or to no further therapy after pancreaticoduodenectomy. The study included patients with resected T1 or T2, N0 or N1a, M0 pancreatic head adenocarcinoma or T1-3, N0 or N1a, M0 periampullary cancer. Of the 207 eligible patients, 108 were in the observation arm and 110 were in the treatment group; 114 patients (55%) had pancreatic cancer and they were well distributed between the treatment and observation arms. Twenty-one patients (20%) in the treatment arm did not undergo any treatment because of postoperative complications or refusal. The median survival durations were 19.0 months and 24.5 months for the observation and (entire) treatment arms, but this difference was not statistically significant ($P = 0.2$). For the subset of patients with pancreatic cancer, the survival durations were 17.1 months for patients in the chemoradiation arm and 12.6 months for patients in the surgery-alone arm ($P = 0.099$). The authors concluded that adjuvant 5-FU-based chemoradiation was safe and well tolerated. However, because the benefit in this study was small, with no statistically significant improvement in median survival, they did not advocate it as a standard therapy for all patients with pancreatic cancer. Criticisms of this trial include the poor survival duration in the pancreaticoduodenectomy arm (12.6 months) and local tumor recurrence as the first site of recurrence in 20% of the patients, suggesting that many patients had an incomplete (R2) resection.

Sohn and colleagues from the Johns Hopkins hospital presented their retrospective single institution data on the role of adjuvant chemoradiation in patients with resected pancreatic cancer [8]. Of the 498 evaluable patients, 366 (74%) underwent adjuvant chemoradiation therapy and 132 (26%) did not undergo therapy for various reasons. In this study, adjuvant treatment resulted in a survival benefit over no treatment (19 months vs. 11 months, respectively; $P < 0.0001$).

These three studies (GITSG, EORTC, and Johns Hopkins Hospital) found consistent results: patients who did not undergo adjuvant therapy survived for 11–12 months, but patients who underwent chemoradiation therapy survived for ≥17 months. Another important finding was that after pancreaticoduodenectomy approximately 20–26% of patients did not undergo adjuvant therapy or had a prolonged period of recovery prior to starting adjuvant therapy.

Neoptolemos and colleagues evaluated the role of adjuvant therapy in a recent randomized postoperative study, the ESPAC-1 trial [23,24]. This trial used a 2×2 factorial design (observation, chemoradiation therapy alone, chemotherapy alone, or chemoradiation therapy and chemotherapy). In contrast to other adjuvant trials, ESPAC-1 did not show any benefit of chemoradiation in an adjuvant setting. Chemoradiation therapy included a split course of 40 Gy and 500 mg/m^2 of 5-FU intravenously on days 1–3, repeated after 2 weeks. Chemotherapy consisted of 425 mg/m^2 of 5-FU and 20 mg/m^2 of folinic acid daily for 5 days, once a month for 6 months. Patients were randomly assigned to one of the 2×2 factorial designs or treatment comparison groups, which included chemoradiation therapy versus no chemoradiation therapy or chemotherapy versus no chemotherapy. Between 1994 and 2000, 61 medical centers in 11 countries randomized 541 eligible patients with pancreatic ductal adenocarcinoma: 285 to the 2×2 factorial design (70 to chemoradiation therapy, 74 to chemotherapy, 72 to both, and 69 to observation), 68 to chemoradiation therapy or no chemoradiation therapy, and 188 to chemotherapy or no chemotherapy. The median follow-up time was 47 months.

The median survival duration was 15.5 months for the 175 patients who underwent chemoradiation therapy and 16.1 months for the 178 patients who did not undergo chemoradiation therapy (hazard ratio, 1.18; 95% confidence interval, CI, 0.90–1.55; $P = 0.24$). These results suggest that there was no benefit of adjuvant chemoradiation therapy. The median survival duration of the 238 patients who underwent chemotherapy was 19.7 months, and the survival of the 235 patients who did not undergo chemotherapy was 14.0 months (hazard ratio, 0.66; 95% CI 0.52–0.83; $P = 0.0005$), suggesting a potential benefit for adjuvant chemotherapy alone in pancreatic cancer. The 5-year survival rate was 10% for the chemoradiation therapy group, 20% for the nonchemoradiation therapy group ($P = 0.05$), 21% for the chemotherapy group, and 8% for the nonchemotherapy group ($P = 0.009$). The authors concluded that the results suggest a benefit for chemotherapy alone and a possible harmful effect for chemoradiation therapy.

The ESPAC-1 results have been criticized because 62% of patients enrolled in the trial had local recurrence as the first site of failure. This number is high for a disease with a high propensity for distant spread. High local recurrence suggests that a significant number of patients underwent grossly incomplete resections. Also, a central review of radiation dosimetry was not required, allowing for the possibility of poor quality control given the multiple investigators and sites. Pretreatment (postoperative) CT to exclude obvious gross residual disease was not required in this study. Physicians who enrolled patients outside the 2×2 design had the option of delivering "background" chemotherapy or radiation prior to study entry, and these treatments were not standardized. Also, in this trial, 19% of patients (101 of 541) enrolled were reported to have undergone an R1 resection. These patients had a median survival duration of approximately 11 months compared with 17 months for patients who underwent an R0 resection [11]. The benefit from adjuvant chemotherapy persisted in R1 tumors but was less than that seen in patients with negative margins.

The Radiation Therapy Oncology Group (RTOG) recently completed accrual for an adjuvant trial

(RTOG-9704) in patients with resected pancreatic cancer. Patients have been randomly assigned to receive three cycles of weekly gemcitabine or three cycles of infusional 5-FU to be given before and after 5-FU-based chemoradiation therapy. Early results are expected soon.

A meta-analysis of five randomized, controlled adjuvant therapy trials for pancreatic cancer was recently published, the aim of which was to determine the roles of adjuvant chemoradiation therapy and adjuvant chemotherapy on survival in potentially curatively resected pancreatic cancer. The authors found a 25% reduction in the risk of death with chemotherapy and no significant reduction in the risk of death with chemoradiation therapy. The median survival durations were estimated to be 19 months (95% CI, 16.4–21.1) with chemotherapy and 13.5 months (95% CI, 12.2–15.8) without and 15.8 months (95% CI, 13.9–18.1) with chemoradiation therapy and 15.2 months (95% CI, 13.1–18.2) without. Chemoradiation therapy was more effective than chemotherapy alone in patients with positive surgical margins. Since gemcitabine has been shown to have radiosensitizer properties, gemcitabine-based chemoradiation therapy phase II trials are ongoing.

Even though some promising and provocative results were found in the trials discussed above, there are several barriers to interpreting the results of adjuvant therapy trials. These include poor consistency in most studies with respect to preoperative staging and serum tumor markers (CA19-9), poor surgical quality control without thorough margin assessment, and generally ineffective systemic therapy. Because most patients are able to begin adjuvant therapy only 8–10 weeks after surgery, the presence of metastatic disease should be excluded. Therefore, future adjuvant chemotherapy and chemoradiation therapy trials should incorporate accurate pretreatment (postoperative) staging to exclude patients with gross residual and metastatic disease using imaging and serum tumor marker (CA19-9) studies and evaluation of margin status, with patients randomly assigned and stratified by this important prognostic factor. It is also clear from the results of current adjuvant trials that of all patients who are candidates for adjuvant therapy, approximately 25% will be unable to undergo treatment because of a prolonged postoperative course or complications or will decline therapy. This provides the rationale for the use of preoperative therapy (discussed below).

Role of Chemotherapy Alone in Pancreatic Cancer

Besides the ESPAC-1 trial, Bakkevold and colleagues studied the role of chemotherapy alone in resected pancreatic cancer [19]. They randomly assigned 61 patients with radically resected pancreatic cancer (47 patients) or the papilla of Vater (14 patients) to either postoperative adjuvant combination chemotherapy with 500 mg/m^2 of 5-FU, 40 mg/m^2 of doxorubicin and 6 mg/m^2 of mitomycin-C once every 3 weeks for six cycles or observation alone (no adjuvant chemotherapy). The median survival duration in the treatment group was 23 months compared with 11 months ($P = 0.02$) in the control group. The long-term prognosis in both groups was the same, with an identical survival duration after 2 years, suggesting that adjuvant chemotherapy increases the disease-free survival duration but does not increase the cure rate.

Because gemcitabine has shown superiority to 5-FU in metastatic pancreatic cancer, current randomized trials of adjuvant therapy incorporate gemcitabine in the chemotherapy arm. ESPAC-3 is a multicenter European trial that plans to enroll more than 900 patients. Patients with resected pancreatic cancer will be randomly selected to receive gemcitabine (1000 mg/m^2 for 30 min, weekly ×3, every 28 days) for 6 months or a bolus of 5-FU and leucovorin (as administered in ESPAC-1) for 6 months. A randomized prospective phase III study by Neuhaus and colleagues compared adjuvant gemcitabine (for 6 months) to observation alone [25]. Stratification criteria included positive or negative resection margins, nodal tumor involvement, and tumor stage. One hundred and seventy-nine patients were randomized to receive gemcitabine and 174 were in the observation arm. Preliminary data demonstrates an increased disease-free survival in patients receiving gemcitabine for 6 months after resection vs. observation (14.2 months vs. 7.5 months, respectively; $P < 0.05$).

Role of Immunotherapy with Chemoradiation Therapy in Pancreatic Cancer

Picozzi and colleagues from the Virginia Mason Medical Center have reported encouraging results from their institutional protocol using interferon-α (IFN-α)-based adjuvant therapy [26]. Data on 43 patients have been reported. Adjuvant therapy consisted of 45–54 Gy of EBRT for 5 weeks (25 fractions). This protocol does not use split fractions as in the GITSG study. 5-FU, cisplatin, and IFN-α are given concomitantly with the EBRT; 5-FU is given as a continuous infusion of 200 mg/m^2/day on days 1–35. A bolus of cisplatin is given weekly at a dosage of 30 mg/m^2 on days 1, 8, 15, 22, and 29. IFN-α is given subcutaneously at a dosage of 3×10^6 units every other day for 5 weeks. This 5-week chemoradiation therapy period is followed by a continuous infusion of 5-FU at a dosage of 200 mg/m^2 daily on days 64–105 and 120–161.

For the 43 patients in the initial analysis, the tumor stages were American Joint Committee on Cancer stage I in 2%, II in 12%, III in 72%, and IVa in 14%. Grade 3 or 4 toxicity during chemoradiation therapy was seen in 30 out of 43 patients (70%), and 42% were hospitalized during therapy, mainly because of gastrointestinal toxicity. The median survival had not yet been reached at the time of the last publication of results presented in 2003. At a mean follow-up time of 31.9 months, 67% of the patients were alive. The reported actuarial overall survival rates for the 1-, 2-, and 5-year periods were 95% (95% CI, 91–98%), 64% (95% CI, 56–72%), and 55% (95% CI, 46–65%), respectively.

Given these data, the American College of Surgeons Oncology Group (ACOSOG-Z5006) initiated a study to confirm these encouraging results; toxicity has been substantial, but final efficacy results are pending. At The University of Texas M.D. Anderson Cancer Center, we are currently accruing patients with previously resected pancreatic cancer for a similar phase II institutional adjuvant trial with postoperative cisplatin, IFN-α, 5-FU, and concurrent radiation therapy. The doses and overall treatment plan are similar to those of the Virginia Mason program except that our trial allows a 1-week break in treatment during the chemoradiation therapy phase.

Role of Preoperative (Neoadjuvant) Therapy in Resectable Pancreatic Cancer

The justification for delivering preoperative treatment to patients with potentially resectable pancreatic cancer includes:

1. Early treatment of micrometastatic disease (approximately 80% of patients with potentially resectable pancreatic cancer have systemic disease at presentation).
2. Adjuvant therapy in a "neoadjuvant" setting when it is better tolerated, allowing more patients to undergo and complete the therapy.
3. A reasonable time interval to gauge cancer aggressiveness and thereby select patients for surgery who have the best chance of a favorable outcome.
4. The potential for tumor down-staging to maximize the chances for an R0 or R1 resection.
5. Allowing radiation delivery to well-oxygenated tissues and thus prevent bowel toxicity (which can occur with postoperative radiation when fixed loops of small intestine are within the treatment field).

This approach has been tested in patients with potentially resectable pancreatic cancer in single-institution phase II trials, and the survival durations, local control rates, and patterns of tumor recurrence are similar in patients treated with preoperative therapy and postoperative chemoradiation therapy [27–30].

In most preoperative trials, 15–25% percent of patients who undergo repeat staging before surgery develop clear evidence of metastatic disease on restaging, often in the liver or peritoneum. These patients are spared the potential morbidity of a pancreaticoduodenectomy. All patients require a tissue diagnosis, which can be a barrier to preoperative therapy, but it can be easily achieved by CT-guided or endoscopic-ultrasonography-guided fine-needle aspiration biopsy [31]. Also, endobiliary stent placement is needed if obstructive jaundice is present. In our experience, when the duration of preoperative therapy is less than 6–8 weeks, stent occlusion is uncommon. When the preoperative period exceeds 6–8 weeks, plastic stents have a propensity to occlude; for that reason we favor the insertion of coated expandable metal stents [32]. This has been shown to reduce the rate of stent failure with no evidence to suggest that a metal stent complicates subsequent surgery.

Hoffman and colleagues reported data on the Eastern Cooperative Oncology group multicenter trial of 53 patients with a median follow-up of 52 months [33]. Radiation therapy (50.4 Gy) with mitomycin and a continuous infusion of 5-FU were given as preoperative therapy. Of the 41 patients who underwent surgery, 17 did not undergo resection (11 had hepatic and/or peritoneal metastases and 6 had locally advanced disease). The median survival durations for the entire group and for the 24 patients who had undergone resection were 9.7 and 15.7 months, respectively. Fifty-one percent of patients in this trial were admitted for gastrointestinal toxicities during or within 4 weeks of completing chemoradiation therapy. Given this high rate of hospital admissions and toxicity, subsequent trials have used a shorter hypofractionation course with a radiation dose of approximately 30 Gy, which has been reasonably well tolerated.

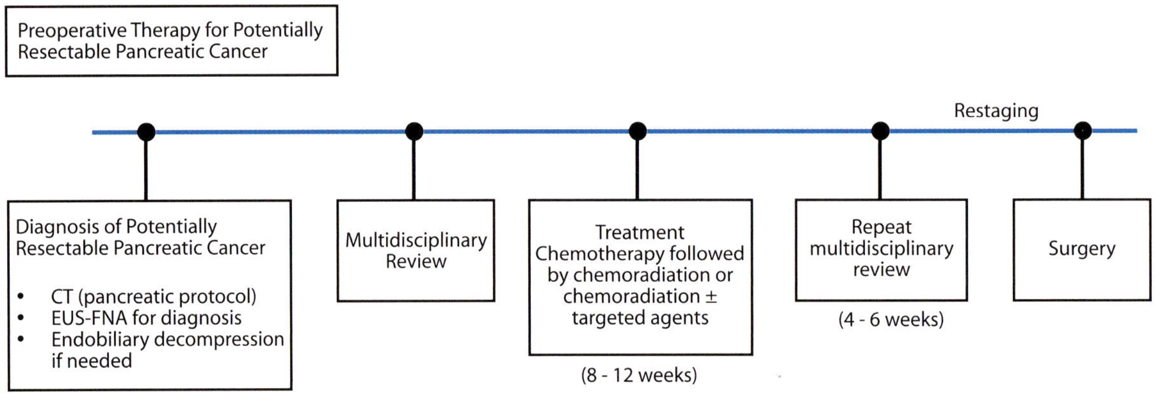

Figure 59.1

Preoperative therapy schema for potentially resectable pancreatic cancer. *CT* Computed tomography, *EUS-FNA* endoscopic-ultrasound-guided fine-needle aspiration

Pisters and colleagues evaluated 35 patients with resectable pancreatic cancer [28]. Patients were treated with 30 Gy of ERBT and concomitant weekly 3-h infusions of paclitaxel (60 mg/m^2). Radiographic restaging was performed 4–6 weeks after chemoradiation therapy, and patients with localized disease underwent pancreatectomy with EBRT–IORT. Sixteen (46%) experienced grade 3 toxicity, and 11% required hospitalization for gastrointestinal toxicities. Twenty of the 25 patients (80%) who underwent surgery underwent pancreatectomy; EBRT–IORT was used in 13 patients. With a median follow-up period of 46 months, the 3-year overall survival rate with chemoradiation therapy and pancreatectomy was 28%. A lower dose of rapid fractionation radiation (30 Gy) was used, and the regimen was better tolerated, without compromise in survival, compared with other preoperative trials as well as standard pancreaticoduodenectomy.

The initial results of our current preoperative trial at M.D. Anderson Cancer Center were recently reported [34]. In this trial, we evaluated the role of initial systemic therapy with four infusions of gemcitabine (750 mg/m^2) and cisplatin (30 mg/m^2) every 2 weeks, followed by 30 Gy of EBRT (3 Gy/fraction over 2 weeks) and 4-weekly doses of gemcitabine during radiation (400 mg/m^2). This study has enrolled 78 patients over 4 years, and of the 77 eligible patients, all completed chemoradiation therapy and received all 10 fractions of EBRT. The hospitalization rate was 47%, mainly because of stent occlusion or other gastrointestinal toxicity. Of the 59 patients (77%) who underwent laparotomy, metastatic disease was found in 13 (22%), and 46 of 77 patients (60%) underwent a successful pancreaticoduodenectomy. Eighty-nine percent (41 of 46) of patients had an R0 resection and 11% had an R1 resection. Eighteen patients (22%) did not undergo surgery; in 12 patients surgery was based on disease progression at restaging. The median survival of resected patients enrolled throughout 2003 was 20.3 months; the final results are not yet available.

Borderline resectable pancreatic cancer is an emerging entity and now seen more often with sophisticated CT imaging [35]. At our institution, tumor abutment of ≤180° (less than or equal to one-half of the circumference) of the SMA, short-segment abutment of the common hepatic artery (usually at the gastroduodenal artery origin), and segmental venous occlusion are used to categorize pancreatic cancer as borderline resectable. These patients are at high risk for margin-positive resection with surgery alone, and most of our patients who meet these criteria undergo preoperative therapy with systemic chemotherapy/chemoradiation therapy. Patients whose tumors show radiographic stability or regression and an improvement in CA19-9, are considered for pancreaticoduodenectomy. A prospective trial by the Eastern Cooperative Oncology Group (ECOG 1200), is evaluating the role of preoperative therapy in this setting.

Figure 59.1 illustrates our institutional preoperative approach to resectable pancreatic cancer. Novel systemic agents are needed to improve systemic and local control in a preoperative and postoperative setting, and the role of targeted agents in this setting is evolving.

Role of Targeted Agents in Neoadjuvant and Adjuvant Therapy for Pancreatic Cancer

Targeted agents have been incorporated into the armamentarium for a variety of cancers including colon, breast, lung, and renal cell cancers. Researchers are enthusiastic to integrate these agents with chemotherapy and/or radiation therapy in the preoperative and postoperative setting in patients with resectable pancreatic cancer.

The epidermal growth factor receptor (EGFR) is overexpressed in up to 95% of patients with pancreatic cancer, and activation of the receptor leads to activation of various downstream signaling molecules, mainly the Ras-Raf-MEK-ERK pathway involved with processes of tumor development, growth, proliferation, metastasis, and angiogenesis [36–39].

The anti-EGFR antibody, cetuximab, and the tyrosine kinase inhibitor, erlotinib, are currently being studied in various stages of pancreatic cancer and may play important roles as radiosensitizers. Cetuximab is a chimeric monoclonal antibody generated from fusion of the variable region of the murine anti-EGFR monoclonal antibody M225 and the human IgG1 constant region. Phase II trial of cetuximab in combination with gemcitabine demonstrates good tolerance and efficacy in advanced pancreatic cancer. Erlotinib is an EGFR tyrosine kinase inhibitor (EGFR-TKI) and like cetuximab, blocks the signal transduction pathways implicated in the growth and proliferation of pancreatic cancer [40]. A phase III trial of the National Cancer Institute of Canada Clinical Trials Group [NCIC-CTG] compared Erlotinib plus gemcitabine compared to gemcitabine alone in patients with advanced pancreatic cancer [41]. Although the improvement in progression-free survival and the overall survival benefit for the combination therapy was modest, given that this was the first phase III trial showing benefit of a combination regimen over single agent gemcitabine, the US Federal Drug Administration recently approved Erlotinib, in combination with gemcitabine for advanced pancreatic cancer [42]. A recent phase I study of Erlotinib with concurrent gemcitabine, paclitaxel, and radiation followed by maintenance erlotinib for patients with locally ad-

Table 59.3. Selected ongoing and planned trials for resectable pancreatic cancer. *NCI* National Cancer Institute, *ACOSOG* American College of Surgical Oncology Group, *SWOG* Southwest Oncology Group, *ECOG* Eastern Cooperative Oncology Group

Sponsor	Study type	Projected accrual/ patients enrolled	Treatment
NCI	Phase III, adjuvant therapy	200	Cetuximab + gemcitabine × 2 cycles followed by cetuximab + capecitabine + RT followed by cetuximab + gemcitabine × 2 cycles vs. Bevacizumab + gemcitabine × 2 cycles followed by bevacizumab + capecitabine + RT followed by bevacizumab + gemcitabine × 2 cycles
ACOSOG Z05031	Phase II, adjuvant	93	RT (50.4 Gy) given concurrently with PVI 5-FU + IFN + CDDP weekly followed by PVI 5-FU for 6 weeks × 2 doses
ACOSOG Z5041	Phase II, preoperative	90	Gemcitabine + bevacizumab followed by surgery and postoperative capecitabine + bevacizumab + RT (45 Gy)
SWOG S0527	Phase II, preoperative	NA	Gemcitabine + oxaliplatin followed by RT (50.4 Gy) with cetuximab followed by surgery and postoperative gemcitabine and oxaliplatin
EORTC 40013	Phase II/III, adjuvant	538	Gemcitabine followed by gemcitabine + RT vs. gemcitabine alone
ESPAC-3	Phase III, adjuvant	660	Gemcitabine vs. 5-FU and leucovorin vs. observation (no radiation)
ECOG 1200	Phase III, preoperative borderline resectable	NA	Gemcitabine + RT vs. gemcitabine + 5-FU + cisplatin followed by RT + 5-FU

vanced pancreatic cancer was reported to be safe and well tolerated [43]. In the 17 patients enrolled, 13 had locally advanced disease and 4 patients had undergone surgery but had positive margins. The median survival of the 13 patients with locally advanced disease was 14.0 months and 46% (6 of the 13) showed a partial response. Studies with EGFR antibodies and EGFR-TKI in the adjuvant and preoperative setting are warranted.

Bevacizumab is a humanized monoclonal antibody that prevents the binding of vascular epithelial growth factor to its receptors [44]. Willet et al. reported the first study using bevacizumab as a radiosensitizer [45]. Crane and colleagues reported on a phase I dose escalation study using capecitabine and bevacizumab in combination with radiation therapy (50.4 Gy) to 47 patients with locally advanced pancreatic cancer, and 9 (20%) of 46 evaluable patients showed an objective partial response to initial therapy. The Radiation Therapy Oncology Group is conducting a phase II trial to evaluate capecitabine-based chemoradiation with bevacizumab (RTOG PA04-11) in locally advanced pancreatic cancer. Table 59.3 outlines selected ongoing or planned studies in potentially resectable or resected pancreatic cancer.

Evolving Role of Vaccines as Adjuvant Therapy for Pancreatic Cancer

Prophylactic vaccines against infectious agents have been in use for decades. These vaccines induce humoral immunity against specific viruses and bacteria; usually before the infection; the general idea is prevention. Because the antigen targets arise during the carcinogenic process in cancer, cancer vaccine research is currently focused on inducing a systemic immune response following the antigenic insult (in the presence of cancer rather than prophylaxis). Considerable effort is being spent in evaluating potential pancreatic antigens as targets that will be recognized by T-cells and antibodies [46,47].

The challenges in creating a superior vaccine include recognition of antigen targets that are expressed on tumor cells and ideally are involved in tumor growth and progression, demonstration of antitumor activity in the presence of immunologic response, development of in vitro and in vivo assays that can prove to be good surrogate markers of such a response, and discovery of novel delivery systems to enhance the immune response. Several pancreatic vaccine approaches have been tested, including peptide-based and gene-modified whole-cell vaccines, both as adjuvant therapy in patients with resected cancer and metastatic disease. Because few pancreatic tumor antigens have been identified, most research has involved the whole tumor cell vaccine approach. Some of the available in vivo assays to evaluate the durability of immunologic response to cancer vaccines include delayed-type hypersensitivity skin reactions, cytotoxic T-cell lymphocyte assay (CTL assay), and in-vitro assays including enzyme-linked immunospot (ELISpot) for measurement of antigen-specific T-cell responses, intracellular cytokine measurement by flow cytometry, and major histocompatibility complex-peptide tetramer analysis (which appears to be the most sensitive of the three) [48].

A phase I clinical trial by Jaffe and colleagues studied a novel granulocyte-macrophage colony-stimulating factor (GM-CSF)-secreting pancreatic tumor vaccine [49]. In this study, 14 patients with stage I–III pancreatic adenocarcinoma were studied with increasing doses of vaccine cells, with the first dose given 8 weeks after pancreatoduodenectomy. Twelve of the 14 patients then went on to receive a 6-month course of adjuvant radiation and chemotherapy. Six of the 12 patients who were still in remission at the end of adjuvant chemotherapy were treated with 3-monthly vaccinations with the same vaccine dose they had originally received. Three patients showed vaccine-induced (dose-dependent) systemic antitumor immunity. This was measured by postvaccination delayed hypersensitivity responses against autologous tumor cells and the authors concluded that this approach is safe and needs further clinical evaluation.

Another study by Gjertsen and colleagues evaluated ex-vivo ras peptide vaccination in patients with advanced pancreatic cancer [50]. Antigen-presenting cells (APC) from peripheral blood of five patients were loaded ex vivo with a synthetic ras peptide, which corresponded to the ras mutation found in the patient's tumor. These APCs were then reinjected into the patients. In two of the five patients treated, an immune response against the immunizing ras peptide could be induced and patients tolerated multiple treatments without side effects. A subsequent phase I/II trial by the same group evaluated tolerability and efficacy in 48 patients (10 surgically resected and 38 with advanced disease) with pancreatic cancer vaccinated by intradermal injection of synthetic mutant ras peptides in combination with GM-CSF [51]. Peptide-specific immunity was induced in 25 of 43 (58%) patients, and patients who were followed for longer periods showed presence of long-lived immunological memory against the ras mutations. Patients with advanced cancer who demonstrated an immune response to the peptide vaccine showed better survival compared to patients without any response (median survival 148 days vs. 61 days, respectively; $P = 0.0002$).

Carcinoembroyonic antigen (CEA) is associated with several malignancies and has been evaluated as the target for tumor vaccine. Early trials using vaccinia and avipox viruses expressing CEA were shown to be safe and T-cell responses to CEA were noted in vaccinated patients [52]. A prime and boost strategy enhanced the immune response. Addition of a triad of costimulatory molecules (B7.1, ICAM-1, and LFA-3 called TRICOM) to these vaccines further enhanced the T-cell responses and this has led to a multicenter phase III study evaluating the efficacy of recombinant vaccinia and avipox vaccine containing five transgenes (CEA, MUC-1, TRICOM) [53]. Further studies with vaccines in the adjuvant setting are warranted.

Summary and Future Direction

Presently, there is no consensus as to the standard management of resectable pancreatic cancer. Neither recent, large, randomized adjuvant trials nor smaller, single-institutional trials of preoperative or adjuvant therapy have helped us decide on the best or preferred therapy. The problem lies with poorly defined eligibility criteria, which hampers interpretation of results from these trials.

Well-defined criteria are required to understand results of preoperative and postoperative treatment trials. These include:

1. Accurate pretreatment staging to assess resectability before surgery and in a postoperative adjuvant trial, a postoperative CT scan to evaluate the presence of metastatic disease prior to delivering "adjuvant" therapy. In the GITSG, EORTC, and ESPAC-1 clinical trials evaluating the role of adjuvant chemoradiation, a postoperative, pretreatment CT scan was not necessary.
2. Accurate margin assessment is essential since there is evidence that patients with positive margins have a shorter survival compared to patients with negative margins. Stratification based on margin status was used in ESPAC-1 and RTOG 97-04 and this should be encouraged for all future prospective trials.
3. Quality control in surgery and delivery of radiation and chemotherapy.
4. High pretreatment serum CA19-9 obtained after pancreaticoduodenectomy is worrisome and persistent elevation after surgery is associated with poor prognosis. Studies evaluating adjuvant therapies should consider a preset level cut-off for this marker level since high levels even in the presence of a normal CT scan may suggest early metastatic disease.

The concept for preoperative therapy is attractive, especially in patients with borderline or marginally resectable pancreatic cancer. The potential for targeted therapies, and immunotherapies including vaccines are currently being exploited in patients with resectable pancreatic cancer. Finally, a better understanding of the pathogenesis of pancreatic cancer and evolving role of molecular profiling in this disease may allow us to develop better therapies.

References

1. Wolff R, Abbruzzese J, Evans D (2003) Neoplasms of the exocrine pancreas. In: Bast RC Jr, Kufe DW, Pollock RE, Weichselbaum RR, Holland JF, Frei E III, Gansler TS (eds) Cancer Medicine. American Cancer Society and BC Decker, pp 1585–1614
2. Sener SF, Fremgen A, Menck HR, Winchester DP (1999) Pancreatic cancer: a report of treatment and survival trends for 100,313 patients diagnosed from 1985–1995, using the National Cancer Database. J Am Coll Surg 189:1–7
3. Millikan KW, Deziel DJ, Silverstein JC, Kanjo TM, Christein JD, Doolas A, et al (1999) Prognostic factors associated with resectable adenocarcinoma of the head of the pancreas. Am Surg 65:618–623; discussion 623–614
4. Kedra B, Popiela T, Sierzega M, Precht A (2001) Prognostic factors of long-term survival after resective procedures for pancreatic cancer. Hepatogastroenterology 48:1762–1766
5. Wenger FA, Peter F, Zieren J, Steiert A, Jacobi CA, Muller JM (2000) Prognosis factors in carcinoma of the head of the pancreas. Dig Surg 17:29–35
6. Lim JE, Chien MW, Earle CC (2003) Prognostic factors following curative resection for pancreatic adenocarcinoma: a population-based, linked database analysis of 396 patients. Ann Surg 237:74–85
7. Yeo CJ, Cameron JL, Lillemoe KD, Sitzmann JV, Hruban RH, Goodman SN, et al (1995) Pancreaticoduodenectomy for cancer of the head of the pancreas in 201 patients. Ann Surg 221:721–731; discussion 731–723
8. Sohn TA, Yeo CJ, Cameron JL, Koniaris L, Kaushal S, Abrams RA, et al (2000) Resected adenocarcinoma of the pancreas – 616 patients: results, outcomes, and prognostic indicators. J Gastrointest Surg 4:567–579
9. Benassai G, Mastrorilli M, Quarto G, Cappiello A, Giani U, Mosella G (2000) Survival after pancreaticoduodenectomy for ductal adenocarcinoma of the head of the pancreas. Chir Ital 52:263–270
10. Benassai G, Mastrorilli M, Quarto G, Cappiello A, Giani U, Forestieri P, et al (2000) Factors influencing survival after resection for ductal adenocarcinoma of the head of the pancreas. J Surg Oncol 73:212–218

11. Neoptolemos JP, Stocken DD, Dunn JA, Almond J, Beger HG, Pederzoli P, et al (2001) Influence of resection margins on survival for patients with pancreatic cancer treated by adjuvant chemoradiation and/or chemotherapy in the ESPAC-1 randomized controlled trial. Ann Surg 234:758–768
12. Takai S, Satoi S, Toyokawa H, Yanagimoto H, Sugimoto N, Tsuji K, et al (2003) Clinicopathologic evaluation after resection for ductal adenocarcinoma of the pancreas: a retrospective, single-institution experience. Pancreas 26:243–249
13. Gunderson LL WC (1997) Pancreas and hepatobiliary tract. In: Perez CA, Brady LW, Halperin EC, Schmidt-Ullrich RK (eds) Principles and Practice of Radiation Oncology. Lippincott-Raven Philadelphia, pp 1467–1488
14. Morganti AG, Valentini V, Macchia G, Alfieri S, Trodella L, Brizi MG, et al (2002) Adjuvant radiotherapy in resectable pancreatic carcinoma. Eur J Surg Oncol 28:523–530
15. Kokubo M, Nishimura Y, Shibamoto Y, Sasai K, Kanamori S, Hosotani R, et al (2000) Analysis of the clinical benefit of intraoperative radiotherapy in patients undergoing macroscopically curative resection for pancreatic cancer. Int J Radiat Oncol Biol Phys 48:1081–1087
16. Sindelar WF, Kinsella TJ (1999) Studies of intraoperative radiotherapy in carcinoma of the pancreas. Ann Oncol 10 Suppl 4:226–230
17. Kalser MH, Ellenberg SS (1985) Pancreatic cancer. Adjuvant combined radiation and chemotherapy following curative resection. Arch Surg 120:899–903
18. Gastrointestinal Tumor Study Group (1987) Further evidence of effective adjuvant combined radiation and chemotherapy following curative resection of pancreatic cancer. Cancer 59:2006–2010
19. Bakkevold KE, Arnesjo B, Dahl O, Kambestad B (1993) Adjuvant combination chemotherapy (AMF) following radical resection of carcinoma of the pancreas and papilla of Vater – results of a controlled, prospective, randomised multicentre study. Eur J Cancer 29A:698–703
20. Demeure MJ, Doffek KM, Komorowski RA, Redlich PN, Zhu YR, Erickson BA, et al (1998) Molecular metastases in stage I pancreatic cancer: improved survival with adjuvant chemoradiation. Surgery 124:663–669
21. Klinkenbijl JH, Jeekel J, Sahmoud T, van Pel R, Couvreur ML, Veenhof CH, et al (1999) Adjuvant radiotherapy and 5-fluorouracil after curative resection of cancer of the pancreas and periampullary region: phase III trial of the EORTC gastrointestinal tract cancer cooperative group. Ann Surg 230:776–782; discussion 782–774
22. Moertel CG, Frytak S, Hahn RG, O'Connell MJ, Reitemeier RJ, Rubin J, et al (1981) Therapy of locally unresectable pancreatic carcinoma: a randomized comparison of high dose (6000 rads) radiation alone, moderate dose radiation (4000 rads + 5-fluorouracil), and high dose radiation + 5-fluorouracil: The Gastrointestinal Tumor Study Group. Cancer 48:1705–1710
23. Neoptolemos JP, Dunn JA, Stocken DD, Almond J, Link K, Beger H, et al (2001) Adjuvant chemoradiotherapy and chemotherapy in resectable pancreatic cancer: a randomised controlled trial. Lancet 358:1576–1585
24. Neoptolemos JP, Stocken DD, Friess H, Bassi C, Dunn JA, Hickey H, et al (2004) A randomized trial of chemoradiotherapy and chemotherapy after resection of pancreatic cancer. N Engl J Med 350:1200–1210
25. Neuhaus P, Oettle H, Post S, Gellert K, Ridwelski K, Schramm H, et al (2005) A randomised, prospective, multicenter, phase III trial of adjuvant chemotherapy with gemcitabine vs. observation in patients with resected pancreatic cancer. Meeting of the American Society of Clinical Oncology, Orlando, May 14–17, 2005; Abstract 4013
26. Picozzi VJ, Kozarek RA, Traverso LW (2003) Interferon-based adjuvant chemoradiation therapy after pancreaticoduodenectomy for pancreatic adenocarcinoma. Am J Surg 185:476–480
27. Breslin TM, Hess KR, Harbison DB, Jean ME, Cleary KR, Dackiw AP, et al (2001) Neoadjuvant chemoradiotherapy for adenocarcinoma of the pancreas: treatment variables and survival duration. Ann Surg Oncol 8:123–132
28. Pisters PW, Wolff RA, Janjan NA, Cleary KR, Charnsangavej C, Crane CN, et al (2002) Preoperative paclitaxel and concurrent rapid-fractionation radiation for resectable pancreatic adenocarcinoma: toxicities, histologic response rates, and event-free outcome. J Clin Oncol 20:2537–2544
29. Spitz FR, Abbruzzese JL, Lee JE, Pisters PW, Lowy AM, Fenoglio CJ, et al (1997) Preoperative and postoperative chemoradiation strategies in patients treated with pancreaticoduodenectomy for adenocarcinoma of the pancreas. J Clin Oncol 15:928–937
30. Wolff R, Evans D, Crane C, Cleary K, Lenzi R, Abbruzzese J, et al (2002) Initial results of preoperative gemcitabine (GEM)-based chemoradiation for resectable pancreatic adenocarcinoma. Presented at the ASCO Annual Meeting, May 18–21, 2002, Orlando, Florida. Abstract 549
31. Raut CP, Grau AM, Staerkel GA, Kaw M, Tamm EP, Wolff RA, et al (2003) Diagnostic accuracy of endoscopic ultrasound-guided fine-needle aspiration in patients with presumed pancreatic cancer. J Gastrointest Surg 7:118–126; discussion 127–118
32. Pisters PW, Hudec WA, Lee JE, Raijman I, Lahoti S, Janjan NA, et al (2000) Preoperative chemoradiation for patients with pancreatic cancer: toxicity of endobiliary stents. J Clin Oncol 18:860–867
33. Hoffman JP, Lipsitz S, Pisansky T, Weese JL, Solin L, Benson AB III (1998) Phase II trial of preoperative radiation therapy and chemotherapy for patients with localized, resectable adenocarcinoma of the pancreas: an Eastern Cooperative Oncology Group Study. J Clin Oncol 16:317–323
34. Varadhachary GR, Evans DE, Crane C, Xiong HQ, Tamm HP, Lee JE, et al (2006) Initial results of preoperative gemcitabine (GEM) plus cisplatin followed by rapid fractionation chemoradiation for resectable pancreatic adenocarcinoma. American Society of Clinical Oncology, Gastrointestinal Cancers Symposium, San Francisco, January 26–28, 2006. Abstract 247
35. Varadhachary GR, Tamm EP, Crane C, Evans DB, Wolff RA (2005) Borderline resectable pancreatic cancer. Curr Treat Options Gastroenterol 8:377–384
36. Bruns CJ, Harbison MT, Davis DW, Portera CA, Tsan R, McConkey DJ, et al (2000) Epidermal growth factor receptor blockade with C225 plus gemcitabine results in regression of human pancreatic carcinoma growing orthotopically in nude mice by antiangiogenic mechanisms. Clin Cancer Res 6:1936–1948
37. Overholser JP, Prewett MC, Hooper AT, Waksal HW, Hicklin DJ (2000) Epidermal growth factor receptor blockade by antibody IMC-C225 inhibits growth of a human pancreatic carcinoma xenograft in nude mice. Cancer 89:74–82

38. Xiong HQ, Abbruzzese JL (2002) Epidermal growth factor receptor–targeted therapy for pancreatic cancer. Semin Oncol 29:31–37
39. Prenzel N, Fischer OM, Streit S, Hart S, Ullrich A (2001) The epidermal growth factor receptor family as a central element for cellular signal transduction and diversification. Endocr Relat Cancer 8:11–31
40. Grunwald V, Hidalgo M (2003) Development of the epidermal growth factor receptor inhibitor OSI–774. Semin Oncol 30:23–31
41. Moore MJ, Goldstein J, Hamm J, Figer A, Hecht J, Gallinger S, Au H, et al (2005) Erlotinib plus gemcitabine compared to gemcitabine alone in patients with advanced pancreatic cancer. A phase III trial of the National Cancer Institute of Canada Clinical Trials Group [NCIC-CTG]. J Clin Oncol 23 (Suppl 16): A-1, 1s
42. Moore MJ (2005) Brief communication: a new combination in the treatment of advanced pancreatic cancer. Semin Oncol 32:5–6
43. Iannitti D, Dipetrillo T, Akerman P, Barnett JM, Maia-Acuna C, Cruff D, et al (2005) Erlotinib and chemoradiation followed by maintenance erlotinib for locally advanced pancreatic cancer: a phase I study. Am J Clin Oncol 28:570–575
44. Jain RK (2005) Normalization of tumor vasculature: an emerging concept in antiangiogenic therapy. Science 307:58–62
45. Willett CG, Boucher Y, di Tomaso E, Duda DG, Munn LL, Tong RT, et al (2004) Direct evidence that the VEGF-specific antibody bevacizumab has antivascular effects in human rectal cancer. Nat Med 10:145–147
46. Jaffee EM, Hruban RH, Canto M, Kern SE (2002) Focus on pancreas cancer. Cancer Cell 2:25–28
47. Greten TF, Jaffee EM (1999) Cancer vaccines. J Clin Oncol 17:1047–1060
48. Laheru D, Jaffee EM (2005) Immunotherapy for pancreatic cancer – science driving clinical progress. Nat Rev Cancer 5:459–467
49. Jaffee EM, Hruban RH, Biedrzycki B, Laheru D, Schepers K, Sauter PR, et al (2001) Novel allogenic granulocyte-macrophage colony-stimulating factor-secreting tumor vaccine for pancreatic cancer: a phase I trial of safety and immune activation. J Clin Oncol 19:145–156
50. Gjertsen MK, Bakka A, Breivik J, Saeterdal I, Solheim BG, Soreide O, et al (1995) Vaccination with mutant ras peptides and induction of T-cell responsiveness in pancreatic carcinoma patients carrying the corresponding RAS mutation. Lancet 346:1399–1400
51. Gjertsen MK, Buanes T, Rosseland AR, Bakka A, Gladhaug I, Soreide O, et al (2001) Intradermal ras peptide vaccination with granulocyte-macrophage colony-stimulating factor as adjuvant: Clinical and immunological responses in patients with pancreatic adenocarcinoma. Int J Cancer 92:441–450
52. Marshall J (2003) Carcinoembryonic antigen-based vaccines. Semin Oncol 30:30–36
53. Marshall JL, Gulley JL, Arlen PM, Beetham PK, Tsang KY, Slack R, et al (2005) Phase I study of sequential vaccinations with fowlpox-CEA(6D)-TRICOM alone and sequentially with vaccini-CEA(6D)-TRICOM, with and without granulocyte-macrophage colony-stimulating factor, in patients with carcinoembryonic antigen-expressing carcinomas. J Clin Oncol 23:720–731
54. Abrams RA, Grochow LB, Chakravarthy A, Sohn TA, Zahurak ML, Haulk TL, Ord S, Hruban RH, Lillemoe KD, Pitt HA, Cameron JL, Yeo CJ (1999) Intensified adjuvant therapy for pancreatic and periampullary adenocarcinoma: survival results and observations regarding patterns of failure, radiotherapy dose and CA19-9 levels. Int J Radiat Oncol Biol Phys 44:1039–1046
55. Takada T, Amano H, Yasuda H, Nimura Y, Matsushiro T, Kato H, Nagakawa T, Nakayama T (2002) Is postoperative adjuvant chemotherapy useful for gallbladder carcinoma? A phase III multicenter prospective randomized controlled trial in patients with resected pancreaticobiliary carcinoma. Cancer 95:1685–1695

Chapter 60

A. Jimeno · M. Hidalgo

Management of Locally Advanced and Recurrent Pancreas Cancer

Pancreatic cancer remains a devastating disease. In 2007 the estimated incidence of the disease in the USA is 37,170 with an expected 33,370 deaths [1]. At the time of diagnosis, 80% of patients have locally advanced or advanced disease for which no curative therapy exist, and 80% of patients treated with curative intent will recur in the first 2 years after surgical resection and will succumb to their disease [2]. Locally advanced pancreatic cancer is usually defined as patients with American Joint Committee on Cancer (6th edition) T4 lesions, where the primary tumor involves branches of the celiac axis or the superior mesenteric artery, indicating an unresectable primary tumor and representing stage III disease. These patients often require operative or nonoperative palliation of disease-related processes such as obstructive jaundice, gastroduodenal obstruction, or abdominal pain. Focused anticancer treatment for such locally advanced pancreatic adenocarcinoma can involve chemoradiation approaches, chemotherapy alone, or locally directed therapy.

Symptoms-Oriented Palliative Treatment

Nonsurgical Interventions

The nonoperative palliative management of patients with pancreatic cancer can be applied to patients with unresectable locally advanced disease, or less frequently to patients with distant metastases. This is also the approach of choice for patients with unresectable disease with acute or chronic debilitating diseases that make anesthesia and surgery prohibitive [3]. One exception to these indications favoring nonoperative management is the patient with symptomatic upper gastrointestinal obstruction (from tumors that obstruct at the duodenal C loop or at the ligament of Treitz) where nonoperative palliation is not reliable, and where gastrojejunostomy may be the best method of palliation. In patients who are to be managed nonoperatively, a tissue diagnosis can be obtained via percutaneous biopsy of distant metastases or of local tumor.

Jaundice is present in the majority of patients with pancreatic adenocarcinoma. If untreated, obstructive jaundice can result in progressive liver dysfunction, hepatic failure and early death [3]. Biliary decompression can be achieved either by endoscopic or by percutaneous transhepatic techniques in nearly all patients who are not candidates for surgical intervention. The available data support the use of an endoscopic endoprosthesis or stent placement method as the primary approach for nonoperative palliation of jaundice in patients with locally advanced pancreatic cancer [3], and a success rate exceeding 90% is expected from skilled teams performing endoscopic stenting on a regular basis. Once biliary cannulation has been accomplished, a guide wire is manipulated above the malignant stricture, and a 7- to 10-Fr plastic endoprosthesis is secured in position, being pushed over the guide wire. Early complications following endoprosthesis placement include cholangitis, pancreatitis, bleeding, and bile duct or duodenal perforation. Late complications include stent obstruction, cholecystitis, and stent migration. Metallic expandable endoprostheses have been developed and have been modified to allow endoscopic placement. Metallic endoprostheses reduce the problem of stent migration, although tumor ingrowth causing late stent occlusion is a potential drawback [3]. A percutaneous transhepatic biliary drainage technique is most typically used when endoscopic placement cannot be performed. A cholangiography serves to both identify the site of obstruction and to guide the advancement of a percutaneous transhepatic biliary catheter through the obstruction, with the tip of the catheter being placed in the duodenum. In most cases biliary drainage with an internal-external catheter is the initial management, with subsequent management including percutaneous placement of a totally indwelling endoprosthesis. Complications of percutaneous transhepatic catheter drainage include stent occlusion, hemobilia related to the transhepatic route, bile peritonitis, bile pleural effusion, cholangitis, pancreatitis, and acute cholecystitis.

In cases of intractable pain despite adequate oral or transdermal treatment, several nonoperative treatment modalities including percutaneous or endoscopic celiac nerve block or external beam radiation therapy (EBRT) directed at the primary tumor and celiac plexus may be considered.

Surgical Interventions

Patients undergoing exploration for a presumed resectable pancreatic adenocarcinoma where unresectability is determined either due to locally advanced or metastatic disease are candidates to undergo palliative procedures such as biliary-enteric bypass, gastrojejunostomy, and chemical (alcohol) nerve block. For a more in-depth analysis, see Chap. 58.

Medical Treatment

Three fundamental questions have been evaluated, but remain largely unanswered. First, no randomized comparisons of radiation and/or chemotherapy versus supportive care (aside from subset analyses in trials for metastatic disease) have been performed in patients with locally advanced disease; the prevalent opinion is that symptom control is better with any treatment than with no treatment at all. Second, EBRT improves the symptoms associated with locally advanced disease, but its high local failure rate and the synergy observed when EBRT is combined with chemotherapy led to trials comparing EBRT versus chemoradiation. Third, the high systemic failure rate led to questioning the real value of EBRT, and this subsequently led to designing studies to compare chemoradiation versus chemotherapy alone. Table 60.1 summarizes the studies discussed hereafter that address these fundamental questions.

Radiation Versus Chemoradiation

Two prospective, randomized studies have demonstrated a modest survival benefit of combined modality therapy over EBRT alone in the management of locally advanced disease, whereas one study showed no such benefit. The first trial included patients with different types of gastrointestinal cancers, 64 of whom had locally unresectable pancreatic cancer randomized to either 5-fluorouracil (5-FU) or placebo, combined with 35–40 Gy of radiation. Median survival in the combined-modality arm was significantly higher than in the radiation-therapy-only arm (10.4 vs. 6.3 months) [4]. The Gastrointestinal Tumor Study Group (GITSG) randomized 194 locally advanced pancreatic cancer patients to receive split-course EBRT, either alone (60 Gy) or combined (either 40 or 60 Gy) with 5-FU (500 mg/m^2) on the first 3 days of each 20 Gy of radiation [5]. The EBRT-alone arm was

Table 60.1. Selected randomized trials in locally advanced pancreatic cancer. Adapted from Earle et al. (2003) [27]. *5-FU*, 5-Fluorouracil, *ECOG* Eastern Cooperative Oncology Group, *GITSG* Gastrointestinal Study Group, *Gy* Gray, *mCCNU* methyl lomustine, *SMF* streptozotocin+mitomycin+5-FU, *SWOG* Southwest Oncology Group

Reference	Radiation (Gy)	Chemotherapy	Number of patients	Median survival (months)	1-year survival (%)
Chemoradiation versus radiation alone					
Moertel et al (1969) [4]	35–40	5-FU	32	10.4*	25*[a]
	35–40	Placebo	32	6.3	6[a]
GITSG (1981) [5]	60	5-FU	111	11.4	44*
	40	5-FU	117	8.4	39*
	60	–	25	5.3	14
Chemoradiation versus chemotherapy alone					
ECOG (1985) [19]	40	5-FU	47	8.3	28[a]
	–	5-FU	44	8.2	31[a]
GITSG (1988) [18]	54	5-FU and SMF	22	9.7*	41*
	–	SMF	21	7.4	19

* $p<0.05$
[a] Calculated from survival curve

discontinued after an interim analysis showed improved median time to progression and overall survival in the combined modality arms. Forty percent of patients treated with the combined regimens were still living at 1 year, compared with 10% of patients treated with radiation only. There were no significant differences between the high- and low-dose EBRT in the chemoradiation arms, although there were trends favoring the higher-dose arm in time to progression and survival. However, a randomized Eastern Cooperative Oncology Group (ECOG) trial that compared EBRT versus EBRT plus 5-FU and mitomycin C in 104 patients showed that chemoradiation increased toxicity without improving disease-free survival or overall survival in patients with locally advanced pancreatic cancer [6].

In an attempt to improve the efficacy of chemoradiation, several agents have been assessed in combination with radiation therapy. In particular, there has been considerable interest in combining EBRT with gemcitabine due to its clinical benefit in the metastatic setting and its potent radiosensitizing properties. Early trials were designed to determine the maximal tolerated dose of gemcitabine when delivered weekly and integrated with radiation therapy consisting of 50.4 Gy in standard 1.8-Gy fractions. The starting dose of gemcitabine was 300 mg/m^2. Hematologic and gastrointestinal toxicities were identified as dose limiting at 700 mg/m^2 [7]. Blackstock et al. examined, in a dose-finding study, gemcitabine (starting at 20 mg/m^2) twice weekly in combination with radiation therapy (total dose 50.4 Gy in 1.8-Gy fractions) in 19 patients with locally advanced pancreatic cancer [8]. Of the 15 patients assessable for response, 3 partial responses were identified. A dose of 40 mg/m^2 twice weekly in combination with radiotherapy to total dose of 50.4 Gy was subsequently examined by the Cancer and Leukemia Group B in a phase II study of 43 patients with locally advanced pancreatic cancer [9]. Following chemoradiotherapy, patients without disease progression received gemcitabine alone (1000 mg/m^2 weekly for 3 weeks and then every 4 weeks for five additional cycles). Grade 3–4 hematologic and gastrointestinal toxicity was significant and identified in 60% and 42% of patients, respectively. With a median follow-up of 10 months, median survival was 8.2 months. The authors acknowledge that although this treatment strategy results in adequate locoregional control, this did not seem to result in a survival advantage. The MD Anderson Cancer Center (MDACC) has published a phase I study of 18 patients with locally advanced disease using rapid fractionation EBRT [10]. Patients received dose escalation gemcitabine from 350 mg/m^2 to 500 mg/m^2 weekly for 7 weeks with concurrent rapid fractionation of 3000 cGy EBRT during the first 2 weeks of therapy. Hematologic and nonhematologic toxicities were significant in all three patient cohorts. There were four partial responses, and one of two patients who were subsequently explored had a resection. The recommended phase II testing dose of gemcitabine was 350 mg/m^2. The authors acknowledged that given the severity of the toxic effects, and until dose and scheduling issues were explored further, concomitant administration of gemcitabine and radiation therapy according to their proposed schedule should still be considered investigational.

Other chemotherapy agents have been added to gemcitabine combined with radiation therapy. The ECOG published a phase I study of seven patients with locally advanced disease using 5-FU/gemcitabine combined with radiation therapy to a maximum dose of 59.4 Gy in 1.8-Gy fractions [11]. 5-FU (200 mg/m^2/day as continuous infusion throughout radiation therapy) was administered with weekly gemcitabine dose escalation beginning at 100 mg/m^2. However, because of dose-limiting toxicities seen both at the starting and at a lower dose level of gemcitabine to 50 mg/m^2, the study was subsequently closed. Gemcitabine has also been combined with cisplatin and radiation in a phase I trial at the Mayo Clinic, which gave twice-weekly gemcitabine and cisplatin for 3 weeks during radiation (50.4 Gy in 28 fractions) [12]. Dose-limiting toxicities consisted of grade 4 nausea and vomiting, and the recommended phase II dose was gemcitabine 300 mg/m^2 and cisplatin 10 mg/m^2. Another trial used gemcitabine (on days 2, 5, 26, and 33) and cisplatin (on days 1–5 and 29–33) combined with radiation, with a recommended phase II dose of 20 mg/m^2 for cisplatin and 300 mg/m^2 for gemcitabine [13]. Interestingly, the response to chemoradiation allowed 10 out of 30 initially unresectable patients to undergo surgery, with an R0 resection in 9 cases and a complete response in 2 cases.

Another agent that has raised Interest has been paclitaxel. In a phase I trial at Brown University (Providence, RI, USA) evaluating paclitaxel and 50 Gy of EBRT for patients with unresectable pancreatic and gastric cancers, the maximum tolerated dose of weekly paclitaxel with conventional irradiation was 50 mg/m^2 [14]. The response rate was 31% among 13 evaluable pancreatic cancer patients. These data have led to a Radiation Therapy Oncology Group (RTOG) phase II study evaluating paclitaxel with EBRT for patients with unresectable pancreatic cancer [15]. The median survival of 109 patients on this study was 11.2 months (95% confidence interval 10.1–12.3) with estimated 1- and 2-year survival rates of 43% and 13%, respectively. External irradiation plus concurrent weekly paclitaxel was well tolerated when administered with large-field radiotherapy, and the median survival seems better than historical results achieved with irradiation and fluoropyrimidines.

Despite the existence of numerous regimens, few trials have compared the use of different chemotherapy agents with radiation therapy in the locally advanced setting. A GITSG study randomized 143 patients to EBRT with either weekly 5-FU or doxorubicin [16]. Median survival was similar in both arms (approximately 8 months), but the doxorubicin arm had more frequent severe toxicity. In a retrospective analysis, the MDACC examined their database of 114 patients with locally advanced disease treated with combination radiation therapy (rapid fractionation 30 Gy in 10 fractions) with either continuous infusion of 5-FU at 200–300 mg/m^2 (61 patients) or gemcitabine at 250–500 mg/m^2 weekly for 7 cycles (53 patients) [17]. Patients receiving gemcitabine developed a higher incidence of severe acute toxicity compared with those patients receiving 5-FU (23% versus 2% $p<0.0001$). Five out of 53 patients treated with gemcitabine plus radiation therapy subsequently underwent surgical resection compared to 1 out of 61 patients treated with 5-FU-based chemoradiation. However, the median survival was similar (11 months vs 9 months; $p=0.19$).

Chemoradiation Versus Chemotherapy Alone

A GITSG study compared streptozotocin, mitomycin, and 5-FU (SMF) alone versus SMF combined with EBRT (54 Gy) in 43 patients, and showed a significant improvement in median survival (9.7 versus 7.4 months) for the chemoradiation arm [18]. Overall survival following this combined-modality treatment program was significantly superior to that following SMF chemotherapy alone (41% vs 19% at 1 year, $p=0.02$). However, an ECOG study of 91 patients comparing 5-FU 600 mg/m^2 weekly with or without EBRT found no significant benefit to combined-modality therapy over chemotherapy alone, although it has been argued that the dose of radiation (40 Gy) was insufficient and a significant proportion of patients were found to be ineligible for analysis [19].

Therefore, and since the benefit of chemoradiation is relatively modest, some oncologists recommend chemotherapy alone for locally advanced disease. The use of gemcitabine is supported by the results of the randomized trial by Burris et al., in which 26% of the study subjects had locally advanced disease [20]. Gemcitabine ameliorated symptoms and modestly improved survival compared to 5-FU, but the results for patients with locally advanced disease were not reported separately. An ECOG phase III trial (E4201) comparing gemcitabine (600 mg/m^2 weekly)/radiation (50.4 Gy in 28 fractions) followed by gemcitabine (1000 mg/m^2 weekly for 3 of 4 weeks) versus gemcitabine, which started in April 2003 will examine this issue. However, accrual has been reported to be poor, and the viability of E4201 is currently in doubt.

Incorporation of Novel Targeted Agents

Erlotinib is a small-molecule quinazoline that is administered orally and selectively and reversibly inhibits the tyrosine kinase activity of the epidermal growth factor receptor. On the basis of extended survival on a trial that compared gemcitabine plus erlotinib or placebo in patients with metastatic pancreas cancer, it has received regulatory approval for that indication. A phase I trial has recently been conducted to determine the maximally tolerated dose of erlotinib with concurrent gemcitabine, paclitaxel, and radiation and to gather preliminary data on maintenance erlotinib after chemoradiation [21]. Patients received gemcitabine (75 mg/m^2) and paclitaxel (40 mg/m^2) weekly for 6 weeks with 50.4 Gy radiation. Erlotinib was administered over three dose levels (50–100 mg/day) with chemoradiation, and then all patients received 150 mg/day until disease progression. Seventeen patients were assessable for toxicity, 13 with locally advanced disease and 4 who had undergone resection but had positive margins. At erlotinib dosages less than or equal to 75 mg/day, the chemoradiation dose-limiting toxicities were diarrhea, dehydration, rash, myelosuppression, and small bowel stricture. The median survival of the 13 patients with locally advanced disease was 14.0 months, and 6 out of the 13 (46%) had a partial response. A prospective phase II trial designed to analyze the feasibility and effectivity of trimodal therapy with gemcitabine-based chemoradiation and cetuximab in locally advanced inoperable pancreatic cancer has been conducted in 55 patients [2]. Preliminary results indicate feasibility without increased toxicity profile, and a promising response rate. However cetuximab failed to improve outcomes in a more broad population [3].

Locally Directed Therapy

Both brachytherapy and intraoperative radiotherapy (IORT) have been employed in the setting of locally advanced disease, with the intent of improving locoregional tumor control. However, and considering the propensity of this disease to disseminate into the liver and adjacent peritoneum as well as systemically, what can be achieved overall for patients by the addition of either modality to EBRT and chemotherapy is not unclear. Mohiuddin et al. reported on 81 patients with localized unresectable carcinoma of the pancreas managed using intraoperative iodine-125 implants, EBRT, and perioperative systemic chemotherapy [22]. Patients were also treated with 50–55 Gy of external beam irradiation and systemic chemotherapy consisting of 5-FU, mitomycin, and occasionally CCNU (lomustine). Implants were performed at laparotomy. There was a 5% mortality rate and a high incidence of both early and late morbidities, including cholangitis, upper gastrointestinal bleeding, and radiation enteritis. Local control was obtained in 39 of 53 (71%) of evaluable patients, but 52 of 81 patients (62%) failed with intra-abdominal disease, primarily hepatic and peritoneal. With a minimum follow-up of 2 years at the time of publication, the median survival for the total group was 12 months, the 2-year survival was 21% and the 5-year survival was 7%.

The use of IORT using single-fraction electron beam treatment has also been extensively studied, usually in combination with EBRT in the range of 45–50.4 Gy with 5-FU alone or 5-FU-based combination chemotherapy. The RTOG reported on 51 patients with unresected nonmetastatic pancreatic cancer treated with IORT and EBRT/5-FU, and found a major postoperative complication rate of 12% [23]. Two patients had major morbidity that led to death. The authors acknowledge that although this study does demonstrate the feasibility of IORT in a multi-institutional setting, it does not demonstrate any advantage of IORT over conventional therapy for this disease. In experienced hands, IORT can be given with acceptable morbidity, although there are occasional reports of unacceptably high complication rates.

In addition to local radiation delivery, a variety of other techniques and agents are under development for the treatment of locally advanced pancreatic cancer. One example is intratumoral injection via endoscopic ultrasound (EUS) of ONYX-015, an engineered adenovirus that selectively replicates in tumor cells. In a phase I/II trial of this agent combined with gemcitabine, 21 patients with locally advanced adenocarcinoma of the pancreas or with metastatic disease, but minimal or absent liver metastases, underwent 8 sessions of ONYX-015 delivered by EUS injection into the primary pancreatic tumor over 8 weeks [24]. After combination therapy, two patients had partial regressions of the injected tumor, two had minor responses and six had stable disease. This study indicated that ONYX-015 injection via EUS into pancreatic carcinomas by the transgastric route with prophylactic antibiotics is feasible and generally well tolerated, either alone or in combination with gemcitabine. Another novel biological agent in development is TNFerade, which is a replication-deficient adenovector carrying a transgene encoding for human tumor necrosis factor alpha regulated by a radiation-inducible promoter. Weekly intratumoral injections have been given in combination with chemoradiation (50.4 Gy along with continuous infusion of 5-FU 200 mg/m^2 daily) [25]. Two of 17 patients in a phase I trial converted from unresectable to resectable, and one of these had a pathologic complete response. A prospective phase II/III trial designed to analyze the feasibilitiy and effectivity of TNFerade denominated the Pancreatic Cancer Clinical Trial with TNFerade (PACT) study is being conducted; patients are randomized to standard of care chemoradiation plus/minus TNFerade [4]. The interim analyses met criteria to continue the study showing a median survival for TNFerade patients of 515 days compared to 335 days. The logrank statistic for comparison between the two arms is X^2=2.014 (p00.16).

Conclusions

The optimal treatment for locally advanced pancreatic cancer remains controversial, and the key questions regarding its management remain unanswered. What is more preoccupying, however, is that the odds that they will be addressed seem at best low. There have been no adequately powered, randomized trials comparing chemoradiation strategies versus best supportive care or chemotherapy alone, and the survival benefit from combined modality therapy for locally advanced disease has been modest in various trials. Nonetheless, most practitioners in the United States employ radiation therapy (typically 54 Gy in 1.8-Gy fractions) with simultaneous chemotherapy, the standard being 5-FU. Although several chemotherapy regimens have been compared to 5-FU in randomized trials, none have proven more efficacious, and they are typically more toxic. Various ways of giving 5-FU have been used in these trials, but most practitioners choose either continuous-infusion 200 mg/m^2/day during radiation therapy, or a 500-mg/m^2 bolus given on the first 3 days and last 3 days of radiation. It will be particularly interesting to see how capecitabine and oral fluoropyrimidine with activity in advanced pancreas cancer [26], is incorporated to chemoradiation schedules. Studies are underway that will examine the role of gemcitabine (both alone, and combined with radiation) for locally advanced disease. In addition, given the limited success of current treatments and the rapidly expanding knowledge of the pathogenesis of cancer at the molecular level, several biologically directed approaches are being actively explored, with the aim of allowing patients who present with unresectable disease to undergo curative surgery.

References

1. Jemal A, Siegel R, Ward E et al. (2007) Cancer statistics 2007. CA Cancer J Clin 57:43–66
2. R. Krempien MW Munter, C. Timke et al. (2007) Journal of Clinical Oncology, ASCO Annual Meeting Proceedings Part I. Vol 25, No. 18S (June 20 Supplement), 2007:4573
3. PA Philip, J Benedetti, C Fenoglio-Preiser, M Zalupski et al. Journal of Clinical Oncology, ASCO Annual Meeting Proceedings Part I Vol 25, No. 18S (June 20 Supplement), 2007: LBA4509
4. M Posner, KJ Chang, A Rosemurgy et al. (2007) Journal of Clinical Oncology, ASCO Annual Meeting Proceedings Part I Vol 25, No. 18S (June 20 Supplement), 2007:4518
5. Moertel CG, Frytak S, Hahn RG, et al (1981) Therapy of locally unresectable pancreatic carcinoma: a randomized comparison of high dose (6000 rads) radiation alone, moderate dose radiation (4000 rads + 5-fluorouracil), and high dose radiation + 5-fluorouracil: The Gastrointestinal Tumor Study Group. Cancer 48:1705–1710
6. Cohen SJ, Dobelbower R Jr, Lipsitz S, et al (2005) A randomized phase III study of radiotherapy alone or with 5-fluorouracil and mitomycin-C in patients with locally advanced adenocarcinoma of the pancreas: Eastern Cooperative Oncology Group study E8282. Int J Radiat Oncol Biol Phys 62:1345–1350
7. McGinn CJ, Zalupski MM (2003) Radiation therapy with once-weekly gemcitabine in pancreatic cancer: current status of clinical trials. Int J Radiat Oncol Biol Phys 56:10–15
8. Blackstock AW, Bernard SA, Richards F, et al (1999) Phase I trial of twice-weekly gemcitabine and concurrent radiation in patients with advanced pancreatic cancer. J Clin Oncol 17:2208–2212
9. Blackstock AW, Tepper JE, Niedwiecki D, Hollis DR, Mayer RJ, Tempero MA (2003) Cancer and leukemia group B (CALGB) 89805: phase II chemoradiation trial using gemcitabine in patients with locoregional adenocarcinoma of the pancreas. Int J Gastrointest Cancer 34:107–116
10. Wolff RA, Evans DB, Gravel DM, et al (2001) Phase I trial of gemcitabine combined with radiation for the treatment of locally advanced pancreatic adenocarcinoma. Clin Cancer Res 7:2246–2253
11. Talamonti MS, Catalano PJ, Vaughn DJ, et al (2000) Eastern Cooperative Oncology Group Phase I trial of protracted venous infusion fluorouracil plus weekly gemcitabine with concurrent radiation therapy in patients with locally advanced pancreas cancer: a regimen with unexpected early toxicity. J Clin Oncol 18:3384–3389
12. Martenson JA, Vigliotti AP, Pitot HC, et al (2003) A phase I study of radiation therapy and twice-weekly gemcitabine and cisplatin in patients with locally advanced pancreatic cancer. Int J Radiat Oncol Biol Phys 55:1305–1310
13. Brunner TB, Grabenbauer GG, Klein P, et al (2003) Phase I trial of strictly time-scheduled gemcitabine and cisplatin with concurrent radiotherapy in patients with locally advanced pancreatic cancer. Int J Radiat Oncol Biol Phys 55:144–153
14. Safran H, Akerman P, Cioffi W, et al (1999) Paclitaxel and concurrent radiation therapy for locally advanced adenocarcinomas of the pancreas, stomach, and gastroesophageal junction. Semin Radiat Oncol 9:53–57
15. Rich T, Harris J, Abrams R, et al (2004) Phase II study of external irradiation and weekly paclitaxel for nonmetastatic, unresectable pancreatic cancer: RTOG-98-12. Am J Clin Oncol 27:51–56
16. Gastrointestinal Tumor Study Group (1985) Radiation therapy combined with adriamycin or 5-fluorouracil for the treatment of locally unresectable pancreatic carcinoma. Cancer 56:2563–2568
17. Crane CH, Abbruzzese JL, Evans DB, et al (2002) Is the therapeutic index better with gemcitabine-based chemoradiation than with 5-fluorouracil-based chemoradiation in locally advanced pancreatic cancer? Int J Radiat Oncol Biol Phys 52:1293–1302
18. Gastrointestinal Tumor Study Group (1988) Treatment of locally unresectable carcinoma of the pancreas: comparison of combined-modality therapy (chemotherapy plus radiotherapy) to chemotherapy alone. J Natl Cancer Inst 80:751–755
19. Klaassen DJ, MacIntyre JM, Catton GE, Engstrom PF, Moertel CG (1985) Treatment of locally unresectable cancer of the stomach and pancreas: a randomized comparison of 5-fluorouracil alone with radiation plus concurrent and maintenance 5-fluorouracil – an Eastern Cooperative Oncology Group study. J Clin Oncol 3:373–378
20. Burris HA III, Moore MJ, Andersen J, et al (1997) Improvements in survival and clinical benefit with gemcitabine as first-line therapy for patients with advanced pancreas cancer: a randomized trial. J Clin Oncol 15:2403–2413
21. Iannitti D, Dipetrillo T, Akerman P, et al (2005) Erlotinib and chemoradiation followed by maintenance erlotinib for locally advanced pancreatic cancer: a phase I study. Am J Clin Oncol 28:570–575
22. Mohiuddin M, Rosato F, Barbot D, Schuricht A, Biermann W, Cantor R (1992) Long-term results of combined modality treatment with I-125 implantation for carcinoma of the pancreas. Int J Radiat Oncol Biol Phys 23:305–311
23. Tepper JE, Noyes D, Krall JM, et al (1991) Intraoperative radiation therapy of pancreatic carcinoma: a report of RTOG-8505. Radiation Therapy Oncology Group. Int J Radiat Oncol Biol Phys 21:1145–1149
24. Hecht JR, Bedford R, Abbruzzese JL, et al (2003) A phase I/II trial of intratumoral endoscopic ultrasound injection of ONYX-015 with intravenous gemcitabine in unresectable pancreatic carcinoma. Clin Cancer Res 9:555–561
25. Hanna N CT, Hecht R, et al (2003) TNFerade in pancreatic cancer: results of a run-in phase of a major randomized study in patients with locally advanced pancreatic cancer. Proc ASCO 22:271, abstract 1086
26. Cartwright TH, Cohn A, Varkey JA, et al (2002) Phase II study of oral capecitabine in patients with advanced or metastatic pancreatic cancer. J Clin Oncol 20:160–164
27. Earle CC, Agboola O, Maroun J, and Zuraw L (2003) The treatment of locally advanced pancreatic cancer: a practice guideline. Can J Gastroenterol 17:161–167

Chapter 61

J.F. Tseng · C. Fernandez-del Castillo · A.L. Warshaw

Survival After Medical and Surgical Treatment of Pancreatic Adenocarcinoma

Pancreatic adenocarcinoma is known for its poor prognosis; the incidence of new cases roughly equals the mortality per year. In the USA, in 2005, it is estimated that there will have been 32,180 new cases of pancreatic cancer, and that 31,800 people will have died of the disease [1]. Pancreatic cancer is the fourth most common cause of cancer death among USA men, and the fifth most common cause of cancer death among USA women [1]. A major factor in the lethality of pancreatic cancer remains its generally advanced stage at diagnosis: 80% of patients present with locally advanced or metastatic disease, and overall survival for all stages combined is 19% at 1 year and 4% at 5 years [2, 3]. This chapter reviews some of the major factors that influence survival in patients with pancreatic cancer. It is to be hoped that our increasing knowledge of which variables alter survival duration will translate into evidence-based medical decision-making to maximize the quality lifespan of future patients with this disease.

Because of their different presentations and operative management, it is useful to divide patients with pancreatic adenocarcinoma into those who have tumors of the pancreatic head (i.e., to the right of the mesenteric vessels) and those who have tumors of the body and tail of the pancreas (i.e., to the left of the mesenteric vessels) [4]. Patients with pancreatic adenocarcinoma of either the head or body and tail can then be further divided into three groups: those with resectable tumors, those with locally advanced, unresectable tumors, and those with metastatic disease. Patients in each group have different natural histories, treatment options, and survival durations.

Approximately 60% of patients present with tumors of the head of the pancreas, of which 20% are resectable at presentation; of patients who undergo pancreaticoduodenectomy for tumors of the head, actuarial 5-year survival is around 20% [3]. The remaining 40% of patients present with tumors of the body and tail of the pancreas, of which <5% are resectable. Survival in patients with tumors of the body and tail of the pancreas is poor due largely to the later stage at diagnosis [5–7]. Even the minority of patients with tumors of the body and tail who have resectable disease and undergo operation appear to have somewhat poorer survival than patients with resected tumors of the pancreatic head, with a 5-year survival of 4–15% [7, 8]. However, a 5-year survival rate of 22% in a small group of patients who were able to undergo "extended" resections has been described [9]. In any case, the poorer prognosis for patients with tail lesions generally reflects the fact that these patients often present with nonspecific, insidious symptoms, and thus frequently have unresectable or metastatic disease, rather than the painless jaundice that heralds pancreatic head lesions, which may still be confined to the pancreas at presentation. Thus, it is important to note that patients should not be denied surgery because of the location of their tumor per se; patients with resectable lesions in the head or body and tail should be treated accordingly regardless of tumor location.

Overall, resectable patients who undergo pancreatectomy for pancreatic adenocarcinoma have been reported to have 5-year survival of approximately 20%, with a median survival of around 20 months [10–14]. Patients with locally advanced tumors have a median survival of 10–12 months with aggressive medical treatment [15]; patients with metastatic pancreatic cancer have a median survival of 4–6 months in published clinical trials [16, 17]. For all patients who present with pancreatic adenocarcinoma at any stage, regardless of tumor location, <3% will be alive 5 years after diagnosis [3, 11, 18].

Although disease stage at presentation has the most profound impact on survival, patient characteristics including demographics, comorbidities, and tumor antigens such as CA19-9 have also been noted to correlate with survival [19–21]. Recently, treatment factors including type of chemotherapy or chemoradiation, and surgical variables beyond the simple occurrence of resection have been demonstrated to correlate significantly with differences in survival.

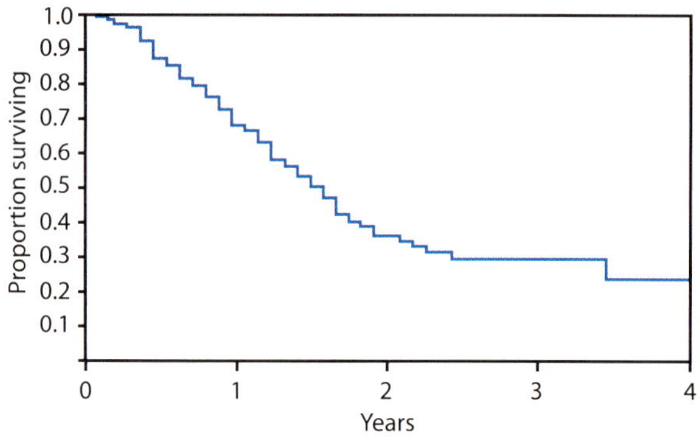

Figure 61.1

The actuarial Kaplan-Meier survival curve for all patients undergoing pancreaticoduodenectomy for pancreatic adenocarcinoma ($n = 174$) between October 1991 and September 1995 (inclusive) at the Johns Hopkins Hospital (with permission from [23])

Resectable Tumors

Survival after Pancreatic Resection

At the present time, surgical resection is the only potentially curative treatment for pancreatic cancer [22]. In a large single-institution series, patients undergoing pancreatic resection for cancer at a major center had an estimated 5-year survival in the range of 20%, with a median survival of 19 months (Fig. 61.1) [23]. Patients who chose not to undergo adjuvant therapy had a median survival of 13.5 months, which was significantly different from the 19.5-month median survival seen in patients who chose adjuvant therapy with two different 5-fluorouracil (FU)-based chemoradiation regimens [23]. The 5-year survival rates after resection of pancreatic adenocarcinoma were found to be predicted by tumor size, DNA content, and lymph node metastases at the time of resection, and a select group of 10-year survivors were found in patients with biologically favorable tumors, suggesting potential surgical cures of pancreatic cancer [24]. Another single-institution study recently demonstrated a median survival of 25 months in 291 patients who underwent pancreaticoduodenectomy for pancreatic adenocarcinoma between 1990 and 2002 [14].

Decreasing Mortality of Pancreatic Resection

Over the last few decades, pancreatic surgery has been performed with decreasing mortality, as reported in several large series. Pancreatic resections are complex and technically challenging operations with significant personal and institutional learning curves [25]. We and others have shown that the perioperative mortality rate for pancreaticoduodenectomy ranges from 1–20%, with a morbidity of 15–60% [14, 26–30]. Recent data from the National Inpatient Sample database demonstrates a significant decrease in nationwide perioperative mortality for pancreatectomy for neoplasm between 1998 and 2003 ranging from 7.7% in 1998 to 4.4% in 2003 [31].

Volume Effects on Survival

In the past two decades, an increasing body of literature has suggested that patients who undergo complex surgery at large-volume centers have superior outcomes. In 1999, Birkmeyer et al. used the Medicare claims database to demonstrate that patients who underwent pancreaticoduodenectomy at high-volume hospitals had improved 3-year survival [32]. In 2002, Kotwall et al. used the Nationwide Inpatient Sample database to show a 50% excess mortality after pancreaticoduodenectomy at low-volume centers [33]. Patients older than 60 years, men, and patients admitted urgently were at highest risk for in-hospital death at low-volume centers, and the authors proposed transfer to high-volume centers for these subgroups of patients. In 2003, Finlayson and Birkmeyer performed a decision analysis to estimate life expectancy for patients undergoing surgical resections for pancreas, lung, or colon cancer [34]. Estimated life expectancy after pancreatic resection varied with volume, with patients undergoing surgery at high-volume centers predicted to have nearly double the life expectancy of those at low volume centers. And more recently, Fong et al. have reported data from the national Medicare database that confirmed this projection. Patients undergoing pancreatectomy at high-volume centers, defined as >25 cases/year, demonstrated higher long-term overall survival compared to patients at low-volume centers (Fig. 61.2) [35].

Recently, investigators have focused on the individual surgeon's effects on surgical outcomes. In 2003, Birkmeyer demonstrated that individual surgeon volume was inversely related to operative mortality for all procedures studied, with the largest difference occurring for pancreatic surgery. Furthermore, using regression analyses, much of the protective effect of high hospital volume could be explained by high individual surgeon volume [36]. The authors suggested that patients could maximize survival by choosing a high-volume surgeon at a high-volume center for operations such as pancreatic resection.

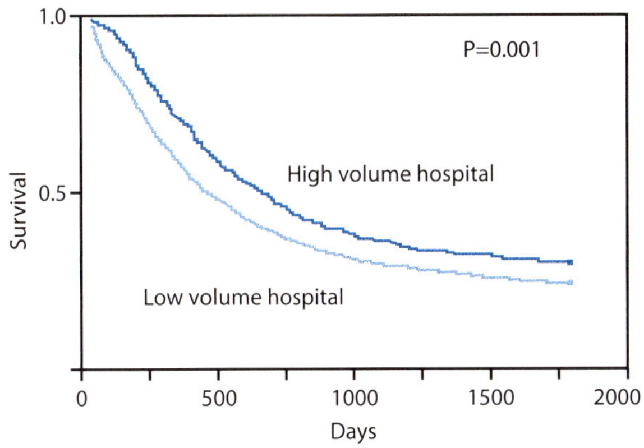

Figure 61.2

Overall survival of patients undergoing pancreatic resection for cancer (with permission from [35])

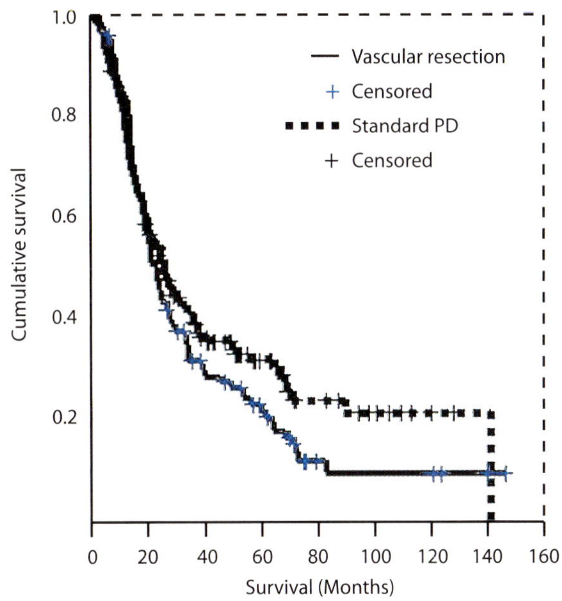

Figure 61.3

Kaplan-Meier survival curves in patients with pancreatic ductal adenocarcinoma who underwent standard pancreaticoduodenectomy (*PD; dashed line*) or pancreaticoduodenectomy with vascular resection and reconstruction (*solid line*). The median survival for standard pancreaticoduodenectomy was 26.5 months. The median survival for vascular resection pancreaticoduodenectomy was 23.43 months. Log-rank test: $P = 0.18$. Reprinted with permission from [14]

Extended Lymphadenectomy

Extended lymphadenectomy and portal vein (PV) resection at the time of pancreaticoduodenectomy was initially performed in an attempt to improve survival duration by performing an en bloc resection of the pancreas and surrounding structures [37]. In 1973, Fortner proposed "regional pancreatectomy," which involved the systematic resection of major peripancreatic vascular structures together with wide soft tissue clearance [38]. The rationale for extended lymphadenectomy has been based in part on autopsy studies demonstrating rates of nodal metastasis of up to 80% in patients with pancreatic cancer [39, 40]. However, radical or extended pancreaticoduodenectomy has not been demonstrated to confer a survival benefit [41]. The 2005 National Comprehensive Cancer Network guidelines state that extended node dissection, in the absence of evidence for improved survival, should not be considered a routine part of pancreatectomy, and should be reserved for patients in whom such a dissection is justified by patient-specific technical details (e.g., higher likelihood of obtaining a margin-negative resection in a reoperative field) or in the setting of a clinical trial [22].

Vascular Resection

PV resection at the time of pancreaticoduodenectomy was initially performed in an attempt to improve survival duration via extended pancreatectomy, as described above [37]. Many clinicians have been led to believe that that the negative experience with regional pancreatectomy also applies to patients with isolated tumor extension to involve a short segment or small portion of the superior mesenteric vein (SMV) or PV; in such patients the only thing preventing complete tumor resection is the area of venous involvement. Because of this, many physicians classify patients with suspected isolated tumor involvement of the SMV, PV, or their confluence as having locally advanced disease. Such patients have a median survival of 10–12 months in contemporary series [15].

A recent large series from the M.D. Anderson Cancer Center included 291 patients who underwent pancreaticoduodenectomy for pancreatic adenocarcinoma, of whom 110 underwent vascular resection and reconstruction [14]. The median overall survival by Kaplan-Meier for the 291 patients was 24.9 months. For the 110 patients that required vascular resection, the median survival was 23.4 months, compared to 26.5 months for the 181 patients who underwent standard pancreaticoduodenectomy, which was not statistically different (Fig. 61.3). Multivariate analysis of the effect of all potential prognostic factors on survival in patients who underwent pancreaticoduodenectomy for pancreatic ductal adenocarcinoma demonstrated that the presence of nodal metastasis and the occurrence of one or more major perioperative complication(s) were significant predictors of decreased survival. In contrast, vascular resection was not associated with decreased survival. These data led the authors to propose that vascular resection and reconstruction should be performed by experienced clinicians in patients with otherwise resectable tumors with isolated venous involvement.

Biliary Stenting

Preoperative biliary stenting before pancreaticoduodenectomy remains the subject of some controversy, as previous reports have described increased morbidity and mortality. However, recent reports have demonstrated no significant difference in morbidity between stented and nonstented patients [42], and that even metal stents can be used to decompress patients with biliary obstruction without affecting perioperative morbidity and mortality [43].

Biopsy

Another controversial area is that of the possible effect of biopsy on patient outcome. Needle tract implantation and tumor seeding has been well described after percutaneous biopsy and drainage procedures in patients with pancreatic and other adenocarcinomas [44–46]; we recommend avoiding percutaneous biopsies, especially in patients who have potentially resectable tumors. Endoscopic ultrasound (EUS)-guided biopsy through the gastrointestinal tract is thought to be safer, as tumor cells should not traverse the peritoneal cavity with this technique. However, the first report of tumor seeding from EUS-guided fine needle aspiration of a pancreatic adenocarcinoma was recently reported [47].

Cytology

Some patients with apparently resectable disease on radiographic imaging will have evidence of metastatic disease on laparoscopy, including patients found to have peritoneal cytology positive for malignant cells with no gross evidence of metastasis [48, 49]. Patients with positive peritoneal cytology share the same poor prognosis as patients with macroscopic metastatic disease [50–52]. This percentage of patients with occult macroscopic or microscopic metastases, reported at 31% in 2000 [49], may be decreasing with more precise imaging techniques.

Adjuvant Treatment

Patients who undergo pancreatic resection are generally offered adjuvant or neoadjuvant treatment with chemotherapy or chemoradiation. In 1985, the Gastrointestinal Tumor Study Group (GITSG) reported that the median survival of patients undergoing pancreaticoduodenectomy could be nearly doubled using chemoradiation consisting of 4,000 cGy with intermittent bolus 5-FU [53]. This regimen produced a 2-year actuarial survival of 43% in the experimental arm, as opposed to 18% in the control arm. Since that time, single-institution studies have shown adjuvant treatment to provide a survival advantage [23]. The European Organization for Research and Treatment of Cancer (EORTC) conducted a randomized trial that showed a trend toward improved survival in the chemoradiation arm [54]. The Radiation Therapy Oncology Group (RTOG) conducted a phase III study comparing chemoradiation with either gemcitabine or infusional fluorouracil; its results are anticipated shortly. The European Study Group for Pancreatic Cancer (ESPAC-1) suggested that 5-FU produced superior results to observation and, controversially, that chemoradiation may have a deleterious effect [55]. The ESPAC-1 study was felt by some observers to lack quality control for radiation therapy [56]. ESPAC-3, a prospective randomized study of 5-FU versus gemcitabine in the adjuvant setting, should further define the results of chemotherapy in the absence of chemoradiation.

A novel approach to adjuvant chemoradiation based on interferon-α (IFNα) pioneered at the Virginia Mason Medical Center has demonstrated remarkable results [57, 58]. The initial report in 2000 stated that 2-year overall survival was superior in the IFNα cohort (84%) versus the cohort that received standard chemoradiation using the GITSG regimen (54%) [58]. With a mean follow-up of 26 months in both cohorts, actuarial survival curves significantly favored the IFNα group ($P = 0.04$). The authors concluded that their interferon/cisplatin/5-FU-based adjuvant chemoradiation protocol might be a promising adjuvant treatment for patients who have undergone pancreaticoduodenectomy for adenocarcinoma of the pancreatic head. A follow-up report in 2003 demonstrated a relatively high rate of hospitalization for toxicity, but confirmed the encouraging survival results of the preliminary paper [57]. With a mean follow-up time of 31.9 months, 67% of the patients were alive and the median survivorship had not been reached. Actuarial overall survival for the 1-, 2-, and 5-year periods was 95%, 64%, and 55%, respectively. IFNα-based adjuvant therapy is currently the subject of confirmatory single-institutional trials such as one ongoing at the M.D. Anderson Cancer Center, as well as a recent American College of Surgeons Oncology Group (ACOSOG) multicenter trial.

Intraoperative Radiation Therapy

Intraoperative Radiation Therapy (IORT) has been promoted in the hopes of improving the high (up to 60%) local recurrence rate in resected pancreatic adenocarcinoma [10]. Thus far, investigators have generally not been able to demonstrate additional benefit of IORT on survival in patients undergoing resection for pancreatic adenocarcinoma [59, 60].

Neoadjuvant Therapy

Neoadjuvant therapy has several theoretical advantages [61, 62]. First, since the majority of apparently localized pancreatic adenocarcinoma patients will have metastasis present in lymph nodes at resection or autopsy [39, 40], it can be argued that above all, these patients require systemic therapy. After initial surgery, a substantial proportion of patients may not recover their performance status sufficiently to receive chemotherapy in a timely fashion. Second, neoadjuvant therapy allows patients with occult metastatic disease or heretofore unrecognized poor performance status to be identified; such patients will do poorly at operation. Third, at present, neoadjuvant therapy may offer theoretical advantages in achieving a margin-negative resection, or even more provocatively, may abrogate the effect of a microscopically positive margin at final pathology [14].

In a nonrandomized study at the M.D. Anderson Cancer Center, 142 patients who underwent pancreaticoduodenectomy for pancreatic adenocarcinoma underwent either neoadjuvant or adjuvant chemoradiation [62]. Preoperative and postoperative chemoradiation resulted in similar treatment toxicity, patterns of tumor recurrence, and survival. The authors found that rapid-fractionation preoperative chemoradiation allowed the delivery of all components of therapy to patients with a shorter treatment timecourse than with standard-fractionation chemoradiation given either before or after pancreaticoduodenectomy. Based on their results, the authors also proposed that prolonged recovery after pancreaticoduodenectomy might prevent the delivery of postoperative adjuvant chemoradiation in up to one-fourth of eligible patients, although more recent reports have suggested that this number is on the decline (unpublished observation, PWT Pisters). Some authors have suggested that chemoradiation may improve resectability in locally advanced or borderline resectable tumors in selected cases [63, 64]. At this time, no randomized trials have been performed comparing adjuvant versus neoadjuvant therapy; thus, no direct comparison of preoperative and postoperative treatment can be made.

Locally Advanced Tumors

Patients with locally advanced, nonmetastatic pancreatic adenocarcinoma are generally managed by chemoradiation. Using contemporary protocols, such patients have a median survival of 10–12 months [15]. The GITSG study initially demonstrated a near doubling of median survival (42.2 vs. 22.9 weeks) when a regimen of bolus 5-FU and 4,000 cGy was compared with radiation alone [65]. Current protocols generally include radiation doses of 50–60 Gy with concomitant 5-FU. Although other radiosensitizing agents have been studied, none have been shown to be superior to GITSG in randomized trials. After completion of radiation therapy, additional gemcitabine-based chemotherapy can be administered to patients with acceptable performance status. Single-agent gemcitabine without radiation is being studied for primary definitive treatment in locally unresectable pancreatic adenocarcinoma by the Eastern Cooperative Oncology Group (ECOG-4201). Intriguingly, a recent phase II study reported at the 2004 American Society of Clinical Oncology meeting found that a patients with locally advanced, unresectable pancreatic cancer treated with gemcitabine and docetaxel had a 69% actuarial 3-year survival, and that 79% of patients were rendered resectable after chemotherapy [66]. Furthermore, a treatment strategy employing intraoperative electron beam radiotherapy has been reported to help achieve long-term survival of at least 3 years in 8 out of 150 patients with unresectable pancreatic cancer. The survival benefit was noted only patients with small tumors [67].

Metastatic Disease

Advanced pancreatic adenocarcinoma cannot be cured with current therapy. The goals of treatment of metastatic pancreatic cancer are twofold: (1) palliation (i.e., to increase quality of life), and (2) survival (i.e., to increase quantity of life). The first goal of palliation is usually foremost due to the limited efficacy of current regimens in patients with large volumes of disease, and the poor performance status of many such patients. The survival benefits of systemic chemotherapy are usually limited to patients with reasonable performance status (EGOG classes 0–2) [22].

For patients with metastatic (as well as locally advanced) pancreatic adenocarcinoma, gemcitabine has been demonstrated to produce clinical responses and has a moderate survival advantage compared to bolus 5-FU [68]. Thus gemcitabine single-drug therapy is standard first-line therapy in patients with metastatic pancreatic adenocarcinoma [22]. The specifics of gemcitabine administration, including fixed-dose rate administration and combinations with other potentially synergistic agents, are currently under investigation, particularly in patients with good performance status (ECOG 0 or 1).

New targeted drugs administered in conjunction with gemcitabine have shown exciting results in early phase clinical trials. The combination of gemcitabine and bevacizumab (antivascular endothelial growth factor antibody, trade name Avastin) is currently being studied in a phase III trial by the Cancer and Leukemia Group B (CALGB). Cetuximab (anti-epidermal-growth-factor receptor, trade name Erbitux) and gemcitabine are being compared with gemcitabine monotherapy in a phase III trial administered by the Southwestern Oncology Group (SWOG). An ongoing phase III trial of erlotinib (epidermal growth factor tyrosine kinase inhibitor, trade name Tarceva) and gemcitabine in patients with locally advanced or metastatic pancreatic cancer has shown a median survival of 6.4 months (1-year survival 25.6%) in the experimental arm, compared with 5.9 months (1-year survival 19.7%) in the control gemictabine-alone arm. Other targeted compounds being used with gemcitabine include ISIS-2503, an antisense compound against H-ras [69].

Other drugs used in combination for first-line therapy with or without gemcitabine include docetaxel, irinotecan, capecitabine, and oxaliplatin. Second-line therapy for metastatic pancreatic adenocarcinoma, depending on the patient's first-line treatment, may include gemcitabine-based therapy, investigational drugs, and capecitabine or infusional 5-FU in patients previously treated with gemcitabine. Due to the grim natural history of pancreatic cancer, all patients with pancreatic adenocarcinoma should be considered for inclusion in appropriate clinical trials, with the goal of eventually extending survival in patients at all stages of disease.

Other Factors Influencing Survival

The previous discussion has centered on the clinical categories of resectable (clinical T1-3 M0, AJCC 6th Edition), locally advanced (clinical T4 M0), and metastatic (M1) tumors [70]. Partial or total pancreatectomy allows the patient to be staged pathologically, with pathologic determination of T, N, and M stages. Regional lymph node involvement, poorly differentiated histology, and larger size of primary tumor have been found to be associated with decreased survival [71]. The factor most associated with decreased survival is incomplete, or R2 resection; such a grossly positive margin provides no survival advantage from resection compared to patients who receive chemoradiation alone [70]. DNA content and the presence of perivascular and perineural invasion are also known clinicopathologic prognostic parameters [24]. Recently, a postoperative decrease in CA19-9 level and a postoperative CA19-9 level of <200 U/ml were both found to independently predict increased survival after pancreatectomy [21].

Molecular genetic studies in pancreatic cancer have yielded information regarding specific oncogenes and tumor suppressors. K-ras mutations occur in >90% of pancreatic adenocarcinomas [72], and sequential accumulation of K-ras mutations and p53 overexpression have been found in the progression of pancreatic mucinous cystic neoplasms to malignancy, which may mimic the path toward ductal adenocarcinoma [73]. Studies using immunohistochemical analysis of p53 and Bcl-2 significantly predicted survival duration; patients whose tumors stained positively for p53 and/or overexpressed Bcl-2 had a significantly longer survival than those whose tumors stained negative for both proteins [74]. Mutations have also been described in APC, MCC, DCC, c-erb B-2, RB-1, and mismatch repair genes, with unclear effects on survival [75]. In 2000, an analysis of potentially useful molecular markers in a large patient population was published, demonstrating that K-ras oncogene subtype mutations were associated with survival but not expression of p53, p16(INK4A), p21(WAF-1), cyclin D1, erbB-2, and erbB-3 in resected pancreatic ductal adenocarcinoma [76]. Telomerase activity has been found to correlate with aggressiveness in pancreatic adenocarcinoma [77]. Recently, cDNA microarrays and DNA methylation studies have been used to identify genes that are differentially expressed in pancreatic cancer, producing a large number of potentially new molecular markers for the possible detection and treatment of pancreatic cancer [78, 79]. Finally, proteonomic technology is being used to identify differentially expressed proteins in malignancies such as pancreatic adenocarcinoma [80].

This chapter has focused on ductal pancreatic adenocarcinoma. In the variant of mucin-producing pancreatic tumors, an analysis of nuclear DNA content suggested that DNA diploid patterns are associated with a favorable prognosis, whereas aneuploidy is associated with invasion of the surrounding organs [81]. Other carcinomas of the pancreas have very different survival curves; invasive intraductal papillary neoplasms have been found to have a 5-year survival of 43% [82].

In the near future, the background in which pancreatic adenocarcinoma arises may be of increasing importance in the diagnosis, treatment, and eventual survival of patients with these tumors. Conditions such as familial pancreatic cancer, the newly described pancreatic epithelial neoplasias (PanINs) and conditions such as chronic pancreatitis may imply a "field defect" in which multifocal or aggressive early tumors can arise [83].

It is hoped that with the advent of targeted therapies and strategies for earlier diagnosis of pancreatic adenocarcinoma, the gloomy outlook for survival in pancreatic cancer patients can be improved in the future.

References

1. Jemal A, Murray T, Ward E, Samuels A, Tiwari RC, Ghafoor A, Feuer EJ, Thun MJ (2005) Cancer Statistics, 2005. CA Cancer J Clin 55:10–30
2. Society AC (2005) Facts and Figures. American Cancer Society, Atlanta, GA
3. Warshaw AL, Fernandez-del Castillo C (1992) Pancreatic carcinoma. N Engl J Med 326:455–465
4. Kalser MH, Barkin J, MacIntyre JM (1985) Pancreatic cancer. Assessment of prognosis by clinical presentation. Cancer 56:397–402
5. Nordback IH, Hruban RH, Boitnott JK, Pitt HA, Cameron JL (1992) Carcinoma of the body and tail of the pancreas. Am J Surg 164:26–31
6. Johnson CD, Schwall G, Flechtenmacher J, Trede M (1993) Resection for adenocarcinoma of the body and tail of the pancreas. Br J Surg 80:1177–1179
7. Dalton RR, Sarr MG, van Heerden JA, Colby TV (1992) Carcinoma of the body and tail of the pancreas: is curative resection justified? Surgery 111:489–494
8. Christein JD, Kendrick ML, Iqbal CW, Nagorney DM, Farnell MB (2005) Distal pancreatectomy for resectable adenocarcinoma of the body and tail of the pancreas. J Gastrointest Surg 9:922–927
9. Shoup M, Conlon KC, Klimstra D, Brennan MF (2003) Is extended resection for adenocarcinoma of the body or tail of the pancreas justified? J Gastrointest Surg 7:946–952
10. Willett CG, Lewandrowski K, Warshaw AL, Efird J, Compton CC (1993) Resection margins in carcinoma of the head of the pancreas. Implications for radiation therapy. Ann Surg 217:144–148
11. Clark JW, Glicksman AS, Wanebo HJ (1996) Systemic and adjuvant therapy for patients with pancreatic carcinoma. Cancer 78 (Suppl 3):688–693
12. Yeo CJ, Cameron JL, Lillemoe KD, Sitzmann JV, Hruban RH, Goodman SN, Dooley WC, Coleman J, Pitt HA (1995) Pancreaticoduodenectomy for cancer of the head of the pancreas. 201 patients. Ann Surg 221:721–731
13. Yeo CJ, Sohn TA, Cameron JL, Hruban RH, Lillemoe KD, Pitt HA (1998) Periampullary adenocarcinoma: analysis of 5-year survivors. Ann Surg 227:821–831
14. Tseng JF, Raut CP, Lee JE, Pisters PW, Vauthey JN, Abdalla EK, Gomez HF, Sun CC, Crane CH, Wolff RA, Evans DB (2004) Pancreaticoduodenectomy with vascular resection: margin status and survival duration. J Gastrointest Surg 8:935–949
15. Wolff RA, Abruzzesse JL, Evans DB (2003) Neoplasms of the exocrine pancreas. In: Kufe DW, Pollock RE, Weichselbaum RR, et al (eds) Holland-Frei Cancer Medicine, vol 2, 6th edn. BC Decker, Ontario, Canada, pp 1585–1614
16. Crane C, Janjan N, Evans D, Wolff R, Ballo M, Milas L, Mason K, Charnsangavej C, Pisters P, Lee J, Lenzi R, Vauthey J, Wong A, Phan T, Nguyen Q, Abbruzzese J (2001) Toxicity and efficacy of concurrent gemcitabine and radiotherapy for locally advanced pancreatic cancer. Int J Gastrointest Cancer 29:9–18
17. Sporn JR, Buzaid AC, Slater D, Cohen N, Greenberg BR (1997) Treatment of advanced pancreatic adenocarcinoma with 5-FU, leucovorin, interferon-alpha-2b, and cisplatin. Am J Clin Oncol 20:81–83
18. Alexakis N, Halloran C, Raraty M, Ghaneh P, Sutton R, Neoptolemos JP (2004) Current standards of surgery for pancreatic cancer. Br J Surg 91:1410–1427
19. Glenn J, Steinberg WM, Kurtzman SH, Steinberg SM, Sindelar WF (1988) Evaluation of the utility of a radioimmunoassay for serum CA19-9 levels in patients before and after treatment of carcinoma of the pancreas. J Clin Oncol 6:462–468
20. Halm U, Schumann T, Schiefke I, Witzigmann H, Mossner J, Keim V (2000) Decrease of CA 19-9 during chemotherapy with gemcitabine predicts survival time in patients with advanced pancreatic cancer. Br J Cancer 82:1013–1016
21. Ferrone CR, Finkelstine DM, Thayer SP, Muzinkansky A, Fernandez-del Castillo C, Warshaw AL (2006) Peri-operative CA19-9 levels can predict stage and survival in patients with resectable pancreatic adenocarcinoma. J Clin Oncol 24(18):2897–902
22. Tempero MA, Behrman S, Ben-Josef E, Benson AB III, Cameron JL, Casper ES, Hoffman JP, Karl RC, Kim P, Koh WJ, Kuvshinoff BW II, Melvin WS, Muscarella P III, Sasson AR, Shibata S, Shrieve DC, Talamonti MS, Tyler DS, Vickers SM, Warren RS, Willett C, Wolff RA (2005) Pancreatic adenocarcinoma: clinical practice guidelines in oncology. J Natl Compr Canc Netw 3:598–626
23. Yeo CJ, Abrams RA, Grochow LB, Sohn TA, Ord SE, Hruban RH, Zahurak ML, Dooley WC, Coleman J, Sauter PK, Pitt HA, Lillemoe KD, Cameron JL (1997) Pancreaticoduodenectomy for pancreatic adenocarcinoma: postoperative adjuvant chemoradiation improves survival. A prospective, single-institution experience. Ann Surg 225:621–633

24. Allison DC, Piantadosi S, Hruban RH, Dooley WC, Fishman EK, Yeo CJ, Lillemoe KD, Pitt HA, Lin P, Cameron JL (1998) DNA content and other factors associated with ten-year survival after resection of pancreatic carcinoma. J Surg Oncol 67:151–159
25. Tseng JF, Lee JE, Pisters PWT, Gomez HF, Sun CC, Evans DB (2007) The learning curve in pancreatic surgery. Surgery141(5):694–701
26. Balcom JH, Rattner DW, Warshaw AL, Chang Y, Fernandez-del Castillo C (2001) Ten-year experience with 733 pancreatic resections: changing indications, older patients, and decreasing length of hospitalization. Arch Surg 136:391–398
27. Yeo CJ, Cameron JL, Sohn TA, Lillemoe KD, Pitt HA, Talamini MA, Hruban RH, Ord SE, Sauter PK, Coleman J, Zahurak ML, Grochow LB, Abrams RA (1997) Six hundred fifty consecutive pancreaticoduodenectomies in the 1990s: pathology, complications, and outcomes. Ann Surg 226:248–257
28. Finlayson EV, Goodney PP, Birkmeyer JD (2003) Hospital volume and operative mortality in cancer surgery: a national study. Arch Surg 138:721–725
29. Gouma DJ, van Geenen RC, van Gulik TM, de Haan RJ, de Wit LT, Busch OR, Obertop H (2000) Rates of complications and death after pancreaticoduodenectomy: risk factors and the impact of hospital volume. Ann Surg 232:786–795
30. Lieberman MD, Kilburn H, Lindsey M, Brennan MF (1995) Relation of perioperative deaths to hospital volume among patients undergoing pancreatic resection for malignancy. Ann Surg 222:638–645
31. McPhee JT, Zayruzny M, Whalen GF, Litwin DE, Sullivan ME, Anderson FA, Tseng JF (2007) Perioperative mortality for pancreatectomy: a national perspective. Ann Surg 246(2):246–253
32. Birkmeyer JD, Finlayson SR, Tosteson AN, Sharp SM, Warshaw AL, Fisher ES (1999) Effect of hospital volume on in-hospital mortality with pancreaticoduodenectomy. Surgery 125:250–256
33. Kotwall CA, Maxwell JG, Brinker CC, Koch GG, Covington DL (2002) National estimates of mortality rates for radical pancreaticoduodenectomy in 25,000 patients. Ann Surg Oncol 9:847–854
34. Finlayson EV, Birkmeyer JD (2003) Effects of hospital volume on life expectancy after selected cancer operations in older adults: a decision analysis. J Am Coll Surg 196:410–417
35. Fong Y, Gonen M, Rubin D, Radzyner M, Brennan MF (2005) Long-term survival is superior after resection for cancer in high-volume centers. Ann Surg 242:540–544
36. Birkmeyer JD, Stukel TA, Siewers AE, Goodney PP, Wennberg DE, Lucas FL (2003) Surgeon volume and operative mortality in the United States. N Engl J Med 349):2117–2127
37. Asada S, Itaya H, Nakamura K, Isohashi T, Masuoka S (1963) Radical pancreatectomy and portal vein resection. Arch Surg 87:609–613
38. Fortner JG (1973) Regional resection of cancer of the pancreas: a new surgical approach. Surgery 73:307–320
39. Cubilla AL, Fortner J, Fitzgerald PJ (1978) Lymph node involvement in carcinoma of the head of the pancreas area. Cancer 41:880–887
40. Nagai H, Kuroda A, Morioka Y (1986) Lymphatic and local spread of T1 and T2 pancreatic cancer. A study of autopsy material. Ann Surg 204:65–71
41. Yeo CJ, Cameron JL, Lillemoe KD, Sohn TA, Campbell KA, Sauter PK, Coleman J, Abrams RA, Hruban RH (2002) Pancreaticoduodenectomy with or without distal gastrectomy and extended retroperitoneal lymphadenectomy for periampullary adenocarcinoma, part 2: randomized controlled trial evaluating survival, morbidity, and mortality. Ann Surg 236:355–368
42. Jagannath P, Dhir V, Shrikhande S, Shah RC, Mullerpatan P, Mohandas KM (2005) Effect of preoperative biliary stenting on immediate outcome after pancreaticoduodenectomy. Br J Surg 92:356–361
43. Mullen JT, Lee JH, Gomez HF, Ross WA, Fukami N, Wolff RA, Abdalla EK, Vauthey JN, Lee JE, Pisters PW, Evans DB (2005) Pancreaticoduodenectomy after placement of endobiliary metal stents. J Gastrointest Surg 9:1094–1105
44. Cutherell L, Wanebo HJ, Tegtmeyer CJ (1986) Catheter tract seeding after percutaneous biliary drainage for pancreatic cancer. Cancer 57:2057–2060
45. Bergenfeldt M, Genell S, Lindholm K, Ekberg O, Aspelin P (1988) Needle-tract seeding after percutaneous fine-needle biopsy of pancreatic adenocarcinoma. Acta Chir Scand 154:77–79
46. Kosugi C, Furuse J, Ishii H, Maru Y, Yoshino M, Kinoshita T, Konishi M, Nakagohri T, Inoue K, Oda T (2004) Needle tract implantation of hepatocellular carcinoma and pancreatic carcinoma after ultrasound-guided percutaneous puncture. World J Surg 28:29–32
47. Paquin SC, Gariepy G, Lepanto L, Bourdages R, Raymond G, Sahai AV (2005) A first report of tumor seeding because of EUS-guided FNA of a pancreatic adenocarcinoma. Gastointest Endosc 61:610–611
48. Fernandez-del Castillo C, Rattner DW, Warshaw AL (1995) Further experience with laparoscopy and peritoneal cytology in the staging of pancreatic cancer. Br J Surg 82:1127–1129
49. Jimenez RE, Warshaw AL, Rattner DW, Willett CG, McGrath D, Fernandez-del Castillo C (2000) Impact of laparoscopic staging in the treatment of pancreatic cancer. Arch Surg 135:409–414
50. Leach SD, Rose JA, Lowy AM, Lee JE, Charnsangavej C, Abbruzzese JL, Katz RL, Evans DB (1995) Significance of peritoneal cytology in patients with potentially resectable adenocarcinoma of the pancreatic head. Surgery 118:472–478
51. Warshaw AL (1991) Implications of peritoneal cytology for staging of early pancreatic cancer. Am J Surg 161:26–29; discussion 29–30
52. Fernandez-del Castillo CL, Warshaw AL (1998) Pancreatic cancer. Laparoscopic staging and peritoneal cytology. Surg Oncol Clin N Am 7:135–142
53. Kalser MH, Ellenberg SS (1985) Pancreatic cancer. Adjuvant combined radiation and chemotherapy following curative resection. Arch Surg 120:899–903
54. Klinkenbijl JH, Jeekel J, Sahmoud T, van Pel R, Couvreur ML, Veenhof CH, Arnaud JP, Gonzalez DG, de Wit LT, Hennipman A, Wils J (1999) Adjuvant radiotherapy and 5-fluorouracil after curative resection of cancer of the pancreas and periampullary region: phase III trial of the EORTC gastrointestinal tract cancer cooperative group. Ann Surg 230:776–782
55. Neoptolemos JP, Dunn JA, Stocken DD, Almond J, Link K, Beger H, Bassi C, Falconi M, Pederzoli P, Dervenis C, Fernandez-Cruz L, Lacaine F, Pap A, Spooner D, Kerr DJ, Friess H, Buchler MW (2001) Adjuvant chemoradiotherapy and chemotherapy in resectable pancreatic cancer: a randomised controlled trial. Lancet 358:1576–1585

56. Choti MA (2004) Adjuvant therapy for pancreatic cancer – the debate continues. N Engl J Med 350:1249–1251
57. Picozzi VJ, Kozarek RA, Traverso LW (2003) Interferon-based adjuvant chemoradiation therapy after pancreaticoduodenectomy for pancreatic adenocarcinoma. Am J Surg 185:476–480
58. Nukui Y, Picozzi VJ, Traverso LW (2000) Interferon-based adjuvant chemoradiation therapy improves survival after pancreaticoduodenectomy for pancreatic adenocarcinoma. Am J Surg 179:367–371
59. Okamoto A, Matsumoto G, Tsuruta K, Baba H, Karasawa K, Kamisawa T, Egawa N (2004) Intraoperative radiation therapy for pancreatic adenocarcinoma: the Komagome hospital experience. Pancreas 28:296–300
60. Schwarz RE, Smith DD, Keny H, Ikle DN, Shibata SI, Chu DZ, Pezner RD (2003) Impact of intraoperative radiation on postoperative and disease-specific outcome after pancreatoduodenectomy for adenocarcinoma: a propensity score analysis. Am J Clin Oncol 26:16–21
61. Evans DB, Rich TA, Byrd DR, Cleary KR, Connelly JH, Levin B, Charnsangavej C, Fenoglio CJ, Ames FC (1992) Preoperative chemoradiation and pancreaticoduodenectomy for adenocarcinoma of the pancreas. Arch Surg 127:1335–1339
62. Spitz FR, Abbruzzese JL, Lee JE, Pisters PW, Lowy AM, Fenoglio CJ, Cleary KR, Janjan NA, Goswitz MS, Rich TA, Evans DB (1997) Preoperative and postoperative chemoradiation strategies in patients treated with pancreaticoduodenectomy for adenocarcinoma of the pancreas. J Clin Oncol 15:928–937
63. Hoffman JP, Lipsitz S, Pisansky T, Weese JL, Solin L, Benson AB III (1998) Phase II trial of preoperative radiation therapy and chemotherapy for patients with localized, resectable adenocarcinoma of the pancreas: an Eastern Cooperative Oncology Group Study. J Clin Oncol 16:317–323
64. Hoffman JP, Weese JL, Solin LJ, Engstrom P, Agarwal P, Barber LW, Guttmann MC, Litwin S, Salazar H, Eisenberg BL (1995) A pilot study of preoperative chemoradiation for patients with localized adenocarcinoma of the pancreas. Am J Surg 169:71–77
65. Moertel CG, Frytak S, Hahn RG, O'Connell MJ, Reitemeier RJ, Rubin J, Schutt AJ, Weiland LH, Childs DS, Holbrook MA, Lavin PT, Livstone E, Spiro H, Knowlton A, Kalser M, Barkin J, Lessner H, Mann-Kaplan R, Ramming K, Douglas HO Jr, Thomas P, Nave H, Bateman J, Lokich J, Brooks J, Chaffey J, Corson JM, Zamcheck N, Novak JW (1981) Therapy of locally unresectable pancreatic carcinoma: a randomized comparison of high dose (6000 rads) radiation alone, moderate dose radiation (4000 rads + 5-fluorouracil), and high dose radiation + 5-fluorouracil: The Gastrointestinal Tumor Study Group. Cancer 48:1705–1710
66. Gnant M, Kuehrer I, Telky B, Goetzinger P, Penz M, Sedivy R, Scheithauer W, Sautner T, Zielinksi C, Jakesz R (2004) Effect of neoadjuvant chemotherapy and docetaxel and 3-year survival and resection rate in previously unresectable locally advanced pancreatic cancer. J Clin Oncol 22(Suppl 14S):4234
67. Willett CG, Del Castillo CF, Shih HA, Goldberg S, Biggs P, Clark JW, Lauwers G, Ryan DP, Zhu AX, Warshaw AL (2005) Long-term results of intraoperative electron beam irradiation (IOERT) for patients with unresectable pancreatic cancer. Ann Surg 241:295–299
68. Burris HA III, Moore MJ, Andersen J, Green MR, Rothenberg ML, Modiano MR, Cripps MC, Portenoy RK, Storniolo AM, Tarassoff P, Nelson R, Dorr FA, Stephens CD, Von Hoff DD (1997) Improvements in survival and clinical benefit with gemcitabine as first-line therapy for patients with advanced pancreas cancer: a randomized trial. J Clin Oncol 15:2403–2413
69. Alberts SR, Schroeder M, Erlichman C, Steen PD, Foster NR, Moore DF Jr, Rowland KM Jr, Nair S, Tschetter LK, Fitch TR (2004) Gemcitabine and ISIS-2503 for patients with locally advanced or metastatic pancreatic adenocarcinoma: a North Central Cancer Treatment Group phase II trial. J Clin Oncol 22:4944–4950
70. American Joint Committee on Cancer (2002) AJCC Staging Manual, 6th edn. Springer, New York
71. Geer RJ, Brennan MF (1993) Prognostic indicators for survival after resection of pancreatic adenocarcinoma. Am J Surg 165:68–72
72. Almoguera C, Shibata D, Forrester K, Martin J, Arnheim N, Perucho M (1988) Most human carcinomas of the exocrine pancreas contain mutant c-K-ras genes. Cell 53:549–554
73. Jimenez RE, Warshaw AL, Z'Graggen K, Hartwig W, Taylor DZ, Compton CC, Fernandez-del Castillo C (1999) Sequential accumulation of K-ras mutations and p53 overexpression in the progression of pancreatic mucinous cystic neoplasms to malignancy. Ann Surg 230:501–511
74. Bold RJ, Hess KR, Pearson AS, Grau AM, Sinicrope FA, Jennings M, McConkey DJ, Bucana CD, Cleary KR, Hallin PA, Chiao PJ, Abbruzzese JL, Evans DB (1999) Prognostic factors in resectable pancreatic cancer: p53 and bcl-2. J Gastrointest Surg 3:263–277
75. Howe JR, Conlon KC (1997) The molecular genetics of pancreatic cancer. Surg Oncol 6:1–18
76. Kawesha A, Ghaneh P, Andren-Sandberg A, Ograed D, Skar R, Dawiskiba S, Evans JD, Campbell F, Lemoine N, Neoptolemos JP (2000) K-ras oncogene subtype mutations are associated with survival but not expression of p53, p16(INK4A), p21(WAF-1), cyclin D1, erbB-2 and erbB-3 in resected pancreatic ductal adenocarcinoma. Int J Cancer 89:469–474
77. Balcom JH, Keck T, Warshaw AL, Antoniu B, Graeme-Cook F, Fernandez-del Castillo C (2001) Telomerase activity in periampullary tumors correlates with aggressive malignancy. Ann Surg 234:344–351
78. Iacobuzio-Donahue CA, Maitra A, Olsen M, Lowe AW, van Heek NT, Rosty C, Walter K, Sato N, Parker A, Ashfaq R, Jaffee E, Ryu B, Jones J, Eshleman JR, Yeo CJ, Cameron JL, Kern SE, Hruban RH, Brown PO, Goggins M (2003) Exploration of global gene expression patterns in pancreatic adenocarcinoma using cDNA microarrays. Am J Pathol 162:1151–1162
79. Goggins M (2005) Molecular markers of early pancreatic cancer. J Clin Oncol 23:4524–4531
80. Chen R, Yi EC, Donohoe S, Pan S, Eng J, Cooke K, Crispin DA, Lane Z, Goodlett DR, Bronner MP, Aebersold R, Brentnall TA (2005) Pancreatic cancer proteome: the proteins that underlie invasion, metastasis, and immunologic escape. Gastroenterology 129:1187–1197
81. Murakami Y, Yokoyama T, Kodama T, Takesue Y, Okita M, Nakamitsu A, Inamura Y, Santo T, Tsumura H, Miyamoto K, et al (1993) Mucin-producing pancreatic tumors: a study of nuclear DNA content by flow cytometry. Surg Today 23:491–495

82. Sohn TA, Yeo CJ, Cameron JL, Hruban RH, Fukushima N, Campbell KA, Lillemoe KD (2004) Intraductal papillary mucinous neoplasms of the pancreas: an updated experience. Ann Surg 239:788–799
83. Brentnall TA (2005) Management strategies for patients with hereditary pancreatic cancer. Curr Treat Options Oncol 6:437–445

Section 7

Endocrine Tumors of the Pancreas

Chapter 62 Pancreatic Endocrine Tumors: Epidemiology, Pathology, Pathophysiology, and Diagnosis *707*
C. Shibata, Y. Funayama, I. Sasaki

Chapter 63 Surgical Treatment of Insulinomas *715*
M. Sunamura, S. Fukuyama

Chapter 64 Surgical Treatment of the Gastrinoma *723*
M. Imamura, I. Komoto

Chapter 65 Surgical Treatment of Rare Endocrine Tumors *735*
S. Egawa, M. Sunamura, S. Matsuno, M. Unno

Chapter 66 Outcome after Surgical Treatment of Endocrine Pancreatic Tumors *749*
S. Fukuyama, S. Matsuno, S. Egawa, M. Sunamura

Chapter 62

C. Shibata · Y. Funayama · I. Sasaki

Pancreatic Endocrine Tumors: Epidemiology, Pathology, Pathophysiology, and Diagnosis

Pancreatic endocrine tumors (PETs) occupy only 2–3% of pancreatic neoplasms and can be divided into two classes depending on whether or not the tumor secretes peptides (functioning or nonfunctioning). Patients with a functioning tumor, in particular, require specific examinations including hormonal tests. Nonfunctioning tumors comprise 30–40% of PETs [1, 2] and are believed to be the most common class of PETs. In this chapter, we overview the history, epidemiology and pathology, clinical manifestations, diagnosis, and treatment of functioning [insulinoma, gastrinoma, glucagonoma, vasoactive intestinal peptide (VIP)-oma, and somatostatinoma) and nonfunctioning PETs.

History, Epidemiology, Pathology

Functioning PETs

Insulinoma

Although approximately three-quarters of functioning PETs are insulinomas, its frequency is as low as 1/million (Table 62.1). Approximately 90% of insulinomas are benign, solitary, and located within the pancreas; multiple, malignant, or extrapancreatic insulinomas are rare [3]. Table 62.2 summarizes the results of an insulinoma series treated at our university. The distribution of insulinomas is equal throughout the pancreas, being less than 2 cm in more than 70% of patients. Multiple insulinomas are often found in complication with multiple endocrine neoplasm (MEN) type I.

Gastrinoma

Gastrinoma is the second most common class of PETs. The clinical characteristics of gastrinomas are high malignancy rate (more than 50%) and high multiplicity (approximately 75%). Ninety percent of gastrinomas are found in a so called "gastrinoma triangle" [4], surrounded by the junction between the pancreatic head and body, the junction between the second and third portions of the duodenum, and the junction between the cystic duct and choledochus. Although it is reported that 60% of gastrinomas are in the pancreas and 30% are located in the duodenum [5], some say that pancreatic gastrinomas are less common and more aggressive than duodenal ones [6]. Gastrinoma are also often found in complication with MEN type-I.

Glucagonoma

Most glucagonomas are solitary and located in the pancreas, especially in the pancreatic body and tail [7]. Approximately 80% of glucagonomas are larger than 3 cm and malignant [8]. More than 50% patients with glucagonomas represent hepatic metastases when the diagnosis is made [9].

VIPoma

VIPomas arise in the pancreas in about 80–90% of cases, especially in the pancreatic tail [10]. VIPomas are usually solitary and larger than 3 cm in diameter, and 40–80% of VIPomas are malignant [11].

Somatostatinoma

More than half of somatostatinomas are located in the pancreas, and two-thirds of pancreatic somatostatinomas are found in the head region [4]. The duodenum is the most common site for extrapancreatic somatostatinoma. Somatostatinomas are generally greater than 5 cm in diameter with a rate of malignancy as high as 75–85% [12].

Table 62.1. Clinicopathological features of functioning pancreatic endocrine tumors (PETs). *MEN-I* Multiple endocrine neoplasm type I, *VIP* vasoactive intestinal peptide

PET	Percentile in functioning PETs (prevalence)	Malignancy	Extra-pancreatic localization	Symptoms	Laboratory data	Complication with MEN-I
Insulinoma	75% (1/million)	<10%	1%	Apathy, amnesia, dizziness, confusion, coma	Hyperinsulinemia, hypoglycemia	0–8%
Gastrinoma	15–20% (1/2.5million)	>50%	20–40%	Intractable peptic ulcer, diarrhea,	Hypergastrinemia	18–24%
Glucagonoma	1–2% (rare)	>50%	Rare	Diabetes, weight loss, eczema	Hyperglucagonemia, anemia,	Sometimes
VIPoma	1–2% (rare)	>70%	5–20%	Watery diarrhea, skin rush	Hypercalcemia,, hypokalemia, hyperVIPemia	Sometimes
Somatostatinoma	<1% (very rare)	>50%	Frequent	Diabetes, gallstone, steatorrhea	Hypersomatostatinemia	?

Table 62.2. Clinical features of 41 patients with insulinoma in our institution

Clinical feature		Number of patients	(%)
Site	Pancreatic head	16[a]	(35)
	Pancreatic body	9	(20)
	Pancreatic tail	20[a]	(43)
	Extrapancreas	1	(2)
Size	Less than 1 cm	9[a]	(20)
	1–2 cm	24[a]	(52)
	More than 2 cm	13	(28)
Number	Solitary	36	(88)
	Multiple	3	(7)
	Complication with MEN	2	(5)
Character of tumor	Benign	28	(68)
	Malignant metastasis (+)	6	(15)
	metastasis (–)	7	(17)

[a] Including patients with multiple insulinomas

Nonfunctioning PETs

Nonfunctioning tumors are the most common class of PETs, with an incidence as high as about 50% [13]. Nonfunctioning PETs usually are larger than functioning PETs at the time of diagnosis [13].

Clinical Manifestations

Functioning PETs

Insulinoma

Most patients with insulinomas have neuroglycopenic symptoms such as apathy, amnesia, dizziness, confusion, and coma [14]. Therefore, patients with insulinomas are often diagnosed as having a neurological disease. Differential diagnosis from other causes of hypoglycemia is important. Other than showing pancreatic tumor with increased serum insulin levels, the ratio of serum insulin (μU/ml):blood glucose (mg/dl) is of help in differential diagnosis [15]; this ratio is around 0.3–0.4 in patients without insulinoma, while it is close to 1.0 in patients with insulinoma [16].

Gastrinoma

In the past, patients with gastrinoma often had a history of intractable peptic ulcer of more than 1 year and were diagnosed after undergoing several surgeries for peptic ulcer, especially in the era when there was no good agent to inhibit gastric acid secretion. The development of histamine-2 receptor (H2) blockers and proton pump inhibitors (PPIs) has made it possible to effectively inhibit gastric acid secretion. Therefore, patients with gastrinoma do not always have a very intractable peptic ulcer as long as they take PPIs. Measurement of fasting gastrin should be attempted if a patient has an intractable peptic ulcer. Although peptic ulcers in patients with gastrinoma are often believed to exist in the descending portion of the duodenum, it is not rare that patients with gastrinoma have duodenal ulcers in the bulb [17, 18]. Other than upper abdominal pain associated with peptic ulcer due to hypersecretion of gastric acid, symptoms for patients with gastrinoma are hematoemesis, bloody stool, vomiting, and watery diarrhea. Although serum gastrin in patients with gastrinoma often rises up to several hundreds to one thousand picograms per milliliter, we need to know that serum gastrin also increases in patients with pernicious anemia, atrophic gastritis, and patients taking PPIs.

Glucagonoma

Symptoms in patients with glucagonoma arise from hypersecretion of glucagon due to alpha cell tumor in the pancreas. Their clinical symptoms are diabetes mellitus, body weight loss, dermatitis, deep vein thrombosis, anemia, and hypoaminoacidemia. Diabetes mellitus is observed in approximately 75–95% of patients, and the degree of diabetes mellitus is often mild and controllable with oral hypoglycemics or insulin [9]. Weight loss is identified in 60–70% of patients. Skin rash in glucagonoma is termed necrolytic migrating erythema [19]. This rash with various stages such as erythema, erosion, and crust appears on the face, groin, and extremities. Anemia in glucagonoma is usually mild. An association between skin rash and hypoaminoacidemia has been suggested [20].

VIPoma

As symptoms other than watery diarrhea, hypokalemia, and achlorhydria (WDHA), patients with VIPoma complain of weight loss, dehydration, general fatigue, and skin flushing. Watery diarrhea in VIPoma is described as “tea-like,” and stool volume is greater than 3 l/day and odorless in VIPoma patients [21]. Due to massive diarrhea, hypokalemia, dehydration, and weight loss are marked, and is accompanied by renal failure in severe patients. Some say that hypochlorhydria rather than achlorhydria is frequently observed in VIPoma patients. Skin flushing is identified in 75% of patients. It is important to measure fasting plasma VIP levels if a patient is suspected to have VIPoma.

Somatostatinoma

Clinical symptoms of somatostatinoma are diabetes, gallstones, anemia, steatorrhea, weight loss, and abdominal pain. Diabetes, considered to be associated with an inhibitory effect of somatostatin on insulin release, is found in about 80% of patients. Gallstones in patients with somatostatinoma must be related to decreased gallbladder contractile activity due to the inhibitory effect of somatostatin on cholecystokinin release. Steatorrhea is associated with the inhibitory effects of somatostatin on pancreatic enzyme secretion [22]. It is not rare that a tumor in the pancreas was incidentally found during surgery for gallstones.

Nonfunctioning PETs

Symptoms in patients with nonfunctioning PETs are abdominal pain, weight loss, and jaundice [13]. All of these symptoms are related to space-occupying or invasive lesions in the pancreas. Tumors may be palpated by the patients themselves or found occasionally by computed tomography or magnetic resonance imaging.

Diagnosis

Ultrasonography

Ultrasonography (US) is important as a screening examination for PETs because of its low cost and noninvasiveness. Most PETs represent hypoechoic lesions with clear margins. The sensitivity of US for PETs is 66–80% [4]. In our insulinoma series, localization of the tumor was feasible by US in approximately 50% patients (Table 62.2).

Endoscopic Ultrasound

Endoscopic ultrasound (EUS) is advantageous in detecting small tumors and examining the fine structure inside the tumor. In particular, this technique can visualize tumors with a diameter of less than 3 cm in the pancreatic head and duodenum [23].

Intraoperative Ultrasound

As an examination during operation, intraoperative ultrasound (IUS) combined with surgical exploration including palpation is useful for detecting small tumors and determining the operative procedure, especially when the tumor could not be visualized by preoperative examinations.

Computed Tomography

Computed tomography (CT) scans are advantageous in diagnosing hypervascular tumors. Because PETs are hypervascular tumors with clear margins, most PETs are detected as a low-density tumor in plain CT and stained with contrast-enhanced imaging. In our insulinoma series, localization of tumor was feasible by CT scans in approximately 50% patients (Table 62.2). In general, the sensitivity of CT scans is about 80% [24] and dependent on the size of the tumor; the sensitivity increases as the size increases [25].

Magnetic Resonance Imaging

Magnetic resonance imaging (MRI) is useful in examining the characteristics of the inside of the tumor. Most PETs exhibit low signal intensity on T1-weighted images and a high signal intensity on T2-weighted images. The latter is considered to be attributable to blood inside the tumor. PETs were detectable in approximately 85% of patients by MRI in one study [26]. The sensitivity of MRI depends on the size of the tumor.

Celiac Angiography

As PETs are hypervascular, angiogenesis and tumor stain is observed on celiac angiography. Celiac angiography was able to localize insulinomas in about 70% of patients in our series (Table 62.2). Intra-arterial injection of stimulation material with blood sampling in the hepatic vein is very useful in localizing peripancreatic small PETs, and this technique is described in the later part of this chapter.

Somatostatin Receptor Scintigraphy

Somatostatin receptor scintigraphy (SRS) utilizes a somatostatin analogue labeled with a radioisotope that binds tissues expressing a significant concentration of somatostatin receptor subtype 2. Somatostatin receptors are present in almost 100% of patients with gastrinoma, 67% of those with insulinoma, and 80–90% of those with other functioning PETs [27]. The sensitivity of SRS in the detection of PETs is approximately 80%, and is as good as other modalities including US, CT scan, MRI, and celiac angiography [27, 28].

Hormonal Examinations

Intravenous Stimulation Test

Showing an increase in fasting plasma levels of the hormone is important in making a diagnosis. However, differential diagnosis is often difficult in PETs. In these patients, a different response to hormonal stimulation between tumors and normal endocrine cells is useful in making a diagnosis. Increase in serum insulin levels after intravenous injection of secretin, which is observed in normal subjects, is abolished in patients with insulinoma [29]. In patients with gastrinomas, increase in serum gastrin levels after an intravenous bolus injection of secretin is very significant compared with normal subjects [30]. This phenomenon is referred to as a "paradoxical increase" of gastrin. We have reported previously that glucagon is also useful as a stimulant instead of secretin [31]. These abnormal hormonal responses are of great help in making a diagnosis in insulinoma and gastrinoma.

Moreover, performing an intraoperative stimulation test with secretin and measuring serum gastrin with a rapid assay is very important in judging the curability during surgery [32]. We can measure serum gastrin by rapid radioimmunoassay in about 2 h. If serum gastrin still increases when secretin is injected intravenously after resecting the tumor, that means tumor-secreting gastrin remains somewhere. Regarding insulinomas, intraoperatively monitoring serum insulin before and after resection of the tumor is also important [33].

Table 62.3. Sensitivity of each imaging modality. *US* Ultrasound, *CT* computed tomography, *MRI* magnetic resonance imaging, *PTPVS* B. percutaneous transhepatic portal venous sampling, *ASVS* arterial stimulation with venous sampling

Examination	Gastrinoma		Insulinoma	
	True positive rate (%)	False positive rate (%)	True positive rate (%)	False positive rate (%)
US	4/20 (20)	1/12 (8)	3/23 (26)	0/23 (0)
CT scan	22/37 (59)	1/19 (5)	4/23 (17)	1/23 (4)
MRI	8/32 (25)	0/19 (0)	2/8 (25)	0/8 (0)
Celiac Angiography	30/44 (68)	1/17 (6)	9/26 (35)	2/26 (8)
PTPVS	11/15 (73)	8/12 (67)	17/22 (77)	0/22 (0)
ASVS	32/38 (85)	0/38 (0)	16/16 (100)	0/4 (0)

Percutaneous Transhepatic Portal Venous Sampling

Percutaneous transhepatic portal venous sampling is a hormonal examination that is used to measure plasma peptides in samples taken from the portal, splenic, and superior mesenteric veins. Localization of the tumor is speculated by comparing plasma peptide concentrations in each vein, and we were able to localize insulinomas in 10 out of 12 patients in our series [34]. However, this examination is being avoided because of its invasiveness.

Arterial Stimulation with Venous Sampling

Arterial stimulation with venous sampling (ASVS), which utilizes an angiographic technique, is very useful in determining the release of peptides from the tumor found in imaging modalities. The most representative ASVS is the selective arterial secretin injection (SASI) test for gastrinoma proposed by Imamura et al. [35]. In this examination, secretin is injected into the peripancreatic arteries (gastroduodenal, splenic, and superior mesenteric arteries) and a blood sample is drawn from the hepatic vein 20, 40, and 60 s after each intra-arterial injection. Serum levels of gastrin in the hepatic vein are measured for diagnosis. If the increase in serum gastrin level 40 s after the injection into an artery exceeds 20% of the basal value and 80 pg/ml, that artery is judged as feeding the tumor. In patients with insulinomas, the plasma concentration of insulin in the hepatic vein is increased after injection of calcium into peripancreatic arteries [36]. Intra-arterial injection of calcium is also available for localization of gastrinoma as an alternative method for the SASI test [37]. Table 62.3 shows the sensitivity of each examination [38]. ASVS has high rate of true-positive and low rate of false-positive results compared with other imaging modalities. Imamura et al. reported that the specificity of the SASI test was 100% [39]. We also showed that the SASI test was able to localize a tumor in four out of five patients [40]. ASVS has an advantage in terms of being able to localize very small tumors that are not visible with conventional imaging modalities. Another advantage of ASVS is that we can say that there is no tumor in the region fed by the artery when no serum gastrin response is seen. This fact is very important in performing curative resection of PETs.

Conservative Treatment

Conservative treatments are: (1) antihormonal treatment for symptoms and complications associated with hypersecertion of peptides, and (2) chemotherapy for malignant tumor. Although the administration of glucose is generally effective for hypoglycemic attack in patients with insulinomas, diazoxide, which inhibits the release of insulin from the tumor, is applied for patients with severe and frequent attacks. H2 blockers are very effective in controlling hypersecretion of gastric acid in gastrinoma. PPIs are more effective than H2 blockers, and the rate of effectiveness is as high as for H2 blockers. The doses of those agents necessary to effectively inhibit gastric acid secretion are generally higher than the normal doses [41, 42]. Use of antidiarrheic agents such as loepramide, as well as supplementation of water and electrolites is important for watery diarrhea due to VIPoma, and steroid hormone is effective for the short term. Insulin is necessary for the treatment of diabetes mellitus associated with glucagonoma. Correction of hypoaminoacidemia with intravenous amino acid administration is effective for skin lesions in glucagonoma. A long-acting somatostatin analogue, Sandostatin, specifically binds somatostatin receptor-2 and inhibits the release of various hormones [43]. This agent has weak tumoricidal effects but stabilizes the tumor

[44]. Glucagonomas, VIPomas, and, to a lesser extent, gastrinomas and metastatic insulinomas are examples of functioning PETs that are amenable to treatment with octreotide [45].

The effective rate of chemotherapy for malignant PETs is generally 40–70% [46]. Streptozocin in combination with other chemotherapy agents such as 5-fluorouracil or doxorubicin is considered the best treatment for malignant PETs [47]. Dacarbazine is also believed to be effective, especially for glucagonomas.

A radiolabeled somatostatin analogue, 111Indium-DTPA-octreotide, reduced the tumor size in 30% of patients with advanced neuroendocrine tumors [48]. Treatment with alpha interferons, which stimulate natural killer cell function, should be attempted unless other treatments are effective [49].

References

1. Kloppel G, Heitz PU (1988) Pancreatic endocrine tumors. Pathol Res Pract 183:155–168
2. Liu TH, Zhu Y, Cui QC, Cai LX, Ye SF, Zhong SX, Jia HP (1992) Nonfunctioning pancreatic endocrine tumors. An immunohistochemical and electron microscopic analysis of 26 cases. Pathol Res Pract 188:191–198
3. Boden G. Glucagonomas and insulinomas (1989) Gastroenterol Clin North Am 18:831–845
4. Mansour JC, Chen H (2004) Pancreatic endocrine tumors. J Surg Res 120:139–161
5. Ectors N (1999) Pancreatic endocrine tumors: Diagnostic pitfalls. Hepatogastroenterology 46:679–690
6. Modlin IM, Lawton GP (1994) Duodenal gastrinoma: the solution to the pancreatic paradox. J Clin Gastroenterol 19:184 188
7. Stacpoole PW (1981) The glucagonoma syndrome: clinical features, diagnosis, and treatment. Endocr Rev 2:347–361
8. Tanaka K, Chokai M, Ito Y, Ogino Y, Noguchi K, Osada M (1996) Glucagonoma syndrome and glucagon producing tumor. J Bil Pancreat 17:33–42 (in Japanese)
9. Wermers RA, Fatourechi V, Kvols LK (1996) Clinical spectrum of hyperglucagonemia associated with malignant neuroendocrine tumors. Mayo Clin Proc 71:1030–1038
10. Doherty GM (2005) Rare endocrine tumours of the GI tract. Best Pract Res Clin Gastroenterol 19:807–817
11. Morrison AB (1980) Islet cell tumors and the diarrheogenic syndrome. In: Fitzgerald PJ, Morrison AB (eds) The Pancreas. Williams and Wilkins, Baltimore, pp185–207
12. Snow N, Liddle R (1995) Neuroendocrine tumors. In Rusygi A (ed) Gastrointestinal Cancers: Biology, Diagnosis, and Therapy. Lippincott-Raven, Philadelphia, p 585
13. Phan GQ, Yeo CJ, Hruban RH, Lillemoe KD, Pittha, Cameron JL (1998) Surgical experience with pancreatic and peripancreatic neuroendocrine tumors: Review of 125 patients. J Gastrointest Surg 2:472–482
14. Dizon AM, Kowalyk S, Hoogwerf BJ (1999) Neuroglycopenic and other symptoms in patients with insulinomas. Am J Med 106:307–310
15. Fajans SS, Floyd JC Jr (1976) Fasting hypoglycemia in adults. N Engl J Med 294:766–772
16. Seregni E, Ferrari L, Stivanello M, Dogliotti L (2000) Laboratory tests for neuroendocrine tumors. Q J Nucl Med 44:22–41
17. Ellison EH, Wilson SD (1964) The Zollinger-Ellison syndrome: re-appraisal and evaluation of 260 registered cases. Ann Surg 160:512–530
18. Bonfils S, Bader JP (1970) The diagnosis of Zollinger-Ellison syndrome with special reference to the multiple endocrine adenomas. In: Jerzy-Glass GB (ed) Progress in Gastroenterology, vol. 2. Grune & Stratton, New York, pp 332–355
19. Wilkinson DS (1973) Necrolytic migrating erythema with carcinoma of the pancreas. Trans St. Johns Hospital Dermatol Soc 59:244–250
20. Klein S, Jahoor F, Baba H, Townsend CM, Shepherd M, Wolfe RR (1992) In vivo assessment of the metabolic alterations in glucagonoma syndrome. Metabolism 41:1171–1175
21. Krejs GJ (1987) VIPoma syndrome. Am J Med 82:37–48
22. Jensen RT, Norton JA (1995) Endocrine neoplasms of the pancreas. In: Yamada T (ed) Textbook of Gastroenterology. JB Lippincott, Philadelphia, pp 2131
23. Muller MF, Meyenberger C, Bertschinger P, Schaer R, Marincek B (1994) Pancreatic tumors: Evaluation with endoscopic US, CT, and MR imaging. Radiology 190:745–751
24. Legmann P, Vignaux O, Dousset B, Baraza AJ, Palazzo L, Dumontier I, Coste J, Louvel A, Roseau G, Couturier D, Bonnin A (1998) Pancreatic tumors: comparison of dual-phase helical CT and endoscopic sonography. Am J Roentgenol 170:1315–1322
25. Orbuch M, Doppman JL, Jensen RT (1995) Localization of pancreatic endocrine tumors. Semin Gastrointestinal Dis 6:90–101
26. Thoeni RF, Mueller-Lisse UG, Chan R, Do NK, Shyn PB (2000) Detection of small, functional islet cell tumors in the pancreas: selection of MR imaging sequences for optimal sensitivity. Radiology 214:483–490
27. Krenning EP, Kweekkeboom DJ, Oei HY, de Jong RJ, Dop FJ, Reubi JC, Lamberts SW (1994) Somatostatin-receptor scintigraphy in gastroenteropancreatic tumors: an overview of European results. Ann N Y Acad Sci 733:416–424
28. Gibril F, Reynolds JC, Doppman JL, Chen CC, Venzon DJ, Termanini B, Weber HC, Stewart CA, Jensen RT (1996) Somatostatin receptor scintigraphy: its sensitivity compared with that of other imaging methods in detecting primary and metastatic gastrinomas. A prospective study. Ann Intern Med 125:26–34
29. Imamura M, Hattori Y, Nishida O, Honda T, Shimada Y, Miyahara T, Wagata T, Baba N, Tobe T (1990) Unresponsiveness of insulinoma cells to secretin: significance of the secretin test in patients with insulinoma. Pancreas 5:467–473
30. Isenberg JI, Walsh JH, Passaro E Jr, Moore EW, Grossman MI (1972) Unusual effect of secretin on serum gastrin, serum calcium and gastric acid secretion of patients with suspected Zollinger-Ellison syndrome. Gastroenterology 62:626–631
31. Imamura M, Kameyama J, Sasaki I, Narui H, Naito H, Tsuchiya T (1984) Zollinger-Ellison syndrome: a study of four cases with special reference to gut hormones. Jpn J Gastroenterol 81:1181–1190 (in Japanese)
32. Shibata C, Sasaki I, Naito H, Funayama Y, Kamiyama Y, Takahashi M, Fukushima K, Segami H, Doi T, Iwatsuki A, Ohtani N, Furukawa T, Matsuno S, Nomura T, Unno M, Okamoto H (1991) A completely resected case of intraduodenal malignant gastrinoma by utilizing selective arterial secretin injection test and intra-operative secretin test. Jpn J Gastroenterol Surg 24:2414–2418 (in Japanese)

33. Amikura K, Nakamura R, Arai K, Kobari M, Matsuno S (2001) Role of intraoperative insulin monitoring in surgical management of insulinoma. J Laparoendosc Adv Surg Tech A 11:193–199
34. Nakamura R, Kobari M, Takeda K, Kimura M, Matsuno S (1994) Role of intraoperative ultrasonography in the surgical management of insulinomas. J Hepatobiliary Pancreat Surg 1:535–541
35. Imamura M, Takahashi K, Adachi H, Minematsu S, Shimada Y, Naito M, Suzuki T, Tobe T, Azuma T (1987) Usefulness of selective arterial secretin injection test for localization of gastrinoma in the Zollinger-Ellison syndrome. Ann Surg 205:230–239
36. Doppman JL, Miller DL, Chang R, Shawker TH, Gorden P, Norton JA (1991) Insulinomas: localization with selective intraarterial injection of calcium. Radiology 178:237–241
37. Wada M, Komoto I, Doi R, Imamura M (2002) Intravenous calcium injection test is a novel complementary procedure in differential diagnosis for gastrinoma. World J Surg 26:1291–1296
38. Meko JB, Norton JA. Gastrinoma (1998) The Pancreas. Blackwell Science, p 1228
39. Imamura M, Takahashi K (1993) Use of selective arterial secretin injection test to guide surgery in patients with Zollinger-Ellison syndrome. World J Surg 17:433–438
40. Shibata C, Funayama Y, Fukushima K, Takahashi K, Ueno T, Nagao M, Haneda S, Watanabe K, Kudoh K, Kohyama A, Naito H, Sasaki I (2006) Role of selective arterial secretin test in diagnosis and treatment of Zollinger-Ellison syndrome. Hepatogastroenterology (in press)
41. McCarthy DM, Olinger EJ, May RJ, Long BW, Gardner JD (1977) H2-Histamine receptor blocking agents in the Zollinger-Ellison syndrome. Experience in seven cases and implications for long-term therapy. Ann Intern Med 87:668–675
42. McArthur KE, Collen MJ, Maton PN, Cherner JA, Howard JM, Ciarleglio CA, Cornelius MJ, Jensen RT, Gardner JD (1989) Omeprazole: effective, convenient therapy for Zollinger-Ellison syndrome. Gastroenterology 88:939–944
43. Reubi JC, Schar JC, Waser B, Wenger S, Heppeler A, Schmitt JS, Macke HR (2000) Affinity profiles for human somatostatin receptor subtypes SST1-SST5 of somatostatin radiotracers selected for scintigraphic and radiotherapeutic use. Eur J Nucl Med 27:273–282
44. Angeletti S, Corleto VD, Schillaci O, Moretti A, Panzuto F, Annibale B, Delle Fave G (1999) Single dose of octreotide stabilize metastatic gastro-entero-pancreatic endocrine tumours. Ital J Gastroenterol Hepatol 31:23–27
45. Oberg K, Kvols L, Caplin M, Delle Fave G, de Herder W, Rindi G, Ruszniewski P, Woltering EA, Wiedenmann B (2004) Consensus report on the use of somatostatin analogs for the management of neuroendocrine tumors of the gastroenteropancreatic system. Ann Oncol 15:966–973
46. Pelley RJ, Bukowski RM (1999) Recent advances in systemic therapy for gastrointestinal neuroendocrine tumors. Curr Opin Oncol 11:32–37
47. Moertel CG, Lefkopoulo M, Lipsitz S, Hahn RG, Klaassen D (1992) Streptozocin-doxorubicin, streptozocin-fluorouracil or chlorozotocin in the treatment of advanced islet-cell carcinoma. N Engl J Med 326:519–523
48. Krenning EP, Valkema R, Pauwels S (1999) Radiolabeled somatostatin analogue(s): Peptide receptor scintigraphy and radionucleotide therapy. In: Mignon M, Colombel JF (eds) Recent Advances in the Pathophysiology and Management of Inflammatory Bowel Diseases and Digestive Endocrine Tumors. John Libbey Eurotext Publishing, Paris, p 220
49. Oberg K (1999) Neuroendocrine gastrointestinal tumors – a condensed overview of diagnosis and treatment. Ann Oncol 10 suppl 2:S3–S8

Chapter 63

M. Sunamura · S. Fukuyama

Surgical Treatment of Insulinomas

Introduction

Insulinomas are the most frequent endocrine tumors of the pancreas (approximately 75% of all endocrine pancreatic neoplasms), causing recurrent episodes of fasting hypoglycemia and giving rise to substantial morbidity [1]. The demonstration of low plasma glucose levels (less than 2.5 mmol/l or 45 mg/dl) in the presence of a high serum insulin (>6 mU/ml) is regarded as being diagnostic of hypoglycemia secondary to an insulinoma [2]. Insulinomas are rare tumors that occur in about 1 in 250,000 persons per year [3] and the majority has a lower malignancy rate [4] than other islet cell tumors such as gastrinomas [5] or glucagonomas [6], and solitary lesions. About 10% of all insulinomas are malignant (with metastases) and 10% are multiple, with 50% of the latter being associated with the multiple endocrine neoplasia syndrome-1 [7].

Surgical resection is the only available cure for insulinomas. Thus, an accurate biochemical diagnosis is warranted prior to surgical exploration. Once biochemical diagnosis is made, our approach is to use computed tomography (CT), magnetic resonance imaging, and/or endoscopic ultrasound for localization. Nearly 80% of these tumors are less than 2 cm in size and may not be easily seen on preoperative imaging [8,9]. Small tumors might require additional diagnostic procedures for preoperative localization. Intra-arterial calcium stimulation with right-hepatic-vein sampling for insulin gradients [10] will confirm the diagnosis and allow for localization of the autonomous focus by showing an incremental response after selective intra-arterial injections of calcium gluconate as a secretagogue. This test is based on the principle that intracellular free calcium release might be important in insulin release from insulinoma cells after they are exposed to a high level of extracellular calcium levels. The human parathyroid calcium receptor could be involved in this mechanism [11]. The detection rate obtained using this test has been evaluated by several groups and found to reach 80–90% [12,13].

When a team of experts reaches a diagnosis, the surgeon can perform a laparotomy with a good certainty of identifying the tumor. Intraoperative manual palpation of the pancreas by an experienced surgeon and intraoperative ultrasound (IOUS) are both sensitive tools (>80%) for the localization of insulinomas [14,15]. Insulinomas appear visually as grey-reddish masses, with a greater density in comparison to the surrounding parenchyma. The reason for inability to detect the pancreatic tumor intraoperatively is probably that the tumor is small, as suggested by the preoperative imaging, and that the tissue density may be similar to that of the surrounding pancreatic parenchyma, diminishing the sensitivity of manual palpation and IOUS to detect the location of the tumor.

Open Laparotomy

After identification, there is no doubt that surgery is indicated in all localized tumors. The choice of procedure will depend on the risk of malignancy based on parameters such as type, size, and features of the mass. Atypical resection (enucleation or middle pancreatectomy) has the advantage of preserving the pancreatic parenchyma as much as possible, thereby reducing the risk of late exocrine/endocrine insufficiency. A lymphadenectomy is not usually performed, since this procedure is not foolproof for this disease. Enucleation can usually be indicated in those cases where the lesion is single, capsulated, of limited dimensions (less than 3 cm in diameter) and does not involve, or is sufficiently far from the main pancreatic duct [16]. When the lesion is in the body and/or nearby the Wirsung duct, a middle pancreatectomy should be the procedure of choice. In these instances, enucleation would be at very high risk for a postoperative fistula. Insulinomas and small, nonfunctioning tumors are the most indicated cases.

Laparoscopic Distal Pancreatectomy

Advancing technology and increasing experience with laparoscopic surgery have led surgeons to perform laparoscopic pancreatic resections. Neuroendocrine and cystic tumors of the pancreas represent the best indications for laparoscopic distal pancreatic resection. Minimally invasive surgery is favored for this pathology. The history of minimally invasive resection of the pancreas is a brief one. Gagner and Pomp [17] reported their initial experience with laparoscopic resections of the pancreas in 1992, and since then others have reported their experience in a variety of settings. Sussman et al. [18] reported a case of sporadic occult insulinoma treated by laparoscopic distal pancreatectomy (LDP) using a laparoscopic ultrasound probe to facilitate localization of the insulinoma, and a laparoscopic surgical stapler to transect the pancreas is presented. This is believed to be the first description of a laparoscopic pancreatic resection. Although clinical experience with these procedures remains limited, an early consensus appears to have emerged. On the other hand, very limited experience reported with laparoscopic pancreaticoduodenectomy suggests that it is not a procedure that confers any patient benefit when compared to open surgical techniques. Benign insulinomas are generally solitary, small, and two-thirds of these lesions are located in the body or tail of the pancreas. These favorable features make insulinomas amenable to the laparoscopic approach. However, only a few authors have reported laparoscopic resection of pancreatic insulinomas. Laparoscopic surgery contrasts greatly with the large size of the abdominal incision required to access this retroperitoneal gland at open surgery; furthermore, there are no anastomoses to fashion. Indeed, in selected patients and in experienced hands, laparoscopic surgery (enucleation and distal pancreatectomy) appears to be associated with a short postoperative hospital stay and rapid recovery coupled with acceptable perioperative morbidity and complication rates [19]. Preservation of the splenic vessels and spleen during distal pancreatectomy is often possible. The risk of pancreatic fistula, however, is not reduced.

The early results with LDP reported by Park and Heniford are encouraging as compared to open distal pancreatectomy [20]. In 25 cases (23 completed laparoscopically), there was no perioperative mortality, and the complication rate was 16%. Mean operative time was 3.7 h, mean blood loss was 270 ml, and mean postoperative length of stay (LOS) was 4.1 days. On the other hand, Lillemoe et al. reported their experience with 235 cases performed at a single institution over a 14-year period [21]. Their perioperative mortality rate was 0.9%, and the overall complication rate was 31%. Mean operative time in this series was 4.7 h (median 4.3 h), mean blood loss was 879 ml (median 450 ml), and mean LOS was reportedly 15 days (median 10 days). Fernandez-del Castillo et al. reported their experience with 71 cases of conventional distal pancreatectomy in which they observed a perioperative mortality rate of 1.4% and a 20% incidence of complications [22]. This also demonstrates the feasibility of employing a spleen-preserving technique when performing LDP; 48% of LDP patients retained their spleens [20]. The advantages to the patient, including eliminating the risk of overwhelming postsplenectomy sepsis, are obvious. Extensive preoperative and even intraoperative studies (including IOUS) failed to identify the insulinoma; there remains no minimally invasive substitute for manual palpation and exploration of the pancreas, particularly the head and neck. Recent advances in hand-assisted laparoscopic surgery have helped address this limitation of purely laparoscopic surgery.

The reported experience with laparoscopic pancreatic resections remains limited to case reports or small series of patients. A retrospective multicenter study was conducted in 25 European surgical centers concerning their experience with laparoscopic pancreatic resections [23]. During the study period, 127 patients with presumed pancreatic neoplasms were enrolled in this series and 89% of tumors were located in the left pancreas. Laparoscopically successful procedures included 21 enucleations, 24 distal splenopancreatectomies, 58 distal pancreatectomies with splenic preservation, and 3 pancreaticoduodenal resections. The overall conversion rate was 14%. There were no postoperative deaths. The rate of overall postoperative pancreatic-related complications was 31%, including a 17% rate of clinical pancreatic fistula. The surgical reoperation rate was 6.3%. In laparoscopically successful operations, the median postoperative LOS was 7 days (range, 3–67 days). These results suggest that laparoscopic pancreatic surgery is feasible and safe in selected patients with presumed benign and distal pancreatic tumors.

Laparoscopic Enucleation

Gagner and his colleagues reported the first laparoscopic enucleation in the treatment of insulinoma [24]. To date, however, the laparoscopic approach for solitary insulinoma has not been compared with the open approach. Sa Cunha et al. reported a study aimed to assess the results from laparoscopic resection (LG) of insulinomas and to compare them with the results from open surgery (OG) of insulinomas [25]. Fifty-six LGs were performed for selected patients, including 12 laparoscopic resections of insulinomas. The results were compared with those of patients who underwent OGs of insulinomas selected from the authors' pancreatic database. There were no deaths in either group, and the morbidity rates were 25% (3/12) for LG and 55% (5/9) for OG (nonsignificant difference). The pancreatic fistula rate after laparoscopic enucleation was statistically lower than after open enucleation (14% vs 100%; $p=0.015$). The mean postoperative LOS was 13±5.9 days for LG and 17.6±7.5 days for OG (no significant difference). After exclusion of the patients who underwent conversion to laparotomy, the mean postoperative hospital stay was 11.5±5.8 days for LG and 17.6±7.5 days for OG ($p=0.04$). This study demonstrates the feasibility and safety of laparoscopic resection of insulinomas. The laparoscopic approach was associated with a decrease in hospital stay and pancreatic fistula after enucleation.

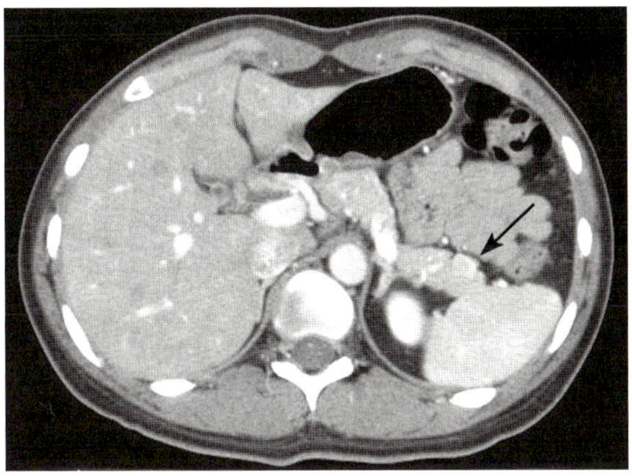

Figure 63.1

Preoperative enhanced computed tomography scan revealing a mass in the pancreatic tail (*arrow*)

It may prove to be more feasible to orchestrate a prospective randomized trial comparing minimally invasive with endoscopic treatments of patients with neuroendocrine pancreatic tumors, and cystic or other benign masses in the body and tail of the pancreas may benefit from laparoscopic extirpation of such lesions. LDP and enucleation of insulinomas performed in selected patients can result in a rapid postoperative recuperation with no mortality and few complications.

We present a clinical case of insulinoma approached by laparoscopy with intraoperative laparoscopic ultrasonography and insulin assay. A 23-year-old woman presented with episodic hypoglycemia. A CT scan identified a 1-cm lesion in the tail of the pancreas (Fig. 63.1). From these findings, the patient was diagnosed with insulinoma. During surgical exploration, after dividing the gastrocolic ligament with electrocautery scissors, a tumor was found in the tail of the pancreas by means of laparoscopy, at the location

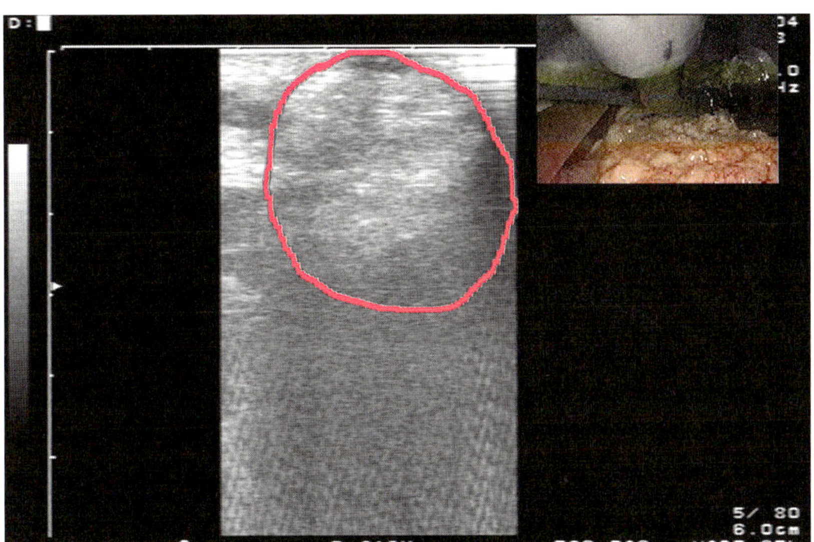

Figure 63.2

The tumor was confirmed (circumscribed by the *pink circle*) using laparoscopic ultrasonography with a 10-mm flexible probe

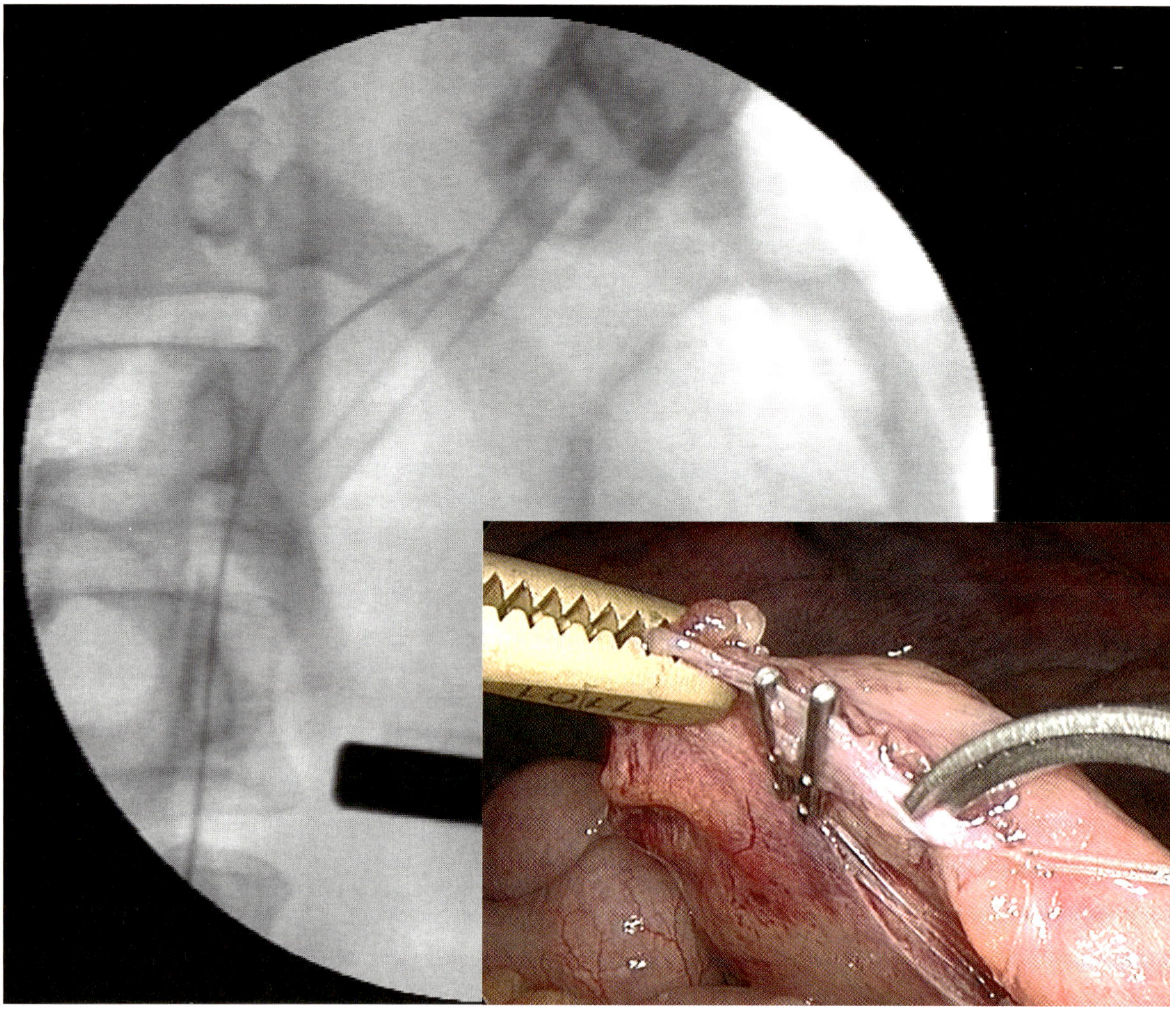

Figure 63.3

The catheter was inserted into the portal system in order to measure intraoperative insulin levels for effective diagnosis of complete removal of the tumor

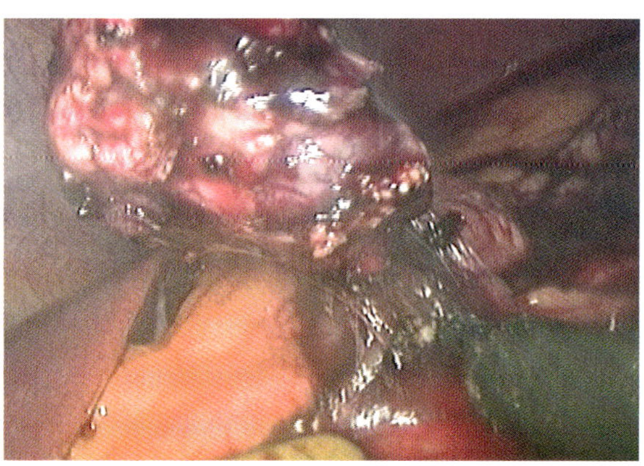

Figure 63.4

Laparoscopic enucleation was performed with electrocautery scissors, and the tumor was excised from the surrounding normal pancreatic tissue

identified preoperatively by abdominal CT. We then confirmed the presence of a tumor using laparoscopic ultrasonography with a 10-mm flexible probe (Fig. 63.2). The catheter was inserted into the portal system, and an intraoperative insulin assay was proposed for effective diagnosis of complete removal of the tumor (Fig. 63.3). Laparoscopic enucleation was performed with electrocautery scissors, and the tumor was excised from the surrounding normal pancreatic tissue (Fig. 63.4) and extracted directly into a plastic bag to avoid tumor spilling or seeding. The tumor was found to be well encapsulated, and there was no evidence of local invasion. A silicone drain was left in the bed of the insulinoma. Serum insulin level of portal vein dropped from 147.2 IU/ml at the beginning of the operation to 48.6 IU/ml after the removal of tumor. Immunohistochemical studies demonstrated that the tumor cells were positive for insulin. The postoperative LOS was 7 days.

According to our experience with open surgery for insulinoma, we monitored intraoperative glucose and insulin levels before and after laparoscopic resection of insulinoma. We believe that this is very important for estimating whether or not tumors have been completely removed. Since serum glucose levels were controlled well during surgery, serum insulin levels in the portal vein system provide helpful information whether no tumor fragments remain. It should be noted that reports have indicated that about 25% of laparoscopic resection of insulinoma cases are eventually converted to open surgery.

Recurrence of Insulinoma

The recurrence rate is very low after complete resection of insulinoma. One confusing factor is that malignant and benign tumors are difficult to distinguish histologically, and often, the diagnosis of malignant insulinoma is made only when metastases occur. The best estimate of the incidence of malignant insulinomas is probably four cases per million people/year [26], which is higher than previously reported. Insulinomas have a lower malignancy rate [4] than other islet cell tumors such as gastrinomas [5] or glucagonomas [6]. It is very difficult to distinguish between malignant and benign insulinomas, since endocrine carcinomas generally show mild nuclear and structural atypia. Most patients with malignant insulinoma have lymph node or liver metastasis [27,28], and only rarely other sites such as bone involvement [29]. Service et al. [26] followed up 196 patients with insulinomas for an average period of 20 years. Recurrences were noted from 4 to 18.5 years after the initial removal of an insulinoma. The cumulative incidence of recurrence was 6% at 10 years and 8% at 20 years after the initial surgical resection. In spite of the therapies in these patients that have been used with some short-term benefits, including surgery, chemotherapy, embolization, radiofrequency ablation, and somatostatin analogs, their prognosis is relatively poor, with a median survival period of approximately 2 years [28,30,31].

There were no distinguishing morphologic features of pancreatic tumors that would predict a subsequent metastasis or a lymph node metastasis. All patients had the characteristic inappropriate elevation of insulin and proinsulin levels at the time of diagnosis, but the more aggressive and less aggressive groups could not be distinguished, nor could either be distinguished from the more common benign insulinoma. Even if the primary tumor is small and histologically benign, insulinomas should be regarded as potentially malignant.

We experienced an interesting case of malignant insulinoma with liver metastasis. A 57-year-old lady underwent enucleation of a 2.7-cm tumor that was diagnosed as subsequent liver metastasis 8 years after the initial operation. The specimen shown in Fig. 63.5 is the removed segment of lobe VI of the liver. Anti-insulin immunostaining revealed that there was no insulin secretion in the metastatic tumor, although this patient was diagnosed with hypoglycemia at the first operation. It is speculated that the biological characteristic of the insulinoma might have changed or the tumor was heterogeneous, containing endocrine cells with a highly malignant potential.

It is clear that when all patients with malignant insulinoma are considered, the initial surgery for tumor removal or diagnosis is the most important factor in their management. After this, the biological behavior of the tumor is the major determinant of long-term survival. All other modalities of therapy are, therefore, palliative and usually of short-term value.

It is essential that we should seek other ways of predicting the metastatic potential of insulinomas, since it is not possible to do so using histopathology alone. Jonkers et al. [32] investigated 62 sporadic insulinomas (44 benign and 18 tumors with metastases) for the identification of reliable indicators of metastatic disease by means of comparative genomic hybridization (CGH). CGH analysis revealed that the total number of aberrations per tumor differs greatly between the benign and the malignant groups (4.2 vs. 14.1; $p<0.0001$). Furthermore, loss of chromosome 6q and gains of 12q, 14q, and 17pq are strongly associated with metastatic disease.

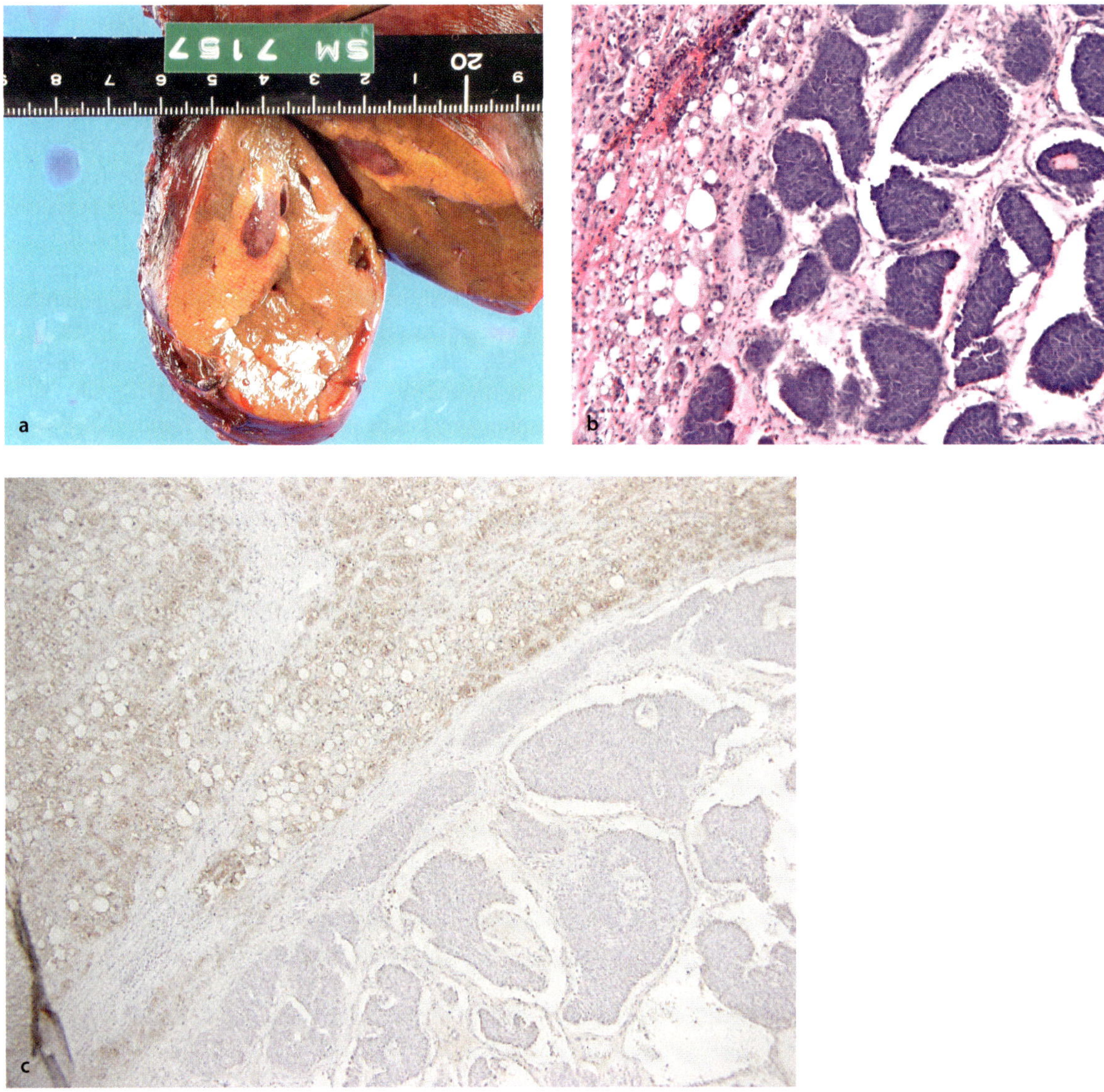

Figure 63.5

a The metastatic tumor was located in the liver of segment VI. b Hematoxylin-eosin staining revealed a tumor of the endocrine cells; however, insulin immunostaining revealed that there was no insulin secretion in the metastatic tumor (c)

References

1. Service FJ (1995) Hypoglycemic disorders. N Engl J Med 332:1144–1152
2. Service FJ (1993) Hypoglycemias (clinical review). J Clin Endocrinol Metab 76:269–272
3. Modlin IM, Lye KD, Kidd M (2003) A 5-decade analysis of 13,715 carcinoid tumors. Cancer 97:934–959
4. Broughan TA, Leslie JD, Soto JM, Hermann RE (1986) Pancreatic islet cell tumors. Surgery 99:671–678
5. Deveney CW, Deveney KS, Way LW (1978) The Zollinger–Ellison syndrome – 23 years later. Ann Surg 188:384–891
6. Prinz RA, Badrinath K, Banerji M, Sparagana M, Dorsch TR, Lawrence AM (1981) Operative and chemotherapeutic management of malignant glucagon-producing tumors. Surgery 90:713–719
7. Waickus CM, de Bustros A, Shakil A (1999) Recognizing factitious hypoglycemia in the family practice setting. J Am Board Fam Pract 12:133–136
8. Service FJ (1999) Diagnostic approach to adults with hypoglycemic disorders. Endocrinol Metab Clin North Am 28:519–532
9. Perry RR, Vinik AI (1995) Clinical Review 72: diagnosis and management of functioning islet cell tumors. J Clin Endocrinol Metab 80:2273–2278

10. Doppman JL, Chang R, Fraker DL, Norton JA, Alexander HR, Miller DL, Collier E, Skarulis MC, Gorden P (1995) Localization of insulinomas to regions of the pancreas by intra-arterial stimulation with calcium. Ann Intern Med 123:269–273
11. Kato M, Doi R, Imamura M, Furutani M, Hosotani R, Shimada Y (1997) Calcium-evoked insulin release from insulinoma cells is mediated via calcium-sensing receptor. Surgery 122:1203–1211
12. Lo CY, Chan FL, Tam SC, Cheng PW, Fan ST, Lam KS (2000) Value of intra-arterial calcium stimulated venous sampling for regionalization of pancreatic insulinomas. Surgery 128:903–909
13. Won JG, Tseng HS, Yang AH, Tang KT, Jap TS, Kwok CF, Lee CH, Lin HD (2003) Intra-arterial calcium stimulation test for detection of insulinomas: detection rate, responses of pancreatic peptides, and its relationship to differentiation of tumor cells. Metabolism 52:1320–1329
14. Norton JA, Shawker TH, Doppman JL, Miller DL, Fraker DL, Cromack DT, Gorden P, Jensen RT (1990) Localization and surgical treatment of occult insulinomas. Ann Surg 212:615–620
15. Doherty GM, Doppman JL, Shawker TH, Miller DL, Eastman RC, Gorden P, Norton JA (1991) Results of a prospective strategy to diagnose, localize, and resect insulinomas. Surgery 110:989–996
16. Park BJ, Alexander HR, Libutti SK, Huang J, Royalty D, Skarulis MC, et al (1998) Operative management of islet-cell tumors arising in the head of the pancreas. Surgery 124:1056–1061
17. Gagner M, Pomp A (1997) Laparoscopic pancreatic resection: is it worthwhile? J Gastrointest Surg 1:20–26
18. Sussman LA, Christie R, Whittle DE (1996) Laparoscopic excision of distal pancreas including insulinoma. Aust NZ J Surg 66:414–416
19. Fernandez-Cruz L, Saenz A, Astudillo E, Martinez I, Hoyos S, Pantoja JP, et al (2002) Outcome of laparoscopic pancreatic surgery: endocrine and nonendocrine tumors. World J Surg 26:1057–1065
20. Park AE, Heniford BT (2002) Therapeutic laparoscopy of the pancreas. Ann Surg 236:149–158
21. Lillemoe KD, Kaushal S, Cameron JL, et al (1999) Distal pancreatectomy: indications and outcomes in 235 patients. Ann Surg 229:673–700
22. Fernandez-del Castillo C, Fattner DW, Warshaw AL (1995) Standards for pancreatic resection in the 1990s. Arch Surg 130:295–300
23. Mabrut JY, Fernandez-Cruz L, Azagra JS, Bassi C, Delvaux G, Weerts J, Fabre JM, Boulez J, Baulieux J, Peix JL, Gigot JF (2005) Hepatobiliary and Pancreatic Section (HBPS) of the Royal Belgian Society of Surgery; Belgian Group for Endoscopic Surgery (BGES); Club Coelio. Laparoscopic pancreatic resection: results of a multicenter European study of 127 patients. Surgery 137:597–605
24. Gagner M, Pomp A, Herrera MF (1996) Early experience with laparoscopic resections of islet cell tumors. Surgery 120:1051 1054
25. Sa Cunha A, Beau C, Rault A, Catargi B, Collet D, Masson B (2007) Laparoscopic versus open approach for solitary insulinoma. Surg Endosc 21:103–108
26. Service FJ, McMahon MM, O'Brien PC, Ballard DJ (1991) Functioning insulinoma – incidence, recurrence, and long-term survival of patients: a 60-year study. Mayo Clin Proc 66:711–719
27. Sarmiento JM, Que FG, Grant CS, Thompson GB, Farnell MB, Nagorney DM (2002) Concurrent resections of pancreatic islet cell cancers with synchronous hepatic metastases: outcomes of an aggressive approach. Surgery 132:976–982
28. Danforth DN Jr, Gorden P, Brennan MF (1984) Metastatic insulin-secreting carcinoma of the pancreas: clinical course and the role of surgery. Surgery 96:1027–1037
29. Hesdorffer CS, Stoopler M, Javitch J (1989) Aggressive insulinoma with bone metastases. Am J Clin Oncol 12:498–501
30. Grama D, Eriksson B, Martensson H, et al (1992) Clinical characteristics, treatment and survival in patients with pancreatic tumors causing hormonal syndromes. World J Surg 16:632–639
31. Hirshberg B, Cochran C, Skarulis MC, Libutti SK, Alexander HR, Wood BJ, Chang R, Kleiner DE, Gorden P (2005) Malignant insulinoma: spectrum of unusual clinical features. Cancer 104:264–72
32. Jonkers YM, Claessen SM, Perren A, Schmid S, Komminoth P, Verhofstad AA, et al (2005) Chromosomal instability predicts metastatic disease in patients with insulinomas. Endocr Relat Cancer 12:435–447

Chapter 64

M. Imamura · I. Komoto

Surgical Treatment of the Gastrinoma

Curative resection of the gastrinoma in patients with Zollinger-Ellison Syndrome (ZES) has been unsuccessful for a long time, mainly due to the difficulty in preoperative localization of the gastrinoma [1–4]. Symptoms of ZES, such as persistent peptic ulcer, esophagitis, or diarrhea, appear even when the gastrinoma is too small to be recognized by imaging techniques [2–9]. The gastrinoma is potentially metastatic, and once metastasized to the liver, prognosis of the patient is usually limited to less than 3 years [4–10]. Liver metastasis is the major prognostic factor in patients with gastrinoma and only R0 resection can achieve an excellent prognosis [2–15]. So, curative resection guided by accurate localization is recommended before developing distant metastases [2–5,11–15].

Curative resection of the gastrinoma has become possible, aided by correct localization with the aid of the selective arterial secretagogue injection (SASI) test with secretin or calcium, and somatostatin receptor scintigraphy (SRS) [2–4,9–18]. Several patients have since received curative resection of gastrinomas, and accordingly new pathological characteristics of gastrinomas have been elucidated [5–22]. One of the most important finding is that gastrinomas develop in a different location depending on whether or not the patient also has multiple endocrine neoplasm type 1 (MEN-1) [5–19]. These findings are summarized below and are helpful in treating patients with ZES.

1. In patients with ZES without MEN-1, single duodenal gastrinoma has been found more often compared to a pancreatic gastrinoma [2–10].
2. In patients with ZES and MEN-1, there are several endocrine tumors in the pancreas, but the gastrinomas are located mostly in the duodenum. About a half of them are multiple, and sometimes they are numerous [5,8,9,11–22].
3. The incidence of lymph node metastases from either a duodenal or pancreatic gastrinoma is more than 40% [19–22].
4. The incidence of hepatic metastases is more than 60% for pancreatic gastrinoma, although it is less than 10% for duodenal gastrinoma [9,19–23].
5. Liver metastases are the most important prognostic factor. Curative resection before they occur is essential for long survival [6–23].

Preoperative Localization

Computed tomography (CT), ultrasound (US), magnetic resonance imaging (MRI), and abdominal arteriography have long been used, but their sensitivity is reported to be between 40 and 70% [2–10]. With these tools it is almost impossible to detect duodenal gastrinomas less than 5 mm in diameter, and only 15–30% of pancreatic gastrinomas between 1 and 3 cm in diameter are visualized [24]. Thus, they are not adequate for the preoperative localization of gastrinomas [2,9,11]. Portal venous sampling (PVS) may not provide any clear data, and its accuracy rate is between 30 and 70% [4,11].

The SASI test and SRS are the most reliable localizing techniques. [2–4,9–14] The principle of the SASI test is to localize gastrinomas by demonstrating their feeding artery utilizing the fact that gastrinoma cells release gastrin when stimulated with secretin or calcium [25–28]. With this test, a gastrinoma more than 1 mm in diameter can be localized, and more than 90% of gastrinomas less than 5 mm in diameter have been localized [11,13,25–28]. SRS visualizes gastrinomas by utilizing the fact that there are somatostatin receptors on the cell membrane in almost all gastrinoma cells. By injecting the radiolabeled anti-somatostatin-receptor antibody intravenously, gastrinomas throughout the whole body can be visualized with scintigraphy [17] The sensitivity of SRS is correlated with the size of the gastrinoma, so only 30% of gastrinomas less than 1 cm are visualized. SRS is the most convenient method to detect the distribution of distant metastases in the whole body [9,23].

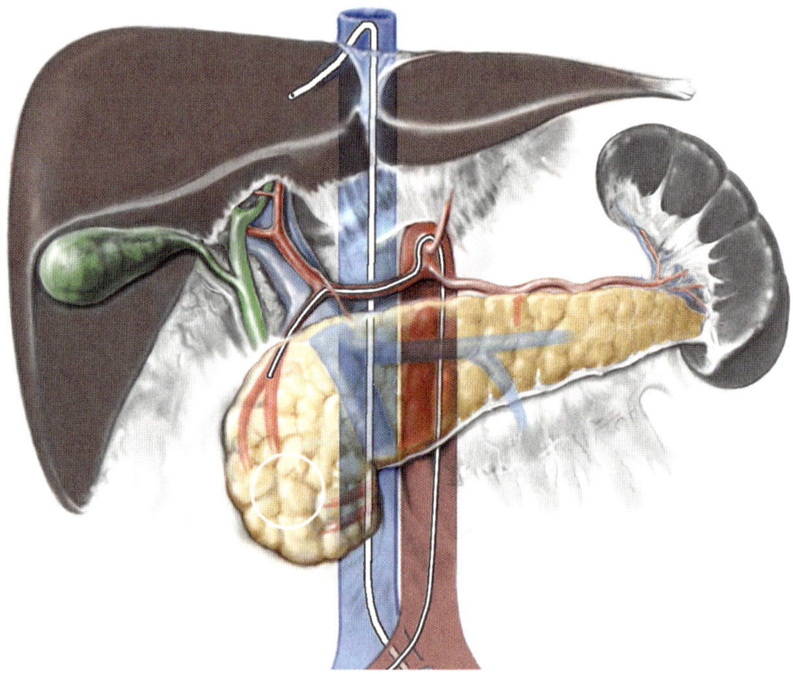

Figure 64.1

Selective arterial secretagogue injection (SASI) test for localization of functioning gastroenteropancreatic endocrine tumors (GEPET). A secretin or calcium solution is injected into the splenic artery, gastroduodenal artery, or superior mesenteric artery through an arteriography catheter. Blood samples are taken from the hepatic vein, before and 20, 40, and 60 s after injection for the measurement of serum hormone levels. In patients with Zollinger-Ellison syndrome (ZES), secretin (rarely calcium) is used as a secretagogue, while calcium is used as the secretagogue for patients with insulinoma or other GEPET

Patients with ZES and MEN-1 usually have various kinds of endocrine tumors in the pancreas, the larger of which are visualized with SRS providing they have somatostatin receptors. However, differentiation of the gastrinomas from other endocrine tumors is not possible with SRS, only with the SASI test [2–4,11–14].

Selective Arterial Secretagoue Injection Test (with Secretin or Calcium)

The SASI test, which was developed at Kyoto University, was first described in 1987 [2]. At the time of abdominal arteriography, 30 units of secretin in 2 ml of solution is injected into the splenic or the gastroduodenal or the superior mesenteric artery and 2-ml blood samples are drawn from the hepatic vein through a catheter inserted via the femoral vein before the injection, immediately and 20, 40, and 60 s after the injection (Figs. 64.1–64.3). The changes of hepatic venous serum immunoreactive gastrin level (IRG, HV-IRG) are measured. When the HV-IRG rises by more than 80 pg/ml within 40 s to at least 120% of the basal IRG, the artery is determined to be the feeding artery of the gastrinoma. The splenic artery feeds the body and tail of the pancreas. The gastroduodenal artery feeds the upper half of the head of the pancreas and the duodenum. The superior mesenteric artery feeds the lower half of the head of the pancreas and the duodenum. Thus, we can diagnose the location of gastrinoma(s) by demonstrating the feeding artery of the gastrinoma. More precise localization is possible by injecting secretin into each branch of the superior mesenteric or the gastroduodenal arteries. When the splenic artery is the feeder, more precise localization is possible by changing the injection point in the splenic artery.

In most patients with ZES, secretin is a useful secretagogue, but in less than 10% of patients with ZES, secretin fails to stimulate the gastrinoma to release gastrin [29]. In this case, calcium solution (2 ml of 8.5% calcium gluconate) is used as the second secretagogue, although the extent of response to calcium is milder than that to secretin in most patients with the gastrinoma [29,30]. Both the specificity and sensitiv-

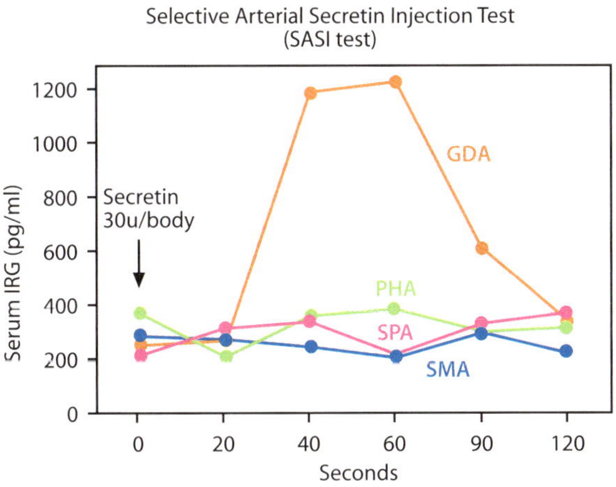

Figure 64.2

SASI test in a patient with ZES. After injection of 30 units of secretin into the gastroduodenal artery (*GDA*, *orange line*), hepatic venous immunoreactive gastrin (*IRG*) rose significantly at 40 s, but it did not increase after injection of secretin into the superior mesenteric artery (*SMA*, *blue line*), splenic artery (*SPA*, *pink line*), or proper hepatic artery (*PHA*, *green line*). From these results, the gastrinoma is located in the proximal duodenum or the head of the pancreas, and not in other parts of the duodenum or pancreas. Surgery revealed a gastrinoma in the proximal duodenum. The patient has remained eugastrinemic and free of disease since resection of the tumor and metastatic lymph nodes

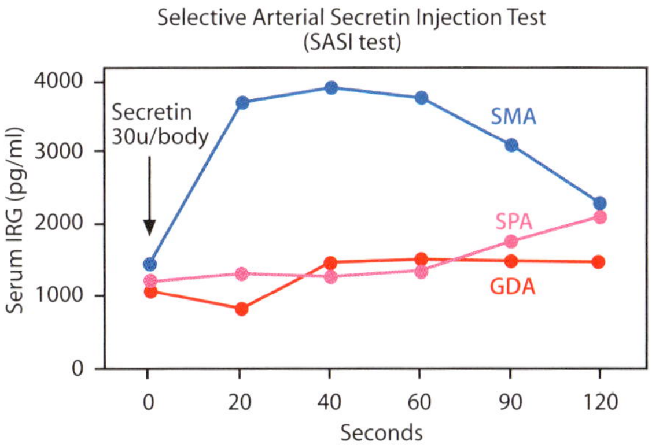

Figure 64.3

SASI test in another patient with ZES. Since only the superior mesenteric artery (*blue line*) is positive, the gastrinoma was expected to be located in the distal duodenum or the head of the pancreas. Laparotomy revealed two gastrinomas in the distal second part of the duodenum and one metastatic lymph node along the inferior pancreaticoduodenal artery. After partial resection of the distal duodenum combined with aggressive dissection of the regional lymph nodes, the patient has remained eugastrinemic and free of disease

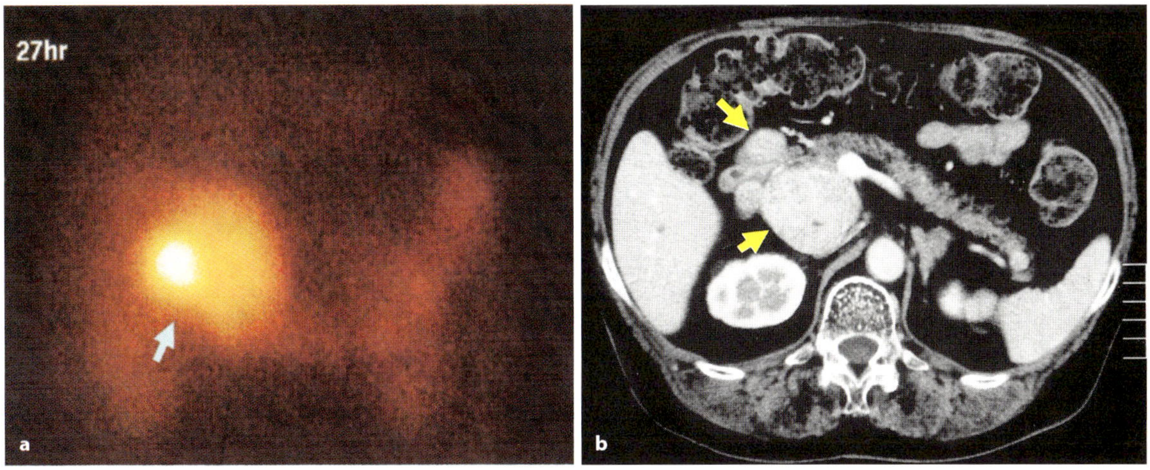

Figure 64.4 a, b

Somatostatin receptor scintigraphy (SRS; a) and computed tomography (CT; b) in a patient with ZES. a SRS displays several endocrine tumors in the right upper quadrant of the abdomen (arrow). b CT shows at least three large metastatic lymph nodes around the head of the pancreas (yellow arrows), although it is unclear where the main tumor is located ity of the SASI test are more than 90%, which makes it an indispensable preoperative localization technique for curative resection of gastrinoma.

Somatostatin Receptor Scintigraphy

Gastrinoma cells have somatostatin receptors in more than 90%. The development of radiolabeled octreotide has enabled visualization of endocrine tumors with somatostatin receptors [17]. SRS visualizes gastrinomas and metastatic lymph nodes that are more than 3 cm in diameter, but rarely visualizes duodenal gastrinomas (Fig. 64.4). SRS is very useful for the detection of some ectopic gastrinomas and for the evaluation of distant metastases. It is an indispensable test for the staging of advanced endocrine tumors [31].

Endoscopic Ultrasonography

Endoscopic ultrasonography is being used with increasing frequency and detects nearly all gastrinomas 1 cm or larger within the pancreas, but does not rule out duodenal gastrinomas, which are rarely imaged.

Intraoperative Localization Methods

The final decision as to the modus of the operation should be performed intraoperatively, based on confirmation of the location and the stage of the tumor, and estimation for surgical curability.

Intraoperative Ultrasonography

Pancreatic tumors more than 5 mm in diameter can be localized with intraoperative ultrasonography (IOUS) by skillful hands [4–6]. During surgery we are apt to believe that the visualized tumor is a gastrinoma, but we should wait with the absolute diagnosis until obtaining pathological confirmation. In addition, gastrinomas are often multiple and metastatic, so we should perform the intraoperative secretin (IOS) test (see below), which is the only test that assures the curability of the operation during surgery. The resection of just one or two tumors may not be enough for a curative resection, particularly in MEN-1 patients [11–15].

Intraoperative Duodenoscopy

Preoperative endoscopic examination of the whole duodenum is usually too uncomfortable for the patient to allow examination for all of the duodenal gastrinomas. More precise endoscopic examination of the whole duodenum using intraoperative duodenoscopy (IDS) is possible if assisted by a surgeon (Fig. 64.5) [9,14]. The duodenal gastrinoma is observed as a minute submucosal tumor with a central depression. Following IDS, a longitudinal duodenotomy is performed for palpation and resection of the minute submucosal tumors [4,5,21]. As there are various kinds of submucosal lesions other than gastrinomas in the duodenum (e.g., ectopic pancreas, enlarged Brunner's glands, or ulcer scars), each of the resected tumors should be sent for pathological examination intraoperatively.

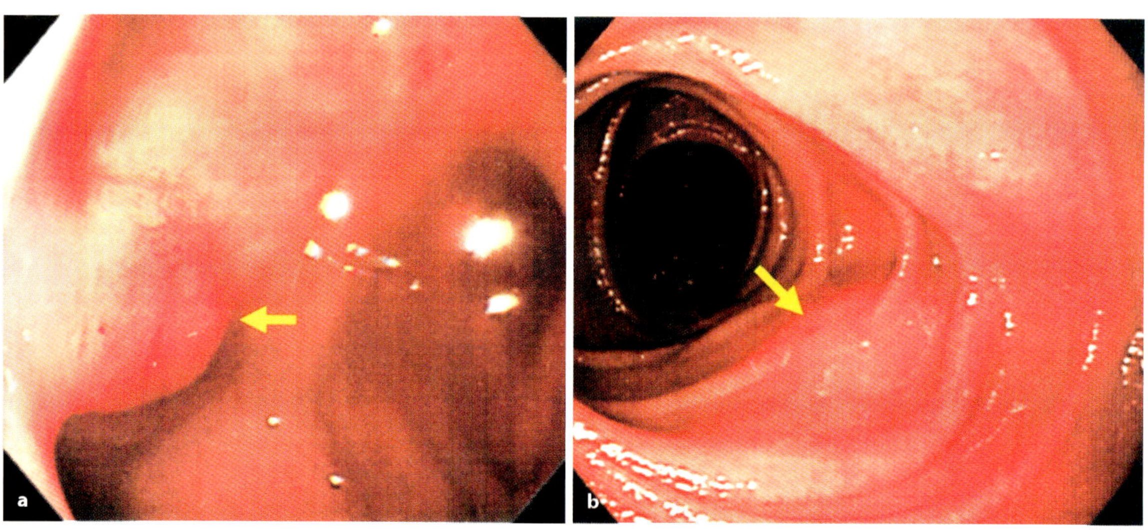

Figure 64.5 a, b

Intraoperative duodenoscopy reveals a tiny submucosal tumor in the proximal second part of the duodenum (*yellow arrows*), which was pathologically diagnosed to be a gastrinoma

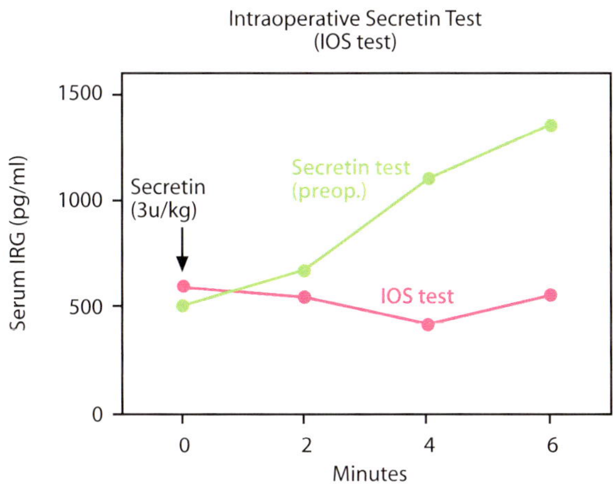

Figure 64.6

Intraoperative secretin (IOS) test. The intravenous secretin test with 2 units/kg of SecrepanR became negative after the enucleation of duodenal tumors and lymph node dissection, although it was positive when surgery started. This suggests that the operation was curative. *preop.* Preoperative

Intraoperative Secretin Test

The IOS test is useful for estimating the curability of the resection [11,14,32]. This test is performed before and after the resection. Secretin (3 units/kg body weight) is injected intravenously, and 2 ml of peripheral venous blood is drawn before the injection and 2, 4, and 6 min afterwards. When the postresection result of IOS becomes negative and the preresection IOS was positive, we can confirm that the resection was a curative one (Fig. 64.6).

Indication for Surgical Resection

Surgical resection of gastrinomas is indicated when CT and/or SRS do not reveal distant metastasis in the lung or bone [5,13,14]. For the countable numbers of metastases to the liver or the brain, aggressive resection or gamma-knife therapy is recommended, because the long-term survivors have been reported by surgical resection from several institutes [33,34]. When multiple gastrinomas are located diffusely in the duodenum in patients with MEN-1, pancreas-preserving total duodenectomy (PPTD) is indicated [35].

Curative Surgery

Curative resection of gastrinomas should be guided by localization with SASI testing, since this test is the most sensitive localization method for gastrinomas [2,3,4,13,14].

Surgery for Gastrinomas in Patients without MEN-1 (Sporadic Gastrinoma)

In these patients, gastrinomas are located either in the pancreas or the duodenum. According to recent reports, the incidence of duodenal gastrinoma is higher than for pancreatic gastrinoma [5,6,8,17]. The rate of liver metastases is much higher with pancreatic gastrinoma than with duodenal gastrinoma. Both of them show high rates of lymph node metastases, accounting for more than 40% [5,6,8,13]. When a duodenal gastrinoma is found in a patient with sporadic ZES, in 80% of patients the resection of a single duodenal gastrinoma with the dissection of regional lymph nodes is sufficient for curative surgery. However in 20%, the duodenal gastrinoma is multiple with or without a pancreatic gastrinoma [2,3,5–13,]. So preoperative SASI Test and IOS is indispensable for curative resection of gastrinomas (Fig. 64.7) [11–14]

Gastrinomas in the Head of the Pancreas or the Duodenum Localized by SASI Test

When the SASI test localizes gastrinomas in the head of the pancreas or the duodenum, a laparotomy is performed and the head of the pancreas is examined carefully by palpation and with US. The duodenum is also examined by palpation after Kocher's mobilization and with IDS. When a tumor is confirmed in the head of the pancreas, pancreatoduodenectomy (PD) or pancreas-preserving pancreatoduodenectomy (PPPD) is performed depending on the status of regional lymph node metastasis. We have experienced a few patients who had both duodenal and pancreatic gastrinomas [2,3,11,15,22]. For these patients, PD is indicated. The lymph node dissection should be performed similar to D2 for pancreatic ductal cancer, with sampling of the para-aortic lymph nodes [2,3,9,11,15,22].

When no tumor is found in the head of the pancreas by palpation and US, the duodenum is examined with IDS and is mobilized for careful examination. The duodenum is then opened along the axis to examine the whole duodenal mucosa with an index finger [5]. Any suspected duodenal tumor is enucle-

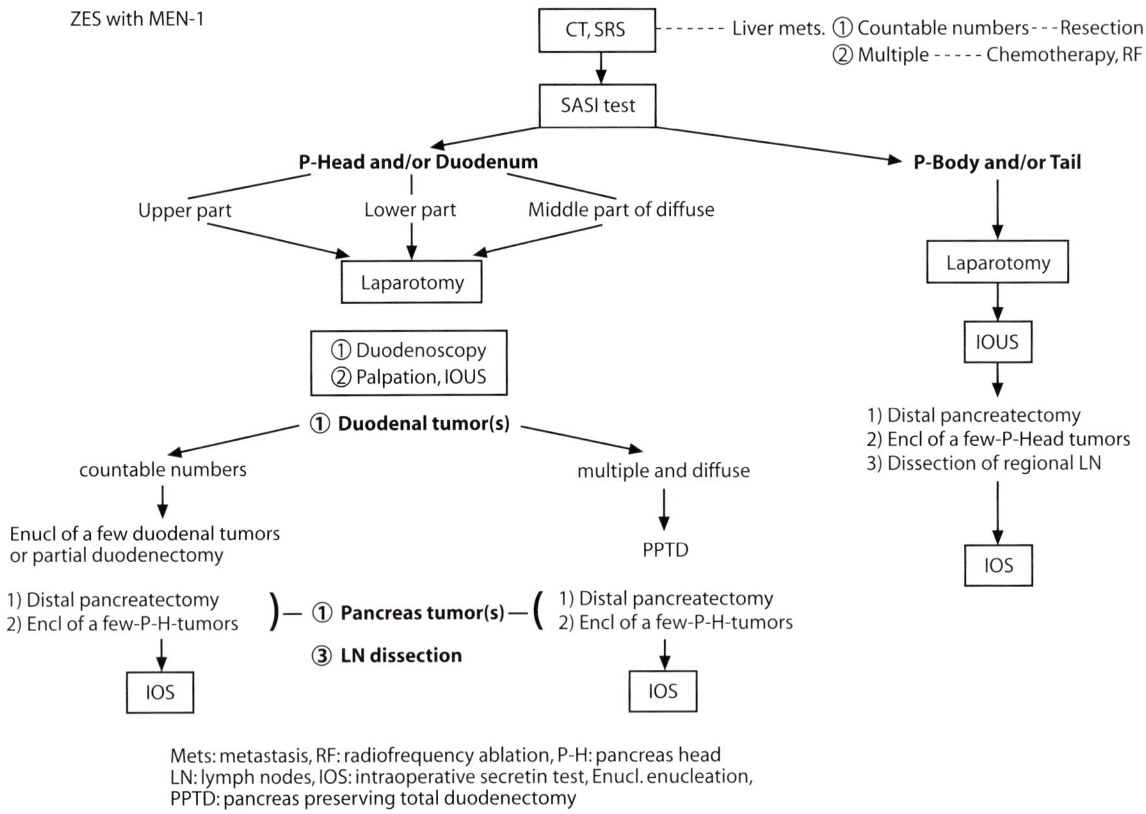

Figure 64.7

A flow chart showing the localization and treatment of sporadic gastrinoma. CT and/or SRS are performed initially for the detection of distant metastases. In patients with liver metastasis, surgical resection and/or radiofrequency ablation (*RF*) are recommended for prolongation of survival. In patients without liver metastasis, the SASI test is performed. When the gastrinoma is localized to either the head of the pancreas or the duodenum, laparotomy is performed and the pancreas is examined by palpation or ultrasound. When a pancreatic tumor is identified, pancreatoduodenectomy (*PD*) or pancreas-preserving pancreatoduodenectomy (*PPPD*) is performed. If no tumor is detected in the head of the pancreas, the duodenum is examined carefully by duodenoscopy (*D-scopy*) and any duodenal gastrinomas are excised by enucleation (*Enucl*) through a duodenotomy or partial resection. When the SASI test suggests that gastrinomas involve the whole area of the duodenum or the head of the pancreas, the pancreas is first examined. If a tumor is detected in the head of the pancreas, PD or PPPD is performed. If no tumor is found in the pancreatic head, the duodenum is carefully examined by duodenoscopy and any duodenal gastrinomas are enucleated. If widespread multiple duodenal tumors are detected, pancreas-preserving total duodenectomy (*PPTD*) is performed. When the SASI test localizes the gastrinoma to the body or tail of the pancreas, distal pancreatectomy is performed. Aggressive dissection of the regional lymph nodes should also be performed in all cases, and the IOS test is recommended for estimating the curability of surgery. *Mets* Metastasis, *P* pancreas, *IOUS* intraoperative ultrasonography, *LN* lymph nodes

ated and the specimens are sent to the pathologist for diagnostic confirmation of endocrine tumor [5–11]. After the resection, curability is confirmed with an IOS test [33]. In the period 1981–1988, when no tumor was identified with these procedures in spite of localization with SASI test, we performed PD [2,3]. In those days, duodenal gastrinoma as a cause of ZES was not well recognized [2–8]. In four of these early patients who underwent PD in our department, one to seven minute duodenal gastrinomas that were not detected during surgery were proved pathologically in the resected specimen. These patients have been cured. At that time there were many surgeons who hesitated to perform PD for these patients because the procedure seemed to be too invasive for this disease [16]. Some aggressive surgeons, however, reported that PD has contributed to a high rate of curability with low morbidity [2,3,6–10,15]. The experience of PD has taught us the difficulty of intraoperative identification of both duodenal gastrinomas and the metastatic lymph nodes.

Since only microscopic duodenal gastrinomas had been revealed in these specimens after PD, we changed our strategy from PD to transduodenal enucleation. But even after this change, PD or PPPD had to be performed for three patients, because identification of duodenal gastrinomas was so difficult. In summary, 18 out of 19 patients who received PD (8 cases), transduodenal enucleations (7), distal pancreatectomy (1), extirpation of the gastrinoma on the upper edge of the pancreatic body (1), and PPTD (1) have been cured during a follow-up of between 3 and 14 years. Only one patient with a metastatic para-aortic lymph node at the time of surgery has not been cured [35].

Gastrinomas in the Body or Tail of the Pancreas Localized by SASI Test

When the SASI test localizes gastrinomas in the body or tail of the pancreas, a distal pancreatectomy with dissection of the regional lymph nodes is performed after the identification of the tumor by palpation or with IOUS. The IOS test is performed before closing the abdomen.

Surgery for Gastrinomas in Patients with MEN-1

In patients with MEN-1 and ZES, there are usually several microscopic or macroscopic endocrine tumors in the pancreas, some of which may be visualized with CT or SRS (Fig. 64.8) [19–21]. Until recently, these tumors have been resected under the misdiagnosis of gastrinoma. Recent studies have revealed that in MEN-1 patients most of these pancreatic tumors are endocrine tumors other than the gastrinoma, and the gastrinomas are predominantly located in the duodenum and often multiple (Fig. 64.9) [19–22].

Before 1990 it was written that more than 30% of gastrinomas were located in the pancreas in patients with MEN-1. Since the recognition of duodenal gastrinomas as the cause of ZES in patients with MEN-1, the incidence of pancreatic gastrinoma has been reported as less than 10% [19–21]. We should be careful about this point when reading the collected literature reporting patients with MEN-1 before 1987 [23].

So, there are two important issues in dealing with patients with ZES and MEN-1, one is how to perform curative resection for duodenal gastrinomas and the other is how to treat pancreatic endocrine tumors.

How to Perform Curative Resection of Duodenal Gastrinomas Before the Development of Liver Metastasis

Enucleation of duodenal gastrinomas through a duodenotomy has been successfully performed at many institutes. However a study at the National Institutes of Health (NIH; Bethesda, USA) reported that none of their ten consecutive patients with MEN-1 and ZES were cured by transduodenal resection. They report that this was attributable to a high rate (86%) of lymph node metastases and the fact that 30% of the patients had more than 20 duodenal gastrinomas [9]. They have not performed PD and did not follow those patients who underwent noncurative resection for long because the natural history of these patients remained unclear and surgical resection of all gastrinomas may not prolong survival [9,16]. Recently Gibril at the NIH reported the results of 57 patients with MEN-1 and ZES who had been followed for 8 years without receiving surgery until the pancreatic endocrine tumors grew larger than 2.5 cm [23]. As a result, 13 patients (23%) developed liver metastasis and 3 of them died of the disease; they suggested that a more aggressive surgical strategy should be applied to patients with aggressive-type tumors [23].

Thompson, who has applied aggressive transduodenal enucleations of duodenal gastrinomas combined with enucleation of any endocrine tumors in the head or uncinate process, and subtotal distal pancreatectomy for multiple microscopic or macroscopic tumors, reported that surgery has contributed to survival in 40 patients with MEN-1 and ZES, hypoglycemia, or both [21]. Of 34 patients with ZES, 23 (68%) remained eugastrinemic for as long as 19 years. One patient developed a single liver metastasis that was excised without any recurrence [21]. Thus, two-thirds of these patients may have the chance to be cured of ZES using aggressive resection of duodenal gastrinomas and dissection of the regional lymph nodes.

We have experienced 14 patients with MEN-1, including two patients with diffuse liver metastasis. We have successfully performed curative resections of gastrinomas for 12 patients who did not have distant metastasis. We have carried out PD for the first four patients between 1986 and 1989 after localization with the SASI test. In all of these patients, the duodenal gastrinoma (seven gastrinomas in one case, two gastrinomas in one, and one gastrinoma in two) was proved in the resected specimen, and in three of them regional lymph node metastases were proved, but no pancreatic gastrinoma was detected. They have been cured for as long as 18 years.

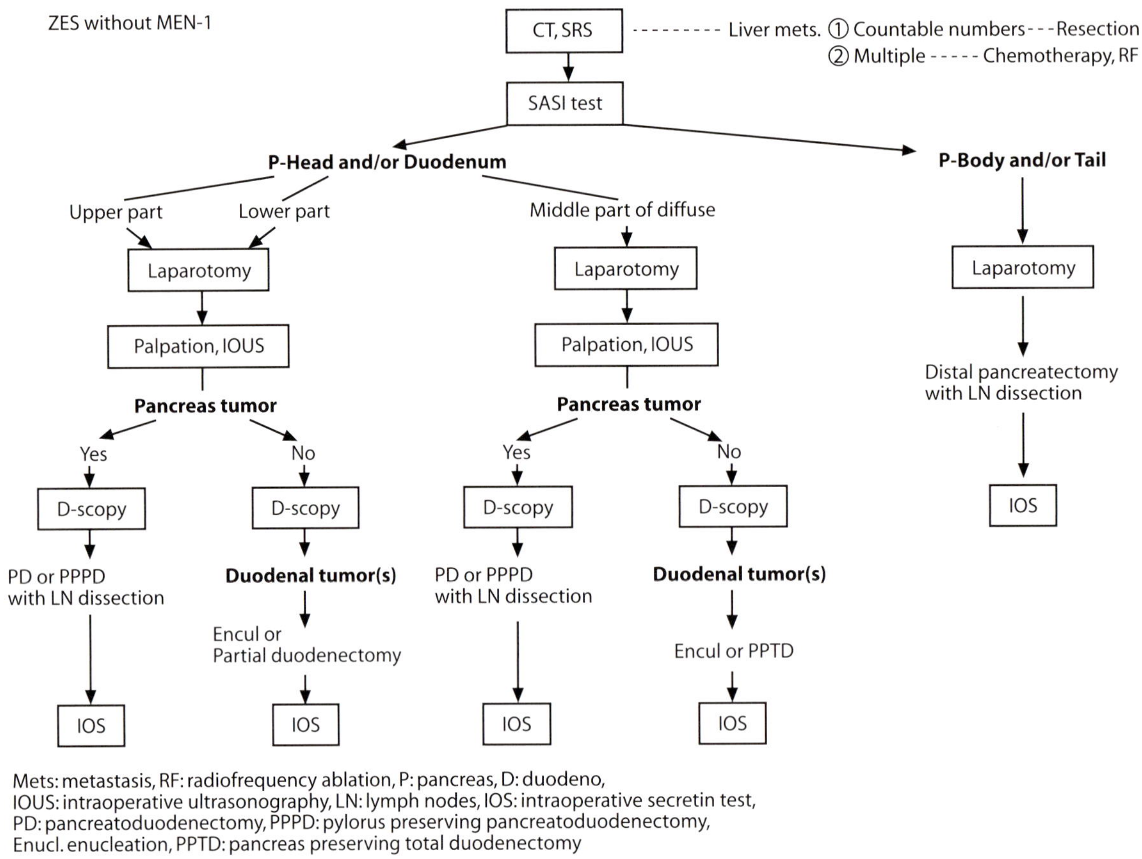

Figure 64.8

A flow chart showing the localization and treatment of tumors in patients with ZES and multiple endocrine neoplasm type 1 (MEN-1). CT and/or SRS are performed initially for the detection of distant metastases, and not for localization of the main tumor. In patients with ZES and MEN-1, there are usually multiple microscopic or macroscopic endocrine tumors scattered throughout the whole pancreas, the larger ones of which may be visualized by CT or SRS. Recent studies have revealed that few of these tumors are gastrinomas, and have shown that gastrinomas are predominantly located in the duodenum. For the localization of gastrinoma(s) and metastatic lymph nodes, we perform the SASI test, which is a reliable and essential study before curative resection of gastrinoma. When the SASI test localizes gastrinomas in either the duodenum or the pancreas, laparotomy is performed to search for the duodenal gastrinoma(s) by palpation and duodenoscopy. If several duodenal gastrinomas are detected, enucleation or partial duodenectomy is performed along with distal pancreatectomy and enucleation to remove the multiple pancreatic endocrine tumors and dissection of the regional lymph nodes. If there are widespread multiple gastrinomas in the duodenum, pancreas-preserving total duodenectomy (PPTD) is performed with dissection of the regional lymph nodes, as well as distal pancreatectomy and enucleation for the pancreatic endocrine tumors. When a gastrinoma is located in the body or tail of the pancreas, distal pancreatectomy is performed along with lymph node dissection and enucleation of the pancreatic head tumors

After these experiences, we changed our operation from PD to the enucleation of duodenal gastrinomas in 1990. Four patients underwent transduodenal enucleations and/or partial resection of the duodenum. Three of them had multiple duodenal gastrinomas and two of them had lymph node metastasis; all of them have been cured for 5–15 years. We encountered a patient in whom duodenoscopy revealed more than seven duodenal tumors. We performed PPTD instead of PD, and a pathological study revealed numerous microscopic duodenal gastrinomas in the resected specimen (Fig. 64.10). He has been cured for 1 year [35]. Since then, two patients have undergone PPTD and one partial resection of the duodenum.

Now, we believe that patients with a single duodenal gastrinoma will be cured by transduodenal enucleation with the dissection of regional lymph nodes. For patients with a few duodenal gastrinomas, partial resection of the duodenum is indicated when their location is deviated in either the upper or the lower part

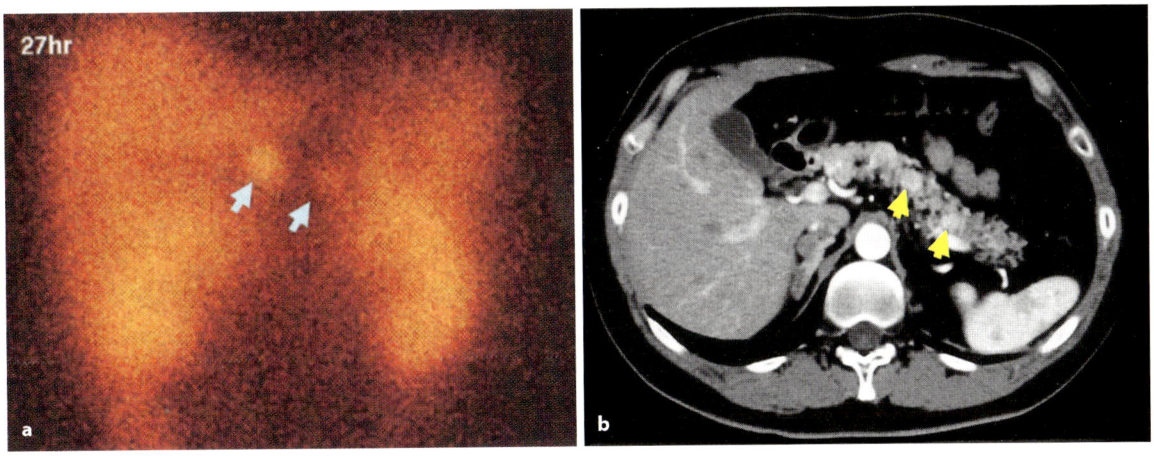

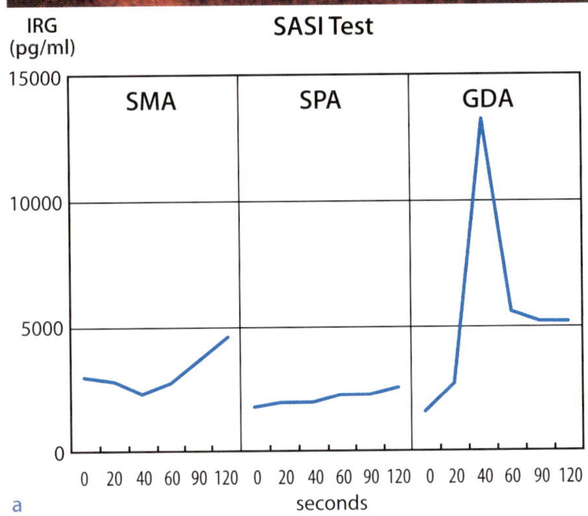

Figure 64.9

In this patient (case A) with ZES and MEN-1, SRS (a) and CT (b) visualized several endocrine tumors scattered throughout the whole pancreas (*arrows*). However, the SASI test (c) showed that the gastroduodenal artery was the only feeder for the gastrinoma(s). This indicated that the gastrinoma(s) were located in the proximal duodenum or head of the pancreas (more probably in the duodenum), while the pancreatic lesions visualized by CT and SRS were other endocrine tumors. Multiple duodenal gastrinomas were detected by preoperative duodenoscopy, and PPTD was performed

of the duodenum. For patients in whom multiple gastrinomas are located diffusely throughout the duodenum, PPTD is indicated. In either case, IOS should be performed for confirmation of the curability of the operation [32].

How to Treat Pancreatic Endocrine Tumors

As to the treatment of the pancreatic endocrine tumors other than the gastrinoma, there remain controversies [7–11,16,21]. The main issue is the prevention of liver metastases from these pancreatic tumors, because once it takes place the prognosis is limited [6–12]. Thompson reported a good result by performing subtotal distal pancreatectomy [21], although surgeons at the NIH had recommend local resection of pancreatic tumors larger than 2 or 3 cm in diameter, because the rate of liver metastasis is related to the size of the tumor [9,16]. As described above, Gibril at the NIH reported recently that their strategy has resulted in a high rate (23%) of liver metastasis in 8 years, which suggest that liver metastasis can take place regardless of the tumor size [23]. Lairmore et al., who performed prospective genetic testing on large numbers of MEN-1 families, also suggested that in a subset of these patients, endocrine tumors metastasize to the liver or distant sites more rapidly than had been expected. Future genetic testing may contribute to early recognition of the rapidly growing tumors [12]. Thus, subtotal distal pancreatectomy should be applied more often for preventing liver metastasis from the numerous microscopic or macroscopic pancreatic tumors [21,35]. Total pancreatectomy seems to be too invasive now. In the future, genetic testing might suggest to us the necessity for this operation for the aggressive type [12]. In any case, strict surveillance of the pancreatic tumors every 4–6 months with MRI or CT is important when treating MEN-1 patients [9].

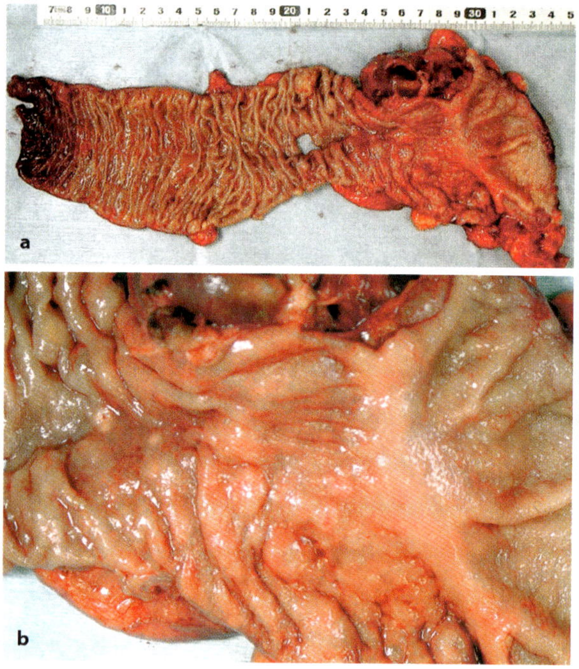

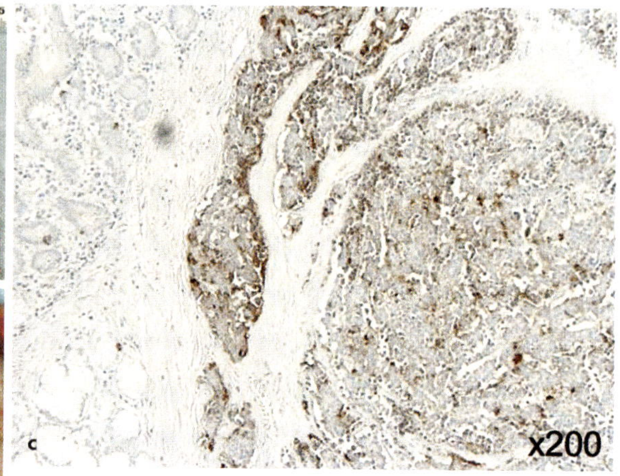

Figure 64.10

a En bloc surgical specimen obtained from case A (shown in Fig. 64.9) by PPTD. There are numerous minute submucosal tumors spread diffusely throughout the duodenum (b), which were confirmed to be gastrinomas by antigastrin antibody staining (c). The patient has been disease free for 2 years postoperatively

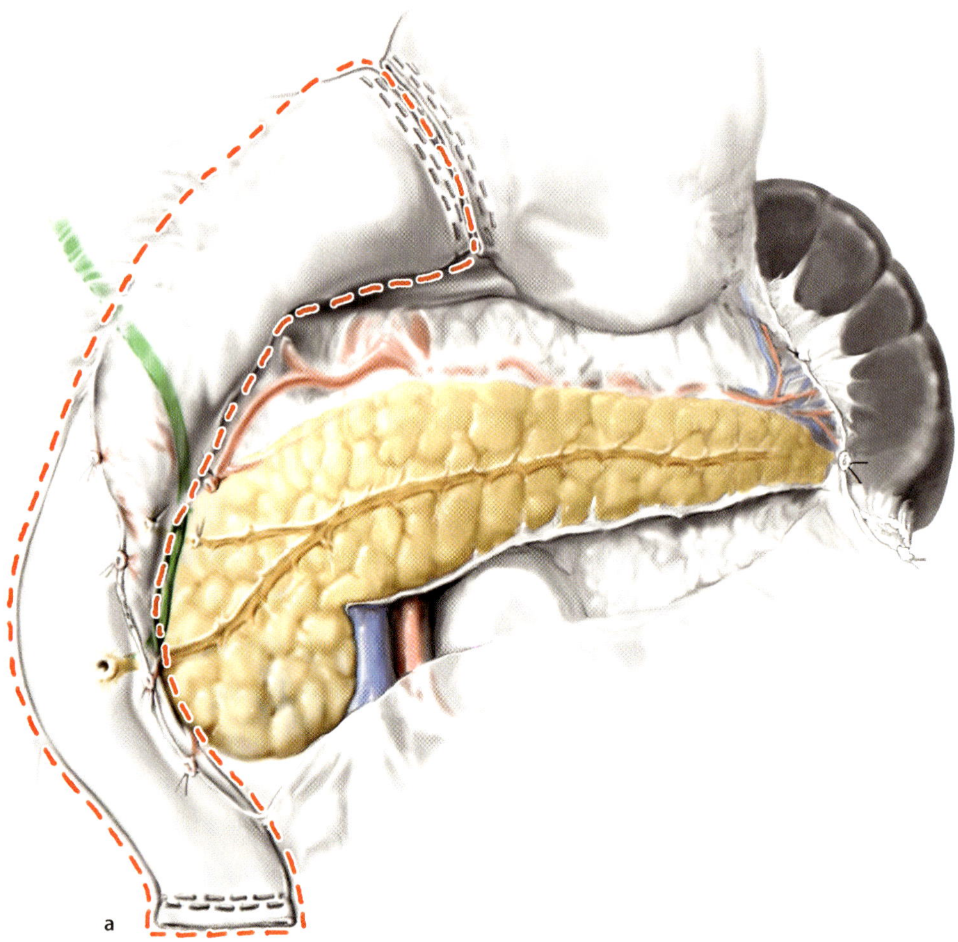

Figure 64.11 a

PPTD. The entire duodenum is resected, while preserving the whole pancreas. A functional major papilla is preserved by only stripping off the mucosa (a).

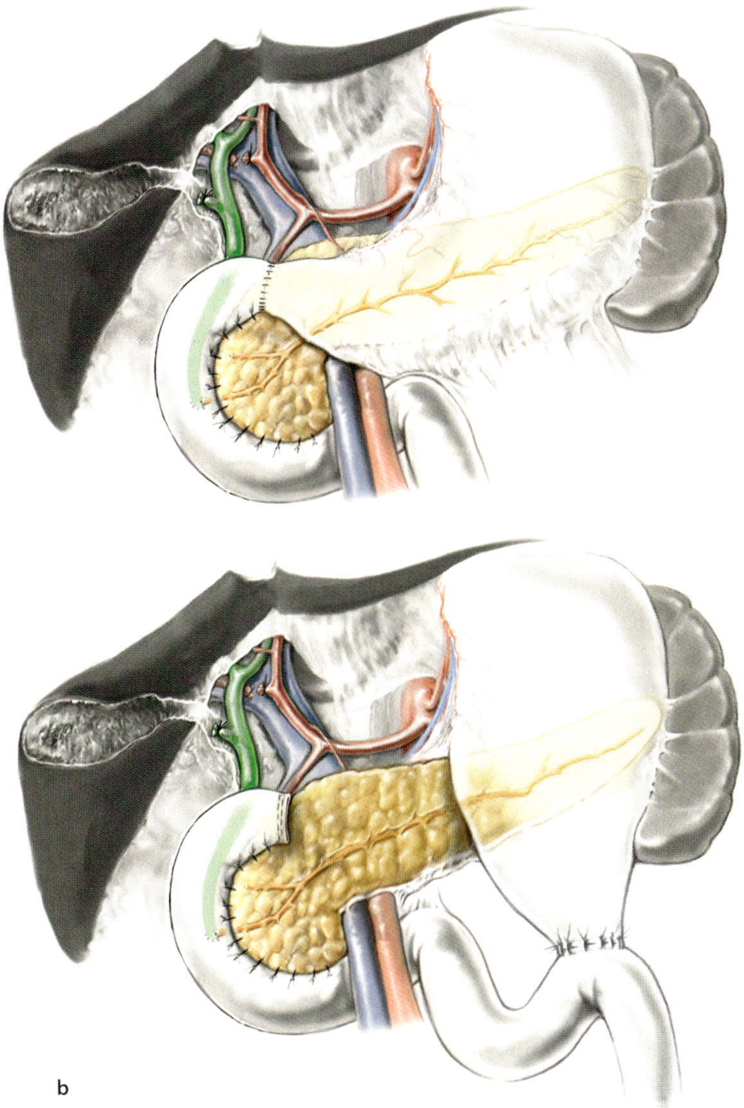

b

Figure 64.11 b

PPTD. The entire duodenum is resected, while preserving the whole pancreas. After incisional papillotomy, the opened papilla is anastomosed to a small incision in the jejunum for reconstruction. The alimentary tract is reconstructed by either a Billroth-1 or Billroth-2 technique (b)

A new PPTD Technique

PPTD was first performed for a patient with familiar adenomatous polyposis (FAP) by Chung et al. in 1995 [36]. PPTD is less invasive than PD. PPTD was first performed by us in 2004 for a patient with MEN-1 and numerous duodenal gastrinomas (Figs. 64.10 and 64.11). We improved Chung's technique and developed a new technique, that is, preservation of the papilla of Vater, stripping off only its mucosal layer, and after the papillotomy, the opened papilla is anastomosed with the jejunal small incision for biliopancreatic reconstruction [35]. We have applied this method to two additional patients with ZES and MEN-1 and three patients with other diseases (intestinal amyloidosis, gastrointestinal stromal tumor, and FAP). None of them had postoperative biliary or pancreatic complications, and all have been well postoperatively. This is a safe and less invasive surgery and could be applied more often to diffuse duodenal diseases including duodenal multiple gastrinomas.

References

1. Zollinger RM (1984) Treatment of gastrinoma. Mount Sinai J Med 51:401–403
2. Imamura M, Takahashi K, Adachi H, et al (1987) Usefulness of selective arterial secretin injection test for localization of gastrinoma in Zollinger-Ellison syndrome. Ann Surg 205:230–239
3. Rosato FE, Bonn J, Shapiro M, Barbot DJ, Furnary AM, Gardiner GA (1990) Selective arterial stimulation of secretin in localization of gastrinomas. Surg Gynecol Obstet 171:196–200
4. Doppman JL (1992) Pancreatic endocrine tumors – the search goes on. New Engl J Med 326:1770–1772
5. Thompson NW, Vinik AI, Eckhauser FE (1989) Microgastrinoma of the duodenum a cause of failed operations for the Zollinger–Ellison syndrome. Ann Surg 209:396–404
6. Schroder W, Hoelscher AH, Beckurts KT, Schusdziarra V, Hofler H, Siewelt Jr (1996) Surgical therapy of gastrinoma with associated Zolinger-Ellison syndrome. Z Gastroenterol 34:465–472
7. Thodiyil PA, El-Masry NS, Williamson RC (2001) Achieving eugastrinaemia in Zollinger-Ellison syndrome: resection or enucleation? Dig Surg 18:118–123
8. Plockinger U, Wiedenmann (2002) Neuroendocrine tumors of the gastro-entero-pancreatic system: the role of early diagnosis, genetic testing and preventive surgery. Dig Dis 20:49–60
9. Jensen RT (2001) Zollinger-Ellison syndrome. In: Doherty GM, Skogseid B (eds) Surgical Endocrinology. Lippincott Williams &Wilkins, Philadelphia, pp 291–343
10. Madeira I, Terris M, Voss M, et al (1998) Prognostic factors in patients with endocrine tumors of the duodenopancreatic area. Gut 43:422–427
11. Imamura M, Takahashi K, Isobe Y, Hattori Y, Tobe T (1989) Curative resection of multiple gastrinomas aided by selective arterial secretin injection test and intraoperative secretin test. Ann Surg 210:710–718
12. Lairmore TC, Piersall LD, DeBenedetti MK, et al (2004) Clinical genetic testing and early surgical intervention in patients with multiple endocrine neoplasia type 1 (MEN1). Ann Surg 239:637–647
13. Imamura M, Takahashi K (1993) Use of selective arterial secretin injection test to guide surgery in patients with Zollinger-Ellison syndrome. World J Surg 17:433–438
14. Imamura M (1999) Establishment of a new strategy for gastrinomas based on the basic research on endocrine tumors. Formos J Surg 32:197–201
15. Sarmiento JM, Farnell MB, Que FG, Nagorney DM (2002) Pancreaticoduodenectomy for islet tumors of the head of the pancreas, World J Surg 26:1267–1271
16. Norton JA, Jensen RT (2004) Resolved and unsolved controversies in the surgical management of patients with Zolinger-Ellison syndrome. Ann Surg 240:757–773
17. Krenning EP, Kwekkeboom DJ, Bakker WH (1993) Somatostatin receptor scintigraphy with [^{111}In-DTPA-D-Phen 1]- and [^{123}Ityr3]-octreotide: the Rotterdam experience with more than 1000 patients. Eur J Nucl Med 20:716–7317
18. Clark OH (1997) What's new in endocrine surgery J Am Coll Surg 184:126–136
19. Imamura M, Kanda M, Takahashi K, et al (1992) Clinicopathological characteristics of duodenal microgastrinomas. World J Surg 16:703–709
20. Pipeleers-Marichal M, Donow C, Heiz PU, Kloppel G (1993) Pathological aspects of gastrinomas in patients with Zollinger-Ellison syndrome with and without multiple endocrine neoplasia type 1. World J Surg 17:481–488
21. Thompson NW (1998) Current concepts in the surgical management of multiple endocrine neoplasia type 1 pancreatic–duodenal disease. Results in the treatment of 40 patients with Zollinger-Ellison syndrome, hypoglycaemia or both. J Intern Med 243:495–500
22. Delcore R, Cheung LY, Friesen SR (1988) Outcome of lymph node involvement in patients with the Zollinger-Ellison syndrome. Ann Surg 208:291–298
23. Gibril F, Venzon DJ, Ojeaburu JV, Bashir S, Jensen RT (2001) Prospective study of the natural history of gastrinoma in patients with MEN-1: definition of an aggressive and a nonaggressive form. J Clin Endocrinol Metab 86:5282–5293
24. Zogakis TG, Gibril F, Libutti SK, et al (2003) Management and outcome of patients with sporadic gastrinoma arising in the duodenum. Ann Surg 238:42–48
25. Imamura M, Adachi H, Takahashi K, Noguchi M, Mizutani N, Nakagawa M (1982) Gastrin release from gastrinoma cells stimulated with secretin. Dig Dis Sci 27:1130–1136
26. Passaro Ejr, Basso N, Walsh JH (1972) Calcium challenge in the Zollinger-Ellison syndrome. Surgery 72:60–67
27. Itami A, Kato M, Komoto I, Doi R, Imamura M (2001) Human gastrinoma cells express calcium-sensing receptor. Life Sci 70:119–127
28. Doppman JL, Miller DL, Chang R, et al (1990) Gastrinomas: localization by means of selective intraarterial injection of secretin. Radiology 174:25–29
29. Wada M, Komoto I, Doi R, Imamura M (2002) Intravenous calcium injection test is a novel complementary procedure in differential diagnosis for gastrinoma. World J Surg 26:1291–129
30. Turner LLO, Wren AM, Jackson JE, Thakker RV, Meeran K (2002) Localization of gastrinomas by selective intra-arterial calcium injection Clin Endocrinol 57:821–825
31. Noda S, Norton JA, Jensen RT, Gay WA Jr (1999) Surgical resection of intracardiac gastrinoma. Ann Thorac Surg 67:532–533
32. Kato M, Imamura M, Hosotani R, et al (2000) Curative resection of microgastrinomas based on the intraoperative secretin test. World J Surg 24:1425–1430
33. Chen H, Hardare JM, Uzar A, Cameron JL, Choti MA (1998) Isolated liver metastases from neuroendocrine tumors: does resection prolong survival? J Am Coll Surg 187:88–93
34. Okuzawa A, Kobayashi S, Sakamoto K, et al (2000) Metastatic gastrinoma to the liver after primary resection. J Gastroenterology 35:717–720
35. Imamura M, Komoto I, Doi R, Onodera H, Kobayashi H, Kawai Y (2005) New pancreas-preserving total duodenectomy technique. World J Surg 29:203–207
36. Chung RS, Church JM, Stolk R (1995) Pancreas-sparing duodenectomy: indications, surgical technique, and results. Surgery 117:254–259

Chapter 65

S. Egawa · M. Sunamura · S. Matsuno · M. Unno

Surgical Treatment of Rare Endocrine Tumors

Neoplasms of the endocrine pancreas are rare, with an incidence approximating five cases per one million person-years. The nationwide registration of the pancreatic neoplasm in Japan (Table 65.1) shows that the most frequent is nonfunctioning tumors, followed by insulinoma, glucagonoma, gastrinoma, pancreatic endocrine tumor associated with multiple endocrine neoplasia-1 (MEN-1) and others [1]. Out of 5,432 registered patients in leading hospitals in Japan, 100 cases (1.8%) harbored nonfunctioning tumors. Other types of endocrine tumors represent less than 1% of all cases. Since a limited number of referral hospitals have the experience of treating islet cell tumors, it is very important to draw a whole picture using a nationwide registry. The locus of the tumor does not correlate with the histological or hormonal characteristics, as shown in Table 65.2. Although the islets are distributed throughout the pancreas, the tumor does

Table 65.1. Endocrine tumors registered by the National Pancreatic Cancer Registry in Japan. MEN-1 Multiple endocrine neoplasia type 1

Tumor type	Resection 2001	Year 2002	2003	2004	Total
Insulinoma	12	11	14	8	45 (0.8%)
Gastrinoma	1	1	1	2	5 (0.1%)
Glucagonoma	3	2	0	2	7 (0.1%)
Somatostatinoma	0	0	1	0	1 (0.0%)
MEN-1	0	2	0	3	5 (0.1%)
Nonfunctioning tumor	16	27	28	29	100 (1.8%)
Other endocrine tumors	3	6	2	3	14 (0.3%)
Total pancreatic neoplasms	**1,289**	**1,267**	**1,436**	**1,440**	**5,432 (100.0%)**

Table 65.2. Correlation between the histology and the number and locus of the tumor

Number and Locus	Single	Multiple	Head	Body	Tail	Whole	Two regions	Undefined	Total
Insulinoma	42	2	15	15	13	0	2	0	45
Gastrinoma	4	1	2	1	1	0	1	0	5
Glucagonoma	6	1	1	5	0	1	0	0	7
Somatostatinoma	1	0	1	0	0	0	0	0	1
MEN-1	3	2	2	0	1	0	2	0	5
Nonfunctioning	86	11	41	23	28	1	4	2	99
Other	12	1	5	5	4	0	0	0	14
Total	**154**	**18**	**67**	**49**	**47**	**2**	**9**	**2**	**176**

Table 65.3. Histology and symptoms (National Pancreatic Cancer Registry in Japan 2001–2004)

Locus	None	Abdominal pain	Jaundice	Weight loss	Back pain	Diabetes Mellitus	Fatigue	Abdominal tumor	Other	Total
Insulinoma	4	0	0	0	0	3	1	0	37	45
Gastrinoma	2	1	0	1	0	0	0	0	1	5
Glucagonoma	4	1	0	1	1	0	0	0	0	7
Somatostatinoma	0	0	1	0	0	0	0	0	0	1
MEN-1	2	0	1	0	0	0	0	0	2	5
Nonfunctioning	50	23	3	5	7	4	3	1	4	100
Other	9	2	1	0	0	0	0	0	2	14
Total	71	27	6	7	8	7	4	1	45	177

not always show a multifocal nature even in hereditary MEN-1, suggesting a multistep tumorigenesis rather than a simple genetic alteration. As shown in Table 65.3, the clinical symptoms of rare endocrine tumors tend to be very subtle or nonspecific compared to insulinoma, resulting in the silent growth of the tumor.

In this chapter, surgical treatment based on the pathophysiological background of the rare endocrine tumors including two inherited types (MEN-1 and Von Hippel-Lindau, VHL) and nonfunctioning tumors will be described. Every type of pancreatectomy, including enucleation, should be applied to minimize the surgical risk, but we will focus on the case of an advanced endocrine tumor in the head of the pancreas to show the typical surgical treatment.

Pathophysiological Backgrounds

VIPoma (Watery Diarrhea, Hypokalemia and Achlorhydria syndrome)

Pathophysiology

Vasoactive intestinal peptide (VIP) is secreted by cells in the pancreatic islet and has a considerable degree of amino acid homology with secretin, pancreatic glucagons, and gastric inhibitory polypeptide [2]. In VIPoma patients, significant amounts of the macromolecular form of VIP were reported in the plasma [3]. VIP induces vasodilatation in most vascular beds and inhibits both acid and pepsin secretion. On the other hand, VIP stimulates intestinal secretion 1,000 times stronger than secretin. Considerable fecal loss of potassium (up to 300–400 Meq/day compared to healthy control 6–12 Meq/day) causes hypokalemia.

Symptoms

Patients with VIPoma characteristically present with intermittent severe diarrhea, averaging 5 l/day; the frequency of the bowel movement is, however, 4–5 times a day. The excretion looks like café au lait and does not contain blood, mucus, or fat. Hypokalemia results in muscular weakness, lethargy, and nausea. Patients sometimes present with glucose intolerance, hypercalcemia, flushing, and hypotension.

Glucagonoma

Pathophysiology

Glucagon causes hyperglycemia and decreases glucose oxidation. As glucagon exerts its action through the liver and fatty tissue, glucagon may be ineffective in cases of hepatic glycogen depletion. Glucagon has a well-known inhibitory action against gastric acid secretion in normal subjects and in patients with gastric ulcers through the inhibition of gastrin release. Glucagon also relaxes and dilates the stomach and duodenum as well as the choledochal sphincter, but induces rapid transit through the small intestine [4, 5].

Symptoms

The clinical syndrome associated with glucagonoma is characterized by severe dermatitis (termed necrolytic migratory erythema), mild diabetes, stomatitis (cheilitis), anemia, weight loss, and an increased tendency to thrombosis [6, 7]. Necrolytic migratory erythema may affect any site, but it most often affects the genital and anal region, the buttocks, groin, and lower legs. The rash fluctuates in severity. Initially there is a ring-shaped red area that blisters, erodes, and crusts over. It can be quite itchy and painful. It also results in a sore smooth tongue, a sore mouth, cracked dry lips, and ridging of the nails. It is not known how the rash arises. It may be due to a relative deficiency of zinc and essential fatty acids because the tumor reduces the amount of albumin. Excessive glucagon may increase the amount of inflammation in the skin, particularly in friction sites. It also raises blood glucose levels, which eventually leads to diabetes mellitus. It destroys protein and fat, resulting in weight loss, anemia, and low levels of amino acids.

Somatostatinoma

Pathophysiology and Symptoms

Somatostatin has effects on the gastrointestinal, cardiovascular, endocrine, hematologic, and genitourinary systems. The actions of somatostatin on the gastrointestinal tract are numerous. Somatostatin inhibits the secretion of the saliva, gastric acid, pepsin, and intrinsic factor [8]. Somatostatin significantly increases gastric mucus production in humans. Somatostatin inhibits the release of all known gastrointestinal hormones including gastrin, secretin, cholecystokinin, gastic inhibitory peptide, motilin, enteroglucagon, VIP and pancreatic polypeptide, insulin, and glucagon. Somatostatin is also known to decrease the release of thyroid hormones in humans. Gastric and gall bladder emptying is delayed by somatostatin. These inhibitory effects result in the nonspecific features of somatostatinoma syndrome including steatorrhea, diabetes, hypochlorhydria, and cholelithiasis.

Multiple Endocrine Neoplasia type 1

Pathophysiology

MEN-1 syndrome is caused by a point mutation in the *MEN-1* gene in an autosomal dominant trait [9]. The mutations are spread over the entire genome including introns, and there are no apparent "hot spots." About 70% of the mutations are non-sense and frameshift mutations resulting in truncation of the protein product, menin. Despite detailed study, no correlation between the genetic mutation and the phenotypic expression has been identified. About 20% of MEN-1 kindred lack an identified mutation in the *MEN-1* gene. Endocrine tumors from MEN-1 patients have loss of heterozygosity. The allelic loss is always from the normal chromosome belonging to the unaffected parent. The mutation of *MEN-1* gene has been identified in 31% of sporadic gastrinoma and less frequently (17% or less) in insulinoma. Approximately, one-third of patients with gastrinoma are associated with MEN-1. Thus, the *MEN-1* gene appears to play an important role in the tumorigenesis of both sporadic and familial endocrine tumors [10].

Symptoms

The clinical manifestations of MEN-1 depends on the individual tumors that are present in the patient, and their functionality. Since the most frequent islet cell neoplasm in MEN-1 is gastrinoma, hypergastrinemia can be detected in early stages of life. More than one clinical symptom may develop in the same patient either synchronously or metachronously. The pituitary adenoma in MEN-1 patients often secretes prolactin. In some patients, hypersecretion of adrenocorticotrophic hormone (ACTH) leads to Cushing's syndrome, or hypersecretion of growth hormone leads to acromegaly.

Von Hippel-Lindau Disease

Pathophysiology

VHL demonstrates an autosomal dominant pattern of inheritance. Germline inactivation of the VHL tumor suppressor gene causes VHL cancer syndrome, and somatic mutations of this gene have been linked to the development of sporadic hemangioblastomas and clear cell renal carcinomas. The VHL protein plays a central role in the mammalian oxygen-sensing pathway through its oxygen-dependent polyubiquitylation of hypoxia-inducible factors [11]. There are supposed to be "hot spots" or fragile sites within the gene associated with particular tumors such as renal carcinoma [12].

Symptoms

Other than retinal, cerebellar, spinal, and medullary hemangioblastomas, patients with VHL syndrome may develop renal cysts and carcinoma, pancreatic cysts, pancreatic tumors, pheochromocytoma, and papillary cystadenoma of the epididymis. The pancreatic tumors in VHL are usually nonfunctioning [13]. About 50% of VHL patients will only have one manifestation of VHL.

Nonfunctioning Islet Cell Tumor

Pathophysiology

The clinical features result from space-occupying or invasive lesions in the pancreas, including abdominal pain, weight loss, and jaundice (Table 65.3). Tumors may be palpated by the patients themselves or found occasionally by the abdominal ultrasound at the health check. The malignant potential of these tumors is 50–90%. However, the growth tends to be slow, with more favorable survival than invasive ductal carcinoma of the pancreas.

Resected specimens frequently show intracellular production of hormones, indicating the islet cell origin. Currently, the tumorigenesis of nonfunctioning islet cell tumors is not well known. *DPC4/smad 4* gene mutation does not play a central role [14].

Diagnosis

Tumor localization and staging begins with abdominal ultrasonography and computed tomography (CT) scan with intravenous contrast because these tumors are usually large and solitary. If the CT scan cannot detect the tumor in the pancreas, extrapancreatic lesion including neural crest tumor should be examined. Endoscopic ultrasonography is useful for detecting small-size lesions in the duodenal wall and pancreas. Angiography has a relatively low positive-predictive value (60–80%) [15], but is useful for the selective infusion of secretin (selective arterial secretagogue injection test) or calcium (selective arterial calcium injection test) for the functional localization of the tumor [16]. Somatostatin analogue scintigraphy is useful for detecting small tumors and extrapancreatic lesions, since the tumor overexpresses the receptor [17–19], however, the false negative rate is considerable [20].

In VIPoma, exclusion of other common cases of diarrhea should be made. Elevation of serum VIP (healthy control <50 pg/ml) should be proved. In glucagonoma, the diagnosis may be suggested by the clinical presentation and biopsy sampling of the skin lesions. The elevated levels of serum glucagon should be documented. The malignant potential of glucagonoma is high, and metastases to the liver or lymph nodes have been found in the majority of patients.

In somatostatinoma, elevated blood levels of somatostatin have been found. However, elevated plasma somatostatin levels can be found in other types of tumor, including thyroid medullary carcinoma, pheochromocytoma, small-cell carcinoma of the lung, bronchial tumor, and thymic tumor. These patients do not exhibit so-called somatostatinoma syndrome. The liver is a frequent metastatic site, followed by bone and other organs. Some patients may show the excess secretion of ACTH, calcitonin, insulin, and gastrin. Somatostatin analogue scintigraphy is reported to be useful in the diagnosis of somatostatinoma [21].

The hormonal assessment of MEN-1 comprises of the assessment of affected glands. Hyperparathyroidism is diagnosed by the presence of hypercalcemia associated with elevated parathyroid hormone levels. Pituitary adenomas are usually associated with elevated serum prolactin or somatomedin C. The imaging modalities often meet challenges since the tumor size in MEN-1 syndrome is relatively small, the location is frequently duodenal, and it may be multifocal. Once MEN-1 is diagnosed in the proband, careful and skilled genetic counseling and genetic testing should be considered in all family members. Those family members who carry the mutated MEN-1 gene should undergo yearly biochemical screening from childhood. Early detection and treatment should reduce the morbidity and mortality.

With respect to VHL, if a family history of retinal or central nervous system hemangioblastoma exists, only one hemangioblastoma or visceral lesion is required to make the diagnosis. The age of onset of VHL is variable and depends on the expression of the disease within an individual, within a family, and the intensity with which asymptomatic lesions are sought.

An intensive screening program can greatly increase the number of known affected individuals in a family. Retinal lesions generally occur first. The mean ages of diagnosis of retinal hemangioblastoma, cerebellar hemangioblastoma, and renal cell carcinoma are 25 years, 30 years, and 37 years, respectively [22]; however, only a minority of patients are discovered before age 10 years. Families with pheochromocytoma as a principle feature of their disease often develop pheochromocytomas before other manifestations of VHL.

The psychological and financial impact of hereditary syndromes like MEN-1 and VHL on individuals and families can be devastating. Denial, anxiety, guilt, isolation, overprotectiveness, and general personality disturbances can be observed. These represent adaptations to the severe chronic stress imposed upon individuals and families. Fortunately, with careful and early medical attention many complications can either be avoided or ameliorated. There is growing optimism that the diagnosis can be made earlier and more accurately with genetic testing. It should be noted that the exact gene mutation has not been identified in certain patients. Thus, patients with negative genetic tests should still be tested periodically for the major complications.

In nonfunctioning tumors, imaging studies for localization and staging with hormonal assays should be performed to exclude functional tumors. Nonfunctioning islet cell tumors frequently retain the ability to secrete significant amounts of chromogranin A. Peracchi et al. reported the elevated plasma chromogranin A levels in gastro-entero-pancreatic neuroendocrine tumors, including nonfunctioning ones, with 92% sensitivity and 83% specificity when taking 20 U/l as a cutoff [23]. In their study, plasma chromogranin A levels were significantly higher in patients with functioning tumors than in patients with nonfunctioning tumors.

For somatostatinoma, administration of a somatostatin analogue is effective for improving the diabetes and diarrhea of somatostatinoma syndrome [21]. MEN-1, the most life-threatening tumor, should be considered as the first candidate to be resected. The operations are performed metachronously rather than synchronously. Radiation may be indicated for the treatment of pituitary tumor. Understanding of the pathophysiological basis of this syndrome and coordination of physicians and surgeons is critically important to treat the patient successfully. Most patients can be managed successfully by medical treatment including proton pump inhibitors and somatostatin analogues. Patients with prolactinoma should initially be treated with bromocriptine or other dopamine analogs. Octreotide reduces pituitary adenoma size and growth hormone secretion in a significant number of patients. There is no universal agreement as to the indications for surgery for pancreatic disease in MEN-1 patients. Many believe that patients with gastrinoma should be explored because of the high risk of malignancy. Since all MEN-1 patients have diffuse islet cell dysplasia, microadenomatosis, and/or discrete islet cell tumors, a cure can only be achieved in a minority of patients.

In VHL, hemangioblastoma in the central nervous system and pheochromocytoma can be life threatening and should be treated first. The hormonal assessment and imaging diagnosis of islet cell tumors should be employed to determine the nature, location, and extent of the pancreatic tumors. In hereditary syndromes, genetic counseling has to be based on individual medical experience of the doctor adjusted to common guidelines and the findings in the family. Paramedics who have been trained in counseling are required as a network that will guarantee periodic clinical examination and secure optimal prevention [26].

Preparation for Surgical Procedure

The preparation for surgical exploration depends on the mediators that alternate the general conditions. In VIPoma, it must include correction of fluid and electrolyte losses. Preoperative administration of octreotide can be an important adjunct, as octreotide leads to a reduction in circulating VIP levels and decrease of the volume of diarrhea. In glucagonoma, while waiting for surgery, administration of a somatostatin analogue may be helpful in controlling hyperglycemia and dermatitis [24, 25]. Zinc supplements can result in complete resolution of the rash in some patients.

Rationale for the procedure

Once the diagnosis of endocrine tumor has been made, the resection should be considered as the first choice. The malignant potential of rare endocrine tumors is high, but their aggressiveness is far better than that of invasive ductal carcinoma of the pancreas. If there are distant metastases, the resection is controversial. As shown in Fig. 65.1, the 2-year survival of Japanese patients with nonfunctioning tumor is 90.5% if there is no liver metastasis at the time of operation, while that of patients with liver metastasis is 83.3% when the primary tumor is resected and 27.3% without resection.

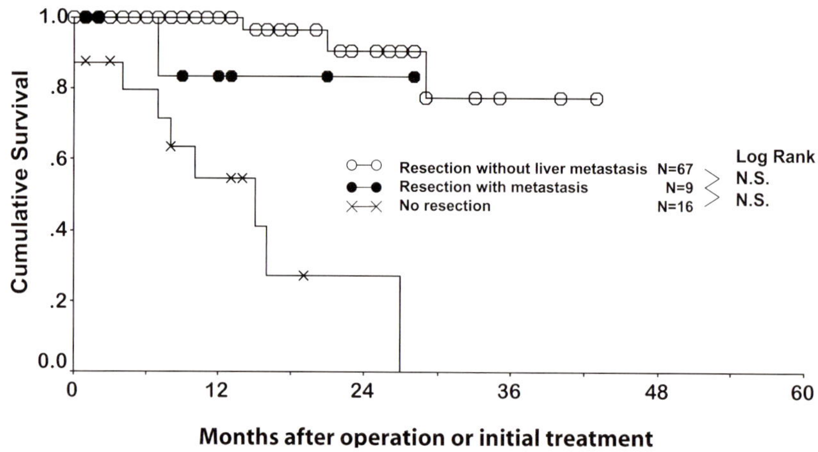

Figure 65.1

Liver metastases and resection affecting the survival of nonfunctioning islet cell tumors. The cumulative survival of patients with nonfunctioning islet cell tumors in Japan was calculated using the Kaplan-Meier method and tested with the log-rank method. The patients were treated in leading hospitals in Japan during the period 2001–2004 and registered to the national pancreatic cancer registry. *Open circles* Patients who did not have any metastasis and underwent pancreatectomy; *closed circles* patients who underwent pancreatectomy even though they had liver metastases at the time of operation; *crosses* patients who did not undergo pancreatectomy mainly because they had liver metastases. *N.S.* Not significant

Depending on the location and the extent of tumor, every kind of pancreatectomy procedure can be employed. If the tumor is larger than 3 cm in size, an appropriate pancreatectomy should be performed since the development of a postenucleation pancreatic fistula is highly likely. Even in a smaller-sized tumor, injury to the main pancreatic duct should be avoided. Once the tumor surface is exposed, traction suture should be placed to help fine dissection along with the tumor capsule to avoid duct injury. In larger tumors, such as nonfunctioning tumor or somatostatinoma, combined resection of the portal vein or other organs may be required due to the invasive nature. Since islet cell tumors are slow growing, safe debulking procedures and/or bypass procedures may be performed.

In this chapter, a VHL case with an advanced tumor in the head with another lesion in the tail of the pancreas and multiple liver metastases is shown as an example. This 35-year-old man had a past history of a bleeding duodenal ulcer and retinal hemangioma when he was 19 years old and underwent the resection of bilateral pheochromocytoma when he was 20 years old followed by steroid coverage. Follow-up ultrasound detected the tumor in the head of the pancreas without any hormonal excess. CT scan with contrast enhancement revealed a large tumor with peripheral vascular enhancement in the head of the pancreas that had invaded the superior mesenteric vein (Fig. 65.2A). There were hypervascular tumors in the tail (Fig. 65.2B) and multiple small hypervascular liver metastases (Fig. 65.2C). A positron emission tomography scan shows the uptake of the primary tumor but fails to show the small liver metastases. After debating with gastroenterologists, pancreaticoduodenectomy with partial resection of the portal vein was selected to reduce the possible source of liver metastasis.

Procedures

Access and Intra-abdominal Examination

A bilateral subcostal incision is preferable since careful evaluation of the whole pancreas and peripancreatic lesions should be performed. The liver is carefully assessed for metastatic disease. Potential extrapancreatic tumor sites should be evaluated carefully in all cases. In particular, the duodenum, splenic hilum, and small bowel and its mesentery, peripancreatic lymph nodes and retroperitoneum should be carefully examined. Intraoperative ultrasonography helps to identify the tumor and to decide to enucleate the tumor or to resect by pancreatectomy. In functional tumor settings, intraportal catheterization from ileocolic vein is carried out to measure the portal venous concentration of the hormone and/or chromogranin A.

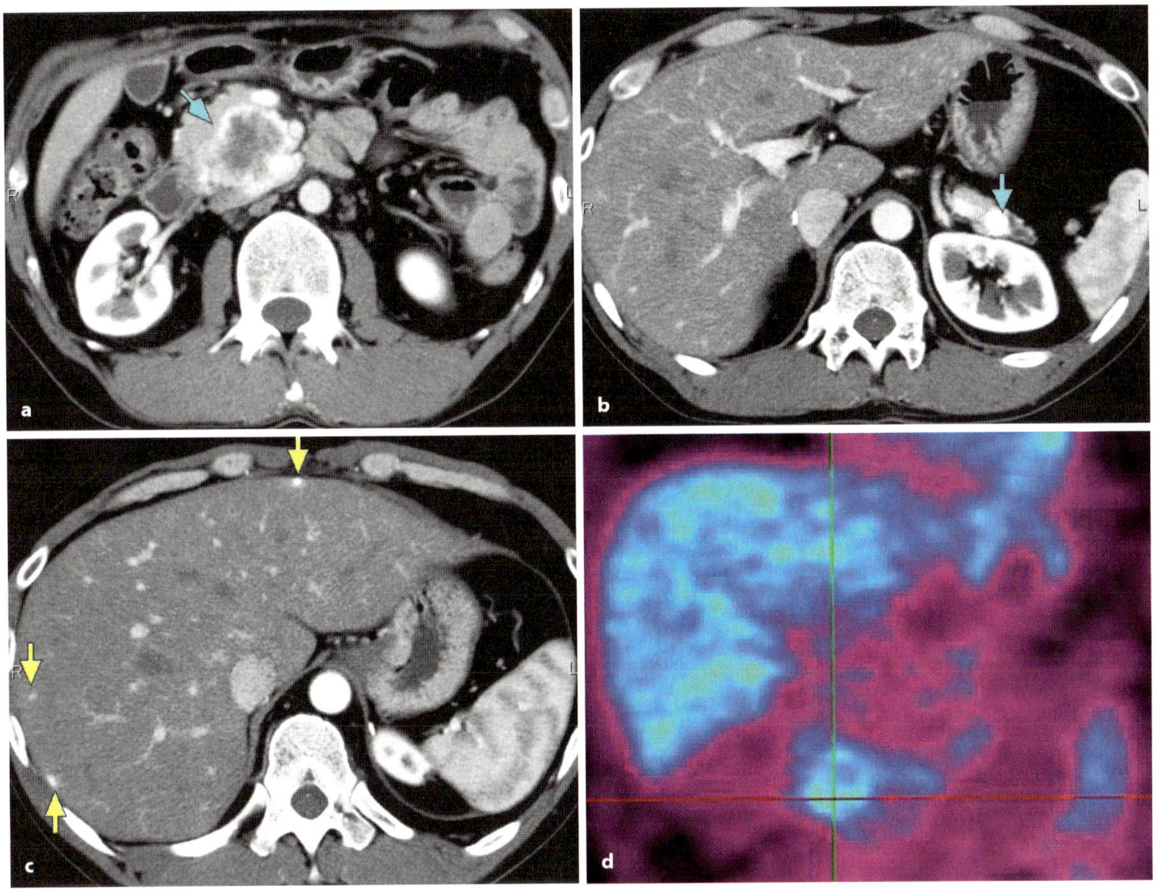

Figure 65.2

Computed tomography (a–c) and positron emission tomography (PET; d) scans of a patient with Von Hippel-Lindau disease. A 35-year-old man showed a hypervascular tumor invading to the superior mesenteric vein (*blue arrow* in a). There was a hypervascular tumor in the tail of the pancreas (*blue arrow* in b). There were multiple hypervascular liver metastases (*yellow arrows* in c). The PET scan depicts the primary tumor in the head, but failed to show the tumor in the tail, and the liver metastases (d)

Principal Surgical Steps

Mobilization of the Duodenum and the Head of the Pancreas

The lateral peritoneal attachments of the duodenum are incised, and the duodenum, head of the pancreas, common bile duct, and portal vein are mobilized by sharp and blunt dissection posteriorly. If possible, the root of superior mesenteric artery (SMA) is taped. The hepatic flexure of the colon may need to be mobilized.

Prepyloric Division of the Stomach

The gastrocolic omentum is divided to expose the anterior surface of the pancreas. The points for resection at 4 cm proximal from the pyloric ring are selected on both greater and lesser curves and the necessary dissection in both the gastrohepatic and gastrocolic omenta is done. The stomach is divided with a stapler.

Cholecystectomy and Dissection of Choledochus

The gall bladder is dissected from its fundus and the common bile duct is divided, and a noncrushing clip is placed to occlude the proximal portion temporarily.

Transection of the Pancreas

The proper hepatic artery and common hepatic artery are identified and taped to identify the gastroduodenal artery. The root of gastroduodenal artery should be double ligated with one free tie and a suture

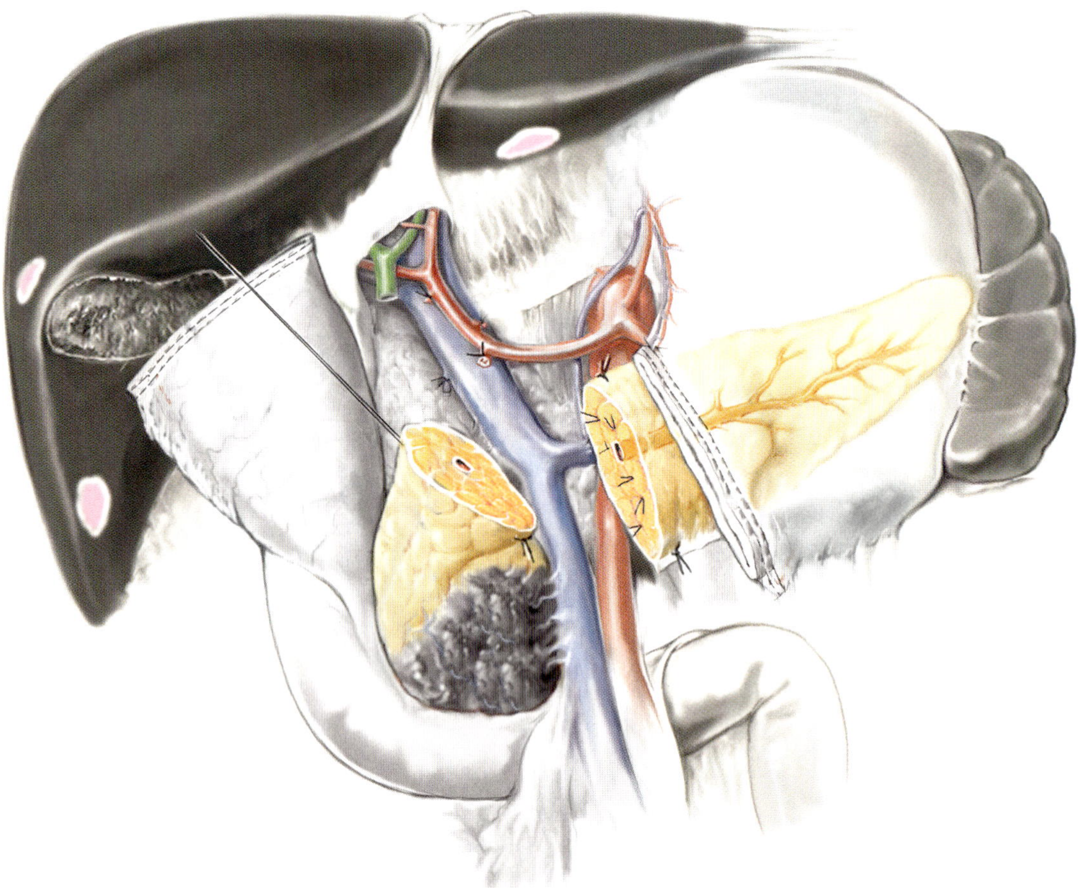

Figure 65.3

Transection of the pancreas

ligature with 5-0 non-absorbable Pronova, since postoperative bleeding from this source can be fatal. The SMV is identified as it course under the pancreas (Fig. 65.3). The dissection of the neck of the pancreas from the superior mesenteric and portal veins behind it should be carried out from the inferior border of the pancreas. When resistance is encountered, however, it may be useful to alternate the dissection between the superior and inferior borders. It is unusual to encounter any vessels during this dissection, since most of the tributaries enter the vein from its lateral and posterior aspects. When the dissection is complete, the neck of the pancreas is taped. Next, hemostatic transfixion sutures are placed through the pancreatic tissue to occlude the transverse arteries in the superior border and two in the inferior border of the gland on either side of the proposed line of transection. The pancreas is then divided sharply and bleeders are controlled with suture ligatures of 6-0 polydioxanone (PDS). The pancreatic duct is identified.

Dissection of the Jejunum

The peritoneal attachments of the first 15 cm of the jejunum is incised. The proximal jejunum is divided with a stapler at a point where the vascular arcades will allow the creation of adequate length of bowel for the subsequent anastomoses. The third and fourth portions of the duodenum are dissected bluntly from the posterior abdominal wall, and the transected proximal jejunum is then passed under the superior mesenteric vessels and delivered to the area of previous dissection.

Division of the Portal Vein and En Bloc Resection of the Pancreatic Head

During the separation of the pancreas from the lateral aspect of the SMV and portal veins, the small vessels should be ligated in continuity and then divided. This is safer than the application of clamps, which should be avoided. The mesoduodenum and the mesentery

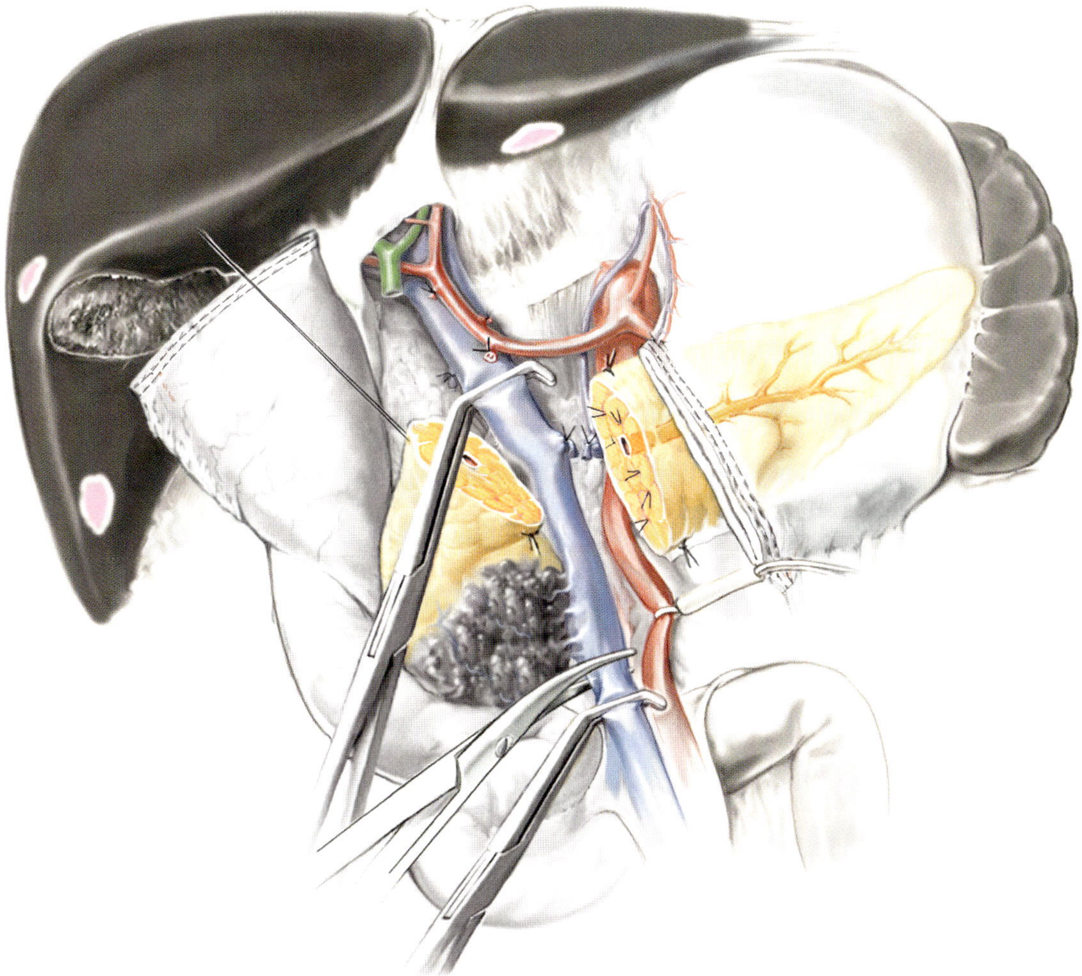

Figure 65.4

Resection of the portal vein

of the uncinate process, which include inferior pancreaticoduodenal arteries and peripancreatic nerve plexus, are dissected so that the portal invasion becomes the last attachment. The splenic vein can be divided and ligated if it is difficult to preserve. The portal invasion is clamped with vascular clamps and resected after clamping the SMA to avoid congestion (Fig. 65.4). The length of the resected portal vein should be less than 4 cm when no vascular graft is prepared. the saphena magna vein or left renal vein can be used as a graft if the resection exceeds 4 cm. Intraoperative frozen sections should be made to confirm that an appropriate resection was performed.

End-to-End Anastomosis of the Portal Vein

The portal vein is reconstructed with end-to-end vascular anastomosis (Fig. 65.5). Two vascular clamps are placed in parallel and a running suture with 5-0 Pronova is made with 1 mm bite and 1 mm pitch. The knot should be placed outside of the lumen. Another 5-0 Pronova is placed to retract the other end. Heparinized saline should be applied intermittently. When the suture reaches the other end, the two strings are ligated to remain a growth factor for the blood flow. Then the clamps are inverted to the other side so that the suture can be continued on the anterior surface of the vessels. After completing the anastomosis, the distal clamp should be removed first to inflate the anastomosis to see if there is any leakage; these can be fixed with transfixing suture.

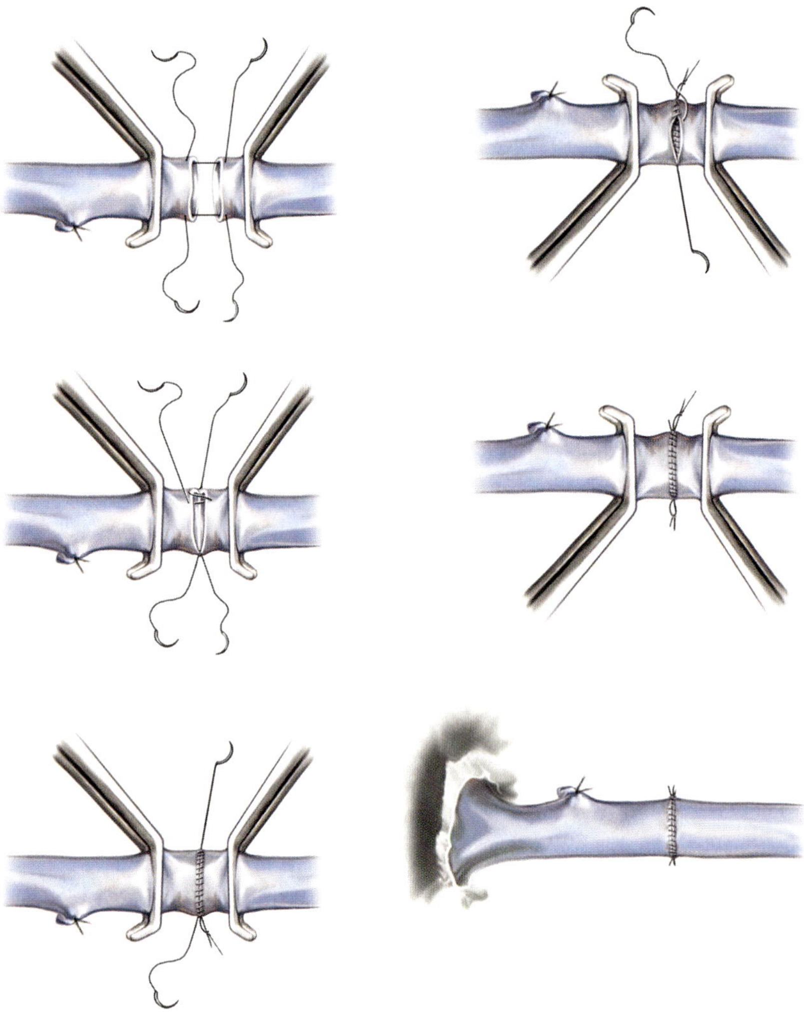

Figure 65.5

End-to-end anastomosis of the portal vein. The vascular clamps are rotated to the left side of the body and the anterior wall is sutured from the left end. After ligation with growth factor, the clamps are inverted and the suture is again continued on the anterior wall

Pancreaticojejunostomy

A pancreaticojejunostomy is performed first (Fig. 65.6). The jejunal limb can be passed through posterior of superior mesenteric vessels or through a hole opened in the mesocolon. The serosa of the jejunal limb is incised with a fine scalpel to create a serosal island surrounding the anastomotic opening and outer exposure of the subserosal layer to fit the transected end of the pancreas. A meticulous mucosa-to-mucosa anastomosis by 6-0 PDS interrupted suture is made between the duct and a small opening in the jejunum. The pancreas is approximated to the jejunal subserosal by an anterior and a posterior row of interrupted sutures of Pronova. No pancreatic duct stent is necessary

Choledochojejunostomy

The choledochojejunal anastomosis is performed next at a sufficient distance from the pancreas to avoid tension on the suture lines, but not far enough to allow kinking of the bowel. A single layer of interrupted 4-0 Biosyn sutures of is performed. No bile duct stent is necessary. When the duct is not thickened, thinner suture material may be used.

Gastrojejunostomy

Finally, an antecolic gastrojejunostomy is constructed about 40 cm distal to the choledochojejunostomy in a standard layer-to-layer fashion. If the pancreatic parenchyma is normal and the possibility of pancreatic fistula is expected, a tube jejunostomy can be placed distal to gastrojejunostomy.

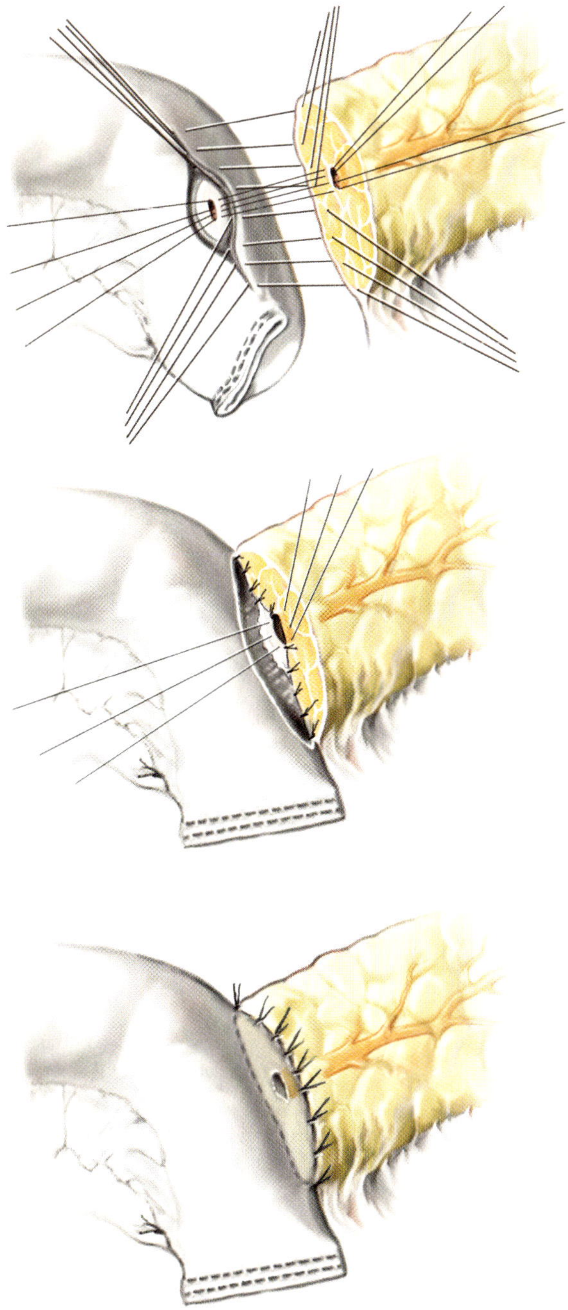

Figure 65.6

Mucosa-to-mucosa pancreaticojejunostomy. Prior to the posterior wall of the pancreatic parenchyma, the anterior wall of the pancreatic duct is retracted with three 6-0 polydioxanone sutures. The ligation will be done after all of the posterior wall of the parenchyma-serosa suture and duct-mucosa suture is placed. The anterior wall of the pancreatic duct is sewn using the retraction sutures. The anterior parenchyma and serosa is sutured with 5-0 Pronova

Closure of the Abdomen

A set of Penrose and Duple drains is placed at the superior border of the pancreaticojejunostomy for the postoperative suction (Fig. 65.7). Two closed suction drains are placed in the right subphrenic space and subhepatic space. A nasogastric tube is placed in the stomach. After the abdomen is irrigated, it is closed in layers.

Early Postoperative Course

The suction of the pancreaticojejunostomy can be stopped if the output is serous and less than 100 ml/day. The gastric tube can be removed if the output is serous and less than 100 ml/day. The first oral water intake is allowed after the first bowel movement without any sign of intestinal obstruction. Oral food intake is allowed if the amylase concentration of the pancreaticojejunostomy is less than 1,000 IU/ml and the discharge is serous at postoperative day (POD) 5 or up to POD 7. If a pancreatic fistula occurs, the oral intake should be postponed and the appropriate drainage and irrigation is required to avoid intra-abdominal abscess formation, which could be fatal.

If there is no leakage, the Penrose drain can be removed on POD 6 and the Duple drain can be removed on POD 7 after confirming that oral food intake did not cause any harm to the anastomosis.

Late Outcomes

The malignant potential of rare islet cell tumors is relatively higher than insulinoma. In MEN-1 and VHL patients, the lesions are multicentric and lifelong follow up is required. The cumulative 5-year survival of the patients after pancreatectomy for islet cell tumor in Japan is 74.3% [1], while that of the patients with nonfunctioning islet cell tumor is 50% [27].

Administration of a somatostatin analogue is effective in most of the recurrent and metastatic cases. Although even with optimal management, symptomatic neuroendocrine tumors may metastasize to the liver, but Chung et al. reported that hepatic cytoreduction can palliate progressive symptoms and postoperative administration of octreotide long-acting release (LAR) achieved 60 months median symptom-free interval, compared to 16 months achieved using other chemotherapeutic agents [28].

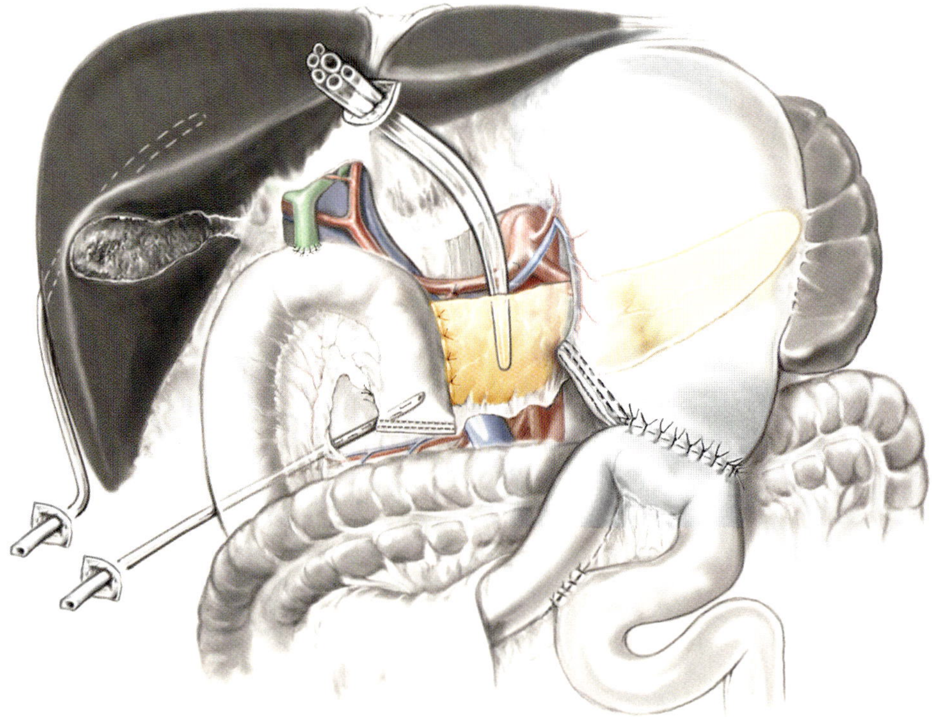

Figure 65.7

Placement of drains. After completion of all anastomoses, the peritoneal cavities are irrigated. A set of Penrose and Duple drains is placed at the superior border of the pancreaticojejunostomy. Two suction drains are placed in the right subphrenic and subhepatic spaces

References

1. Matsuno S, Egawa S, Fukuyama S, Motoi F, Sunamura M, Isaji S, Imaizumi T, Okada S, Kato H, Suda K, Nakao A, Hiraoka T, Hosotani R, Takeda K (2004) Pancreatic Cancer Registry in Japan: 20 years of experience. Pancreas 28:219–230
2. Said SI, Mutt V (1972) Isolation from porcine-intestinal wall of a vasoactive octacosapeptide related to secretin and to glucagons. Eur J Biochem 28:199–204
3. Yamaguchi K, Abe K, Miyakawa S, Ohnami S, Sakagami M, Yanaihara N (1980) The presence of macromolecular vasoactive intestinal polypeptide (VIP) in VIP-producing tumors. Gastroenterology 79:687–694
4. Miller RE, Chernish SM, Greenman GF, Maglinte DD, Rosenak BD, Brunelle RL (1982) Gastrointestinal response to minute doses of glucagon. Radiology 143:317–320
5. Carr-Locke DL, Gregg JA, Aoki TT (1983) Effects of exogenous glucagon on pancreatic and biliary ductal and sphincteric pressures in man demonstrated by endoscopic manometry and correlation with plasma glucagon. Dig Dis Sci 28:312–320
6. Higgins GA, Recant L, Fischman AB (1979) The glucagonoma syndrome: surgically curable diabetes. Am J Surg 137:142–148
7. Marx M, Newman JB, Guice KS, Nealon WH, Townsend CM, Thompson JC (1987) Clinical significance of gastrointestinal hormones. In: Thompson JC, Greeley GH, Rayford PL, Townsend CM Jr (eds) Gastrointestinal Endocrinology. McGraw-Hill, New York, pp 409–428
8. Arnold R, Lankisch PG (1980) Somatostatin and the gastrointestinal tract. Clin Gastroenterol 9:733–753
9. Chandrasekharappa SC, Guru SC, Manickam P, Olufemi SE, Collins FS, Emmert-Buck MR, Debelenko LV, Zhuang ZP, Lubensky IA, Liotta LA, Crabtree JS, Wang Y, Roe BA, Weisemann, J, Boguski MS, Agarwal SK, Kester MB, Kim YS, Heppner C, Dong Q, Spiegel AM, Lee Burns A, Marx SJ (1997) Positional cloning of the gene for multiple endocrine neoplasia type 1. Science 276:404–407
10. Zhuang Z, Vortmeyer AO, Pack S, Huang S, Pham TA, Wang C, Park WS, Agarwal SK, Debelenko LV, Kester M, Guru SC, Manickam P, Olufemi SE, Yu F, Heppner C, Crabtree JS, Skarulis MC, Venzon DJ, Emmert-Buck MR, Spiegel AM, Chandrasekharappa SC, Collins FS, Burns AL, Marx SJ, Jensen RT, Liotta LA, Lubensky IA (1997) Somatic mutations in the MEN1 tumor suppressor gene in sporadic gastrinomas and insulinomas. Cancer Res 57:4682–4686
11. Kim WY, Kaelin WG (2005) Role of VHL gene mutation in human cancer. J Clin Oncol 22:4991–5004
12. Chen F, Kishida T, Yao M, Hustad T, Glavac D, Dean M, Gnarra JR, Orcutt ML, Duh FM, Glenn G (1995) Germline mutations in the von Hippel-Lindau disease tumor suppressor gene: correlations with phenotype. Hum Mutat 5:66–75

13. Melmon KL, Rosen SW (1964) Lindau's disease. Am J Med 36:595–617
14. Perren A, Saremaslani P, Schmid S, Bonvin C, Locher T, Roth J, Heitz PU, Komminoth P (2003) DPC4/Smad4: no mutations, rare allelic imbalances, and retained protein expression in pancreatic endocrine tumors. Diagn Mol Pathol 12:181–186
15. Phan GQ, Yeo CJ, Hruban RH, Lillemoe KD, Pitt HA, Cameron JL (1998) Surgical experience with pancreatic and peripancreatic neuroendocrine tumors: review of 125 patients. J Gastrointest Surg 2:472–482
16. Imamura M, Takahashi K, Adachi H, Minematsu S, Shimada Y, Naito M, Suzuki T, Tobe T, Azuma T (1987) Usefulness of selective arterial secretin injection test for localization of gastrinoma in the Zollinger-Ellison syndrome. Ann Surg 205:230–239
17. Nauck C, Ivancevic V, Emrich D, Creutzfeldt W (1994) 111In-pentetreotide (somatostatin analogue) scintigraphy as an imaging procedure for endocrine gastro-entero-pancreatic tumors. Z Gastroenterol 32:323–327
18. Nikou GC, Toubanakis C, Nikolaou P, Giannatou E, Safioleas M, Mallas E, Polyzos A (2005) VIPomas: an update in diagnosis and management in a series of 11 patients. Hepatogastroenterology 52:1259–1265
19. Virgolini I, Traub-Weidinger T, Decristoforo C (2005) Nuclear medicine in the detection and management of pancreatic islet-cell tumours. Best Pract Res Clin Endocrinol Metab 19:213–227
20. Yim JH, Siegel BA, DeBenedetti MK, Norton JA, Lairmore TC, Doherty GM (1998) Prospective study of the utility of somatostatin-receptor scintigraphy in the evaluation of patients with multiple endocrine neoplasia type 1. Surgery 124:1037–1042
21. Angeletti S, Corleto VD, Schillaci O, Marignani M, Annibale B, Moretti A, Silecchia G, Scopinaro F, Basso N, Bordi C, Delle Fave G (1998) Use of the somatostatin analogue octreotide to localise and manage somatostatin-producing tumours. Gut 42:792–794
22. Choyke PL, Glenn GM, Walther MM, Patronas NJ, Linehan WM, Zbar B (1995) Von Hippel Lindau disease: genetic, clinical and imaging features. Radiology 146:629–642
23. Peracchi M, Conte D, Gebbia C, Penati C, Pizzinelli S, Arosio M, Corbetta S, Spada A (2003) Plasma chromogranin A in patients with sporadic gastro-entero-pancreatic neuroendocrine tumors or multiple endocrine neoplasia type 1. Eur J Endocrinol 148:39–43
24. Boden G, Ryan IG, Eisenschmid BL, Shelmet JJ, Owen OE (1986) Treatment of inoperable glucagonoma with the long-acting somatostatin analogue SMS 201-995. N Engl J Med. 314:1686–1689
25. Altimari AF, Bhoopalam N, O'Dorsio T, Lange CL, Sandberg L, Prinz RA (1986) Use of a somatostatin analog (SMS 201-995) in the glucagonoma syndrome. Surgery 100:989–996
26. Lips CJ, Hoppener JW, Van Nesselrooij BP, Van der Luijt RB (2005) Counselling in multiple endocrine neoplasia syndromes: from individual experience to general guidelines. J Intern Med 257:69–77
27. Evans DB, Skibber JM, Lee JE, Cleary KR, Ajani JA, Gagel RF, Sellin RV, Fenoglio CJ, Merrell RC, Hickey RC (1993) Nonfunctioning islet cell carcinoma of the pancreas. Surgery 114:1175–1181
28. Chung MH, Pisegna J, Spirt M, Giuliano AE, Ye W, Ramming KP, Bilchik AJ (2001) Hepatic cytoreduction followed by a novel long-acting somatostatin analog: a paradigm for intractable neuroendocrine tumors metastatic to the liver. Surgery 130:954–962

Chapter 66

S. Fukuyama · S. Matsuno · S. Egawa · M. Sunamura

Outcome after Surgical Treatment of Endocrine Pancreatic Tumors

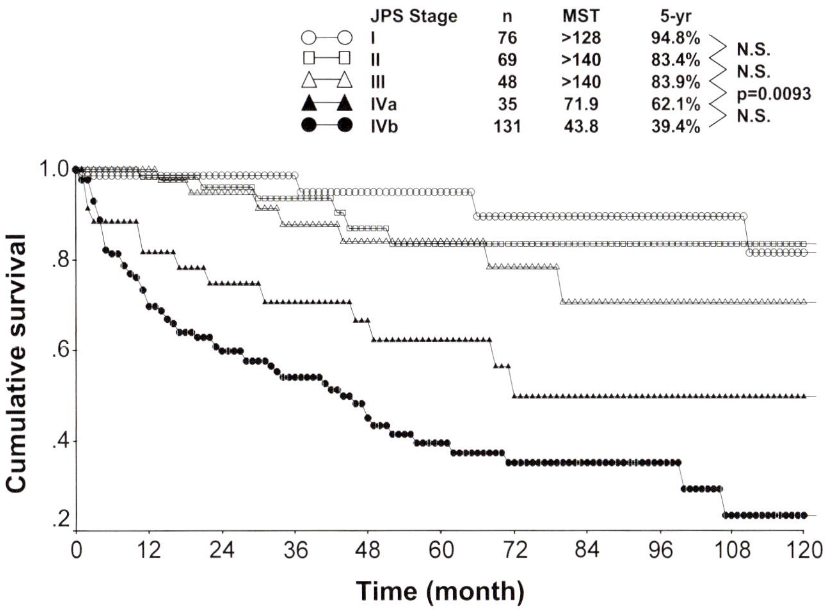

Figure 66.1

Japan Pancreas Society (*JPS*) stage and survival of the patients with islet cell tumor. Courtesy of the Japan Pancreas Society; National Pancreatic Cancer Registry (1981–2004). *N.S.* Not significant, *MST* median survival time (months), *5-yr* 5-year survival rate

Pancreatic endocrine tumors constitute a wide variety of rare lesions that are named according to the hormones that they produce. The most common pancreatic islet cell tumors are insulinoma and gastrinoma, followed in frequency of diagnosis by glucagonomas and vasoactive intestinal peptide (VIP)omas. Somatostatinomas are even more unusual. Nonfunctioning neoplasms with morphological features of islet cell tumors constitute 30% of pancreatic islet cell tumors [1].

According to a report from Japan Pancreas Society (JPS) [2], of 11,819 epithelial tumors, 307 cases were with endocrine tumors and the cumulative 5-year survival of the patients after pancreatectomy for islet cell tumor in Japan is 74.3%, while that of the patients with nonfunctioning islet cell tumor is 50%. The 5-year survival of the patients of stage IVa and IVb (of JPS) were 62.1% and 39.4% and was significantly lower than that of patients disease of other stages (Fig. 66.1). We describe herein details of the surgical outcome of endocrine tumors of pancreas.

Insulinoma

The goals of operation for the patient with insulinoma are fundamentally:

1. To locate and excise, if possible, all abnormally functioning tissue.
2. To differentiate between benign and malignant tumors by searching for the presence of metastatic disease.
3. To accomplish both of the above with minimal concomitant postoperative morbidity and mortality.

In a review by Stefanini of 1,012 cases, it was shown that 10% of patients developed diabetes mellitus and another 16% had persistence or recurrence of hypoglycemia after surgery [3]. In 6.8% of the patients, hypoglycemia was the result of either unresectable metastatic disease or diffuse adenomatosis, but 9.2% of the patients had tumors that were missed at operation. However, these operative failures will be less frequent as new operative techniques gain widespread usage. Hellman et al. reported 65 cases of insulinoma [4]. According to their report, 10.8% of cases were malignant, and 12.3% had multiple tumors. Starke et al. reported the outcome from 10 malignant cases [5]: median survival was 2.6 years, and 40% died after a median survival of 1.8 years from unmanageable hypoglycemia. In general, the long-term outcome for patients after resection of a benign insulinoma is excellent. Minimal data are available in the literature regarding the difficult group of patients undergoing reexploration for persistent hyperinsulinemia following an initial unsuccessful operation. These are indeed a problematic group of patients. Not only is exposure more difficult, but so also is gentle palpation of the pancreas, which is rendered less accurate because of the postoperative changes present. In a study by Thompson et al. [6], 10% of patients surgically explored were undergoing reexploration. Of these patients, eight had multiple tumors (two were multiple endocrine neoplasm type 1 patients) and two had malignant islet cell carcinoma. The surgical difficulties in the reoperative insulinoma patient, as in almost all reoperative situations, emphasize the importance of successful primary operations.

Recent days, laparoscopic approaches are also performed for solitary, small insulinoma, and successful results have been reported in various studies in the literature [7–9]. Even though laparoscopic surgery for pancreatic tumors has still not been defined, laparoscopic surgery offers significant benefit in selected patients, such as reduced trauma to the abdominal wall, short hospital stay, and a quick postoperative recovery.

These results confirm that nowadays patients with insulinomas can be treated with high success and low morbidity and mortality. To achieve this, surgical experience and expertise are a prerequisite, as is a dedicated multidisciplinary team approach.

Nonfunctioning Islet Cell Tumor

Nonfunctioning islet cell tumors are not associated with obvious signs or symptoms of hormone hypersecretion. The goals of operative resection are to improve local disease control and to increase the quality and length of patient survival. These goals must be tempered by the potential operative morbidity and the long-term complications of insulin dependence and gastrointestinal dysfunction. Evans et al. reported that resection of a primary tumor in the presence of metastatic disease does not prolong patient survival [10]. Survival data for 73 patients treated at the M.D. Anderson Cancer Center for nonfunctioning islet cell carcinomas of the pancreas were analyzed based on disease extent and treatment of the primary tumor. A survival advantage was demonstrated for patients who underwent complete resection of the primary tumor in the absence of metastatic disease. In contrast to the short survival in patients with metastatic adenocarcinoma of the pancreas, patients with liver metastases from islet cell carcinoma had a median survival of 3.3–4.5 years. It is important to note that, in the 22 patients with liver metastases who did not undergo resection of the primary tumor, only one patient had symptoms related to the primary pancreatic tumor prior to death. Patients with liver metastases from primary tumors in the pancreatic body and tail achieved no benefit from distal pancreatectomy in the absence of significant symptoms related to the primary tumor. This concept may change as strategies for the management of hepatic metastases become more successful. Guo et al. [11] reported 41 cases of nonfunctioning islet cell tumor in China, and found that the curative resection and complication rates were 88% and 22%, respectively. There was no local recurrence case, 8.3% suffered liver metastases. According to Gullo et al. [12], survival was improved by tumor resection, absence of metastases, and small tumor size (≤3 cm) significantly in 184 cases in Italy.

Gastrinoma

The experienced surgeon does not hesitate to excise one or more tumors from any portion of the pancreas. Such surgeons also tend to favor total gastrectomy if they are certain that the tumor remains either in the pancreas or in metastases. Oberhelman et al. [13] reported that a submucosal tumor located near the pylorus was palpated and removed, and that the patient was cured. Metastases to the lymph nodes produce gastrin, just as the primary tumors do, and their resection is very important. One of the most important factors in a favorable surgical result is to ensure that the patient with gastrinoma is operated on by a surgeon experienced in surgical problems of the pancreas and stomach. The surgical mortality should be very low. Long-term follow up shows that two-thirds of the patients with total gastrectomy will have maintained an ideal weight over the previous 10-year period. As localization techniques have improved and the habits of growth of the gastrinoma become better understood, more and more local excisions have no doubt been successful. Attempts to remove tumors in the head of the pancreas are encouraged, while tumors in the left half of the pancreas may be excised by distal pancreatectomy. The 5-year and 10-year survival rates of all patients with gastrinoma are 62–75% and 47–53%, respectively [14, 15]. In these studies, the extent of tumor is an important prognostic factor. When all of the tumor is completely resected, 5-year survival is 69–100%. If the tumor is incompletely resected or unresectable, or if there is a recurrent tumor, the 5- and 10-year survival rates are 43% and only 25%, respectively. If no tumor is found at laparotomy, these figures are 90–100% and 63–100%, respectively. Metastases occur in 23–90% of patients with gastrinoma and are the most common source of morbidity and mortality. Despite the fact that islet cell tumors are usually considered to be slow growing, 5-year survival of the patients with metastatic gastrinoma is only 20–38%. Slow but inexorable progression of the tumor has been the mode of death in these patients.

Glucagonoma

The only chance for cure in patients with glucagonoma is complete surgical resection, and operation is recommended in essentially all patients. The majority of glucagonomas are malignant, large, and advanced at the time of operation [16, 17]. While most patients with a glucagonoma are incurable, patients undergoing tumor resection for debulking can have dramatic and rapid improvement in many of the symptoms in the weeks following surgery. Glucagonomas, like other neuroendocrine tumors of the pancreas, tend to be slow growing, and the morbidity and mortality of these tumors are often related more to excessive hormone production than to the tumor mass. A marked decrease in serum glucagon is possible with palliative debulking, which often results in a prolonged disappearance or amelioration of the preoperative manifestations for years. A mean response of approximately 1 year, with prolongation of survival, has been shown [18]. Disease-free survival of 6 years or more has been reported with the resection of metastatic nodal spread of a glucagonoma [19]. Surgical debulking may also enhance the medical control of glucagons excess. Multiple operations aimed at re-resection or debulking recurrent or metastatic disease may result in prolonged survivals of 10–15 years [18, 20, 21]. Hepatic transplantation for metastatic disease confined to the liver has been performed in at least four patients with glucagonomas [22–24]. One patient died from immune rejection, but the other three were alive and free from disease at 3 years. This technique offers potential benefit for selected patients with advanced glucagonomas and deserves further study.

VIPoma

The only potentially curative treatment is surgical resection. About 50% of VIPomas are malignant, three-quarters of which have metastasized by the time of initial exploration [25, 26]. There is no curative therapy for tumors that cannot be completely resected, and 1-year survivals average about 40% [27]. Because of their rarity, conclusions about optimal modes of treatment are necessarily limited. Most investigators advise no treatment for asymptomatic patients with advanced metastatic disease, unless the tumor demonstrates aggressive biological behavior [28]. In contrast, in symptomatic patients, an aggressive approach with debulking is indicated, whenever possible, because resection of the majority of the disease can ameliorate or relieve the diarrhea [29] and may even return serum VIP concentrations to normal [30]. Resection of diarrheogenic tumors provides the only effective means for cure or long-lasting remission.

Somatostatinoma

The optimal treatment of somatostatinoma has not been defined, since little term follow up information is available because of the natural history of this disease. Small intestinal tumors are adequately treated by local resection. In one study, patients with proven duodenal somatostatinomas were treated by simple wedge resection [31]. In all of these patients, the tumors were <2 cm and confined to the bowel wall, without evidence of liver metastases.

The treatment of somatostatinomas is surgical resection, whenever possible. Small duodenal tumors can be treated by local excision or wedge resection, while large periampullary duodenal tumors or tumors arising from the head of the pancreas require pancreaticoduodenectomy. Coexisting focal liver metastasis should be resected, whenever feasible. The majority of somatostatinomas are malignant and will ultimately progress, with associated tumor cachexia and death. However, proper patient selection and aggressive but judicious resection will palliate troublesome symptoms related to glucose intolerance or malabsorptions.

References

1. Deveney CW (1998) Islet cell tumors: an overview. In: Beger HG, Warshaw AL, Büchler MW, Carr-Locke DL, Neoptolemos JP, Russell C, et al (eds) The Pancreas. Blackwell Science, Oxford, pp 1183–1186
2. Matsuno S, Egawa S, Fukuyama S, Motoi F, Sunamura M, Isaji S, Imaizumi T, Okada, S, Kato, H, Suda, K, Nakao A, Hiraoka T, Hosotani R, Takeda K (2004) Pancreatic Cancer Registry in Japan: 20 years of experience. Pancreas 28:219–230
3. Stefanini P, Carboni W, Patrassi N, Benedetti-Valentini FJ (1974) Surgical treatment and prognosis of insulinoma. Clin Gastroenterol 3:697
4. Hellman P, Goretzki P, Simon D, Dotzenrath C, Roher HD (2000) Therapeutic experience of 65 cases with organic hyperinsulinism. Langenbecks Arch Surg 385:329–336
5. Starke A, Saddig C, Mansfeld L, Koester R, Tschahargane C, Czygan P, Goretzki P (2005) Malignant metastatic insulinoma-postoperative treatment and follow-up. World J Surg 29:789–793
6. Thompson GB, Service FJ, van Heerden JA, Carney JA, Charboneau JW, O'Brien PC, Grant CS (1993) Reoperative insulinomas, 1927 to 1992: an institutional experience. Surgery 114:1196–1204; discussion 1205–1196
7. Masson B, Sa-Cunha A, Laurent C, Rault A, Collet D [Laparoscopic pancreatectomy: report of 22 cases]. Ann Chir 128:452–456
8. Iihara M, Obara T (2003) Recent advances in minimally invasive pancreatic surgery. Asian J Surg 26:86–91
9. Fernandez-Cruz L, Saenz A, Astudillo E, Martinez I, Hoyos S, Pantoja JP, Navarro S (2002) Outcome of laparoscopic pancreatic surgery: endocrine and nonendocrine tumors. World J Surg 26:1057–1065
10. Evans DB, Skibber JM, Lee JE, Cleary KR, Ajani JA, Gagel RF, Sellin RV, Fenoglio CJ, Merrell RC, Hickey RC (1993) Nonfunctioning islet cell carcinoma of the pancreas. Surgery 114:1175–1181; discussion 1181–1172
11. Guo KJ, Liao HH, Tian YL, Guo RX, He SG, Shen K (2004) Surgical treatment of nonfunctioning islet cell tumor: report of 41 cases. Hepatobiliary Pancreat Dis Int 3:469–472
12. Gullo L, Migliori M, Falconi M, Pederzoli P, Bettini R, Casadei R, Delle Fave G, Corleto VD, Ceccarelli C, Santini D, Tomassetti P (2003) Nonfunctioning pancreatic endocrine tumors: a multicenter clinical study. Am J Gastroenterol 98:2435–2439
13. Oberhelman HA Jr, Nelsen TS, Dragstedt LR (1958) Peptic ulcer associated with tumors of the pancreas. AMA Arch Surg 77:402–415
14. Bonfils S, Landor JH, Mignon M, Hervoir P (1981) Results of surgical management in 92 consecutive patients with Zollinger–Ellison syndrome. Ann Surg 194:692–697
15. Malagelada JR, Edis AJ, Adson MA, van Heerden JA, Go VL (1983) Medical and surgical options in the management of patients with gastrinoma. Gastroenterology 84:1524–1532
16. Holst J (1985) Glucagon-producing tumors. In: Cohen S, Soloway RD (eds) Hormone-Producing Tumors of the Gastrointestinal Tract. Churchill Livingstone, New York, pp 57–84
17. Prinz RA, Dorsch TR, Lawrence AM (1981) Clinical aspects of glucagon–producing islet cell tumors. Am J Gastroenterol 76:125–131
18. Montenegro F, Lawrence GD, Macon W, Pass C (1980) Metastatic glucagonoma. improvement after surgical debulking. Am J Surg 139:424–427
19. Hendry WS, Munro A (1986) Pancreatic glucagonoma with lymph node metastases: disease-free survival six years after resection. J R Coll Surg Edinb 31:115–116
20. Bloom SR, Polak JM (1987) Glucagonoma syndrome. Am J Med 82:25–36
21. Higgins GA, Recant L, Fischman A B (1979) The glucagonoma syndrome: surgically curable diabetes. Am J Surg 137:142–148
22. Alsina AE, Bartus S, Hull D, Rosson R, Schweizer RT (1990) Liver transplant for metastatic neuroendocrine tumor. J Clin Gastroenterol 12:533–537
23. Makowka L, Tzakis AG, Mazzaferro V, Teperman L, Demetris AJ, Iwatsuki S, Starzl TE (1989) Transplantation of the liver for metastatic endocrine tumors of the intestine and pancreas. Surg Gynecol Obstet 168:107–111
24. Arnold JC, O'Grady JG, Bird GL, Calne RY, Williams R (1989) Liver transplantation for primary and secondary hepatic apudomas. Br J Surg 76:248–249
25. Verner JV, Morrison AB (1974) Endocrine pancreatic islet disease with diarrhea. Report of a case due to diffuse hyperplasia of nonbeta islet tissue with a review of 54 additional cases. Arch Intern Med 133:492–499
26. Capella C, Polak JM, Buffa R, Tapia FJ, Heitz P, Usellini L, Bloom SR, Solcia E (1983) Morphologic patterns and diagnostic criteria of VIP-producing endocrine tumors. A histologic, histochemical, ultrastructural, and biochemical study of 32 cases. Cancer 52:1860–1874
27. O'Dorisio TM, Mekjian HS (1985) VIPoma syndrome. In: S Cohen, RD Soloway (eds) Contemporary Issues in Gastroenterology. Churchill-Livingstone, New York, pp 101–116
28. Ajani JA, Levin B, Wallace S (1989) Systemic and regional therapy of advanced islet cell tumors. Gastroenterol Clin North Am, 18:923–930
29. Andersson H, Dotevall G, Fagerberg G, Raotma H, Walan A, Zederfeldt B (1972) Pancreatic tumour with diarrhoea, hypokalemia and hypochlorhydria. Report of a case, with clinical, radiological and histopathological studies. Acta Chir Scand 138:102–107
30. Nagorney DM, Bloom SR, Polak JM, Blumgart LH (1983) Resolution of recurrent Verner-Morrison syndrome by resection of metastatic vipoma. Surgery 93:348–353
31. O'Brien TD, Chejfec G, Prinz RA (1993) Clinical features of duodenal somatostatinomas. Surgery 114:1144–1147

Periampullary Tumors

Chapter 67 Histopathology of Tumors of the Papilla of Vater *755*
W. Kimura

Chapter 68 Clinical Diagnosis of Adenoma of the Papilla of Vater *765*
K. Shiratori

Chapter 69 Clinical Diagnosis of Periampullary Carcinoma *771*
T. Kamisawa, A. Okamoto

Chapter 70 Endoscopic Management of Adenoma *779*
H. Maguchi, M. Osanai, A. Katanuma, K. Takahashi

Chapter 71 Surgical Management of Adenoma *789*
S. Ikeda, Y. Yasunami

Chapter 72 Surgical Treatment of Carcinoma of the Ampulla of Vater *797*
K. Yamaguchi, M. YTanaka

Chapter 73 Surgical Resection of Distal Common Bile Duct Carcinoma *807*
T. Rikiyama, M. Unno, S. Matsuno

Chapter 74 Cancer of the Duodenum – Surgical Treatment *817*
T. Imaizumi, M. Ishii, K. Tobita, S. Douwaki, H. Makuuchi

Chapter 75 Long-Term Outcome After Resection of Periampullary Carcinoma *827*
H. Amano, T. Takada

Chapter 67

W. Kimura

Histopathology of Tumors of the Papilla of Vater

Although it is quite small, the papilla of Vater is an important part of the body. Carcinoma of the papilla may be one of the smallest cancers that can cause death [1]. Therefore, the pathogenesis of carcinoma of the papilla has drawn the attention of many pathologists as well as surgeons.

In the Japanese experience from 1988 to 1994, carcinoma of the papilla of Vater was found in 939 cases, which represents 12.7% of extrahepatic biliary tract carcinoma (7,380 cases; Fig. 67.1) [2]. In the same period, extrahepatic bile duct carcinoma was found in 3,294 cases and gallbladder carcinoma was found in about 3,147 cases. As shown in this survival curve for resected cases of carcinoma of the papilla of Vater (Fig. 67.1), the 5-year survival rate was 51%, which is not satisfactory. If the carcinoma was not resected, most of the patients died within 2 years.

Topics under discussion in this chapter are the pathogenesis, histological characteristics, and molecular biological characteristics of carcinoma of the papilla of Vater.

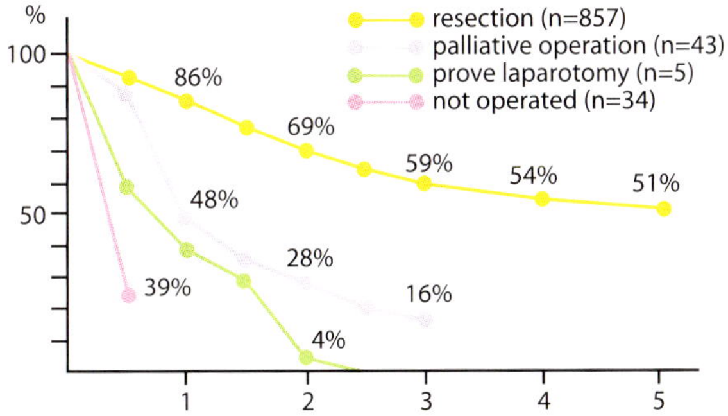

Figure 67.1

Survival curves of patients with carcinoma of the papilla of Vater (1988–1994; with permission from [2])

Pathogenesis of Carcinoma of the Papilla of Vater

Sites of Origin

With regard to the adenoma-carcinoma sequence, Sobol et al. [3] reviewed the literature and analyzed 45 cases of adenoma of the papilla of Vater, and found carcinoma in 12 cases (27%). With regard to the incidence of adenoma surrounding carcinoma of the papilla of Vater, the values have been reported to be 82% by Kozuka et al. [4] and 91% by Baczako et al. [5]. Therefore, the adenoma-carcinoma sequence is very important in the pathogenesis of carcinoma of the papilla of Vater. Some authors have insisted, however, that some carcinoma of the papilla of Vater arise de novo, since adenoma is very rare compared to carcinoma in this region [6,7].

Figure 67.2 is a schematic drawing of the papilla of Vater, which is defined as the area surrounded by the broken line. The papilla of Vater is composed of the common channel, the intraduodenal portion of the common bile duct, the intraduodenal portion of the pancreatic duct, and the duodenal mucosa.

When considering the pathogenesis of carcinoma, it is very important to investigate the site of development. In 1913, Outerbridge [8] reported that carcinoma of the papilla of Vater can theoretically originate from the following sites:

1. Epithelia of the common pancreatico-biliary channel (the common channel; Ac in Fig. 67.3).
2. Epithelia of the common bile duct at its lower end (Ab in Fig. 67.3).
3. Epithelia of the pancreatic duct at its lower end (Ap in Fig. 67.3).
4. Duodenal mucosa covering the papilla (Ad in Fig. 67.3).
5. The glands of Brunner.
6. Aberrant pancreatic acini in the wall of the common duct.

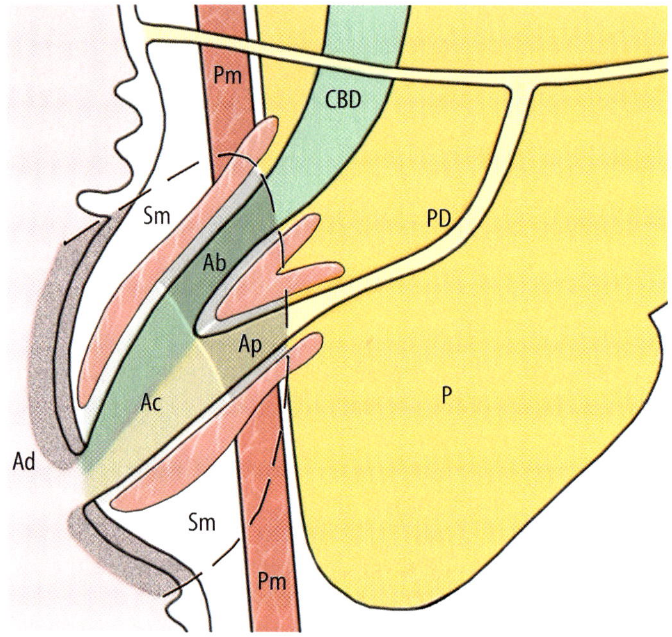

Figure 67.2

A schematic drawing of the papilla of Vater, which is defined as the area surrounded by the *broken line*. The papilla of Vater is composed of the common channel (*Ac*), the intraduodenal portion of the common bile duct (*Ab*), the intraduodenal portion of the pancreatic duct (*Ap*), and the duodenal mucosa (*Ad*). *CBD*, common bile duct *PD*, pancreatic duct, *P* Pancreas, *Sm* submucosa, *Pm* musclaris propria (with permission from [11])

We examined the papilla of Vater histologically in 576 autopsy cases of elderly people [1]. Special attention was paid to the presence of epithelial atypism. After fixation by formalin, serial sections were obtained, as shown in Fig. 67.3. When the papilla is cut between the left and middle diagonal lines in Fig. 67.3a, the epithelia of the common channel could be investigated (Fig. 67.3b). When the papilla is cut between the middle and right diagonal lines in Fig. 67.3a, the epithelia of the intraduodenal bile duct and intraduodenal pancreatic duct could be investigated (Fig. 67.3c).

These are criteria for epithelial atypism of the papilla of Vater. Epithelial atypism was classified into the following five groups according to cellular and structural atypism [1].

1. Group 1. Normal (Fig. 67.4a)
2. Group 2. Mild atypism (Fig. 67.4b).
3. Group 3. Moderate atypism (Fig. 67.5 a, b).
4. Group 4. Severe atypism (Fig. 67.6 a, b).
5. Group 5. Unequivocal carcinoma (Fig. 67.7 a, b).

Table 67.1 shows that group 1 epithelia accounted for 71% of the epithelia of the common channel in 451 cases, while group 2 accounted for 25% of the epithelia of the common channel in 451 cases. Group 3 epithelia accounted for 2.9% of the common channel, 1.7% of the intraduodenal portion of the common bile duct, and 0.6% of the intraduodenal portion of the pancreatic duct. The incidences of groups 3 and 4 in the common channel were significantly higher than those in the intraduodenal portion of the bile duct, pancreatic duct, or duodenal epithelia. These results show that atypical epithelia were most frequently found in the common channel. Thus, this study of autopsy cases suggests that the common channel is the most important site in the pathogenesis of carcinoma of the papilla of Vater.

When we investigated resected specimens from 60 cases, the common channel was the most frequent site for the possible origin of carcinoma (Fig. 67.8) [9]. When 12 cases of early carcinoma of the papilla of Vater were investigated, the results were the same (Fig. 67.9). That is, among all of the sites of the papilla of Vater, carcinoma was most often found in the common channel [9].

In conclusion, atypical epithelium was found most frequently in the common channel, where pancreatic juice and bile mix physiologically.

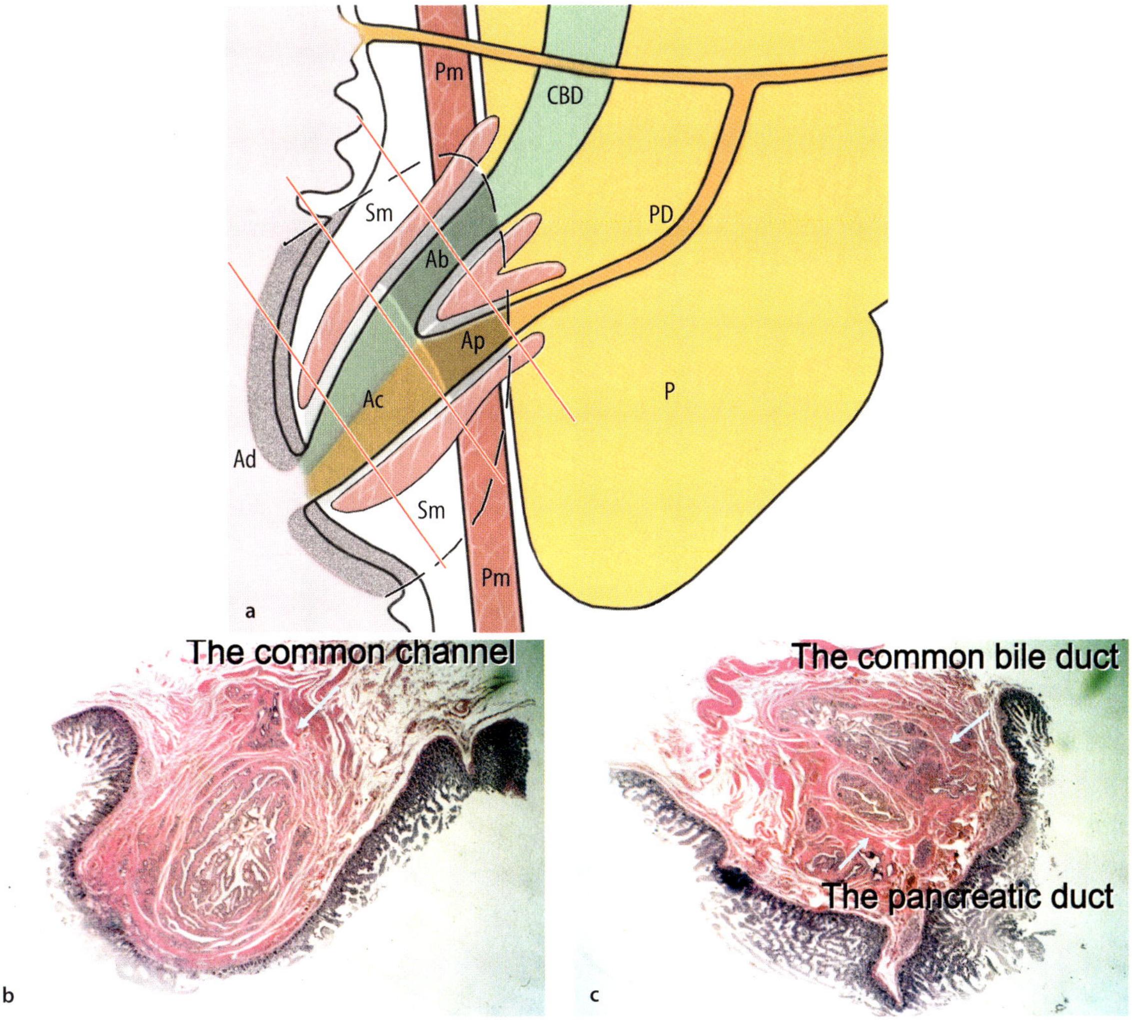

Figure 67.3

Serial sections were obtained, as shown in this figure. When the papilla is cut between the left and middle *diagonal lines* in a, the epithelia of the common channel could be investigated (b). When the papilla is cut between the middle and right *diagonal lines* in a, the epithelia of the intraduodenal bile duct and intraduodenal pancreatic duct could be investigated (c) (with permission from [11])

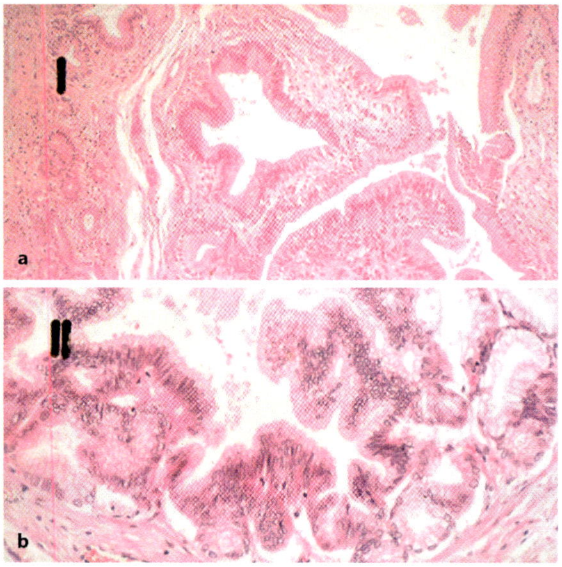

Figure 67.4

a Epithelia of group 1 (normal epithelium that does not show any atypism). b Epithelia of group 2 (mild atypism of benign hyperplasia). Hematoxylin and eosin stain (H&E): a ×100; b ×200 (with permission from [11])

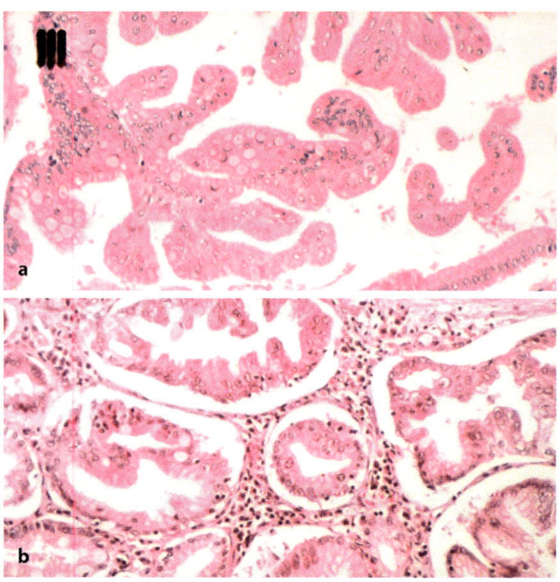

Figure 67.5 a, b

Epithelia of group 3. (moderate atypism; borderline lesion between benign and malignant). H&E: a, b ×200 (with permission from [11])

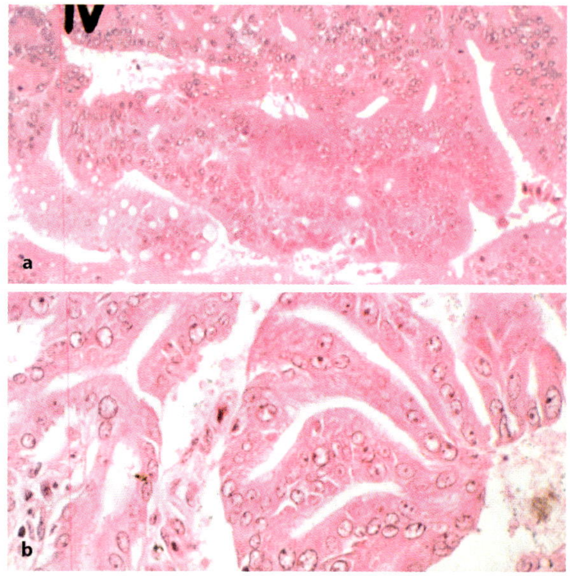

Figure 67.6 a, b

Epithelia of group 4 (severe atypism). This is strongly suggestive of a malignant lesion, but without definite evidence of carcinoma. H&E: a ×100; b ×250 (with permission from [11])

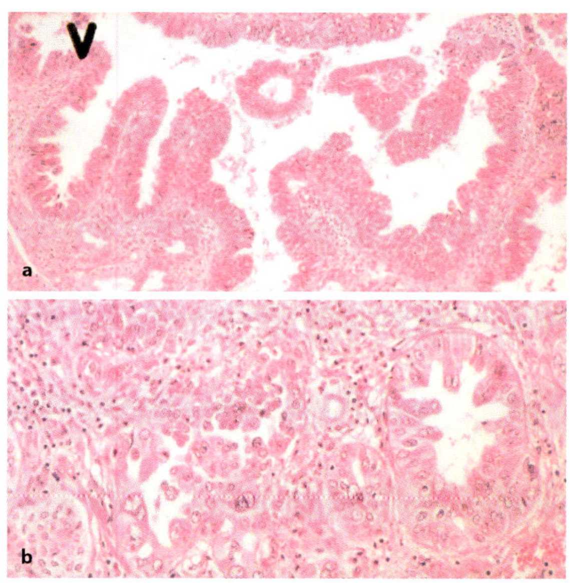

Figure 67.7 a, b

Epithelia of group 5 (unequivocal carcinoma with stromal invasion). H&E: a ×100; b ×250 (with permission from [11])

Table 67.1. Incidence of atypical epithelium in the sites of the papilla of Vater (with permission from [1])

Sites	Total no of cases	% of cases by groups				
		1	2	3	4	5
Commom channel	451	71	25	2.9	0.9	0.2
Bile duct	531	83	15	1.7	0.6	0.2
Pancreatic duct	531	93	6	0.6	0.4	0.2
Duodenal epithelium	481	97	3	0.4	0.2	0

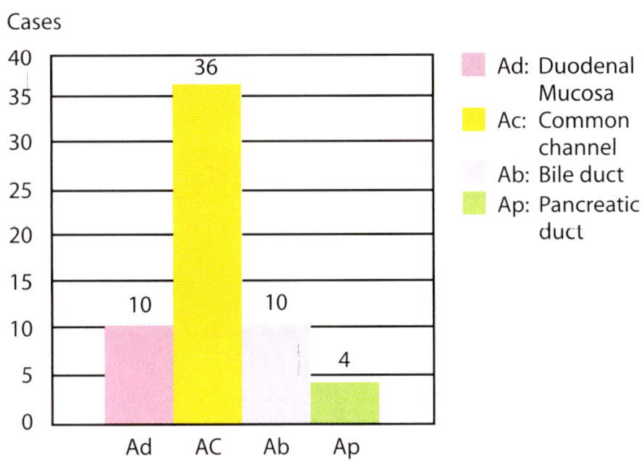

Figure 67.8

Detected site of development of carcinoma of the papilla of Vater (with permission from [9]). Sixty resected cases of carcinoma of the papilla of Vater were studied clinicopathologically. After pancreatoduodenectomy or local resection of the tumor, specimens were fixed in 10% formalin and embedded in paraffin, cut into 40-μm-thick sections, stained with H&E, and the site at which the tumor was believed to have developed in the papilla of Vater was studied histologically

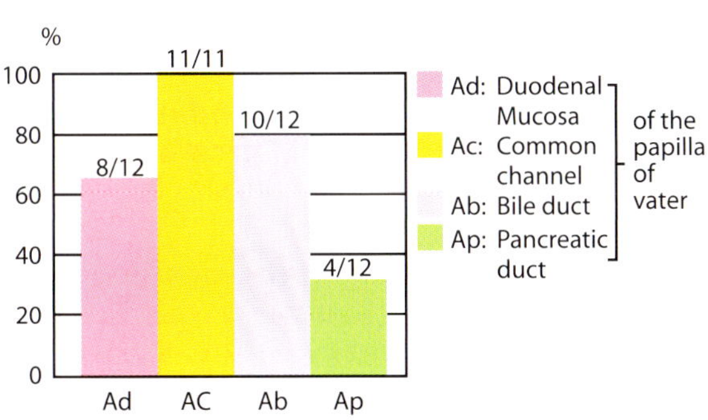

Figure 67.9

Histological spread in patients with early carcinoma of the papilla of Vater (with permission from [9])

The Immunohistochemical and Histochemical Characteristics of the Epithelia

To investigate the immunohistochemical and histochemical characteristics of these epithelia, sections were stained for carbohydrate antigen 19-9 (CA19-9), carcinoembryonic antigen (CEA), and mucin stains such as periodic acid-Schiff and alcian blue (Fig. 67.10) [1]. The incidences of positive staining are shown in Table 67.2. The most definitive results were obtained with CEA and alcian blue (pH 2.5) staining. Most of the carcinoma (79%), but none of the epithelia in groups 1 and 2 were positive for CEA. In contrast, most of the epithelia in groups 1 and 2 (91%), and a few of the carcinoma (7%), were stained positively with alcian blue, pH 2.5. Thus, groups 1 and 2 were characterized by negative CEA and positive alcian blue, groups 3 and 4 were characterized by negative CEA and negative alcian blue, and group 5 was characterized by positive CEA and negative alcian blue (Tables 67.2 and 67.3). Therefore, the type of atypical epithelia was between normal and cancerous. These characteristics of biopsy specimens may be helpful for distinguishing carcinoma of the papilla of Vater before an operation.

Pathogenesis

When we summarized the results of studies of atypical epithelium in autopsy cases with respect to the pathogenesis of carcinoma of the papilla of Vater, group 4 epithelia were found in two out of five cases (40%) with group 3 epithelia [1]. Among 23 cases of groups 3 and 4, so-called adenoma, in the narrow sense, was found in only 3 cases. In other 20 cases, papillary projection with atypia without adenomatous growth was found. In 13 of 18 cases in group 3, group 2 epithelia were found surrounding group 3 epithelia. These atypical epithelia were found most frequently in the common channel. This fact is con-

Table 67.2. Incidence of cancer-associated antigens and mucin-production in groups 1 and 2, groups 3 and 4, and in cases of carcinoma (with permission from [1]). *CEA* Carcinoembryonic antigen, *CA19-9* carbohydrate antigen 19-9, *AB* alcian blue, *PAS* periodic acid-Schiff

Classification	No. of Cases	Cancer-associated antigen staining		Mucinstaining		
		CEA	CA 10-9	AB pH1.0	AB pH2.5	PAS
Groups 1 and 2	23	0	14 (61)	13 (57)	21 (91)	19 (83)
Groups 3 and 4	23	1 (4)	20 (87)	2 (9)	9 (39)	7 (30)
Carcinoma	14	11 (79)	9 (64)	1 (7)	1 (7)	1 (7)

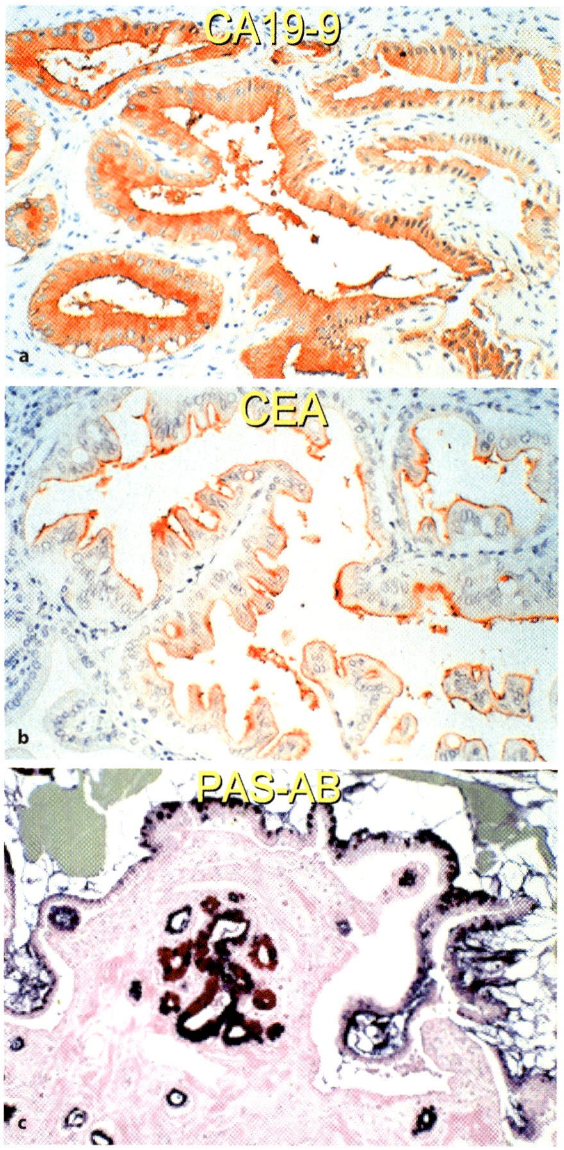

Figure 67.10

To investigate the immunohistochemical and histochemical characteristics of these epithelia, sections were stained for carbohydrate antigen 19-9 (*CA19-9*, a), carcinoembryonic antigen (*CEA*, b), and mucin stains, such as periodic acid-Schiff and alcian blue (*PAS-AB*, **c**) (with permission from [11])

Table 67.3. Normal, atypical and cancerous types of epithelia of the papilla of Vater, stained with a combination combination of carcinoembryonic antigen (*CEA*) and alcian blue (with permission from [1])

	CEA	AB (pH2.5)
Normal Type	–	+
Atypical Type	–	–
Cancerous Type	+	–

sistent with the results of clinical cases. That is, from the investigation of clinical cases, carcinoma was thought to be most frequently found in the common channel. With regard to CEA and alcian blue staining, the type of atypical epithelia was between normal and cancerous. Therefore, we concluded that atypical epithelia may be a precursor of carcinoma of the papilla of Vater.

However, in another three cases in group 4 and in one case in group 5, atypical epithelia were entirely surrounded by group 1 epithelia. These facts also show that atypical epithelium and carcinoma in these cases might arise de novo.

Different Clinicopathologic Findings in Two Histologic Types of Carcinoma of the Papilla of Vater

We were the first group to classify carcinoma of the papilla of Vater into two histological types: intestinal type and pancreaticobiliary type [10]. Figure 67.11a shows carcinoma of an intestinal type, which resembles tubular adenocarcinoma of the colon. The cytoplasm is eosinophilic. These epithelia may originate from the duodenal mucosa. This type of carcinoma was found in 13 cases (25%).

Figure 67.11b shows epithelia of the pancreaticobiliary type, which is characterized by papillary projections with scant fibrous cores. The cytoplasm is clear. These epithelia originate from pancreaticobili-

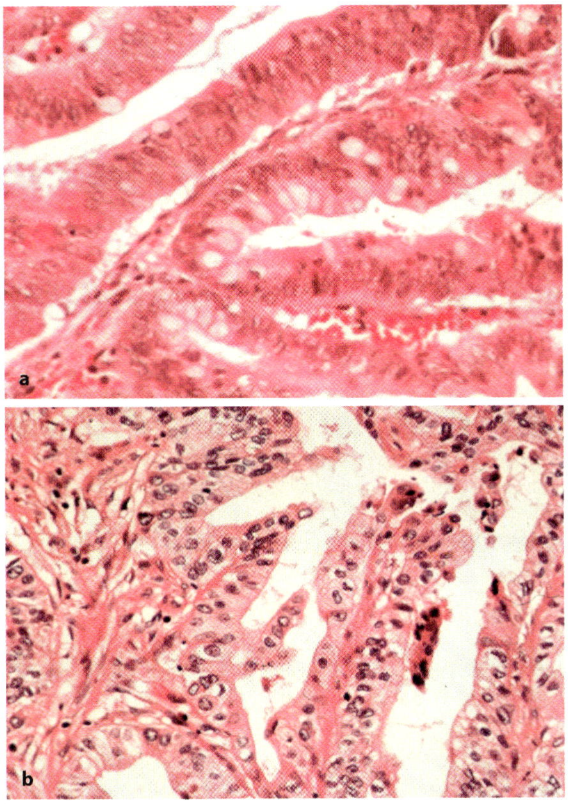

Figure 67.11

a Carcinoma of the intestinal type, which resembles tubular adenocarcinoma of the colon. The cytoplasm is eosinophilic. These epithelia may originate from the duodenal mucosa. b Carcinoma of the pancreaticobiliary type, which is characterized by papillary projections with scant fibrous cores. The cytoplasm is clear. H&E: a, b ×200 (with permission from [11])

ary epithelia, since the epithelia of the pancreatic or bile duct often show papillary growth with a scant fibrous core. This type of carcinoma was found in 38 cases (72%) [10].

Paneth cells, argyrophil cells positively stained with Grimelius stain, and cells that stain positively for the antilysozyme antibody (Fig. 67.12) were found more frequently in the intestinal type than in the pancreaticobiliary type.

The incidences of both gross ulceration and histologic pancreas invasion were more frequent in the pancreaticobiliary type than in the intestinal type (Table 67.4). Although these differences were not statistically significant, the trend is clear. The incidence of histological lymph node metastasis was significantly higher in cases of pancreaticobiliary type than in intestinal type carcinoma.

Survival curves obtained using the Kaplan-Meier method for both types of carcinoma are shown in

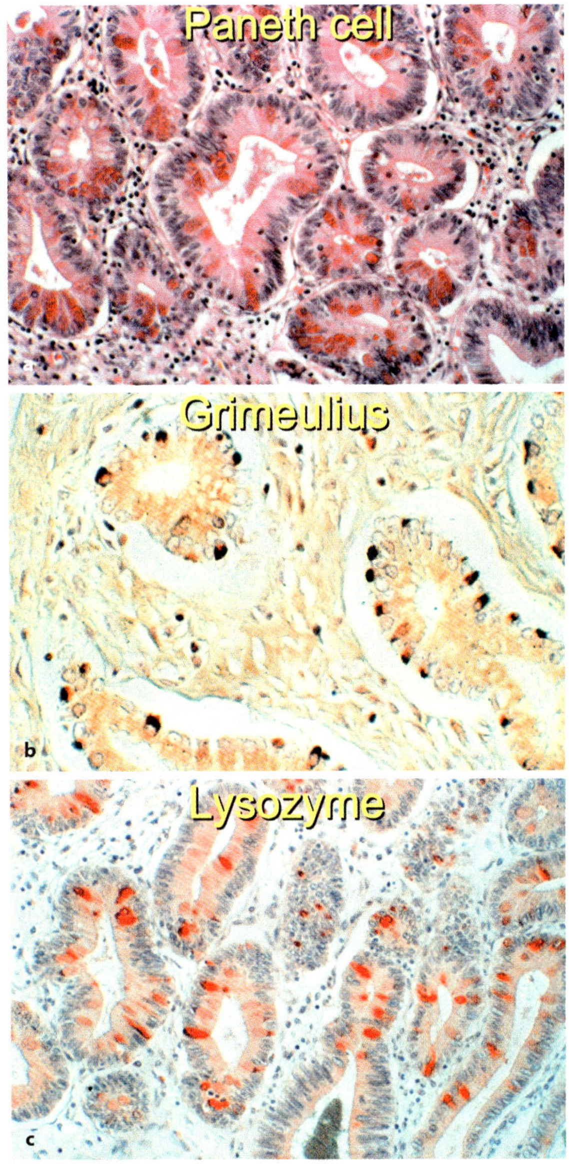

Figure 67.12

Paneth cells (a), argyrophil cells positively stained with Grimelius stain (b), and cells that were positively stained for the antilysozyme antibody (c) (with permission from [11])

Fig. 67.13. Long-term survival after resection of the tumor was significantly greater in cases with the intestinal type than in cases with the pancreaticobiliary type.

In conclusion, these two types of carcinoma should be treated by different operative procedures or adjuvant therapies [10]. When the carcinoma is of the intestinal type, very radical lymph node dissection may not be necessary. However, complete and thorough lymph node dissection during surgery and intensive

Table 67.4. Ulcer formation, histologic pancreas infiltration, and lymph node metastasis in patients with carcinoma of pancreaticobiliary type or intestinal type of the papilla of Vater (with permission from [10]). *Fisher's exact test $P<0.05$. *N.S.* Not significant

	Histologic type of the epithelium Pancreaticobiliary type (*n*=38)	Intestinal type (*n*=13)
Ulcer Formation	20/38 (52.6)	3/12 (23.1)
Histologic pancreas invasion	21/38 (55.3)	4/13 (30.8)
Histologic lymph node metastasis	21/38 (55.3)	2/13 (18.2)

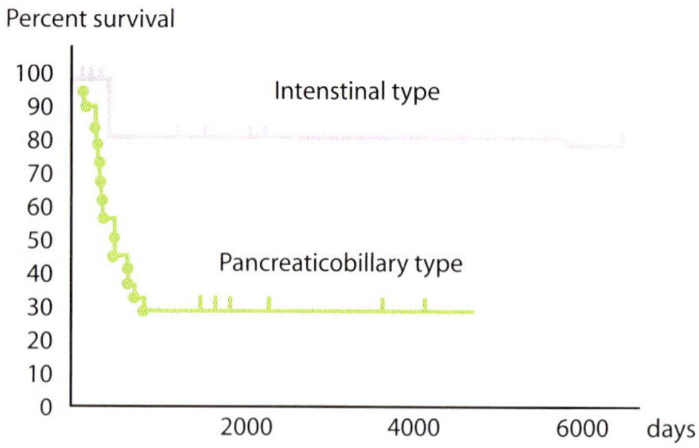

Figure 67.13

Survival curves, obtained by the Kaplan-Meier method, for both types of carcinoma (pancreaticobiliary type and intestinal type; with permission from [10])

Table 67.5. Comparison of K-ras codon 12 mutation in carcinomas of different histological types (with permission from [23])

Histological Type	No. of cases	Type of Mutation		
		GAT	GTT	GCT
Intestinal Type	6	3	3	0
Pancreaticobiliary Type	8	6	1	1
Total	14/37	(38 %)		

adjuvant therapy, such as chemotherapy or radiation, may be required in cases of the pancreaticobiliary type of carcinoma of the papilla of Vater [11].

The significance of classifying carcinoma of the papilla of Vater into two histological types is supported by Fischer and Zhou (Fig. 67.13) [12].

The Molecular Biological Characteristics of Neoplasia of the Papilla of Vater

K-ras gene mutation in carcinoma of the papilla of Vater has been reported in several studies. The incidence of this mutation is reported to be between 0 and 40% [13–16]. Chung et al. [15] concluded that, *K-ras* codon 12 mutations occur in about 40% of ampullary neoplasms at a relatively early stage in tumorigenesis. The pattern of mutations in these tumors resembles that of the adenoma-carcinoma sequence in the colon and rectum (Table 67.5).

Overexpression of p53 protein has been identified in a variety of carcinomas of the papilla of Vater. p53 is a tumor-suppressor gene that is located on chromosome 17p, and is inactivated through mutation or loss of heterozygosity. p53 is also related to apoptosis and progression of the cell cycle.

The incidence is reported to be 0–83% [17–22]. In 1995, Younes et al. [21] reported that p53 overexpression was found in 0% of normal ampullae, 40% of adenomas, and 94% of carcinomas of the papilla of Vater. They concluded that, p53 accumulation in tumors of the ampulla of Vater occurs early in the neoplastic process. Tumors of the ampulla of Vater with biopsy samples that are negative for malignancy but positive for p53 are very likely to be carcinoma.

We investigated p53 and p21/Waf1 protein expression and *K-ras* codon 12 mutation in carcinoma of the papilla of Vater, using 37 cases [23]. The p21/Waf1 gene encodes a cyclin-dependent kinase inhibitor, which inhibits multiple complexes of cyclin and cyclin-dependent kinase in initiating the progression of cells from G1 to S phase. p53 is related to progression of the cell cycle through the regulation of p21.

Paraffin-embedded sections were stained immunohistochemically for p53 and p21. *K-ras* codon 12 mutation was detected by two-step polymerase chain reaction-restriction fragment length polymorphism followed by direct sequencing. On direct sequencing, *K-ras* codon 12 mutation was found in 14 out of 37 cases (38%; Table 67.5) [23]. *K-ras* mutations were mainly GGT to GAT and GGT to GTT. The type of mutation did not correlate with the histological type. The incidence of *K-ras* mutation in cases with ulceration was almost the same as that in cases

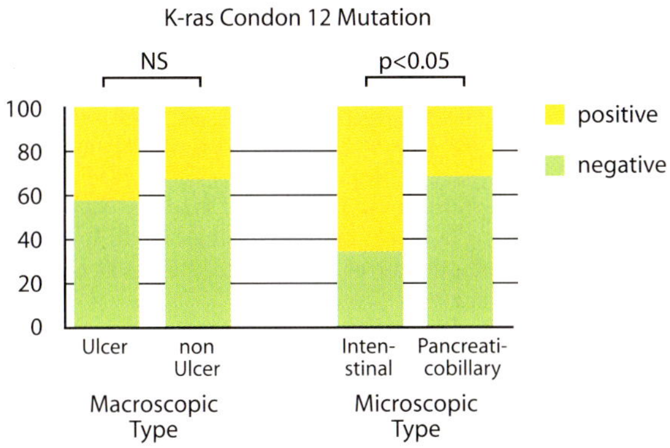

Figure 67.14

The incidence of K-ras mutation in cases with and without ulceration and in cases of the intestinal type and those of the pancreaticobiliary type (with permission from [23]). *NS* Not significant

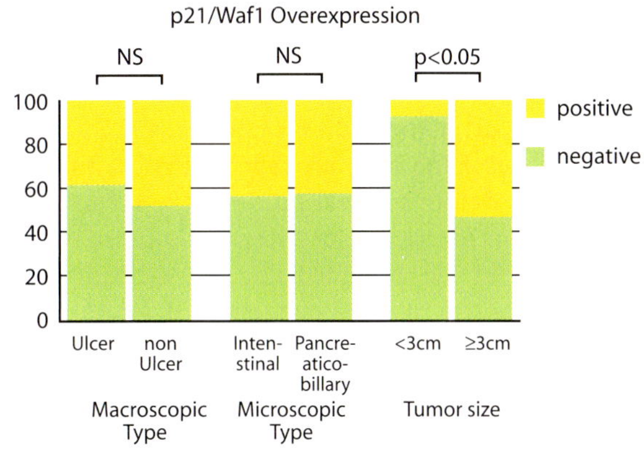

Figure 67.16

The incidence of p21/Waf1 protein expression in cases with and without ulceration, in cases of the intestinal type and those of the pancreaticobiliary type, in cases with tumors larger than 3 cm in diameter, and cases with tumors smaller than 3 cm in diameter (with permission from [11])

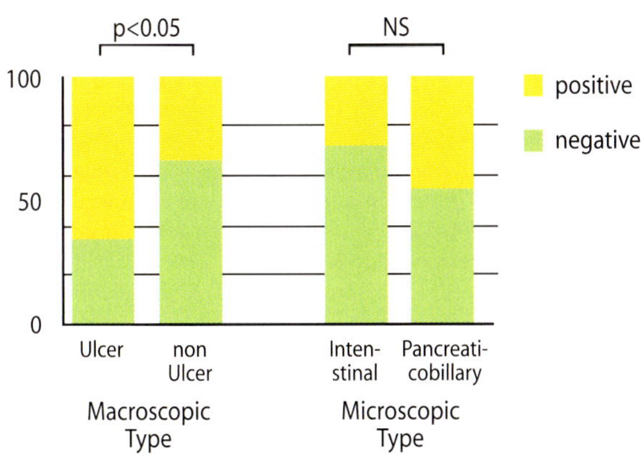

Figure 67.15

The incidence of p53 overexpression in cases with and without ulceration and in cases of the intestinal type and pancreaticobiliary type carcinoma (with permission from [23]

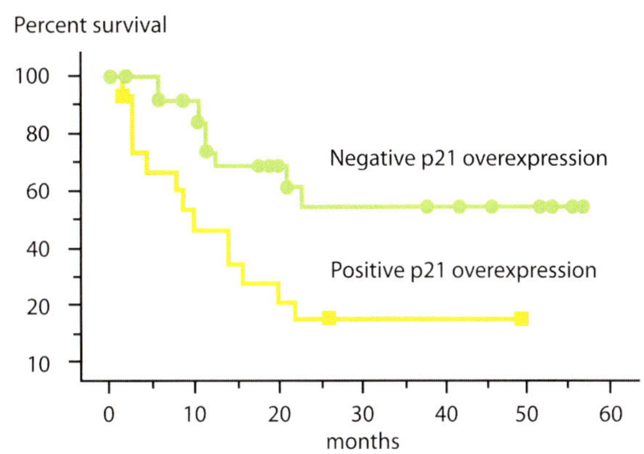

Figure 67.17

Survival curves, obtained by the Kaplan-Meier method, for cases with p21 overexpression and without p21 overexpression. p21 overexpression was significantly correlated with a poor prognosis (with permission from [11])

without ulceration (Fig. 67.14). However, *K-ras* mutation was found significantly more often in carcinomas of the intestinal type than in the pancreaticobiliary type. p53 overexpression was found in 46% and was seen significantly more often in cases with ulcer than in cases without ulcer (Fig. 67.15). p53 overexpression was also seen more often in carcinomas of the pancreaticobiliary type than in intestinal type, but this difference was not statistically significant.

p21/Waf1 protein expression was found in 15 cases (41%). p21/Waf1 expression was seen more frequently in tumors larger than 3 cm in diameter than in tumors smaller than 3 cm (Fig. 67.16). p21/Waf1 expression did not correlate with any other clinicopathological parameter. Cases with p21 overexpression showed worse postoperative survival than cases without p21 overexpression. Thus, p21 overexpression was significantly correlated with a poor prognosis (Fig. 67.17).

Summary

Although it is quite small, the papilla of Vater is an important part of the body. Carcinoma of the papilla may be one of the smallest cancers that can cause death. The 5-year survival rate after resection was 51%, which is not satisfactory. Results obtained by investigation of 576 autopsied and 51 resected cases demonstrate that atypical epithelium is found most frequently in the common channel, where pancreatic juice and bile mix physiologically. Atypical epithelia may be a precursor of carcinoma of the papilla of Vater. Carcinoma of the papilla of Vater could be classified into two histological types, an intestinal type and a pancreaticobiliary type. The prognosis of cases with the intestinal type appears to be much better than that of cases with the pancreaticobiliary type. These two types of carcinoma should be treated by different operative procedures or adjuvant therapies. Regarding the molecular biological characteristics of carcinoma of the papilla of Vater: (1) *K-ras* mutation is mainly associated with the intestinal type, (2) carcinomas of the intestinal and pancreaticobiliary types may develop via different mechanisms, (3) p53 overexpression may play a role in tumor ulceration, and (4) p21/Waf1 overexpression was significantly correlated with a poor prognosis.

References

1. Kimura W, Ohtsubo K (1988) Incidence, sites of origin, and immunohistochemical and histochemical characteristics of atypical epithelium and minute carcinoma of the papilla of Vater. Cancer 61:1394–1402
2. Nagakawa T (ed) (1994) Japanese Society of Carcinoma of the Biliary Tract. Reports of Carcinoma of the Biliary Tract in Japan. Yuki, Ishikawa, Japan
3. Sobol S, Cooperman AM (1978) Villous adenoma of the ampulla of Vater: an unusual cause of biliary colic and obstructive jaundice. Gastroenterology 75:107–109
4. Kozuka S, Tsubone M, Yamaguchi A, Hachisuka K, Yasui A (1981) Adenomatous residue in cancerous papilla of Vater. Gut 22:1031–1034
5. Baczako K, Buchler M, Beger HG, Kirkpatrick CJ, Haferkamp O (1985) Morphogenesis and possible precursor lesions of invasive carcinoma of the papilla of Vater: epithelial dysplasia and adenoma. Hum Pathol 16:305–310
6. Tasaka K (1977) Carcinoma in the region of the duodenal papilla: a histopathologic study. Fukuoka Acta Med 68:20–44
7. Enjoji M, Kido H (1981) Carcinoma of the duodenal papilla; its growth and histogenesis. Tan to Sui (J Biliary Tract Pancreas) 2:1651–1656 (in Japanese)
8. Outerbridge GW (1913) Carcinoma of the papilla of Vater. Surgery 57:402–426
9. Futakawa N, Kimura W, Wada Y, Muto T (1996) Clinicopathological characteristics and surgical procedures for carcinoma of the papilla of Vater. Hepatogastroenterology 43:260–267
10. Kimura W, Futakawa N, Yamagata S, Wada Y, Kuroda A, Muto T (1994) Different clinicopathologic findings in two different histologic types of carcinoma of the papilla of Vater. Jpn J Cancer Res 85:161–166
11. Kimura W, Futakawa N, Zhao B (2004) Neoplastic diseases of the papilla of Vater. J Hepatobiliary Pancreat Surg 11:223–231
12. Fischer HP, Zhou H (2004) Pathogenesis of carcinoma of the papilla of Vater. J Hepatobiliary Pancreat Surg 11:301–309
13. Lee JC, Lin PW, Lin YJ, Lai J, Yang HB, Lai MD (1995) Analysis of K-ras gene mutation in periampullary cancers, gallbladder cancer and cholangio-carcinomas from paraffin-embedded tissue sections. J Formos Med Assoc 94:919–923
14. Motojima K, Tsunoda T, Kanematsu T, Nagata Y, Urano T, Shiku H (1991) Distinguishing pancreatic carcinoma from other periampullary carcinomas by analysis of mutation in the Kirsten-ras oncogene. Ann Surg 241:657–662
15. Chung CH, Wilentz RE, Polak MM, Ramsoekh TB, Noorduyn LA, Gouna DJ, Huibregtse K, Offerhaus GJA, Slebos RJC (1996) Clinical significance of K-ras oncogene activation in ampullary neoplasms. J Clin Pathol 49:460–464
16. MalatsN, Porta M, Pinol JL, Josep M (1995) Ki-ras mutations as a prognostic factor in extrahepatic bile system cancer. J Clin Oncol 13:1679–1686
17. Diamantis I, Karamitopoulou E, Perentes E, Zimmermann A (1995) p53 protein immunoreactivity in extrahepatic bile duct and gallbladder cancer: correlation with tumor grade and survival. Hepatology 22:774–779
18. Scarpa A, Capelli P, Zamboni G, Oda T, Mukai K, Bonetti F, Martignoni G, Lacono C, Serio G, Hirohashi S (1993) Neoplasia of the ampulla of Vater. Ki-ras and p53 mutations. Am J Pathol 142:1163–1172
19. Lee CS, Pirdas A (1995) p53 protein immunoreactivity in cancers of the gallbladder, extrahepatic bile ducts and ampulla of Vater. Pathology 27:117–120
20. Teh M, Wee A, Raju GC (1994) An immunohistochemical study of p53 protein in gallbladder and extrahepatic bile duct/ampullary carcinomas. Cancer 74:1542–1545
21. Younes M, Riley S, Genta RM, Mosharaf M, Mody DR (1995) p53 protein accumulation in tumors of the ampulla of Vater. Cancer 76:1150–1154
22. Zhu L, Kim K, Domenico DR, Appert HE, Howard JM (1996) Adenocarcinoma of duodenum and ampulla of Vater: clinicopathology study and expression of p53, c-neu, TGF-alpha, CEA, and EMA. J Surg Oncol 61:100–105
23. Zhao B, Kimura W, Futakawa N, Muto T, Kubota K, Harihara Y, Takayama T, Makuuchi M (1999) p53 and p21/Waf1 protein expression and K-ras codon 12 mutation in carcinoma of the papilla of Vater. Am J Gastroenterol 94:2128–2134

Chapter 68

K. Shiratori

Clinical Diagnosis of Adenoma of the Papilla of Vater

Various pathological types of benign tumors arise from the papilla of Vater, including lipomas, fibromas, lymphangiomas, leiomyomas, leiomyofibromas, and hamartomas, and the most common types, villous and tubulovillous adenomas. Although classified as benign, ampullary adenomas are actually premalignant neoplasms that arise from the mucosal epithelium of the papilla of Vater.

Adenomas

Adenomas are the most common benign tumors of the major duodenal papilla, and according to the World Health Organization classification of small-bowel tumors, they are classified into tubular, villous, and tubulovillous types on the basis of their histological appearance [1–3]. Adenomas of the major duodenal papilla are more likely to undergo malignant transformation through metaplastic and dysplastic change than adenomas arising elsewhere in the duodenum. An adenoma-carcinoma sequence similar to that in colon cancer has been postulated for Vater adenomas [1,4]. Although classified as benign, ampullary adenomas are truly premalignant neoplasms that arise from the mucosal epithelium of the papilla of Vater.

Villous Adenomas

The incidence of villous adenomas of the ampulla of Vater in autopsy series has been reported to be 0.04–0.12% [5], and it has increased as a result of the recent widespread use of endoscopy examinations. Histological evaluation of forceps biopsy specimens of the papilla of Vater has revealed rates of tubular adenoma, tubulovillous adenoma, and villous adenoma of 53.6%, 36.3%, and 5.5%, respectively [1], whereas histological examination of surgically resected tumors has demonstrated the presence of adenocarcinomas, tubular adenomas, and villous adenomas in 47.5%, 15%, and 17.5%, respectively [6]. Schoenberg et al. [3] also reported final postoperative diagnoses in patients with benign papilla tumors in terms of villous adenoma in 29%, tubulovillous adenoma in 35%, and tubular adenoma in 3%.

Villous adenomas of the papilla of Vater and the duodenum have greater potential for malignant transformation than tumors of the tubulovillous type. Stolte and Pscherer [1] reported observing malignant transformation of adenomas in 83.3% of villous-type adenomas, in 69.7% of the tubulovillous type, and in 34.6% of the tubular type. Motton et al. [7] detected adenocarcinoma in endoscopic biopsy specimens from three out of nine cases of villous adenoma. Thus, the risk of malignant transformation depends on the histological type of the adenoma, including whether it is tubular, tubulovillous, or villous. Villous tumors are considered precursors of malignant degeneration [8, 9].

Familial Adenomatous Polyposis

Some ampullary adenomas occur in association with familial polyposis syndromes. The most common and the best characterized of these syndromes is familial adenomatous polyposis (FAP), an autosomal dominant disease that is characterized by the development of innumerable adenomas in the large intestine. FAP is associated with an inherited defect in the adenomatous polyposis coli gene, which normally suppresses tumor growth. A high rate of progression of adenomatous polyps to cancer is well known to occur in patients with FAP.

The results of several surveys have shown that ampullary adenomas progress to adenocarcinoma in patients with FAP. Peripapillary carcinoma has been found to be the second leading cause of death in FAP, after prophylactic colectomy. The natural course of ampullary adenoma has been documented in only a few reports. Burke et al. [10] reported observing macroscopic and microscopic progression of adenomas of the main duodenal papilla in 14% and 11% of FAP patients, respectively, based on a follow-up study for a mean period of 51 months. A high cumulative risk of periampullary lesions was also been shown in FAP patients [11]. Another follow-up study concluded that aggressive endoscopic or surgical removal is unnecessary because the investigators observed no change in ampullary adenomas in FAP patients over a more than 10-year period [12]. However, endoscopic surveillance is widely recommended in FAP patients, because it is generally accepted that ampullary adenomas have a very high potential to undergo trans-formation into carcinoma.

Clinical Features

Signs and Symptoms

The clinical presentation and evaluation of benign and malignant ampullary tumors overlap [13]. The signs and symptoms of ampullary adenomas depend on their anatomic location, although small tumors may be asymptomatic. The most frequent symptom other than nonspecific upper abdominal discomfort, such as abdominal bloating, epigastric pain, emesis, anorexia, or dyspepsia, is jaundice. Benign tumors are less often initially jaundice, because of their smaller size and the absence of tissue invasion. These symptoms are attributable to ampullary (biliary or pancreatic) obstruction resulting from the mass effect of the adenoma compressing and impeding biliary or pancreatic outflow. A review by Motton et al. [7] reported that epigastric pain (36.3%), jaundice (33.9%), weight loss (20.2%), and anemia (12%) are the most frequent clinical manifestation of benign ampullary adenomas, vomiting (4.8%), and diarrhea (1.6%) being less common. These symptoms may be present alone or in combination. Catalano et al. [14] recently reported jaundice and/or pain (57%), epigastric pain due to pancreatitis (25%), and bleeding (11.7%) as the most common presenting symptoms. Occult gastrointestinal bleeding and iron-deficiency anemia secondary to blood loss are common, but overt bleeding is rare. Biliary tract stones are present in about 20% of patients with ampullary adenoma [15,16], but 25% have no symptoms attributable to the lesion of the papilla [14].

Laboratory Tests

Abnormal laboratory data frequently result from the biliary obstruction caused by ampullary adenomas obstructing biliary drainage. The most common laboratory finding is elevated serum levels of the liver enzymes alkaline phosphatase and gamma-glutamyl transpeptidase [17]. The rises in their levels are disproportionately higher than the corresponding increases in serum bilirubin and transaminase levels. Rarely, the serum amylase and lipase levels are increased if pancreatic juice drainage is obstructed. Anemia and a positive stool test for occult blood may be found. No serum tumor markers specific for ampullary adenomas have ever been identified [5].

Diagnosis

The diagnosis of tumors of the papilla of Vater requires an appropriate level of clinical suspicion based on the history and physical examination, and prompt and accurate evaluation is very important, particularly when jaundice is present. Laboratory tests, diagnostic imaging, including ultrasound (US) and/or computed tomography (CT), should be conducted in any patient with jaundice.

Ultrasound and Computed Tomography

Abdominal US and CT are used frequently as the initial imaging studies for the diagnosis of tumor of the papilla. Conventional US is often used for the initial evaluation of patients presenting with abdominal pain and/or jaundice because it easily visualizes dilated intrahepatic and extrahepatic bile ducts. In patients with biliary obstruction secondary to an ampullary tumor, US demonstrates diffuse dilatation of the entire bile duct at the level of the ampulla of Vater. Other important findings, including gallstones, enlarged lymph nodes, and liver metastases are also routinely detected with US. However, a major limitation of US is its technical inadequacy for detecting ampullary tumors themselves, visualizing ampullary tumors in less than 15% of cases [7].

CT is a more sensitive method for making a differential diagnosis of obstructive jaundice, and can provide important information as to the level of biliary obstruction with respect to the pancreatic parenchyma, because when the CT images rule out a pancreatic mass, the obstruction is likely to be at the papilla. Unfortunately, CT also sometimes fails to

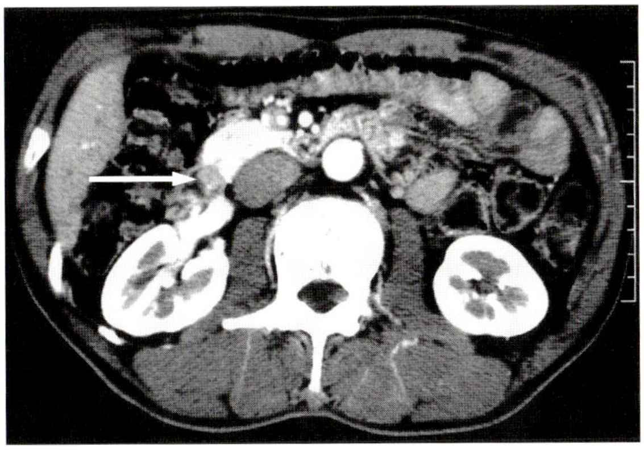

Figure 68.1

Computed tomography (CT) scan of a patient with ampullary tumor. A slightly enhanced and elevated papilla of Vater is seen in the duodenal lumen (*arrow*)

identify ampullary tumors themselves because they tend to be relatively small and be concealed by the adjacent duodenal folds. Tumors of the papilla can be detected with CT when they protrude into the duodenum distended with contrast medium (Fig. 68.1). A recent study showed that helical CT missed small pancreatic cancers 2 cm in diameter, whereas magnetic resonance imaging (MRI) clearly visualized tumors 0.8 cm in diameter [18]. Recent reports of rates of detection of ampullary tumors by CT have ranged between 24 and 29.6% [19, 20], which is a significantly lower range than the rates of detection by endoscopic ultrasound (EUS), intraductal ultrasonography (IDUS), and MRI.

The roles of US and CT are as screening examinations for evidence of biliary or pancreatic duct dilatation that suggests obstruction at the level of the ampulla, although their specificity and sensitivity are relatively low. Schoenberg et al. [3] reported a sensitivity of US and CT for benign ampullary tumors of 43% and 34%, respectively. The specificities of these two methods at 35% and 20%, respectively, were also low [3]. However, CT has an important additional role in preoperative staging [19–21] and prediction of resectability [22], although neither US nor CT is sensitive in detecting the small ampullary tumor.

Endoscopy

Endoscopy is the optimal diagnostic procedure for patients suspected of having an ampullary or duodenal neoplasm, because it enables the extent, size, and gross appearance of the lesion to be determined and

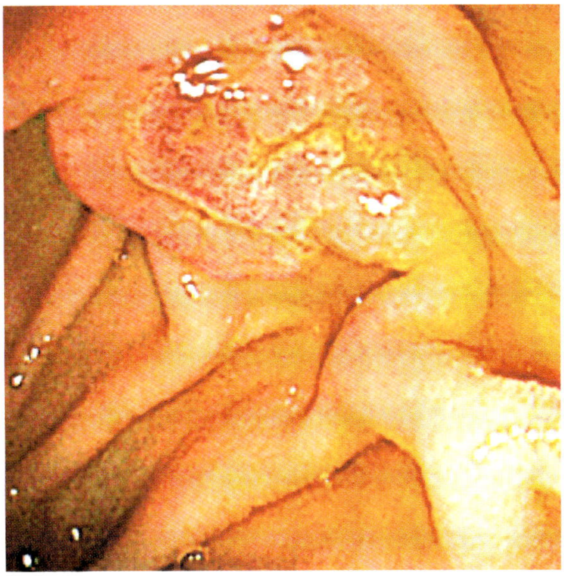

Figure 68.2

Duodenoscopic view of tubular adenoma of the papilla of Vater. The overlying mucosa has an even, granular appearance without ulcer or erosion

allows endoscopic biopsy sampling and cytologic brushing at the same time. Since the endoscopic appearance of benign and malignant ampullary lesions is often similar, detailed observation of the major papilla is very important [17]. Adenomas are manifested by symmetrical enlargement of the papilla with preservation of its normal configuration (Fig. 68.2). The overlying mucosa frequently appears discolored and granular, but there is no evidence of erosion or ulceration. The endoscopic appearance alone is insufficient to differentiate between malignant and benign ampullary tumors. Malignant transformation of ampullary adenomas is manifested by characteristic endoscopic findings, including induration and rigidity of the papilla on probing, ulceration or erosion of the lesion, and a submucosal mass effect that leaves the overlying mucosa intact but indicates tumor extension into the duodenal wall.

The characteristic appearance of villous adenomas of the papilla is a cauliflower-like, lobulated, sessile polypoid mass with no evidence of ulceration or erosion. Villous adenomas often contain foci of adenocarcinoma at the time of diagnosis. Surface nodularity, increased friability, and spontaneous bleeding during endoscopic examination favor the diagnosis of a lesion.

Biopsy/Cytology

Endoscopic forceps biopsy is the most practical modality for making a tissue diagnosis of ampullary neoplasms short of tumor excision. On the other hand, the presence of foci of adenocarcinoma has been reported in 15–50% of excised ampullary adenomas in the endoscopic, pathologic, and surgical literature findings regarding lesions of the ampulla that were diagnosed as benign before treatment [1,3,4,6,7,9]. Sauvanet et al. [23] reported that the accuracy of histologic diagnosis of 26 biopsy samples of papillary tumors was 69%, and the overall accuracy of endoscopic forceps biopsy diagnosis in Menzel's experience in 40 cases, was 62% [6]. Kimchi et al. [24] reported findings that diagnosis of periampullary carcinomas by endoscopic biopsy sampling is less accurate than diagnosis on the basis of their endoscopic appearance (81% vs 90%). Although these results suggest limited reliability of endoscopic biopsy given an incident carcinoma in ampullary tumors, forceps biopsy may be the only way to definitively exclude a focus of malignancy.

Endoscopic brush cytology is also an effective mean of diagnosing ampullary neoplasms. Bardales et al. [25] reported 100% diagnostic sensitivity and specificity, although cytologic diagnosis of an ampullary adenoma does not rule out an underlying malignant neoplasm. It may be difficult to distinguish between villous tumors with severe dysplasia and adenocarcinomas by cytological examination alone.

Stolte et al. [1] performed the follow-up evaluation of patients with a diagnosis of adenoma. Biopsy material from the surface of the tumors revealed that an adenocarcinoma was already present in other parts of the tumor in 60.25% of patients at the time the adenoma was diagnosed. An incidence of cancer in residual adenoma tissue was reported in 30–91% of the cases (1).

Endoscopic Retrograde Cholangiopancreatography, Magnetic Resonance Cholangiopancreatography/MRI

Endoscopic retrograde cholangiopancreatography (ERCP) is highly accurate for detecting small ampullary tumors, because reliable endoscopic signs are observed in the procedure. Since the biliary duct and pancreatic duct are visualized by injection of contrast medium, obstruction or invasion of these ducts can be detected. Although ERCP is invasive and there is a risk of adverse effects, including acute pancreatitis, cholangitis, and perforation, it remains the only method of examining for intraductal extension of adenomas along the bile and pancreatic ducts. Moreover, biopsy specimens can be collected and biliary or pancreatic drainage can be performed by sphincterotomy, or a stent can be inserted during the same procedure.

Magnetic resonance cholangiopancreatography (MRCP) has become competitive with ERCP as a method of diagnosing pancreatobiliary diseases because it is noninvasive and is capable of providing equivalent diagnostic information [26]. However, in contrast to the detection of pancreatic carcinomas [27], MRCP has not been shown to be more useful than CT, US, or ERCP for the detection of small ampullary tumors [28]. Use of MRCP in the process of diagnosis of ampullary tumors has a role in patients, suggesting biliary obstruction at the ampullary level diagnosed by US or CT. MRI is a less accurate method of detecting ampullary neoplasms than EUS, but is more accurate than CT [19].

Endoscopic Ultrasound

EUS provides significant advantages over other imaging methods for evaluation of ampullary tumors. It provides a high tumor detection rate (96% to 100%) for small ampullary tumors that is comparable to the rate obtained by ERCP, and better than the rate obtained by US, CT, and angiography [29]. EUS is particularly useful for the detection of small tumors that may be missed by CT [21]. In addition to its high rate of ampullary tumor detection, EUS is capable of imaging the distal biliary and pancreatic ducts to identify intraductal tumor extension and invasion (Fig. 68.3). EUS is the single most accurate method for determining the T stage of ampullary tumors. The reported accuracy of T staging by EUS ranges from 74% to 83% [19, 23, 30, 31], and the rates have been superior to those obtained with CT or US. The accuracy of EUS in detecting lymph node metastases range from 63 to 100% [19,23,30,31]. EUS is superior to CT and MRI for determining the T stage of ampullary lesions, but not the N stage. EUS more accurately predicts involvement of the portal-mesenteric axis by ampullary tumors than does CT (87% vs 67%) [32], and thus it is a more accurate means of staging and assessing the resectability of ampullary cancer [32,33]. The role of EUS in the process of diagnosing ampullary tumors therefore lies in the preoperative staging of ampullary carcinomas and identification of invasive lesions in suspected benign ampullary neoplasms [32,33].

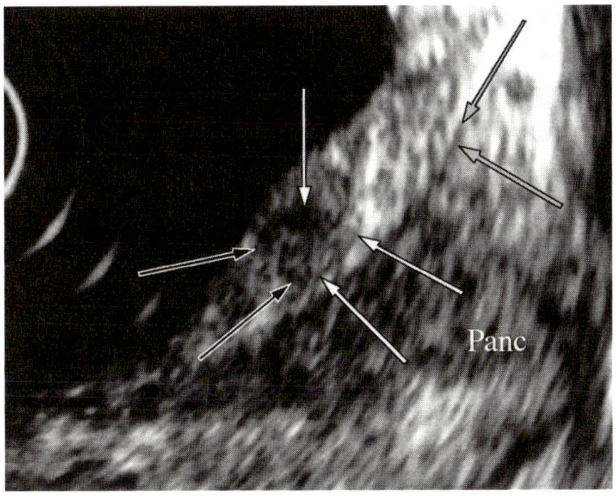

Figure 68.3

Endoscopic ultrasonography of an ampullary adenoma represented by a hypoechoic area with irregular outer margins (*black arrows*). The tumor did not infiltrate beyond the muscle layer of sphincter of Oddi (*white arrows*) into the pancreas (*Panc*) and the duodenal wall (*gray arrows*)

Although EUS is clearly helpful in detecting ampullary tumors, the sonographic images themselves do not allow the differentiation between benign and malignant tumors, and histological evaluation is necessary to demonstrate malignancy. Failure of a lesion to lift after submucosal injection is suggested to be the strongest predictor of malignancy [34]. EUS enables superficial biopsy sampling or guided fine-needle aspiration (FNA) biopsy sampling of neoplasms of the papilla of Vater, but is not helpful in detecting small malignant foci in adenomas of the papilla [1,3,4,6,7,9]. In addition to superficial mucosal biopsy of the papilla itself, EUS also enables FNA biopsy of surrounding deeper structures, including lymph nodes. Defrain et al. [35] reported a high diagnostic accuracy (88.8%) for FNA.

Intraductal Ultrasonography

IDUS, a combination of ERCP and catheter-probe sonography, has provided a new diagnostic method for detecting small tumors in the biliary and pancreatic ducts (Fig. 68.4) [36,37]. Menzel et al. [20] reported 100% tumor visualization by IDUS, and the overall accuracy of ampullary tumor diagnosis by IDUS (88.9%) was significantly superior to EUS (56.3%). The accuracy of IDUS for diagnosing the extension of cancer of the papilla of Vater into the duodenum was markedly high (d0 100%, d1 92.3%, d2 100%, and pancreatic invasion 75%) [38]. IDUS appears to be the most effective imaging tool for visualizing, diagnosing, and staging tumors of the major duodenal papilla.

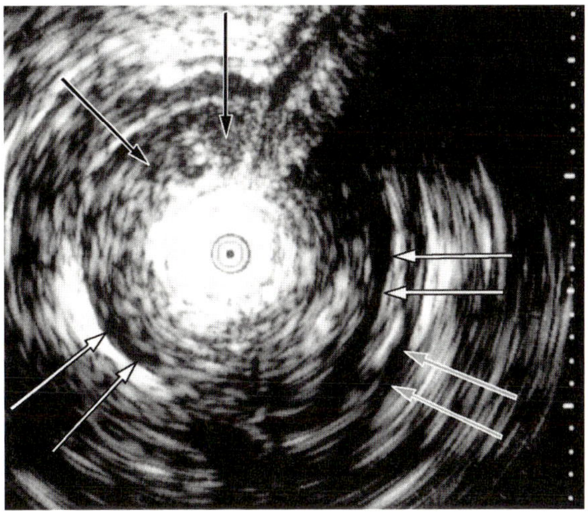

Figure 68.4

Intraductal ultrasonography of an adenoma of the papilla. The adenoma appears with a hypoechoic area (*black arrows*). Irregular margins at the duodenal lumen (at the 10–12 o'clock position indicated with *black arrows*) and a well-demarcated duodenal wall (at the 3 o'clock and 7 o'clock positions indicated with *white arrows*) are evident. The muscle layer of sphincter of Oddi in the duodenal wall is seen (*gray arrows*)

References

1. Stolte M, Pscherer C (1996) Adenoma-carcinoma sequence in the papilla of Vater. Scand J Gastroenterol 31:376–382
2. Treitschke F, Beger HG (1999) Local resection of benign periampullary tumors. Ann Oncol 10:212–214
3. Schoenberg MH, Treitschke F, Harada N, Beger HG (1998) Benign tumour of the ampulla of Vater: surgical treatment and prognosis. Eur J Surg 164:765–770
4. Seifert E, Schulte F, Stolte M (1992) Adenoma and carcinoma of the duodenum and papilla of Vater: a clinicopathologic study. Am J Gastroenterol 87:37–42
5. Martin JA, Haber GB (2003) Ampullary adenoma: clinical manifestations, diagnosis, and treatment. Gastrointest Endosc Clin N Am 13:649–69
6. Menzel J, Poremba C, Dietl KH, Bocker W, Domschke W (1999) Tumors of the papilla of Vater – inadequate diagnostic impact of endoscopic forceps biopsies taken prior to and following sphincterotomy. Ann Oncol 10:1227–1231
7. Motton G, Veraldi GF, Fracastoro G, Ricci F, Laterza E, Dorrucci V, Cordiano C (1996) Vater's papilla and periampullary area villous adenoma: personal experience about nine cases and review of the literature. Hepatogastroenterology 43:448–455
8. Beger HG, Treitschke F, Gansauge F, Harada N, Hiki N, Mattfeldt T (1999) Tumor of the ampulla of Vater: experience with local or radical resection in 171 consecutively treated patients. Arch Surg 134:526–532

9. Sakorafas GH, Friess H, Dervenis CG (2000) Villous tumors of the duodenum: biologic characters and clinical implications. Scand J Gastroenterol 35:337–344
10. Burke CA, Beck GJ, Church JM, van Stolk RU (1999) The natural history of untreated duodenal and ampullary adenomas in patients with familial adenomatous polyposis followed in an endoscopic surveillance program. Gastrointest Endosc 49:358–364
11. Bjork J, Akerbrant H, Iselius L,Bergman A, Engwall Y, Wahlstrom J, Martinsson T, Nordling M, Hultcrantz R (2001) Periampullary adenomas and adenocarcinomas in familial adenomatous polyposis: cumulative risks and APC gene mutations. Gastroenterology 121:1127–1135
12. Matsumoto T, Iida M, Nakamura S, Hizawa K, Yao T, Tsuneyoshi M, Fujishima M (2000) Natural history of ampullary adenoma in familial adenomatous polyposis: reconfirmation of benign nature during extended surveillance. Am J Gastroenterol 95:1557–1562
13. Rivera JA, Rattner DW, Fernandez-del Castillo C, Warshaw AL (1996) Surgical approaches to benign and malignant tumors of the ampulla of Vater. Surg Oncol Clin N Am 5:689–711
14. Catalano MF, Linder JD, Chak A, Sivak MV Jr, Raijman I, Geenen JE, Howell DA (2004) Endoscopic management of adenoma of the major duodenal papilla. Gastrointest Endosc 59:225–232
15. Saurin JC, Chavaillon A, Napoleon B, Descos F, Bory R, Berger F, Ponchon T (2003) Long-term follow-up of patients with endoscopic treatment of sporadic adenomas of the papilla of Vater. Endoscopy 35:402–406
16. Binmoeller KF, Boaventura S, Ramsperger K, Soehendra N (1993) Endoscopic snare excision of benign adenomas of the papilla of Vater. Gastrointest Endosc 39:127–131
17. Kim MH, Lee SK, Seo DW, Won SY, Lee SS, Min YI (2001) Tumors of the major duodenal papilla. Gastrointest Endosc 54:609–620
18. Irie H, Honda H, Kaneko K, Kuroiwa T, Yoshimitsu K, Masuda K (1997) Comparison of helical CT and MR imaging in detecting and staging small pancreatic adenocarcinoma. Abdom Imaging 22:429–433
19. Cannon ME, Carpenter SL, Elta GH, Nostrant TT, Kochman ML, Ginsberg GG, Stotland B, Rosato EF, Morris JB, Eckhauser F, Scheiman JM (1999) EUS compared with CT, magnetic resonance imaging, and angiography and the influence of biliary stenting on staging accuracy of ampullary neoplasms. Gastrointest Endosc 50:27–33
20. Menzel J, Hoepffner N, Sulkowski U, Reimer P, Heinecke A, Poremba C, Domschke W (1999) Polypoid tumors of the major duodenal papilla: preoperative staging with intraductal US, EUS, and CT – a prospective, hisotpathologically controlled study. Gastrointest Endosc 49:349–357
21. Midwinter MJ, Beveridge CJ, Wilsdon JB, Bennett MK, Baudouin CJ, Charnley RM (1999) Correlation between spiral computed tomography, endoscopic ultrasonography and findings at operation in pancreatic and ampullary tumours. Br J Surg 86:189–193
22. Howard TJ, Chin AC, Streib EW, Kopecky KK, Wiebke EA (1997) Value of helical computed tomography, angiography, and endoscopic ultrasound in determining resectability of periampullary carcinoma. Am J Surg 174:237–241
23. Sauvanet A, Chapuis O, Hammel P, Flejou JF, Ponsot P, Bernades P, Belghiti J (1997) Are endoscopic procedures able to predict the benignity of ampullary tumors? Am J Surg 174:355–358
24. Kimchi NA, Mindrul V, Broide E, Scapa E (1998) The contribution of endoscopy and biopsy to the diagnosis of periampullary tumors. Endoscopy 30:538–543
25. Bardales RH, Stanley MW, Simpson DD, Baker SJ, Steele CT, Schaefer RF, Powers CN (1998) Diagnostic value of brush cytology in the diagnosis of duodenal, biliary, and ampullary neoplasms. Am J Clin Pathol 109:540–548
26. Hintze RE, Adler A, Veltzke W, Abou-Rebyeh H, Hammerstingl R, Vogl T, Felix R (1997) Clinical significance of magnetic resonance cholangiopancreatography (MRCP) compared to endoscopic retrograde cholangiopancreatography (ERCP). Endoscopy 29:182–187
27. Adamek HE, Albert J, Breer H, Weitz M, Schilling D, Riemann JF (2000) Pancreatic cancer detection with magnetic resonance cholangiopancreatography and endoscopic retrograde cholangiopancreatography: a prospective controlled study. Lancet 356:190–193
28. Geier A, Nguyen HN, Gartung C, Matern S (2000) MRCP and ERCP to detect small ampullary carcinoma. Lancet 356:1607–1608
29. Mukai H, Nakajima M, Yasuda K, Mizuno S, Kawai K (1992) Evaluation of endoscopic ultrasonography in the pre-operative staging of carcinoma of the ampulla of Vater and common bile duct. Gastrointest Endosc 38:676–683
30. Kubo H, Chijiiwa Y, Akahoshi K, Hamada S, Matsui N, Nawata H (1999) Pre-operative staging of ampullary tumours by endoscopic ultrasound. Br J Radiol 72:443–447
31. Chen CH, Tseng LJ, Yang CC, Yeh YH, Mo LR (2001) The accuracy of endoscopic ultrasound, endoscopic retrograde cholangiopancreatography, computed tomography, and transabdominal ultrasound in the detection and staging of primary ampullary tumors. Hepatogastroenterology 48:1750–1753
32. Maluf-Filho F, Sakai P, Cunha JE, Garrido T, Rocha M, Machado MC, Ishioka S (2004) Radial endoscopic ultrasound and spiral computed tomography in the diagnosis and staging of periampullary tumors. Pancreatology 4:122–128
33. Buscail L, Pages P, Berthelemy P, Fourtanier G, Frexinos J, Escourrou J (1999) Role of EUS in the management of pancreatic and ampullary carcinoma: a prospective study assessing resectability and prognosis. Gastrointest Endosc 50:34–40
34. Kahaleh M, Shami VM, Brock A, Conaway MR, Yoshida C, Moskaluk CA, Adams RB, Tokar J, Yeaton P (2004) Factors predictive of malignancy and endoscopic resectability in ampullary neoplasia. Am J Gastroenterol 99:2335–2339
35. Defrain C, Chang CY, Srikureja W, Nguyen PT, Gu M (2005) Cytologic features and diagnostic pitfalls of primary ampullary tumors by endoscopic ultrasound-guided fine-needle aspiration biopsy. Cancer 105:289–297
36. Furukawa T, Oohashi K, Yamao K, Naitoh Y, Hirooka Y, Taki T, Itoh A, Hayakawa S, Watanabe Y, Goto H, Hayakawa T (1997) Intraductal ultrasonography of the pancreas: development and clinical potential. Endoscopy 29:561–569
37. Ariyama J, Suyama M, Satoh K, Wakabayashi K (1998) Endoscopic ultrasound and intraductal ultrasound in the diagnosis of small pancreatic tumors. Abdom Imaging 23:380–386
38. Itoh A, Goto H, Naitoh Y, Hirooka Y, Furukawa T, Hayakawa T (1997) Intraductal ultrasonography in diagnosing tumor extension of cancer of the papilla of Vater. Gastrointest Endosc 45:251–260

Chapter 69

T. Kamisawa · A. Okamoto

Clinical Diagnosis of Periampullary Carcinoma

Periampullary carcinomas in a broad sense indicate carcinomas arising at or near the ampulla of Vater. They can be divided into four histologies: pancreatic carcinoma, ampullary carcinoma, distal common bile duct carcinoma, and duodenal carcinoma according to their sites of origin [1,2]. They are grouped together because they arise in the almost same area, their exact origin is difficult to ascertain at the time of diagnosis, and their symptoms and surgical treatment are essentially the same. However, it is necessary to separate these carcinomas strictly, because their rate of resectability and prognosis are different. The incidence of the sites of origin in periampullary carcinomas is reportedly different. The most common site of origin is the head of the pancreas, ampullary carcinoma being the second commonest [3]. In a narrow sense, periampullary carcinomas indicate carcinomas originating from the ampulla of Vater and its vicinity, excluding pancreatic head tumors. This chapter describes mainly clinical diagnosis of ampullary carcinoma, but also a brief overview of diagnosis of distal common bile duct carcinoma and periampullary duodenal carcinoma. Diagnosis of pancreatic carcinoma is discussed elsewhere.

Ampullary Carcinoma

Before instituting appropriate treatment, it is important to distinguish benign lesions, including adenoma, from malignant lesions and to differentiate ampullary carcinoma from other periampullary carcinomas. Accurate diagnosis and staging are especially important for ampullary carcinoma because the strategies employed vary according to the staging as follows: endoscopic resection, local resection, pylorus-preserving pancreaticoduodenectomy, radical pancreaticoduodenectomy, bypass procedures, and endoscopic stenting.

Clinical Presentations

Many of the difficulties in the treatment of ampullary carcinoma can be traced to the physician's inability to diagnose the disease in its early stage, because the vague early symptoms of ampullary carcinoma are often minimized by both the patient and physicians. It is ordinarily not until the patient manifests jaundice that the diagnosis is made. Fortunately, ampullary carcinoma will lead to jaundice at an early stage that might be seen in tumors arising from the pancreas. Obstructive jaundice is the most constant symptom and sign, and is present in about 70% of cases [4,5]. Jaundice may fluctuate initially, and is often associated with pruritis. Many patients have constitutional symptoms such as malaise and/or anorexia for several weeks or months prior to the appearance of jaundice [6].

Abdominal pain and weight loss are also common and occur in about half of patients [7,8]. Other general signs of malignant diseases are malaise, anorexia, nausea, vomiting, melena, anemia, and occult blood in the feces. The triad of fluctuating painless jaundice, anemia, with or without symptoms of gastrointestinal bleeding, and a palpable gallbladder has been considered relatively specific for an ampullary tumor [9]. Unfortunately, this classic triad is seldom observed [7]. Some patients with ampullary carcinoma present with pancreatitis. Acute pancreatitis was reported as the presenting picture in 5–18% of cases [8,10]. Cholangitis is an uncommon presentation of ampullary carcinoma, being reported in only 6 out of 102 cases (6%) [7]. However, several authors report fever and chills without specifically mentioning cholangitis [11]. It is reported that those patients with ampullary carcinoma who present without jaundice have a better outcome compared with those who present with jaundice [12]. In this report, multivariate regression analysis revealed that jaundice had no independent prognostic value, but that a greater number of early ampullary carcinomas and papillary-type adenocarcinomas were present in the nonjaundiced group. The observation of the papilla of Vater during routine upper gastrointestinal endoscopy will detect early stage ampullary carcinomas without symptoms.

In addition to the presenting symptoms, the patient's past medical history and family history may also be highly relevant. Patients with the hereditary disorders of Gardner's syndrome and familial polyposis of the colon have more than a 200-fold increased risk of ampullary and duodenal carcinoma compared with the general population [13]. In most of these patients, the polyps will be multiple and involve much of the duodenal mucosa.

The findings on physical examination are usually limited to jaundice, hepatomegaly, and a palpable gallbladder. There are no specific diagnostic laboratory tests for ampullary carcinoma. Laboratory investigation usually shows an increase in liver enzymes consistent with biliary tract obstruction, including increased plasma concentration of bilirubin and alkaline phosphatase. Concentration of serum CA19.9 is sometimes elevated in patients with ampullary carcinoma, but it is frequently normal in the early stage.

Imaging Studies

The prompt evaluation of a patient with jaundice offers the opportunity for early diagnosis of ampullary carcinoma. Any patient presenting jaundice should undergo diagnostic imaging with either ultrasonography (US) or computed tomography (CT). Both diagnostics will confirm the obstructive nature of the jaundice by demonstrating a dilated intra- and extrahepatic bile duct and therefore focus the next steps in evaluation.

Abdominal US, which is a safe and useful noninvasive technique in the evaluation of a jaundiced patient, is helpful as an initial screening examination but lacks specificity in the documentation of ampullary lesions, partly because of the small size of some of ampullary carcinomas. Unfortunately, approximately 20% of pancreatic ultrasound evaluations are technically inadequate because bowel gas or obesity obscure resolution [14].

Thin-slice CT of the abdomen with adequate administration of oral contrast agents to delineate the duodenum demonstrates most often a dilated common bile duct down to the level of the duodenum, absence of a pancreatic mass, and, occasionally, a mass at the ampulla. The presence of dilatation of the intrapancreatic portion of the common bile duct suggests an ampullary or distal common bile duct lesion, even in the absence of a mass.

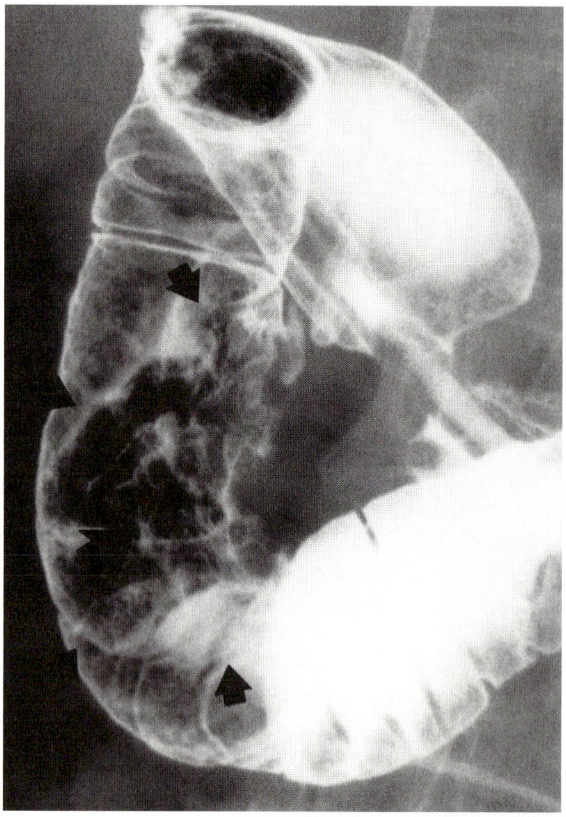

Figure 69.1

Hypotonic duodenography of ampullary carcinoma

Magnetic resonance imaging (MRI) offers almost the same advantages as CT. Irie et al. [15] reported that the signal intensities of the tumor on each image varied, and dynamic study detected most tumors, all of which showed delayed enhancement. Magnetic resonance cholangiopancreatography (MRCP) can provide reliable information that is almost the same as that provided by endoscopic retrograde cholangiopancreatography (ERCP). Classical hypotonic duodenography can demonstrate the appearance of ampullary carcinoma (Fig. 69.1), but this tool has become less significant recently.

Endoscopic Diagnosis

Once biliary obstruction without an obvious pancreatic mass has been confirmed by imaging studies, the next potential step in the evaluation of the jaundiced patient is ERCP. This technique allows not only visualization of the ampullary region, but also examination of the relevant duct systems, and simultaneous performance of an endoscopic biopsy or brush cytology.

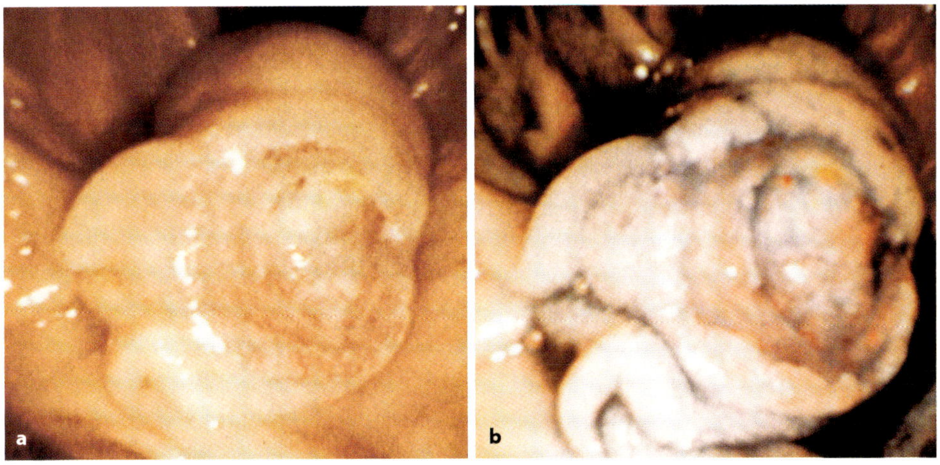

Figure 69.2

Endoscopic appearance of ampullary carcinoma (exposed protruding type) without (a) or with dye spraying (b)

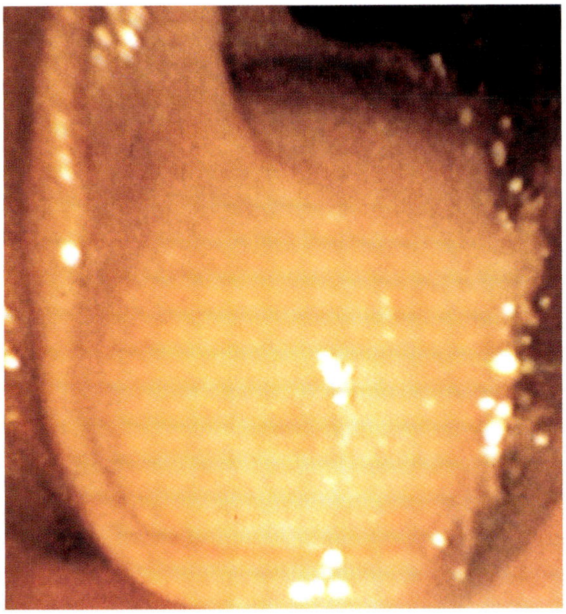

Figure 69.3

Endoscopic appearance of ampullary carcinoma (intramural protruding type)

The major duodenal papilla is seen only in part with a forward-viewing endoscope, so that complete evaluation almost always requires use of a side-viewing endoscope. The endoscopic appearance of an ampullary carcinoma can be divided into three main types: exposed protruding type (Fig. 69.2), intramural protruding type (Fig. 69.3), and ulcerating type (Fig. 69.4) [16,17]. Several rare cases show a peduncular polypoid lesion (Fig. 69.5). The protruding type represents an earlier form of the carcinoma, while the ulcerating type is usually in an advanced stage. Intramural type ampullary carcinoma, which is covered with grossly normal mucosa, requires a sphincterotomy before it can be visualized.

Although endoscopic biopsy sampling is very useful in diagnosing ampullary carcinoma, it may be inaccurate in 10–30% of patients [18–22], yielding false negative results, largely due to sampling error. The demonstration of malignancy on biopsy specimens is definitive, but a diagnosis of a benign adenoma does not rule out the presence of an adenocarcinoma elsewhere in the adenoma. Even without an overt mass lesion, the presence of a generous or enlarged papilla associated with extrahepatic bile duct dilatation should prompt sphincterotomy and intra-ampullary biopsy sampling.

ERCP is indicated in almost all patients presenting with obstructive jaundice or dilated extrahepatic bile duct without an obvious periampullary mass. However, in many cases of ampullary tumors, the orifice of the biliary and/or pancreatic duct cannot be visualized or cannulated for cholangiography. In cases of ampullary carcinoma, cholangiography may demonstrate a supra-ampullary intraductal mass, a focal stricture, or bile duct dilatation proximal to the ampullary area (Fig. 69.6), and pancreatography may demonstrate a normal pancreatic duct, or stenosis of the main pancreatic duct associated with upstream dilatation (Fig. 69.7). ERCP is also the procedure of choice when choledocholithiasis is considered in the differential diagnosis for obstructive jaundice. Calculus impacted in the distal end of common bile duct causes pseudotumor appearance at the papilla. On

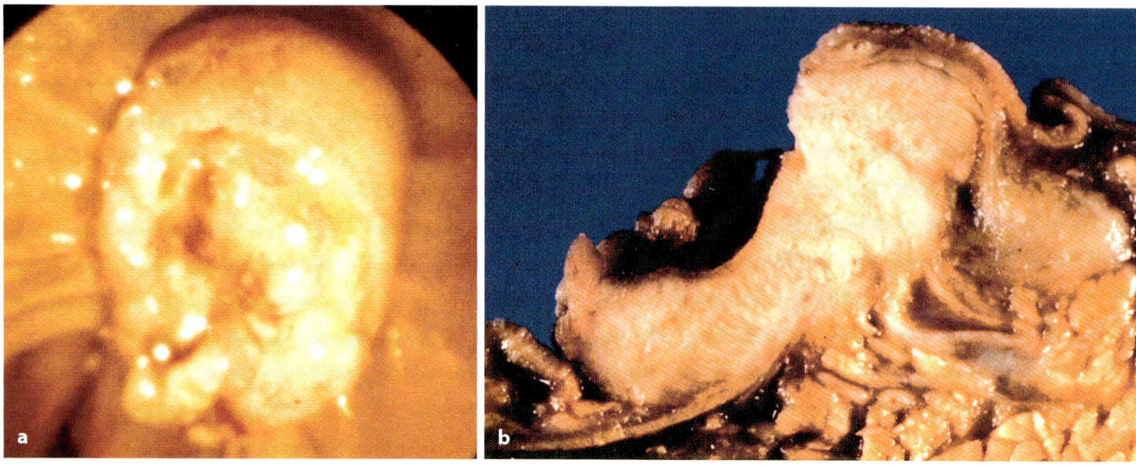

Figure 69.4

a Endoscopic appearance of ampullary carcinoma (ulcerating type), and b cut surface of the resected specimen

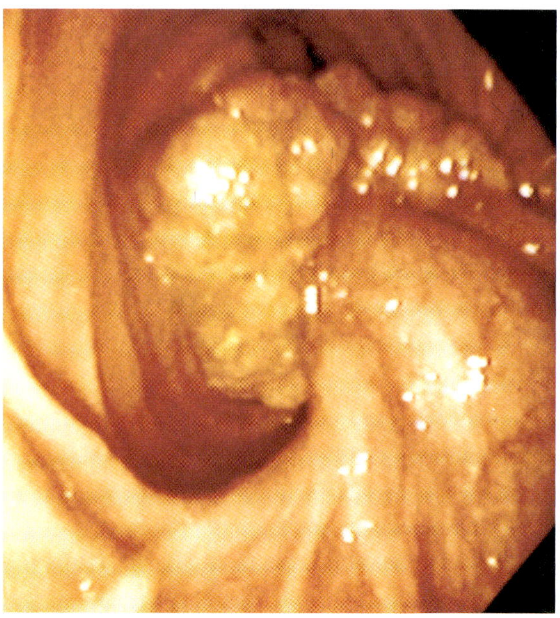

Figure 69.5

Endoscopic appearance of ampullary carcinoma (large polypoid type)

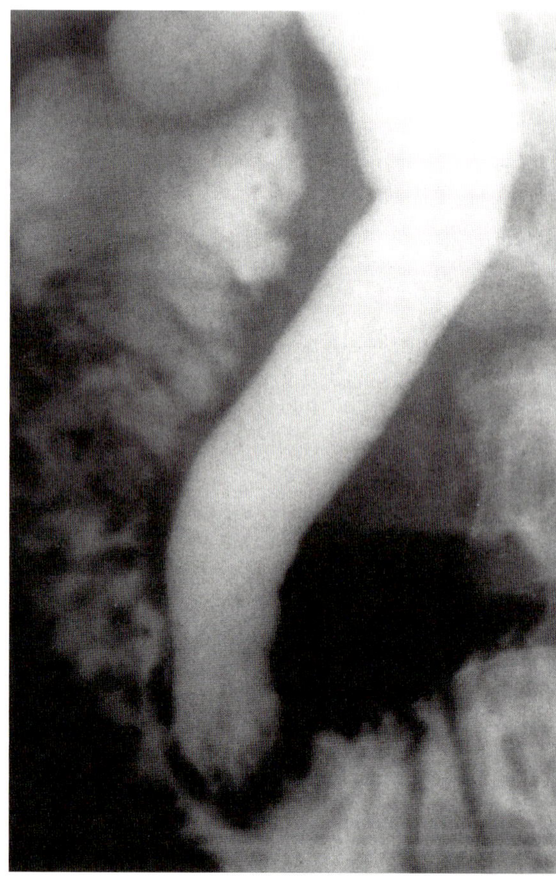

Figure 69.6

Endoscopic retrograde cholangiographic image of advanced ampullary carcinoma showing supra-ampullary mass with bile duct dilatation

the other hand, a relatively large number of patients with ampullary carcinoma also have coexistent calculi in the bile duct and/or gallbladder [23]. Hayes et al. [8] found coexistent calculus disease of the biliary system in 12 out of 37 patients with ampullary carcinoma. The presence of calculi has frequently resulted in errors in diagnosis, since the clinical manifestations of ampullary carcinoma and biliary calculi are similar. After cholangiographic demonstration of the

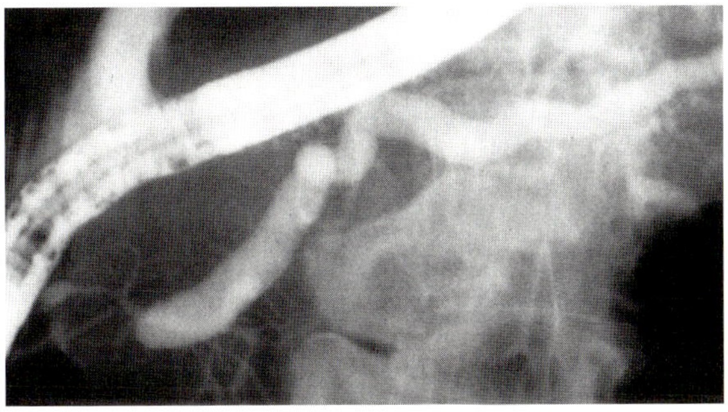

Figure 69.7

Endoscopic retrograde pancreatographic image of advanced ampullary carcinoma showing stenosis of the main pancreatic duct with upstream dilatation

obstructing lesion, a biliary stent or nasobiliary drainage tube can be inserted to alleviate the jaundice. Percutaneous transhepatic biliary drainage is also useful if ERCP is unsuccessful.

Preoperative Staging

The specific aims of preoperative staging are to determine which tumors are potentially resectable and have not already metastasized to distant sites or directly invaded the major peripancreatic vessels, and to determine indications for local resection including endoscopic resection. In general, preoperative staging is less important in patients with ampullary carcinoma, because it has high rate of resectability.

Intravenous and oral contrast-enhanced multidetector row CT can detect some ampullary carcinomas (Fig. 69.8) in addition to hepatic or other distant metastases, ascites, and vascular involvement. Endoscopic ultrasonography (EUS) is currently the optimal technique for evaluation of the periampullary region. EUS can detect rather small ampullary carcinoma (Fig. 69.9). The accuracy of EUS for ampullary carcinoma is significantly better than that of other imaging procedures, including blood vessel invasion and spread to regional lymph nodes. It has been reported that assessment of T and N categories in EUS for ampullary carcinoma has an accuracy of 83% and 100%, respectively [24]. The overall accuracy of EUS in the assessment of tumor categories using the TNM classification in patients with ampullary carcinoma was reported to be 88% [25].

Intraductal ultrasonography (IDUS) performed endoscopically or transhepatically allows the anatomy of the ampulla of Vater to be studied with visualization of the sphincter of Oddi [26]. Therefore, it is

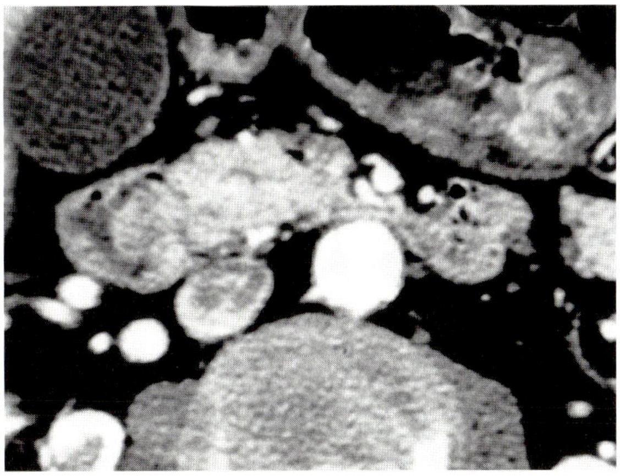

Figure 69.8

Multidetector row computed tomography of ampullary carcinoma showing a tumor protruding into the duodenum

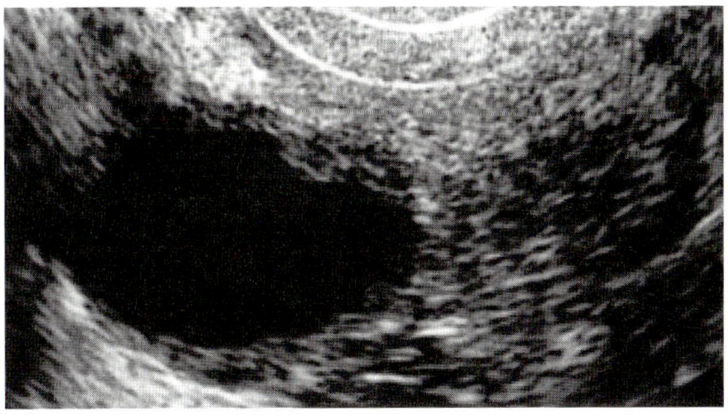

Figure 69.9

Endoscopic ultrasonographic image of ampullary carcinoma showing obstruction of the distal common bile duct by the tumor

possible to identify early ampullary carcinomas that have not crossed the sphincter of Oddi and can be given curative treatment involving endoscopic or local resection. As IDUS is more suited for observing the near field, such as diagnosing whether the tumor has infiltrated beyond Oddi's muscle layer, rather than far-field observation to diagnose the tumor infiltration into the pancreatic parenchyma, diagnostic accuracy is higher for smaller-sized ampullary carcinomas [27].

Given the much lower frequency of major visceral vessel involvement in ampullary carcinoma when compared with pancreatic carcinoma, angiography is seldom warranted in most patients with ampullary carcinoma, unless the suspicion of vessel involvement has been suggested by CT. Recently, it has been demonstrated that CT-angiography offers benefit of displaying an anatomical anomaly in a major visceral artery in preoperative evaluation.

The diagnosis and staging of ampullary lesions has evolved significantly in the past decade. These lesions can now be distinguished from more ominous lesions in the head of the pancreas, and a combination of endoscopic and imaging techniques provides remarkably accurate information about the stage of disease.

Distal Common Bile Duct Carcinoma

Cholangiocarcinomas occur throughout the biliary tree. The spectrum of these tumors is classified into three broad anatomical groups: intrahepatic, perihilar, and distal cholangiocarcinoma. Distal common bile duct carcinoma is the second most common, accounting for 20–30% of bile duct malignancies [28,29]. Distal common bile duct carcinomas are usually small and have a better prognosis than the more central bile duct carcinomas [30]. Obstructive jaundice is present in almost 100% of patients with this disease [29,31]. ERCP usually demonstrates a short stricture or a polypoid mass causing biliary obstruction, but a normal pancreatic duct. Scrape biopsy, and brush or bile cytology are useful for pathohistological assessment. MRCP and percutaneous transhepatic cholangiography also provide obstruction of the distal common bile duct. Cholangiocarcinoma that arises in the intrapancreatic portion of the common bile duct is well depicted as a ringed, enhanced mass on enhanced CT. EUS can demonstrate the extent of this disease. However, it is sometimes difficult to differentiate distal common bile duct carcinoma extending into the duodenum from ampullary carcinoma, even when using multiple imaging modalities. In general, distal common bile duct carcinomas present at an earlier stage are more likely to be resectable, and have a better prognosis.

Duodenal Carcinoma

Primary carcinomas arising in the small bowel are uncommon, but a high portion of those found are in the duodenum. Duodenal carcinoma accounts for less than 1% of all gastrointestinal neoplasms [32]. Almost all of these lesions are located in the postbulbar portion of the duodenum at or below the level of the ampulla of Vater [33,34]. In many reports, differentiation between lesions arising in the duodenal mucosa and those of ampulla itself is not clearly performed. Most authors who have differentiated between these tumors have regarded the lesions as being of duodenal origin only when they have been clearly separated from the ampulla. In Japan and the United Kingdom, the ratio of ampullary to duodenal carcinoma is approximately 9:1 [35,36]. Periampullary duodenal carcinomas are typically small, polypoid, or indurated masses, which present relatively early with biliary or pancreatic obstruction. Tumors occurring at other locations in the duodenum often grow to a larger size, forming either exophytic fungating or annular stenosing lesions [37]. Over half of patients with duodenal carcinoma present with metastatic disease, involving lymph nodes, liver, omentum, mesentery or peritoneum [38]. Weight loss and abdominal pain are the most frequent complaints, followed by nausea, vomiting, anorexia, melena, and duodenal obstruction or clinical gastric outlet obstruction [39,40]. Jaundice may occur where the lesion involves the ampulla of Vater. Upper gastrointestinal endoscopy with biopsy and barium studies are diagnostic. Resectability is evaluated by the lack of vascular encasement, contiguous organ invasion, distant lymphadenopathy, or liver or peritoneal metastases on CT or MRI.

References

1. Wise L, Pizzimbono C, Dehner LP (1976) Periampullary cancer: a clinicopathologic study of sixty-two patients. Am J Surg 131:141–148
2. Michelassi F, Erroi F, Dawson PJ, et al (1989) Experience with 647 consecutive tumors of the duodenum, ampulla of Vater, head of the pancreas, and distal common bile duct. Ann Surg 210:544–556
3. Schmidt CM, Powell ES, Yiannoutsos CT, et al (2004) Pancreaticoduodenectomy A 20-year experience in 516 patients. Arch Surg 139:718–727
4. Todoroki T, Koike N, Morishita Y, et al (2003) Patterns and predictors of failure after curative resections of carcinoma of the ampulla of Vater. Ann Surg Oncol 10:1176–1183
5. Duffy JP, Hines OJ, Liu JH, et al (2003) Improved survival for adenocarcinoma of the ampulla of Vater. Arch Surg 138:941–950
6. Walsh DB, Eckhauser FE, Cronenwett JL, et al (1982) Adenocarcinoma of the ampulla of Vater. Diagnosis and treatment. Ann Surg 195:152–157
7. Yamaguchi K, Enjoji M (1987) Carcinoma of the ampulla of Vater: a clinicopathological study and pathologic staging of 109 cases of carcinoma and 5 cases of adenoma. Cancer 59:506–515
8. Hayes DH, Bolton JS, Willis GW, et al (1987) Carcinoma of the ampulla of Vater. Ann Surg 205:572–577
9. Beall MS, Dyer GA, Stephenson HE (1970) Disappointments in the management of patients with malignancy of pancreas, duodenum and common bile duct. Arch Surg 101:461–465
10. Jones BA, Langer B, Taylor BR, et al (1985) Periampullary tumors: which ones should be resected? Am J Surg 149:46–51

11. Neoptolemos JP, Talbot IC, Carr–Locke DL, et al (1987) Treatment and outcome in 52 cases of ampullary carcinoma. Br J Surg 74:957–961
12. Yamaguchi K, Enjoji M, Kitamura K (1990) Non-icteric ampullary carcinoma with a favorable prognosis. Am J Gastroenterol 85:994–999
13. Iwama T, Tomita H, Kawachi Y, et al (1994) Indications for local excision of ampullary lesions associated with familial adenomatous polyposis. J Am Coll Surg 179:462–464
14. Brambs HJ, Claussen CD (1993) Pancreatic and ampullary carcinoma: ultrasound, computed tomography, magnetic resonance imaging and angiography. Endoscopy 25:58–68
15. Irie H, Honda H, Shinozaki K, et al (2002) MR imaging of ampullary carcinomas. J Comput Assist Tomogr 26:711–717
16. Tasaka K (1977) Carcinoma in the region of the duodenal papilla: a histopathological study. Fukuoka Acta Med 68:20–44
17. Kamisawa T, Fukayama M, Koike M, et al (1988) Carcinoma of the ampulla of Vater: expression of cancer-associated antigens inversely correlated with prognosis. Am J Gastroenterol 83:1118–1123
18. Ryan DP, Schapiro RH, Warshaw AI (1986) Villous tumors of the duodenum. Ann Surg 203:301–306
19. Yamaguchi K, Enjoji M, Kitamura K (1990) Endoscopic biopsy has limited accuracy in diagnosis of ampullary tumors. Gastrointest Endosc 36:588–592
20. Komorowski RA, Beggs BK, Geenan JE, et al (1991) Assessment of ampulla of Vater pathology: an endoscopic approach. Am J Surg Pathol 15:1188–1196
21. Ashbum JH, Rossai RL, Munson JL (1993) Local resection for ampullary tumors: is there a place for it? Arch Surg 128:515–520
22. Kimchi NA, Mindrul V, Broide E, et al (1998) The contribution of endoscopy and biopsy to the diagnosis of periampullary tumors. Endoscopy 30:538–543
23. Mnox RA, Kingston RD (1986) Carcinoma of the ampulla of Vater. Br J Surg 73:72–73
24. Buscail L, Pages P, Berthelemy P, et al (1999) Role of EUS in the management of pancreatic and ampullary carcinoma: a prospective study assessing respectability and prognosis. Gastrointest Endosc 50:34–40
25. Tio TL, Tytgat GNJ, Cikot RJLM, et al (1990) Ampullopancreatic carcinoma: preoperative TNM classification with endosonography. Radiology 175:455–461
26. Palazzo L (1998) Staging of ampullary carcinoma by endoscopic ultrasonography. Endoscopy 30 (Suppl 1):A128–A131
27. Itoh A, Goto H, Naitoh Y, et al (1997) Intraductal ultrasonography in diagnosing tumor extension of cancer of the papilla of Vater. Gastrointest Endosc 45:251–260
28. Pitt HA, Dooley WC, Yeo CJ, et al (1995) Malignancies of the biliary tree. Curr Probl Surg 32:1–100
29. Nakeeb A, Pitt HA, Coleman J, et al (1996) Cholangiocarcinoma: a spectrum of intrahepatic, perihilar and distal tumors. Ann Surg 224:463–473
30. Nichols DA, MacCarty RL, Gaffey TA (1983) Cholangiographic evaluation of bile duct carcinoma. AJR 141:1291–1294
31. Yeo CJ, Cameron JL, Lillemoe KD, et al (1995) Pancreatoduodenectomy for cancer of the head of the pancreas: 201 patients. Ann Surg 221:721–733
32. Spira IH, Ghazi A, Wolff WI (1977) Primary adenocarcinoma of the duodenum. Cancer 39:1721–1726
33. Cortese AF, Cornell GN (1972) Carcinoma of the duodenum, Cancer 29:1010–1015
34. Joesting DR, Beart RW Jr, van Heerden JA, et al (1981) Improving survival in adenocarcinoma of the duodenum. Am J Surg 141:228–231
35. Blumgart LH, Kennedy AC (1973) Carcinoma of the ampulla of Vater and duodenum. Br J Surg 60:33–40
36. Nakase A, Matsumoto Y, Uchida K, et al (1977) Surgical treatment of cancer of the pancreas and periampullary region. Ann Surg 185:52–57
37. Attanoos R, Williams G (1991) Epithelial and neuroendocrine tumors of the duodenum. Semin Diagn Pathol 8:149–162
38. Delcore R, Thomas J, Forster J, et al (1993) Improving respectability and survival in patients with primary duodenal carcinoma. Am J Surg 166:626–631
39. Rotman N, Pezet D, Fagniez PL, et al (1994) Adenocarcinoma of the duodenum: factors influencing survival. Br J Surg 81:83–85
40. Rose DM, Hochwald SN, Klimstra DS, et al (1996) Primary duodenal adenocarcinoma: a ten-year experience with 79 patients. J Am Coll Surg 183:89–96

Chapter 70

H. Maguchi · M. Osanai · A. Katanuma · K. Takahashi

Endoscopic Management of Adenoma

Adenoma of the ampulla of Vater is more likely to undergo malignant transformation than those arising elsewhere in the duodenum [1]. While the optimal management of adenoma has not been established, standard treatment has been complete surgical resection of the lesion. Pancreatoduodenectomy (PD) is effective, but highly invasive, whereas surgical papillectomy is less invasive, but is associated with high local recurrence [2–4]. Regardless of the drawbacks, endoscopic treatment has been introduced as a treatment for adenoma of the ampulla of Vater, arousing controversy with regard to its indications and management of its complications [5–16].

Since it is a rather new treatment modality, it has been described under a variety of names and techniques, such as endoscopic sphincterotomy and fulguration [5], endoscopic snare excision [7], endoscopic snare resection, endoscopic papillectomy [11,12], and endoscopic snare papillectomy [8,10,13,16]. In this chapter, we use the term endoscopic papillectomy (EP).

Indications for EP

EP is most suitably indicated for adenoma of the ampulla of Vater, particularly for cases of familial adenomatous polyposis (FAP). Patients with FAP have an increased risk of developing papillary neoplasm, and their risk of malignancies has been estimated at greater than 100 times that of the general population [17,18]. However, some adenomas remain dormant for a long period of time, and thus the question remains as to whether all adenomas need to be resected [19]. On the other hand, we must also note that there exists the adenoma-carcinoma sequence, and that there is occasionally difficulty in distinguishing between adenoma and adenocarcinoma, even on biopsy specimens [20–23]. Furthermore, it must be discussed whether treatment is indicated for early stage cancer, and if it is, preoperative diagnosis of the tumor progression must be fully taken into account. Even if a lesion is adenoma, it may have horizontal extension within the bile duct or the pancreatic duct; in such a case, endoscopic treatment is excluded (Fig. 70.1). The current guideline is that EP is indicated for adenoma of the ampulla of Vater without infiltration into the bile duct or the pancreatic duct. Accurate preoperative diagnosis is indispensable in this regard [11].

Diagnostic Work-Up

Endoscopic images, biopsy, endoscopic ultrasound (EUS) and endoscopic retrograde cholangiopancreatography (ERCP) are required to differentiate between adenoma and carcinoma, and to evaluate the progression of ampullary tumors. When diagnosing a lesion of the ampulla of Vater, we must be particularly careful because sometimes differentiation between adenoma and carcinoma is very difficult, even on a biopsy specimen [20–23]. Endoscopic findings are of particulary importance; benign features include pale, lobulated, and well-marginated lesion without ulcerated or depressed areas [12].

EUS has a higher diagnostic efficacy for the evaluation of tumor invasion and the detection of tumor extension along the bile and the pancreatic ducts (Figs. 70.2 and 70.3) [11].

ERCP is useful for evaluating the tumor extension not only along the ducts but also the orifice and its direction. Intraductal ultrasonography (IDUS) with an ultrasound probe can also provide precise imaging of the ampulla structure and the tumor extension [11, 24]. However, it is challenging to obtain definitive information about the microinvasion of ampullary tumors even using EUS in conjunction with IDUS. Therefore, EP should be very carefully indicated for carcinoma of the ampulla of Vater.

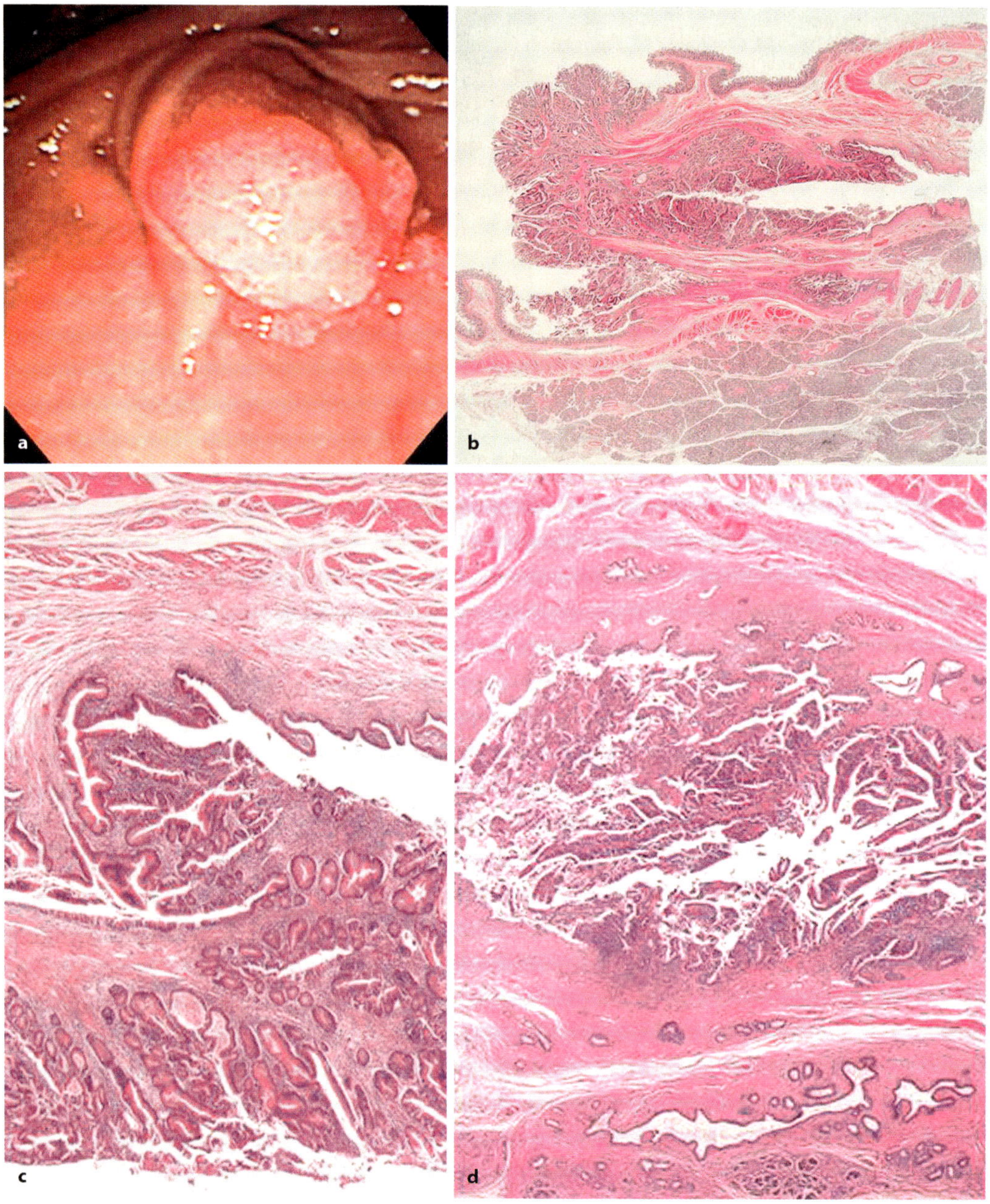

Figure 70.1

Endoscopic view of a protruded type of adenoma of the ampulla of Vater (a). The pathological findings after pancreatoduodenectomy was compatible with tubular adenoma extending into the bile and the pancreatic ducts (b–d)

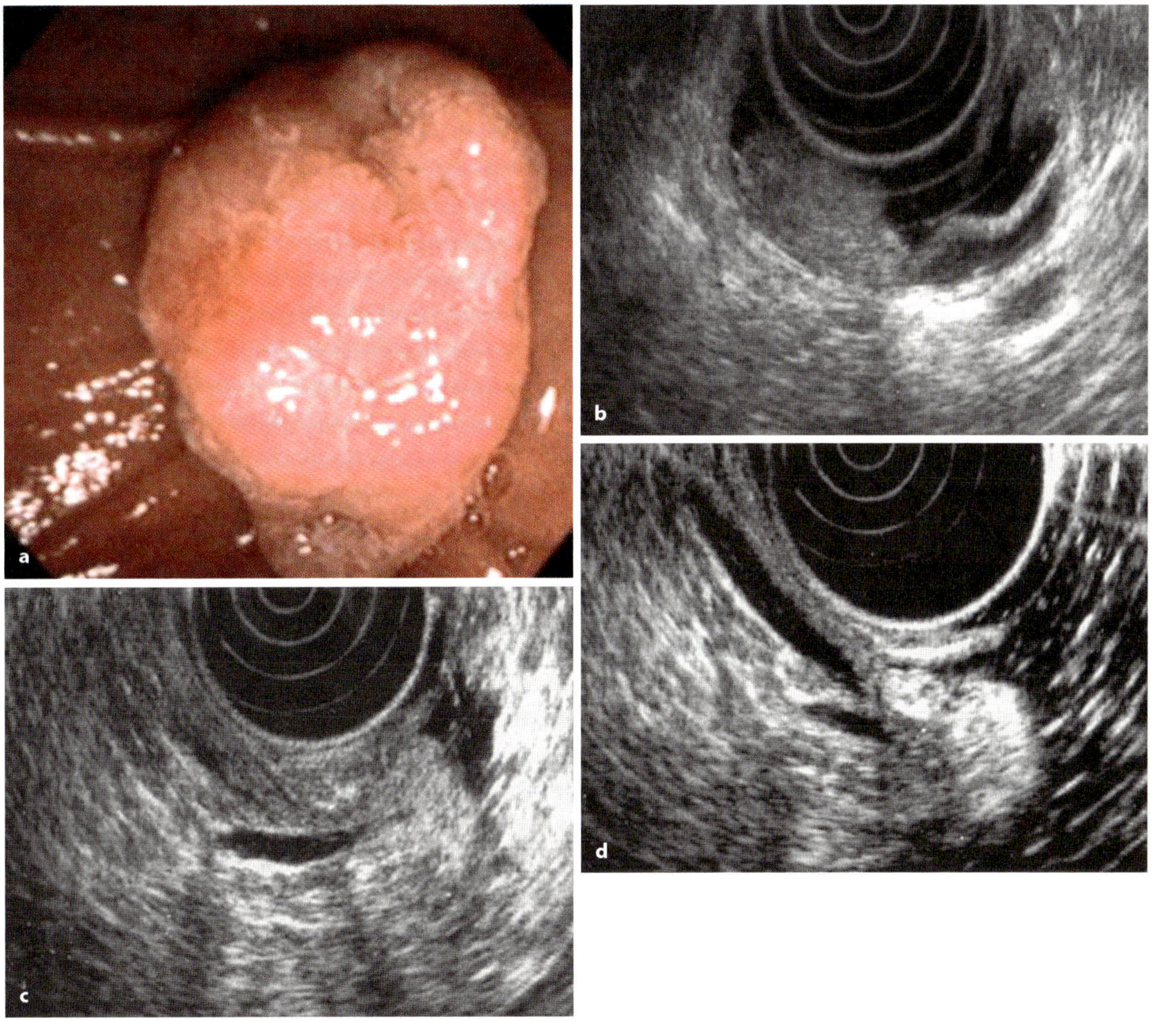

Figure 70.2

Endoscopic view of a protruded type of adenoma of the ampulla (a). Endoscopic ultrasound (EUS) images show a hyperechoic mass of the ampulla (b–d). Tumor invasion is absent in the muscularis propria of the duodenum wall without extent into the bile and the pancreatic ducts

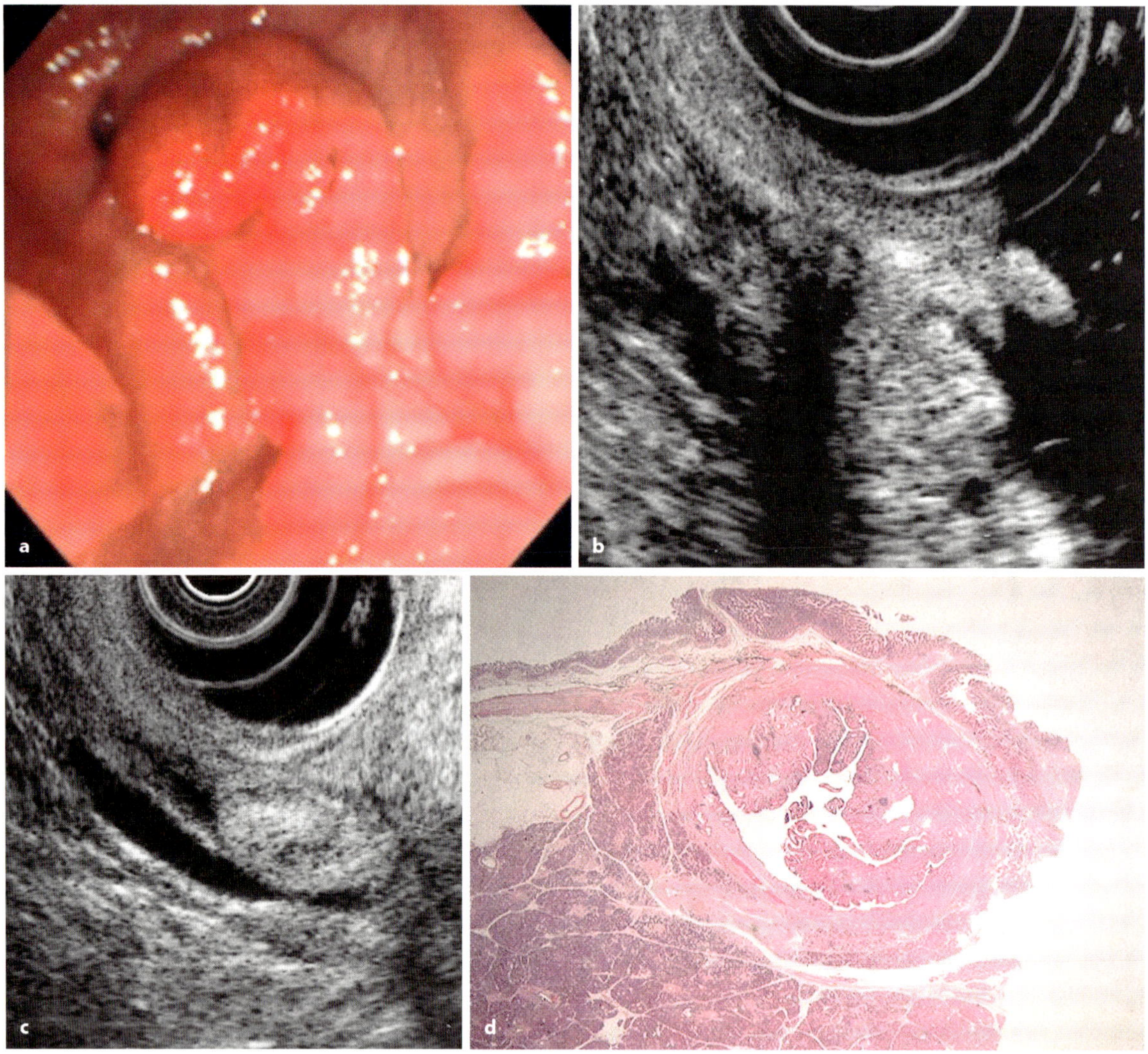

Figure 70.3

Endoscopic finding shows a protruded tumor of the ampulla (a). EUS demonstrates the tumor echo extending into the bile duct (b, c). Pathological findings of resected specimen show the tumor extent into the bile duct (d)

Treatment Technique

Endoscopic resection of adenomas or early gastrointestinal (GI) tract carcinomas has become popular following the development of new techniques and various endoscopic devices. These procedures are called endoscopic mucosal resection (EMR). While the use of this technique is being extended to the resection of adenoma of the ampulla of Vater, there are some difficulties with this method. The technical aspect of endoscopic resection of a lesion at the ampulla of Vater is different from EMR applied to other parts of the GI tract, as the ampulla of Vater is the orifice of biliopancreatic ducts. We have to ensure that we do not create complications such as acute pancreatitis or cholangitis, which can sometimes become lethal.

The basic procedure is to perform a snare excision using a standard polypectomy snare without endoscopic sphincterotomy (EST) or saline injection [11,12]. As shown in Fig. 70.4, a snare is set on the oral side, which is then squeezed after confirming the margin of the anal side; constant tension is applied to the snare loop during electrosurgery until the lesion is transected. Opinions differ, however, regarding this technique. It is very common to inject saline into the submucosal layer beneath the lesion to lift the lesion up to ease mucosal resection in EMR of GI tract. However, for tumors of the ampulla of Vater, there is

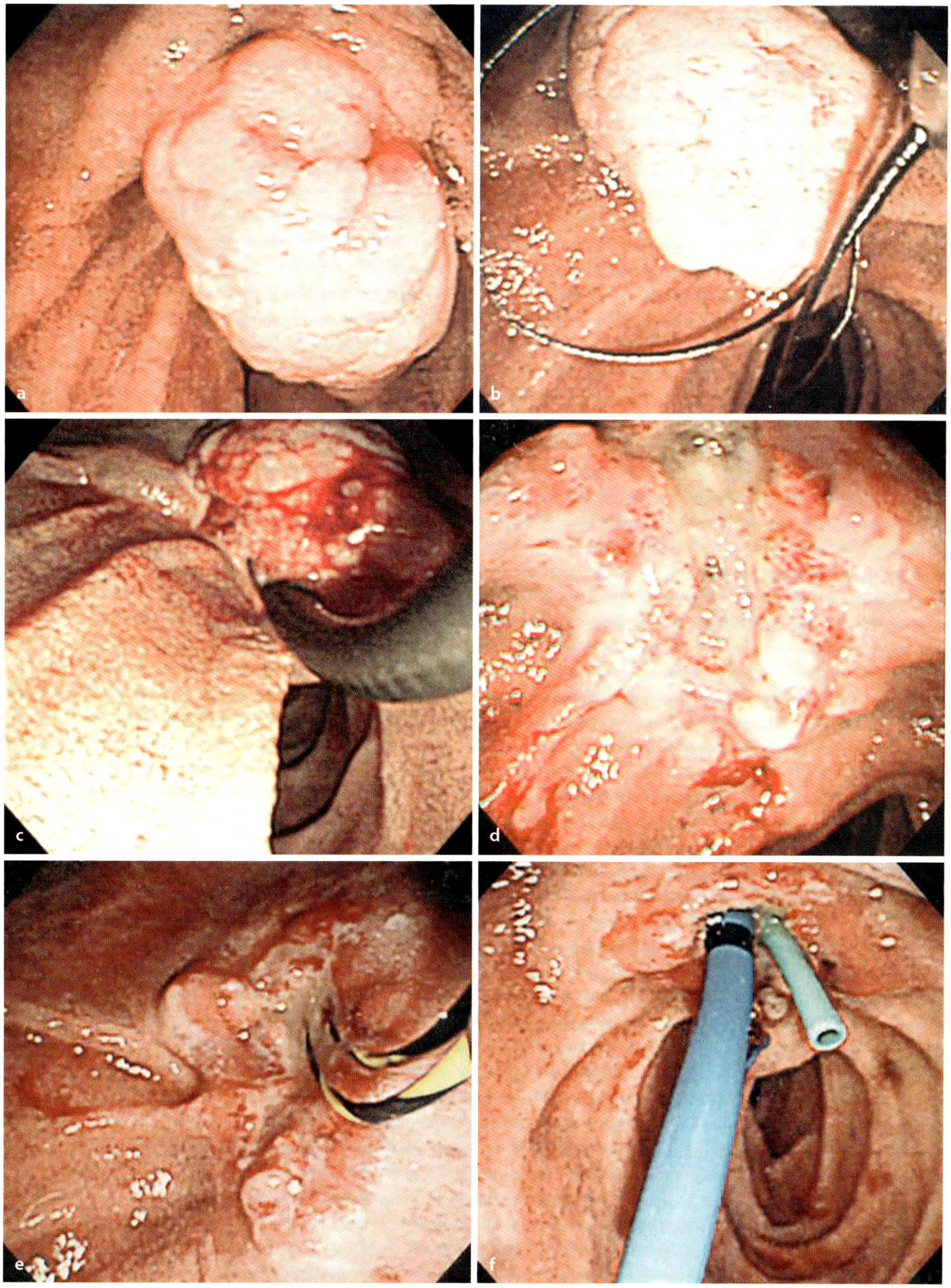

Figure 70.4

Endoscopic papillectomy (EP) procedures. Endoscopic finding shows a protruded adenoma of the ampulla (a). The snare is set on the oral side (b), then squeezed after confirming the margin on the anal side (c). Constant tension is being applied to the snare loop during the electrocautery until the lesion is transected (d). Two stents are inserted into the pancreatic and bile ducts (e, f)

Table. 70.1. Success rate of endoscopic papillectomy (EP)

References	*n*	Single session (*n*)	Piecemeal resection and/or ablation	Overall
Binmoeller et al. [7]	25	92% (23)	8% (2)	92% (23)
Zadorova et al. [9]	16	69% (11)	31% (5)	94% (16)
Norton et al. [10]	26	46% (12)	54% (14)	96% (25)
Maguchi et al. [11]	12	92% (11)	8% (1)	100% (12)
Catalano et al. [12]	108	50% (52)	30% (31)	80% (83)
Cheng et al. [13]	55	55% (30)	13% (7)	67% (37)

no reason to inject saline into the submucosa of the duodenal wall because at the papilla of Vater, saline injection tends to elevate the lesion with a low angle, which could make it difficult to snare the lesion. The pros and cons of the injection must be further discussed. Another problem is that EST inevitably incises into the tumor, which may make if difficult for the pathologist to evaluate the resected margin. For this reason, EST should be avoided, but a consensus has yet to be reached on this issue. Other techniques such as balloon retraction and wire-guided papillectomy have been reported [15,16], and these may be useful in selected cases. Complete en bloc resection of the tumor is recommended. Positive efforts should be made to retrieve all existing tumor tissues that may contain focal high-grade dysplasia or carcinoma. When piecemeal resection is inevitable (e.g., in the case of a large neoplasm), additional thermal ablation is highly recommended to destroy any residual adenomatous tissue (Table 70.1).

Opinions are also diverse on the current that should be used. In Japan, a pure cutting current is recommended for the prevention of postoperative pancreatitis, whereas in Western countries, a blended current is used. Further discussions are needed to resolve this issue. It is recommended that stents are placed in the pancreatic duct and the bile duct after excision of the tumor to prevent postoperative pancreatitis and cholangitis; a 5- to 7-Fr stent should be used for the pancreatic duct and a 7- to 10-Fr stent for the bile duct. Several reports suggest that pancreatic stent placement is recommended for the prevention of postoperative pancreatitis or late-stage stricture of the pancreatic duct orifice. Conversely, some are of the opinion that bile duct stenting is not necessary since the incidence of cholangitis or late-stage bile duct stricture is low.

Pathological Evaluation of Specimens

It is important to handle excised specimens appropriately because they sometimes contain focally grown high-grade dysplasia or carcinoma. For evaluation of the horizontal margin of a specimen, "oral side" and "anal side" must be clearly marked, and for evaluation of the vertical margin, the orifices of bile duct and pancreatic duct must be sectioned vertically. For this reason, en bloc resection instead of piecemeal resection has been highly recommended.

Postoperative Testing

Patients must rest in bed for at least initial 24 h with NPO, and be hospitalized for 48 h after EP. During the initial 24 h, they are kept under instillation management, and vital signs must be checked. Opinions are divided on the use of protease inhibitors for prevention of pancreatitis, and on the use of antibiotics, H2 blockers or proton pump inhibitors.

During the 1st day post-EP, signs and symptoms suggesting complications must be checked in conjunction with the blood test.

Early Postoperative Course

Patients resume eating if there is no sign of complications 24 h after EP. The major complications of EP include hemorrhage, pancreatitis, cholangitis, and perforation. The prevalence of these complications has been reported to be moderately high, ranging from 10 to 42% (Table 70.2). The most prevalent complications are hemorrhage and pancreatitis. Hemorrhage occurs mostly within 24 h after EP, frequently at the anal side of the ampulla and the excised margin. Bleeding is usually mild and can be treated endoscopically by using standard techniques (injection of epinephrine, electrocoagulation, or hemoclip placement; Fig. 70.5).

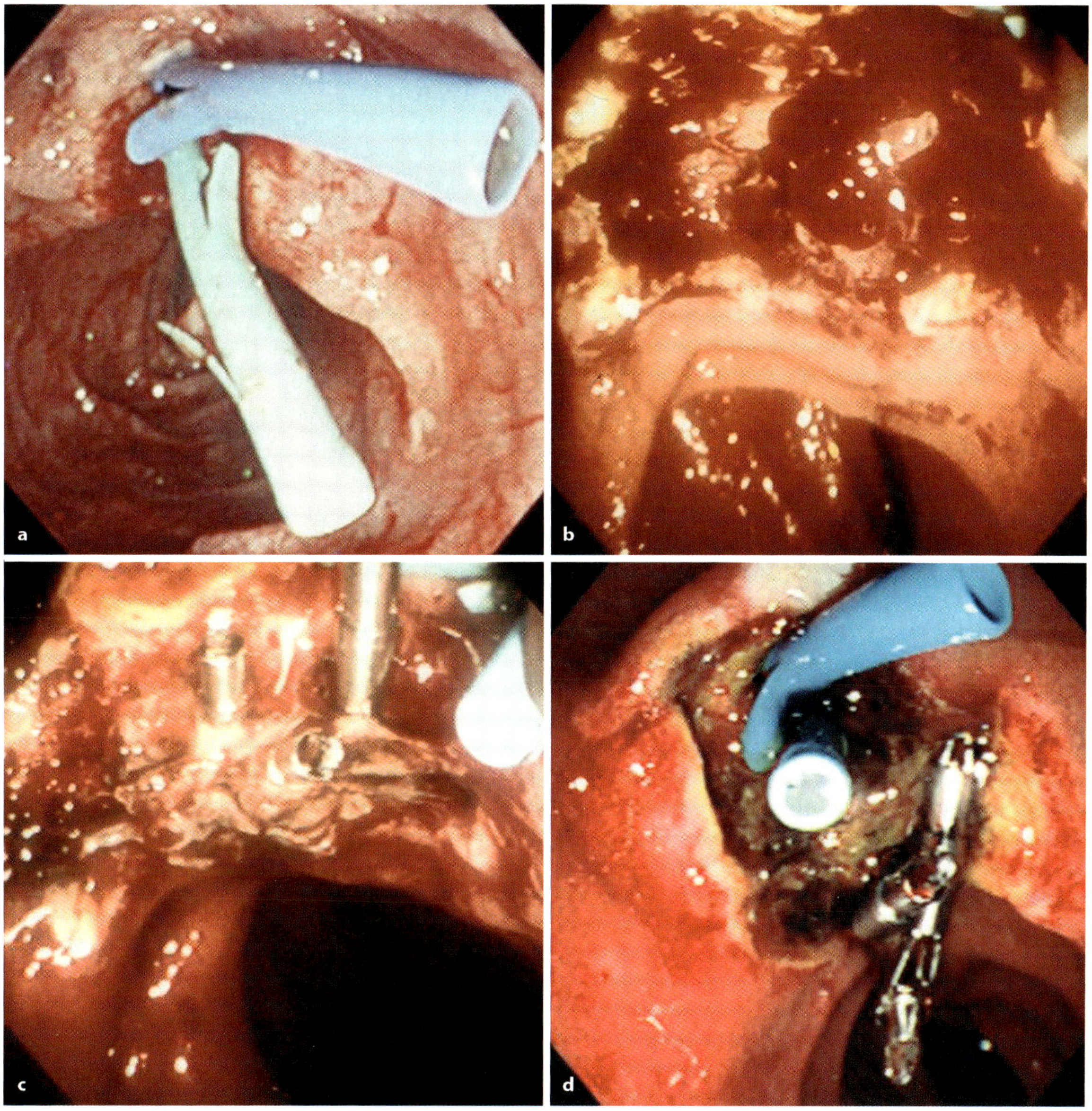

Figure 70.5

Endoscopic findings revealed spurting bleeding from a visible vessel after EP (a, b).The bleeding was stopped by heater probe coagulation and hemoclipping (c, d)

Table 70.2. EP-related complications

References	*n*	Bleeding (*n*)	Pancreatitis	Overall
Binmoeller et al. [7]	25	8% (2)	12% (3)	20% (5)
Zadorova et al. [9]	16	13% (2)	13% (2)	25% (4)
Norton et al. [10]	26	8% (2)	15% (4)	27% (7)
Maguchi et al. [11]	12	25% (3)	25% (3)	42% (5)
Catalano et al. [12]	103	2% (2)	5% (5)	10% (10)
Cheng et al. [13]	55	7% (4)	9% (5)	18% (10)

Table 70.3. Recurrence rate after EP. *NR* Not recorded

References	*n*	Recurrence rate	Mean Follow-up period (months)
Binmoeller et al. [7]	25	26% (6/23)	37
Zadorova et al. [9]	16	19% (3/16)	NR
Norton et al. [10]	26	8% (2/21)	13
Maguchi et al. [11]	12	0% (0/12)	21
Catalano et al. [12]	103	24% (20/83)	36
Cheng et al. [13]	55	33% (9/27)	30

If pancreatitis has developed, oral intake is suspended and protease inhibitors and antibiotics are administered.

In the sole mortality case that has been reported after EP so far, the cause of death was severe necrotizing pancreatitis. This is the problem we must watch for in the management of post-EP patients.

Table 70.4 Late complication after EP

References	Papillary stenosis
Norton et al. [10]	8% (2/25)
Maguchi et al. [11]	8.3% (1/12)
Catalano et al. [12]	3.6% (3/83)
Cheng et al. [13]	7.4% (2/27)

Long-Term Outcome After EP

Tumor recurrence rates after EP have been reported at 0–33% (Table 70.3). The risk factors for recurrence are said to be large-size tumor, genetic background, young age, and positive margins. It should be noted that most of the recurrences reported so far were found within the 1st year after EP. Therefore, it is strongly recommended that patients who had adenomas removed completely undergo endoscopic surveillance at 6-month intervals for a minimum of 2 years. If a neoplasm was incompletely removed at the initial treatment, EP and thermal ablation should be repeated at 2- to 3-month intervals until ablation has been completed [12]. Subsequently, endoscopic surveillance should be performed every 6 months for a minimum of 2 years. After the initial surveillance period of 2 years, an annual follow-up examination is recommended; in Western countries it is recommended that patients with FAP should undergo surveillance at 3-year intervals, and those with sporadic adenoma should be re-examined endoscopically only when any sign is clinically manifested. If recurrence is detected, it can be managed usually by endoscopic ablation, but in some cases surgical resection is required. Such recurrent adenoma requiring surgical treatment occurs more frequently among patients with FAP, suggesting that these patients may be less suitable candidates for endoscopic therapy.

The periods of stent placement for the prevention of pancreatitis or cholangitis vary from 1 week to 12 weeks. This variation depends partly on the diameter of the stent used. In any case, the development of secondary pancreatitis due to stent occlusion must be watched carefully. If using a 5-Fr stent, it should be removed within 8 weeks. However, papillary stenosis can occur as a late-stage complication after EP, and is seen particularly at the pancreatic duct (Table 70.4), and its occurrence is said to be closely related to the use of pancreatic duct stents.

References

1. Seifert E, Schulte F, Stolte M (1992) Adenoma and carcinoma of the duodenum and papilla of Vater: a clinicopathologic study. Am J Gastroenterol 87:37–42
2. Neoptolemos JP, Talbot IC, Carr-Locke DL (1987) Treatment and outcome in 52 cases of ampullary carcinomas. Br J Surg 74:957–961
3. Farouk M, Niotis M, Braunum GD (1991) Indications for and the technique of local resection of tumors of the papilla of Vater. Arch Surg 126:650–652
4. Cahen DL, Fockens P, de Wit DLT, et al (1997) Local resection or pancreaticoduodenectomy for villous adenoma of Vater diagnosed before operation. Br J Surg 84:948–951
5. Shemesh E, Nass S, Czerniak A (1989) Endoscopic sphincterotomy and endoscopic fulguration in the management of adenoma of the papilla of Vater. Surg Gynecol Obstet 169:445–448
6. Ponchon T, Berger F, Chavaillon A, et al (1989) Contribution of endoscopy to diagnosis and treatment of tumors of the ampulla of Vater. Cancer 64:161–167
7. Binmoeller KF, Boaventura S, Ramsperger K, et al (1993) Endoscopic snare excision of benign adenomas of the papilla of Vater. Gastrointest Endosc 39:127–131

8. Silvis SE (1993) Endoscopic snare papillectomy. Gastrointest Endosc 39:205–207
9. Zadorova Z, Dvofak M, Hajor J (2001) Endoscopic therapy of benign tumors of the papilla of Vater. Endoscopy 33:345–347
10. Norton ID, Gostout CJ, Baron TH, et al (2002) Safety and outcome of endoscopic snare excision of the major duodenal papilla. Gastrointest Endosc 56:239–243
11. Maguchi H, Takahashi K, Katanuma A, et al (2003) Indication of endoscopic papillectomy for tumors of the papilla of Vater and its problems. Dig Endosc 15:S33–S35
12. Catalano MF, Linder JD, Chak A, et al (2004) Endoscopic management of adenoma of the major duodenal papilla. Gastrointest Endosc 59:225–232
13. Cheng CL, Sherman S, Fogel EL, et al (2004) Endoscopic snare papillectomy for tumors of duodenal papillae. Gastrointest Endosc 60:757–764
14. Charton JP, Deinert K, Schumacher B, et al (2004) Endoscopic resection for neoplastic diseases of the papilla of Vater. J Hepatobiliary Pancreat Surg 11:245–251
15. Aiura K, Imaeda H, Kitajima M, et al (2003) Ballon-cater-assisted endoscopic snare papillectomy for benign tumors of the major duodenal papilla. Gastrointest Endosc 57:743–747
16. Moon JH, Cha SW, Cho YD, et al (2005) Wire-guided endoscopic snare papillectomy for tumors of the major duodenal papilla. Gastrointest Endosc 61:461-466
17. Yao T, Iida M, Watanabe H (1977) Duodenal lesions in familial polyposis of the colon. Gastroenterology 73:1086–1092
18. Jones TR, Nance FC (1977) Periampullary malignancy in Gardner's syndrome. Ann Surg 185:165–173
19. Matumoto T, Iida M, Nakamura S, et al (2000) Natural history of ampullary adenoma in familial adenomatous polyposis: reconfirmation of benign nature during extended surveillance. Am J Gastroenterol 95:1557–1562
20. Oh C, Jemerin FE (1965) Benign adenomatous polyps of the papilla of Vater. Surgery 57:495–503
21. Baczako K, Buchler M, Beger HG (1985) Morphogenesis and possible precursor lesions of invasive carcinoma of the papilla of Vater: epithelial dysplasia and adenoma. Hum Pathol 16:307–310
22. Gouma DJ, Obertop H, Visman J (1987) Progression of a benign epithelial ampullary tumor to adenocarcinoma. Surgery 101:501–504
23. Yamaguchi K, Nishihara K (1992) Long- and short-term survivors after pancreatoduodenectomy for ampullary carcinoma. J Surg Oncol 50:195–200
24. Itoh A, Goto H, Naitoh Y, et al (1997) Intraductal ultrasonography in diagnosing tumor extension of cancer of the papilla of Vater. Gastrointest Endosc 45:251–260

Chapter 71

S. Ikeda · Y. Yasunami

Surgical Management of Adenoma

Local excision is considered for the treatment of benign ampullary tumors. The procedure of choice for local excision includes surgical or endoscopic ampullectomy depending upon the size and spread of tumors, based on the feasibility of the procedures. The first local resection of an ampullary tumor was performed by William S. Halsted in 1899 [1]. Binmoeller et al. first reported endoscopic excision of benign adenomas of the papilla of Vater in 1993 [2]. In this chapter, the procedure for surgical resection of ampullary tumors is described.

Indications and Inclusion Criteria

Surgical resection is indicated for benign ampullary tumors including adenomas, neuroendocrine tumors, and nonepithelial lesions. In addition, local resection is considered in patients who are at high risk of malignancy or those who refuse major operations and those in whom endoscopic resection cannot be performed due to technical reasons.

Work-up of Diagnostic Measures

Since major signs and symptoms in patients with ampullary tumors are caused by stenosis or obstruction of the common bile duct and the main pancreatic duct [3,4], laboratory data to define obstructive jaundice and pancreatitis is required. Abdominal ultrasound and magnetic resonance cholangiopancreatography (MRCP) are the initial examinations to be indicated for patients with suggestive ampullary tumors because the dilatation of the ducts, which is the indirect finding of ampullary tumors, is visualized by both examinations. Computed tomography scan is also indicated providing the similar findings of dilated ducts to those obtained by ultrasound and MRCP, and can occasionally detect the tumor itself. Endoscopic retrograde cholangiopancreatography is essential for the diagnosis of an ampullary tumor since the procedure enables biopsy sampling of a tumor, facilitating the pathological diagnosis. Endoscopic ultrasound is also essential to determine the depth of lesions as well as to differentiate benign from malignant tumors.

Preparation Prior to Surgery

In patients with high risk due to other medical morbidities and with obstructive jaundice, percutaneous transhepatic biliary drainage (PTBD) is indicated prior to surgery. In general, PTBD is not required in patients with a benign ampullary tumor since jaundice is mild in intensity in these patients. In patients with acute pancreatitis associated with an ampullary tumor, surgery is considered when pancreatitis subsides by conservative treatments.

Procedures

The duodenum is mobilized by the Kocher maneuver. Cholecystectomy is performed since there is a potential risk for development of postoperative cholecystitis caused by the duodenobiliary regurgitation after excision of the papilla. After dissecting the gallbladder free from its bed, a metallic probe is introduced into the common bile duct through the cystic duct, facilitating identification of the location of the papilla by digital palpation (Fig. 71.1). A transverse or oblique duodenotomy is then made opposite the region of the papilla is made, and a tumor of the papilla is exposed (Fig. 71.2a).

A suture is placed into the posterior wall of the duodenum with adequate margin to the tumor (Fig. 71.2a), which is retracted downward, facilitating creation of a fenestration of the common bile duct through posterior wall of the duodenum (Fig. 71.2b). It is essential to confirm that the distal portion of the common bile duct is not involved by the tumor. An approximation is made by a suture ligature between the posterior wall of the duodenum and the common

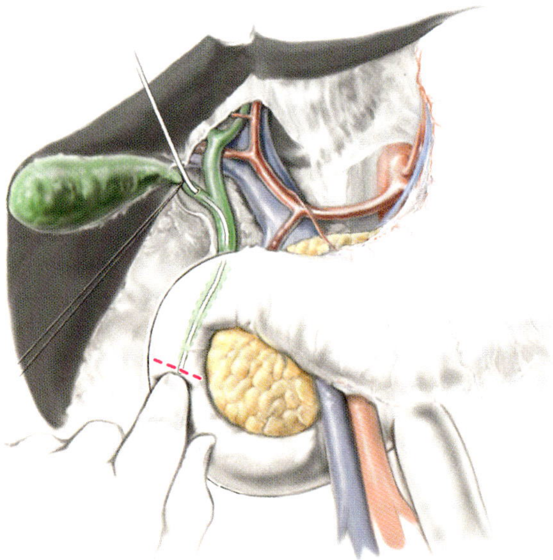

Figure 71.1

Digital palpation of the metallic probe introduced into the common bile duct facilitates identification of the location of the papilla

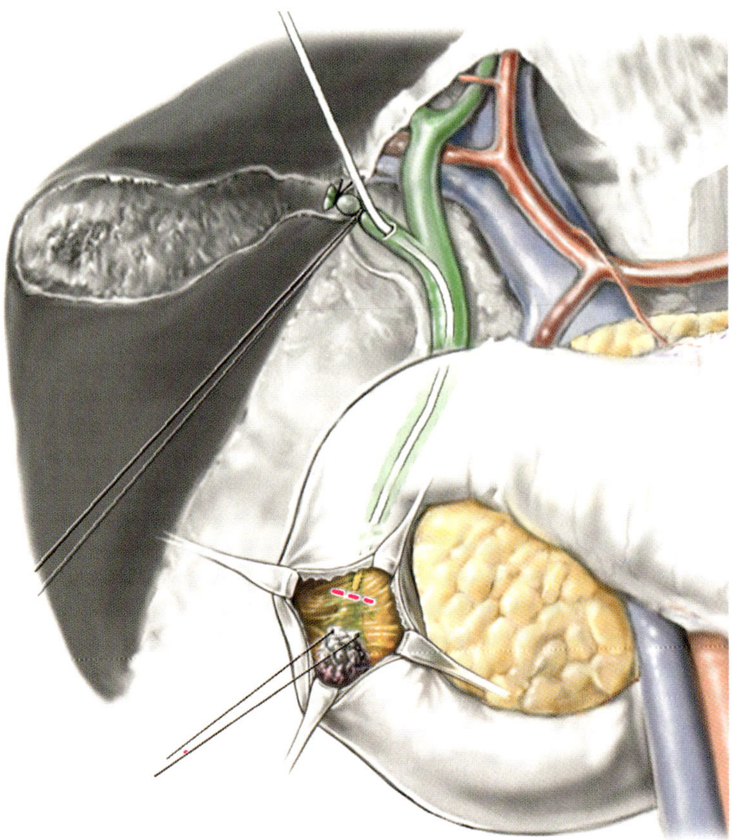

Figure 71.2 a

A tumor of the papilla is exposed by an oblique duodenotomy (a).

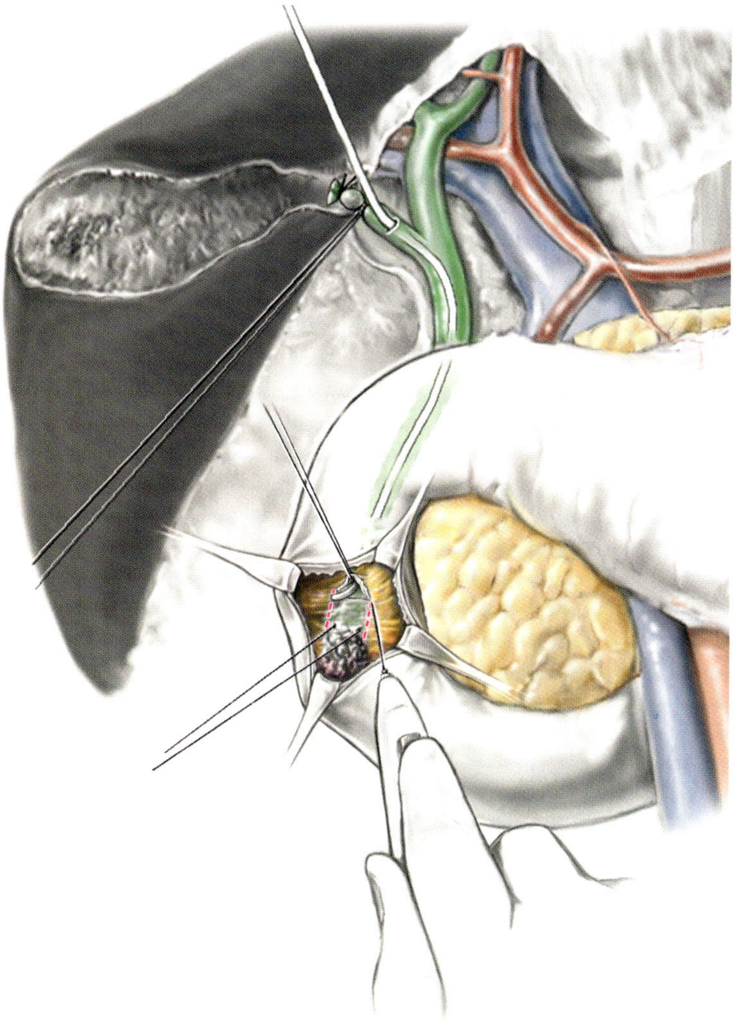

Figure 71.2 b

The common bile duct is fenestrated through the posterior wall of the duodenum (b)

bile duct (Fig. 71.2b) and electrocautery is used to make a circumferential incision on the posterior wall of the duodenum along the periphery of the papilla (Fig. 71.3a, b). The main pancreatic duct and the common bile duct are then transected. Note that the cut surfaces of both ducts are approximated by interrupted sutures to prevent the main pancreatic duct from becoming buried within the pancreatic parenchyma (Fig. 71.4a). Finally, an anastomosis between both ducts and the duodenum is made with interrupted sutures (Fig. 71.4b). The metallic probe placed through the cystic duct is replaced with a catheter, which will be used for bile drainage. Another catheter equipped with a flexible tip made of aluminum is used for drainage of the pancreatic juice as follows. The catheter is inserted and placed into the main pancreatic duct through the orifice of the anastomosis. The other side of the catheter with an aluminum tip is introduced from the duodenum to the anterior wall of the stomach where the catheter is brought outside the stomach (Fig. 71.5). The duodenotomy is closed with interrupted sutures.

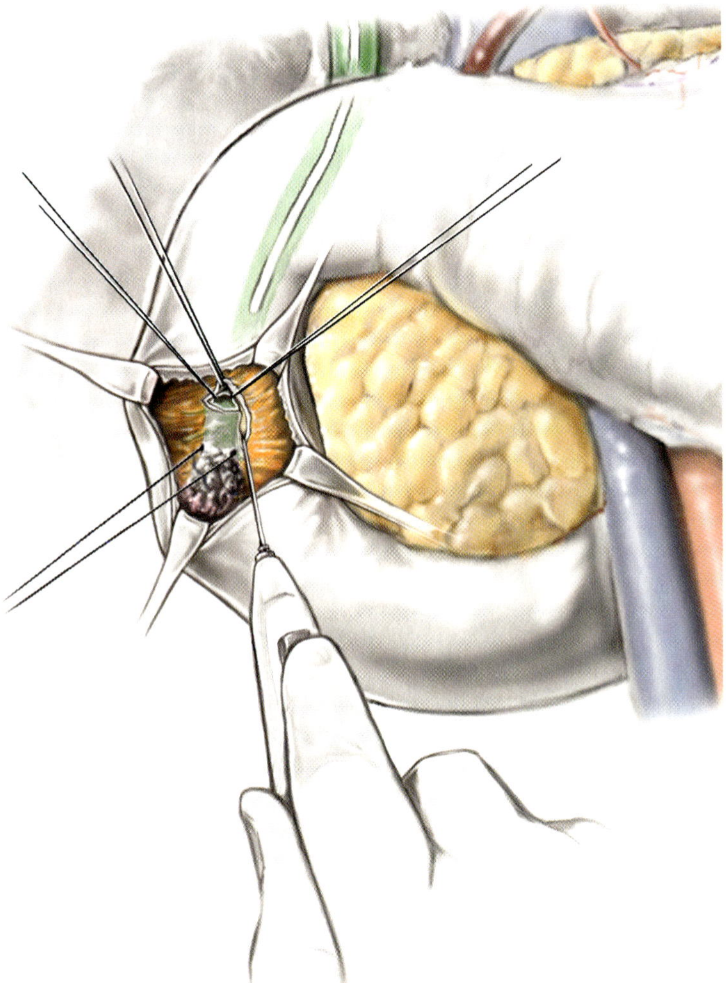

Figure 71.3 a

The posterior wall of the duodenum is incised circumferentially with electrocautery to expose both the common bile duct and the main pancreatic duct

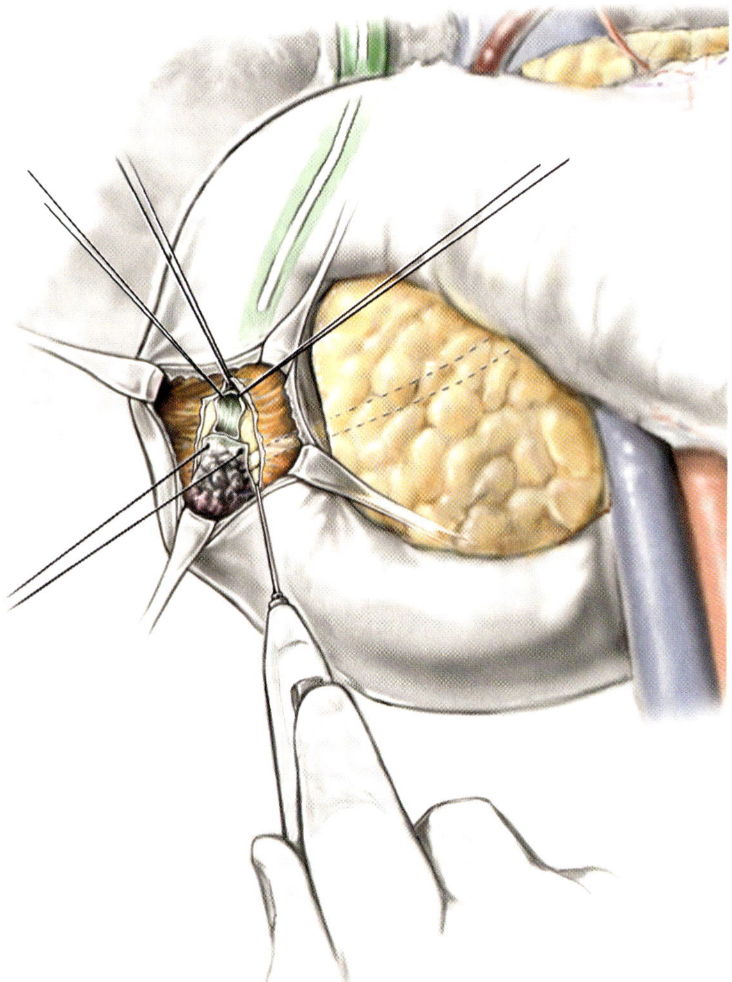

Figure 71.3 b

After opening the anterior wall of the common bile duct, the main pancreatic duct is going to be exposed

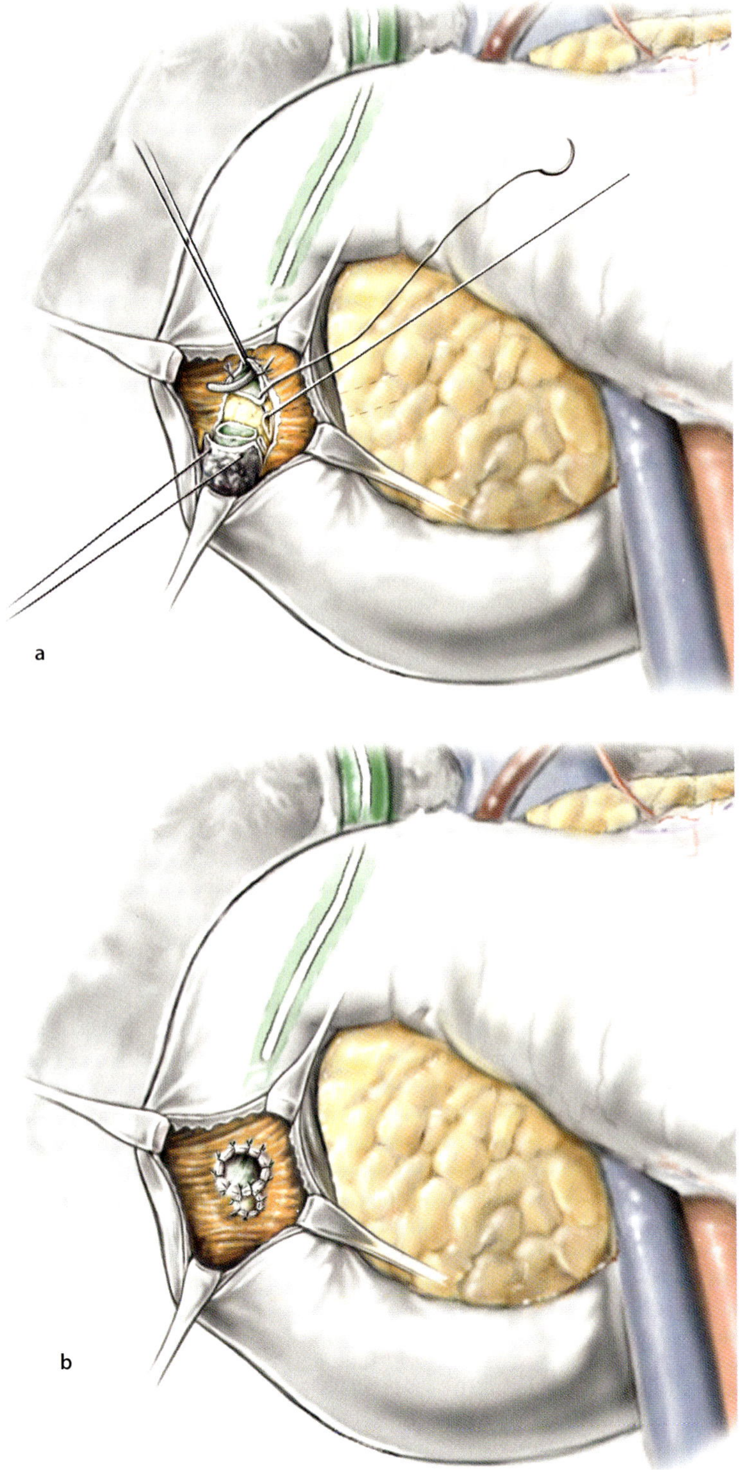

Figure 71.4

Both the common bile and main pancreatic ducts are approximated by interrupted sutures prior to transection (a). Anastomoses between both ducts and the duodenum are completed (b)

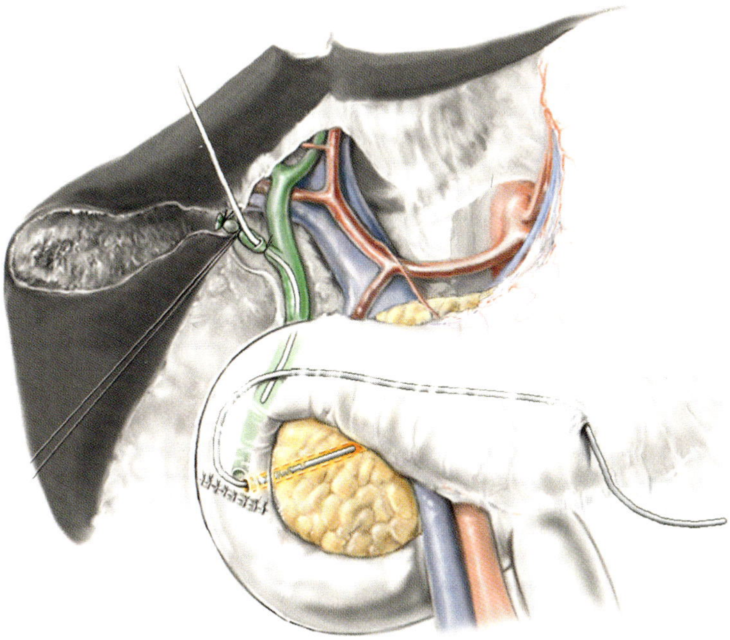

Figure 71.5

A bile drainage tube is placed through the cystic duct. A catheter placed into the main pancreatic duct is brought outside to the anterior wall of the stomach

Postoperative Management

The gastric tube is removed at 3–5 days after surgery. First food intake is initiated approximately at 5–7 days and the tubes for the drainage of bile and pancreatic juice are removed 2–3 weeks after surgery when there is no longer any leakage from the anastomosis.

Postoperative Complications

Major complications after surgery include the leakage of the anastomosis and acute pancreatitis, which are usually treated conservatively.

Late Outcome

The outcome of surgical resection of an ampullary tumor is satisfactory as long as the lesion is benign. When the resection of a tumor is incomplete, the residual tumor may cause recurrence of symptoms.

References

1. Halsted WS (1899) Contributions of the surgery of the bile passages, especially of the common bile duct. Boston Med Surg J 141:645–654
2. Binmoeller KF, Boaventura S, Ramsperger K, Soehendra N (1993) Endoscopic snare excision of benign adenomas of the papilla of Vater. Gastrointest Endosc 39:127–131
3. Ratter DW, Fernandez-del Castillo C, Brugge WR, Warshow AL (1996) Defining the criteria for local resection of ampullary neoplasms. Arch Surg 131:366–371
4. Branum GD, Pappas TN, Meyers WC (1996) The management of tumors of the ampulla of Vater by local resection. Ann Surg 224:621–627
5. Clary BM, Tyler DS, Dematos P, Gottfield M, Pappas TN (2000) Local ampullary resection with careful intraoperative frozen section evaluation for presumed benign ampullary neoplasms. Surgery 127:628–633

Chapter 72

K. Yamaguchi · M. Tanaka

Surgical Treatment of Carcinoma of the Ampulla of Vater

Carcinoma of the ampulla of Vater is a rare gastrointestinal tumor, comprising 0.063–0.21% of all routine autopsy cases [1]; however, accounts for 10.2–36% of all surgically operable periampullary cancer [2]. The clinical course of patients with carcinoma of the ampulla of Vater is more favorable than that of carcinoma of the other pancreatoduodenal components such as pancreatic head cancer and bile duct cancer [2,3]. In 1912, Walter Kausch [4] was the first to perform a successful partial pancreatoduodenectomy. Pancreatoduodenectomy was a standard operation for this tumor for a long time, and pylorus-preserving pancreatoduodenectomy (PPPD) has been widely introduced on the basis of preservation of organ function. Transduodenal ampullectomy or endoscopic amupllectomy has been performed experimentally in patients with adenoma of the ampulla of Vater, in situ carcinoma of the ampulla of Vater, or high-risk patients.

Pattern of Lymph Node Involvement

With the progression of ampullary carcinoma, the tumor infiltrates the lymphatic and vascular channels locally and further develops lymph node metastasis, hematogenous metastasis, and peritoneal dissemination. Cancer-cell dissemination in the lymphatic channels is observed in 25% and 45% of stage I and II cancer of the ampulla of Vater, respectively [1]. Venous invasion is present in 15–20% of stage I and II lesions; however, selective perineural cancer infiltration has been observed only in the advanced cancer stages. Of the investigated patients, 25–55% have absence of lymph node metastasis. In pT1 cancer, no lymph node metastasis is usually evident. In pT2 cancer, 27–67% are lymph-node-positive and in pT3 cancer, lymph node metastases are present in 40–80%, as assessed histomorphologically.

Prognosis relates to the extent of local spread, the involvement of lymph nodes, and tumor differentiation. Of these factors, only lymph node metastasis is potentially controlled by surgery. In carcinoma of the papilla, lymph node metastases have been reported at the incidences of between 40% and 80% [5]. Investigations of the pattern of lymphatic dissemination of ampullary cancer have revealed that the posterior pancreaticoduodenal lymph node groups (no. 13) were involved in more than half of the patients (Table 72.1) [6]. Kayahara et al. [7] found that the posterior inferior pancreaticoduodenal lymph node group was most frequently involved in cancer dissemination. All patients with metastases of the lymph nodes around the superior mesenteric artery showed lymph node metastases in the posterior inferior pancreaticoduodenal nodes. It can be concluded that the primary lymph nodes involved in cancer of the papilla of Vater are the no. 13 nodes, being classified as n1 according to the Japanese Society of Biliary Surgery (JSBS) classification system [8]. Similar to pancreatic head cancer, the lymph nodes around the superior mesenteric artery (no. 14) are involved in advanced ampullary cancers. Nakao et al. [9] reported that no. 14 lymph node involvement was identified in 11%.

Regarding the perigastric lymph node, Nakao et al. [9] found that only 1 of 27 patients had lymph node metastases. The lymph node involvement around the left gastric artery and the celiac trunk was 0% and 2%, respectively. Kayahara et al. [7] were unable to identify any lymph node involvement in the perigastric, celiac, and para-aortic lymph node compartments in 36 patients.

Based on the pattern of positive lymph nodes after radical lymphadenectomy for cancer of the ampulla of Vater, the goals of an extended lymph node dissection include the posterior pancreatoduodenal lymph nodes, the anterior pancreatoduodenal lymph nodes, and the lymph nodes on the right side of the superior mesenteric artery. The retroportal lymph nodes and the lymph nodes along the common bile duct in the lower segment of the ligament hepatoduodenal are N2 nodes and have to be considered as additional dissection targets (D2 lymph node dissection) according to the JSBS classification [8]. In more advanced disease, stage III and IV, the interaortocaval lymph node groups and the para-aortal lymph nodes can be involved.

Table 72.1 Pattern of lymph node metastasis in ampullary carcinoma. Modified from [6]

No.		Yes	No	Incidence(%)
8a	Anterior hepatic artery	19	896	2.1
8p	Posterior hepatic artery	11	753	1.4
9	Celiac artery	2	389	0.5
12h	Hepatic hilum	0	429	0
12a1	Superior hepatic artery	3	702	0.4
12a2	Inferior hepatic artery	7	856	0.8
12b1	Superior bile duct	1	749	0.1
12b2	Inferior bile duct	37	931	3.8
12c	Cystic duct	3	823	0.4
12p1	Superior portal vein	1	688	0.1
12p2	Inferior portal vein	10	869	1.1
13a	Superior retropancreatic lymph nodes	241	813	22.9
13b	Inferior retropancreatic lymph nodes	220	774	22.1
14a	Origin of the superior mesenteric artery	42	684	5.8
14b	Origin of the inferior pancreatoduodenal artery	55	691	7.4
14c	Origin of the middle colic artery	17	565	2.9
14d	First jejunal branch	45	565	7.4
16	Para-aortic lymph nodes	48	425	10.1
17a	Superior anterior pancreatic	49	801	5.8
17b	Inferior anterior pancreatic	61	755	7.5

Indication for Oncological Resection

In ampullary tumor, preoperative endoscopic biopsy sampling has its limitations [10]. In ampullary carcinoma, superficial areas show only dysplasia similar to adenoma, and unequivocal carcinoma is located in the deep portion [11]. It is difficult to obtain specimens under endoscopy that can be diagnosed as carcinoma. Thus, surgical resection of the ampullary tumor is justified even if preoperative endoscopic diagnosis is adenoma.

Because of the survival benefits regarding long-term outcome, each patient with cancer of the papilla stage I–III has to be considered as a candidate for resection. The resection rate at experienced institutions is about 70–80% [5]. Based on the standardization of surgical techniques for pancreatoduodenectomy, the operative risk regarding surgical morbidity and hospital mortality is low.

For patients who are suffering from cancer with metastasis in the liver, or peritoneal dissemination with malignant ascites and unequivocal and massive para-aortic lymph node metastases, a major resection is not recommended. Infiltration of the portal vein with a long narrowing or complete occlusion with collateral drainages is a contraindication for surgical treatment. Many patients with an advanced cancer of the papilla are of an older age, above 70 years, and the age-related commodity has to be taken into account in the decision-making. In high-risk patients who are in poor condition, transduodenal ampullectomy or endoscopic ampullectomy may be indicated, although the resection margin may be affected by cancer cells.

Surgical Techniques

In 1912, Walter Kausch [4] performed the first successful two-stage pancreatic head resection in a patient suffering from a carcinoma of the papilla of Vater in Berlin. The Kausch-Whipple resection has become the standard technique for periampullary carcinoma. The Kausch-Whipple resection includes the pancreatic head, duodenum up to the flexure duodenojejunalis, extrahepatic biliary duct, and gastric antrum; reconstruction necessitates pancreatojejunostomy, hepaticojejunostomy, and additional gastrojejunostomy.

Today, the PPPD has become the surgical procedure of choice in the treatment of cancer of the am-

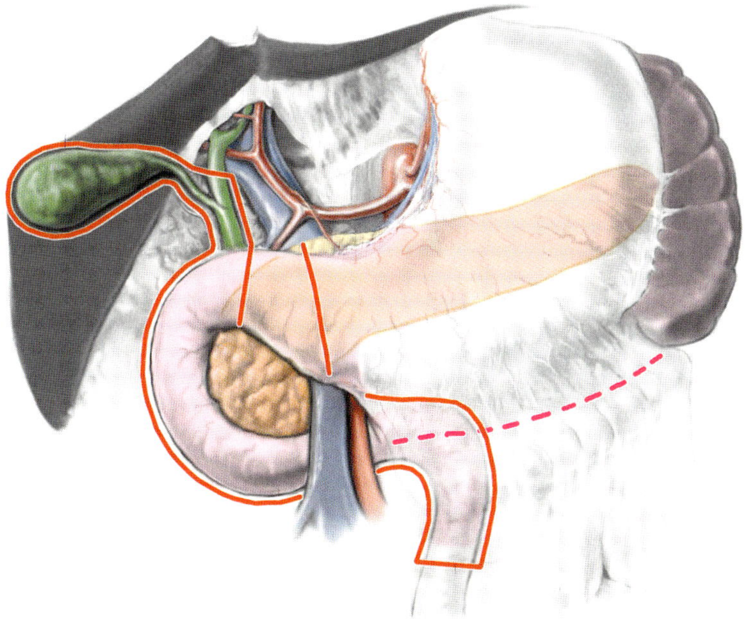

Figure 72.1

Pylorus-preserving pancreatoduodenectomy comprises the *shaded areas*

Table 72.2. Survival of cancer of the ampulla of Vater

Author	Reference	Year	Patients (*n*)	5-year survival (%) Overall	Stage I	Stage II	Stage III	Stage IV
Yamaguchi and Enjoji	1	1987	109	28	85	11	25	24
Monson et al.	15	1991	104	34				
Yamaguchi et al.	5	1993	36	30	50	40	18	20
Chareton et al.	16	1996	43	40	85	65	44	8
Talamini et al.	17	1997	106	38				
Beger et al.	18	1999	126	50	84	70	27	0
De Castro et al.	19	2004	178	46	75	66	35	0

pulla of Vater (Fig. 72.1). The hospital mortality after PPPD at high-volume centers is below 5%, as is that for the Kausch-Whipple resection, as evidenced by randomized clinical trials [12–14]. The advantages of the pylorus-preserving resection in comparison to the Kausch-Whipple procedure are a shorter time for operation [13], lower intraoperative blood loss [13], and a better nutritional state at postoperative late phase, such as a faster gain of weight in the first postoperative year. However, in the early postoperative course, the pylorus-preserving technique may have the disadvantage of delayed gastric emptying [12].

Patients with stage I or II cancer have a significantly better prognosis after partial pancreaticoduodenectomy than patients with cancer stages III and IV (Table 72.2) [1,15–19]. With respect to the results of PPPD, the reported short- and long-term survival times are equal to those achieved after Kausch-Whipple resection [13,14] and recurrence rate [13]. Because the incidence of lymph node metastases of the infrapyloric lymph nodes is only 3–6% in patients with carcinoma of the ampulla [7,9], the risk of incomplete cancer resection while preserving the gastric antrum and a segment of the postpyloric duodenum is very low. Lymph nodes in the pyloric and gastroepiploic compartments should be checked intraoperatively by frozen section, when enlarged. The preservation of a 4-cm segment of the postpyloric duodenum is optional for a resection.

Resection Techniques

Incision and Laparotomy

A long midline incision starting from the xiphoid process and extending below the umbilicus is used to explore the abdomen. After opening the abdomen, distant metastases including liver metastasis and peritoneal dissemination should be immediately checked. When obviously present, resection is contraindicated. Two less apparent sites of involvement should be examined; the root of the transverse mesocolon and the celiac axis. The fixity of the mesocolon indicates unresectability, whereas minimal puckering alone may be amenable to resection of a segment of the mesocolon and, if necessary, the attached transverse colon is removed en bloc with the pancreas specimen. Obvious extensions of the tumor around the celiac axis or the superior mesenteric vessels indicate that the tumor is incurable.

Mobilization of the Duodenum

The peritoneal reflection lateral to the second part of the duodenum is incised near the right renal capsule and the duodenum and pancreatic head are mobilized anteriorly and to the left of the patient. This plane of dissection is continued until the left renal vein is displayed exposing in turn the right renal vein, inferior vena cava, and the aorta. During this dissection, the para-aortic lymph nodes (no. 16) can be examined by palpation. Next, the lesser omentum is explored. The gastrocolic omentum is divided along the avascular plane close to its attachment with the transverse colon. The stomach and attached greater omentum are then reflected superiorly and the transverse colon and mesocolon are refracted inferiorly. The anterior aspect of the pancreatic head can then be explored.

Mobilization of the Pancreatic Neck

The superior mesenteric vein is identified emerging from beneath the neck of the pancreas by tracing the middle colic vein down the mesocolon to its point of entry into the superior mesenteric vein. The pancreas is isolated free from the superior mesenteric vein (Fig. 72.2). Because the majority of pancreatic venous tributaries enter the major veins on their lateral aspects, there exists a "safe" plane anterior to the portal vein along which instruments or fingers may be passed beneath the neck of the pancreas.

Cholecystectomy and Dissection of the Hepatoduodenal Ligament

The gallbladder is dissected from the liver "fundus first" and the cystic artery clearly defined, ligated, and divided. The hepatoduodenal ligament is skeletonized (Fig. 72.3). Using blunt dissection, the common hepatic duct is isolated from the portal vein and hepatic artery. The common hepatic duct is transected just above the entrance of the cystic duct. The proximal end of the duct is occluded with a bulldog clamp to prevent bile spillage, and the distal end is sutured and ligated. The right hepatic artery is usually present transversely just beneath the division. Traction along this suture will allow further access to the anterior aspect of the portal vein. The gallbladder, distal common bile duct, and the surrounding lymphatic and connective tissues are then stripped inferiorly, thus skeletonizing the portal vein and proper hepatic artery. The dissection is continued until the hepatic artery has been followed to its origin from the celiac axis. When the right hepatic artery is supplied from the superior mesenteric artery, the right hepatic artery runs at the right side of the bile duct. This anatomical anomaly should be carefully considered in skeletonization of the hepatoduodenal ligament. During the procedure, the lymph nodes around the lower part of the hepatoduodenal ligament (no. 12) and the common hepatic artery (no. 8) are dissected completely.

Division of the Duodenum and Neck of the Pancreas

For a PPPD, the proximal gastrointestinal tract is divided 2–3 cm distal to the pylorus using a linear stapler. The right gastric artery is spared but can be taken if it allows better mobilization of the retained duodenal stump. The right gastroepiploic artery is divided at its origin from the gastroduodenal artery. Routine lymph node dissection of the perigastric lymph nodes is not performed; when swollen, however, these lymph nodes can be removed with the preservation of the pylorus ring and a 3- to 4-cm cuff of the duodenum.

The neck of the pancreas is carefully transected to the left side of the portal vein. Noncrushing clamps are placed on the head and tail sites of the pancreas to minimize blood loss. The division is completed using a sharp knife blade. Individual bleeding vessels are ligated as they are visualized using single through-and-through 4-0 silk sutures. The main pancreatic duct is identified during the procedure.

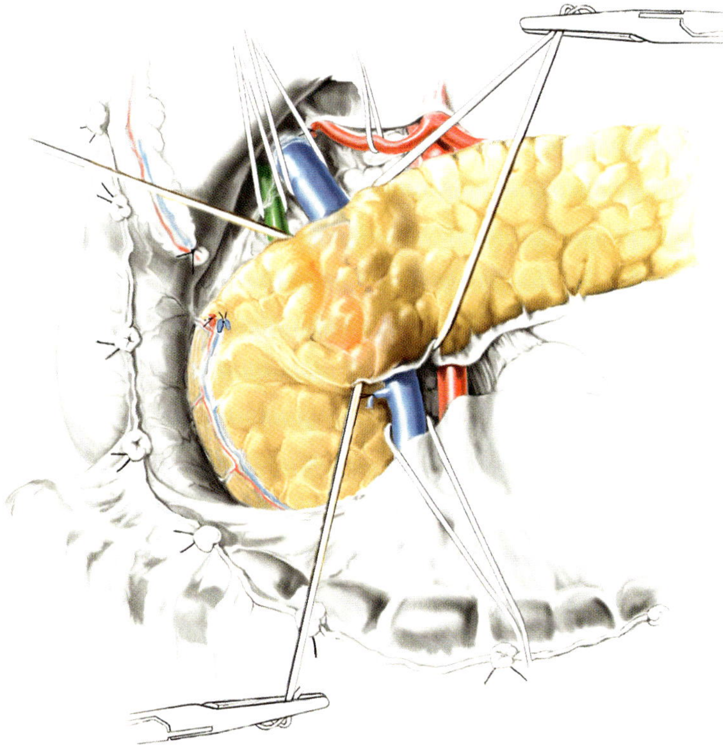

Figure 72.2

The neck of the pancreas is isolated from the portal vein (tunneling)

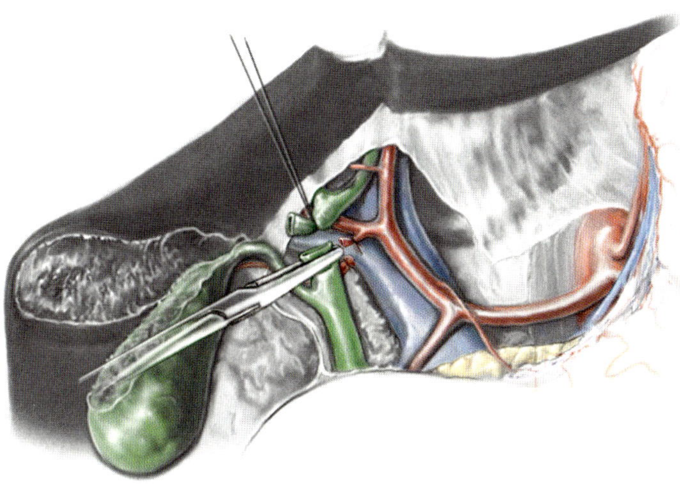

Figure 72.3

The hepatoduodenal ligament is skeletonized and the common hepatic duct is divided

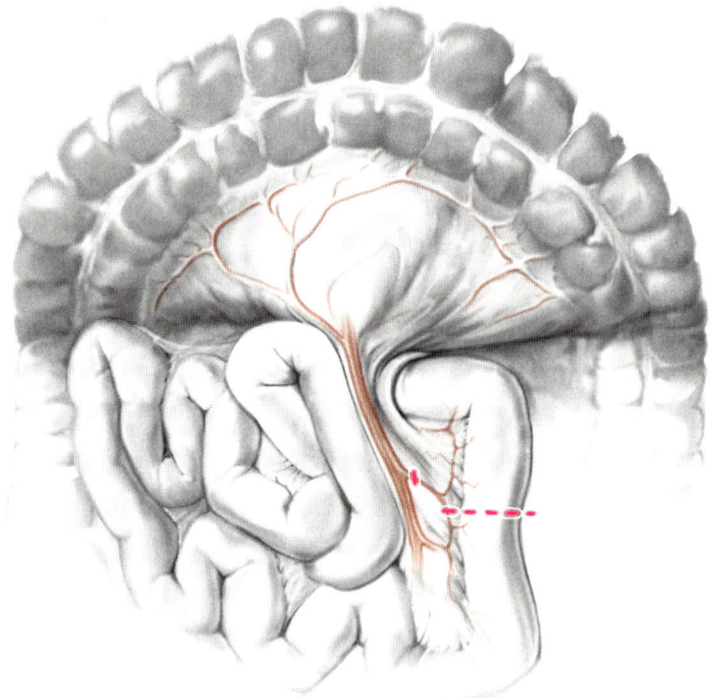

Figure 72.4

The first jejunal artery is divided and the proximal jejunum is divided

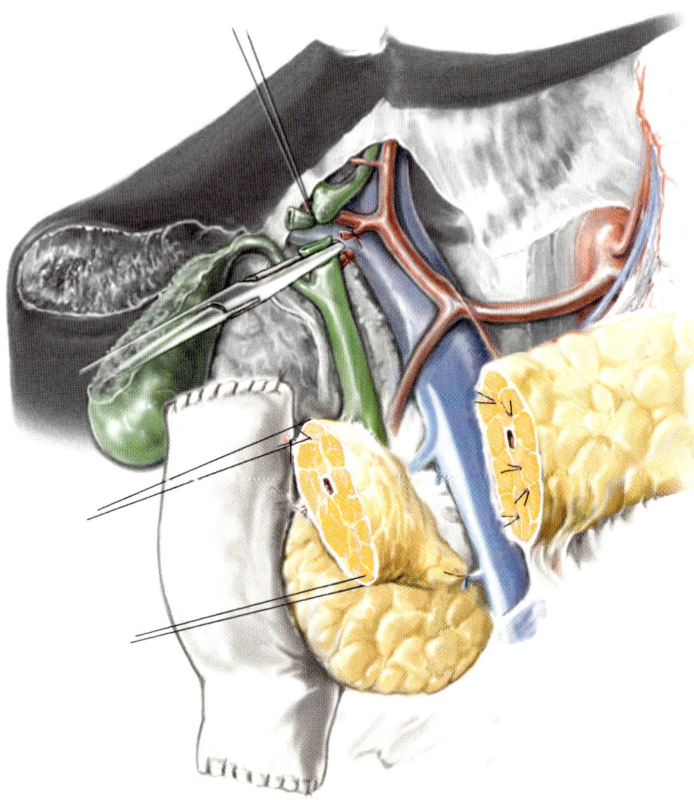

Figure 72.5

The pancreas head is dissected from the portal vein and superior mesenteric artery

Division of the Jejunum

With the transverse colon is pulled upwards and the first jejunal loop retracted down, the duodenojejunal junction is freed by division of the adhesions including the ligament of Treitz. The peritoneum of the proximal jejunum is dissected and the first jejunal and superior mesenteric vessels are identified (Fig. 72.4). The first jejunal vessels are divided at the origin and the color of the drained proximal jejunum turns pale and ischemic. The proximal jejunum is divided along the ischemic line with a stapler. The upper jejunum is herniated beneath the superior mesenteric vascular pedicle into the right upper quadrant of the abdomen.

Dissection of the Retropancreatic Vessels

The specimen now remains attached only by the uncinate process, the small bowel, and the midgut vascular pedicle. The head of the pancreas is then grasped by the surgeon's left hand and folded over to the patient's right side. Venous tributaries from the uncinate process are visualized and isolated, doubly ligated and divided. The portal vein is retracted to the patient's left using a vein retractor, and the dissection continued at a deeper level on the bridge of tissue that exists between the uncinate process and the superior mesenteric artery (Fig. 72.5). The inferior pancreatoduodenal artery is identified within the wedge of the tissue remaining between the specimen and the superior mesenteric artery. After its ligation and division, the uppermost jejunal vessels are ligated and served from the superior mesenteric artery. The right side of the superior mesenteric artery is almost completely explored.

The Reconstruction

Pancreatojejunostomy

Prior to the reconstruction, the entire operative field is thoroughly irrigated with warm saline, and active bleeding points that have been overlooked are carefully ligated. The closed upper end of the jejunum is usually brought up retrocolically. The end-to-side pancreatcojejunal anastomosis is carried out first. To minimize leakage of the anastomosis, we usually perform a close contact method, modifying Kakita's original procedure (Fig. 72.6) [20]. At first, a 3-0 nonabsorbable suture with straight needle is introduced

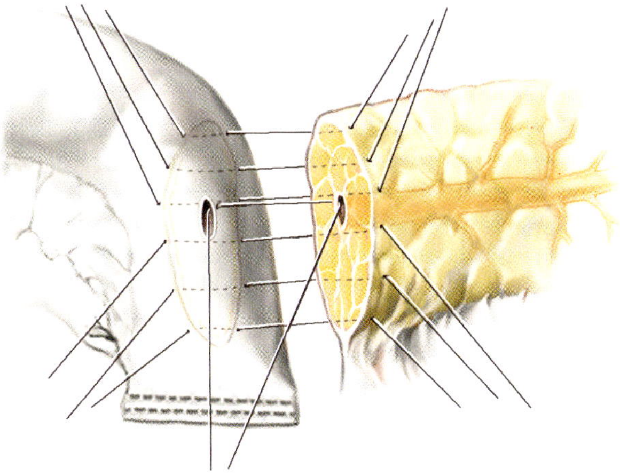

Figure 72.6

End-to-side pancreatojejunostomy using the close contact method (modified Kakita's procedure)

through the full thickness of the pancreas just near the main pancreatic duct. The needle is then through the seromuscular layer of the jejunum. Six to eight sutures are placed in the same manner and left untied. Before the ligation, duct-to-duct anastomosis is carried out. The main pancreatic duct and the surrounding pancreatic parenchyma and the whole thickness of the jejunum are ligated with interrupting sutures of 5-0 absorbable sutures, five sutures in the posterior aspect and three in the anterior aspect in case of the normal pancreas and more than eight sutures when the main pancreatic duct is dilated. The duct-to-duct anastomosis sutures are ligated. A plastic catheter is used to stent the pancreatic duct and is sutured to the pancreas using a 5-0 absorbable suture. This tube is inserted from the closed jejunal stump. The whole layer sutures, which were previously placed, are then ligated.

Hepaticojejunostomy

The common hepatic duct is implanted distal to the pancreatojejunostomy on the antimesenteric border of the jejunum using single layers of interrupted absorbable sutures. A tube stent is placed to stent the anastomosis and is sutured to the bile duct using an absorbable suture. It is inserted from the closed jejunal stump. The pancreatic and biliary drainage tubes are exteriorized through the jejunal stump using a Witzel type tunnel in the jejunal wall and brought to the outside through separate small stab incisions.

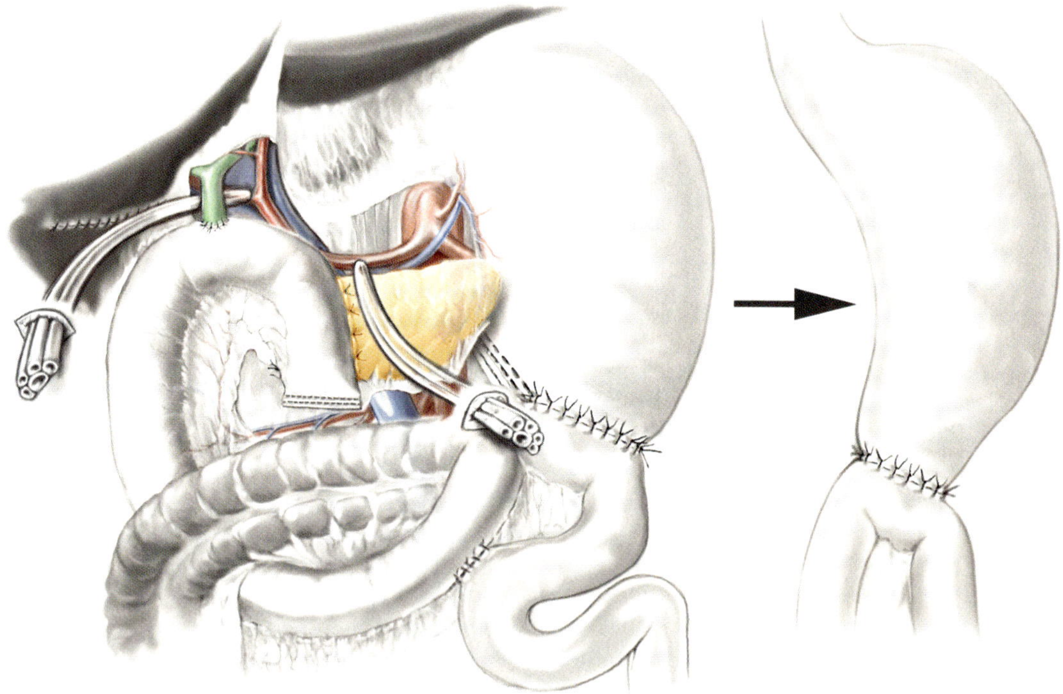

Figure 72.7

Reconstruction after pylorus-preserving pancreatoduodenectomy and placement of drainages

Duodenojejunostomy with Braun Anastomosis

An end-to-side duodenojejunostomy is made using a two-layer anastomosis (inner layer: continuous absorbable sutures; outer layer: interrupted silk sutures) about 40 cm distal to the hepaticojejunostomy above the transverse colon. A Braun side-to-side jejunojejunostomy is also completed using the two-layer method to ensure decompression of the proximal jejunal loop (carrying bile and pancreatic juice).

Two separate pleat drainage tubes are placed behind and posterior to the hepaticojejunostomy and anterior and superior to the pancreatojejunostomy, respectively (Fig. 72.7). The two drainage tubes are exteriorized through separate stab incisions.

After irrigation of the abdomen with warm saline a final check is made to ensure the complete hemostasis. The abdomen is closed in one layer using interrupted sutures of nonabsorbable sutures and the skin is approximated with interrupted nylon sutures.

Postoperative Morbidity an Mortality after Pancreatoduodenectomy

Hospital mortality after the Kasch-Whipple resection (or PPPD) has been declining recently, the incidence being less than 5%. In the past 5 years, in most institutions with a high-volume case load, the morbidity is less than 20%, and the mortality is below 5% at experienced centers (Table 72.3) [1,15,17–19,21]. Intra-abdominal abscess causing sepsis and severe gastrointestinal tract hemorrhage are early postoperative complications [22]. The most frequently observed local complication is pancreatic fistula, which occurs in about 20% of cases (Table 72.4) [15–17,23]. The pancreatojejunostomy has to be performed with the soft tissue of the pancreatic remnant, and so pancreatic fistula is frequently a consequence of surgical techniques. To lower the local complications derived from the pancreatic anastomosis, we perform a close contact (modified-Kakita's) method. This technique is an easy and safe anastomosis procedure. In most patients with pancreatic fistula the hospitalization is prolonged but it can be cured by conservative methods.

Table 72.3. Carcinoma of the ampulla of Vater: hospital mortality and morbidity after pancreaticoduodenectomy

Author	Reference	Year	Patients (*n*)	Mortality (%)	Morbidity (%)
Yamaguchi and Enjoji	1	1987	107	5.8	
Monson et al.	15	1991	104	5.7	
Yamaguchi et al.	5	1993	36	7.5	
Klempnauer et al.	21	1995	85	9	
Talamini et al.	17	1997	106	3.8	47
Berger et al.	18	1999	98	3.2	
De Castro et al.	19	2004	107	5.7	62

Table 72.4. Postoperative complications

Author	Reference	Year	Patients (*n*)	Pancreatic fistula (%)	Hemorrhage (%)	Biliary fistula (%)
Monson	15	1991	104		4.8	
Chareton	16	1996	43	5	5	
Talamini	17	1997	106	25	7	3
Yamaguchi	22	1999	1,066	16	3.7	4.7
Farnell	23	2000	20	20		20

Delay of gastric emptying has been reported after the pylorus-preserving reconstruction technique [12,22]. Clinical observation [12,24] and animal experiments [25,26] have demonstrated that the preservation of a segment of the postpyloric duodenum relates to the delayed gastric emptying in the early postoperative period. This phenomenon may be explained by motilin in the duodenal mucosa [26–28].

Long-Term Outcome after Partial Pancreatoduodenectomy

The chance of experiencing long-term survival after the application of an oncological pancreatoduodenectomy ampullary carcinoma including lymph node dissection is about 50%. The overall 5-year survival is between 38% and 63% (Table 72.2). In recently published series from experienced centers, the 1-year survival is above 80%, and the 3-year survival is between more than 50%. In stage I ampullary carcinoma, the 5-year survival probability is about 65%; in stage II ampullary carcinoma, the 5-year survival probability is above 60%; and even in stage III ampullary carcinoma, the 5-year survival probability is between 25% and 45%.

Diabetes mellitus and malabsorption are late complications after PPPD [22].

Independent Prognostic Factors

The poor prognosis of cancer of the papilla associates with ulceration of ampullary carcinoma, poorly differentiation of carcinoma, the presence of lymph node metastasis and the infiltration of the cancer into the pancreatic head tissue [29]. The presence or absence of jaundice [30], and age of the patient with ampullary carcinoma [31] are also prognostic factors. The application of an R0-resection is the surgeons' contribution to the increase of 5-year survival rates or sure rates. The survival probability after the application of R0 resection is between 53% and 64%. After resection with a cancer-positive margin or an incomplete lymph node dissection, only a minority of the patients has the chance of a long-term survival.

References

1. Yamaguchi K, Enjoji M (1987) Carcinoma of the ampulla of Vater. A clinicopathologic study and pathologic staging of 109 cases of carcinoma and 5 cases of adenoma. Cancer 1987 59:506–515
2. Yamaguchi K, Enjoji M, Tsuneyoshi M (1991) Pancreatoduodenal carcinoma: a clinicopathologic study of 304 patients and immunohistochemical observation for CEA and CA19-9. J Surg Oncol 47:148–154

3. Yamaguchi K, Chijiiwa K, Yamashita H, et al (1995) Pancreatoduodenectomy for periampullary tumors: A univariate and multivariate analysis of the pancreas influencing the morbidity, mortality and survival rates. Int Surg 80:211–214
4. Kausch W (1912) Das Carcinoma der Papilla duodeni und seine radikale Entfernung. Beitr Klin Chir 78:439–451
5. Yamaguchi K, Nagai E, Ueki T, et al (1993) Carcinoma of the ampulla of Vater. Aust N Z J Surg 63:256–262
6. Nagakawa T, Kayahara M (2005) Diagnosis and Treatment of Bile Duct Cancer: Results from the Biliary Tract Cancer Statistics Registry in Japan. Kanahara, Tokyo, Japan
7. Kayahara M, Nagakawa T, Ohta T, et al (1997) Surgical strategy for carcinoma of the papilla of Vater on the basis of lymphatic spread and mode of recurrence. Surgery 121:611–617
8. Japanese Society of Biliary Surgery (JSBS) (2001) Classification of Biliary Tract Carcinoma. Kanahara, Tokyo, Japan
9. Nakao A, Harada A, Nonami T, et al (1994) Prognosis of cancer of the duodenal papilla of Vater in relation to clinicopathological tumor extension. Hepatogastroenterology 41:73–78
10. Yamaguchi K, Enjoji M, Kitamura K (1990) Endoscopic biopsy has limited accuracy in diagnosis of ampullary tumors. Gastrointest Endosc 36:588–592
11. Yamaguchi K, Enjoji M (1991) Adenoma of the ampulla of Vater: putative precancerous lesion. Gut 1991 32:1558–1561
12. Lin P, Lin Y (1999) Prospective randomized comparison between pylorus preserving and standard pancreaticoduodenectomy. Br J Surg 86:603–607
13. Seiler C, Wagner M, Sadorwski C, et al (2000) Randomized prospective trial of pylorus-preserving vs. classic duodenopancreatectomy (Whipple procedure): initial clinical results. J Gastrointest Surg 4:443–452
14. Tran KT, Smeenk HG, van Eijck CH, et al (2004) Pylorus preserving pancreaticoduodenectomy versus standard Whipple procedure: a prospective, randomized, multicenter analysis of 170 patients with pancreatic and periampullary tumors. Ann Surg 240:738–745
15. Monson JR, Donohue JH, McEntee GP, et al (1991) Radical resection for carcinoma of the ampulla of Vater. Arch Surg 126:353–357
16. Chareton B, Coiffic J, Landen S, et al (1996) Diagnosis and therapy for ampullary tumors: 63 cases. World J Surg 20:707–712
17. Talamini MA, Moesinger RC, Pitt HA, et al (1997) Adenocarcinoma of the ampulla of Vater. A 28-year experience. Ann Surg 225:590–599; discussion 599–600
18. Beger HG, Treitschke F, Gansauge F, et al (1999) Tumor of the ampulla of Vater: experience with local or radical resection in 171 consecutively treated patients. Arch Surg 134:526–532
19. de Castro SM, van Heek NT, Kuhlmann KF, et al (2004) Surgical management of neoplasms of the ampulla of Vater: local resection or pancreatoduodenectomy and prognostic factors for survival. Surgery 136:994–1002
20. Kakita A, Yoshida M, Takahashi T (1996) New devices of pancreatic surgery: close contact pancreacreatojejunostomy. Shujyutu 50:1867–1873
21. Klempnauer J, Ridder GJ, Pichlmayr R (1995) Prognostic factors after resection of ampullary carcinoma: multivariate survival analysis in comparison with ductal cancer of the pancreatic head. Br J Surg 82:1686–1691
22. Yamaguchi K, Tanaka M, Chijiiwa K, et al (1999) Early and late complications of pylorus-preserving pancreatoduodenectomy in Japan 1998. J Hepatobiliary Pancreat Surg 6:303–311
23. Farnell MB, Sakorafas GH, Sarr MG, et al (2000) Villous tumors of the duodenum: reappraisal of local vs. extended resection. J Gastrointest Surg 4:13–21, discussion 22–23
24. Naritomi G, Tanaka M, Matsunaga H, et al (1996) Pancreatic head resection with and without preservation of the duodenum: different postoperative gastric motility. Surgery 120:831–837
25. Tanaka M, Sarr MG (1987) Total duodenectomy: effect on canine gastrointestinal motility. J Surg Res 42:483–493
26. Tanaka M, Sarr MG (1988) Effects of exogenous motilin and morphine on interdigestive gastrointestinal motor activity after total duodenectomy in dogs. Surgery 104:317–325
27. Matsunaga H, Tanaka M, Naritomi G, et al (1998) Effect of leucine 13-motilin (KW5139) on early gastric stasis after pylorus-preserving pancreatoduodenectomy. Ann Surg 227:507–512
28. Matsunaga H, Tanaka M, Takahata S, et al (2000) Manometric evidence of improved early gastric stasis by erythromycin after pylorus-preserving pancreatoduodenectomy. World J Surg 24:1236–241 discussion 1242
29. Yamaguchi K, Nishihara K (1992) Long- and short-term survivors after pancreatoduodenectomy for ampullary carcinoma. J Surg Oncol 50:195–200
30. Yamaguchi K, Enjoji M, Kitamura K (1990) Non-icteric ampullary carcinoma with a favorable prognosis. Am J Gastroenterol 85:994–999
31. Yamaguchi K, Enjoji M (1990) Ampullary carcinoma in patients under 50 years of age with a poor prognosis. J Surg Oncol 45:201–206

Chapter 73

T. Rikiyama · M. Unno · S. Matsuno

Surgical Resection of Distal Common Bile Duct Carcinoma

Adenocarcinoma of the extrahepatic bile ducts is a relatively rare malignant neoplasm. Despite the recent progress of diagnostic and therapeutic modalities, the prognosis for patients with middle and distal bile duct carcinoma remains poor. Even in recent reports, the 5-year survival rate after resection of the middle-distal bile duct carcinoma is still not satisfactory (at around 35%) [1–7]. On the other hand, although the recent several phase II trials of chemotherapy for biliary carcinoma with novel agents, such as the combination of gemcitabine and capecitabine [8], capecitabine and cisplatin [9], and gemcitabine and oxaliplatin [10], show both improvements in response rates in the range of 21–33% and prolonged median survivals in the range of 9.1–15.4 months when compared with older series, these results are still far from satisfactory.

Despite the poor prognosis, surgical resection remains the only potentially curative treatment for bile duct carcinoma. We describe herein the surgical treatment and outcome of distal common bile duct carcinoma.

Rationale of Pylorus-Preserving Pancreaticoduodenectomy for Distal Common Bile Duct Carcinoma

Bile duct carcinoma is likely to spread outside the wall, followed by neural invasion, lymph node metastasis, and direct invasion to peripheral tissue. Distal common bile duct carcinoma tends to invade the pancreatic head directly, and pancreatoduodenectomy (PD), the classical operation described by Kausch [11] and Whipple [12], has been used as the standard surgical procedure for distal bile duct carcinoma. In fact, 64 patients with distal bile duct carcinoma, excluding periampullary carcinoma, underwent PD between 1960 and 1997 at our institute, and of those, 38 patients (59.4%) had cancerous invasion that extended to the pancreatic parenchyma [4].

On the other hand, Watson [13] performed the first pylorus-preserving pancreatoduodenectomy (PpPD) in 1944, and Traverso and Longmire [14] reported their experience of PpPD in 1978. The major concern about PpPD is represented by the oncological radicality of this procedure for the treatment of distal bile duct carcinoma. One of the criticisms is the limitation of performing an adequate lymphadenectomy, because distal bile duct carcinoma tends to be associated with lymph node metastasis. However, preservation of the pylorus does not prevent dissection of the pyloric nodes. The only lymph nodes that are not removed in PpPD, as opposed to PD, are those along the lesser and greater gastric curvatures. The involvement of these lymph nodes by periampullary cancer is extremely rare [15]. In our study, more than 30% of patients with middle and distal bile duct carcinoma who underwent PD had positive lymph nodes, but the percentage of those patients who tested positive for metastasis in perigastric lymph nodes was only 1.3% (1/76) [4]. Therefore, we believe that the radicality of PD for distal bile duct carcinoma is usually not affected by the persistence of perigastric nodes.

The critical question is whether the preservation of distal stomach and pylorus reduces the survival in patients operated for malignancies. Some randomized clinical trials of PD with or without pylorus preservation for periampullary or pancreatic cancer show similar survival outcomes [16–19]. We introduced PpPD for distal bile duct carcinoma from 1996, and show the Kaplan-Meier analysis of overall survival in 80 patients who underwent PD or 38 patients who underwent PpPD, even though it is a retrospective study at our institute from 1960 to 2004 (Fig. 73.1). The median survival and the 5-year survival rates were 36 months and 36.8%, respectively, for patients having PpPD, compared with 38 months and 37.6%, respectively, for those having PD. There was no significant difference in the long-term outcome between PD and PpPD.

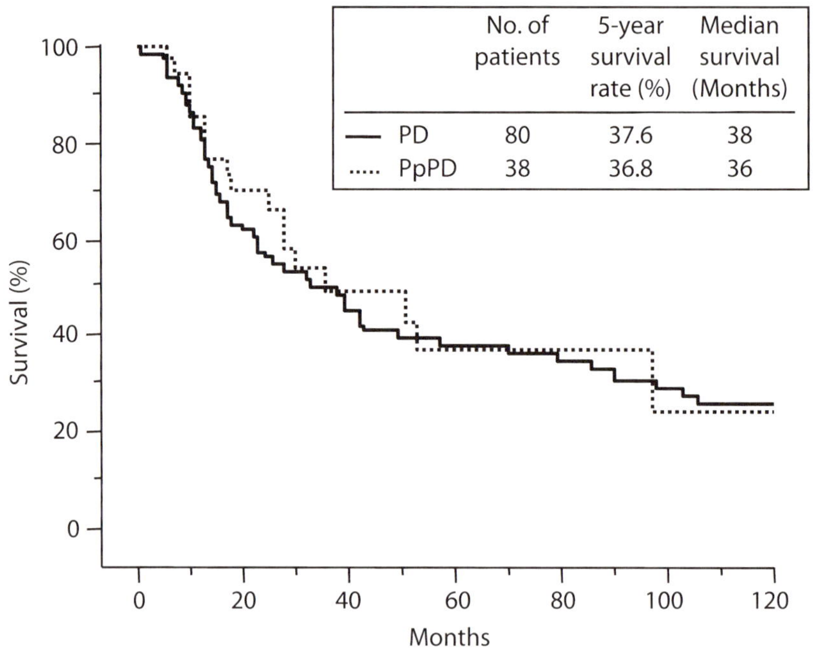

Figure 73.1

Kaplan-Meier survival curves after resection of middle and distal bile duct carcinoma in accordance with pancreatoduodenectomy (*PD*) or pylorus-preserving pancreatoduodenectomy (*PpPD*) grouping. P=0.8329 (log-rank test)

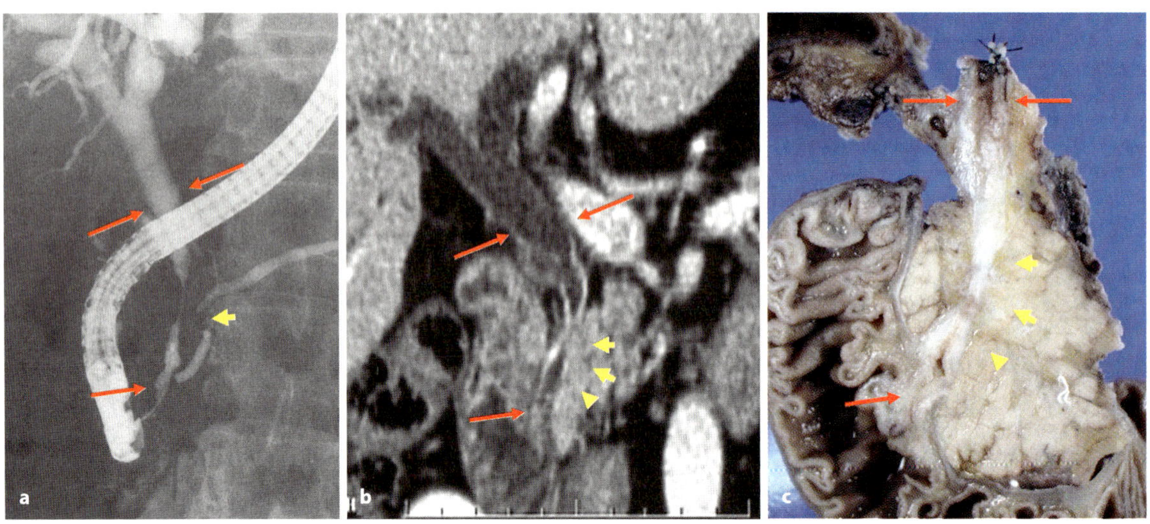

Figure 73.2

Imaging of a 63-year-old man with distal common bile duct carcinoma. a Endoscopic retrograde cholangiopancreatography image showing a distal bile duct stricture (*red arrows*) and main pancreatic duct stricture (*yellow arrowheads*). b Late arterial phase multidetector row computed tomography (MDCT) showing enhanced, hypertrophic wall of the bile duct (*red arrows*), which resulted in bile-duct carcinoma, and an ill-defined, slightly enhanced mass in the pancreatic head (*yellow arrowheads*), which resulted in direct invasion to the pancreatic parenchyma. c Surgical specimen after PpPD shows much the same extent of carcinoma as MDCT

Although there are many randomized clinical trials of PD or PpPD with or without extended lymphadenectomy for periampullary or pancreatic head cancer, there is no evidence of extended lymphadenectomy for distal bile duct cancer. In our personal experience, the percentages of patients having positive nodes were 10% in the lymph node along the celiac artery, 14.8% along the superior mesenteric artery, and 7.7% around the aorta [4].

Therefore, as mentioned above, PpPD with lymphadenectomy is now accepted as the standard surgical procedure for distal common bile duct carcinoma.

Diagnostic Work-Up

The recent introduction of multidetector row computed tomography (MDCT), with a great gain in spatial and temporal resolution if compared with single-detector computed tomography, allowed better results in terms of sensitivity and specificity for bile duct carcinoma in the assessment of both its longitudinal and vertical extent, and changed the strategy of the examination for it. Patients who are suspected of having cholangiocarcinoma should, first of all, undergo a serial multiphase MDCT examination before undergoing biliary drainage (Fig. 73.2). There is no evidence of either a positive or adverse effect of preoperative biliary drainage on the outcome of surgery in patients with periampullary or pancreatic head cancer [20]. Whether a biliary stent should be inserted before an intended PpPD for distal bile duct carcinoma may be decided based upon individual patient characteristics, such as severe cholestasis with pruritus or cholangitis. Upper gastrointestinal endoscopy as well as an endoscopic retrograde cholangiopancreatography or magnetic resonance imaging with reconstruction of the bile ducts must be performed.

Surgical Technique

A combination of upper midline and bilateral subcostal incisions is preferred for resection of the head of the pancreas, duodenum, and lymph nodes of the hepatoduodenal ligament. Very good exposure of the hepatic hilum is needed because distal common bile duct carcinoma often extends to the proximal or hepatohilar bile duct. The round ligament is ligated and divided. Further mobility of the liver can be obtained if the falciform ligament is divided. After the round ligament has been divided, a self-retaining retractor can be inserted.

The head of the pancreas is exposed by dividing the gastrocolic and duodenocolic ligaments. Mobilization of the duodenum and the head of the pancreas is performed using the Kocher maneuver, and the inferior vena cava and abdominal aorta are exposed. After taping the left renal vein and right renal artery, the para-aortic lymph nodes, such as the precaval, interaortico-caval, and preaortic lymph nodes from the celiac artery to the inferior mesenteric artery, are dissected.

The superior mesenteric vein below the pancreatic head is identified. The gastrocolic trunk, the accessory right colic vein, the right gastroepiploic vein and its branches from the duodenum, preserving the branches from the stomach, are ligated and divided. The right gastroepiploic artery and its branches to the duodenum, preserving the gastroepiploic arcade along the greater curvature, are also ligated and cut to dissect the infrapyloric lymph nodes (Fig. 73.3). Originally, it was recommended that the right gastric artery be preserved [14]; however, we usually divide the right gastric artery and its branches to the duodenum, preserving the branches to the stomach and the nerves of Latarjet, to dissect the suprapyloric lymph nodes (Fig. 73.4). We have never noticed ischemic damage to the preserved portion of the duodenum, which is supplied by the major gastroepiploic arcade. The right gastric artery will be divided again close to its origin later. The proximal duodenum is divided 2 cm from the pylorus.

The gastroduodenal artery, the common hepatic artery, and the proper hepatic artery are exposed and banded, and the lymph nodes along the celiac artery and the common hepatic artery are dissected. The right and left hepatic arteries are also exposed and banded. The gastroduodenal artery is double-ligated with a transfixing suture and cut close to its origin from the common hepatic artery; the right gastric artery and the cystic artery are also divided close to their origin. After cholecystectomy, the common hepatic duct is identified and cut around the bifurcation (Fig. 73.5). To avoid possible seeding of malignant cells from the opening of the common hepatic duct, the distal side of the common bile duct is ligated before cutting, and the proximal end is controlled with a noncrushing clamp. A frozen-section examination of the resection line is mandatory. If the tumor spreads to the transection line, the bile duct resection must be extended until a negative margin is found. The additional hepatectomy with caudate lobectomy should be considered, depending on the situation. After the portal vein is exposed and banded, the lymph nodes in the hepatoduodenal ligament are dissected en bloc with the common bile duct.

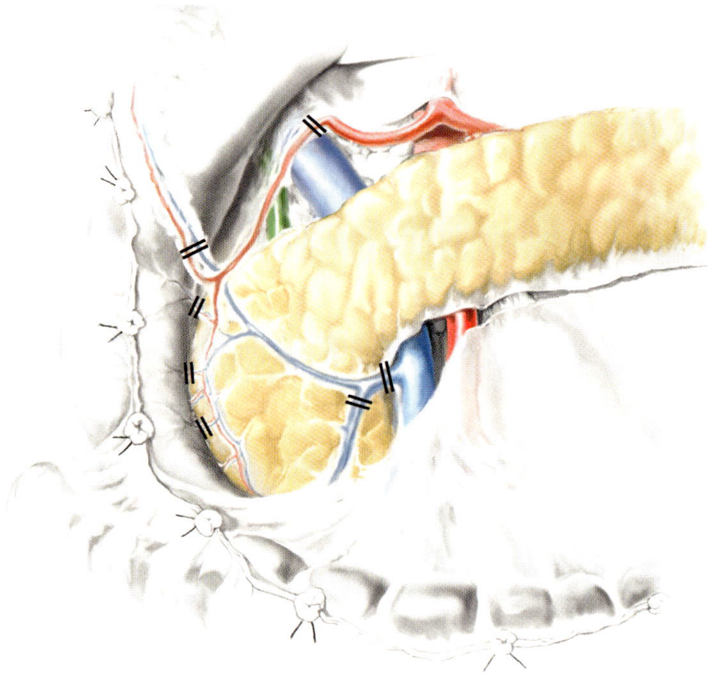

Figure 73.3

The gastrocolic trunk, the accessory right colic vein, the right gastroepiploic vein, and its branches from the duodenum, preserving the branches from the stomach, are ligated and divided. The right gastroepiploic artery and its branches to the duodenum, preserving the gastroepiploic arcade along the greater curvature, are also ligated and cut to dissect the infrapyloric lymph nodes

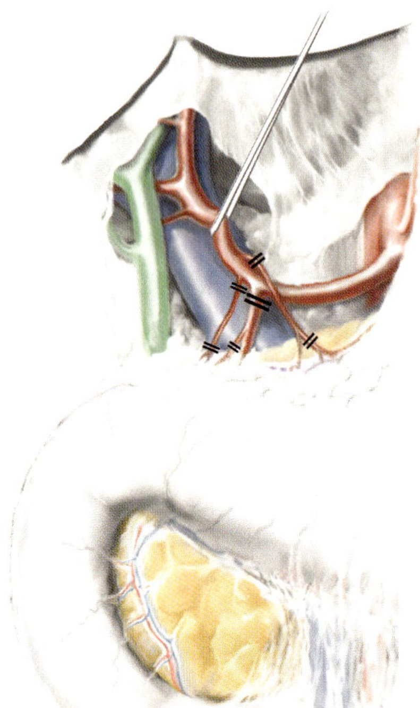

Figure 73.4

The right gastric artery and its branches to the duodenum, preserving the branches to the stomach, are ligated and divided to dissect the suprapyloric lymph nodes

Starting at the anterior surface of the superior mesenteric vein below the pancreatic head, a blunt instrument is carefully inserted to develop the avascular plane between the anterior surface of the superior mesenteric vein or the portal vein and the posterior capsule of the pancreas. After finishing the dissection of the portal vein from the dorsal pancreatic tissue, a silk ribbon is positioned and ligated around the neck of the pancreas to reduce bleeding and to lift the neck of the pancreas. Sutures, 4-0 absorbable monofilament, are placed distal to the proposed line of transection of the pancreas in both the superior and inferior longitudinal pancreatic arteries, and the neck of the gland is transected with a knife. Small bleeding vessels in the left side of the pancreas are immediately sutured and can be controlled. After identification of the pancreatic main duct, transection is completed (Fig. 73.6). The branches entering the superior mesenteric vein and the portal vein from the head of the pancreas and the uncinate process, such as the posterior superior pancreaticoduodenal vein, the anterior inferior pancreaticoduodenal vein, and the posterior inferior pancreaticoduodenal vein, are ligated and cut. The inferior pancreaticoduodenal artery and some small branches from the superior mesenteric ar-

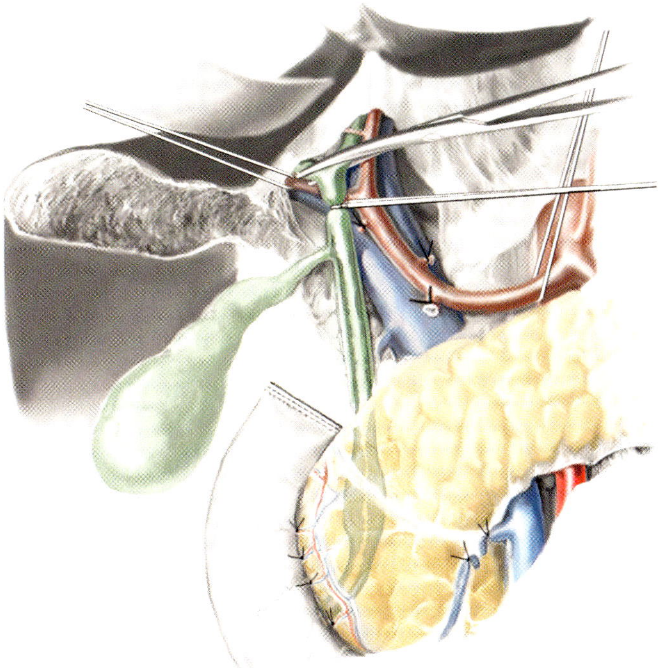

Figure 73.5

After cholecystectomy, the common hepatic duct is identified and cut around the bifurcation. To avoid a possible seeding of malignant cells from the opening of the common hepatic duct, the distal side of the common bile duct is ligated before cutting

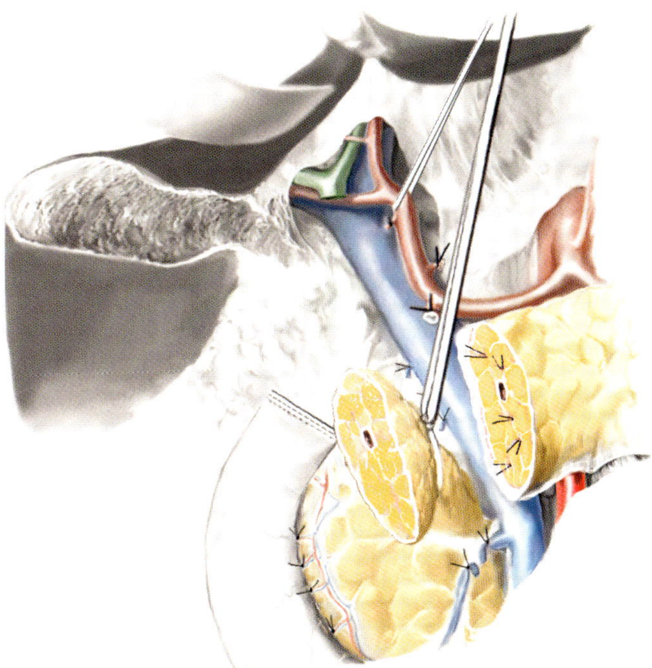

Figure 73.6

A silk ribbon is ligated around the neck of the pancreas to lift the neck of the pancreas. The neck of the gland is transected with a knife. After identification of the pancreatic main duct, transection is completed

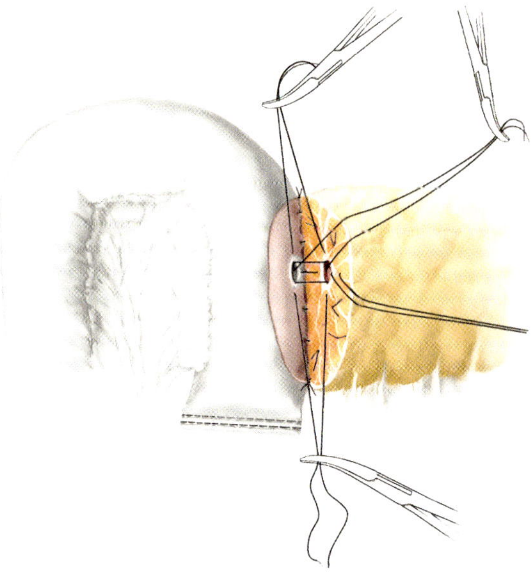

Figure 73.7

The serosa of the jejunum is removed in order to obtain good adaptation of this anastomosis. After interrupted, 5-0, non-absorbable monofilament sutures of the posterior side, interrupted, 6-0 absorbable sutures are placed between the main pancreatic duct and the small opening of the jejunum. The supporting suture for traction at the center of the anterior side of the main pancreatic duct is very useful for following the sutures

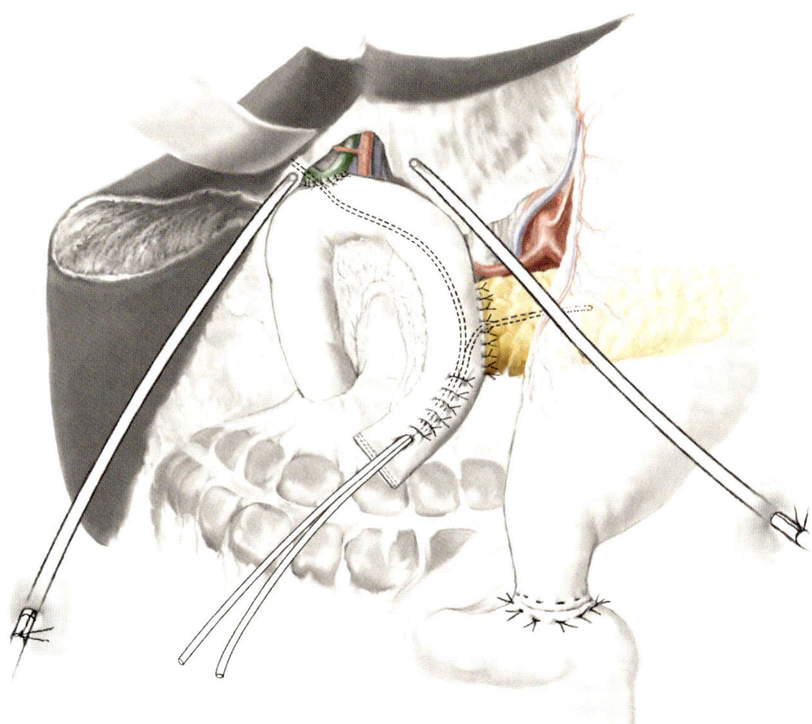

Figure 73.8

An end-to-side hepaticojejunostomy is performed 5 cm distal to the pancreaticojejunostomy with one layer of interrupted, 4-0 absorbable monofilament sutures, and an end-to side duodenojejunostomy is performed using an Albert-Lembert anastomosis

tery to the pancreas are ligated and cut. The jejunum is cut using an autosuture kit at a point about 5 cm distal to the ligament of Treitz. The first jejunal artery is ligated and cut close to its origin from the superior mesenteric artery to dissect the lymph nodes along the superior mesenteric artery. Finally, PpPD with lymphadenectomy is completed.

The pancreaticojejunostomy and hepaticojejunostomy are usually placed proximal to the duodenal anastomosis, to help to neutralize gastric acid secretion. The jejunum is brought to the pancreatic region through a small opening in the transverse mesocolon. Although the gland is soft and the duct is small in most patients, we prefer a two-layer end-to-side mucosa-to-mucosa pancreaticojejunostomy with a stent tube. An area of the serosa of the jejunum, the same size as the cut end of the pancreas, is removed in order to obtain good adaptation of this anastomosis at a point 10 cm distal to the end of the jejunum. The posterior side of the pancreatic parenchyma is sutured to the transmural layer of the jejunum with interrupted, 5-0, nonabsorbable monofilament sutures. A small opening is made at the center of the jejunum, and interrupted, 6-0 absorbable sutures are placed between the main pancreatic duct and the small opening of the jejunum. The supporting suture for traction at the center of the anterior side of the main pancreatic duct is very useful for following the sutures. The first suture is placed at the center of the posterior side, and at least five sutures are placed along the posterior side (Fig. 73.7). At least three sutures, including the supporting suture, are placed along the anterior side. While these sutures are being placed, this anastomosis is stented with a polypropylene tube. This tube is brought out through the end of the jejunum. The anterior suture line is placed on the anterior cut surface of the pancreas and jejunal layer with interrupted, 5-0 nonabsorbable monofilament sutures.

An end-to-side hepaticojejunostomy (two or more anastomoses are necessary depending on the situation) is performed 5 cm distal to the pancreaticojejunostomy with one layer of interrupted, 4-0, absorbable monofilament sutures. A biliary drainage tube is placed through the anastomosis and brought out through the end of the jejunum. The jejunum, about 40 cm distal to the hepaticojejunostomy, is brought by means of antecolic approach, and an end-to side duodenojejunostomy is performed using an Albert-Lembert anastomosis (Fig. 73.8). We prefer wrapping up the pancreatic anastomosis with an omental flap. External drains are placed around the biliary and pancreatic anastomoses, as well as in the left and right subphrenic space.

Long-Term Outcome

Table 73.1 lists a survey of the published series with middle-distal bile duct carcinoma since 1996 demonstrating rates of patient survival. We also show the 5-year survival rate and the median survival after surgery in the 118 patients who were diagnosed with middle or distal bile duct carcinoma, excluding periampullary carcinoma, and underwent PD or PpPD from 1960 to 2004 in our institute in Table 73.1. The 5-year survival rates ranged from 26% to 39% and the median survival ranged from 22 months to 38 months in these reports.

Suzuki et al. [4] reported that the degree of surgical curability, the t-category, and the comprehensive stage were prognostic factors related to survival after PD for middle and distal bile duct carcinoma. The prognostic significance of each clinicopathological variable following resection was calculated in the 118 patients in our institute. T and N categories significantly influenced survival, as well as TNM stage and R status (Table 73.2). Primary tumor (T) [6], lymph node involvement (N) [1, 5], surgical margin or residual tumor (R) [1, 3], TNM stage [6], and histological grade (G) [1] have been identified by multivariate analysis as independent predictors of survival after surgical resection of middle and distal bile duct cancers.

Table 73.1. Published series on resectional treatment of middle-distal bile duct carcinoma

Author	Year	No. of Patients	Np. of curative resections (Rate, %)	Lymph node involvement (Rate, %)	5-year survival rate (%)	Median survival (months)
Nakeeb [1]	1996	73	66 (90 %)	35 (48 %)	28	22
Fong [2]	1996	45	37 (82 %)	19 (42 %)	27	33
Kayahara [3]	1999	50	36 /72 %)	34 (68 %)	35	–
Sasaki [5]	2001	59	50 (85 %)	23 (39 %)	34	–
Todoroki [6]	2001	57	26 (46 %)	36 (63 %)	39	37
Sakamoto [7]	2005	55	–	27 (53 %)	26	38
Our institute	–	118	77 (65 %)	48 (41 %)	38	38

Table 73.2. Prognostic factors related to survival after resection in 118 patients (univariate analysis)

Prognostic factor	No. of patients	5-year survival	Median survival	p*
Primary turmor (t)				
T1	32	73.5	131.3	<0.0001
T2	29	38.1	42.0	
T3	28	20.6	22.0	
T4	29	10.7	13.6	
Lymph node involvement (N)				
N0	70	53.2	79.0	<0.0001
N1	48	15.5	17.0	
TNM stage				
Ia	29	73.1	106.0	<0.0001
Ib	18	56.5	98.0	
IIa	12	24.4	31.8	
IIb	31	20.4	28.0	
III	28	11.1	13.6	
IV	0	–	–	
Residual tumor (R)				
R0	77	49.1	57.0	<0.0001
R1	41	8.2	17.0	

* Log-rank test

Conclusions

We have discussed herein the surgical treatment and outcome of distal common bile duct carcinoma. Although surgical resection provides the only chance of cure, the survival of patients with distal bile duct carcinoma, even those who had an R0 resection, is far from satisfactory. Therefore, more effective preoperative and/or postoperative systematic multidisciplinary therapeutic strategies should be developed without delay, and effective early detection methods need to be established for the successful treatment of distal bile duct cancer.

References

1. Nakeeb A, Pitt HA, Sohn TA, et al (1996) Cholangiocarcinoma. A spectrum of intrahepatic, perihilar, and distal tumors. Ann Surg 224:463–473
2. Fong Y, Blumgart LH, Lin E, et al (1996) Outcome of treatment for distal bile duct cancer. Br J Surg 83:1712–1715
3. Kayahara M, Nagakawa T, Ohta T, et al (1999) Role of nodal involvement and periductal soft-tissue margin in middle and distal bile duct cancer. Ann Surg 229:76–83
4. Suzuki M, Unno M, Oikawa M, et al (2000) Surgical treatment and postoperative outcomes for middle and lower bile duct carcinoma in Japan – experience of a single institute. Hepatogastroenterology 47:650–657
5. Sasaki R, Takahashi M, Funato O, et al (2001) Prognostic significance of lymph node involvement in middle and distal bile duct cancer. Surgery 129:677–683
6. Todoroki T, Kawamoto T, Koike N, et al (2001) Treatment strategy for patients with middle and lower third bile duct cancer. Br J Surg 88:364–370
7. Sakamoto Y, Kosuge T, Shimada K, et al (2005) Prognostic factors of surgical resection in middle and distal bile duct cancer: an analysis of 55 patients concerning the significance of ductal and radial margins. Surgery 137:396–402
8. Knox JJ, Hedley D, Oza A, et al (2005) Combining gemcitabine and capecitabine in patients with advanced biliary cancer: A phase II trial. J Clin Oncol 23:2332–2338
9. Kim TW, Chang HM, Kang HJ, et al (2003) Phase II study of capecitabine plus cisplatin as first-line chemotherapy in advanced biliary cancer. Ann Oncol 14:1115–1120
10. Andre T, Tournigand C, Rosmorduc O, et al (2004) Gemcitabine combined with oxaliplatin (GEMOX) in advanced biliary tract adenocarcinoma: A GERCOR study. Ann Oncol 15:1339–1343
11. Kausch W (1912) Das Carcinom der Papilla duodeni und seine radikale Entfernung. Beirt Klin Chir 78:439–486
12. Whipple A (1942) Present day surgery of the pancreas. N Engl J Med 226:515–518
13. Watson K (1944) Carcinoma of the ampulla of Vater: successful radical resection. Br J Surg 31:368–373

14. Traverso LW, Lomgmire WP Jr (1978) Preservation of the pylorus in pancreaticoduodenectomy. Surg Gynecol Obstet 146:959–962
15. Mu DQ, Peng YS, Wang FG, et al (2004) Significance of perigastric lymph node involvement in periampullary malignant tumor. World J Gastroenterol 10:614–616
16. Seiler CA, Wagner M, Bachmann T (2005) Randomized clinical trial of pylorus-preserving duodenopancreatectomy versus classical Whipple resection – long term results. Br J Surg 92:547–556
17. Tran KTC, Smeenk HG, van Eijck CHJ, et al (2004) Pylorus preserving pancreaticoduodenectomy versus standard Whipple procedure – a prospective, randomized, multicenter analysis of 170 patients with pancreatic and periampullary tumors. Ann Surg 240:738–745
18. Nguyen TC, Sohn TA, Cameron JL, et al (2003) Standard vs. radical pancreaticoduodenectomy for periampullary adenocarcinoma: a prospective, randomized trial evaluating quality of life in pancreaticoduodenectomy survivors. J Gastrointest Surg 7:1–11
19. Mosca F, Giulianotti PC, Balestracci T, et al (1997) Long-term survival in pancreatic cancer: pylorus-preserving versus Whipple pancreatoduodenectomy. Surgery 122:553–566
20. Saleh MMA, Norregaard P, Jorgensen HL, et al (2002) Preoperative endoscopic stent placement before pancreaticoduodenectomy: a meta-analysis of the effect on morbidity and mortality. Gastrointest Endosc 56:529–534

Chapter 74

T. Imaizumi · M. Ishii · K. Tobita · S. Douwaki · H. Makuuchi

Cancer of the Duodenum – Surgical Treatment

The incidence of duodenal cancer is extremely low and collected clinicopathological data are scarce. The duodenum is anatomically closely connected with the stomach, upper small intestine, and pancreaticobiliary tract. In particular, the bile duct and pancreatic duct open into the second part of the duodenum. The sphincter of Oddi's exquisite physiology exerts a great effect on hepatobiliary drainage and the pancreas above it. Although it is just called duodenal cancer, the clinical picture differs greatly depending on its location and level of advancement, and how to deal with the duodenal papilla is a great problem surgically. Until now, pancreaticoduodenectomy (PD) has been the standard surgical procedure for duodenal cancer, but recent advances in various diagnostic methods have enabled us to grasp the cancer's invasion depth and extent of development, and various pancreas-sparing reduction surgeries are being performed on benign tumors and early-stage cancers [1–6]. We describe here some surgical techniques for duodenectomy to eliminate duodenal papillary cancers.

Overview of Duodenal Cancer

The incidence of duodenal cancers is altogether 0.3–0.4% or less of all cancers of the alimentary canal. However, among cancers of the small intestine they hold the highest frequency, at 30–50% [7–11]. Duodenal cancers are commonly located in the upper part of the papilla, and most occur in the second part (descending portion) of the duodenum with 0–16% being found in the first part, 52–74% in the second part, 22–39% each in the third and fourth parts, 13% in the bulb, 57% in the upper part of the papilla in the descending portion, 22% in the lower part of the papilla in the descending portion, and 9% in the horizontal portion [3–5,12–16]. Table 74.1 presents the sites of occurrence reported by familial adenomatous polyposis (FAP) and Gardner's syndrome patients. While there is the opinion that a PD should be conducted prophylactically for adenomatous polyposis, reports that careful follow-up observation is enough can also be found [17,18]. On the other hand, villous adenoma is know to be a precancerous lesion with cancer rates of 30–47%, and complete resections is desirable because the tumors are a mixture of malignant and benign, and diagnosis by biopsy sampling is difficult [19–21].

Clinical manifestations include decreased body weight, abdominal pain, and vomiting, which resemble those of a benign tumor; this lack of distinctive symptoms makes early diagnosis more difficult in the further inferior parts [4,22]. Since duodenal cancer of the papilla constricts the biliary/pancreatic duct system and causes dilatation, finding clues for its detection is not difficult. Duodenal cancer of the papilla located inferiorly can be detected because the duodenum becomes constricted as the cancer advances, especially in the third and fourth parts. However, it is almost asymptomatic in the early stage and, since it cannot be observed during routine examination by upper gastrointestinal endoscopy, X-ray imaging of the entire duodenum is vital. Therefore, detecting duodenal cancer in the early stage is extremely difficult [23–26].

The five-year survival rate for primary duodenal cancer was reported in a recent large series of reports to be 23–33% [4,5,13–16,22]. The basic therapy is surgical resection, and there are almost no cases of 5-year survival with noncurative resection (Table 74.1). Prognostic factors for duodenal cancer include lymph node metastasis, tumor depth, positive margin, tumor diameter, histological tumor differentiation, and infiltration outside the intestinal wall [12], with lymph node metastasis considered to be the most closely related to prognosis [6,8,27], and lymphadenectomy with en bloc resection being reportedly beneficial [7,28,29]. On the other hand, it is reported that the presence or absence of lymph node metastasis is unrelated to prognosis [13,14,22,30,31], but the handling of lymph node metastasis remains controversial today.

Table 74.1. Summary of major recent reviews of duodenal cancer. *PD* Pancreaticoduodenectomy, *PPPD* pylorus-preserving pancreatoduodenectomy

First author	Kakla-manos	Ryder	Bakaeen	Santoro	Rose	Barnes	Rotmano
Year	2000	2000	2000	1997	1996	1994	1994
Publication	Am J Surg	Arch Surg	Arch Surg	Hepatogastro-enterology	J Am Coll Surg	Ann Surg Oncol	Br J Surg
Reference number	[4]	[5]	[12]	[16]	[22]	[15]	[13]
No. of patients	63	49	101	89	79	67	66
Rate of curative resection	59%	51%	67%	73%	53%	61%	69%
Five-year survival overall	23%	33%	37%	25%	31%	29%	33%
Lymph node metastasis		41%	32%	24%	38%	36%	42%
Five-year survival with lymph node metastasis	15%	10%	22%		38%	47%	
Five-year survival without lymph node metastasis	60%	40%	68%		62%	59%	
Mortality	3%	4%	1%	10.1%.			8%
Complications	18%	48%	60%				
PD, PPPD	68%	87%	45%	42%	90%	76%	58%
Segmental resection	30%	13%	22%	17%	10%		10%
Local resection			4%	12%		34%	
Pancreatic site							
Supra	–	–	–	16%	–	5%	–
Peri			53%	63%		60%	
Infra				21%		35%	
First part	13%	0%	4%				13%
Second part	52%	61%	74%				52%
Third, fourth part	35%	39%	22%	–	–	–	35%

Conventionally, the basic surgical procedure for duodenal cancer, in which advanced cases are common, has been PD [7,28,29], but there are reports from overseas recommending partial duodenectomy. In a segmental resection, sufficient lymphadenectomy is possible if the mesoduodenum is separated and the duodenum is mobilized, and the incidence of complications is smaller compared to PD. Particularly for tumors on the anal side of the papilla, there are increasing reports that PD and segmental resection do not differ in prognosis, and segmental resection is recommended from the point of view of mortality and complications [4–6,13,15,22,31,32].

Bibliographic Considerations on Early Duodenal Cancer

In Japan, it has come to be thought that even for early cancer, improved prognosis should be attempted by conducting a complete lymphadenectomy [33]. However, reports of early cancer are increasing in Japan together with recent developments in endoscopy; up to 1994 there were 249 cases of early cancer reported [34], while from 1998 to 2002 there were 69 reported cases [35]. The known details of 35 cases in the period 2000–2004 (excluding data on endoscopic resections) are given in Table 74.2. Of particular note is that 48% were detected without symptoms, and most were detected by upper gastrointestinal endoscopy. Of these cases, 80% were submucosal cancers, 46.9% were polyploidy type, and 45.7% were treated by endoscopic mucosal resection (EMR), and improved diagnostic ability and treatment techniques due to the develop-

Table 74.2. Summary of reported cases of early duodenal cancer in Japan from 2000 to 2005. *EMR* Endoscopic mucosal resection

Age and Sex		Depth	
Age	48-82	Mucosa	20%
Mean age	66	Submucosa	80%
Sex (M:F)	27:8		
		Macroscopic type	
Chief complaint		Polypoid	46.9%
Abdominal discomfort, pain	37%	Flat elevated	21.9%
Asymptomatic	22.9%	Depressed	31.3%
Evidence of other disease	25.7%		
Gastrointestinal bleeding	8.5%	Operation	
Others	5.7%	Distal gastrectomy	
		+ partial resection of duodenum	14.3%
Location in pancreas		PD or PPPD	22.9%
First part	36.3%	Partial resection	17.1%
Second part	60.6%	EMR	45.7%
Third part	4.0%		
Fourth part	0%		

ment of endoscopy equipment enable early detection and treatment. However, PD or pylorus-preserving PD (PPPD) was conducted on 22–29% of cases even though they were diagnosed as early cancers before surgery, and there is a remarkable difference in the operative stress imposed by EMR and PD. It is reported that the rate of lymph node metastasis for early cancers to submucosa is 5% [36], and there are reports of reduction surgeries (segmental resection, pancreas-sparing duodenectomy – PSD) accompanying lymph node sampling as well as local surgery [33,38,39] and we are awaiting the results of treatment outcome.

Location of Duodenal Cancer and Selection of Surgical Procedure

Various surgical procedures are available depending on the location and depth of the duodenal cancer. Surgical procedures appropriate to the location and depth of the duodenal cancer are shown in Table 74.2. For advanced cancers where the tumor extends into the muscula propria (T2) or further, PD is the basic procedure regardless of location. First- and fourth-part duodenal cancers that have invaded the serosa membrane or pancreas are candidates for a circular duodenectomy, which preserves the pancreas, and if the second group of lymph nodes is removed the chance of a permanent cure improves. In early stage cancers where the tumor extends only as far as the submuscosal layer (T1) or less, various surgical procedures that preserve the pancreas are possible. A circular duodenectomy for the first, third, and fourth parts, an outer partial duodenectomy for the outer portions of the second part, and a circular duodenectomy for duodenal cancers in the inner portion of the second part where the duodenal papilla can be preserved can be conducted. When the duodenal papilla must be removed, however, a transduodenal duodenal papillectomy or a pancreas-sparing duodenectomy is conducted and the common bile duct or pancreatic duct must be reconstructed. In this case, a lymphadenectomy is not necessary.

As described above, segmental resection is being used proactively for tumors in the third and fourth parts of the duodenum. However, for tumors near the papilla, there are the problems of infiltration to the pancreas and lymphadenectomy, or reconstruction of the bile duct and pancreas, and segmental resection is not much used.

Recently there are scattered reports of the usefulness of a procedure known as PSD for tumors in the second part of the duodenum [1,2,37–41]. We describe here the pancreas-sparing technique as reduction surgery for early stage duodenal cancer, but first we will discuss the historical background of the procedure.

History of Pancreas-Sparing Duodenectomy

The surgical procedure PSD was named very recently and was first reported clinically in Surgery in 1995 by Chung et al. in "Pancreas-sparing duodenectomy: Indications, surgical techniques and results," describing one case of trauma and four cases of FAP [39]. Removal of the duodenum dates back to 1922, when Mann et al. reported a "duodenectomy" in an animal experiment [42], and "duodenectomy" that preserved the pancreas and "segmental resection of the duodenum" that removed the third and fourth parts of the duodenum were reported even before 1995. The PSD procedure of Chang et al., however, differs from a simple duodenectomy in that the duodenum is removed together with the duodenal papilla. In 1984 Sille et al. (of the same group as Chang et al.) demonstrated the safety of removing the duodenum containing duodenal papilla in animal experiments, and labeled it a "95% duodenectomy" [43].

As reports that preceded 95% duodenectomy from the point of view of separating the duodenum and pancreatic head, in 1965 Fry et al. reported a procedure for removing only the pancreas and leaving the duodenum, labeling it as "95% distal pancreatectomy in chronic pancreatitis" [44], and in 1980 Berger et al. reported "duodenum-preserving pancreatic head resection," then further conducted pancreatic head-preserving pancreatic duodenum resection as reduction surgery [45]. That is, after establishing the safety of and actively conducting procedures for partial resection of the pancreatic head that preserve the duodenum in pancreatic resections for pancreatic disease, they conversely advocated procedures that remove only the duodenum and preserve the pancreatic head in treating duodenal lesions that have not invaded the pancreas.

Historically, in 1968 Newton reported a radical enterectomy for hereditary megaduodenum. In 1984 Sillet reported an experimental PSD using dogs, a technique for 95% duodenectomy that preserves the papillary area, and in 1995, Chang et al. used the term PSD for the first time clinically

Six reports for FAP have been published: (1) in 1996, Ryu et al. conducted the first PSD for early-stage duodenal cancer [1]; (2) in 1996, Maher et al. report 24 cases of PSD, the largest such report [2]; (3) in 1999 Nagai et al. classified PSD as types 1–3, reporting 6 cases [37]; (4) in 2002, Sarmiento reports 8 cases [46]; (5) in 2002, Lundell reports 4 cases of PSD [40]; (6) in 2004, Isenberger reports 4 cases [41].

Features, Schemes, and Results of Our Surgical Procedure

Surgical Technique

The surgical technique is illustrated in Figs. 74.1–74.6.

1. Following abdominal exploration and midline incision, the hepatic flexure of the colon is retracted inferiorly and an extensive Kocher maneuver is performed. The duodenum and the pancreatic head are extensively mobilized from the retroperitoneum well to the left of the midline.
2. The papillae are confirmed by palpation.
3. Lukewarm water is infused from a gastric tube and ultrasound is conducted during the operation. The depth of the tumor is diagnosed.
4. Biopsy samples of the regional lymph nodes around the pancreatic head are taken and examined by frozen section to confirm the absence of metastasis.
5. The duodenum is gently separated from the pancreatic head from the areas anterior and posterior to the papilla area of the duodenum. The blood vessels of the arcade of pancreatic head are preserved. At this time the accessory papilla are preserved as far as possible (Figs. 74.1 and 74.2). The pancreatic and bile ducts are pursued as far as taping is possible for each. If papillary tumors are present, the duodenum and pancreas should not be separated too much (Fig. 74.3).
6. Approximately 2 cm is cut from the papilla at both the oral side and anal side of the duodenum (Fig. 74.4).
7. The pancreatic and bile ducts are transected outside the pancreas and duodenum.
8. The cut ends are examined to confirm that they are free of cancer. Pancreatoduodenectomy is performed if abnormal findings are present at the cut ends. If cancer invasion is found in the intrapancreatic bile duct or pancreatic duct, the procedure should be changed to PD.

Reconstruction

9. The bile duct and pancreatic duct are sutured with nonabsorbable 5-0 monofilament thread and 3, 4 needles (Fig. 74.5)
10. Reconstruction is possible by double tract, interposition, and duodenal anastomosis. If the length of the excised duodenum is short (about 6 cm or less) end-to-end anastomosis of the oral end section and anal end section is possible. In each case,

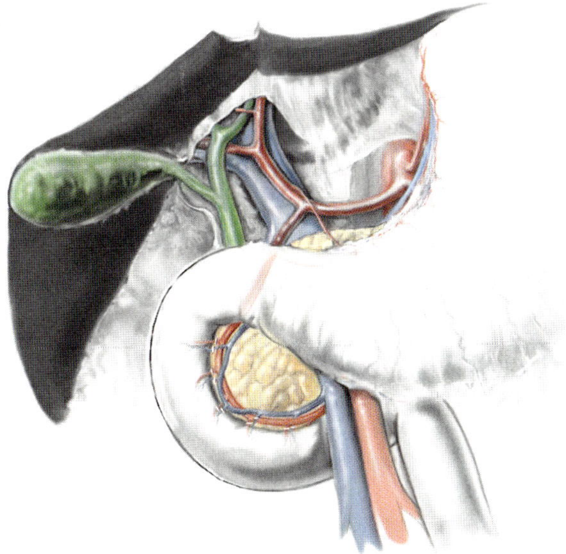

Figure 74.1

The pancreas was extensively mobilized from retroperitoneum. *Du* Duodenum

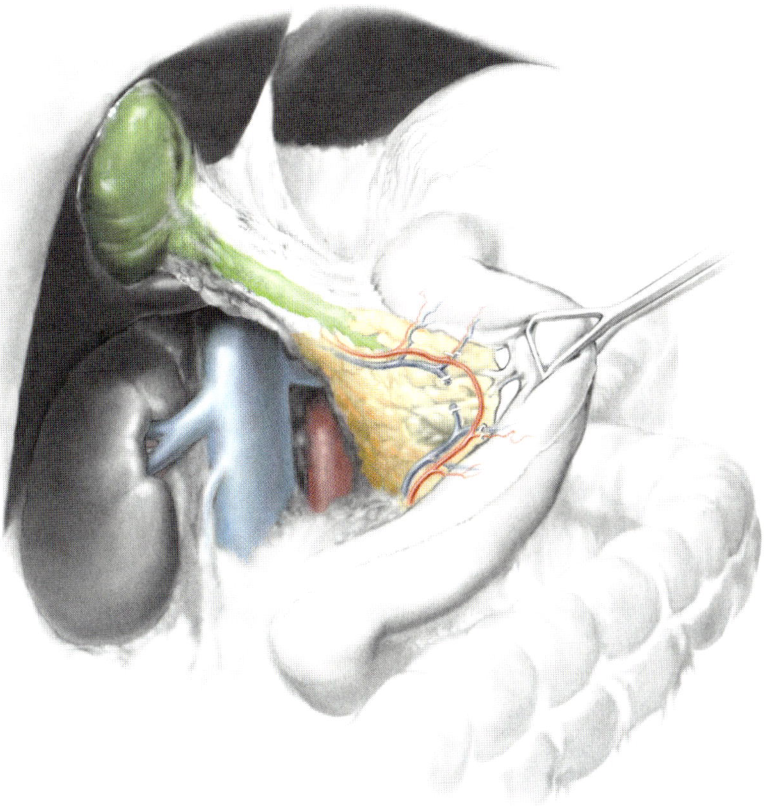

Figure 74.2

Detachment of the duodenum from pancreas with bile duct and main pancreatic duct intact. The minor pancreatic duct was not recognized, but it was ligated with fibrous tissue along the duodenum

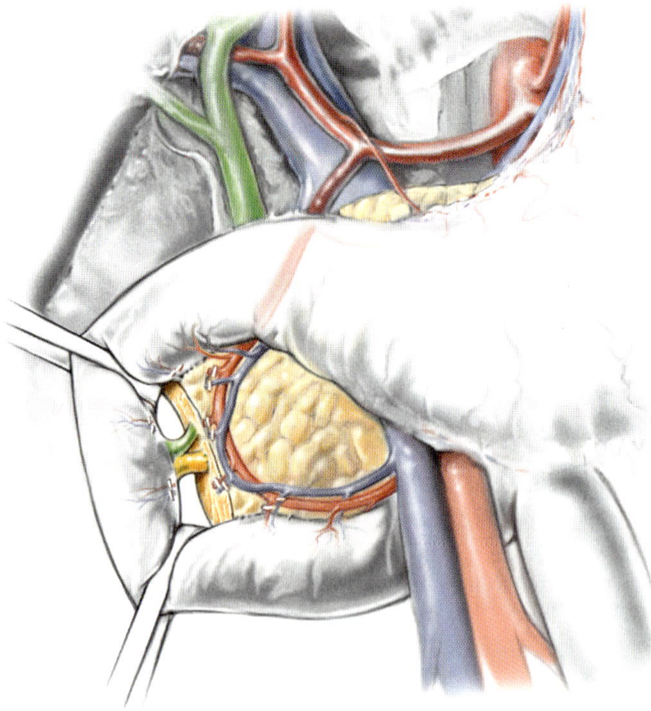

Figure 74.3

The pancreatic and bile ducts were transected outside the pancreas and duodenum

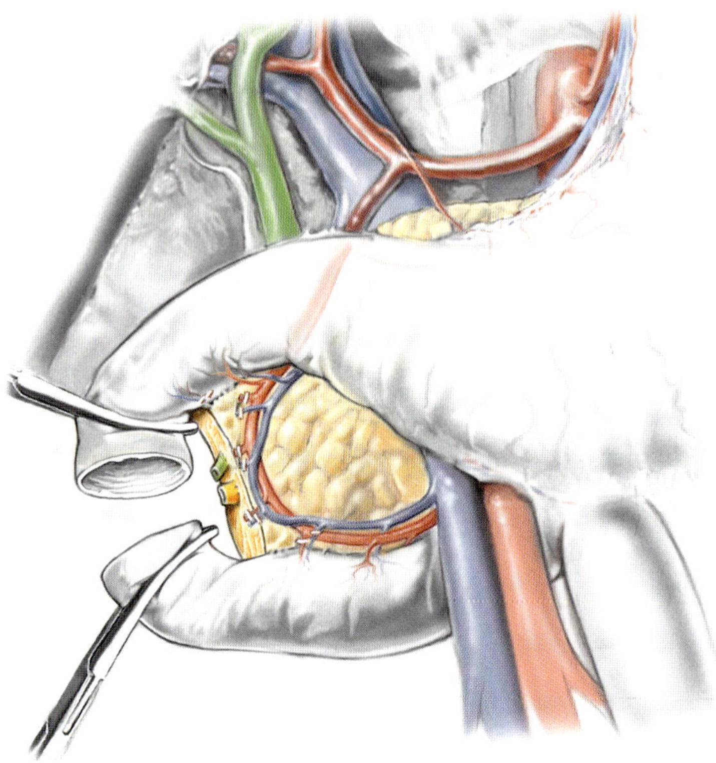

Figure 74.4

Pancreaticocholedochoplasty was performed. The walls of the biliary and pancreatic ducts were sutured together

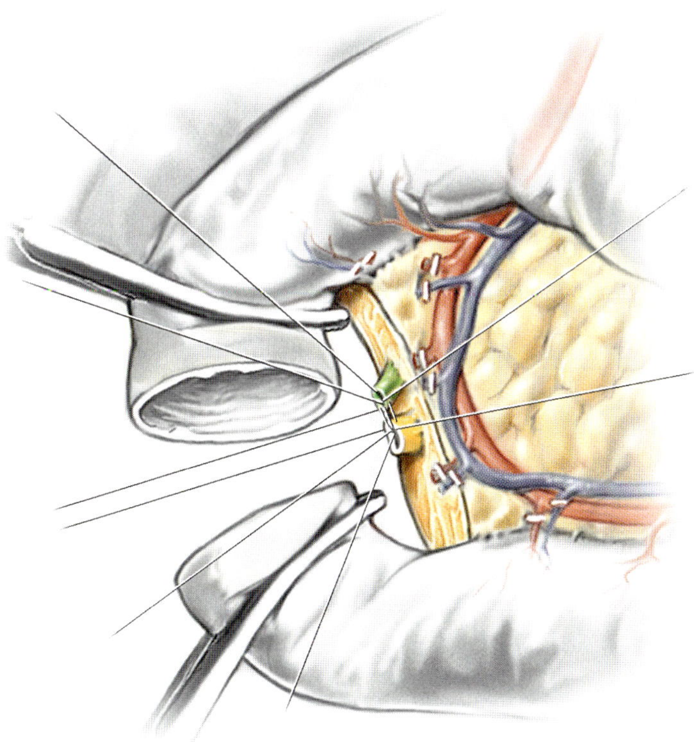

Figure 74.5

Reimplantation of the bile and pancreatic ducts was performed, followed by end-to-side anastomosis into the jejunal loop

by performing anastomosis on the oral side of the duodenum first, excessive tension is avoided at later anastomosis of the pancreatic duct and bile duct.

11. For duodenal anastomosis all layers of the oral and anal sides of the cut duodenum are anastomosed end-to-end and reconstructed with seromuscular suturing on two layers.
12. In each case, after plastic surgery on the left wall of the second part of the neoduodenum, a new common duct was anastomosed side-to-end in one layer. It is usual to anastomose the wall of the anal side of the duodenum (Fig. 74.6).

Advantages and Applications of this Surgical Technique

The following advantages are suggested.

1. Tumors are completely resected including the duodenal papilla while the pancreas can be preserved.
2. The bile duct and pancreatic duct can be severed from the outer wall of the duodenum.
3. Compared to focal excision, excision of the duodenal mucosa is sufficient horizontally.
4. The presence or absence of lymph node metastasis can be confirmed.
5. If quick pathologic diagnosis of the positive margin reveals lymph node metastasis, it is possible to change to PD.
6. Impairment of absorption is considered slight, since the first part of the duodenum and, depending on the case, the third part and below can also be preserved as physiological reconstruction is possible.

In determining candidates for surgery, it is important to diagnose presence or absence of infiltration to the pancreatic bile duct, parenchyma and pancreatic duct, the depth in the duodenal wall and horizontal expansion. Therefore, endoscopic ultrasound and intraductal ultrasound are indispensable tests in addition to the conventional abdominal ultrasound, computed

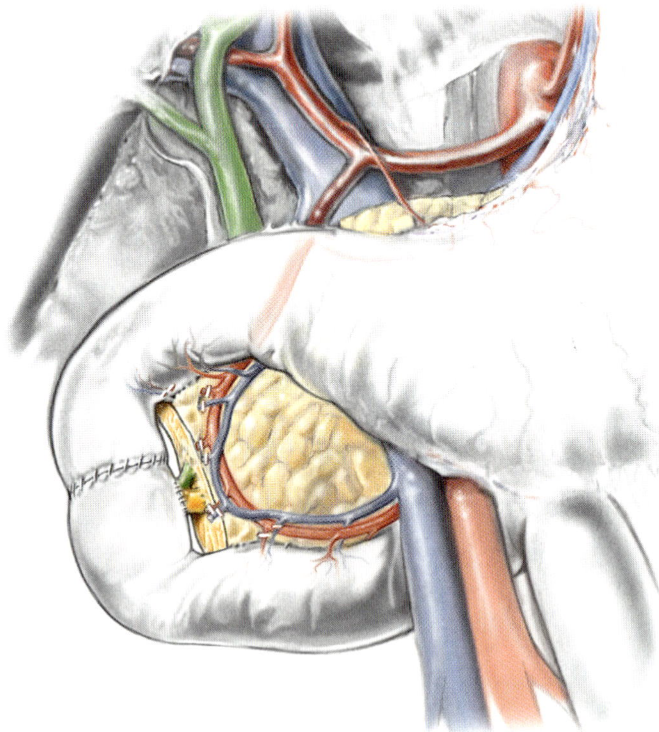

Figure 74.6

Reconstruction with duodenoduodenostomy and pancreaticocholedochoduodenstomy

tomography, endoscopic retrograde cholangiopancreatography, and magnetic resonance cholangiopancreatography.

Indications for seeking a complete cure include duodenal papilla adenoma (including FAP), carcinoma in adenoma, papilla carcinoma, duodenal early stage cancers (infiltration to the submucosa), endocrine tumors, leiomyoma, leiomyosarcoma, lipomas, and carcinoid tumors. In particular, it is reported that cancer rates for villous adenoma in the duodenum are reportedly high at 30–64%, the recurrence rate is low for PSD compared to endoscopic transduodenal focal excision, surgical time is short, the amount of blood loss is less, and recurrence is less compared to PD. To reiterate, if considering the invasion depth, extent, and associated lymph node metastasis the chance for permanent cure has been undermined, this procedure is not indicated as reduction surgery, and PD should be selected. As a disadvantage, the risk of delayed gastric emptying is somewhat high in the early postsurgery period, but in the long term of 3 months or more, decreased body weight is hardly seen.

Early Postsurgical Results

For PSD conducted at our facility, the surgery takes an average of 4 h and blood loss is about 100 ml. Early postsurgical complications such as ruptured sutures were not fatal. However, delayed gastric emptying was seen in all cases, and on this point this surgical method has room for improvement. Decreased body weight was not observed after consuming meals, however, and the entire procedure is considered less invasive than conventional PD. We are now awaiting long-term results including recurrence.

References

1. Ryu M, Kinoshita T, Konishi M, Kawano N, Arai Y (1996) Segmental Resection of the duodenum including the papilla of Vater for focal cancer in adenoma. Hepatogastroenterology 43:835–838
2. Maher MM, FRCSI, Yeo CJ, Lillemoe KD, Roberts JR, Cameron JL (1996) Pancreas-sparing duodenectomy for infra-ampullary duodenal pathology. Am J Surg 171:62–67

3. Oka S, Tanaka S, Nagata S, Hiyama T, Ito M, et al (2000) Clinicopathologic features and endoscopic resection of early primary nonampullary duodenal carcinoma. J Clin Gastroenerol 37:381–386
4. Kaklamanos LG, Bathe OF, Franceschi D, et al (2000) Extent of resection in the management of duodenal adenocarcinoma. Am J Surg 179:37–41
5. Ryder NM, Ko CY, Hincs OJ, Gloor B, Rcber HA (2000) Primary duodenal adenocarcinoma: a 40-year experience. Arch Surg 135:1070–1075
6. Lowell JA, Rossi RL, Munson JL Braasch JW (1992) Primary adenocarcinoma of third portion and fourth portion of duodenum. Favorable prognosis after resection. Arch Surg 127:557–561
7. Spira IA, Ghazi A, Wolff WI (1977) Primary adenocarcinoma of the duodenum. Cancer 39:1721–1726
8. Ouriel K, Adamus JT (1984) Adenocarcinoma of small intestine. Am J Surg 147:66–71
9. Cunningham JD, Aleali R, Aleali M, et al (1997) Malignant small bowel neoplasms: histopthologic determinations of recurrence and survival. Ann Surg 1997 225:300–306
10. Debaja BS, Suki D, Pro B, Bonnen M, Ajani J (2004) Adenocarcinoma of the small bowel. Presentation, prognostic factors, and outcome of 217 patients. Cancer 101:518–526
11. Alwmark A, Anderson A, Lasson A (1980) Primary carcinoma of the duodenum. Ann Surg 191:13–18
12. Bakaeen GB, Murr MM, Sarr MG, Thompson GB, Farnell MB, et al (2000) What prognostic factors are important in duodenal adenocarcinoma? Arch Surg 135:635–642
13. Rotman N, Pezet D, Fagniez PL, Cherqui D, Celicout B (1994) Adenocarcinoma of the duodenum: factors influencing survival. Br J Surg 81:83–86
14. Pickieman J, Koelsch M, Chejfec G (1997) Node-positive duodenal carcinoma is curable. Arch Surg 132:241–244
15. Barnes G Jr, Romero L, Hess KR, Curley SA (1994) Primary adenocarcinoma of the duodenum: management and survival in 67 patients. Ann Surg Oncol 1:73–78
16. Santoro D, Sacchi M, Scutari F, et al (1997) Primary adenocarcinoma of the duodenum: treatment and survival in 89 patients. Hepatogastroenterology 44:1157–1163
17. Schnur PL, David E, Brown PW Jr, et al (1973) Adenocarcinoma of the duodenum and Gardner syndrome. JAMA 223:1229–1232
18. Iida M, Yao T, Itoh H, et al (1989) Natural history of duodenum lesions in Japanese patients with familial adenomatosis coli (Gardner's syndrome). Gastroenterology 961:301–306
19. Farnell MB, Sakorafas GH, Sarr MG, et al (2000) Villous tumors of the duodenum: reappraisal of local vs extended resection. J Gastrointest Surg 4:13–21
20. Pezet D, Rotman N, Slim K, et al (1995) Villous tumors of the duodenum: a retrospective study of 47 cases by the French associations for surgical research. J Am Coll Surg 180:541–544
21. Bjork KJ, Davis CJ, Nagorney DM, et al (1990 Duodenal villous tumors. Arch Surg 125:961–965
22. Rose DM, Hochwald SN, Klimstra DS, Brennan MF (1996) Primary duodenal adenocarcinoma: A ten-year experience with 79 patients. J Am Coll Surg 183:89–96
23. Bradford D, Levine MS, Hoang D (2000) Early duodenal cancer: detection on double contrast upper gastrointestinal radiography. AJR Am J Roentgenol 174:1564–1566
24. Matsuura H, Kuwano H, Kanematsu T, Sugimachi K, Haraguchi Y (1990) Clinicopathological features of elevated lesions of the duodenal bulb. J Surg Oncol 45:79–84
25. Obata S, Suenaga M, Araki K, et al (1992) Use of strip biopsy in a case of early duodenal cancer. Endoscopy 24:232–234
26. Tringali M, Crotta S, Bodrato C, Lolli R, Cerrato C, Cerrato G (1994) Early primary duodenal carcinoma successfully treated by endoscopic polypectomy. Endoscopy 26:709
27. Joesting MD, Beart RW, van Heerden JA, Weiland LH (1981) Improving survival in adenocarcinoma of the duodenum. Am J Surg 141:228–131
28. Cortese AF, Cornel GN (1972) Carcinoma of the duodenum. Cancer 225:300–306
29. Moss WM, McCart PM, Juler G, Miller DR (1974) Primary adenocarcinoma of the duodenum. Arch Surg 108:805–807
30. Scott-Coombes DM, Williamson RCN (1994) Surgical treatment of primary duodenal carcinoma: a personal series. Br J Surg 81:1472–1474
31. Sohn TA, Lillemoe KD, Cameoron JL, et al (1998) Adenocarcinoma of the duodenum: factors influencing long term survival. J Gastrointest Surg 2:79–87
32. Tocchi A, Mazzoni G, Puma F, Miccini M, Cassini D, Betteti E, et al (2003) Adenocarcinoma of the third and fourth portions of the duodenum: results of surgical treatment. Arch Surg 138:80–85
33. Fujisawa T, Tomofuji Y, Kuroda N, Hagino H, Sakamoto N, et al (1995) A case of early duodenal cancer with tublo-vilous adenoma: report of case and clinicopathological review of the Japanese literature. Gastroenterol Endosc 37:2768–2775
34. Ozawa T, Mimuro M, Kitamura K, Endo M, Tsuchida A, et al (2004) A case of early duodenal cancer: review of the surgical therapy reported for past five years in the literature. J Jpn Coll Surg 29:58–63
35. Nagatani K, Takekoshi T, Baba Y, Kaku S, Fujii A, et al (1993) Indications for endoscopic treatment of early duodenal cancer: based on cases reported in the literature. Endosc Digest 7:969–976
36. Ryu M, Watanabe K, Takayama W, Kionshita T, Konishi M, et al (1994) Case report of early duodenal cancer with segmental resection and long term survival. Review of 122 reported Japanese cases. J Hepatobil Pancreat Surg 4:429–434
37. Nagai H, Hyodo M, Kurihara K, Ohki J, Yasuda T, et al (1999) Pancreas-sparing duodenectomy: classification, indication and procedures. Hepatogastroenterology 46:1953–1958
38. Ota T, Takasaki K (2003) Partial resection of para ampulla portion of the duodenum for carcinoma of the ampulla of Vater. Tan to sui 24:33–37
39. Chang RS, Church JM, Rosalind van Stolk (1995) Pancreas-sparing duodenectomy: Indications, surgical technique, and results. Surgery117:254–259
40. Lundell L, Hyltander A, Liedman B (2002) Pancreas-sparing duodenectomy: technique and indications. Eur J Surg 168:74–77
41. Eisenberger CE, Knoefe WTl, Peiper M, Yekebas EF, Hosch SB (2004) Pancreas-sparing duodenectomy in duodenal pathology: indication and results. Hepatogastroenterology 51:727–731
42. Mann FC, Kawamura K (1922) Duodenectomy, an experimental study. Ann Surg 75:208–220
43. Sillen LF, Rosenbloom MS, Chung RS (1984) Ninety-five percent duodenectomy: an experimental study. Am J Surg 148:337–339
44. Fry WJ, Child CG III (1965) Ninety-five percent distal pancreatectomy for chronic pancreatitis. Ann Surg 162:543–549

45. Beger HG, Witte C, Kraas E, Bittner R (1980) Erfahrung mit einer das Duodenum erhltenden Pankreaaskopfresektion bei chonischer Pankreatitis. Chirurg 51:303–309

46. Sarmiento JM, Thompson GB, Nagorney DM, Donohue JH, Farnell MB (2002) Pancreas-sparing duodenectomy for duodenal polyposis. Arch Surg 137:557–563

Chapter 75

H. Amano · T. Takada

Long-Term Outcome After Resection of Periampullary Carcinoma

Periampullary carcinoma, a malignant gastrointestinal tract neoplasm occurs at a frequency of 5% [1]. Pancreatic cancer, carcinoma of the ampulla of Vater, lower bile duct cancer, and duodenal adenocarcinoma are classified as periampullary carcinomas.

Pancreatic cancer has been described in Part 6 of this book (Chaps 44–61), so in this chapter we will we comment on the long-term outcome of carcinoma of the ampulla of Vater and lower bile duct cancer.

Carcinoma of the Ampulla of Vater

Background

Carcinoma of the ampulla of Vater is a rare neoplasm, found at a frequency of 0.063–0.21% during routine autopsies. As for periampullary tumors, we experience cases in the following decreasing order of prevalence: pancreatic cancer, bile duct cancer, and carcinoma of the ampulla of Vater [1, 2].

Carcinoma of ampulla of Vater reportedly accounts for 10–30% of resectable periampullary tumors [1, 2]. A resection rate of carcinoma of the ampulla of Vater of 68.1–95.7%, a 5-year survival rate of 28–67.7%, and a median survival time of 32.5–58.8 months are reported. The resection rate is the highest and outcome is the most favorable among the periampullary carcinomas (Table 75.1) [1–15].

Concerning the operative procedure for carcinoma of the ampulla of Vater, pancreatoduodenectomy (PD)/pylorus-preserving pancreatoduodenectomy (PPPD) is the standard technique. A mortality rate of 0–15.2% has been reported for PD/PPPD [3–13], but in recent years this procedure has become safer because of improvements in surgical and anesthetic techniques, critical care, and institutional specialization [9]. Mortality in a representative institution has been reported at less than 5%. Nagakawa et al. [11] accumulated data on 1,423 cases in Japan, reporting a mortality rate of 1.3%, and Duffy et al. [12] reported 0% in 55 cases. PD/PPPD-related morbidity was reported to be 29–68% (Table 75.1). Pancreatic fistula, intra-abdominal hemorrhage, and delayed gastric emptying are still a serious associated problem.

Local resection (LR) is sometimes performed for cases such as suspicious carcinoma, early carcinoma, refusal of radical operation, and poor performance status [1, 13, 16].

Prognostic factors

Pathological Factors Regarding the Tumor

The following tumor-related pathological factors have been shown to affect outcome (Table 75.2): extent of the primary tumor (T) [1, 2, 4, 6, 13–15], nodal status (N) [1–3, 5, 6, 8–10, 13, 14], stage [4, 6, 10], epithelial origin [5], tumor grade [5, 6, 8–10, 14, 15], microscopic lymphatic invasion [5], and perineural invasion [12, 13].

T-Staging

Prognosis when a tumor is limited to the sphincter of Oddi (T0, Tis, T1) is good, but that of a case with pancreatic infiltration (T3) becomes poor [1, 2, 4, 6, 13–15]. Beger [1, 2] reported 5-year survival rates of positive (+) and negative (–) pancreatic invasion of 24% and 79%, respectively. In addition, lymph node metastasis occurred frequently with progression of the tumor (T) [4].

Nodal Status (N)

The frequency of positive lymph nodes varies among reports from 20.1 to 60%. The 5-year survival rates of N (+) and N (–) cases are 9.5–53.4% and 40–76.5%, respectively. Regarding the site-frequency of lymph node metastasis, posterior pancreaticoduodenal node (no. 13) was the highest at 22% according to Nagakawa et al. [11], and the 5-year survival was 29%. The superior mesenteric artery (SMA) circumference lymph node (no. 14) metastasis frequency was 5.9% and the 5-year survival was 9–23%; the frequency of metastasis at the para-aortic lymph node (no. 16) was 10.1% and the 5-year survival was 4%.

Table 75.1. Carcinoma of ampulla of Vater. *PD* Pancreatoduodenectomy, *PPPD* pylorus-preserving pancreatoduodenectomy, *TP* total pancreatectomy, *LR* local resection

Author	Period	Year	No. of patients	Resection (%)	Procedure	Mortality	Morbidity	Overall 5-year survival	Median survival time
Warren [3]	1942–1971	1975	112	112	PD	11% (recent 10-year, 7.6%)	/	32% (excluding operative death)	/
Yamaguchi [4]	1969–1985	1987	109	109	107 PD, 2 LR	5.5%	/	28.0%	/
Monson [5]	1965–1989	1991	104	104	87 PD, 17 TP	5.7%	/	34.0%	33.6 months
Roder [6]	1983–1994	1995	69	66 (95.7%)	37 PD, 26 PPPD, 3 TP	4.5%	29.0%	34.6%	41 months
Allema [7]	1984–1992	1995	67	67	62 PD, 5 TP	9% (PD 6%, TP 40%)	68.0%	50.0%	/
Talamini [8]	1969–1996	1997	120	106 (88.3%)	103 PD, 2 TP (pylorus-preserving 85, antrectomy 20), 1 LR	3.8%	47.0%	38.0%	46 months
Howe [9]	1983–1995	1998	123	101 (82.1%)	99 PD, 2 LR	5.0%	/	46.0%	58.8 months
Beger [1, 2]	1982–1997	1999	126	98 (77.8%)	50 PPPD, 38 PD, 10 ampullectomy	3.2% (PD) 0% (LR)	/		/
Su [10]	1965–1995	1999	132	132	PD/PPPD	15.2% (5.6% since 1991)	48.5%	37.5% (excluding operative death)	32.5 months
Nagakawa [11]	1987–1997	2002	1423	1298 (91.2%)		1.3%	/	51.0%	/
Duffy [12]	1988–2001	2003	55	55	32 PPPD, 23 PD	0.0%	49.1%	67.7%	not reached
De Castro [13]	1992–2002	2004	126	126	113 PD, 9 LR&PD, 4 LR	6% (PD), 4% (LR)	/	37.0%	
Brown [14]	1991–2004	2005	72	51 (70.8%)	51 PD	2.0%	47.0%	58.0%	42 months
Di Giorgio [15]	1981–2002	2005	94	64 (68.1%)	55 PPPD, 8 PD, 1 TP	9.3%	48.4%	64.4%	54 months

Table 75.2. Carcinoma of ampulla of Vater

Author	N(+)	N(-)	5-year survival		5-year survival				5-year survival		5-year survival		5-year survival					
			N(+)	N(-)	Stage 1	Stage 2	Stage 3	Stage 4	pancreatic invasion (+)	pancreatic invasion (-)	well	poor	perineural invasion (+)	perineural invasion (-)	R0	R1,2	R0	R1,2
Warren [3]	28.0%	72.0%	9.5%	40.0%														
Yamaguchi [4]	52.0%	48.0%			85.0%	11.0%	25.0%	24.0%										
Monson [5]	31.0%	69.0%	16.0%	43.0%														
Roder [6]	42.4%	57.6%													92.4%	7.6%		
Allema [7]	52.2%	47.8%	41.0%	59.0%							56%	44%						
Talamini [8]	40.0%	60.0%	31.0%	43.0%							49%	18%						
Howe [9]	45.5%	54.5%																
Beger [1, 2]	54.8%	45.2%	21.0%	63.0%	84.0%	70.0%	27.0%	0.0%	24%	79%					83.7%	16.3%	64%	15%
Su [10]	20.1%	79.9%	10.1%	44.9%														
Nagakawa [11]	60.0%	40.0%	N1 33% N2 22%	64.0%	75.0%	48.0%	34.0%	19.0%							78.5%	21.5%		
Duffy [12]	41.8%	58.2%	53.4%	76.5%							77.8%	58.4%	29.2%	78.8%				
De Castro [13]	46.4%	53.6%	N1a 40%, N1b, N2 0%	63.0%	70.0%	69.0%	22.0%	0.0%					19.0%	45.0%	86.4%	13.6%	48%	0%
Brown [14]	47.1%	52.9%	25.0%	78.0%							82%	37%						
Di Giorgio [15]	28.1%	71.9%	53.2%	68.6%	92.3%	61.4%	66.2%	25.2%										

Table 75.3. Carcinoma of ampulla of Vater. *Hct* Hematocrit, *BUN* blood urea nitrogen

Author	Prognostic factors Univariate analysis	Multivariate analysis
Warren [3]	Nodal involvement	
Yamaguchi [4]	Stage 1, Oddi	
Monson [5]	Microscopic lymphatic invasion, regional nodal metastasis, tumor grade, epithelium of origin	Microscopic lymphatic invasion
Roder [6]	T, N, Stage, G, 0-2 positive lymph nodes	
Allema [7]	Resection margin	Free margins
Talamini [8]	Resection, negative nodes, blood transfusion, moderately or well differentiated	Blood transfusion
Howe [9]	Resection, negative nodes, negative margin, moderately or well differentiated	Negative nodes, negative margin
Beger [1, 2]	Negative nodes, infiltration into the pancreatic head tissue, G, R0	Negative nodes, infiltration into pancreatic head tissue, R0
Su [10]	Age<75, Hct>30%, BUN<20, stage, tumor size, nodal metastasis, well differentiated	Negative nodes, Hct>30%
Duffy [12]		Perineural invasion
De Castro [13]	R, T, N, Stage, perineural invasion	pT4, nodal status
Brown [14]	Lymph node, T, histology	Node-negative
Di Giorgio [15]	Resection, tumor size, tumor grade, tumor infiltration	Depth of tumor infiltration

Nagakawa et al. also reported 5-year survival rates of n1 at 33% and n2 at 22%. De Castro et al. [13] reported a 5-year survival of N1a at 40% and N1b and N2 at 0%. Prognosis becomes poor if lymph node metastasis has spread to distant lymph node groups.

According to Roder et al. [6], a metastasis number between 0 and 2 is significantly better in terms of prognosis than more than 2 for positive lymph nodes.

Stage

The 5-year survival rate for stage 1 ampulla of Vater tumors is 70–85%, with good results. However, survival worsens with stage progression, and 5-year survival of stage 4 is a poor at 0–24% [2, 4, 11, 13, 15].

Tumor Differentiation, Epithelial Origin

The 5-year survival of well-differentiated adenocarcinoma is 49–77.8%, while that of poorly differentiated cases is 18–58.4%. Some studies report that tumor differentiation is a pathological factor [5, 6, 8–10, 14, 15]. Monson et al. [5] reported that the median survival time of ampullary epithelial origin is two times that of nonampullary epithelial origin. Kimura compared the intestinal type with pancreatobiliary type, and reported that the intestinal type had significantly lower frequency of lymph node metastasis and significantly better prognosis [17].

Multivariate Analysis

On the basis of multivariate regression analysis, negative nodes, infiltration into pancreatic head tissue, microscopic lymphatic invasion, and perineural invasion are significant independent pathological factors (Table 75.3) [7, 9, 10, 12–15].

Factors of Resection – Operative Procedure and Lymph Node Dissection

PD/PPPD is the standard operative procedure for carcinoma of the ampulla of Vater, and local resection (LR) is performed for selected cases [2, 13, 16] such as suspicious carcinoma, refusal of radical operation, and high-risk patients. De Castro et al. [13] performed 13 LRs for carcinoma of the ampulla of Vater, but 10 cases were R1, and PPPD was then added to 9 cases. Beger [2] performed ten LRs, six of which were R1. Among the R1 cases, there were no 3-year survivors. Therefore, we need to consider the possibility of changing the operative procedure to PD/PPPD. PD is an adequate treatment for patients who are found to have invasive adenocarcinoma during or after LR. Furthermore, periodic follow-up for local recurrence is essential after LR.

More recently, PPPD has been performed for periampullary tumor and malignancy. Reports comparing PPPD with PD for carcinoma of the ampulla of

Vater showed no difference in survival [6, 12]. The frequency of PPPD for carcinoma of ampulla of Vater is increasing and becoming the standard technique.

The appropriate range of lymph node dissection is still uncertain, but the lymph nodes considered as regional might be the posterior pancreaticoduodenal (no. 13), anterior pancreaticoduodenal (no. 17), common and proper hepatic artery (nos. 8, 12), hepatoduodenal ligament (no. 12), and the right side of the superior mesenteric artery (no. 14), based on the frequency of lymph node metastasis [1, 2].

By multivariate analysis, negative margin and R0 were shown to be significant independent factors affecting prognosis (Table 75.3) [2, 7, 9]. The percentage of R0 tumors is reportedly in the range of 78.5–92.4%, with a 5-year survival rate of 48–64% [1, 2, 7, 11]. On the other hand, the 5-year survival of R1, R2 tumors is only 0–15%. It is clear that the operative procedure that can achieve a negative margin and R0 is necessary for a longer survival.

Lower Bile Duct Cancer

Background

Bile duct cancer varies in its manner of development with tumor localization, and the operative procedure must be adaptable to its localization. On the other hand, there have been few reports limited to lower bile duct cancer; so we reviewed reports that included middle, upper, and hilar bile duct cancer [11, 18–27]. The frequency of bile duct cancer among periampullary tumors is 5–10%, and the cases of lower bile duct cancer account for about 20% of the total bile duct cancer cases [19].

The standard surgical procedure for lower bile duct cancer is PD/PPPD. The reported resection, mortality, and morbidity rates are 43–91%, 0–5.2%, and 22–37.8%, respectively. Nagakawa et al. [11] reported that there were 3328 resected cases of bile duct cancer in Japan between 1987 and 1997, and that mortality after resection of middle or lower bile duct tumors was 2.1%. The 5-year survival rate of lower bile duct cancer is 26–40%, with a median survival time of 20.5–37.1 months (Table 75.4).

Prognostic factors

Pathological Factors Regarding the Tumor

Nodal status (N) [18–20, 22–27], stage [18, 24, 27], histology [18, 20, 24, 27], and depth of tumor are factors that will affect the prognosis (Table 75.5).

Nodal Status (N)

The frequency of N (+) lower bile duct tumors varies among reports, ranging from 39 to 71% [11, 19–22, 24–26]. The reported 5-year survival rates of N (+) and N (–) lower bile duct tumors are 0–50% and 30–65%, respectively [11, 19–26]. According to Nagakawa et al. [11], lymph nodes along the bile duct (no. 12) and posterior pancreaticoduodenal nodes (no. 13) had significantly higher metastatic rates than other lymph node sites. The para-aortic lymph node (no. 16) metastasis rate was 9.3%, and the 5-year survival rate of metastatic cases was 0%. The 5-year survival rate of metastatic cases of lymph nodes around the SMA (no. 14) was 11%.

Kayahara et al. reported a lymph node metastasis rate of 71% (25/36) in lower bile duct cancer [22]. The metastatic rate was 3% for 8, 22% for 12, 50% for 13a, 11% for 13b, 28% for 14, 8% for 16, 3% for 17a, and 0% for 17b. There are some reports that the lymph node metastasis number influences prognosis [25, 26, 28]. Yoshida et al. [26] reported that prognosis was significantly different with a metastasis number greater than three, while Hong et al. [28] reported that more than five metastasized lymph nodes significantly affected prognosis.

Kayahara et al. [22] reported that the frequency of lymph node metastasis increases with increasing tumor depth.

Stage

The 5-year survival rate of stage 1 lower bile duct cancer is 54–86%, and the results are relatively good. But the ratio of R0 tumors decreases with stage progression, and the 5-year survival of stage 4 cancer is reduced to 0–15% [11, 23, 24].

Multivariate Analysis

On the basis of multivariate regression analysis of the pathological factors, negative nodes [19, 20, 22, 27, 28], tumor differentiation [18, 20, 28], and stage [24] are significant independent pathological factors (Table 75.6).

Table 75.4. Mortality, morbidity, and survival associated with lower bile duct cancer. *BDR* Bile duct resection, *HBR* hilar bile duct resection

Author	Period	Year	No. of Patients	Resection (%)	Procedure	Mortality	Morbidity	Overall 5-year survival	Median survival time
Nagorney [18]	1976–1985	1993	39	22 (56.4%)	PD 21, TP 1	/	/	40.0%	24 months
Fong [19]	1983 –1993	1996	104	45 (43.3%)	PD 39, BDR 6	4.4%	37.8%	27.0%	32.9 months
Nakeeb [20]	1973–1995	1996	80	73 (91%)	PD 11, PPPD 62	0.0%	35.0%	28.0%	22 months
Kurosaki [21]	1981–1995	1998	24	24	PD 24				
Kayahara [22]	1973–1997	1999	50 (14 middle and 36 lower)	50	PD 43, BDR 7	2.0%	30.0%	35.0%	
Suzuki [23]	1960–1997	2000	99 (29 middle and 70 lower)	99	PD 74, PPPD 6, TP 1, BDR 18	3.0%	/	37.4% (excluding operative death)	
Todoroki [24]	1977–2000	2001	67 (middle and lower)	57 (85%)	PD 49, PPPD 1, TP 1, BDR 6	5.2%	/	39.1%	37.1 months
Sasaki [25]	1985–1988	2001	59 (33 middle and 26 lower)	59	PD 28, PPPD 28, BDR 3	/	/	33.6%	
Nagakawa [11]	1987–1997	2002	4833 (lower and hilar)	3328 (67%)		2.4% (2.1% middle or lower, 3.0% hilar or upper)	/	26% (lower-hilar)	/
Yoshida [26]	1995–1999	2002	27	27	PD 16, PPPD 11	3.7%	22.0%	37.0%	20.5 months
Jang [27]	1986–1997	2005	282 (lower and hilar)	151	HBR 23, BDR 25, PD 103	4.9% (PD)	32% (PD)	30.1% (PD)	

Table 75.5. Influence of nodal involvement (*N*), stage, and completeness of resection (*R*) on 5-year survival in lower bile duct cancer

			5-year survival		5-year survival						5-year survival				5-year survival	
Author	**N(+)**	**N(-)**	**N(+)**	**N(-)**	**Stage 1**	**Stage 2**	**Stage 3**	**Stage 4**	**Margin +**	**Margin -**	**Margin +**	**Margin -**	**R0**	**R1,2**	**R0**	**R1,2**
Nagorney [18]													56.0%			
Fong [19]	44.2%	55.8%	0.0%	54.0%					14.0%	86.0%						
Nakeeb [20]	52.0%	48.0%	/	30.0%					10.0%	90.0%		29.0%				
Kurosaki [21]	60.0%	40.0%	50.0%	64.0%					16.7%	83.3%	25.0%	63.0%				
Kayahara [22]	71% (lower)	29% (lower)	21.0%	65.0%					0% (lower)	100% (lower)			86% (lower)	14% (lower)		
Suzuki [23]					81.9%	57.1%	0.0%	0.0%					56.7%	43.3%	51.6%	22.9%, 7.8%
Todoroki [24]	67.3%	32.7%	41%, 9%	61.0%	86.0%	67.0%	49.0%	34%, 0%					45.6%	54.4%	63.0%	16%, 0%
Sasaki [25]	39.0%	61.0%	0.0%	53.0%												
Nagakawa [11]	40.0%	60.0%	17% (n1)	35.0%	54% (middle or lower)	33% (middle or lower)	20% (middle or lower)	15% (middle or lower)					55.6%	44.4%		
Yoshida [26]	58.0%	42.0%	20.0%	61.0%					15.4%	84.6%	0.0%	44.0%				

Table 75.6. Prognostic factors associated with lower bile duct cancer. *TNM* tumor-node-metastasis

Author	Prognostic factors Univariate analysis	Multivariate analysis
Nagorney [18]	Gross pathology, tumor grade, lymph node, stage, etc.	Curative resection, performance status, total bilirubin concentration, tumor grade
Fong [19]	Resection, lymph node	Lymph node
Nakeeb [20]	Resection, lymph node, poor tumor differentiation	Lymph node, poor tumor differentiation
Kurosaki [21]	Surgical margin	
Kayahara [22]	Depth of tumor, lymph node, surgical margin	Lymph node, surgical margin
Suzuki [23]	Duodenal invasion, depth of tumor, lymph node, surgical margin	/
Todoroki [24]	Sex, TNM, stage, histological grade, R	T, stage
Sasaki [25]	Lymph node, number of lymph nodes	
Yoshida [26]	Absence of lymph node metastasis, no more than two involved nodes, surgical margin	Up to two positive nodes, surgical margin, postoperative adjuvant chemotherapy
Jang [27]	Histology, lymph node, stage	Histology, lymph node

Factors of Resection – Operative Procedure and Lymph Node Dissection

PD/PPPD is the procedure of choice for lower bile duct cancer, and the frequency of the performance of PPPDs has been increasing. Based on the reported frequency of lymph node metastasis, posterior pancreaticoduodenal node (no. 13), anterior pancreaticoduodenal node (no. 17), common and proper hepatic artery (nos. 8, 12), hepatoduodenal ligament (no. 12), and the right side of the superior mesenteric artery (no. 14) were thought to be regional lymph nodes.

A negative surgical margin [22, 26] and curative resection [18] are significant independent factors affecting prognosis, as assessed by multivariate analysis. The percentage of negative surgical margins was reported to be 83.3–100%, with a 29–63% 5-year survival rate. In contrast, the 5-year survival rate of positive surgical margins was 0–25%. The percentage of achieving R0 was reported to be 45.6–86%, with 5-year survival of 51.6–63% [19–22]. The 5-year survival rate of R1, R2 has a poor range of 0–22.9%. Improved survival will depend on a surgical technique that can achieve negative surgical margins and R0.

References

1. Beger HG, Treitschke F, Gansauge F, Harada N, Hiki N, Mattfeldt T (1999) Tumor of the ampulla of Vater: experience with local or radical resection in 171 consecutively treated patients. Arch Surg 134:526–532
2. Beger HG, Thorab FC, Liu Z, Harada N, Rau BM (2004) Pathogenesis and treatment of neoplastic diseases of the papilla of Vater: Kausch-Whipple procedure with lymph node dissection in cancer of the papilla of Vater. J Hepatobiliary Pancreat Surg 11:232–238
3. Warren KW, Choe DS, Plaza J, Relihan M (1975) Results of radical resection for periampullary cancer. Ann Surg 181:534–540
4. Yamaguchi K, Enjoji M (1987) Carcinoma of the ampulla of Vater. A clinicopathologic study and pathologic staging of 109 cases of carcinoma and 5 cases of adenoma. Cancer 59:506–515
5. Monson JR, Donohue JH, McEntee GP, McIlrath DC, van Heerden JA, Shorter RG, Nagorney DM, Ilstrup DM (1991) Radical resection for carcinoma of the ampulla of Vater. Arch Surg 126: 353–357
6. Roder JD, Schneider PM, Stein HJ, Siewert JR (1995) Number of lymph node metastases is significantly associated with survival in patients with radically resected carcinoma of the ampulla of Vater. Br J Surg 82:1693–1696
7. Allema JH, Reinders ME, van Gulik TM, van Leeuwen DJ, Verbeek PC, de Wit LT, Gouma DJ (1995) Results of pancreaticoduodenectomy for ampullary carcinoma and analysis of prognostic factors for survival. Surgery 117:247–253
8. Talamini MA, Moesinger RC, Pitt HA, Sohn TA, Hruban RH, Lillemoe KD, Yeo CJ, Cameron JL (1997) Adenocarcinoma of the ampulla of Vater. A 28-year experience. Ann Surg 225:590–600
9. Howe JR, Klimstra DS, Moccia RD, Conlon KC, Brennan MF (1998) Factors predictive of survival in ampullary carcinoma. Ann Surg 228:87–94
10. Su CH, Shyr YM, Lui WY, P'eng FK (1999) Factors affecting morbidity, mortality and survival after pancreaticoduodenectomy for carcinoma of the ampulla of Vater. Hepatogastroenterology 46:1973–1979
11. Nagakawa T, Kayahara M, Ikeda S, Futakawa S, Kakita A, Kawarada H, Matsuno M, Takada T, Takasaki K, Tanimura H, Tashiro S, Yamaoka Y (2002) Biliary tract cancer treatment: results from the Biliary Tract Cancer Statistics Registry in Japan. J Hepatobiliary Pancreat Surg 9:569–575

12. Duffy JP, Hines OJ, Liu JH, Ko CY, Cortina G, Isacoff WH, Nguyen H, Leonardi M, Tompkins RK, Reber HA (2003) Improved survival for adenocarcinoma of the ampulla of Vater: fifty-five consecutive resections. Arch Surg 138:941–950
13. De Castro SM, Van Heek NT, Kuhlmann KF, Busch OR, Offerhaus GJ, Van Gulik TM, Obertop H, Gouma DJ (2004) Surgical management of neoplasms of the ampulla of Vater: Local resection or pancreatoduodenectomy and prognostic factors for survival. Surgery 136:994–1002
14. Brown KM, Tompkins AJ, Yong S, Aranha GV, Shoup M (2005) Pancreaticoduodenectomy is curative in the majority of patients with node-negative ampullary cancer. Arch Surg 140:529–523
15. Di Giorgio A, Alfieri S, Rotondi F, Prete F, Di Miceli D, Ridolfini MP, Rosa F, Covino M, Doglietto GB (2005) Pancreatoduodenectomy for tumors of Vater's ampulla: report on 94 consecutive patients. World J Surg 29:513–518
16. Posner S, Colletti L, Knol J, Mulholland M, Eckhauser F (2000) Safety and long-term efficacy of transduodenal excision for tumors of the ampulla of Vater. Surgery 128:694–701
17. Kimura W, Futakawa N, Zhao B (2004) Neoplastic diseases of the papilla of Vater. J Hepatobiliary Pancreat Surg 11:223–231
18. Nagorney DM, Donohue JH, Farnell MB, Schleck CD, Ilstrup DM (1993) Outcomes after curative resections of cholangiocarcinoma. Arch Surg 128:871–879
19. Fong Y, Blumgart LH, Lin E, Fortner JG, Brennan MF (1996) Outcome of treatment for distal bile duct cancer. Br J Surg 83:1712–1715
20. Nakeeb A, Pitt HA, Sohn TA, Coleman J, Abrams RA, Piantadosi S, Hruban RH, Lillemoe KD, Yeo CJ, Cameron JL (1996) Cholangiocarcinoma. A spectrum of intrahepatic, perihilar, and distal tumors. Ann Surg 224:463–465
21. Kurosaki I, Tsukada K, Watanabe H, Hatakeyama K (1998) Prognostic determinants in extrahepatic bile duct cancer. Hepatogastroenterology 45:905–909
22. Kayahara M, Nagakawa T, Ohta T, Kitagawa H, Tajima H, Miwa K (1999) Role of nodal involvement and the periductal soft-tissue margin in middle and distal bile duct cancer. Ann Surg 229:76–83
23. Suzuki M, Unno M, Oikawa M, Endo K, Katayose Y, Matsuno S (2000) Surgical treatment and postoperative outcomes for middle and lower bile duct carcinoma in Japan – experience of a single institute. Hepatogastroenterology 47:650–657
24. Todoroki T, Kawamoto T, Koike N, Fukao K, Shoda J, Takahashi H (2001) Treatment strategy for patients with middle and lower third bile duct cancer. Br J Surg 88:364–370
25. Sasaki R, Takahashi M, Funato O, Nitta H, Murakami M, Kawamura H, Suto T, Kanno S, Saito K (2001) Prognostic significance of lymph node involvement in middle and distal bile duct cancer. Surgery 129:677–683
26. Yoshida T, Matsumoto T, Sasaki A, Morii Y, Aramaki M, Kitano S (2002) Prognostic factors after pancreatoduodenectomy with extended lymphadenectomy for distal bile duct cancer. Arch Surg 137:69–73
27. Jang JY, Kim SW, Park do J, Ahn YJ, Yoon YS, Choi MG, Suh KS, Lee KU, Park YH (2005) Actual long-term outcome of extrahepatic bile duct cancer after surgical resection. Ann Surg 241:77–84
28. Hong SM, Cho H, Lee OJ, Ro JY (2005) The number of metastatic lymph nodes in extrahepatic bile duct carcinoma as a prognostic factor. Am J Surg Pathol 29:1177–1183

Cystic Neoplasia of the Pancreas

Chapter 76 Cystic Neoplasms of the Pancreas – Pathological Aspects *839*
T. Furukawa

Chapter 77 Clinical Diagnosis and Staging *843*
M. Tanaka

Chapter 78 Surgical Treatment of Cystic Tumors of the Pancreas *849*
T. Mori, N. Abe, M. Sugiyama, Y. Atomi

T. Furukawa

Cystic Neoplasms of the Pancreas – Pathological Aspects

Cystic neoplasms of the pancreas can be pathologically classified into the following groups: serous cystic neoplasms (SCNs), mucinous cystic neoplasms (MCNs), solid-pseudopapillary neoplasms (SPNs), intraductal papillary-mucinous neoplasms (IPMNs), and miscellaneous. Each group shows distinct clinicopathological features.

Serous Cystic Neoplasm

On gross examination, SCNs usually appear as single, round, well-circumscribed tumors involving the body and tail of the pancreas [1]. They are composed of multiple small cysts filled with serous fluid and have a honeycomb-like appearance on the cut surface (Fig. 76.1). Communication between the cysts and the pancreatic ductal system is usually not demonstrated [2]. Microscopically, the cysts are lined by cuboidal cells with clear cytoplasm that is rich in glycogen, and are positive for periodic acid Schiff staining, which is abolished by digestion with diastase [1]. The cells contain centrally located, small, round nuclei and show little cytological atypia, which leads to the diagnosis of serous cystadenoma. SCNs predominantly affect women of a relatively young age and reveal an invariably benign clinical course when treated by complete resection [1]. Malignant cases are extremely rare [3, 4]. Mutation of *KRAS2* is rarely observed [5, 6]. Associations of a mutation of *VHL*, a predisposing gene for the von Hipple-Lindau disease, with these neoplasms have been reported [7, 8].

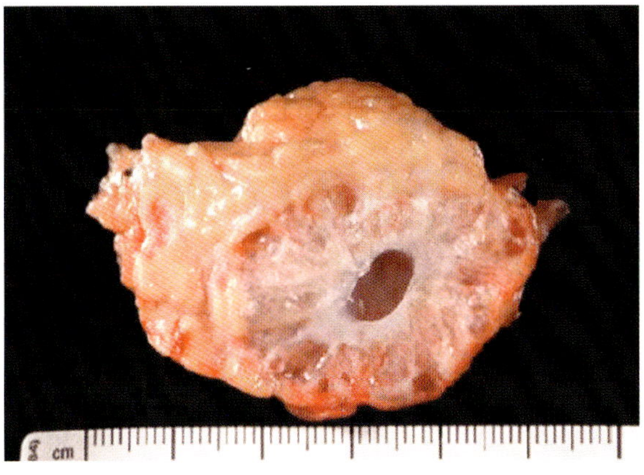

Figure 76.1

Cut surface of a serous cystic neoplasm. Note the multiple small cysts giving the appearance of a honeycomb

Mucinous Cystic Neoplasm

On gross examination, MCNs appear as large and single cysts, often oligocysts, filled with mucus. The cyst has a thick fibrous wall, which demarcates the cyst from surrounding pancreatic parenchyma (Fig. 76.2). MCNs usually involve the tail of the pancreas [9]. Communication between the cyst and the pancreatic ductal system is usually not demonstrated, which is one of the major features that distinguish it from IPMNs, which often show mucinous cystic lesions [10]. Microscopically, the cysts are lined with mucus-containing tall, columnar cells, often showing papillary projections and various degrees of cytological as well as architectural atypia. An ovarian-type stroma showing a thick layer of spindle-shaped cells is seen characteristically beneath the neoplastic epithelial cells, which has been defined as a necessary component for a diagnosis of mucinous cystic neoplasm [11]. The neoplasms are diagnosed as cystadenoma, cystic neoplasms with moderate dysplasia, and cystadenocarcinoma (noninvasive) according to the degree of atypia. Neoplasms accompanied by invasive components usually showing features of conventional ductal adenocarcinoma are diagnosed as invasive mucinous cystadenocarcinoma [12]. The neoplasms develop preferentially in middle-aged women. Malignant phenotypes are associated with older age [12]. The prognosis usually depends on the extent of invasion. Molecular alterations in *KRAS2*, *TP53*, or *SMAD4* are observed in some fractions of the neoplasms [6, 13].

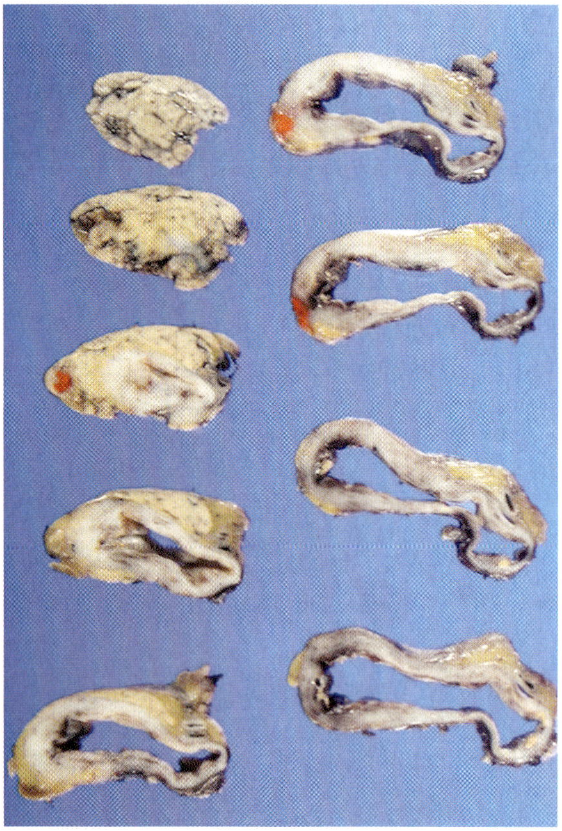

Figure 76.2

Gross serial sections of a mucinous cystic neoplasm. Note the unilocular cyst well demarcated by a thick fibrous capsule

Solid-Pseudopapillary Neoplasm

SPNs usually present as a large, solitary, and well-demarcated mass [14]. On gross examination they appear as solid tumors with hemorrhage and cystic degeneration on the cut surfaces, for which reason they are referred as solid and cystic tumors (Fig. 76.3). Microscopically, the neoplasms consist of cells with small and round nuclei and eosinophilic cytoplasm arranged in a pseudopapillary pattern along fibrovascular cores. Necrosis and hemorrhage are often seen, and are occasionally is extensive enough to involve the whole tumor [14]. Cholesterin clefts and foreign body giant cells are also often seen. They occur predominantly in young women (20–30 years of age), but may occasionally also be encountered in men [9]. They seldom cause symptoms and are usually found incidentally [9]. Patients are generally cured by complete resection of the tumor, which leads to an excellent prognosis [14]. A small fraction of patients have metastases at the time of diagnosis or later after removal of the primary tumors. Even if metastases have developed, many of them are amenable to resection, usually resulting in long-term survival of the affected patients [9]. Mutations of *CTNNB1/beta-catenin* are known to be associated with the neoplasms [15].

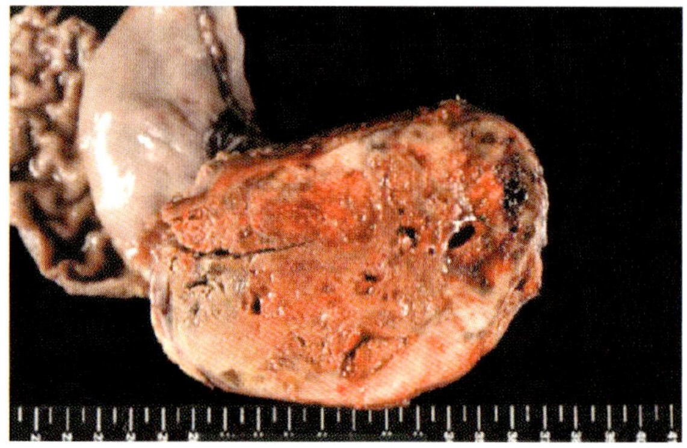

Figure 76.3

Cut surface of a solid-pseudopapillary neoplasm. Note the solid and cystic appearance

Intraductal Papillary-Mucinous Neoplasm

IPMNs show visible cystic dilated ducts filled with mucus on gross examination (Fig. 76.4) [16]. They may show small cysts involving a few branch ducts or large multicystic lesions involving the main duct and several connecting branches [16]. The former represents the branch duct-type and the latter the main duct type. Neoplasms of the main duct type harbor carcinoma more often than do those of the branch duct type [17]. Sometimes, the neoplasm presents as a large single cyst in the pancreas, resembling a mucinous cystic neoplasm. In this situation, communication with the ductal system and the lack of ovarian-type stroma can be important features for differential diagnosis [18]. The neoplasms occur in elderly men more frequently than in women [19]. Patients with neoplasms may have pancreatitis-like symptoms including abdominal pain, digestive insufficiency, and diabetes mellitus. These symptoms are associated with obstructive pancreatitis caused by the clogging of the ducts with mucus [20]. Microscopically, they are composed of tall columnar, mucin-producing, papillary epithelial cells that exhibit a spectrum of cytologic and architectural atypia [16]. According to the degree of atypia, IPMNs are diagnosed as adenoma, borderline, or noninvasive carcinoma [21]. They may show a variety of cell types: the gastric (null) type, the intestinal type, the pancreatobiliary type, or the on-

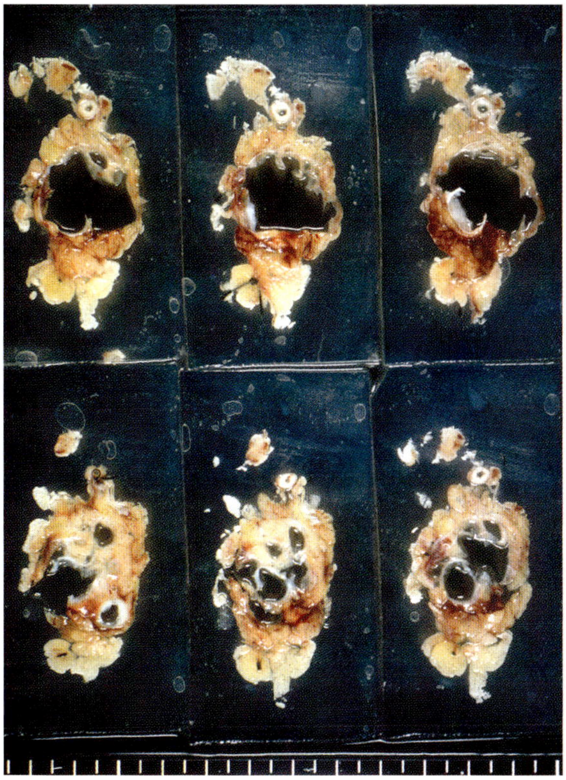

Figure 76.4

Gross serial sections of the intraductal papillary-mucinous neoplasm. Note the multiple cystic dilatations of the ducts

cocytic type [22, 23]. They may be accompanied by invasive components consisting of tubular adenocarcinoma or mucinous, colloid, noncystic carcinoma, which leads to a diagnosis of invasive adenocarcinoma associated with IPMN [24]. The prognosis depends on the presence of invasive carcinoma, which would lead to a poor prognosis [18]. Patients with noninvasive carcinomas usually have a fair prognosis after complete resection [20]. Mutations of *KRAS2* or *TP53* are occasionally observed [25, 26]. The expression of SMAD4 is usually retained regardless of the grade of atypia [27].

Miscellaneous

Mature Cystic Teratoma

Mature cystic teratomas are, on gross examination, unilocular or multilocular cysts filled with thick yellowish fluid. The cyst is lined with columnar cells or squamous epidermoid cells. They are referred to as dermoid cysts [28].

Acinar Cell Cystadenocarcinoma

Acinar cell cystadenocarcinomas appear as cystic neoplasms with acinar cellular features [29].

Pancreatoblastoma (Cystic Variant)

Pancreatoblastomas usually present as solid tumors on gross examination. Rarely, they present as cystic neoplasms, which are known to be associated with Beckwith-Wiedeman syndrome [30].

Metastatic Carcinoma

Metastatic carcinomas in the pancreas may exhibit cystic neoplasms. Common origins of the metastases are kidney, lung, breast, colon, and skin (melanoma) [31].

References

1. Capella C, Solcia E, Klöppel G, Hruban RH (2000) Serous cystic neoplasms of the pancreas. In: Aaltonen LA, Hamilton SR (eds) Pathology and Genetics of Tumours of the Digestive System. IARC Press, Oxford, pp 231–233
2. Fernandez-del Castillo C, Warshaw AL (2001) Cystic neo plasms of the pancreas. Pancreatology 1:641–647
3. Eriguchi N, Aoyagi S, Nakayama T, et al (1998) Serous cystadenocarcinoma of the pancreas with liver metastases. J Hepatobiliary Pancreat Surg 5:467–470
4. Strobel O, Z'Graggen K, Schmitz-Winnenthal FH, et al (2003) Risk of malignancy in serous cystic neoplasms of the pancreas. Digestion 68:24–33
5. Ishikawa T, Nakao A, Nomoto S, et al (1998) Immunohistochemical and molecular biological studies of serous cystadenoma of the pancreas. Pancreas 16:40–44
6. Kim SG, Wu TT, Lee JH, et al (2003) Comparison of epigenetic and genetic alterations in mucinous cystic neoplasm and serous microcystic adenoma of pancreas. Mod Pathol 16:1086–1094
7. Vortmeyer AO, Lubensky IA, Fogt F, Linehan WM, Khettry U, Zhuang Z (1997) Allelic deletion and mutation of the von Hippel-Lindau (VHL) tumor suppressor gene in pancreatic microcystic adenomas. Am J Pathol 151:951–956
8. Moore PS, Zamboni G, Brighenti A, et al (2001) Molecular characterization of pancreatic serous microcystic adenomas: evidence for a tumor suppressor gene on chromosome 10q. Am J Pathol 158:317–321
9. Klöppel G, Kosmahl M (2001) Cystic lesions and neoplasms of the pancreas. The features are becoming clearer. Pancreatology 1:648–655
10. Sarr MG, Murr M, Smyrk TC, et al (2003) Primary cystic neoplasms of the pancreas. Neoplastic disorders of emerging importance – current state-of-the-art and unanswered questions. J Gastrointest Surg 7:417–428

11. Klöppel G, Gibson JB, World Health Organization (1996) Histological Typing of Tumours of the Exocrine Pancreas, 2nd edn. Springer, Berlin, New York
12. Zamboni G, Klöppel G, Hruban RH, Longnecker DS, Adler G (2000) Mucinous cystic neoplasms of the pancreas. In: Aaltonen LA, Hamilton SR (eds) Pathology and Genetics of Tumours of the Digestive System. IARC Press, Oxford, pp 234–236
13. Gerdes B, Wild A, Wittenberg J, et al (2003) Tumor-suppressing pathways in cystic pancreatic tumors. Pancreas 26:42–48
14. Klöppel G, Lüttges J, Klimstra D, Hruban R, Kern S, Adler G (2000) Solid-pseudopapillary neoplasm. In: Aaltonen LA, Hamilton SR (eds) Pathology and Genetics of Tumours of the Digestive System. IARC Press, Oxford, pp 246–248
15. Tanaka Y, Kato K, Notohara K, et al (2001) Frequent beta-catenin mutation and cytoplasmic/nuclear accumulation in pancreatic solid-pseudopapillary neoplasm. Cancer Res 61:8401–404
16. Furukawa T, Takahashi T, Kobari M, Matsuno S (1992) The mucus-hypersecreting tumor of the pancreas. Development and extension visualized by three-dimensional computerized mapping. Cancer 70:1505–1513
17. Kobari M, Egawa S, Shibuya K, et al (1999) Intraductal papillary mucinous tumors of the pancreas comprise 2 clinical subtypes: differences in clinical characteristics and surgical management. Arch Surg 134:1131–1136
18. Suzuki Y, Atomi Y, Sugiyama M, et al (2004) Cystic neoplasm of the pancreas: a Japanese multiinstitutional study of intraductal papillary mucinous tumor and mucinous cystic tumor. Pancreas 28:241–246
19. Kimura W, Sasahira N, Yoshikawa T, Muto T, Makuuchi M (1996) Duct-ectatic type of mucin producing tumor of the pancreas – new concept of pancreatic neoplasia. Hepatogastroenterology 43:692–709
20. Tanaka M (2004) Intraductal papillary mucinous neoplasm of the pancreas: diagnosis and treatment. Pancreas 28:282–288
21. Longnecker DS, Adler G, Hruban RH, Klöppel G (2000) Intraductal papillary-mucinous neoplasms of the pancreas. In: Aaltonen LA, Hamilton SR (eds) Pathology and Genetics of Tumours of the Digestive System. IARC Press, Oxford, pp 237–240
22. Hruban RH, Takaori K, Klimstra DS, et al (2004) An Illustrated consensus on the classification of pancreatic intraepithelial neoplasia and intraductal papillary mucinous neoplasms. Am J Surg Pathol 28:977–987
23. Adsay NV, Merati K, Basturk O, et al (2004) Pathologically and biologically distinct types of epithelium in intraductal papillary mucinous neoplasms: delineation of an "intestinal" pathway of carcinogenesis in the pancreas. Am J Surg Pathol 28:839–848
24. Adsay NV, Conlon KC, Zee SY, Brennan MF, Klimstra DS (2002) Intraductal papillary-mucinous neoplasms of the pancreas: an analysis of in situ and invasive carcinomas in 28 patients. Cancer 94:62–77
25. Sessa F, Solcia E, Capella C, et al (1994) Intraductal papillary-mucinous tumours represent a distinct group of pancreatic neoplasms: an investigation of tumour cell differentiation and K-ras, p53 and c-erbB-2 abnormalities in 26 patients. Virchows Arch 425:357–367
26. Satoh K, Shimosegawa T, Moriizumi S, Koizumi M, Toyota T (1996) K-ras mutation and p53 protein accumulation in intraductal mucin-hypersecreting neoplasms of the pancreas. Pancreas 12:362–368
27. Iacobuzio-Donahue CA, Klimstra DS, Adsay NV, et al (2000) Dpc-4 protein is expressed in virtually all human intraductal papillary mucinous neoplasms of the pancreas: comparison with conventional ductal adenocarcinomas. Am J Pathol 157:755–761
28. Solcia E, Capella C, Klèoppel G, Armed Forces Institute of Pathology (U.S.), Universities Associated for Research and Education in Pathology (1997) Tumors of the Pancreas. Armed Forces Institute of Pathology, Washington, DC
29. Klimstra DS, Longnecker D (2000) Acinar cell carcinoma. In: Aaltonen LA, Hamilton SR (eds) Pathology and Genetics of Tumours of the Digestive System. IARC Press, Oxford, pp 241–243
30. Klöppel G, Longnecker D (2000) Pancreatoblastoma. In: Aaltonen LA, Hamilton SR (eds) Pathology and Genetics of Tumours of the Digestive System. IARC Press, Oxford, pp 244–245
31. Minni F, Casadei R, Perenze B, et al (2004) Pancreatic metastases: observations of three cases and review of the literature. Pancreatology 4:509–520

Chapter 77

M. Tanaka

Clinical Diagnosis and Staging

It is now well known that cystic tumors of the pancreas consist of two major entities, intraductal papillary mucinous neoplasms (IPMNs) and mucinous cystic neoplasms (MCNs), although serous cystadenomas, solid-pseudopapillary tumors, acinar cell carcinomas, and endocrine neoplasms may also take a cystic form due to their inherent nature and/or central necrosis [1]. IPMNs are characterized by an intraductal proliferation of mucinous cells usually forming a prominent papillary structure. IPMNs cause cystic dilatation of the main and/or branch pancreatic ducts due to profuse secretion of mucin. IPMNs are clinically classified into three types; main-duct type, branch-duct type, and combined type. Main-duct IPMNs are sometimes difficult to distinguish from chronic pancreatitis. If a branch-duct IPMN forms a multilocular spherical cyst in the tail of the pancreas, it may be reminiscent of an MCN.

In fact, branch-duct IPMNs and MCNs have several common characteristics that include formation of cystic masses with or without mural nodules and histological progression from adenoma to carcinoma, previously causing considerable confusion. The definition and classification proposed by the World Health Organization [2] and the Armed Forces Institute of Pathology [3] have contributed to better clarification of the distinction of these two entities. Appreciation of the similarities and distinguishing characteristics between IPMN and MCN is important, although clear distinction may still be impossible in some patients (Table 77.1). In the latter case, we still need an "indeterminate category of the cystic neoplasm of the pancreas" with imaging, and even histopathological features that do not enable us to make a distinctive diagnosis.

Clinical Diagnosis

Symptoms

MCNs are almost invariably diagnosed incidentally by imaging studies such as ultrasonography (US) and computed tomography (CT) taken for other purposes. Compression by a huge MCN may possibly cause dilatation of the main pancreatic duct, but the appearance of clinical symptoms is exceptional.

In IPMNs, obstruction of the main pancreatic duct with mucin may cause acute pancreatitis. Approximately one-quarter of patients with IPMNs present with symptoms such as epigastric pain, discomfort, and/or backache [4, 5]. Some patients have hyperamylasemia for many years [5, 6]. Long-standing occlusion of the main pancreatic duct may lead to pancreatic in-

Table 77.1. Characteristics that can be used to distinguish between mucinous cyst neoplasm (MCN) and branch-duct intraductal papillary mucinous neoplasm (IPMN)

Feature	MCN	Branch-duct IPMN
Age	erimenopausal	Elderly
Sex (% female)	>95%	–30%
Location (% head)	5%	>60%
Calcification	Rare	No
Common capsule	Yes	No
Gross macroscopic appearance	Orange-like	Grape-like
Internal structure	Cysts in cyst	Cyst by cyst
Communication with pancreatic duct	Infrequent	Yes
Main pancreatic duct	Normal or deviated	Normal or dilated

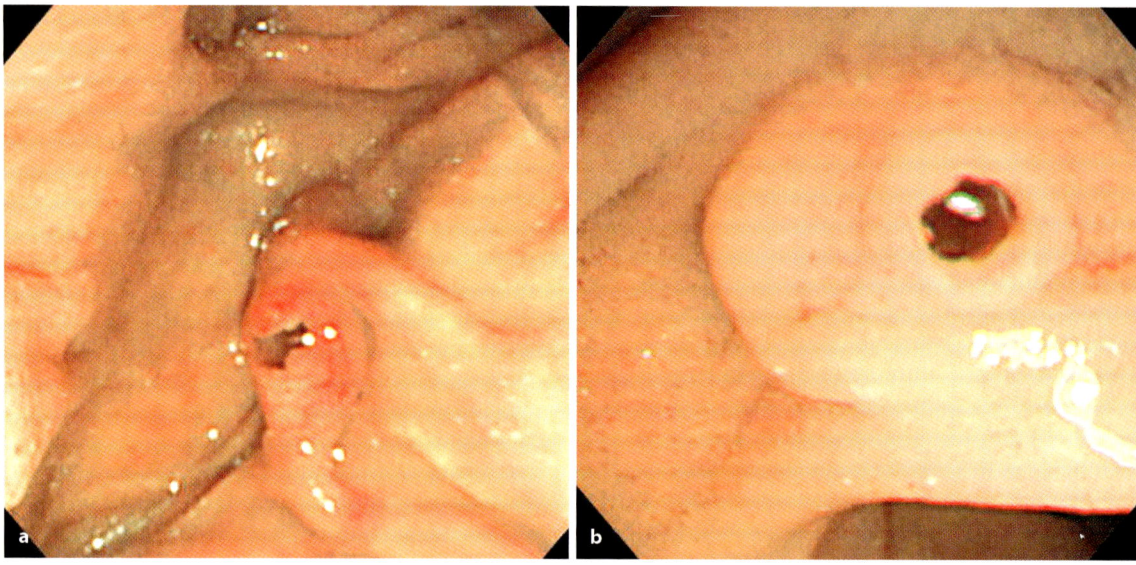

Figure 77.1

Patulous orifices of the major (a) and minor (b) duodenal papillae with profuse mucin extrusion

sufficiency presenting with diabetes, steatorrhea, or both. In advanced stages of IPMNs, jaundice may appear when mucin occludes the ampulla, when the IPMN compresses the common bile duct, or when the common bile duct or ampulla becomes involved by mural nodules frequently representing carcinoma.

Two-thirds of patients with IPMNs do not have any symptoms. Asymptomatic IPMNs are diagnosed by chance by imaging studies or endoscopy conducted for some other reason or at autopsy. Profuse secretion of mucin may dilate the ampulla. This finding in main-duct IPMNs originally drew our attention to this entity (Fig. 77.1a) [7–9]. This unique widening of the orifice is sometimes also observed at the minor papilla (Fig. 77.1b).

Imaging Studies

MCNs and IPMNs have several distinct characteristics shown by a variety of imaging studies (Table 77.1) [10, 11]. MCNs usually form a thick-walled, orange-like cystic lesion in the pancreatic tail of perimenopausal women, having no communication with the pancreatic ducts [12, 13]. In contrast, IPMNs are more frequently found in the pancreatic head of elderly men. The collective review of 259 patients with IPMN of the pancreas reported by Kimura et al. [14] showed distinct male preponderance (M:F = 2.2) and a mean age of 65.5 years (range 30–94 years). Yamaguchi and Tanaka [1] also reported a similar age and sex distribution.

Magnetic resonance cholangiopancreatography is the best method with which to visualize the entire outline of both MCNs and IPMNs (Fig. 77.2a, b). US, endoscopic ultrasonography (EUS), and CT show one or more cystic dilatations of pancreatic duct branches (branch-duct IPMN), segmental or diffuse dilatation of the main pancreatic duct (main-duct IPMN), or a multilocular thick-walled spherical mass with or without mural nodules in the pancreas (MCN) [5, 11, 15–17]. Endoscopic retrograde cholangiopancreatography (ERCP) may demonstrate deviation of the main pancreatic duct, if any, caused by compression by an MCN, but the presence of communication between the pancreatic duct and MCN is exceptional (Fig. 77.3a). In contrast, in patients with IPMN, ERCP shows dilatation of the main pancreatic duct (main-duct IPMN) or branches (branch-duct IPMN) frequently with filling defects due to the presence of either mural nodules or mucin (Fig. 77.3b) [11].

Communication between branch-duct IPMNs and the main pancreatic duct is usually present, being evident in 85% of 53 patients in our previously reported series, although not always demonstrable by ERCP due to the presence of viscid mucin filling the cyst and communication [1]. Such communication with the pancreatic duct is usually absent in patients with MCN, but is rarely reported to be present when contrast medium is injected under pressure [11]. This type of communication is likely to be rather a sort of fistula formed between the cystic lesion and the pancreatic duct than a real connection.

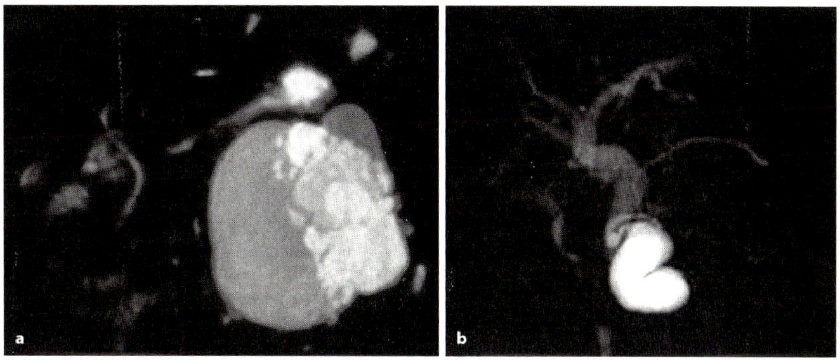

Figure 77.2

Magnetic resonance cholangiopancreatography (MRCP) showing a mucinous cystic neoplasm (MCN; a) and a branch-duct intraductal papillary mucinous neoplasm (IPMN; b)

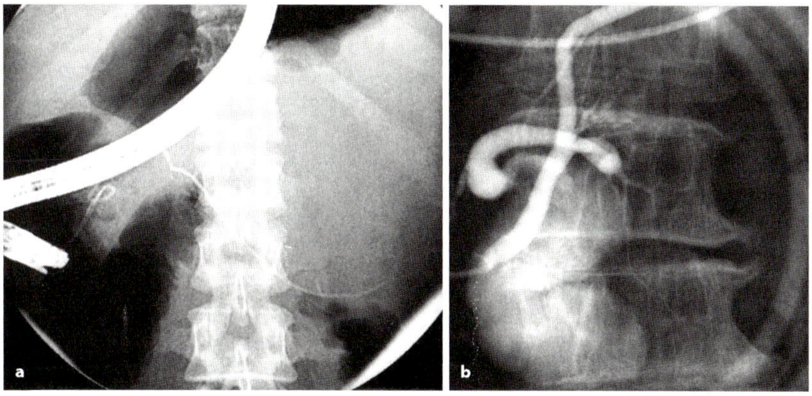

Figure 77.3

Endoscopic retrograde pancreatograms demonstrating deviation of the main pancreatic duct caused by a huge MCN (a) and a branch-duct IPMN communicating with the main pancreatic duct (b)

Clinical Diagnosis of Malignancy

For the preoperative diagnosis of malignancy associated with IPMN or MCN, serum levels of carcinoembryonic antigen (CEA) and CA19-9 may sometimes be elevated and helpful to indicate the presence of malignancy. Pancreatic juice may also show high levels of CEA and CA19-9 [18].

Most branch-duct IPMNs are benign, while the main-duct type is frequently malignant. Thus, the presence of main-duct IPMN per se often indicates malignancy. The combined type is generally similar to main-duct IPMN rather than branch-duct IPMN. The existence of large mural nodules increases the possibility of malignancy in both branch-duct and main-duct IPMNs, and also in MCNs. Yamaguchi et al. [4] reported that marked dilatation of >1 cm of the main pancreatic duct and the presence of mural nodules of >1 cm are highly suggestive of malignancy in patients with IPMNs.

The main duct is generally larger in patients with malignant IPMNs than in those with benign IPMNs due to more profuse secretion of mucin, and therefore a dilated main duct is a simple and reliable indicator of malignancy [19, 20]. The presence or absence of mural nodules and extent of the involvement are best confirmed by EUS. Intraductal ultrasonography (IDUS) provides high-quality images within a short distance and appears to be useful to demonstrate mural nodules, especially in main-duct IPMN [21]. However, differentiation between mucin plugs and mural nodules sometimes remains difficult. Peroral pancreatoscopy may reveal a fish-egg-like appearance of IPMN in the main pancreatic duct and be helpful in distinguishing mural nodules from mucin.

Cytology of pancreatic juice aspirates from the main pancreatic duct during ERCP sometimes confirms the diagnosis when positive for malignant cells, although the rate of positive cytology in those with malignant IPMNs is less than 50% [22, 23]. Extrapancreatic invasion and resectability of invasive malignant IPMN and MCN is best determined by contrast-enhanced CT.

Synchronous or metachronous malignancy may develop in various organs including the pancreas in IPMNs but not in MCNs. The rate of association of IPMN with extrapancreatic malignant neoplasms was reported to range from 23.6% to 32% [1, 24, 25]. Yamaguchi et al. [1] found extrapancreatic malignancies in 18 out of 56 patients (32%) with surgically resected IPMNs. Sugiyama et al. [24] also reported that 15 out of 42 patients (32%) with benign and malignant IPMNs had synchronous or metachronous colorectal, gastric, or bile duct cancer. Osanai et al. [25] reported that 35 out of 148 patients (23.6%) with IPMNs had malignancies of the colon, stomach, or lung.

The high prevalence of pancreatic cancer independent of IPMN in patients with branch-duct IPMN is worthy of note. We previously reported that 7 out of 76 patients (9.2%) with resected IPMN had synchronous and/or metachronous pancreatic cancer [26]. In particular, the presence of IPMN led to the diagnosis of concomitant pancreatic cancer in four of the seven patients. Of particular interest is the fact that two of the patients were diagnosed as having carcinoma in situ (CIS) [27] and another minimally invasive carcinoma. All of the branch-duct IPMNs associated with pancreatic carcinoma in this series were adenomas with mild dysplasia. Nakaizumi et al. [28] also reported the same combination of branch-duct IPMN and pancreatic carcinoma in five patients.

Clinical Staging

Prognosis is excellent after complete resection of benign and noninvasive malignant IPMN and MCN [29–32]. Since only ~40% of malignant IPMNs are invasive [33], ~80% of patients with malignant IPMN survive for more than 5 years overall [13]. Even for invasive malignant IPMN, the prognosis is relatively good compared to pancreatic cancer. The 3-year survival rate for 10 patients with invasive malignant IPMN was 48% after curative resection in our series [1]. Nonetheless, incomplete and/or inadequate resection may lead to recurrence. In addition, the prognosis of invasive malignant IPMN depends on its histological type and the extent of invasion and metastasis [34].

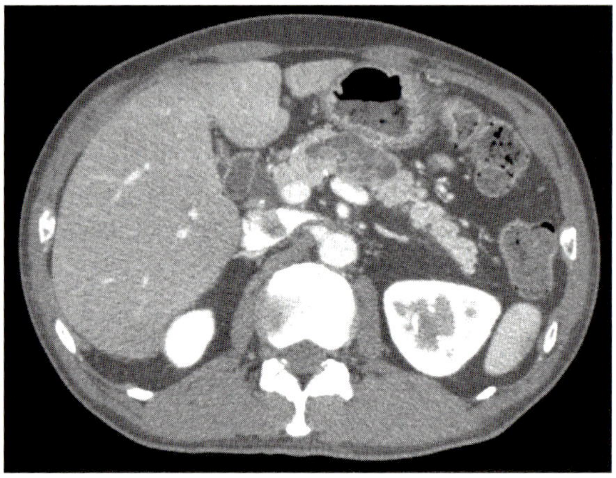

Figure 77.4

Computed tomogram clearly showing the presence of invasive carcinoma derived from a main-duct IPMN. A mass consisting of mural nodules and parenchymal invasion extends to the retropancreatic tissue and splenic vein

Clinical staging and determination of the extent of involvement are therefore of paramount importance in the management of malignant IPMN and MCN. Carcinoma derived from IPMN or MCN is classified into three stages: (1) CIS, (2) minimally invasive carcinoma, and (3) invasive carcinoma. The Japan Pancreas Society (JPS) defined noninvasive intraductal papillary mucinous carcinoma (IPMC) as carcinoma limited to the pancreatic duct, and minimally invasive IPMC as having invaded slightly beyond the ductal wall [35]. However, it is impossible to preoperatively diagnose CIS by any diagnostic imaging modality, although pancreatic juice cytology may incidentally prove positive and suggest the presence of carcinoma.

Current interests are concentrating on the possibility of preoperative diagnosis of minimally invasive carcinoma derived from IPMN. However, it is currently practically impossible to diagnose the minimally invasive IPMC or mucinous cystadenocarcinoma preoperatively even by EUS or IDUS, if the minimal invasion is defined as microscopic invasion to the pancreatic parenchyma [36]. A more sophisticated high-resolution imaging modality needs to be developed for this purpose.

On the other hand, invasive carcinoma derived from IPMN and MCN is relatively easy to diagnose by CT, magnetic resonance imaging, and EUS (Fig. 77.4).

When IPMN is large enough to cause compression to the main pancreatic duct or common bile duct, obstructive pancreatitis or jaundice, respectively, may result. Furthermore, IPMN may produce fistulae into the stomach, duodenum, colon, or common bile duct depending on the site of the involvement. These phenomena are mostly a sign of invasive malignancy. When IPMN is associated with far-advanced invasive carcinoma, the presence of the IPMN may be obscure on gross appearance. Malignant IPMN would acquire aggressive behavior similar to pancreatic carcinoma once it has invaded the pancreatic parenchyma [37].

References

1. Yamaguchi K, Tanaka M (2000) Atlas of Cystic Neoplasms of the Pancreas. Kyushu University Press/Kager, Fukuoka, Japan
2. Kloeppel G, Solcia E, Longnecker DS, Capella C, Sobin LH (1996) World Health Organization International Histological Classification of Tumours. Histological typing of tumours of the exocrine pancreas, 2nd edn. Springer-Verlag, Berlin, pp 1–61
3. Solcia E, Capella C, Kloeppel G (1997) Tumors of the exocrine pancreas. In: Rosai J (ed) Atlas of Tumor Pathology. Fascicle 20, 3rd Series. Armed Forces Institute of Pathology, Washington DC, pp 31–41
4. Yamaguchi K, Ogawa Y, Chijiiwa K, Tanaka M (1996) Mucin-hypersecreting tumors of the pancreas: assessing the grade of malignancy preoperatively. Am J Surg 171:427–431
5. Obara T, Maguchi H, Saitoh Y, Ura H, Koike Y, Kitazawa S, Namiki M (1991) Mucin-producing tumor of the pancreas: a unique clinical entity. Am J Gastroenterol 86:1619–1625
6. Rogers PN, Seywright MM, Murray WR (1987) Diffuse villous adenoma of the pancreatic duct. Pancreas 2:727–730
7. Ohhashi K, Murakami F, Maruyama M (1982) Four cases of mucous secreting pancreatic cancer. Progr Dig Endosc 203:348–351 (in Japanese with English abstract)
8. Yamaguchi K, Tanaka M (1991) Mucin-hypersecreting tumor of the pancreas with mucin extrusion through enlarged papilla. Am J Gastroenterol 86:835–839
9. Yamao K, Nakazawa S, Naito Y, Kimoto E, Morita K, Inui K, Ohnuma T, Funakawa T, Hayashi Y (1986) Clinicopathological sutyd of mucus-producing pancreatic tumors. Jpn J Gastroenterol 83:2588–2597
10. Kimura W (2003) IHPBA in Tokyo, 2002: Surgical treatment of IPMT vs MCT: a Japanese experience. J Hepatobiliary Pancreat Surg 10:156–162
11. Yamao K, Nakamura T, Suzuki T, Sawaki A, Hara K, Kato T, Okubo K, Matsumoto K, Shimizu Y (2003) Endoscopic diagnosis and staging of mucinous cystic neoplasms and intraductal papillary-mucinous tumors. J Hepatobiliary Pancreat Surg 10:142–146
12. Sugiyama M, Atomi Y, Kuroda A (1997) Two types of mucin-producing cystic tumors of the pancreas: diagnosis and treatment. Surgery 122:617–625
13. Cross MR (1980) Mucinous cystadenoma of the pancreas. Endoscopy as an aid to diagnosis. Gastroenterology 78:944–947
14. Kimura W, Sasahira N, Yoshikawa T, Muto T, Makuuchi M (1996) Duct-ectatic type of mucin producing tumor of the pancreas – new concept of pancreatic neoplasia. Hepatogastroenterology 43:692–709
15. Itai Y, Kokubo T, Atomi Y (1987) Mucin-hypersecreting carcinoma of the pancreas. Radiology 165:51–55
16. Sahani D, Prasad S, Saini S, Mueller P (2002) Cystic pancreatic neoplasms evaluation by CT and magnetic resonance cholangiopancreatography. Gastrointest Endosc Clin N Am 12:657–672
17. Itai Y, Minami M (2001) Intraductal papillary-mucinous tumor and mucinous cystic neoplasm: CT and MR findings. Int J Gastrointest Cancer 30:47–63
18. Bastid C, Bernard JP, Sarles H, Payan MJ, Sahel J (1991) Mucinous ductal ectasia of the pancreas: a premalignant disease and a cause of obstructive pancreatitis. Pancreas 6:15–22
19. Yamaguchi K, Chijiiwa K, Shimizu S, Yokohata K, Morisaki T, Yonemasu H, Tanaka M (1999) Intraductal papillary neoplasm of the pancreas: a clinical review of 13 benign and four malignant tumors. Eur J Surg 165:223–229
20. Yamaguchi K, Sugitani, Chijiiwa K, Tanaka M (2001) Intraductal papillary-mucinous tumor of the pancreas: assessing the grade of malignancy from natural history. Am Surg 67:400–406
21. Taki T, Goto H, Naitoh Y, Hirooka Y, Furukawa T, Hayakawa T (1997) Diagnosis of mucin-producing tumor of the pancreas with an intraductal ultrasonographic system. J Ultrasound Med 16:1–6
22. Rogers PN, Seywright MM, Murray WR (1987) Diffuse villous adenoma of the pancreatic duct. Pancreas 2:727–730
23. Ito Y, Blackstone MO, Frank PH, Skinner DB (1977) Mucinous biliary obstruction associated with a cystic adenocarcinoma of the pancreas. Gastroenterology 73:1410–1412
24. Sugiyama M, Atomi Y (1999) Extrapancreatic neoplasms occur with unusual frequency in patients with intraductal papillary mucinous tumors of the pancreas. Am J Gastroenterol 94:470–473
25. Osanai M, Tannno S, Nakano Y, Koizumi K, Habiro A, Kohgo Y (2003) Extrapancreatic neoplasms in patients with intraductal papillary mucinous tumors of the pancreas: analysis in surgical and follow-up series. J Jpn Pancreas Soc 18:565–569 (in Japanese with English abstract)
26. Yamaguchi K, Ohuchida J, Ohtsuka T, Nakano K, Tanaka M (2002) Intraductal papillary-mucinous tumor of the pancreas concomitant with ductal carcinoma of the pancreas. Pancreatology 2:484–490
27. Yamaguchi K, Nakamura K, Yokohata K, Shimizu S, Chijiiwa K, Tanaka M (1997) Pancreatic cyst as a sentinel of in situ carcinoma of the pancreas: report of two cases. Int J Pancreatol 22:227–231
28. Nakaizumi A, Tanaka S, Oshikawa O, Takakura R, Ioka T, Mitani K, Higashino A, Uehara H, Iiishi H, Yokoyama S, Ohigashi H, Ishikawa O, Takenaka A, Kasugai T, Tatsuta M (2002) Synchronous and metachronous occurrence of branch type IPMT and invasive ductal carcinoma of the pancreas. Tan to Sui (Biliary Tract and Pancreas) 23:1013–1019 (in Japanese)
29. Rickaert F, Cremer M, Deviere J, Tavares L, Lambiolliotte JP, Schroeder S, Wurbs D, Kloeppel G (1991) Intraductal mucin-hypersecreting neoplasms of the pancreas. Gastroenterology 101:512–519
30. Warshaw AL, Compton CC, Lewandrowski K, Cardenosa G, Mueller PR (1990) Cystic tumors of the pancreas: new clinical, radiologic, and pathologic observations in 67 patients. Ann Surg 212:432–445

31. Morohoshi T, Kanada M, Asanuma M, Kloeppel G (1989) Intraductal papillary neoplasms of the pancreas. A clinico-pathologic study of six patients. Cancer 64:1329–1335
32. Loftus ED Jr, Olivares-Pakad BA, Batts KP, Adkins MC, Stephens DH, Sarr MG, DiMagno EP (1996) Intraductal papillary-mucinous tumors of the pancreas: Clinicopathologic features, outcome, and nomenclature. Gastroenterology 110:1909–1918
33. Kimura W, Sasahira N, Yoshikawa T, Muto T, Makuuchi M (1996) Duct-ectatic type of mucin producing tumor of the pancreas – new concept of pancreatic neoplasia. Hepatogastroenterology 43:692–709
34. Sessa F, Solcia E, Capella C, Bonato M, Scarpa A, Zamboni G, Pellegata NS, Ranzani GN, Rickaert F, Kloeppel G (1994) Intraductal papillary-mucinous tumours represent a distinct group of pancreatic neoplasms: an investigation of tumour cell differentiation and K-ras, p53 and c-erbB2 abnormalities in 26 patients. Virchows Arch Pathol Anat 425:357–367
35. Japan Pancreas Society (2003) Classification of Pancreatic Carcinoma, Second English edition, Kanehara, Tokyo
36. Yamao K, Ohashi K, Nakamura T, Suzuki T, Watanabe Y, Shimizu Y, Nakamura Y, Ozden I (2001) Evaluation of various imaging methods in the differential diagnosis of intraductal papillary-mucinous tumor (IPMT) of the pancreas. Hepatogastroenterology 48:962–966
37. Seki M, Yanagisawa A, Ohta H, Ninomiya Y, Sakamoto Y, Yamamoto J, Yamaguchi T, Ninomiya E, Takano K, Aruga A, Yamada K, Sasaki K, Kato Y (2003) Surgical treatment of intraductal papillary-mucinous tumor (IPMT) of the pancreas: operative indications based on surgico-pathologic study focusing on invasive carcinoma derived from IPMT. J Hepatobiliary Pancreat Surg 10:147–155

Chapter 78

T. Mori · N. Abe · M. Sugiyama · Y. Atomi

Surgical Treatment of Cystic Tumors of the Pancreas

Cystic tumors and tumor-like lesions of the pancreas are rare, but have attracted a great deal of attention because they are easily recognized with modern imaging methods and, in contrast to ductal adenocarcinoma, they can potentially be cured surgically. The increasing resection rate of these tumors in recent years has also enhanced our understanding of cystic pancreatic tumors by conspicuously enlarging their morphological spectrum. Known entities have been better characterized (i.e., solid pseudopapillary neoplasm) [1], intraductal papillary mucinous neoplasm [2, 3], and new ones have been described (i.e., serous oligocystic adenoma, mucinous nonneoplastic cyst, acinar cell cystadenoma, and cystic hamartoma) [4]. This chapter discusses the most important cystic tumors with regard to their nature, indication, and outcome of the surgical treatment.

Cystic Lesion of the Pancreas

Cystic lesions in the pancreas come in a variety of pathologies (Table 78.1). For decades, it has been clear that correctly differentiating between a cystic neoplasm and a pseudocyst is vital to avoid incorrect treatment. More recently, as the divergent natural histories and malignant potentials of different cystic neoplasms have been elucidated, it has become increasingly important to be able to differentiate between mucinous cystic tumors (MCTs), intraductal papillary mucinous neoplasms (IPMNs), serous cystadenomas (SCAs), and other less common tumors [5–8]. As opposed to pancreatic pseudocysts, neoplastic cystic tumors have an epithelial lining. The epithelium of IPMNs and MCTs consists of columnar, mucin-producing epithelium. However, MCTs, which occur almost exclusively in women, are devoid of communication with the ductal system and are supported by ovarian-type stroma, whereas IPMNs arise in the main pancreatic duct or its major branches. The copious amount of mucin produced by IPMNs results in a hugely dilated and frequently mucus-filled main pancreatic duct, whereas the main pancreatic duct in MCTs is basically normal. Imaging studies reflect the morphologic characteristics of these neoplasms.

Table 78.1. Clinical features of intraductal papillary mucinous neoplasms (IPMNs) and mucinous cystic tumors (MCTs)

Congenital true cysts
Single cysts
Polycystic disease of the pancreas without related anomalies
Pancreatic macrocysts associated with cystic fibrosis
Pancreatic cysts associated with cerebellar tumors and retinal angiomas (von Hippel-Lindau's disease)
Pancreatic cysts associated with polycystic disease of the kidneys (Potter type I or II)
Enterogenous cysts
Dermoid cysts
Acquired cysts
Pseudocysts, in association with either acute or chronic pancreatitis
Parasitic cysts (Echinococcus, Taenia solium)
Retention cysts
Mucinous nonneoplastic cyst
Angiomatous cysts
Simple or proliferative cysts
Proliferative cysts (cystic neoplasms)
Serous cystadenoma or adenocarcinoma
Mucinous cystadenoma or adenocarcinoma
IPMNs
Solid pseudopapillary neoplasms
Acinar cell cystadenoma
Cystic hamartoma
Ductal adenocarcinoma with cystic necrosis
Teratomatous cysts
Cystic choriocarcinoma
Neuroendocrine cystic tumors of the pancreas

MCT of the Pancreas

General Considerations

In 1978, Compagno and Oertel differentiated MCTs from serous cystic tumors (SCTs) [5, 6] because the former was of overt or latent malignancy and the latter was almost perfectly benign. In their series of 41 cases, all of the MCTs were considered potentially or obviously malignant based on the following observations: (1) recurrence of mucinous cystadenoma as cystadenocarcinoma after an incomplete resection or internal drainage, and (2) histopathological concomitance of a benign columnar epithelium and severe dysplasia or obvious invasive carcinoma. Consequently, they introduced the term "mucinous cystic neoplasm with overt or latent malignancy" for all MCTs. This implies that all MCTs, regardless of their individual morphologic features, fall into one group without any further differentiation and should be resected surgically. However, some small MCTs that are found incidentally at radiological examination, surgery, or autopsy show no evidence of severe dysplasia even after a complete histological workup. Although the basic concept that even the benign-looking tumors of this category have the potential to transform into carcinoma cannot be denied, some mucinous cystadenomas with a perfectly benign nature are certainly considered to exist. At present, it is impossible to differentiate between mucinous cystadenoma of such a perfectly benign nature and those of malignant potential [7, 8].

MCTs of the pancreas are classified according to their grade of dysplasia and represent a spectrum of lesions that include mucinous cystadenoma, MCT of borderline malignant potential, and mucinous cystadenocarcinoma. This separation follows the idea of mucinous cystic neoplasms of the ovary, which closely resemble MCTs of the pancreas with regard to both biological behavior and cell lineage differentiation. Thomson et al. from the Armed Forces Institute of Pathology (AFIP) proposed the use of the term of mucinous cystadenocarcinoma [9] of low-grade malignant potential for all mucinous cystic neoplasms of the pancreas irrespective of the histological appearance of the epithelial component and with or without stromal invasion. This was based on the experiences that MCTs of the pancreas cannot be reliably and reproducibly separated into benign, borderline, and malignant categories.

It is also important to note that the close resemblance of the MCTs of the pancreas to hepatobiliary cystadenomas and cystadenocarcinomas with mesenchymal stroma of the hepatobiliary duct [10] and retroperitoneal counterparts, with regard to both their morphology and biology [11, 12]. MCTs are almost exclusively found in women. In addition, both pancreatic and hepatobiliary MCTs usually have an ovarian-type stroma, which makes them comparable to ovarian MCTs. It therefore seems that tumors of this type, regardless of the different organs of origin (i.e., ovary, pancreas, liver or retroperitoneum) may have a common cellular origin that is determined by gender and is characterized by differentiation toward gastroenteropancreatic cells.

From the discussion above, MCT of the pancreas is defined as a large multicystic tumor lined by mucus-secreting epithelial cells, showing gastroenteropancreatic differentiation and subtended by an "ovarian-type stroma." It develops almost exclusively in the body or tail of the pancreas in middle-aged women. According to the degree of epithelial dysplasia, the tumor is classified into adenoma, borderline tumor, and adenocarcinoma.

Clinicopathologic Features of MCTs

MCTs are uncommon variations of pancreatic neoplasms, representing from 2 to 5.7% of all exocrine pancreatic tumors. The biological behavior of invasive mucinous cystadenocarcinoma resembles that of ductal adenocarcinoma. Local spread is often detected in the interstitial tissue, perineural sheaths, vascular and lymphatic channels, and peripancreatic fatty tissue. As MCTs are commonly located in the body and tail of the pancreas, direct invasion of the adjacent organs are seen in the stomach, duodenum, spleen, left adrenal gland, left kidney, and colon. Metastases to the regional peripancreatic lymph nodes are common in cyst adenocarcinoma, and distant metastasis may be first detected in the liver or bone. The incidence of mucinous cystadenocarcinoma is about 50% [13] or less than one half of MCTs of the pancreas [14]. In Thompson's current review of 130 patients with MCTs of the pancreas, the definition included an ovarian-type stroma and the patients were all women [9]. In a current Japanese multi-institutional study, 171 patients with MCTs were all women (Table 78.1) [14]. MCTs can develop in all races [5, 15]. The etiology of the tumor remains unknown, but the predominance in women and presence of ovarian-type stroma suggest that some genetic or hormonal factors are involved in its pathogenesis. Smoking and alcohol abuse do not seem to play a significant role [9]. Albores-Saavedra et al. postulated that the tumors originate from "endodermal stem cells" that differentiate into cells with an intestinal phenotype, from their ultrastructural and immunohistochemical observations [16].

Patients with MCTs may present symptoms (43.6%, Table 78.1), including upper abdominal pain and discomfort, pancreatitis, weight loss, and weakness. Symptoms can usually be attributable to direct compression of adjacent organs and the clinical presentation depends on the size of the tumor. Jaundice due to obstruction of the common bile duct is unusual even in those tumors located in the head of the pancreas. In Thompson's series, gallbladder disease was seen in 12.3% and diabetes mellitus (postoperative diabetes was excluded) were evident in 3.8% [9].

Macroscopic Findings

More than 70% of the MCTs affect the body or tail of the pancreas [6, 14]. Small MCTs are usually located in the peripheral portion of the pancreas. The tumors are usually solitary, with a diameter of 2–35 cm in its greatest dimension. In a multi-institutional study from Japan, the mean diameter of benign tumors measured 53.5 mm, whereas that of adenocarcinoma was significantly larger at 71.8 mm. In Thompson's series, a cut-off of 15 cm was used and larger tumors tended to have a worse clinical outcome. The mean age of patients with benign tumors was 52 years (range 19–80 years), whereas that of adenocarcinoma was significantly higher at 61 years (range 61–85 years) [14]. Other concomitant neoplasms may be seen in patients with MCTs, 12% of which will be benign tumors and 9.4% malignant ones (Table 78.2). Elevation of serum tumor markers such as CEA or CA19-9 suggests the presence of cystadenocarcinoma [15].

On cut sections, the tumor is a multilocular cyst consisting of large cysts separated by fibrous septa (Figs. 78.1 and 78.2). Some peripheral small cysts are seen in the capsule. The inner surface is smooth in benign tumors, while sometimes, especially in large and malignant tumors, macroscopic papillary excrescences, solid nodules, or protuberances can be seen (Fig. 78.2). In some tumors, the contents of the cyst are hemorrhagic or necrotic. The tumor capsule may contain small focal areas of calcification (peripheral calcification) or ossification. It may adhere to the adjacent organs by inflammation, or may directly invade the pancreatic parenchyma or further the adjacent organs. A mucinous fistula formation into the duodenum, stomach, bile duct, or colon has been described [17]. Communication between the cyst and the pancreatic duct system is uncommon. Rarely, a tumor may be found attached to the pancreas by only a narrow tissue stalk, or retroperitoneal or intrasplenic MCTs may arise from the heterotopic pancreatic tissue [18].

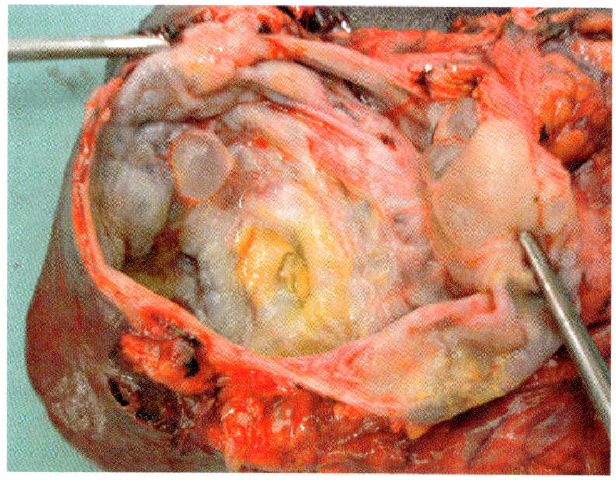

Figure 78.1

Surgical specimen of mucinous cystic tumors (MCTs, adenoma). Note a multilocular cyst consisting of large cysts separated by fibrous septa. Some peripheral small cysts are seen in the capsule

Table 78.2. Clinicopathologic features of benign tumors and adenocarcinoma in surgical cases of MCTs. *NS* Not significant

	Benign tumor n=118	Adenocarcinoma n=53	p value
Age (years; mean±SD)	52±16	61±16	<0.0001
Range	19–80	61–85	
Symptoms (%)	43 (36.4)	30 (56.6)	0.0195
Other pancreatic disorders (%)	17 (14.4)	14 (26.4)	0.0133
Other malignant neoplasms (%)	12 (10.2)	5 (9.4)	NS
Enlarged orifice of the papilla (%)	4 (3.4)	4 (7.5)	NS
Mural nodule (%)	20 (16.9)	28 (52.8)	<0.0001
Size (mm; mean±SD)	13.2±12.9	28.2±26.3	NS
Cyst diameter (mm, mean±SD)	53.5±38.0	71.8±50.1	<0.0001
Main pancreatic duct diameter (mm, mean±SD)	6.7±2.1	12.7±10.9	NS

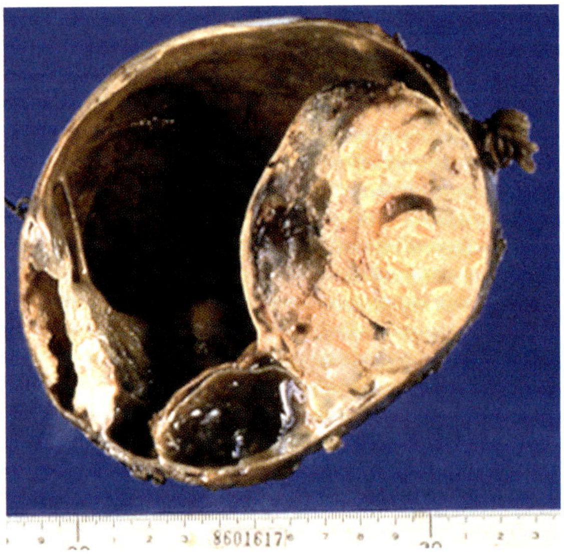

Figure 78.2

Surgical specimen of an MCT (adenocarcinoma). Note a solid nodule in the adenocarcinoma

Imaging Studies of MCTs

A plain abdominal roentgenogram may demonstrate tumor contour, or rough, nodular calcification or ossification in the capsule, or septa of the tumor and compression or displacement of the stomach, duodenum, or colon. The rate of calcification is reportedly 16% [19]. Computed tomography (CT) and ultrasound (US) can demonstrate the morphologic characteristics of the tumor and are excellent tools for both detection and differential diagnosis. CT and US usually reveal a sharply demarcated, low-density or hypoechoic mass with one or more loculations (Fig. 78.3a). Structural complexities including irregular thickening of the cyst wall or septa and papillary excrescences protruding into the cyst cavity are indicative of malignant transformation (Fig. 78.3b) [20–23]. The tumor is usually located in the peripheral area of the body or tail of the pancreas. Upper gastrointestinal series may reveal external compression of the stomach or duodenum by the pancreatic mass. Endoscopic US (EUS) also demonstrates unilocular or multilocular lesions of the pancreas and is the most useful for detecting structural complexities, such as a solid component or mural nodule (also indicative of malignancy; Fig. 78.4). Endoscopic retrograde pancreatography (ERP) shows no communication between the cystic tumor and ductal system of the pancreas, in contrast to the case in IPMNs, where this communication is usually proven. Enlargement of the orifice of the ampulla and excretion of copious mucin, which are characteristics of IPMNs, are uncommon in MCTs. Angiography usually demonstrates a hypovascular or avascular lesion with vessels stretched over the surface in benign cystadenomas. In an advanced case of cystadenocarcinoma, hypervascularity and vascular encasement or obstruction may be demonstrated. Aspirated fluid from the cyst frequently contains high levels of CEA and CA19-9 and only low levels of amylase and elastase [24]. Determination of CEA and CA19-9 levels in the cyst fluid has also been reported to be useful in the differential diagnosis of cystadenoma and cystadenocarcinoma. Determination of CA 72-4, pS2, and tissue polypep-

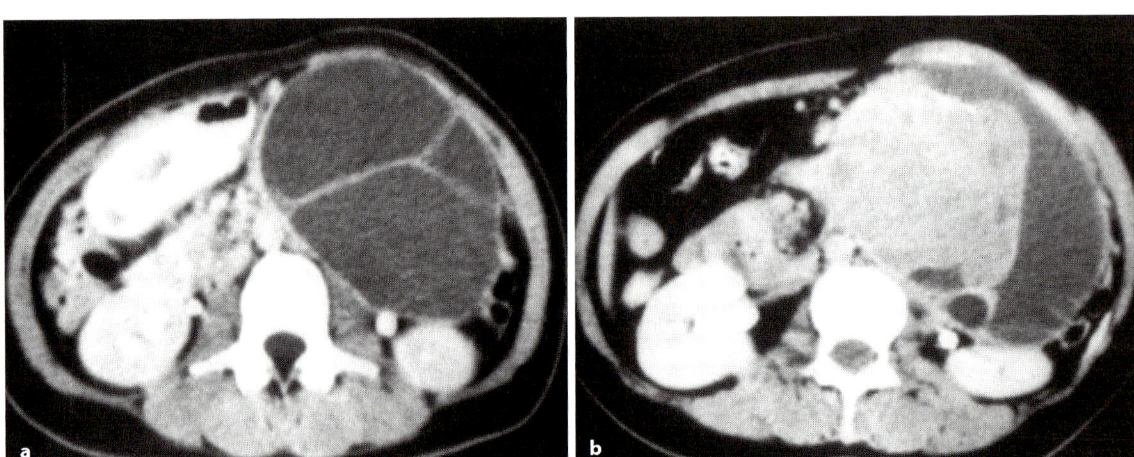

Figure 78.3 a, b

MCT (computed tomography, CT). a CT usually reveals a sharply demarcated, low-density mass with one or more loculations. b Structural complexities including irregular thickening of the cyst wall or septa and a papillary excrescences protruding into the cyst cavity are indicative of malignant transformation

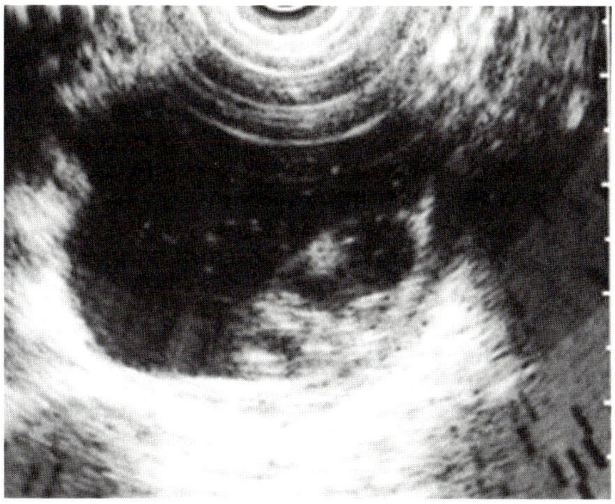

Figure 78.4

MCT (endoscopic ultrasound, EUS). EUS also demonstrates a unilocular or multilocular lesion of the pancreas and is the most useful tool for detecting structural complexities

tide antigen in the cystic fluid in combination with or without cytology may also be useful for predicting malignancy [25].

Differential Diagnosis

It is important to differentiate MCTs from postinflammatory pseudocysts with hemorrhage or necrotic debris. Other pancreatic cystic neoplasms including IPMNs, SCA, solid and pseudopapillary tumor (SPT), acinar cell cystadenocarcinoma, mucinous noncystic adenocarcinoma, cystic endocrine tumor, and nonneoplastic cysts such as lymphoepithelial cyst, should also be in the list of differential diagnoses.

Pseudocysts represent 70–90% of all cystic lesions in the pancreas and are usually preceded by a history of acute and chronic pancreatitis or abdominal trauma. Needle aspiration may yield brownish fluid with high amylase contents, whereas in MCTs, high CEA levels are found. Histological, pseudocysts lack an epithelial lining, an ovarian-type stroma, and mucoid contents. Instead, pseudocysts are lined with granulation tissue with hemosiderin deposits and occasional foreign body giant-cell reactions, and contain hemorrhagic necrotic debris. It should be noted, however, that the epithelial lining of MCTs may be partially absent or denuded and the results obtained from a small biopsy should, therefore, be interpreted with some caution in assessing the neoplastic nature as well as the malignant potential.

IPMNs develop predominantly in elderly male patients and are most frequently located in the head of the pancreas, in contrast to MCTs, which as mentioned earlier are found in the body and tail of the pancreas in middle-aged women. IPMNs involve cystic dilatation of the pancreatic ductal tree. Histologically, IPMNs are characterized by intraductal growth of mucin-producing columnar cells and do not form cysts other than in the duct system. As a result, communication between the cyst and ductal system is usually proven in IPMNs, while it is rarely seen in MCTs (Tables 78.3 and 78.4). As the cells of IPMNs also display a wide range of differentiation, cytology cannot be used to differentiate between MCTs and IPMNs. In IPMNs, the ampulla of Vater is enlarged and the orifice sometimes opens widely, excreting copious amounts of mucin.

Table 78.3. Pathologic features of IPMNs and MCTs

	IPMN (*n*=1024)	MCT (*n*=173)	*p* value
Location			
Pancreas head (%)	588 (57.4)	32 (18.5)	<0.0001
Pancreas body (%)	220 (21.4)	45 (25.0)	
Pancreas tail (%)	85 (8.3)	80 (46.2)	
Total pancreas (%)	30 (2.9)	0 (0.0)	
Multiple (%)	83 (8.1)	15 (8.7)	
Adenocarcinoma (%)	445 (43.5)	53 (30.6)	0.0015
Secondary pancreatitis (%)	140 (13.7)	2 (1.2)	<0.0001
Fibrous capsule (%)	160 (16.5)	130 (75.1)	<0.0001
Communication between cyst and duct (%)	626 (61.3)	21 (12.1)	<0.0001
Ovarian-type stroma (%)	0 (0.0)	73 (42.2)	<0.0001

Table 78.4. Diagnostic criteria for IPMTs and MCTs. Proposed by the working group studying pancreatic cystic tumors (Japan Pancreatic Society)

	IPMT	MCT
Fibrous capsule	Hardly present	Present
Ovarian-type stroma	Absent	Usually present
Communication between cyst and duct	Present	Usually absent
Intraductal growth	Present	Usually absent
Secondary pancreatitis	Frequently present	Usually absent
Age	Middle-aged to elderly	Middle-aged
Gender	For the most part men	Exclusively women

Surgical Treatment

As discussed above, it is difficult to assess the grade of dysplasia by imaging studies or with a small biopsy specimen, and so all MCTs should be completely resected when possible. Because of the potential to transform from a benign lesion to a malignant neoplasm, MCTs that appear to be histologically benign at biopsy or are discovered incidentally should be resected. One exception includes cysts less than 3 cm in diameter that do not display the findings indicative of malignancy, such as mural nodules or a thick septum. These cysts can be carefully followed until a possible progression sign is identified (i.e., increase in cyst diameter, development of a mural nodule).

Pancreatic resection is performed in relation to the site of the tumor. The cut end of the pancreas should include normal pancreatic tissue (i.e., a surgical margin of 5 mm or more), since local recurrence is reportedly not rare. In the resected margins, intraoperative radiation therapy may be indicated to control local recurrence. Postoperatively, external and/or chemotherapy may improve the clinical outcome in malignant cases. The peripancreatic lymph nodes should be dissected in cases of adenocarcinoma. Sugiyama et al. advocated wider range lymph node dissection (i.e., D2) [26]. Internal enteric drainage of MCTs (cyst–enteric anastomosis) should be avoided since there are many well-documented cases of apparently histologically benign MCTs that have recurred as invasive cystadenocarcinomas after the drainage procedure [13, 21–23].

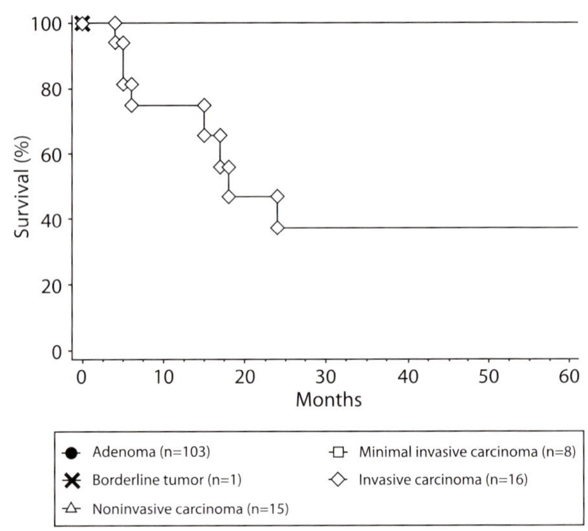

Figure 78.5

Postoperative survival curves for 143 cases of MCT (Kaplan-Meier)

Prognosis

Patients with mucinous cystadenoma, borderline MCT, and mucinous cystadenocarcinoma without stromal invasion, regardless of the degree of cellular dysplasia, far excellently if the tumor is completely resected. In a multi-institutional study from Japan, a postoperative survival rate of 100% was observed after surgery to remove an adenoma (n=103), borderline tumor (n=1), noninvasive carcinoma (n=15), and minimal invasive carcinoma (n=8; Fig. 78.5) [14]. In contrast, for invasive cystadenocarcinoma, the 1-year, 2-year, and 5-year survival rates were 75.0%, 37.5%, and 37.5%, respectively. According to a report from the AFIP [9], the presence of an aneuploid tumor, a reduction in or no progesterone immunoreactivity in stromal cells, tumor size (with 15 cm as a cut-off), and p53 immunoreactivity were significant potential prognostic factors. Incomplete resection or formation of a tumor fistula into adjacent organs almost inevitably leads to malignant transformation of the remnant tumor tissue [27–29], and leads to death of the patient as a result of metastatic adenocarcinoma within months or a few years, similar to the case for noncystic pancreatic adenocarcinomas [23]. In the study of Compagno and Oertel [2], the mean interval between diagnosis and death in such cases was 30 months. The resectability of mucinous cystadenocarcinomas is reported to be around 70%. The clinical course of mucinous cystadenocarcinoma with massive invasion is as poor as that of typical ductal adenocarcinoma of the pancreas, even after a surgical resection. For mucinous cystadenocarcinomas that are unresectable as a result of advanced local extension or distant metastasis, patient survival is similar to that of unresected typical ductal adenocarcinoma [30].

Intraductal Papillary Mucinous Neoplasm

General Considerations

The concept of mucinous papillary cystic neoplasms with ductal ectasia was introduced recently. Ohashi and Takagi first reported a patient with a polypoid cancer inside a markedly dilated main pancreatic duct [19]. With the increasingly wider-spread use of US and CT, an increasing number of patients with dilated pancreatic ducts have been observed, treated, and reported using various terminologies. As cases accumulated, confusion surrounding the terminology was further increased since these reports included cases with various morphologies and degrees of tumor cell dysplasia. Synonyms included mucin-producing cancer of the pancreas [31], ductectatic mucinous cystadenoma and cystadenocarcinoma [32], intraductal papillary neoplasms [33], mucinous pancreatic duct ectasia [34], intraductal mucin-hypersecreting neoplasms [35], mucin-hypersecreting tumor [36], mucin-producing tumor [37, 38], mucinous ductal ectasia [39], mucin-producing cystic adenocarcinoma [40], intraductal mucin-producing tumor [41], papillary adenoma of the pancreas with excessive mucin secretion [42], intraductal papillary adenocarcinoma [43], ductectatic-type mucinous cystadenoma and cystadenocarcinoma [44], mucin-secreting tumor [45], and mucin-producing neoplasms [46]. This has led to much confusion concerning the terminology, nature, and biology of these lesions. Some interpreted the lesions as reactive changes of the duct system and accordingly described them as atypical papillary hyperplasia [47–49], some regarded the lesions as precursors of typical ductal adenocarcinoma [50–52], yet others regarded them as variants of MCTs [32, 53, 54].

Currently, the definition of these tumors has been approached from two different perspectives, a clinical standpoint (narrow view) [36, 37, 55, 56], and a pathological or clinicopathologic context (broad view) [57, 58]. The narrow and classical view of this tumor was originally described by Ohashi et al. [31]. This definition is based on a clinical concept and, more specifically, on the characteristic endoscopic features of the papilla of Vater (excretion of mucin through the patulous orifice and accumulation of mucin in the dilated pancreatic duct; Fig. 78.6). In contrast, the broad view, first defined by Kato and Yanagiswa [59], is based on the mucin-secreting nature of tumor cells, and naturally included a heterogeneous group of lesions, intraductal papillary tumor of the mucin-producing type, MCTs, and mucinous adenocarcinoma. Although there are no cytological difference between IPMNs and MCTs, IPMNs are morphologically different and clinicopathologically distinct from ductal adenocarcinoma, MCT, and ductal papillary hyperplasia. If "mucin-hypersecreting tumor" is divided into the main pancreatic duct type, branch duct type, and peripheral type according to the main site of the tumor, IPMNs correspond mainly to the main pancreatic duct and branch duct types, and MCTs roughly to the peripheral type.

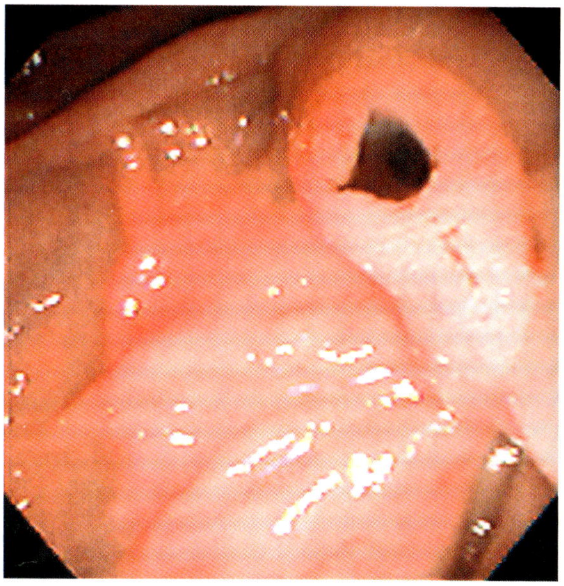

Figure 78.6

Characteristic endoscopic features of the papilla of Vater in intraductal papillary mucinous neoplasms (IPMNs). Note the excretion of copious amounts of mucin through the patulous orifice of the ampulla

Like MCTs, IPMNs show a spectrum of epithelial dysplasias from almost benign-looking epithelium (mild dysplasia) through to moderate to severe dysplasia, and further carcinoma in situ [60, 61]. Overt invasive tumors have also been reported [38, 60, 62],

Table 78.5. Clinicopathologic features of benign tumors and adenocarcinoma in surgical cases of IPMNs

	Benign tumor *n*=564	Adenocarcinoma *n*=445	*p* value
Gender			
No. of males (%)	403 (71.5%)	298 (67.0)	NS
No. of females (%)	157 (27.8)	166 (37.3)	
Age (years; mean±SD)	65±9	67±9	0.0002
Range	(27–87)	(29–91)	
Symptoms (%)	200 (35.5)	217 (48.8)	<0.0001
Other pancreatic disorders (%)	166 (29.4)	189 (42.5)	<0.0001
Other malignant neoplasms (%)	96 (17.0)	81 (18.2)	
Subtype			
Main duct type (%)	81 (14.4)	120 (27.0)	<0.0001
Branch duct type (%)	359 (63.6)	150 (33.7)	<0.0001
Combined type (%)	80 (14.2)	148 (33.3)	<0.0001
Enlarged orifice of the papilla (%)	193 (34.2)	213 (47.9)	<0.0001
Mural nodule (%)	159 (28.4)	281 (63.0)	<0.0001
Size (mm; mean±SD)	4.6±3.3	11.7±10.5	<0.0001
Cyst diameter (branch duct type, in mm; mean±SD)	27.5±14.3	34.6±18.4	<0.0001
Main pancreatic duct diameter (main duct and combined type, in mm; mean±SD)	9.3±5.4	12.6±9.5	0.0005

and there is presumably an adenoma–carcinoma sequence. IPMNs are classified according to the grade of dysplasia, into adenoma, tumor of borderline lesion, intraductal carcinoma, and invasive carcinoma. Invasive carcinomas derived from IPMN are known as papillary mucinous carcinomas (Table 78.5) [14]. IPMNs are divided morphologically into the main duct type and branch duct type according to the site of the tumor (for further discussion see the sections in this chapter on macroscopic findings and on imaging studies).

Clinicopathologic Features of IPMNs

IPMN is an uncommon tumor of the pancreas that accounts for 0.5% of all pancreatic tumors found at autopsy, 7.5% of clinically diagnosed tumors, and 16.3% of tumors in resected cases [63]. Kimura et al. reviewed a total of 269 cases of mucin-producing tumor of the pancreas collected from Japanese, European, and American literature. In the collection of 259 patients, there were 177 males and 82 females (male:female ratio=2.2) with a mean age of 65.5 years. In a multi-institutional study from Japan, a total of 1379 cases of IPMN were collected, comprising 919 males and 460 females (male:female ratio=2.0) with a mean age 67.0 years (range 27–95 years) [14]. IPMN develops in all races, but the largest number of cases has been accumulated in Japan.

The etiology of the tumor is not known. Yamada et al. noted that most patients in their series were smokers [64]. Patients often have synchronous or metachronous malignancies in other organs, at a rate of 19–32% [14, 57]. This suggests the occurrence of frequent genetic alterations in IPMNs of the pancreas shared with that of malignant conditions in other organs. This fact, however, may be biased since IPMNs are often detected by a follow-up imaging study for other previously treated malignancies.

Patients with IPMNs may present symptoms (32.9%, Table 78.1), including upper abdominal pain and back pain. About one-quarter of the patients will have experienced pancreatitis-like manifestations (e.g., epigastric discomfort, episodes of heavy pain, and hyperamylasemia) for many years [55, 59]. Eventually, about half of these patients develop pancreatic insufficiency with diabetes and steatorrhea, or both. All of these symptoms are attributable to occlusion of the main duct by either proliferation of the tumor or accumulation of viscous mucin. When the papillary tumor involves the ampulla or viscous mucin in the ampulla, the common bile duct becomes compressed and obstructive jaundice may develop. When the tumor is located in the body or tail of the pancreas, the

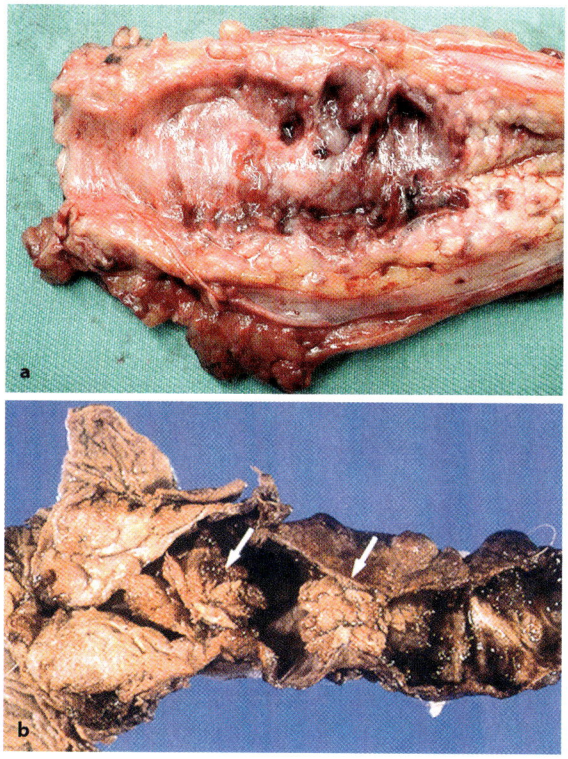

Figure 78.7 a, b

IPMN (main pancreatic duct type). a Note the cystic dilatation of the main pancreatic duct. The inner surface of the dilated duct may display papillary excrescence: villous tumor, polypoid tumor, granulous mucosa, localized mucosal thickening, or rough mucosa. b Invasive IPMN carcinoma

presentation of symptoms is less common. In noninvasive variants, two-third of the patients were asymptomatic and most of the tumors were discovered during a routine check-up or at autopsy.

Macroscopic Findings of IPMNs

The majority of the IPMNs develop in the head (57.4%) and the body (21.4%) of the pancreas (Table 78.4). Although IPMNs are usually classified into two groups according to the main tumor location (branch duct type and main pancreatic duct type), some tumors display both components of the tumor, namely the combined type. In the branch duct type, the ecstatic branch duct appears gray in color and forms grape-like clusters in the peripheral portion of the pancreas. The ectatic pancreatic duct may contain viscous mucin, and solitary or multiple sessile polyps on the inner surface may be noted. These cystic lesions may display hard nodules. In the main duct type, the main pancreatic duct measures 1–8 cm in diameter. The distal pancreas may also be accompanied by chronic obstructive pancreatitis. The inner surface of the dilated duct may display papillary excrescences: villous tumor, polypoid tumor, granulous mucosa, localized mucosal thickening, or rough mucosa (Fig. 78.7). The average size of the tumors in the main duct is 2–4 cm. They are soft, friable, and tan-to-grey/white in color. In a few instances, the entire main pancreatic duct is studded with tumor tissue that may involve the ampulla of Vater and the minor papilla. In such cases, the protruded tumor can be seen from the duodenum. Malignant tumors in the head of the pancreas may form a fistula into the duodenum and distal bile duct.

Extreme intraductal mucin accumulation in the absence of a grossly visible tumor characterizes the ductectatic mucin-hypersecreting variant of the IPMN. This variant develops predominantly in the head of the pancreas and only occasionally in the tail or one of a few secondary ducts in the uncinate process. The inner surface of the dilated mucin-filled duct is smooth, but may exhibit tiny microscopic papillary excrescences. The pancreatic tissue surrounding the dilated ducts occluded by the tumor or viscous mucin shows marked fibrosis, and thus invasive carcinoma is difficult to recognize. Thick capsule is usually absent in IPMNs, in contrast to the capsule that is almost always present in MCTs.

Imaging Studies of IPMNs

US, CT, and magnetic resonance imaging (MRI) can be used to demonstrate the typical morphologic characteristics of the tumor and are excellent tools for both detection and differential diagnosis. In the main pancreatic duct type, a diffuse dilatation or segmental cystic ectasia of the main pancreatic duct filled with mucin shown by US, CT, and MRI is diagnostic. Imaging studies may also detect a polypoid lesion (or lesions), in the main pancreatic duct. In branch duct types, imaging studies display a cystic mass, usually in the uncinate process of the pancreas. Ectatic branch ducts form grape-like clusters in the peripheral portion of the pancreas. In some cases, both components of the main pancreatic and branch duct types can be seen simultaneously, namely a combined type (CT Fig. 78.8; magnetic resonance cholangiopancreatography, MRCP Fig. 78.9; endoscopic retrograde cholangiopancreatography, ERCP Fig 78.10; EUS Fig.78.11).

In patients presenting with mucin hypersecretion, an enlarged papilla with a wide-open orifice and copious mucin excretion may be observed at duodenos-

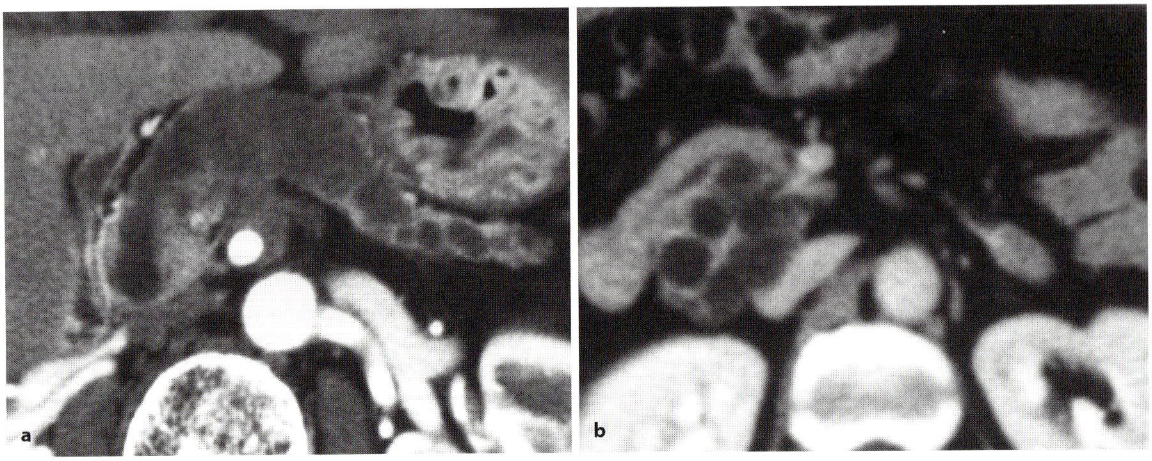

Figure 78.8 a, b

IPMN (CT). a Main pancreatic duct type: note the diffuse dilatation and segmental cystic ectasia of the main pancreatic duct. b Branch duct type: note the ecstatic branch ducts forming grape-like clusters in the peripheral portion of the pancreas

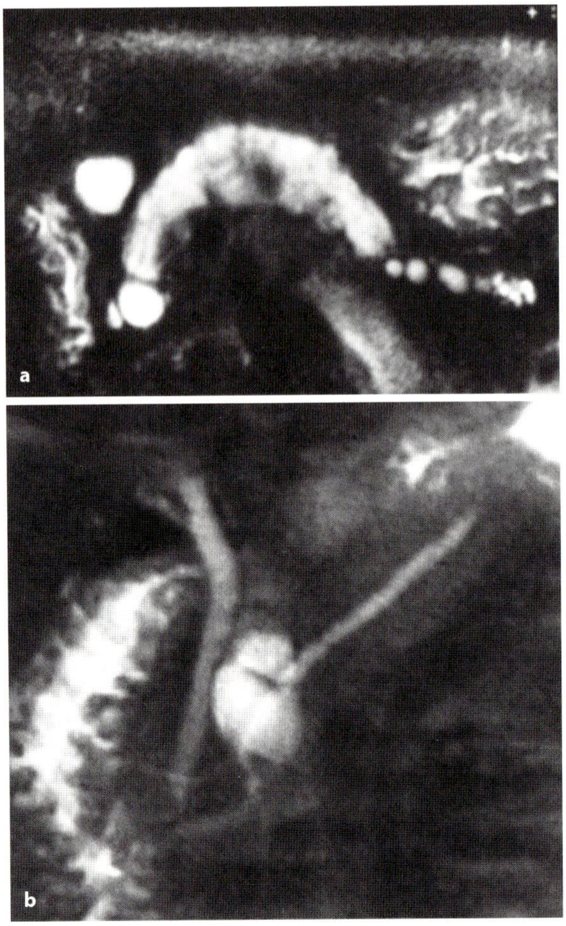

Figure 78.9 a, b

IPMN (magnetic resonance cholangiopancreatography, MRCP). a Main pancreatic duct type. b Branch duct type

copy (Fig 78.6). This feature is characteristic of IPMNs, but the positive rate for this findings is reportedly about 50% [26, 36]. These characteristic features are sometimes also observed at the accessory papilla. Aspirated secretion or mucin from the dilated duct may contain malignant cells or high levels of CEA and CA19-9. The positive rate of transpapillary biopsy is reportedly only 50% or lower [36]. ERP displays diffuse dilatation of the main pancreatic duct or the dilated branch duct with filling defects caused by either papillary tumors or mucin plugs. Pancreatography may display a papillary tumor with a fish-egg appearance, granular mucosa, polyp, or rough mucosa. It should, however, be noted that full visualization of the pancreatic duct system in IPMN by ERP is sometimes difficult due to excessive mucin in the duct. Structural complexities, such as a solid component or mural nodule, are indicative of malignancy, but the pancreatogram should be interpreted with some caution, because differentiation of these structural complexities from the cluster or aggregation of mucin is sometimes impossible. The communication of the lesion to the pancreatic ductal system is usually evident in IPMNs in 61–85% of cases, in contrast to the case of MCTs, where this communication is usually absent.

EUS and intraductal US employ high-frequency US and are invaluable tools for detecting the structural complexities indicative of malignancy (Fig. 78.12). The use of intraoperative US or intraductal US is also advocated for making the surgical cut-line decision.

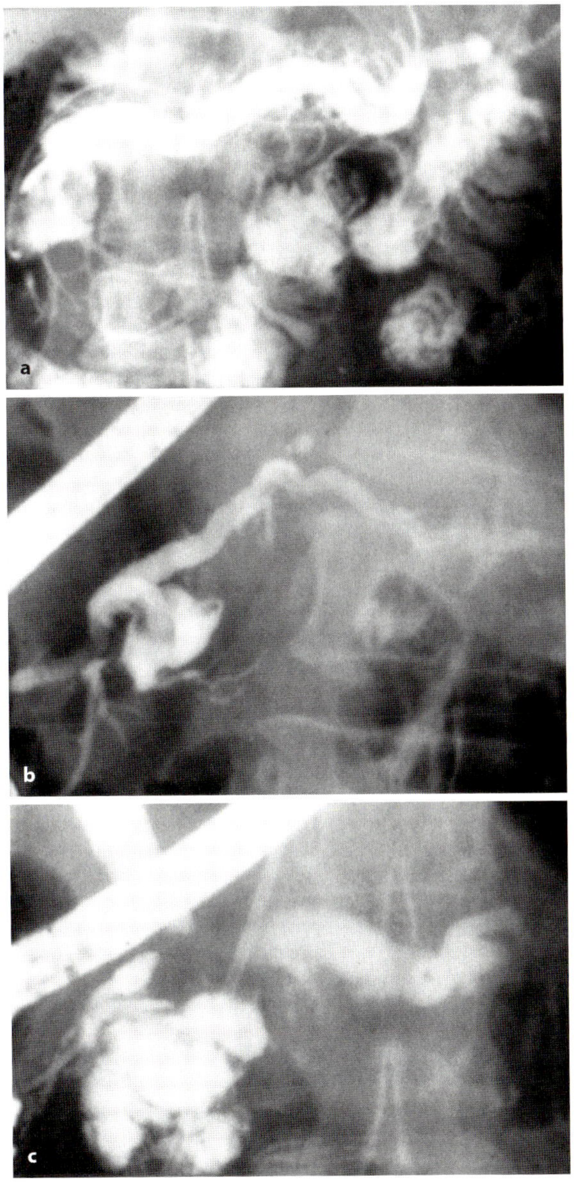

Figure 78.10 a–c

Endoscopic retrograde pancreatography. a Main pancreatic duct type. b Branch duct type. c Combined type

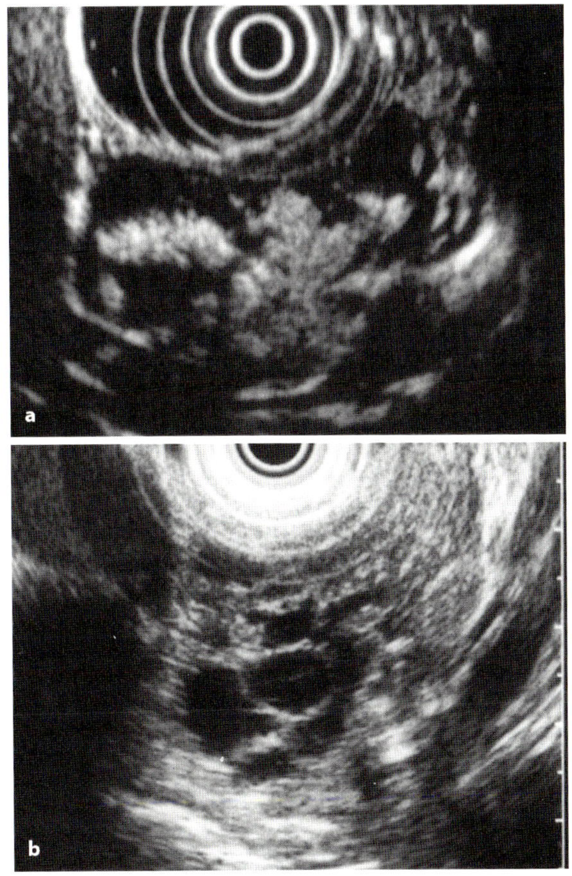

Figure 78.11 a, b

IPMN (endoscopic ultrasound, EUS). a Combined type: note that EUS can effectively display papillary excrescences in the dilated duct. b Branch duct type

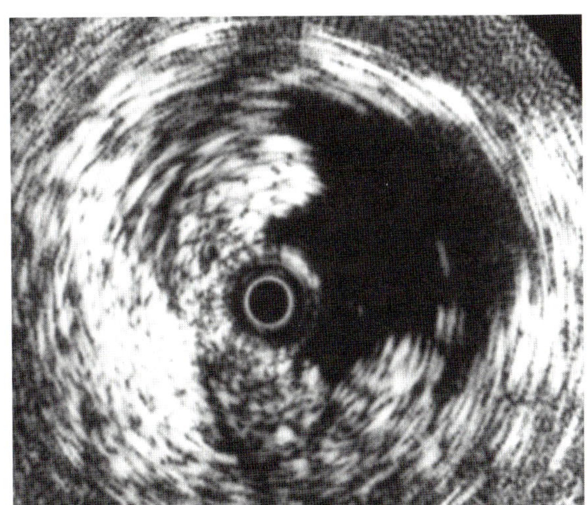

Figure 78.12

Intraductal ultrasound (US) of an IPMN. Intraductal US is an invaluable tool for detecting mucosal changes indicative of malignancy

Angiography is usually noncontributing in benign small lesions and there may be stretching and displacement of the intrapancreatic or peripancreatic vessels in large tumors. In malignant cases, vascular encasement and obstruction of the vessels may be demonstrated, as seen in ordinary invasive ductal carcinomas.

It is of greatest importance to distinguish benign from malignant IPMNs, since the appropriate management differs. Sugiyama et al. reported predictive factors for malignancy: mural nodules and a main pancreatic duct diameter of 7 mm or more. Mural nodules in the main duct or combined types, and mural nodules and a tumor diameter of 30 mm or more in the branch duct type were particularly indicative of malignancy. Mural nodules, jaundice, and main duct or combined types were predictors of invasive carcinoma in a multivariate analysis [65].

Differential Diagnosis

It is important to differentiate IPMNs from MCTs, ductal carcinoma, and ductal papillary hyperplasia. There is usually no difficulty in distinguishing IPMN from other pancreatic tumors including SCA, SPT, acinar cell cystadenocarcinoma, cystic endocrine tumor, and nonneoplastic cysts. The discrimination between IPMN from chronic pancreatitis is of clinical significance rather than being a morphological problem.

IPMNs develop predominantly in elderly male patients and are most frequently located in the head of the pancreas. In contrast, MCTs are found in the body and tail of the pancreas in middle-aged women. IPMNs involve cystic dilatation of the pancreatic ductal tree. Histologically, IPMNs are characterized by intraductal growth of mucin-producing columnar cells and do not form cysts apart from in the duct system. As a result, communication between the cyst and ductal system is usually proven in IPMNs, while communication is hardly seen in MCTs (Tables 78.3 and 78.4). As the cells of IPMNs display a wide range of differentiation, cytology can not be used to differentiate them from MCTs. In IPMNs, the ampulla of Vater is enlarged and the orifice sometimes wide open, excreting copious amounts of mucin.

Because of its poor prognosis, common invasive ductal carcinoma has to be clearly distinguished from IPMN. This is usually not difficult because of the grossly obvious and solid and invasive tumor growth of the former. The difficulty lies in differentiating invasive papillary-mucinous carcinoma from ductal adenocarcinoma with intraductal spread. This differentiation is usually made on the basis of predominance of tumor location. In ductal adenocarcinomas, the invasive component of the tumor is predominant, and the reverse is true for papillary-mucinous carcinomas. Interestingly, there is evidence to indicate that some pancreatic papillary-mucinous cancers are derived from IPMNs [66].

The nonneoplastic pancreatic duct change known as ductal papillary hyperplasia has similar cytological and histological features to those of IPMNs. Ductal papillary hyperplasia, however, is usually a small lesion in the secondary branch and does not give rise to interval change or clinical symptoms.

Chronic pancreatitis is characterized by uneven scarring of the pancreas parenchyma. The duct system, particularly the main pancreatic duct, is irregularly distorted as well as developing strictures (chain and lakes), and in advanced cases contains pancreatic stones. Chain and lakes observed by imaging sometimes resemble diffuse dilatation of the main pancreatic duct in IPMNs. Pseudocysts may also mimic the cystic dilation of the branch duct. It is rare for these cystic lesions to be dominant, and careful interpretation of the pancreatogram is a key to differential diagnosis.

Surgical Treatment

Owing to the malignant potential of the tumors and their effects on pancreatic function, IPMNs should be completely resected surgically. This is only possible, however, in tumors confined to the head or body-tail of the pancreas. It should also be noted that the extent of tumors could be unexpectedly wider than the area defined by preoperative imaging studies. Intraoperative frozen-section diagnosis or intraoperative pancreatoscopy should be considered, especially in main pancreatic duct types, although the diagnosis is not always definite. Some cases may thus necessitate a total pancreatectomy [67]. Such an aggressive approach, however, has to be evaluated carefully against the risk associated with the surgery and the problems arising from resultant endocrine and exocrine pancreatic insufficiency. As most tumors are slow-growing neoplasms with a favorable prognosis and affect the older-aged man, a conservative option should be considered in cases without evident cancer. Although the natural history of adenomas in main duct type IPMN is not yet precisely known, there is accumulating evidence of observed cases without surgery, which favors the observation policy, especially in the elderly [68]. In addition, in the branch duct type observation may be justified in the elderly when the parameters indicative of malignancy (i.e., main pancreatic duct diameter >7 mm, cyst diameter >30 mm, presence of mural nodules) are absent.

Concerning lymph-node dissection at the time of surgery, Sugiyama et al. recently reported that peri-pancreatic lymph node dissection, namely D1, is sufficient for intraductal papillary carcinoma, in contrast to the case for MCTs, for which extensive dissection, namely D2, is required [26].

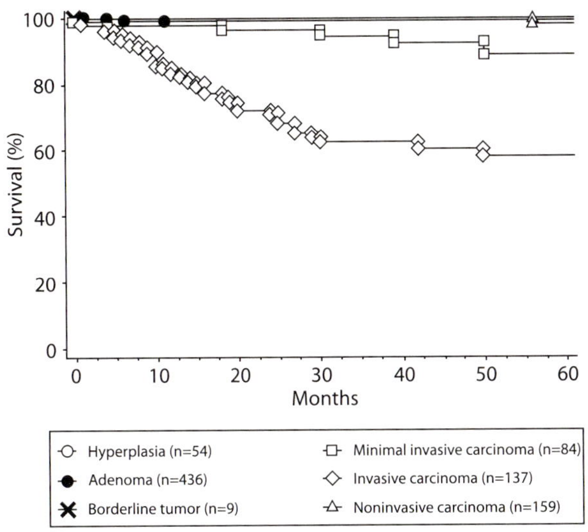

Figure 78.13

Postoperative survival curves for 879 cases of IPMNs (Kaplan-Meier)

Prognosis

Survival following resection of IPMNs without invasive cancer (regardless of degree of dysplasia) is good. Sohn et al. reported an overall 5-year survival for patients with IPMNs without invasive cancer of 77% (several deaths were secondary to metachronous invasive cancer) [68]. In a multi-institutional study from Japan, no death of the recurrent disease was observed after surgery for hyperplasia (n=54), adenoma (n=436), borderline tumor (n=9), and noninvasive carcinoma (n=159) [14]. Similarly, there were no statistically significant differences in survival when comparing branch duct, main duct, and combined variants; however, the branch duct variants were more often noninvasive. In contrast, Sohn et al. also reported an overall 5-year survival rate of 43% for patients with IPMNs including an invasive component. In this report, for those patients with invasive IPMNs, 2-year survival was 40% when the cut end was positive for IPMN regardless of the presence of invasive cancer, or for IPMNs without invasive cancer, and 60% when the cut end was tumor free (p=0.15). Those patients with colloid carcinomas (n=14) had a better survival rate compared to those with tubular carcinomas (n=31), with 5-year survival rates of 83% and 24%, respectively. IPMN recurrences and deaths of cancer occurred in patients with both invasive and noninvasive IPMNs at initial resection. Recurrent disease in the residual pancreas suggests that long-term surveillance is critical. Also in the Japanese study, the postoperative 3-year survival rate was 62.2% for patients with invasive carcinoma; the 5-year survival rate was 57.7%. In general, the survival rates for the patients with IPMNs with an invasive cancer component after surgery compare better than those for patients with cystadenocarcinoma, for whom the 1-year, 2-year, and 5-year survival rates were 75.0%, 37.5%, and 37.5%, respectively (Fig. 78.13) [14].

SCT of the Pancreas

General Considerations

SCTs alone account for about 1–2% of all exocrine pancreatic neoplasms [69], and for about 25% of all cystic tumors of the pancreas [15, 23]. More recently, SCTs have been reported with increasing frequency, probably due to the increased awareness of the disease and increased sophistication of diagnostic procedures [70].

In the past, SCTs were classified merely as cystadenomas, a category that included both SCTs and MCTs. In 1978, Compagno and Oertel described 34 cases of SCTs (SCAs) and made the differences clear between this benign lesion (SCT) and the MCT with malignant potential [5]. SCTs have gained attention in the diagnosis and treatment of cystic tumors of the pancreas because they have little or no malignant potential. SCTs are basically benign in nature, but since George's first report of a malignant case displaying locally invasive growth and apparent metastases in 1989 [71], more than 20 cases of malignant SCTs (serous cystadenocarcinomas, SCACs) have been reported in the world literature [72–89]. Although the true incidence of malignancy SCTs is difficult to determine, Strobel et al. estimated that they have malignant potential, with a risk of malignancy of 3% [86].

SCT is defined as a cystic tumor lined by cuboidal or flattened epithelial cells containing glycogen in the cytoplasm. Most SCTs are microcystic, forming a honeycomb-like appearance, and have therefore also been called microcystic adenomas or glycogen-rich cystadenomas. The current World Health Organization (WHO) classification of pancreatic tumors has defined two categories of SCTs: SCAs and SCACs [90]. Macrocystic or oligocystic variants that are composed of only a few relatively large cysts have been described [91]. Thus, the WHO subclassifies SCAs into serous microcystic adenomas and serous oligocystic adenomas [91]. The incidence of serous oligocystic adenomas is reported to be 7% [92]. A rare variant of SCA, which poses an additional diagnostic pitfall, lacks cysts [93]. This variant has been termed simply solid serous adenoma of the pancreas [70]; they are cytologically identical to SCAs and have the same immunohistochemical profile [70].

Clinicopathologic Features of SCTs

SCTs develop predominantly in women in the sixth decade of life (75% in women, mean age 61.5 years) [92]. Like many pancreatic cystic neoplasms, the typical clinical scenario is that of an incidentally discovered pancreatic mass [94]. In a series of SCAs (n=106) at Massachusetts General Hospital, 47% of patients were asymptomatic and the tumor was identified as part of the workup for a different problem [92]. In another large series (n=100), 56% of patients were asymptomatic [95]. Clinical symptoms, when they are present, include abdominal pain, anorexia, mass or fullness, nausea/vomiting, weight loss, jaundice, and fatigue and/or malaise [92, 95]. Rare clinical manifestations include portal hypertension, hemoperitoneum, and acute gastrointestinal hemorrhage [94]. Patients with small SCAs are less likely to be symptomatic than are the patients with large SCAs [92]. The mean size of SCTs at surgical resection is reportedly 6–11 cm (range 1–30 cm) [70]. SCTs occur anywhere in the pancreas; however, the aforementioned recent large-series report indicates that SCAs may develop predominantly in the body or tail of the pancreas (44% in head, 56% in the body or tail of the pancreas) [92].

Macroscopic and Microscopic Findings of SCTs

Gross examination of SCAs shows a well-circumscribed lesion. The appearance of the cut surface varies markedly depending on the tumor subtype. Serous microcystic adenomas are usually composed of innumerable tiny (often <0.1 cm in diameter) cysts filled with clear fluid that give the tumor a sponge-like or honeycomb appearance on cross-section (Fig. 78.14) [70]. They often contain a central stellate scar, usually containing calcium deposits [70]. In contrast, serous oligocystic adenomas are composed of a single or a few relatively large cysts. Histologically, serous microcystic adenoma is a multicystic mass. The fibrous stroma is composed of dense collagenized tissue. The central stellate core is composed of hyalinized tissue with a few clusters of minute cysts. The epithelial lining of the cysts is composed of cuboidal or flattened epithelial cells. Substantial nuclear atypia is absent, and mitoses are extremely rare [70]. The cytoplasm of the cells is filled with glycogen, and, as such, will stain positively with periodic acid Schiff and is diastase-sensitive. Serous oligocystic adenomas present identical histology to microcystic adenomas. Differential diagnosis between SCACs and SCAs may be difficult or impossible on histological or cytological basis alone and may be established by the presence of metastatic deposits and/or invasive growth [70].

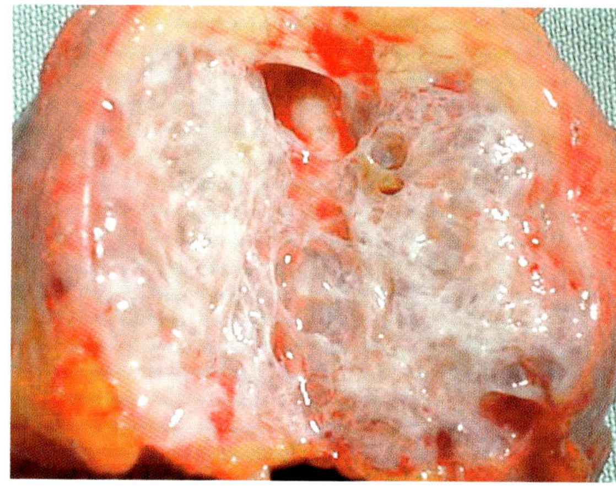

Figure 78.14

Surgical specimen of a serous cystadenoma (SCA). The cut surface of the specimen shows innumerable tiny cysts, giving the cystic tumor a sponge-like appearance

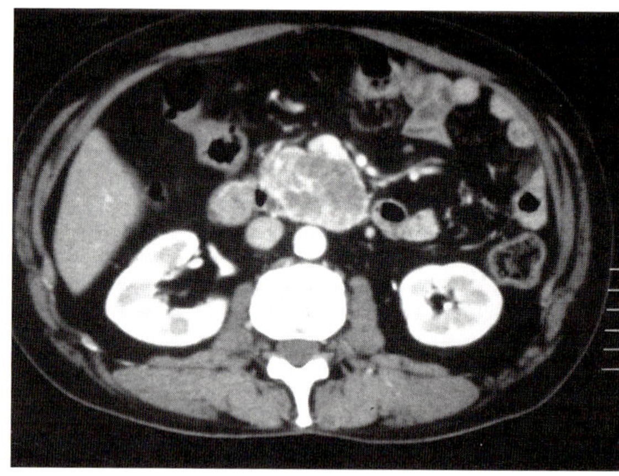

Figure 78.15

SCA (CT). Enhanced CT shows clearly a sharply demarcated, multilocular cyst separated by enhanced thin septa

Imaging Studies of SCTs

CT in particular (Fig. 78.15) and EUS (Fig. 78.16) can be used to demonstrate the morphologic characteristics of the tumor. These reveal a sharply demarcated, multilocular cyst, occasionally with a clearly recognized central stellate scar and a calcification of sunburst type. In 10–30% of cases, plain CT shows a low-density mass with a classic sunburst pattern of calcification within a central scar, but some tumors may show peripheral calcification [70]. On enhanced CT, SCAs show a honeycomb pattern of microlacunae separated by thin septa. Angiography usually demonstrates a hypervascular lesion, a feature that distinguishes SCTs from pseudocysts or MCTs [70]. EUS

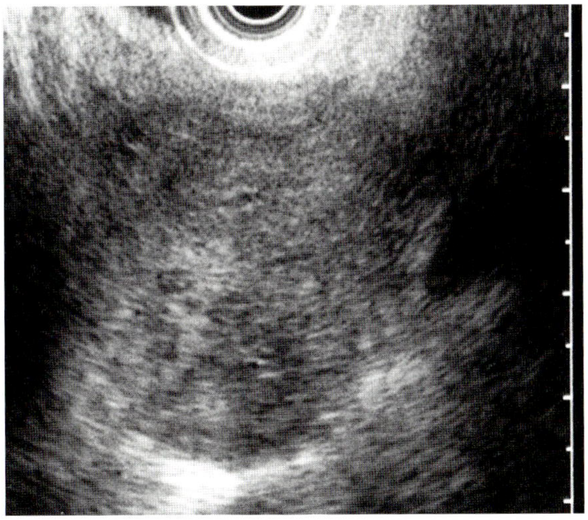

Figure 78.16

SCA (EUS). EUS demonstrates the characteristic honeycomb mesh network pattern of morphology and is the most useful tool for detecting structural complexities

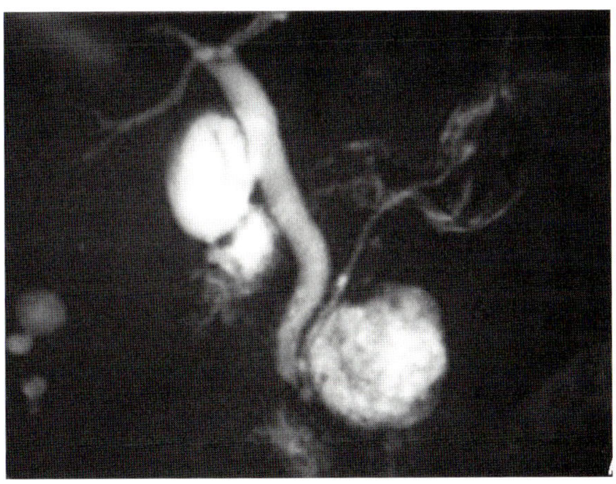

Figure 78.17

SCA (MRCP). On T2-weighted images, a serous cystic tumor is demonstrated as a high-intensity mass. MRCP shows no communication between the cystic tumor and the ductal system of the pancreas

demonstrates the characteristic honeycomb morphology and is the most useful tool for detecting structural complexities. MRI shows multilocular cystic lesion containing characteristic hyperintensity areas on T2-weighted images (Fig. 78.17). On T1-weighted images, SCTs are demonstrated as a low-intensity mass. ERP and MRCP show no communication between the cystic tumor and ductal system of the pancreas (Fig. 78.17).

It is of great importance to be able to distinguish SCAs from SCACs, since the appropriate management may differ. However, this is generally not possible [87]. There are no radiological criteria that allow the precise diagnosis of an SCAC unless tumor infiltration or metastasis is obvious [87].

Differential Diagnosis

In typical situations, it is not difficult to make a diagnosis of SCTs because of their specific imaging findings. However, image interpretation is complicated by morphological variations in SPTs and by overlap of their radiological features with those of other cystic neoplasms [70]. Misdiagnosis by EUS or CT occurs in as many as 20–50% of cases [70]. Misdiagnosis of SCTs is most commonly related to the misinterpretation of serous oligocystic cystadenomas as either MCTs or as pseudocysts, because all of these lesions are either oligocystic or unilocular. Serous microcystic cystadenomas are sometimes misdiagnosed as solid lesions on EUS or CT because a homogeneous image results either from small uniform locules without visualization of septa or hemorrhage into the cysts [70]. In a solid serous adenoma, islet cell tumors should be differentiated. In addition to other cystic neoplasms, the differential diagnosis for SCTs includes metastatic renal cell carcinoma and lymphangioma [94].

Surgical Treatment and Prognosis

Although natural history, diagnostic criteria, potential for growth or malignancy, and outcomes are not well defined, surgical resection is generally performed only for symptoms, large size, or the inability to distinguish an SCT from other cystic neoplasms that have greater malignant potential, such as MCTs or IPMNs [92]. SCTs may be treated conservatively (followed and observed), particularly in elderly patients or those who are a poor operative risks [70]. This is because SCTs are clearly benign in the vast majority of cases, with rare exceptions. On the other hand, Strobel et al. [86] have recommended surgical resection for all cases in consideration of their malignant potential (risk of malignancy of 3%). Others advocate a more selective approach. Tseng et al. [92] recently reported that patients who are asymptomatic and have tumors less than 4 cm are candidates for nonoperative management with clinical follow-up and serial imaging, and that patients with symptoms, patients in whom other potentially malignant cystic neoplasms cannot be excluded, and patients with tumors measuring 4 cm or more who are reasonable surgical candidates should be offered surgical resection. These recommendations are based on both the growth rate of SCTs on the prevalence of developing symptoms depending on the tumor size.

Complete surgical resection of SCAs is definitive treatment [70]. Pancreatectomy is performed according to the tumor location. The prognosis of SCTs is excellent because there is only a minimal risk of malignant transformation. It seems that SCACs are relatively low-malignant tumors with a slow rate of tumor progression, and therefore, a palliative resection may be helpful even if a curative resection is not possible.

Solid and Pseudopapillary Tumor

General Considerations

The pancreatic SPT tumor has been documented since the 1950s [96, 97], and various names have been applied to it [98–101], including benign and malignant papillary neoplasms, papillary-cystic tumors of the pancreas, papillary epithelial neoplasms, solid and papillary epithelial neoplasms, and solid and cystic acinar cell tumors. Since Kloppel's review of five cases in 1981 [102], this tumor has gained increasing attention among clinicians. SPT has been reported recently with an increasing frequency, probably due to the increased awareness of the disease and sophistication of diagnostic procedures. To date, more than 700 cases have been reported in the English literature [103]. To reflect the two histological features of this tumor: the solid areas and pseudopapillary region, both WHO and AFIP classifications have proposed the name "solid and pseudopapillary tumor" of the pancreas [90, 104].

As has been reported repeatedly, SPT of the pancreas has borderline malignant potential [105]. Nevertheless, only a small number of the cases recur or develop metastasis after a potentially curative resection [106]. Even in the metastatic lesions, SPTs tend to proliferate slowly. The histopathological criteria to distinguish malignant tumors from benign ones include the presence of angioinvasion, perineural invasion, and deep infiltration of the surrounding pancreatic parenchyma in the resected specimen. It should be noted that tumors without these findings might as well behave in a malignant manner.

Cells of SPTs express various markers, including epithelial as well as parenchymal, and occasionally exocrine and endocrine markers. This diversity may suggest that SPT originates from the multipotential cells such as ductular-centroacinar cell. The predominance of this tumor in women suggests that genetic and hormonal factors play a role in its etiology. Interestingly, Landanyi et al. first reported an increased level of both estrogen and progesterone receptors in an 18-year old patient with SPT [107]. Morales et al. reported a very rapid growth of SPT enhanced by concurrence of pregnancy in a 21-year-old woman [108].

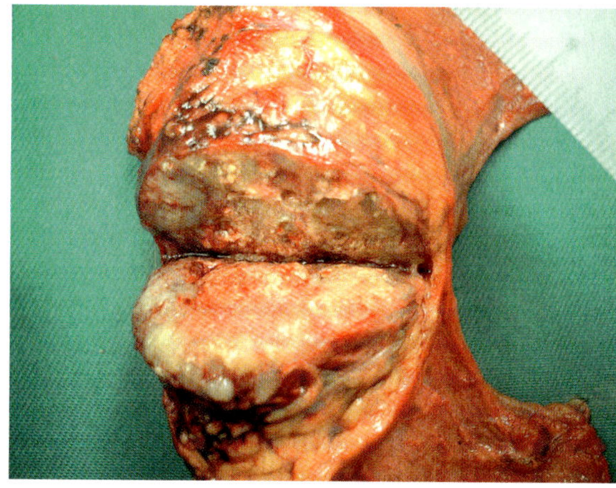

Figure 78.18

Surgical specimen of solid and pseudopapillary tumor (SPT). The cut surface of the resected tumor displays solid monomorphous tumor tissue in the periphery accompanied by sclerosis, hemorrhage, and cyst formation in the center

SPTs account for approximately 1–2% of all exocrine pancreatic tumors. It develops predominantly in adolescent girls and young women (mean age 23.9 years, ranging from 2 to 72 years) [109]. SPTs develop in all races.

Clinicopathologic Features of SPTs

The tumors more frequently develop in the body and tail of the pancreas. They present as large, round, solitary masses measuring 3–8 cm in diameter. Direct invasion of surrounding organs (the stomach, duodenum, spleen, or transverse colon) or the portal vein is rarely evident. The cut surface of the encapsulated and often fluctuant tumors exhibits lobulated, light brown solid areas admixed with hemorrhagic and necrotic areas as well as cystic spaces filled with necrotic debris. The hemorrhagic–cystic change occasionally involves almost all of the tumor tissue (cystic type), so that the tumor should be differentiated from a pseudocyst. The capsule, but also in inner portion of mass, may contain calcification or ossification. A few extrapancreatic SPTs are also reported.

In small tumors, all tumor tissue is preserved without secondary changes, while in large tumors, the tissue is preserved only in the tumor periphery under

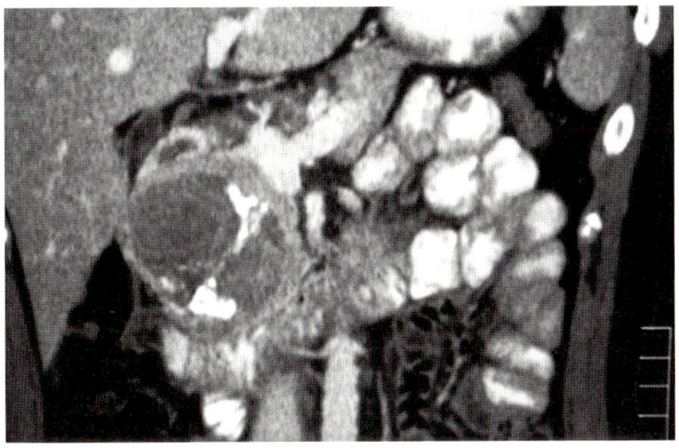

Figure 78.19

SPT (CT). Note an encapsulated tumor with variably solid and cystic changes inside. Calcification or ossification is reportedly seen in 30% of cases

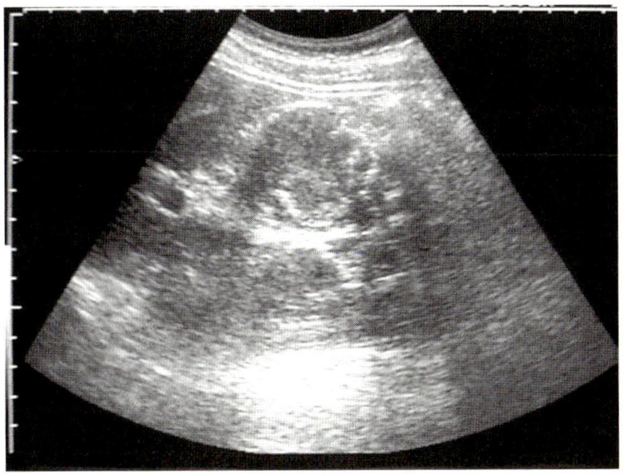

Figure 78.20

SPT (US). US also demonstrates a sharply demarcated tumor, the inside of which exhibits variable echogenicity

the fibrous capsule. This tissue exhibits a solid monomorphous pattern with various degrees of sclerosis, and more centrally, a pseudopapillary pattern (Fig. 78.18).

Imaging studies for nonspecific abdominal pain and abdominal trauma usually identify SPTs as incidental findings. Jaundice is rare, even in tumors in the pancreatic head. Endocrine syndrome has not been reported. A rapture of the capsule may take place, resulting in hemoperitoneum in 8 of 292 cases of a cumulative review of the world's literature. All known tumor markers are reportedly within normal limits.

There have been only a few reports of metastasized SPTs. Of 18 patients reported, metastatic tumors were seen in the liver in 11, peritoneum and greater omentum in 5, regional lymph nodes and subcutis in 4.

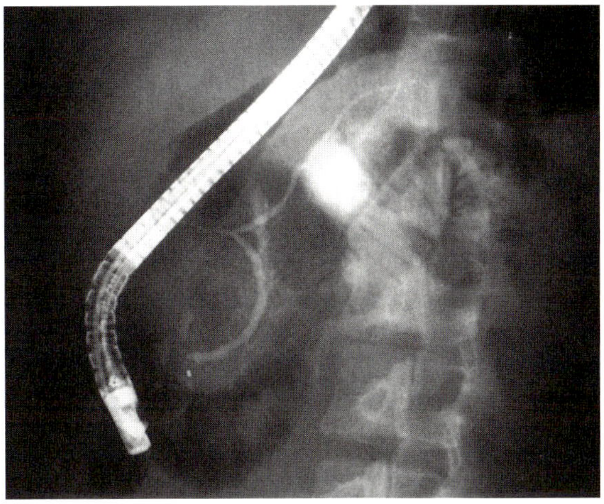

Figure 78.21

SPT (endoscopic retrograde cholangiopancreatography, ERCP). Communication of the tumor to the ductal system is absent on ERCP, and displacement of the duct may be the only finding

Metastatic liver lesions are usually solitary, and imaging findings resemble that of the original pancreatic tumor. Local recurrence of the tumor 3–10 years after a potentially curative operation is also reported [104].

Imaging studies of SPTs

Abdominal plain X-ray film may show the tumor contour and reveal calcification or ossification attributable to the tumor in about 30% of cases. CT and US demonstrate a sharply demarcated, solid and cystic mass without any internal septation (CT Fig. 78.19; US Fig. 78.20). In accordance with the predominance of a solid and cystic component, SPTs are divided into three types: solid, mixed, and cystic types. MRI may show an inhomogeneous mass with high-intensity areas on T2-weighted images, corresponding to the cystic component of the tumor. Communication of the tumor to the ductal system is absent on ERCP (Fig. 78.21), and displacement of the duct may be the only findings. Angiography may depict a hypo- to mildly hypervascular mass that displaces the surrounding vessels. Encasement or obstruction of the vessels is not seen [103].

Differential Diagnosis

In typical situations, it is not difficult to make diagnosis of SPT because of its predominance in young women and specific imaging findings. In a solid type of SPT, islet cell tumors or solid pancreatic tumors should be differentiated. It is sometimes difficult because the monomorphous appearance of endocrine cell tumors really resembles the solid component of SPTs. It may be of help that endocrine tumors usually lack widespread hemorrhagic-degenerative changes, while these are common in SPTs, resulting in the pseudopapillary pattern associated with this tumor.

Acinar cell carcinoma should also be differentiated, but it develops more frequently in men aged over 50 years of age.

When an SPT is found in children less than 10 years of age, it should be distinguished from pancreatoblastoma. Pancreatoblastoma is predominantly seen in boys, in contrast to SPTs, which occur predominantly in girls. Serum alpha fetoprotein levels are reportedly elevated in 70% of pancreatoblastoma cases.

Surgical Treatment and Prognosis

SPTs should be resected surgically in consideration of its malignant potential. Pancreatectomy is performed according to the tumor location. After a complete tumor removal, more than 95% patients are cured [103]. Long disease-free periods have been reported after surgery even in patients with tumors with local spread or metastasis. Only a few cases of death as a result of malignant SPT have been reported [110].

References

1. Papavramidis T, Papavramidis S (2005) Solid pseudopapillary tumors of the pancreas: review of 718 patients reported in English literature. J Am Coll Surg 200:965–972
2. Tanaka M, Kobayashi K, Mizumoto K, Yamaguchi K (2005) Clinical aspects of intraductal papillary mucinous neoplasm of the pancreas. J Gastroenterol 40:669–675
3. Conlon KC (2005) Intraductal papillary mucinous tumors of the pancreas. J Clin Oncol 23:4518–4523
4. Kosmahl M, Pauser U, Anlauf M, Sipos B, Peters K, Luttges J, Kloppel G (2005) Cystic pancreas tumors and their classification: features old and new. Pathologe 26:22–30
5. Compagno J, Oertel JE (1978) Microcystic adenomas of the pancreas (glycogen-rich cystadenoma): a clinicopathologic study of 34 cases. Am J Clin Pathol 69:289–298
6. Compagno J, Oertel JE (1978) Mucinous cystic neoplasms of the pancreas with overt and latent malignancy (cystadenocarcinoma and cystadenoma). A clinicopathologic study of 41 cases. Am J Clin Pathol 69:573–580
7. Fernandez-del Castillo C, Warshaw AL (1995) Cystic tumors of the pancreas. Surg Clin North Am 75:1001–1016
8. Sarr MG, Murr M, Smyrk TC, Yeo CJ, Fernandez-del Castillo C, Hawes RH, Freeny PC (2003) Primary cystic neoplasms of the pancreas. Neoplastic disorders of emerging importance-current state-of-the-art and unanswered questions. J Gastrointest Surg 7:417–428
9. Thompson LDR, Becker RC, Prygodzki RM, Adair CF, Heffess CS (1999) Mucinous cystic neoplasm (mucinous cystadenocarcinoma of low-grade malignant potential) of the pancreas. Am J Pathol 23:1–16
10. Wheeler DA, Edmondson HA (1985) Cystadenoma with mesenchymal stroma (CMS) in the liver and bile ducts. A clinicopathologic study of 17 cases, 4 with malignant change. Cancer 56:1434–1445
11. Ishak KG, Willis GW, Cummins SD, Bullock AA (1977) Biliary cystadenoma and cystadenocarcinoma: report of 14 cases and review of the literature. Cancer 38:322–328
12. Akwari OE, Tucker A, Seilger HF, Itani KM (1990) Hepatobiliary cystadenoma with mesenchymal stroma. Ann Surg 211:18–27
13. Hodgikinson DJ, ReMine WH, Weland LH (1978) Clinicopathologic study of 21 cases of pancreatic cystadenocarcinoma. Ann Surg 188:679–684
14. Suzuki Y, Atomi Y, Sugiyama M, Isaji S, Inui K, Kimura W, Sunamura M, Furukawa T, Yanagisawa A, Ariyama J, Takada T, Watanabe H, Suda K (2004) Cystic neoplasm of the pancreas. A Japanese multi-institutional study of intraductal papillary mucinous tumor and mucinous cystic tumor. Pancreas 28:241–246
15. Yamaguchi K, Enjoji M (1987) Cystic neoplasms of the pancreas. Gastroenterology 92:1934–1943
16. Albores-Saavedra J, Angeles-Angeles A, Nadji M, Henson DE, Alvarez L (1987) Mucinous cystadenocarcinoma of the pancreas. Morphologic and immunohistochemical observations. Am J Surg Pathol 11:11–20
17. Ito Y, Blackstone MO, Frank PH, Skinner DB (1977) Mucinous biliary obstruction associated with a cystic adenocarcinoma of the pancreas. Gastroenterology 73:1410–1412
18. Morinaga S, Ohyama R, Koizumi J (1992) Low grade mucinous cystadenocarcinoma in the spleen. Am J Surg Pathol 16:903–908
19. Ohashi K, Takagi K (1980) ERCP and imaging diagnosis of pancreatic cancer (in Japanese). Gastrointestinal Endosc 77:1493–1495
20. Friedman AC, Lichtenstein JE, Dachman AH (1983) Cystic neoplasm of the pancreas. Radiological-pathological correlation. Radiology 149:45–50
21. Yamaguchi K, Hirakata R, Kitamura K (1990) Mucinous cystic neoplasm of the pancreas: radiological and pathological characteristics in 11 cases. Br J Surg 70:1000–1003
22. Mathieu D, Guigui B, Valette PJ, Dao TH, Bruneton JN, Bruel JM, Pringot J, Vasile N (1989) Pancreatic cystic neoplasms. Radiol Clin North Am 27:163–176
23. Warshaw AL, Compton CC, Lewandrowski K, Cardenosa G, Mueller PR (1990) Cystic tumors of the pancreas: new clinical, radiologic, and pathologic observations in 67 patients. Ann Surg 212:432–445
24. Tatsuta M, Ishii H, Ichii M, Noguchi S, Yamamoto R, Yamamura H, Okuda S (1986) Values of carcinoembryonic antigen, elastase I, and carbohydrate antigen determinant in aspirated pancreatic cyst fluid in the diagnosis of cysts of the pancreas. Cancer 57:1836–1839
25. Yang JM, Lee J, Southern JF, Warshaw AL, Dhanak E, Lewandroski KB (1998) Measurement of pS2 protein in pancreatic cyst fluid. Evidence of a potential role of pS2 protein in the pathogenesis of mucinous cystic tumors. Int J Pancreatol 24:181–186
26. Sugiyama M, Atomi Y, Kuroda A (1997) Two types of mucin-producing cystic tumors of the pancreas: diagnosis and treatment. Surgery 122:617–625

27. Becker WF, Welsh RA, Pratt HS (1965) Cystadenoma and cystadenocarcinoma of the pancreas. Ann Surg 161:845–863
28. Warren KW, Hardy KJ (1968) Cystadenoma of the pancreas. Surg Gynecol Obstet 127:734–736
29. ReMine FG, Frey D, Rossi RL, Mazzoleni G, Campione O, Marrano D (1987) Cystic neoplasms of the pancreas. Arch Surg 122:443–446
30. Warshaw AL, Rutledge PL (1987) Cystic tumors mistaken for pancreatic pseudocysts. Ann Surg 205:393–398
31. Ohashi K, Murakami Y, Maruyama M (1982) Four cases of mucin-producing cancer of the pancreas on specific findings of the papilla of Vater (in Japanese). Prog Digest Endosc 20:348–351
32. Itai Y, Ohashi K, Nagai H, Murakami Y, Kokubo T, Makita K, Ohtomo K (1986) "Ductectatic" mucinous cystadenoma and cystadenocarcinoma of the pancreas. Radiology 161:697–700
33. Morohoshi T, Kanda M, Asanuma K, Klopel G (1986) Intraductal papillary neoplasms of the pancreas. Radiology 161:697–700
34. Agostini S, Choux R, Payan MJ, Sastre B, Sahel J, Clement JP (1989) Mucinous pancreatic duct ectasia in the body of the pancreas. Radiology 170:815–816
35. Rickaert F, Cremer M, Deviere J, Tavares L, Lambilliotte JP, Schroder S, Wurbs D, Kloppel G (1991) Intraductal mucin-hypersecreting neoplasms of the pancreas. A clinicopathologic study of eight patients. Gastroenterology 101:512–519
36. Yamaguchi Y, Tanaka M (1991) Mucin-hypersecreting tumor of the pancreas with mucin extrusion through an enlarged papilla. Am J Gastroenterol 86:835–839
37. Obara T, Maguchi H, Saitoh Y, Ura H, Koike Y, Kitazawa S, Namiki M (1991) Mucin-producing tumor of the pancreas: a unique clinical entity. Am J Gastroenterol 86:1619–1625
38. Yamada M, Kazika S, Yamao K, Nakazawa S, Naitoh Y, Tsukamoto Y (1991) Mucin-producing tumor of the pancreas. Cancer 68:159–168
39. Bastid C, Bernard P, Sarles H, Payan MJ, Sahel J (1991) Mucinous ductal ectasia of the pancreas: a premalignant disease and a cause of obstructive pancreatitis. Pancreas 6:15–22
40. Kawarada Y, Yano T, Yokoi H, Maruyama T, Nakano T, Mizumoto R (1992) Mucin-producing cystic adenocarcinoma of the pancreas a case report, 7 year follow-up period. Hepatogastroenterology 39:478–480
41. Kawarada Y, Yano T, Yamamoto T, Yokoi H, Imai T, Ogura Y, Mizumoto R (1992) Intraductal mucin-producing tumors of the pancreas. Am J Gastroenterol 87:634–638
42. Obara T, Saitoh Y, Maguchi H, Ura H, Yokota K, Okamura K, Namiki M (1992) Papillary adenoma of the pancreas with excessive mucin secretion. Pancreas 7:114–117
43. Kojima Y, Akiyama T, Saitoh H, Kosaka T, Kita I, Takashima S, Kinami Y, Konishi F, Matsunou H (1993) Multifocal intraductal papillary adenocarcinoma of the pancreas: report of a case. Surg Today 23:471–475
44. Yanagisawa A, Ohashi K, Hori M, Takagi K, Kitagawa T, Sugano H, Kato Y (1993) Ductectatic-type mucinous cystadenomas and cystadenocarcinoma of the human pancreas: a novel clinicopathological entity. Jpn J Cancer Res 84:474–479
45. Lichtenstein JR, Carr-Locke DL (1995) Mucin-secreting tumors of the pancreas Gastrointest Endosc Clin North Am 5:237–258
46. Shyr YM, Su CH, Tsay SH, Lui WY (1996) Mucin-producing neoplasms of the pancreas. Intraductal papillary and mucinous cystic neoplasms. Ann Surg 223:141–146
47. Ferrari BT, O'Halloran RL, Longmire WP Jr, Lewin KJ (1979) Atypical papillary hyperplasia the duct mimicking obstructing pancreatic carcinoma. N Engl J Med 301:531–530
48. Obara T, Saitoh Y, Maguchi H, Ura H, Kitazawa S, Koike Y, Okamura K, Namiki M (1992) Multicentric development of pancreatic intraductal carcinoma through atypical papillary hyperplasia. Hum Pathol 23:82–85
49. Shimizu M, Itoh H, Okumura S, Hashimoto K, Hanioka K, Ohyanagi H, Yamamoto M, Kuroda Y, Tanaka T, Saitoh Y (1989) Papillary hyperplasia of the pancreas. Hum Pathol 20:806–807
50. Smith RC, Kreale K, Goulston K (1986) In situ carcinoma of the pancreas. Aust NZ J Surg 56:369–373
51. Mizumoto K, Inagaki K, Kizumi M, Uemura M, Ogawa M, Kitazawa S, Tsutsumi M, Toyokawa M, Konishi Y (1988) Early pancreatic adenocarcinoma. Hum Pathol 19:242–244
52. Conley CR, Scheithauer BW, Weiland LH, van Heerden JA (1987) Diffuse intraductal papillary adenocarcinoma of the pancreas. Ann Surg 205:246–249
53. Loeler B, Koeler G, Rieman J (1990) Pancreoscopic diagnosis of inraductal cystadenoma of the pancreas. Dig Dis Sci 35:382–384
54. Nicki NJ, Lawson JM Cotton PB (1991) Mucinous pancreatic tumors: ERCP findings. Gastrointest Endosc 37:133–138
55. Yamaguchi K, Ogawa Y, Chiziiwa K Tanaka M (1996) Mucin-hypersecreting tumors of the pancreas: assessing the grade of malignancy preoperatively. Am J Surg 171:427–431
56. Yamao K, Nakazawa S, Naito Y, Kimoto E, Morita K, Inui K, Ohnuma T, Funakawa T, Hayashi Y (1986) Clinicopathological study of mucus-producing pancreatic tumors. Jpn J Gastroenterol 83:2588–2597
57. Yamaguchi K, Chijiiwa K, Shimizu Y, Yokohata K, Tanaka M (1999) Intraductal papillary neoplasms of the pancreas: a clinical review of 13 benign and four malignant conditions. Eur J Surg 165:223–229
58. Morohoshi T, Kanda M, Asanuma M, Kloppel G (1989) Intraductal papillary neoplasms of the pancreas. A clinicopathologic study of six patients. Cancer 64:1329–1335
59. Kato Y, Yanagisawa A (1986) Mucus producing carcinoma of the pancreas. Its concept and classification (in Japanese). Tan to Sui 7:731–737
60. Sessa F, Solcia E, Capella C, Bonato M, Scarpa A, Zamboni G, Pellegata NS, Razani GN, Rickaert F, Kloeppel G (1994) Intraductal papillary-mucinous tumors represent a distinct group of pancreatic neoplasms: an investigation of tumor cell differentiation and K-ras, p53 and c-erbB2 abnormalities in 26 patients. Virchows Arch Pathol Anat 425:357–367
61. Furukawa T, Takahashi T, Kobari M, Matsuno S (1992) The mucin-hypersecreting tumor of the pancreas. Development and extension visualized by three-dimensional computerized mapping. Cancer 70:1505–1513
62. Milchgrub S, Campuzano M, Casillas J, Albores-Saaverdra J (1992) Intraductal carcinoma of the pancreas. Cancer 69:651–656
63. Furuta K, Watanabe H, Ikeda S (1992) Differences between solid and duct-ectatic types of pancreatic duct carcinomas Cancer 69:1327–1333
64. Yamada , Kozuka S, Yamao K, Nakazawa S, Naitoh Y, Tsukamoto Y (1991) Mucin-producing tumor of the pancreas. Cancer 68:159–168

65. Sugiyama M, Izumisato Y, Abe N, Masaki T, Mori T, Atomi Y (2003) Predictive factors for malignancy in intraductal papillary-mucinous tumours of the pancreas. Br J Surg 90:1244–1249
66. Takahashi H, Oda T, Hasebe T, Aoyagi Y, Kinoshita T, Konishi M, Nakagohri T, Inoue K, Takahashi S, Kawahira H, Monden M, Ochiai A (2004) Biologically different subgroups of invasive ductal carcinoma of the pancreas: Dpc4 status according to the ratio of intraductal carcinoma components. Clin Cancer Res 10:3772–3779
67. Sohn TA, Yeo CJ, Cameron JL, Hruban RH, Fukushima N, Campbell KA, Lillemoe KD (2004) Intraductal papillary mucinous neoplasms of the pancreas: an updated experience. Ann Surg 239:788–797
68. Kamisawa T, Fujiwara T, Tu Y, Egawa N, Tanaka T, Sakai N, Funata N, Koike M (2002) Long-term follow-up of intraductal papillary adenoma of the pancreas. J Gastroenterol 37:868–873
69. Morohashi T, Held G, Kloppel G (1983) Exocrine pancreatic tumours and their histological classification. A study based on 167 autopsy and 97 surgical cases. Histopathology 7:645–661
70. Compton CC (2000) Serous cystic tumors of the pancreas. Semin Diagn Pathol 17:43–55
71. George DH, Murphy F, Michalski R, Ulmer BG (1989) Serous cystadenocarcinoma of the pancreas: a new entity? Am J Surg Pathol 13:61–66
72. Friedman HD (1990) Nonmucinous, glycogen-poor cystadenocarcinoma of the pancreas. Arch Pathol Lab Med 114:888–891
73. Okada T, Nonami T, Miwa T, Yamada F, Ando K, Tatematsu A, Sugie S, Kondo T (1991) Hepatic metastasis of serous cystadenocarcinoma resected 4 years after operation of primary tumors – a case report. Nippon Shokakibyo Gakkai Zasshi 88:283–289
74. Kamei K, Funabiki T, Ochiai M, Amano H, Kasahara M, Sakamoto T (1991) Multifocal pancreatic serous cystadenoma with atypical cells and focal perineural invasion. Int J Pancreatol 10:161–172
75. Yoshimi N, Sugie S, Tanaka T, Aijin W, Bunai Y, Tatematsu A, Okada T, Mori H (1992) A rare case of serous cystadenocarcinoma of the pancreas. Cancer 69:2449–2453
76. Ohta T, Nagakawa T, Itoh H, Fonsecal L, Miyazaki I, Terada T (1993) A case of serous cystadenocarcinoma of the pancreas with focal malignant changes. Int J Pancreatol 14:283–289
77. Widmaier U, Mattfeldt T, Siech M, Beger HG (1996) Serous cystadenocarcinoma of the pancreas. Int J Pancreatol 20:135–139
78. Eriguchi N, Aoyagi S, Nakayama T, Hara M, Miyazaki T, Kutami R, Jimi A (1998) Serous cystadenocarcinoma of the pancreas with liver metastases. J Hepatobiliary Pancreat Surg 5:467–470
79. Abe H, Kubota K, Mori M, Miki K, Minagawa M, Noie T, Kimura W, Makuuchi M (1998) Serous cystadenoma of the pancreas with invasive growth: benign or malignant? Am J Gastroenterol 93:1963–1966
80. Ishikawa T, Nakao A, Nomoto S, Hosono J, Harada A, Nonami T, Takagi H (1998) Immunohistochemical and molecular biological studies of serous cystadenoma of the pancreas. Pancreas 16:40–44
81. Siech M, Tripp K, Schmidt-Rohlfing B, Mattfeldt T, Widmaier U, Gansauge F, Gorich J, Beger HG (1998) Cystic tumours of the pancreas: diagnostic accuracy, pathologic observations and surgical consequences. Langenbecks Arch Surg 383:56–61
82. Wu CM, Fishman EK, Hruban RK, Schlott WD, Cameron JL (1999) Serous cystic neoplasm involving the pancreas and liver: an unusual clinical entity. Abdom Imaging 24:75–77
83. Kimura W, Makuuchi M (1999) Operative indications for cystic lesions of the pancreas with malignant potential – our experience. Hepatogastroenterology 46:483–491
84. Horvath KD, Chabot JA (1999) An aggressive resectional approach to cystic neoplasms of the pancreas. Am J Surg 178:269–274
85. Schmidt-Rohlfing B, Siech M, Mattfeldt T, Schoenberg MH, Beger HG (1998) Cystic neoplasms of the pancreas: surgical therapy and chances for cure. Z Gastroenterol 36:939–945
86. Strobel O, Z'graggen K, Schmitz-Winnenthal FH, Friess H, Kappeler A, Zimmermann A, Uhl W, Buchler MW (2003) Risk of malignancy in serous cystic neoplasms of the pancreas. Digestion 68:24–33
87. Friebe V, Keck T, Mattern D, Schmitt-Graeff A, Werner M, Mikami Y, Adam U, Hopt UT (2005) Serous cystadenocarcinoma of the pancreas: management of a rare entity. Pancreas 31:182–187
88. Matsumoto T, Hirano S, Yada K, Shibata K, Sasaki A, Kamimura T, Ohta M, Kitano S, Kashima K (2005) Malignant serous cystic neoplasm of the pancreas: report of a case and review of the literature. J Clin Gastroenterol 39:253–256
89. Shintaku M, Arimoto A, Sakita N (2005) Serous cystadenocarcinoma of the pancreas. Pathol Int 55:436–439
90. Klöppel G, Solcia E, Longnecker DS, Capella C, Sobin LH (1996) Histological Typing of Tumors of the Exocrine Pancreas. In: Jass JR, Sobin LH (eds) World Health Organization International Histological Classification of Tumours (2nd edition). Springer-Verlag, Berlin, pp 1–61
91. Lewandrowski K, Warshaw A, Compton C (1992) Macrocystic serous cystadenoma of the pancreas: a morphologic variant differing from microcystic adenoma. Hum Pathol 23:871–875
92. Tseng JF, Warshaw AL, Sahani DV, Lauwers GY, Rattner DW, Fernandez-del Castillo C (2005) Serous cystadenoma of the pancreas. Tumor growth rates and recommendations for treatment. Ann Surg 242:413–421
93. Perez-Ordonez B, Naseem A, Lieberman PH, Klimstra DS (1996) Solid serous adenoma of the pancreas. The solid variant of serous cystadenoma? Am J Surg Pathol 20:1401–1405
94. Goldsmith JD (2003) Cystic neoplasms of the pancreas. Am J Clin Pathol 119:3–16
95. Bassi C, Salvia R, Molinari E, Biasutti C, Falconi M, Pederzoli P (2003) Management of 100 consecutive cases of pancreatic serous cystadenoma: wait for symptoms and see at imaging or vice versa? World J Surg 27:319–323
96. Franz VK (1959) Tumors of the pancreas. In: Stout AP (ed) Atlas of Tumor Pathology, Section VII, Fascicles 27 and 28, 1st series. Armed Forces Institute of Pathology, Washington DC, pp 32–33
97. Nanson EM (1945) An unusual case of carcinoma of the pancreas. Br J Surg 41:439–441
98. Frable WJ, Still WJS, Kay S (1971) Carcinoma of the pancreas. Infantile type. A light and electron microscopic study. Cancer 27:667–673
99. Taxy JB (1976) Adenocarcinoma of the pancreas in childhood. Report of a case and a review of the English literature. Cancer 37:1508–1518
100. Boor PJ, Swanson MR (1979) Papillary-cystic neoplasm of the pancreas. Am J Pathol 3:69–75

101. Benjamin E, Wright DH (1980) Adenocarcinoma of the pancreas of childhood: a report of two cases. Histopathology 4:87–104
102. Kloppel G, Morohoshi T, John HD, Oehmichen W, Opitz K, Angekort A, Lietz H, Ruckert K (1981) Solid and cystic acinar cell tumour of the pancreas. A tumour in young women with favorable prognosis. Virchows Arch A Pathol Anat Histol 392:171–183
103. Papavramidis T, Papavramidis S (2005) Solid pseudopapillary tumors of the pancreas: review of 718 patients reported in English literature. J Am Coll Surg 200:965–972
104. Solcia E, Capella C, Kloppel G (1997) Tumors of the pancreas. In: Rosai J (ed) Atlas of Tumor Pathology. Fascicle 20, 3rd Series. Armed Forces Institute of Pathology, Washington DC, pp 1–262
105. Compagno J, Oertel JE, Kremzar M (1979) Solid and papillary epithelial neoplasm of the pancreas. Lab Invest 40:248–249
106. Nishihara K, Nagoshi M, Tsuneyoshi M, Yamaguchi K, Hayashi I (1993) Papillary cystic tumors of the pancreas. Assessment of their grade of malignant potential. Cancer 70:82–92
107. Ladanyi M, Mulay S, Areneau J, Bettez P (1987) Estrogen and progesterone receptor determination in the papillary cystic neoplasm of the pancreas. Cancer 60:1604–1611
108. Morales A, Ruiz Molina JM, Esteves HE, Robles-Diaz G, Diaz Sanches V (1998) Papillary-cystic neoplasm of the pancreas. A sex-steroid dependent tumor Int J Pancreatol 24:219–225
109. Mao C, Guvendi M, Domenico DR, Kim K, Thomford NR, Howard JM (1995) Papillary cystic and solid tumors of the pancreas. A pancreatic embryonic tumor? Studies of three cases and cumulative review of word literature. Surgery 118:821–828
110. Matsunou H, Konishi F (1990) papillary-cystic neoplasm of the pancreas. A clinicopathologic study concerning the tumor aging and malignancy of nine cases. Cancer 65:283–291

Section 10

Congenital Anomalies of the Pancreas

Chapter 79 Congenital Cysts: Diagnosis, Clinical Impact, and Management *873*
G. Klöppel, H. D. Saeger

Chapter 80 Pancreas Divisum – Diagnosis and Endoscopic Management *881*
N. Soehendra, T. L. Ang, Y. Zhong, S. Seewald

Chapter 81 Surgical Treatment of Pancreas Divisum *891*
H. G. Beger, P. Poch

Chapter 82 Biliopancreatic Maljunction: Classification, Diagnosis, and Treatment *895*
T. Onogawa, T. Rikiyama, M. Unno, S. Matsuno

Chapter 79

G. Klöppel · H. D. Saeger

Congenital Cysts: Diagnosis, Clinical Impact, and Management

Cystic lesions in the pancreas differ very much in origin. As a result of their improved recognition by modern imaging techniques and their successful and uncomplicated surgical treatment, they increasingly occupy gastroenterologists, surgeons, and pathologists, although their incidence is low. The identification and definition of pancreatic cysts has improved, however 5–10% of these lesions still remain undiagnosed prior to surgical intervention and assessment by the pathologist. The final diagnosis is not trivial or only of scientific interest, because of the major problem underlying all of these lesions, that of ruling out malignancy. The uncertainty related to cystic lesions for which all available preoperative diagnostic procedures have failed to definitely rule out the suspicion of cancer usually makes resection necessary. Of course, surgical or invasive treatment is obviously called for if symptoms or complications such as severe pain, intestinal obstruction or infection potentially leading to abscess formation or sepsis are present.

These considerations relating to cystic lesions of the pancreas are also valid for congenital cysts. Only few of them can be diagnosed and specifically classified pre- or intraoperatively. Mechanical complications are not uncommon with these lesions. Regarding the decision whether to operate or to wait and watch, it is extremely valuable to know all about these lesions, their nature, and their potential for complications.

Classification

For practical purposes cystic neoplasms and lesions of the pancreas need to have a classification system of their own. A classification system has recently been proposed that has both morphological and biological relevance and includes all new entities [1].

The most common cystic neoplasms of the pancreas are intraductal papillary mucinous neoplasms [2–4], mucinous cystic neoplasms [5], serous cystic neoplasms [1], and solid pseudopapillary neoplasms [6]. Whereas the vast majority of serous cystic neoplasms and solid pseudopapillary neoplasms are benign, mucinous cystic neoplasms and intraductal papillary mucinous neoplasms have a malignant potential and may be associated with invasive carcinomas. Apart from these cystic neoplasms, there are a several rare entities, which include the so-called congenital cysts.

Congenital cysts are by definition already present at birth, if not morphologically, at least genetically. According to this definition, the following cystic changes of the pancreas may be discussed under the term congenital cyst: solitary cysts in infants, cysts found in association with genetic syndromes such as Von Hippel-Lindau syndrome (VHL) and Gruber-Meckel syndrome, enterogenous cysts (foregut cysts, duplication cyst), cystic transformation of acini (so-called acinar cell cystadenoma), lymphoepithelial cysts, and dermoid cysts. Some other rare cystic changes of the pancreas such as paraduodenal wall cysts, mucinous nonneoplastic cysts, endometrial cysts, and cystic hamartomas, which might also have a congenital background, are also included in this chapter.

Solitary Cysts in Infants

There are several reports on children who presented with single, sometimes large cysts that were unassociated with cystic lesions in other organs [7–13]. Neither were they associated with any malformation syndrome. The cysts were several centimeters in diameter, unilocular, and lined by a columnar or cuboidal epithelium (Fig. 79.1). A few, however, that had the appearance of serous cystadenomas have been described in association with cytomegalovirus infection [14, 15].

The symptoms resulting from these cysts are usually related to compression of adjacent structures. Because these cysts usually show no communication with the duct system of the pancreas, excision is the treatment of choice.

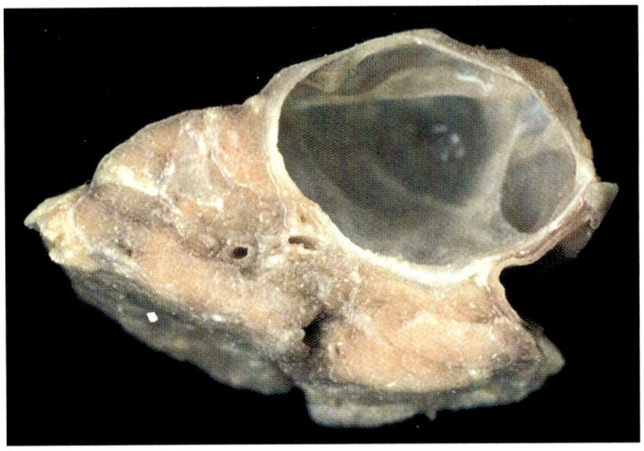

Figure 79.1

Congenital cyst of the pancreas: pancreatic tissue with a peripheral thin-walled solitary cyst

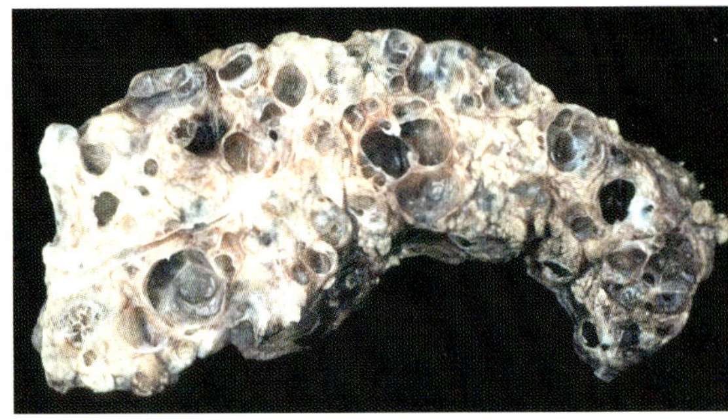

Figure 79.2

Multiple cysts in a left-sided resection specimen from a patient with von Hippel-Lindau disease

VHL-Associated Serous Cystic Lesions and Neoplasms

The pancreas of VHL patients commonly (15–75%) exhibits multiple serous cysts distributed randomly in the organ (Fig. 79.2). Some patients may have focal aggregates of cysts that resemble serous cystic adenoma in non-VHL patients [16, 17]. These cystic lesions and neoplasms are closely related to serous microcystic adenomas and serous oligocystic and ill-demarcated adenomas [18]. All of these tumors are composed of the same cell type, a cuboidal or flattened epithelial cell with pale to clear cytoplasm and a small oval nucleus. The cells produce serous fluid and lack any signs of cellular atypia. A single layer of these cells lines the cysts. Immunohistochemically, they stain for cytokeratin [7, 11, 19, 20], alpha-inhibin, MUC6, and usually also for neuron-specific enolase (NSE) [21].

In addition to cystic changes VHL patients may develop pancreatic endocrine neoplasms that typically show a clear cell cytology and are nonfunctioning [16, 22]. Because of obstruction of adjacent structures and/or the presence of associated endocrine neoplasms, selected VHL patients may require specific treatment.

Malformation Syndromes

Cystic dysplasia of the pancreas is found in several malformation syndromes such as Meckel-Gruber syndrome, trisomy 13, tuberous sclerosis, asphyxiating thoracic dysplasia, short-rib polydactyly syndrome, and, very rarely, polycystic kidney disease [11, 19, 23, 24].

Acinar Cystic Transformation (So-Called Acinar Cell Cystadenoma)

This is a usually multiloculated cystic change of the pancreas that may form a cystic tumor (without a preferential localization) or diffusely involve the gland (Fig. 79.3) [25]. The size of the single cysts varies considerably, ranging from a few millimeters to several centimeters. They contain watery fluid. The single cysts seem to develop from single acini and are therefore lined by normal-appearing flattened acinar cells. These acinar cells stain for trypsin and also express cytokeratin 7, in contrast to the surrounding normal acinar cells, which only stain for cytokeratins 8 and 18. The lining cells of the cysts are negative for alpha-inhibin, NSE, carcinoembryonic antigen, synaptophysin, and vimentin. Cellular atypia and increased proliferative activity are lacking.

These lesions are rare. Children (G.K. personal observation) as well as adults may be affected. There is no gender predilection. The symptoms are unspecific and related to the expansion of the cysts. So far, follow-up in these patients did not reveal any malignant change [25].

The pathogenesis of this peculiar cystic change of the pancreas is not known. The name acinar cystic transformation denotes that it might be an alteration of the microarchitecture of the pancreas that results in cyst formation. However, because a neoplastic cause of the lesion can yet not be excluded, the term acinar cell cystadenoma is also appropriate [25]. In the absence of compression of adjacent structures, the lesion requires no treatment.

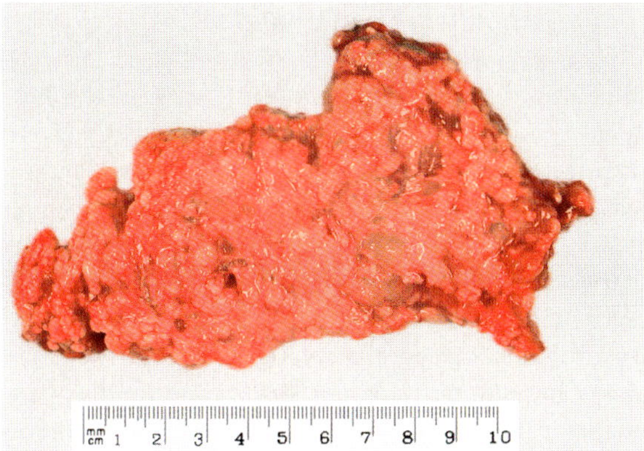

Figure 79.3

Acinar cystic transformation (acinar cell cystadenoma): multiple scattered cysts in the pancreatic parenchyma

Dermoid and Epidermoid Cysts

Dermoid cysts are monodermal teratomas. Only few examples have been observed in the pancreas [26]. These cysts are often more retroperitoneal than pancreatic. They are well-circumscribed cystic and also solid masses, the cysts often containing hair and the solid parts calcifications. Microscopically, they show a squamous lining and sebaceous differentiation; occasionally also columnar mucinous epithelium and respiratory-type mucosa. Malignant changes are lacking.

Clinically, patients, who are generally young (mean age 29 years), present with abdominal and back pain and sometimes vomiting. There is no gender predilection. Complete resection of the cystic mass is the treatment of choice.

An epidermoid cyst may occur in an intrapancreatic accessory spleen, which are mostly located in the tail of the pancreas [26, 27]. The squamous-lined cysts are surrounded by splenic tissue that has to be distinguished from the lymphoid tissue in lymphoepithelial cysts.

Enterogenous Cysts (Ciliated Foregut Cysts and Duplication Cysts)

The term "enterogenous cysts" usually includes ciliated foregut cysts as well as (enteric) duplication cysts. Ciliated foregut cysts can occur at various sites such as the tracheobronchial tree, the esophagus, and the liver. They occur only exceedingly rarely in the pancreas, where they seem to occur in the tail [28–30]. They are lined by ciliated columnar epithelium, as it occurs in the fetal esophagus from the 10th to the 20th week of gestation. An origin from a detached remnant of the pancreatic outpouching of the embryonic foregut is discussed.

Duplications are more common and are mostly found in young children of both genders [31, 32]. They occur in any portion of the gastrointestinal tract, including the duodenum, and usually contain the epithelium of the intestine supported by a bilayer of smooth muscle cells. The duplication cysts present either as cystic lesions within the wall of the original bowel or hang free as a pedunculated structure. Duplication cysts of the pancreas may be included in the parenchyma of the head–body region. The size of the often unilocular cystic lesions varies from 2 to 7 cm. The cysts contain clear-to-reddish brown fluid or thick mucinous material. Microscopically, the mucosal lining resembles that of the duodenum or any other gastrointestinal structure.

Clinically, patients may suffer from nausea and vomiting due to partial duodenal obstruction. In children, a large palpable mass may be identified that may cause pancreatitis [11, 33, 34]. The treatment of choice is a resection of the mass.

The cause of the enterogenous cysts is probably that the foregut-derived multipotential epithelium of early embryogenesis persists at sites where it is normally replaced by the topospecific cells that form the later organs.

Lymphoepithelial Cysts

Lymphoepithelial cysts are uncommon [35]. They are multilocular or unilocular and may be located in any part of the pancreas; some are attached to its surface. They are well delineated from the pancreatic parenchyma and their size ranges from 1 to several centimeters (mean 4 cm). The cyst content is caseous. Microscopically, the lymphoepithelial cysts are lined by stratified squamous epithelium that is supported by a band of dense lymphoid tissue, which often contains germinal centers (Fig. 79.4). Immunohistochemically, the bulk of lymphoid cells are T-cells, with lymphoid cells populating the follicles.

Clinically, most patients are men between 40 and 70 years of age. They may complain about epigastric pain, but some lesions are detected incidentally. Simple resection is the treatment of choice.

Pathogenetically, the development of lymphoepithelial cysts probably shares the same mechanisms that underlie the development of branchial cleft cysts and Warthin's tumors, since the latter lesions have a similar, if not identical morphology. One mechanism

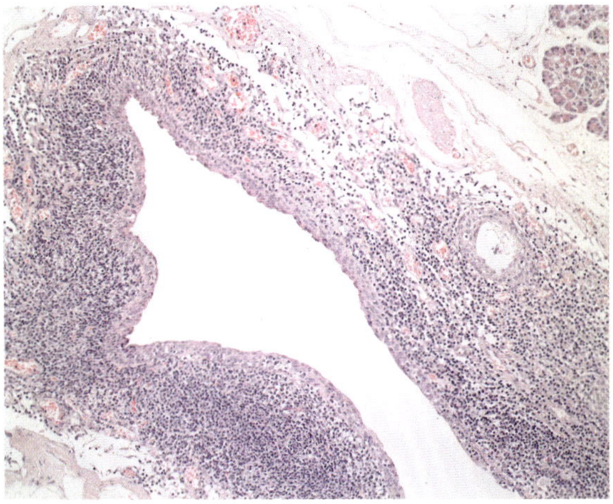

Figure 79.4

Lymphoepithelial cyst: squamous-lined cyst with a well-defined rim of lymphoid tissue

is the development from epithelial remnants in lymph nodes. A more modern view is that these lesions are the result of an interplay of lymphoid cells and ductal epithelia to which these lymphocytes are attracted [35].

Mucinous Nonneoplastic Cysts

Mucinous nonneoplastic cysts occur mainly in the head region of the pancreas [36]. The size of the cysts varies from 3 to 12 cm. They do not communicate with the duct system. Microscopically, the cysts are lined with columnar or flat mucin-producing epithelial cells without atypia, which are supported by a small rim of almost cellular connective tissue. Immunohistochemically, they are positive for cytokeratins, Ca 19-9 and MUC5AC. There has been no report of malignant transformation (mean follow-up period 2 years) [36].

Clinically, the lesions occur in men and women alike (mean age 58 years). Patients may present with obstructive jaundice caused by compression and dislocation of the common bile duct by the cystic lesion. So far, follow-up has not revealed any malignant transition. As these cystic tumors are often difficult to distinguish preoperatively from mucinous cystic neoplasms and intraductal papillary mucinous neoplasms [37], resection is required.

The pathogenesis of this cyst is not known.

Para-ampullary Duodenal Wall Cysts

Para-ampullary duodenal wall cysts occur in the duodenal submucosa and muscular layer, usually at the site of the minor papilla (Fig. 79.5) and in association with chronically inflamed pancreatic tissue. This lesion has been described under various names in the literature, which represent the different facets of this cystic and/or inflammatory change in the duodenal wall and the adjacent pancreatic tissue: cystic dystrophy of heterotopic pancreas [38], para-ampullary duodenal wall cyst [4], groove pancreatitis [39], pancreatic hamartoma of the duodenal wall [40], and, recently, paraduodenal pancreatitis [41].

Grossly, there are sieve-like cystic changes in the duodenal wall, particularly in the area corresponding to the minor papilla (Fig. 79.5), often combined with thickening and scarring of the duodenal wall that extend to the adjacent pancreatic head tissue. The cysts, the diameter of which range between 1 and several centimeters, contain clear fluid, but others may contain more granular white material and even stones. In several cases, there is only fibrotic thickening of the duodenal wall and the adjacent tissue, while cystic changes are not visible. The fibrotic tissue that develops in the wall of the pancreas and also involves the groove between the wall and the pancreatic tissue may compress and indent the common bile duct. Microscopically, the chronic inflammatory process resides in the duodenal submucosa, the duodenal wall, and the adjacent pancreatic tissue. Typically, there are several small foci of necrosis surrounded by a dense proliferation of myoid cells that show all the features of myofibroblasts and are positive for muscle markers. Between the myoid proliferations there may be cystic ductal elements, acinar lobules, some islets, and nerves. Apart from cystically dilated ducts there are often pseudocystic lesions filled with acidophilic material and lined by granulation tissue with a foreign body giant cell reaction. Occasionally, there are also clusters of eosinophils. A common finding associated with the cystic and inflammatory changes is Brunner's gland hyperplasia, which contributes to the thickening of the duodenal mucosa. If the inflammatory process in the duodenal wall extends to the adjacent pancreas, the cellular and fibrotic reaction becomes less intense so that the central parts of the pancreatic head are usually not involved.

Clinically, this particular pancreatic inflammation is found predominantly in male patients (40–50 years) with a history of alcohol abuse. The main symptoms are severe upper abdominal pain, postprandial vomiting and nausea due to stenosis of the duodenum,

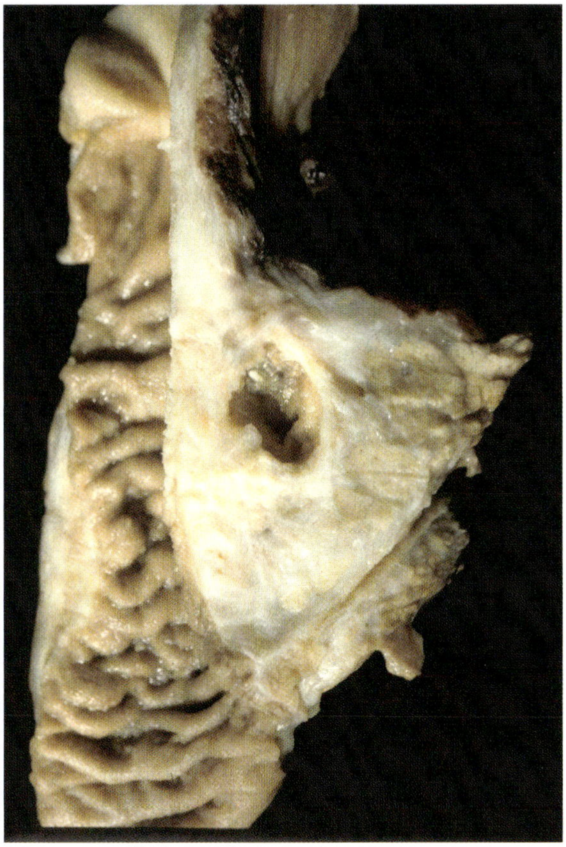

Figure 79.5

Para-ampullary duodenal wall cyst: cystic lesion in the duodenal wall with perifocal chronic pancreatitis (paraduodenal chronic pancreatitis)

and weight loss. Jaundice develops in approximately 20% of patients, suggesting pancreatic cancer. Imaging may reveal cystic changes in the duodenal wall, calcifications in the paraduodenal pancreatic tissue, pseudocysts at the duodenal wall, a tumor in the region between the duodenum and the pancreas, and irregularities in the pancreatic ducts in the head of the pancreas.

Pathogenetically, alcohol abuse appears to be a precipitating factor, since most of the patients with paraduodenal pancreatitis are alcoholics. The location of the inflammatory process suggests that there may be some anatomic variation in the region of the minor papilla that makes this appear particularly susceptible to injury by alcohol. It is therefore conceivable that the outflow is obstructed at the level of the minor papilla, as may be seen in some cases of pancreas divisum, a condition in which a fetal-type ductal drainage system persists in the adult pancreas. The fact that the duodenal wall often contains so-called heterotopic pancreatic tissue may reflect the incomplete involution of the dorsal pancreas in this region and contribute to an obstruction of outflow in this area.

Treatment is related to the most prominent changes. In cases of duodenal narrowing by large para-ampullary cysts in the duodenal submucosa, internal endoscopic cyst drainage can resolve the clinical problems. If the patient has pain and vomiting because of pseudocystic and chronic inflammatory changes of the duodenal wall, or if he develops jaundice, resection of the duodenum and the pancreatic head is necessary.

Endometrial Cysts

Endometrial cysts are a manifestation of extrauterine endometriosis. It is exceptionally rare in the pancreas [1, 42]. They have been described as single or multiple cysts (up to 5 cm in diameter) in the tail of the pancreas. The cyst wall was smooth and gray-brown, with focal areas of hemorrhage. Microscopically the cysts showed endometrial glands and stroma in the cyst wall, with extended areas of epithelial denudation, hemorrhage, and hemosiderin deposits in macrophages.

Cystic Hamartomas

These well-demarcated solid tumors show focal cystic changes with diameters of up to 10 cm. The cysts in the hamartomas show cystic ductal structures lined by cuboidal or flattened epithelium, surrounded by well-differentiated acini embedded in inflammatory fibroblast-rich or paucicellular stroma. They are accompanied by distorted and haphazardly organized small ducts, acini, and single endocrine cells embedded in fibrotic tissue. The surrounding pancreatic parenchyma displays no specific abnormalities and lacks significant chronic pancreatitis. Lesions of this kind have been described in adults [20, 43, 44] and in children [45].

Hamartomas are defined as a localized excessive overgrowth of mature normal cells and tissues in an organ composed of identical cellular elements. Although the cellular elements are mature and identical to those found in the remainder of the organ, they do not reproduce the normal architecture of the surrounding tissue. The frequency of some of these lesions in infancy and childhood gives credence to the belief that they are developmental aberrations.

Clinically, if they are young, patients may present with abdominal distension due to a mass in the pancreas. Adults usually have symptoms of abdominal discomfort. Resection is required because of the size of the lesions or the uncertainty of their nature.

References

1. Kosmahl M, Pauser U, Peters K, et al (2004) Cystic neoplasms of the pancreas and tumor-like lesions with cystic features: a review of 418 cases and a classification proposal. Virchows Arch 445:168–178
2. Adsay NV, Klimstra DS (eds) (2000) Cystic Lesions of the Pancreas. Vol. 17. Saunders, Philadelphia
3. Klöppel G (1998) Clinicopathologic view of intraductal papillary-mucinous tumor of the pancreas. Hepatogastroenterology 45:1981–1985
4. Solcia E, Capella C, Klöppel G (eds) (1997) Tumors of the Pancreas. AFIP Atlas of Tumor Pathology, third series, fascicle 20. Armed Forces Institute of Pathology, Washington, DC
5. Zamboni G, Scarpa A, Bogina G, et al (1999) Mucinous cystic tumors of the pancreas. Clinicopathological features, prognosis and relationship to other mucinous cystic tumors. Am J Surg Pathol 23:410–422
6. Klimstra DS, Wenig BM, Heffess CS (2000) Solid-pseudopapillary tumor of the pancreas: a typically cystic carcinoma of low malignant potential. Semin Diagn Pathol 17:66–80
7. Auringer ST, Ulmer JL, Sumner TE, et al (1993) Congenital cyst of the pancreas. J Pediatr Surg 28:1570–1571
8. Casadei R, Campione O, Greco VM, et al (1996) Congenital true pancreatic cysts in young adults: case report and literature review. Pancreas 12:419–421
9. Gundersen AE, Janis JF (1969) Pancreatic cystadenoma in childhood. Report of a case. J Pediatr Surg 4:478–481
10. Howard JM (1989) Cystic neoplasms and true cysts of the pancreas. Surg Clin North Am 69:651–655
11. Jaffe R (1992) The pancreas. In: Stocker JT, Dehner LP (eds) Pediatric Pathology, Vol. 2. Lippincott, Philadelphia, PA, pp 791–823
12. Mares AJ, Hirsch M (1977) Congenital cysts of the head of the pancreas. J Pediatr Surg 12:547–552
13. Olurin EO (1971) Pancreatic cysts: a report of 10 cases. Br J Surg 58:502–508
14. Amir G, Hurvitz H, Neeman Z, et al (1986) Neonatal cytomegalovirus infection with pancreatic cystadenoma and nephrotic syndrome. Pediatr Pathol 6:393–401
15. Chang CH, Perrin EV, Hertzler J, et al (1980) Cystadenoma of the pancreas with cytomegalovirus infection in a female infant. Arch Pathol Lab Med 104:7–8
16. Hammel PR, Vilgrain V, Terris B, et al (2000) Pancreatic involvement in von Hippel-Lindau disease. The Groupe Francophone d'Etude de la Maladie de von Hippel-Lindau. Gastroenterology 119:1087–1095
17. Vortmeyer AO, Lubensky IA, Fogt F, et al (1997) Allelic deletion and mutation of the von Hippel-Lindau (VHL) tumor suppressor gene in pancreatic microcystic adenomas. Am J Pathol 151:951–956
18. Kosmahl M, Klöppel G (2004) Pancreatic cystic lesions and neoplasms. In: Johnson CD, Imrie CW (eds) Pancreatic Disease. Basic Science and Clinical Management. Springer, London, pp 133–143
19. Bronstein M, Reichler A, Borochowitz Z, et al (1994) Early prenatal diagnosis of polycystic pancreas with narrow thorax and short limb dwarfism. Am J Med Genet 49:6–9
20. Izbicki JR, Knoefel WT, Müller-Höcker J, et al (1994) Pancreatic hamartoma: a benign tumor of the pancreas. Am J Gastroenterol 89:1261–1262
21. Kosmahl M, Wagner J, Peters K, et al (2004) Serous cystic neoplasms of the pancreas: an immunohistochemical analysis revealing alpha-inhibin, neuron-specific enolase, and MUC6 as new markers. Am J Surg Pathol 28:339–346
22. Lubensky IA, Pack S, Ault D, et al (1998) Multiple neuroendocrine tumors of the pancreas in von Hippel-Lindau disease patients: histopathological and molecular genetic analysis. Am J Pathol 153:223–231
23. Carles D, Serville F, Dubecq JP, et al (1988) Renal, pancreatic and hepatic dysplasia sequence. Eur J Pediatr 147:431–432
24. Milutinovic J, Schabel SI, Ainsworth SK (1989) Autosomal dominant polycystic kidney disease with liver and pancreatic involvement in early childhood. Am J Kidney Dis 4:340–344
25. Zamboni G, Terris B, Scarpa A, et al (2002) Acinar cell cystadenoma of the pancreas. A new entity? Am J Surg Pathol 26:698–704
26. Adsay NV, Hasteh F, Cheng JD, et al (2000) Squamous-lined cysts of the pancreas: lymphoepithelial cysts, dermoid cysts (teratomas) and accessory-splenic epidermoid cysts. Semin Diagn Pathol 17:56–65
27. Morohoshi T, Hamamoto T, Kunimara T, et al (1991) Epidermoid cyst derived from an accessory spleen in the pancreas. A case report with literature survey. Acta Pathol Jpn 41:916–921
28. Kohzaki S, Fukuda T, Fujimoto T, et al (1994) Case report: ciliated foregut cyst of the pancreas mimicking teratomatous tumour. Br J Radiol 67:601–604
29. Pappas S, Diaz L, Talamonti M (2002) A cystic pancreatic mass discovered in a patient with ileocecal carcinoid (pathologic quiz case). Arch Pathol Lab Med 126:229–230
30. Pilcher CS, Bradley EL III, Majmudar B (1982) Enterogenous cyst of the pancreas. Am J Gastroenterol 77:576–577
31. Ackerman NB (1974) Duodenal duplication cysts: diagnosis and operative management. Surgery 76:330–333
32. Luckmann KF, Welch RW, Schwesinger W, et al (1979) Symptomatic duodenal duplication cyst in an adult demonstrated by endoscopic retrograde cholangiopancreatography. Case report and literature review. Am J Gastroenterol 72:153–159
33. Lavine JE, Harrison M, Heyman MB (1989) Gastrointestinal duplications causing relapsing pancreatitis in children. Gastroenterology 97:1556–1558
34. Mahmood K, Butt MM, Haleem A (1989) Duplication of the duodenum exhibiting heterotopia in the pancreas: report of a case. Ann Saudi Med 9:602–604
35. Adsay NV, Hasteh F, Cheng JD, et al (2002) Lymphoepithelial cysts of the pancreas: a report of 12 cases and a review of the literature. Mod Pathol 15:492–501
36. Kosmahl M, Egawa N, Schröder S, et al (2002) Mucinous nonneoplastic cyst of the pancreas: a novel nonneoplastic cystic change? Mod Pathol 15:154–158
37. Goh BK, Tan YM, Tan PH, et al (2005) Mucinous nonneoplastic cyst of the pancreas: a truly novel pathological entity? World J Gastroenterol 11:2045–2047

38. Fléjou JF, Potet F, Molas G, et al (1993) Cystic dystrophy of the gastric and duodenal wall developing in heterotopic pancreas: an unrecognized entity. Gut 34:343–347
39. Stolte M, Weiss W, Volkholz H, et al (1982) A special form of segmental pancreatitis: "groove pancreatitis". Hepatogastroenterology 29:198–208
40. McFaul CD, Vitone LJ, Campbell F, et al (2004) Pancreatic hamartoma. Pancreatology 4:533–537
41. Adsay NV, Zamboni G (2004) Paraduodenal pancreatitis: a clinico0pathologically distinct entity unifying "cystic dystrophy of heterotopic pancreas," "paraduodenal wall cyst," and "groove pancreatitis". Semin Diagn Pathol 21:247–254
42. Marchevsky AM, Zimmerman MJ, Aufses AH Jr, et al (1984) Endometrial cyst of the pancreas. Gastroenterology 86:1589–1591
43. Pauser U, Kosmahl M, Kruslin B, et al (2005) Pancreatic solid and cystic hamartoma in adults: characterization of a new tumorous lesion. Am J Surg Pathol 29:797–800
44. Wu SS, Vargas HI, French SW (1998) Pancreatic hamartoma with Langerhans cell histiocytosis in a draining lymph node. Histopathology 33:485–487
45. Flaherty MJ, Benjamin DR (1992) Multicystic pancreatic hamartoma: a distinctive lesion with immunohistochemical and ultrastructural study. Hum Pathol 23:1309–1312

Chapter 80

N. Soehendra · T.L. Ang · Y. Zhong · S. Seewald

Pancreas Divisum – Diagnosis and Endoscopic Management

Pancreas divisum is the most common congenital variant of pancreatic ductal development. It results from the failure of fusion of the ventral and dorsal anlagen of the embryonic pancreas during organogenesis (Fig. 80.1). As a consequence, the dorsal duct drains via the minor papilla, and the short ventral duct drains the inferior portion of the head via the major papilla. It occurs in approximately 10% of individuals [1]. The frequency is lower in endoscopic retrograde cholangiopancreatography (ERCP) series (0.3–7.5%), depending on the success of minor papilla cannulation [2]. Pancreas divisum is classified into complete and incomplete forms (Fig. 80.2). In complete pancreas divisum, the anatomy consists of a small ventral duct, which drains through the major papilla, and the larger dorsal duct, which drains through the minor papilla; in incomplete pancreas divisum, which comprises about 15% of cases of pancreas divisum, a filamentous branch of the ventral duct communicates with the dorsal duct.

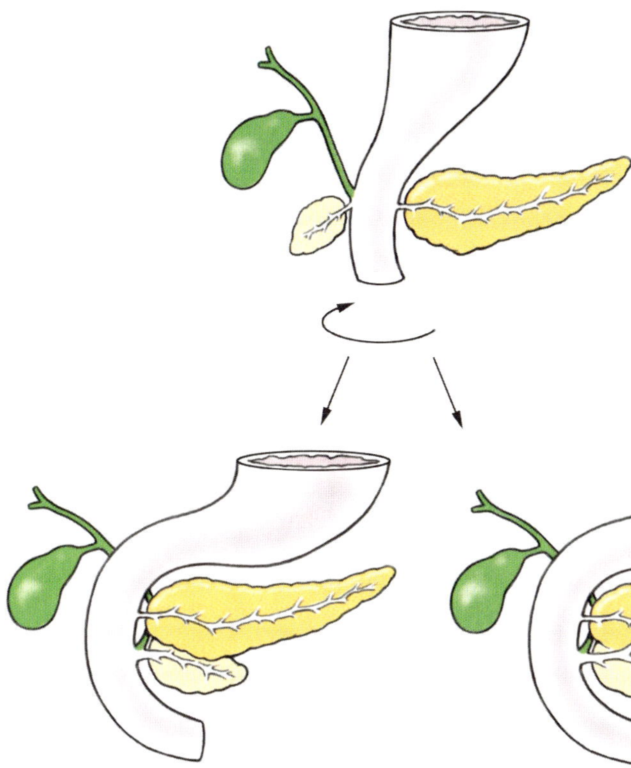

Figure 80.1

Pancreas divisum arises due to a failure of fusion of the ventral and dorsal buds of the embryonic pancreas during organogenesis

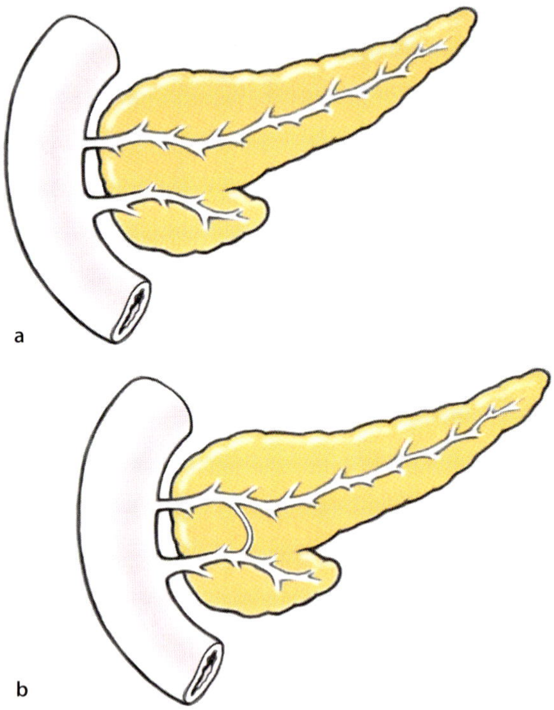

Figure 80.2

Classification of pancreas divisum. a Complete pancreas divisum. b Incomplete pancreas divisum

Clinical Significance of Pancreas Divisum

It is estimated that less than 5% of individuals with pancreas divisum develop pancreatic symptoms; this low frequency of symptoms has created a controversy as to whether pancreas divisum is ever a cause of obstructive pancreatitis. Although the majority of individuals with pancreas divisum are asymptomatic, a subset of them has acute recurrent pancreatitis, chronic pancreatitis, or pancreatic-type pain. This is postulated to be due to a stenotic minor papilla impeding dorsal pancreatic duct drainage. Clinical evidence supports the role of pancreas divisum as a cause for recurrent pancreatitis or pain. Cotton [3] found that 25.6% of patients with unexplained pancreatitis had pancreas divisum, compared to 3.6% of patients with biliary tract disease. In a cohort of patients with chronic calcific pancreatitis who underwent treatment with extracorporeal shockwave lithotripsy, we found the prevalence of pancreas divisum to be 23% [4], which is similar to that reported by Cotton. Surgical specimens from patients with pancreas divisum and pancreatitis have shown pathologic changes confined to dorsal duct distribution. Dilatation of only the terminal portion of the dorsal duct at the duodenal wall (the so-called Santorinicele) is thought to reflect obstruction at the minor papilla [5]. Intraductal pressures in patients with pancreas divisum and pancreatitis are higher compared to controls [6]. Importantly, symptoms may be effectively relieved after endoscopic or surgical dorsal duct drainage [7]. The clinical implication is similar between complete and partial pancreatic divisum [8].

Diagnostic Work-Up

Abdominal ultrasound and computed tomography performed in patients with pancreas divisum who presented with unclear upper abdominal discomfort often reveal enlargement of the pancreatic head, which may be misinterpreted as a tumor. ERCP is the reference standard for the diagnosis of pancreas divisum. When cannulation of the major papilla reveals a short ventral duct, the possibility of pancreas divisum must be considered. Identification and cannulation of the minor papilla is then pursued to demonstrate the presence of a dominant dorsal duct (Fig. 80.3). Differentiation of a seemingly short ventral duct in pancreas divisum from a cut-off in pancreatic cancer (Fig. 80.4) or benign stricture may be difficult until a complete dorsal ductography is obtained. A filamentous connection between both ducts will be seen in the context of incomplete pancreas divisum (Fig. 80.5).

Magnetic resonance cholangiopancreatography allows noninvasive, multiplanar visualization of the biliary and pancreatic ducts without injection of contrast medium. This technique has a similar accuracy to ERCP in identifying pancreas divisum (Fig. 80.6) [9].

Endoscopic ultrasound (EUS) appears promising for the detection of possible pancreas divisum. Bhutani et al. used the absence of a "stack sign" (the simultaneous visualization of both the distal common bile duct and pancreatic duct) in the pancreatic head with radial EUS as an indirect means of confirming the presence of pancreas divisum; the stack sign was present in 33% of patients with pancreas divisum, compared to 83.3% in patients without (Fig. 80.7) [10]. One may also use linear EUS to follow the pancreatic duct in the pancreatic head region. The duct can often be seen crossing a sonographic border between the ventral and dorsal pancreas; if ductal continuity cannot be demonstrated, then pancreas divisum may be present. This diagnostic approach was used by Lai et al. [11]. Unfortunately, adequate visualization of the pancreatic duct was possible in only 78% of cases.

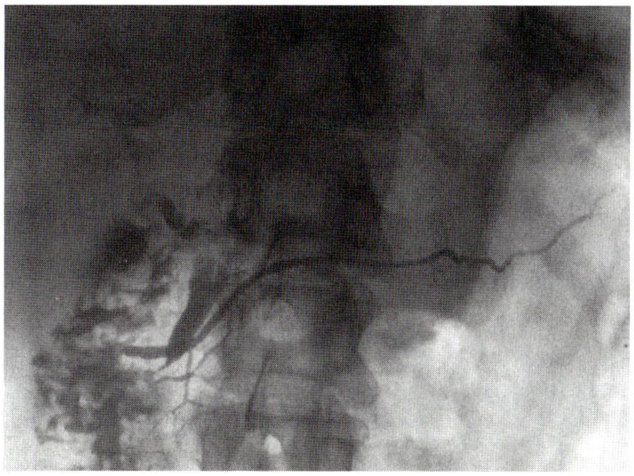

Figure 80.3

Complete pancreas divisum showing a dominant dorsal duct emptying into the minor papilla while the common bile duct (CBD) and ventral pancreatic duct drain via the major papilla. The dorsal duct crosses the distal CBD

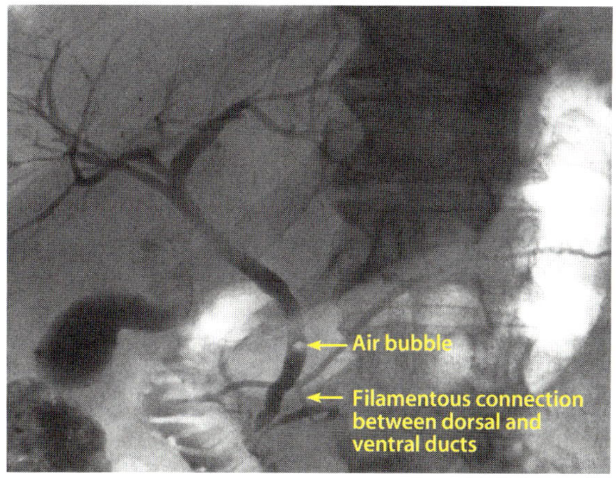

Figure 80.5

Incomplete pancreas divisum. There is a filamentous connection between the ventral and dorsal ducts

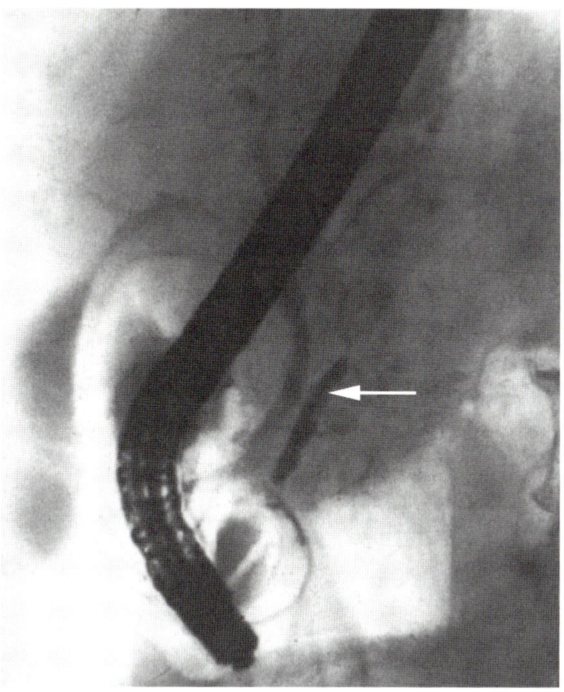

Figure 80.4

"Short" ventral duct *(arrow)* due to the presence of pancreatic cancer proximally

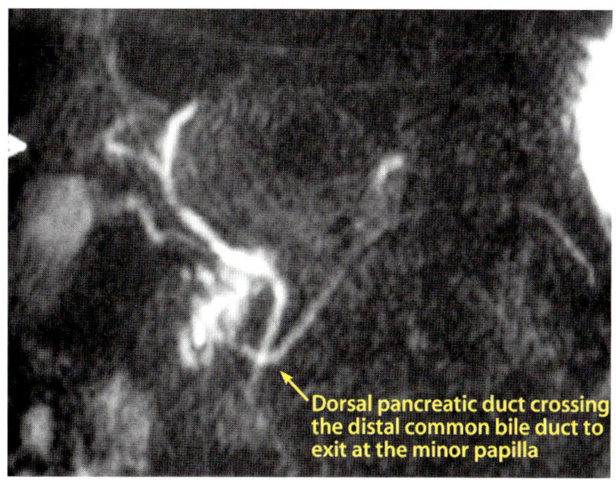

Figure 80.6

Magnetic resonance cholangiopancreatographic diagnosis of complete pancreas divisum

With adequate duct visualization, the positive and negative predictive values were 86% and 97%, respectively. Nonetheless, EUS cannot be used as a sole means of diagnosis; a confirmatory pancreatogram is still required.

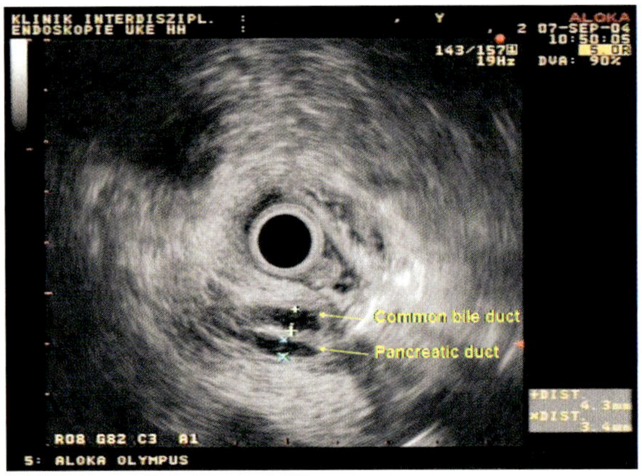

Figure 80.7

The "stack sign," in which the distal CBD is seen above the pancreatic duct, is present in only one-third of patients with pancreas divisum. In contrast, it can be visualized in more than 80% of patients without pancreas divisum

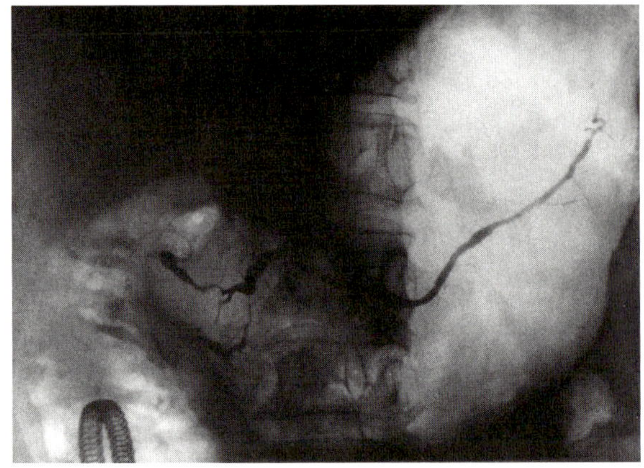

Figure 80.8

Chronic pancreatitis with stricturing in the dorsal pancreatic duct due to pancreas divisum

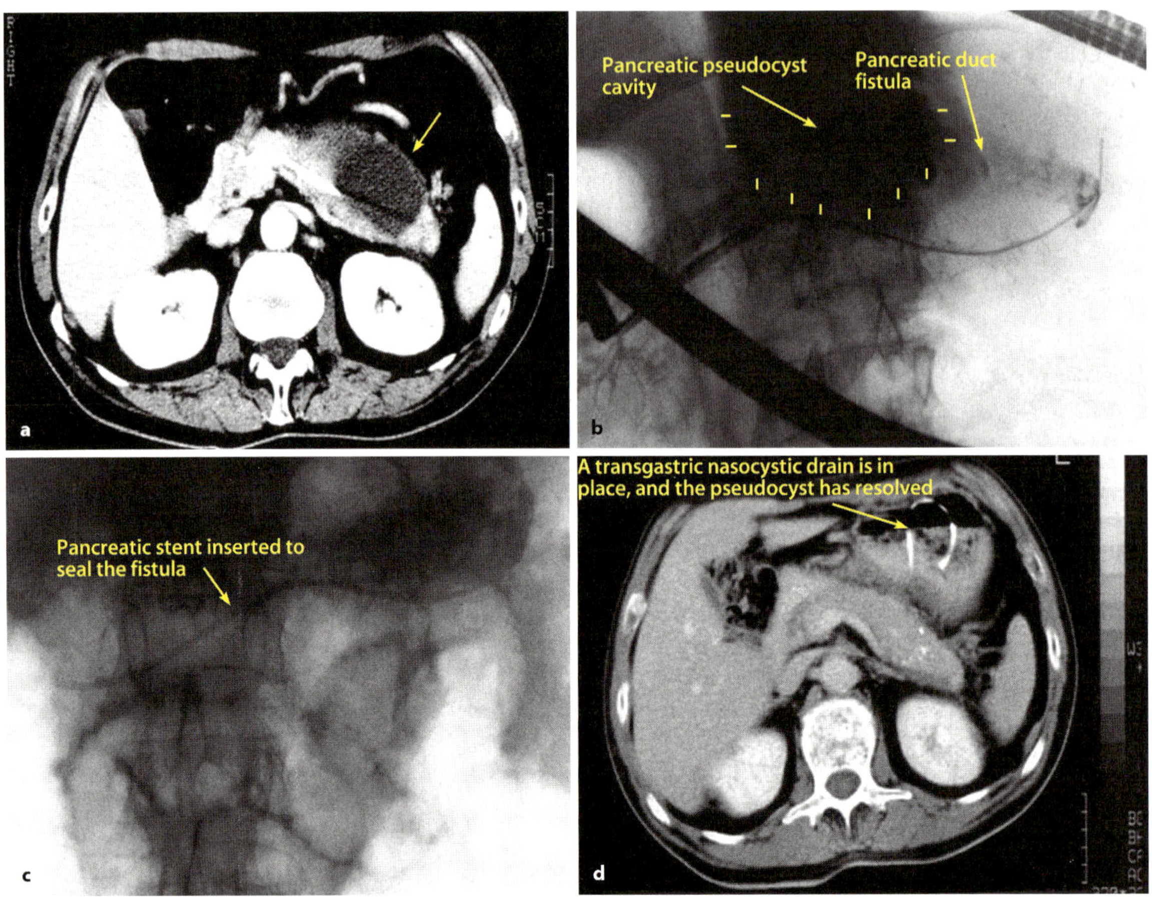

Figure 80.9

a A symptomatic pancreatic pseudocyst *(arrow)* was present in a patient with chronic pancreatitis due to pancreas divisum. b A pancreatic duct fistula communicating with the pseudocyst was diagnosed during pancreatography. c The pancreatic duct fistula was treated by the insertion of a 7-Fr pancreatic stent. d A transgastric nasocystic drain was inserted for the treatment of the pseudocyst. Computed tomography was then repeated and it showed that the pseudocyst had resolved

Indications and Patient Selection for Endoscopic Treatment

The most common clinical presentations of patients who have pancreatic disease related to pancreas divisum include acute recurrent pancreatitis, chronic pancreatitis (Fig. 80.8), and chronic "pancreatic-type" pain without biochemical or radiological evidence of pancreatitis. Other causes of pancreatitis are eliminated by extensive evaluation. A trial of endoscopic therapy is warranted if the patient has recurrent, acute attacks of pancreatitis or significant ongoing pain despite medical management. Endoscopic therapy corrects the minor papilla narrowing, thus preventing excessively high intrapancreatic dorsal duct pressure from occurring during active secretion, which would otherwise result in inadequate drainage, ductal distension, pain, and pancreatitis. Similar to other causes of acute or chronic pancreatitis, patients with pancreas divisum associated with pancreatitis may also develop further complications such as pseudocyst formation or pancreatic duct fistula, and these complications would necessitate additional endoscopic therapies such as pseudocyst drainage and pancreatic duct stenting (Fig. 80.9A–D).

Endoscopic Therapy Technique

When cannulation of the major papilla reveals only a short ventral duct, the possibility of pancreas divisum is considered. Care must be taken not to inject excessive contrast material, as there is a risk of pancreatic acinarization due to the short ventral duct. Cannulation of the minor papilla is then pursued to demonstrate the presence of a dominant dorsal duct. The minor papilla is located about 2–3 cm cephalad and medial to the major papilla (Fig. 80.10). It usually appears as flat and diminutive, and lacks a longitudinal fold with almost no elevation or apparent orifice. Therefore, this tiny minor papilla has customarily offered a special challenge to endoscopic diagnosis and subsequent attempts at endoscopic treatment. When difficulty locating the minor papilla is encountered, secretin can be administered intravenously to stimulate the flow of pancreatic juice, with consequent widening of the papillary orifice. Methylene blue dye can also be used as an adjunct – a dilute solution is sprayed in the area most likely to contain the papilla, and with extended observation, the location may be revealed as the flow of pancreatic juice washes the dye away from the orifice.

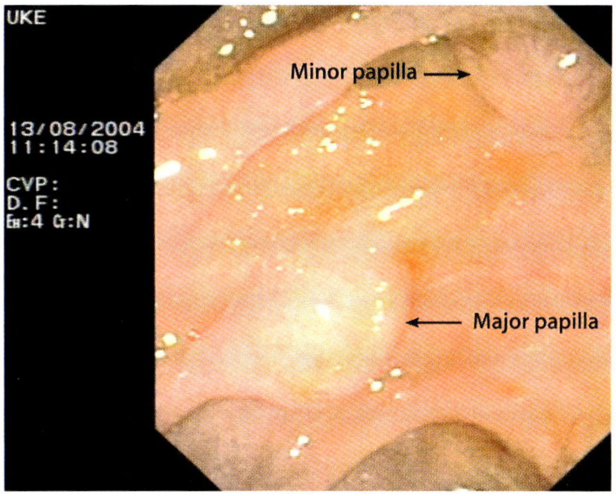

Figure 80.10

Endoscopic view of the major and minor papillae

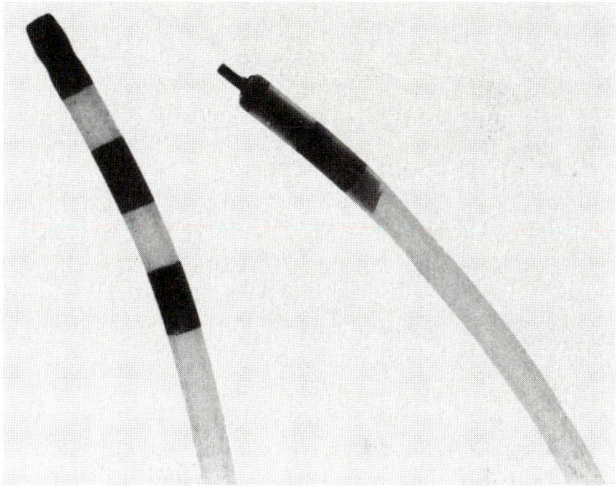

Figure 80.11

A usual 6-Fr catheter (*left*) and a 5-Fr catheter with a blunted 23-gauge needle at the tip (*right*)

Cannulation of the minor papilla is usually best achieved with the endoscope pushed into a semi-long position along the greater curve of the stomach with the tip deflected upward and in left lateral flexion. For cannulation, a standard 5-Fr tapered tip catheter can be used, but a 5-Fr catheter with a blunted 23-gauge needle at its tip is often useful (Fig. 80.11). The catheter is used in conjunction with the 260-cm-long, 0.018- to 0.032-inch (0.046–0.081 cm)-diameter curved-tipped hydrophilic Terumo guidewire. A catheter with a tapered tip is preferable for positioning the guidewire at the orifice of the minor papilla. Santorini's duct is first cannulated with the fine hydrophilic guidewire. The wire is advanced under flu-

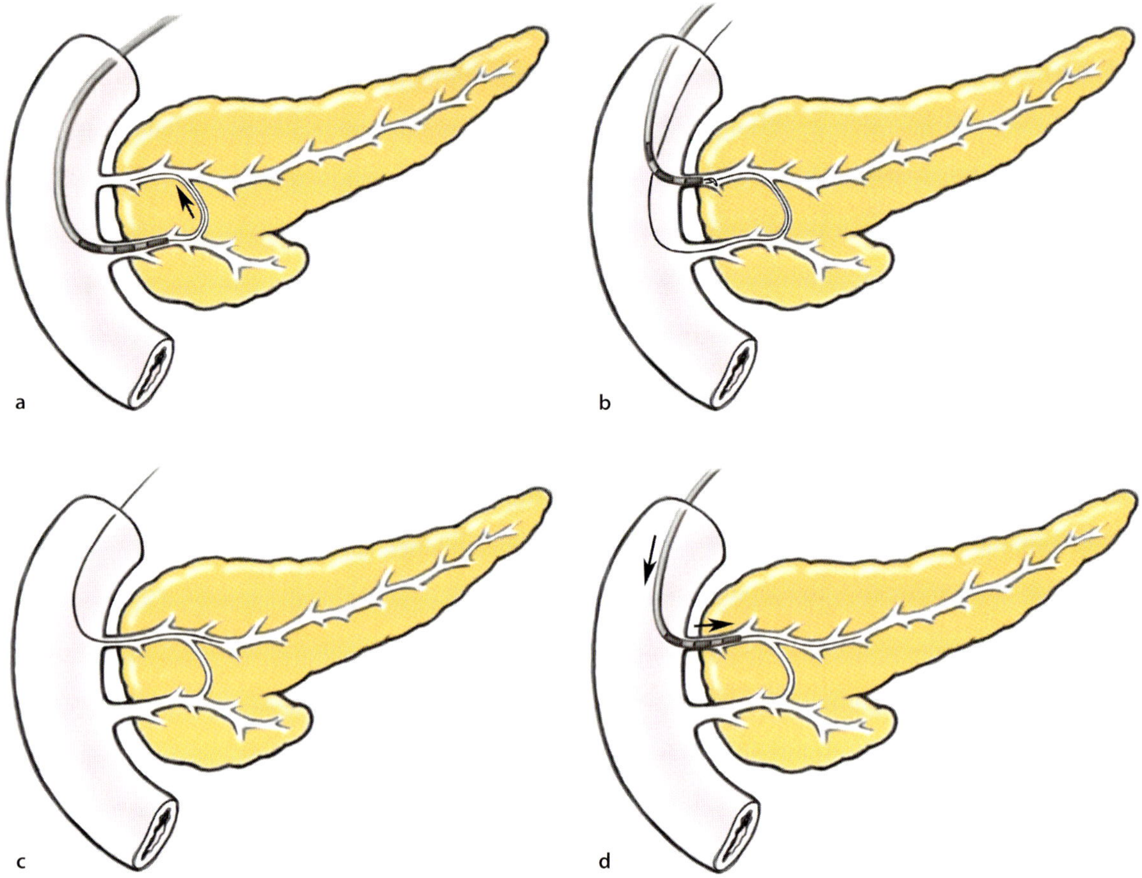

Figure 80.12 a–d

A rendezvous technique of cannulation of the minor papilla may be used for incomplete pancreas divisum. a the major papilla is first cannulated with a hydrophilic guidewire. The guidewire then passes through the filamentous connection between the ventral and dorsal ducts and exits via the minor papilla. b, c The initial catheter is removed and a snare is inserted to pull up the curved end of the guidewire through the working channel of the endoscope such that the other end of the guidewire will pass through the connection and come to reside in the dorsal duct. d A 5-Fr catheter is railroaded over the guidewire through the minor papilla into the dorsal duct. The guidewire is then finally withdrawn and replaced by a conventional guidewire

oroscopic control into the main pancreatic duct using a combination of to-and-fro and twirling movements of the wire. The catheter is then inserted into the pancreatic duct and the hydrophilic wire exchanged for a conventional 400-cm-long, 0.035-inch (0.089 cm) guidewire. In addition, for incomplete pancreas divisum, a rendezvous technique may also be utilized. This is feasible when the connection between the ventral and dorsal ducts is angled toward the minor papilla. In this technique, the major papilla is first cannulated with a hydrophilic guidewire. The guidewire then passes through the filamentous connection between the ventral and dorsal ducts and exits via the minor papilla. The initial catheter is removed and a snare is inserted to pull up the curved end of the guidewire through the working channel of the endoscope such that the other end of the guidewire will pass through the connection and come to reside in the dorsal duct. Next, a 5-Fr catheter is railroaded over the guidewire through the minor papilla into the dorsal duct, and the guidewire is then finally withdrawn and replaced by a conventional guidewire (Fig. 80.12). Sphincterotomy is performed either with a one-step or two-step approach. Using a one-step approach, a double-lumen sphincterotome with a short cutting wire (20 mm long) is advanced over a previously inserted guidewire and a 2- to 3-mm incision made in an approximately 12–13 o'clock position (Fig. 80.13). In the two-step approach, a 5- or 7-Fr stent (5 cm long) is first inserted over the guidewire. The sphincterotomy is performed over the stent using the needle knife (Fig. 80.14). The latter approach has

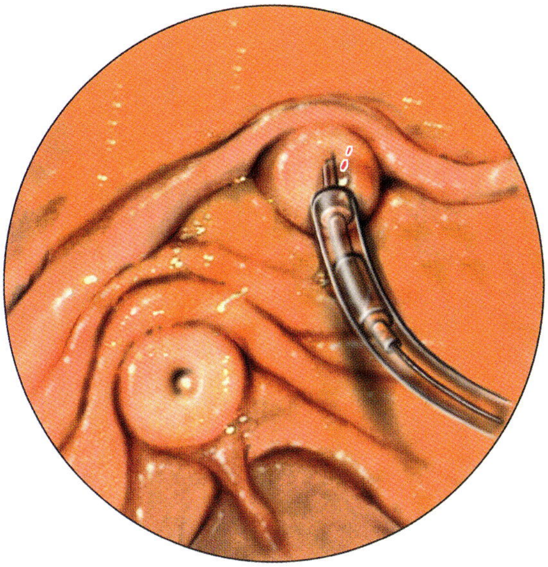

Figure 80.13

One-step approach for performing a sphincterotomy in pancreas divisum

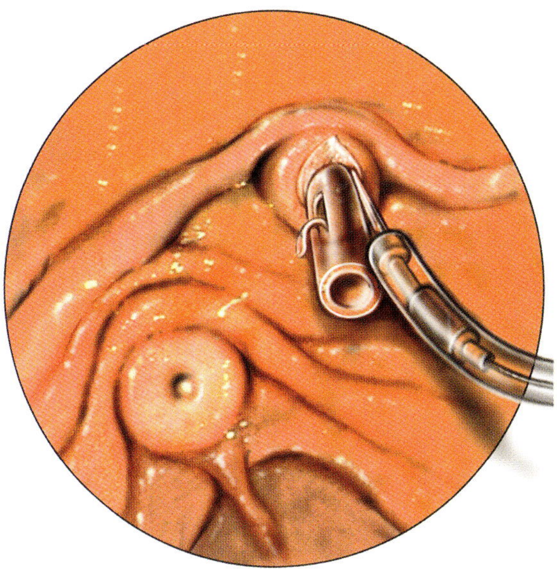

Figure 80.14

Two-step approach for performing a sphincterotomy in pancreas divisum

the advantage that the indication for sphincterotomy can be determined by the therapeutic response to stent drainage alone. After sphincterotomy, the stent can be left in place for several days with a view to minimizing the risk of postprocedure pancreatitis. Strategies for stent use include either short- or long-term placement.

In the context of chronic pancreatitis associated with pancreas divisum, further endoscopic procedures such as stone extraction and dilatation of the pancreatic duct stricture may be required. Extracorporeal shockwave lithotripsy is used as an adjunct to endoscopic stone extraction.

Postprocedure Complications and Management

The short-term complication rate for endoscopic minor papilla sphincterotomy is low and similar to that for the major papilla [12]. These early complications include exacerbation of pancreatitis and bleeding, which can invariably be managed with supportive measures. In the later stage, restenosis may occur, necessitating further endoscopic treatment. Pancreatic stent insertion can lead to complications, including acute pancreatitis, stent migration (either proximally or distally), and stent occlusion, with infectious consequences [13]. Kozarek also reported that pancreatic duct stents may lead to ductal changes ranging from diffuse ductal enlargement to pseudocyst formation and ductal stenosis [14]. To circumvent these stent-related complications, scheduled stent exchange at 3- to 4-month intervals has been advocated should long-term stenting be required.

Long-Term Outcome After Endoscopic Treatment

In terms of long-term clinical response, patients with acute recurrent pancreatitis, normal dorsal ducts, and no chronic pain have the best response rate. About 80% of these patients may achieve symptom resolution [15]. The long-term response rate in the series by Gerke et al. [16] was unusually poor, with a response rate of only 43%; this may be due to the retrospective design of the study as well as the fact that 40% of treated patients were lost to follow up. In patients with chronic pancreatitis, the overall clinical improvement is lower and more variable; the response rates range from 27% to 31% [17,18], but up to 60% may have an improvement in pain score [19]. In patients with chronic pain syndrome, the response to minor papillary drainage is also low, with a response rate of 26–33% [8,17]. In addition, it has been found that repeated endoscopic treatment is of little additional value when the initial effect is unsatisfactory [17]. The results of

Table 80.1. Endoscopic treatment of symptomatic pancreas divisum. *ARP* Acute relapsing pancreatitis, *CP* chronic pancreatitis, *PP* pancreatic-type pain, *ER* emergency room

First Author (year) [reference no.]	Study design (size)	Indications for treatment	Duration of follow up, and outcome
Soehendra (1986) [20]	($n = 6$)	ARP: 2 CP: 2	Follow up: 4–24 weeks Clinical response: ARP: 2/2 CP: 3/4
Satterfeld (1987) [21]	Retrospective case series ($n = 10$)	ARP: 6 CP: 4	Follow up: 18 months Significant improvement in pain/hospitalization for ARP but not CP
Siegel (1990) [15]	Case series ($n = 31$)	ARP	Follow up: 24 months Clinical benefit: 84%
Lans (1992) [22]	Randomized controlled trial ($n = 19$)	ARP	Follow up: 29 months Treatment group: no ER visit or hospitalizations Control: two ER visits and five hospitalizations ($p < 0.05$)
Lehman (1993) [17]	Retrospective case series ($n = 51$)	ARP: 17 CP: 11 PP: 24	Follow up: 20 months Improvement in symptoms and hospitalizations: ARP (76%); CP (27%); PP (26%; $p < 0.01$)
Coleman (1994) [19]	Retrospective case series (PD; $n = 34$)	ARP: 9 CP: 20 PP: 5	Follow up: 23 months Improvement in pain score: ARP (78%); CP (60%); PP (40%)
Kozarek (1994) [14]	Retrospective case series ($n = 39$)	ARP: 15 CP: 19 PP: 5	Follow up: 26 months ARP and CP: significant decrease in pancreatitis episodes; CP: significant improvement in pain. PP: no significant improvement
Jacob (1999) [8]	Retrospective case series (incomplete PD; $n = 18$)	ARP: 10 CP: 5 PP: 3	Follow up: 15.5 months Clinical benefit: ARP: 60%; CP: 80%; PP: 33%
Boerma (2000) [18]	Retrospective case series ($n = 16$)	CP	Follow up: 51 months Pain free: 31%
Ertan (2000) [23]	Retrospective case series ($n = 16$)	ARP	Follow up: 24 months Clinical benefit: 76%
Heyries (2002) [24]	Retrospective case series ($n = 24$)	ARP	Follow up: 39 months Significant decrease in pancreatitis episodes. Trend toward decrease in chronic pain
Gerke (2004) [16]	Retrospective case series ($n = 53$)	ARP: 30 CP: 14 PP: 9	Follow up: 29 months Immediate improvement: ARP: 73.3%; CP: 42.9%; PP: 44.4% Long-term improvement: ARP: 43.3%; 21.4%; 11.1%

publications on treatment outcomes are summarized in Table 80.1.

In conclusion, it appears that when endoscopic therapy for pancreas divisum is being contemplated, patient selection is extremely important, with the outcomes for patients with objective findings of pancreatitis being clearly superior to those with pancreatic-type abdominal pain alone. A trial of endoscopic therapy is warranted if the patient has recurrent, acute attacks of pancreatitis or significant ongoing pain despite medical management, even when ductal dilatation is absent, once other causes have been excluded. Endoscopic treatment performed in the earliest stage of the disease carries the best results.

References

1. Lehman GA, Sherman S (1998) Diagnosis and therapy of pancreas divisum. Gastrointest Endosc Clin Am 8:55–77
2. Delhaye M, Cremer M (1992) Clinical significance of pancreas divisum. Acta Gastroenterol Belg 55:306–313
3. Cotton PB (1980) Congenital anomaly of pancreas divisum as cause of obstructive pain and pancreatitis. Gut 21:105–114
4. Brand B, Kahl M, Sidhu S (2000) Prospective evaluation of morphology, function, and quality of life after extracorporeal shockwave lithotripsy and endoscopic treatment of chronic calcific pancreatitis. Am J Gastroenterol 95:3428–3438
5. Eisen G, Schutz S, Metzler D (1994) Santorinicele: new evidence for obstruction in pancreas divisum. Gastrointest Endosc 40:73–76
6. Staritz M, Meyer zum Buschenfelde KH (1988) Elevated pressure in the dorsal part of pancreas divisum: the cause of chronic pancreatitis? Pancreas 3:108–110
7. Klein SD, Affronti JP (2004) Pancreas divisum, an evidence-based review: part II, patient selection and treatment. Gastrointest Endosc 60:585–589
8. Jacob L, Geenen JE, Catalano MF (1999) Clinical presentation and short-term outcome of endoscopic therapy of patients with symptomatic incomplete pancreas divisum. Gastrointest Endosc 49:53–57
9. Bret PM, Reinhold C, Taourel P (1996) Pancreas divisum: evaluation with MR cholangiopancreatography. Radiology 199:99–103
10. Bhutani MS, Hoffman BJ, Hawes RH (1999) Diagnosis of pancreas divisum by endoscopic ultrasonography. Endoscopy 31:167–169
11. Lai R, Freeman ML, Cass OW (2004) Accurate diagnosis of pancreas divisum by linear-array endoscopic ultrasonography. Endoscopy 36:705–709
12. Sherman S, Lehman GA (1998) Endoscopic pancreatic sphincterotomy: techniques and complications. Gastrointest Endosc Clin N Am 8:115–124
13. Huibregtse K, Schneider B, Vriji AA (1988) Endoscopic pancreatic drainage in chronic pancreatitis. Gastrointest Endosc 34:9–15
14. Kozarek RA (1990) Pancreatic stents can induce ductal changes consistent with chronic pancreatitis. Gastrointest Endosc 36:93–95
15. Siegel JH, Ben-Zvi JS, Pullano W (1990) Effectiveness of endoscopic drainage for pancreas divisum: endoscopic and surgical results in 31 patients. Endoscopy 22:129–133
16. Gerke H, Byrne MF, Stiffler HL (2004) Outcome of endoscopic minor papillotomy in patients with symptomatic pancreas divisum. JOP. J Pancreas (online) 5:122–131
17. Lehman GA, Sherman S, Nisi, Hawes RH (1993) Pancreas divisum: result of minor papilla sphincterotomy. Gastrointest Endosc 39:1–8
18. Boerma D, Huibregtse K, Gulik TM (2000) Long-term outcome of endoscopic stent placement for chronic pancreatitis associated with pancreas divisum. Endoscopy 32:452–456
19. Coleman SD, Gisen GM, Troughton AB (1994) Endoscopic treatment in pancreas divisum. Am J Gastroenterol 89:1152–1155
20. Soehendra N, Kempeneers I, Nam VC (1986) Endoscopic dilatation and papillotomy of the accessory papilla and internal drainage in pancreas divisum. Endoscopy 18:129–32
21. Satterfield ST, McCarthy JH, Geenen JE (1988) Clinical experience in 82 patients with pancreas divisum: preliminary results of manometry and endoscopic therapy. Pancreas 3:248–253
22. Lans JI, Geenen JE, Johanson JF (1992) Endoscopic therapy in patients with patients with pancreas divisum and acute pancreatitis: a prospective, randomized, controlled clinical trial. Gastrointest Endosc 38:430–434
23. Ertan A (2000) Long-term results after endoscopic pancreatic stent placement without pancreatic papillotomy in acute recurrent pancreatitis due to pancreas divisum. Gastrointest Endosc 52:9–14
24. Heyries L, Barthet M, Delvasto C (2002) Long-term results of endoscopic management of pancreas divisum with recurrent acute pancreatitis. Gastrointest Endosc 55:376–381

Chapter 81

H. G. Beger · P. Poch

Surgical Treatment of Pancreas Divisum

Pancreas divisum (PD) is the most common congenital anomaly of the pancreas. In autopsy studies, PD is found in 4–14% of patients [1–3]. Using endoscopic retrograde cholangiopancreatography (ERCP) data, PD has been identified in up to 6% of cases [2,4,5]. In patients with acute idiopathic pancreatitis, however, PD is found in up to 25% [1,6,7].

Clinical Appearance of Pancreas Divisum

The clinical appearance of PD is characterized by the development of pancreatitis in individuals with high-grade PD anomalies [1,8,9]. Most frequently, a dorsal duct hypertension secondary to inadequate pancreatic flow of juice through a narrowed segment of the duct of Santorini and/or the papilla minor finally leads to chronic pancreatitis (CP) [4,10]. In addition, recurrent acute pancreatitis (rAP) without abnormal endocrine and exocrine pancreatic function and pathomorphological signs of CP may be causally linked to the presence of PD [7]. In some patients the presence of PD is the leading pathomorphological factor, but additional injuries such as those caused by alcohol abuse are effective for the development of rAP and, finally, CP.

The pathomorphological changes underlying PD are developed dominantly in the duct system of the pancreatic head. On the basis of computed tomography (CT) investigations, 42% of patients demonstrate an inflammatory mass in the head of the pancreas [11]. The presence of pseudocystic lesions in 28% of the patients and prepapillary stenosis of the duct of Santorini in 44% emphasizes the pancreatic head as the dominant area in this type of CP and rAP.

Clinical Management of Pancreas Divisum

Many endoscopic interventional and surgical procedures, such as endoscopic dilatation, papillotomy, and stent implantation, and sphincteroplastic or even surgical duct drainage have been employed to prevent or improve the acute or chronic inflammatory changes associated with PD [1–4,12–17] (also see Chap. 80). Only a few studies have reported an improvement of pain and reduction of pancreatic episodes after endoscopic interventional treatment [18–22]. In most trials, including recent prospective series, a short-lasting clinical improvement has been reported [18,23,24].

The prevalence of PD in patients who undergo ERCP is about 4–8% in the Western population, and less than 2% among Asians. In most patients, PD is an incidental finding; only a small subset of these patients develop symptoms of acute pancreatitis, and later on recurrent CP with the need of surgical management after failure of endoscopic treatment.

Endoscopic dilatation or papillotomy of the minor papilla are mostly of limited benefit in respect to short-term pain relief and they are burdened with the risk of local complications such as bleeding, pancreatitis, and ductal distraction [25–27].

Pain relief is frequently observed with endoscopic stenting of the minor papilla; however, this procedure necessitates a change of the stents every 3–5 months [28,29]. Reported long-term results suggest a limited benefit in less than 15% of the patients with CP [30,31] and in 60–70% of patients with rAP [14,32].

In a recent published large series with endoscopic minor papillotomy in patients with symptomatic PD, 60% of the patients reported immediate improvement. However, symptoms recurred in about 55%, with the need of endoscopic reinterventions performed in half of those patients. Overall, long-term improvement was effected in only 32% [15].

Transduodenal surgical sphincteroplasty has been performed with a very low morbidity and, in relation to endoscopic sphincterotomy, has a comparable low mortality [14,32]. Almost every patient with PD and attacks of acute pancreatitis diagnosed below the age of 20 years will have an endoscopic sphincterotomy, and 1/3 a surgical sphincteroplasty. However, both techniques have limited benefit. In patients with dilatation of the pancreatic main duct including the duct of Santorini, a drainage procedure using a modification of the Partington-Rochelle duct drainage are of some benefit to reduce the pain and the severity of further attacks of acute pancreatitis.

Surgical Treatment of Pancreas Divisum

Since PD is a disease of the duct system in the pancreatic head that may be responsible for CP, surgical treatment has been applied as an ultimate treatment modality to interrupt the pain syndrome and further attacks of acute pancreatitis.

Since after endoscopic interventional treatment of the narrowed papilla the duct stenosis frequently recurs after a period of disappearance of clinical symptoms, a surgical procedure to interrupt the pain syndrome and the ongoing course of pancreatitis is indicated. Surgical duct drainage has been reported in several series. Patients in whom endoscopic therapy of the dorsal pancreatic duct failed had long-lasting benefits as a result of surgical duct drainage (Table 81.1). Long-lasting pain relief was achieved in children who did not respond to conservative management of CP using the Frey procedure [16]. The outcome after lateral pancreaticojejunostomy in patients with CP associated with PD was beneficial in 90%. Only 10% of the 21 patients who underwent lateral pancreaticojejunostomosis had a further resurgery using a pancreatic head resection procedure [17].

Since the leading pathomorphological changes in PD develop in the duct systems of the pancreatic head,

Table 81.1. Results of surgical treatment of pancreas divisum. *LPJ* Lateral pancreaticojejunostomosis, *Frey* Frey procedure, *DPPHR* duodenum-preserving pancreatic head resection

	Surgical procedure	Patients (*n*)	Follow up	Long-term improvement	Postoperative pain recurrence
Rollins [16]	Frey	8	2.5 years	excellent, good	
Schnelldörfer [17]	LPJ	21	29 months	90%	10%
Schlosser [11]	DPPHR	36	39.3 months	82%	18%

Table 81.2. Pain status after surgery (with permission from [11])

	Patient condition	
Pain status	Preoperative ($n = 36$)	Late postoperative[a] ($n = 32$)
Daily	14 (38%)	3 (9%)
Weekly	7 (19%)	2 (6%)
Monthly	14 (38%)	11 (34%)
No pain	1 (3%)	16 (50%)*
Pancreatic attacks	35 (97%)	6 (19%)*
Periods of hospitalization	63 (1.8 patients)	6 (0,2 patients)*

[a] Late postoperative follow up: 32/32 patients (median follow-up: 39.3 months; range, 5–109 months)
*$p < 0.002$ (McNemar) preoperative vs. postoperative

Table 81.3. Endocrine status (with permission from [11]). *OGTT* Oral glucose tolerance test, *IDDM* insulin-dependent diabetes mellitus

	Patient condition		
	Preoperative ($n = 36$)	Early postoperative ($n = 36$)	Late postoperative[a] ($n = 32$)
Normal OGTT	23 (64%)	27 (75%)	24 (75%)
Impaired OGTT	11 (31%)	5 (14%)	3 (9%)
IDDM	2 (6%)	4 (11%)	5 (16%)

[a] Late postoperative follow up: 32/32 patients (median follow-up: 39.3 months; range, 5–109 months)

many patients present the disease with an inflammatory mass in the head of the pancreas. Using CT criteria, a pancreatic head resection has been used to interrupt the progressive clinical deterioration.

In a recent large surgical series, a duodenum-preserving pancreatic head resection has been applied in patients with symptomatic PD, including rAP in children after failure of endoscopic management of the duct obstructions in the pancreatic head [11]. The major advantage of duodenum-preserving pancreatic head resection in comparison to the pylorus-preserving pancreatic head resection is the preservation of the gastrointestinal tract [33]. This limited surgical resection with preservation of the duodenum has a low postoperative surgical morbidity [34]. In the presented series no hospital death occurred [11]. The surgical procedure can be combined with a drainage procedure of the dilated left pancreatic main duct. The limited resection of the pancreatic head leads to a decompression of the narrowed segment of the intrapancreatic common bile duct and significantly reduces the pain pattern. As demonstrated in Table 81.2, the pain status and the need for rehospitalization was significantly reduced following duodenum-preserving pancreatic head resection. Duodenum-preserving pancreatic head resection, furthermore, preserves the endocrine function in the early and late postoperative period (Table 81.3). The low recurrence rate of acute pancreatitis after duodenum-preserving pancreatic head resection and the preservation of the endocrine function of the duodenum and the pancreas may indicate a slower progression of the disease. However, supplementation is mandatory in most of the patients because of the still-reduced exocrine function capacity of the pancreas in the advanced stages of PD and in the late postoperative period after pancreatic head resection.

References

1. Gregg JA (1997) Pancreas divisum: Its association with pancreatitis. Am J Surg 134:539–543
2. Cotton PB (1980) Congenital anomaly of pancreas divisum as cause of obstructive pain and pancreatitis. Gut 21:105–114
3. Sumanio T (1969) Proposed nomenclature and classification of the human pancreatic ducts and duodenal papillae: study based on 200 post mortems. Int Surg 52:152–154
4. Warshaw AL, Simeone JF, Schapiro RH (1990) Evaluation and treatment of the dominant dorsal duct syndrome (pancreas divisum redefined). Am J Surg 159:59–60
5. Delhaye M, Engelholm L, Cremer M (1985) Pancreas divisum: congenital anatomic variant or anomaly? Gastroenterology 89:951–958
6. Richer JA, Schapiro RH, Mulley A (1981) Association of pancreas divisum and pancreatitis and its treatment by sphincteroplasty of the accessory ampulla. Gastroenterology 81:1104–1110
7. Bernhard J, Sahel J, Giovanni M (1990) Pancreas divisum is a probable cause of acute pancreatitis: a report of 137 cases. Pancreas 5:248–254
8. Varshney S, Johnson CD (1999) Pancreas divisum. Int J Pancreatol 25:135–141
9. Stern CD (1986) A historical perspective on the discovery of the accessory duct of the pancreas, the ampulla of Vater and pancreas divisum. Gut 27:203–212
10. Wind P, Berger A, Chevallier JM (1992) Pancreas divisum, chronic pancreatitis and diabetes mellitus: Improvement by pancreaticojejunostomy. Ann Chir 46:625–629
11. Schlosser W, Rau B, Poch B, Beger HG (2005) Surgical treatment of pancreas divisum causing chronic pancreatitis: the outcome benefits of duodenum-preserving pancreatic head resection. J Gastrointest Surg 9:710–715
12. Alvarez C, Widdison AL, Reber HA (1991) New perspectives in the surgical management of chronic pancreatitis. Pancreas 6:S76–S81
13. Bornman PC, Marks IN, Girdwood AH, et al (1980) Is pancreatic duct obstruction or stricture a major cause of pain in calcific pancreatitis? Br J Surg 67:425–428
14. Cotton PB (1978) Duodenoscopic papillotomy at the minor papilla of Vater for recurrent dorsal pancreatitis. Endosc Digest 3:27–28
15. Gerke H, Byrne M, Stiffler H, Obando J, Mitchell R, Jowell P, Branch M, Baillie J (2004) Outcome of endoscopic minor papillotomy in patients with symptomatic pancreas divisum. JOP J Pancreas 5:122–131
16. Rollins MD, Meyers RL (2004) Frey procedure for surgical management of chronic pancreatitis in children. J Pediatr Surg 39:817–820
17. Schnelldorfer T, Adams DB (2003) Outcome after lateral pancreaticojejunostomy in patients with chronic pancreatitis associated with pancreas divisum. Am Surg 69:1041–1044
18. Lans JI, Geenen JE, Hogan WJ, et al (1992) Endoscopic therapy in patients with pancreas divisum and acute pancreatitis: a prospective, randomized trial. Gastrointest Endosc 38:430–434
19. Prabhu M, Geenen JE, Hogan WJ, et al (1989) Role of endoscopic stent placement in the treatment of acute recurrent pancreatitis associated with pancreas divisum: a prospective assessment. Gastrointest Endosc 35:165
20. McCarthy J, Geenen JE, Hogan WJ (1988) Preliminary experience with endoscopic stent placement in benign pancreatic diseases. Gastrointest Endosc 34:16–18
21. Cohen SA, Siegel JH (2001) Pancreas divisum: endoscopic therapy. Surg Clin North Am 81:467–477
22. Ertan A (2000) Long term results after endoscopic pancreatic stent placement without pancreatic papillotomy in acute recurrent pancreatitis due to pancreas divisum. Gastrointest Endosc 52:134–137
23. Sherman S, Howes R, Nisi R, et al (1994) Randomized controlled trial of minor papilla sphincterotomy in pancreas divisum patients with pain only. Gastroenterology 108:348A
24. Gerke H, Byrne MF, Stiffler HL, et al (2004) Outcome of endoscopic minor papillotomy in patients with symptomatic pancreas divisum. JOP 5:122–131
25. Kozarek RA (1990) Pancreatic stents can induce ductal changes consistent with chronic pancreatitis. Gastrointest Endosc 36:93–95

26. Derfus GA, Geene JE, Hogan WJ (1990) Effect of endoscopic pancreatic duct stent placement on pancreatic ductal morphology. Gastrointest Endosc 36:A206
27. Simmons TC, Henderson DR, Glentten F (1988) Pancreatic abscess associated with pancreas divisum. J Natl Med Assoc 80:453–458
28. Ikkenberg SO, Sherman S, Hawes RH, et al (1994) The occlusion rate of pancreatic stents. Gastrointest Endosc 40:611–613
29. Weiner G, Geenen JE, Hogan WJ, et al (1994) Stent therapy in patients with pancreatic type pain and pancreas divisum: a randomized controlled clinical trial. Gastroenterology 106:330A
30. Kozarek RA, Ball TJ, Patterson DJ, et al (1995) Endoscopic approach to pancreas divisum. Dig Dis Sci 40:1974–1981
31. Siegel JH, Cooperman AM, Pullano W, et al (1993) Pancreas divisum: Observation, endoscopic drainage and surgical treatment results in 65 patients. Surg Laparosc Endosc 3:281–285
32. Bradley EL, Stephan RN (1996) Accessory duct sphincteroplasty is preferred for long term prevention of recurrent acute pancreatitis in patients with pancreas divisum. J Am Coll Surg 183:65–70
33. Beger HG, Büchler M (1990) Duodenum-preserving resection of the head resection in chronic pancreatitis with inflammatory mass in the head. World J Surg 14:83–87
34. Beger HG, Schlosser W, Friess HM, Büchler MW (1999) Duodenum-preserving head resection in chronic pancreatitis changes the natural course of the disease: a single-center 26-year experience. Ann Surg 230:512–519

Chapter 82

T. Onogawa · T. Rikiyama · M. Unno · S. Matsuno

Biliopancreatic Maljunction: Classification, Diagnosis, and Treatment

Biliopancreatic maljunction, also known as pancreaticobiliary maljunction or an anomalous junction between the pancreatic duct and the bile duct (APBDJ) is a congenital anomaly that has been defined as a union of the pancreatic and biliary ducts that is located outside of the duodenal wall. Because the function of the sphincter muscle of the duodenal papilla does not extend the full length of the common channel, this results in the regurgitation of the pancreatic juice and bile. In most cases, since the pressure within the pancreatic duct is higher than that of the biliary tract, the pancreatic juice regurgitates continuously into the biliary tract and the biliary mucosa is continually susceptible to damage as a result of the continued presence of infectious bile and activated pancreatic enzymes. This eventually causes cancer and other pathological changes to occur in the biliary mucosa. Since APBDJ can cause various diseases and conditions in the pancreas as well as the liver, further research is needed in this field.

With developments in endoscopic retrograde cholangiopancreatography (ERCP), the morphology of APBDJ has been clarified and it was soon discovered that some cases of APBDJ are not accompanied by dilatation of the extrahepatic bile duct. APBDJ is very closely related not only to congenital biliary dilatation, but also to the occurrence of cancer in the biliary tract, and so many researchers, including those whose research is focused on the biliary tract and pancreas of adults, have participated in conferences on this subject. Much data have been collected from various groups and fundamental research in a wide range of areas has been conducted.

Classification of APBDJ

Kimura et al. classified APBDJ was into two types [1, 2]. In the first type, the main pancreatic duct joins the common bile duct (CBD) just below the site of cystic dilatation. In the second, the distal end of the cystic dilatation joins the main pancreatic duct through a short, narrow segment.

Another classification of APBDJ, proposed by Komi et al. [3, 4], was based on the results of a Japanese nationwide questionnaire survey of 183 cases of choledochal cyst. APBDJ was classified into three groups as follows:

- Type a: the narrowed CBD joins with the pancreatic duct at a site distant from the papilla of Vater at an approximately right angle.
- Type b: the pancreatic duct joins with the CBD at a site distant from the papilla, usually at an angle of slightly less than 90°.
- Type c: the complex arrangement of the pancreatic duct, the terminal portion of the CBD, and the accessory pancreatic duct; occasionally these ducts form a network.

In order to ensure that surgical dissection of the terminal portion of the CBD does not cause injury to the pancreatic duct, intraoperative selective contact cholangiopancreatography (ISCCP) is used [5, 6]. ISCCP is useful not only for avoiding injuries to the pancreatic duct, but also for detailed visualization of the ductal systems. These findings were used for the new Komi classification of APBDJ (Fig. 82.1) [7].

The new Komi classification of APBDJ seems to be an acceptable amendment and modification of the previous one [3, 8]. Fifty-one cases of choledochal cyst complicated with APBDJ were examined extensively and analyzed for clear visualization of the APBDJ to make this new classification [7, 9].

APBDJ was broadly classified into three types: type I, type II, and type III as in the original Komi classification [8] of types a, b, and c, respectively. Each type of the new Komi classification was divided into subtypes. Type I and type II were divided into a and b subtypes according to whether they were without (a) or with (b) a common channel dorsal pancreatic duct [10].

Of 51 cases of choledochal cyst in which the pancreaticobiliary ductal system was extensively examined, type I APBDJ was seen in 18 cases (35.5%), type

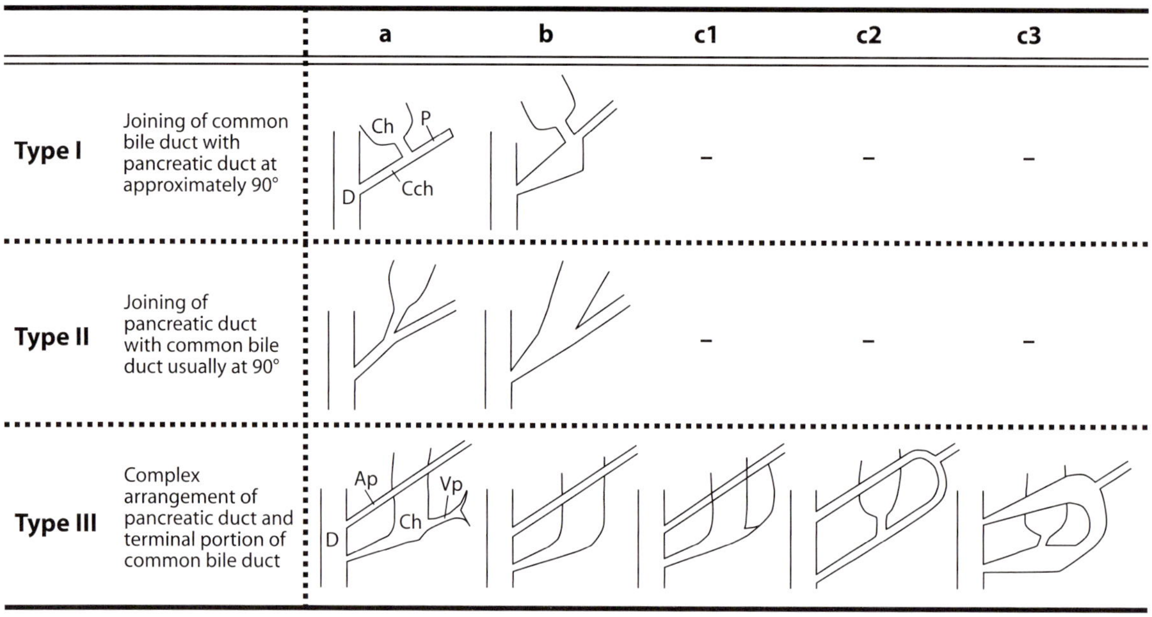

Figure 82.1

The new Komi classification of anomalous junction between the pancreatic duct and the bile duct (APBDJ). *Ch* Choledochus, *P* pancreatic duct, *Cch* common channel, *D* duodenum, *Ap* accessory pancreatic duct, *Vp* ventral pancreatic duct

II in 11 (21.6%), and type III in 22 (43.1%) [7]. In 41 cases of choledochal cyst registered during the period of 1981–2006 by our department, type I was the most common, comprising about 58% (26 cases) of all cases of APBDJ. Type II was also common, comprising about 25% (11 cases). Type III was the least common (17%, 8 cases).

A radical operation, including complete excision of the dilated biliary duct followed by reconstruction of the biliary tract is the surgical treatment of choice, because the reflux of the pancreatic juice into the biliary tract is thereby prevented. However, a dilated common channel or accessory pancreatic duct, according to the new Komi types Ib, IIb, and IIIc3 of APBDJ, could be the cause of relapsing pancreatitis leading to chronic pancreatitis, due to the formation of a protein plug or pancreatic calculus in the dilated duct, even after the radical operation. Pylorus-preserving pancreaticoduodenectomy was reported to be one of the operative methods of choice in complicated cases of type IIIc3 APBDJ with choledochal cyst. Long-term follow up over several decades is essential to evaluate the outcomes of the surgical procedure for choledochal cyst, especially in complicated cases with types Ib, IIb, and IIIc3 of APBDJ according to the new Komi classification [8, 9].

Diagnosis of APBDJ

Although APBDJ occurs most frequently in female Asians, it has been reported to be a very rare disease even in Japan. It has also been reported that APBDJ was present in 1.5–3.2% of patients undergoing ERCP [11–13]. However, since ERCP is always performed for some reason, such cases belong to a very limited population. In contrast, the subjects of some studies were asymptomatic individuals who underwent routine ultrasound examination. Although not all of the subjects who were requested to undergo follow-up examination did so, Kato et al. found APBDJ in at least 1 out of 3,000 persons, indicating that this abnormality is by no means rare [11].

Ultrasonography (US) is the best screening method for the diagnosis of APBDJ associated with congenital choledochal cysts (CCC), revealing extrahepatic and/or intrahepatic bile duct dilatation. The recently developed multidetector row computed tomography (MDCT) can also demonstrate dilatation of the biliary tree. Although US and MDCT can suggest the presence of disease, they do not provide a definitive diagnosis. For confirmation, drip-infusion cholangiography-MDCT or direct cholangiography is necessary. ERCP can give detailed information concerning biliary malignancies, and can also reveal APBDJ. Magnetic resonance cholangiopancreatography (MRCP) is noninvasive and can provide almost the same information obtained by ERCP [14]. Endoscopic US (EUS) can also depict the shape of the extrahepatic biliary tree, pancreatobiliary maljunction, and complications of biliary malignancies on an outpatient basis [15]. Moreover, unlike ERCP it can be performed at an outpatient clinic and is associated with few complications.

In cases of APBDJ not associated with CCC (nondilated type), Yamao et al. revealed that there were more patients without symptoms for a long period than they had expected [16]. Clinical symptoms do not occur from birth, but appear when complications occur. Most adult patients with this anomaly were diagnosed after ERCP was performed for biliary cancer or symptoms such as abdominal pain and jaundice. Unfortunately, this approach is useless for improving the prognosis of biliary cancer complicating APBDJ. Therefore, a correct diagnosis for such patients should be made before the complication of biliary malignancy occurs. A specific diagnosis can be made only with accurate imaging modalities. US can only give clues to the diagnosis in such patients because it reveals sonographic characteristics such as gallbladder wall thickening [16, 17] and/or mild dilatation of the extrahepatic bile duct. EUS has the advantage that it can visualize not only gallbladder lesions, which need to be distinguished as benign or malignant, but also the anatomy of the pancreatobiliary ducts so that APBDJ can be easily delineated on an outpatient basis [15, 16]. Finally, APBDJ should be diagnosed by ERCP. Recently, however, MRCP has been reported to provide almost the same quality cholangiopancreatograms as ERCP [14].

In APBDJ with spindle-like dilatation of the extrahepatic bile duct, US can depict dilatation and/or wall thickening of the gallbladder. A definitive diagnosis of APBDJ and complications can be obtained by EUS or ERCP.

Therefore, early detection of APBDJ and improvement of the prognosis in biliary tract cancer with APBDJ can best be achieved by US, EUS, MRCP, DIC-MDCT, and ERCP serial examinations of asymptomatic individuals.

Malignant Change

It has been noted above that the epithelium of the cysts frequently shows evidence of previous inflammation, and this may lead to areas of dysplasia, which may be the precursor of invasive malignancy. The mechanism is unclear, and its relationship to pancreatic reflux has not been fully defined. Biliary stasis predisposes to the formation of secondary bile acids, which are mutagenic. The risk increases with the duration of exposure: malignancy is hardly ever seen in cysts removed in infancy, and the mean age of presentation is 32 years. Carcinoma in association with bile duct cysts was first reported in 1944 [18]. Tumors may develop anywhere within the biliary tree, but more than one-half occur within the cyst itself [19]. Tumors are most common in type 1 and type 4 cysts [20] (i.e., those with fusiform dilatation of the intrahepatic and/or extrahepatic ducts), but they also occur in type 5 (Caroli's disease) [21]. The commonest tumor type is adenocarcinoma (cholangiocarcinoma), although other types have been reported, including squamous cell carcinoma [20]. It must be noted that cancer in other types of intrahepatic cysts (simple cysts or polycystic disease) is exceedingly rare, and should not direct decisions regarding therapy [22]. The younger the patient at presentation of the choledochal cyst, the lower the incidence of subsequent malignant change: the risk is less than 1% if the choledochal cyst presents within the first decade of life, but increases to 14% if presentation is delayed beyond 20 years of age [23]. The youngest reported patient with adenocarcinoma in a choledochal cyst was 17 years old, and she had undergone biliary bypass 8 years earlier [24]. Preoperative diagnosis of carcinoma is very rare and the prognosis is poor, with less than 10% being resectable [25]. In our department, we experienced a case of adenocarcinoma in a choledochal cyst of a 15 years old female. We performed resection of the extrahepatic bile duct and pancreaticoduodenectomy, but she died 13 months after surgery from liver metastasis.

Ishibashi et al. [26] reported biliary carcinoma in 9 of 48 patients presenting with choledochal cysts. Six of these died from recurrence with a mean survival time of 13 months, while three patients were alive and free from recurrence 2 months, 1 year, and 7 years after operation. While early drainage may have beneficial results by reducing biliary stasis and cholangitis and reducing contact with possible carcinogens, it would be logical to perform resection to reduce the incidence further, not only by removing the most vulnerable part of the mucosa, but also by providing better biliary drainage and preventing the reflux of pancreatic juice. In Ishibashi's series of 48 patients managed over a 21-year period [26], 39 had no carcinoma at first admission, and 37 of these underwent complete or near-complete cyst excision with hepaticojejunostomy. In these 37 patients, no carcinoma developed in the remnant proximal hepatic duct or the terminal bile duct after a mean follow-up of 9.1 years.

Hopkins et al. reported a series of seven patients with complications of choledochal cysts in adulthood: one had malignant change and was typical in presentation, age, gender, extent of tumor, and outcome [27].

Pathogenesis of Malignant Change

Experimental studies in dogs have simulated an APBDJ by means of a pancreaticocholecystostomy [28]. After 24–41 days, cylindrical CBD dilatation, up to 3.28±2.48 times the ordinary diameter, was found in 23/29 (79%) of the dogs, with biliary stones in 3/29 (10%). The amylase level and levels of phospholipase A2 in the bile were elevated in all 25 dogs tested. Inflammatory changes were observed in all specimens, with intramural glandular structures in 17/25 (68%) of gallbladder specimens and 10/25 (40%) of CBD specimens. DNA ploidy abnormalities were found by cytofluorometry in both gallbladder and bile duct epithelium. Similar ploidy abnormalities were found by the same workers in two clinical cases of choledochal cyst without malignant change [29]. Dot-blot hybridization and immunohistochemical studies did not reveal any mutations in the *c-K-ras* gene, or any overexpression of the p53 protein in the specimens. Using a similar model, gallbladder bile acids were studied 14 months after pancreaticocholecystostomy, with or without pancreatic duct ligation as a control. The fraction of cholic acid tended to be lower, and that of deoxycholic acid slightly higher in APBDJ dogs, while the percentage of ursodeoxycholic acid in APBDJ dogs was significantly decreased compared with that in the control and normal dogs. A high frequency of DNA strand breaks was shown in only two out of seven APBDJ dogs, and in these two dogs, the cholic acid percentage was decreased and that of deoxycholic acid greatly increased. These findings suggest that an alteration of the bile composition in APBDJ may cause frequent DNA strand breaks and repair, which might lead to gene mutation and biliary tract carcinoma. Further studies have suggested that pancreatic juice enzymes and bacteria infecting the biliary duct can deconjugate detoxified mutagens in the bile and induce the mutagenicity of the bile in APBDJ dogs or patients [30]. The same group carried out immunohistochemical studies on excised specimens of choledochal cysts. An APBDJ was observed in all 39 cases examined. Among the total of 47 patients, 5 (10.6%) had biliary carcinoma. Among 24 adults, 81.8% exhibited mucous glands in the cyst wall, 41.7% exhibited goblet cells, and 27.3% exhibited argyrophil cells. In 23 children, the incidence of these metaplastic changes was lower (27.3% mucous glands, 13.0% goblet cells, and 9.5% argyrophil cells). Immunoreactivity to gastrin or somatostatin was evident immunohistochemically in four adults.

Surgical Treatment for APBDJ

The necessity of surgical treatment for APBDJ is evident, irrespective of the presence of associated diseases. When biliary tract cancer is already present, the surgical procedure of choice depends primarily upon the location and stage of the cancer.

For patients who have APBDJ without biliary dilatation or cancer, prophylactic cholecystectomy is considered to be indicated because of the high prevalence of gallbladder cancer [31]. Sugihara et al. reported a 78% incidence of gallbladder cancer associated with cancer of APBDJ without biliary dilatation [32]. Laparoscopic cholecystectomy is a recommended procedure because it is minimally invasive. The indication for bile duct resection in patients without biliary dilatation remains controversial. Some investigators have shown genetic abnormalities in the biliary epithelia, such as *p53* and *K-ras* mutations [33]. Because Nakano et al. [34] reported that they had had no experience with bile duct cancer in their 40 APBDJ patients without biliary dilatation, and because the frequency of bile duct cancer is very low (2/181 cases) in other institutions, they do not add resection of the bile duct, but only follow up the condition of the bile duct carefully.

Since Babitt first reported APBDJ [35], the correlation between congenital dilatation of the bile duct and APBDJ has been noted and discussed. Surgical treatment for patients who have both APBDJ and biliary dilatation has two important roles. One is to treat the symptoms of cholangitis or pancreatitis caused by APBDJ, such as pyrexia and abdominal pain. The other is to prevent the development of biliary malignancy, because APBDJ is known to be a risk factor for the biliary carcinomas [36–39]. Complete excision of a dilated bile duct, the epithelium of which has already developed the mutation of genes, is essential to prevent the onset of biliary carcinomas as well as to terminate the reflux of pancreatic juice into the bile duct. Since postoperative complications from reconstruction of the bile duct develop frequently, the reconstruction or anastomosis method should be carefully selected. Kenmochi et al. [40] reported that the frequency of complications was higher with reconstruction by interposition of the jejunum as compared to the Roux-en Y reconstruction. Interposition of the

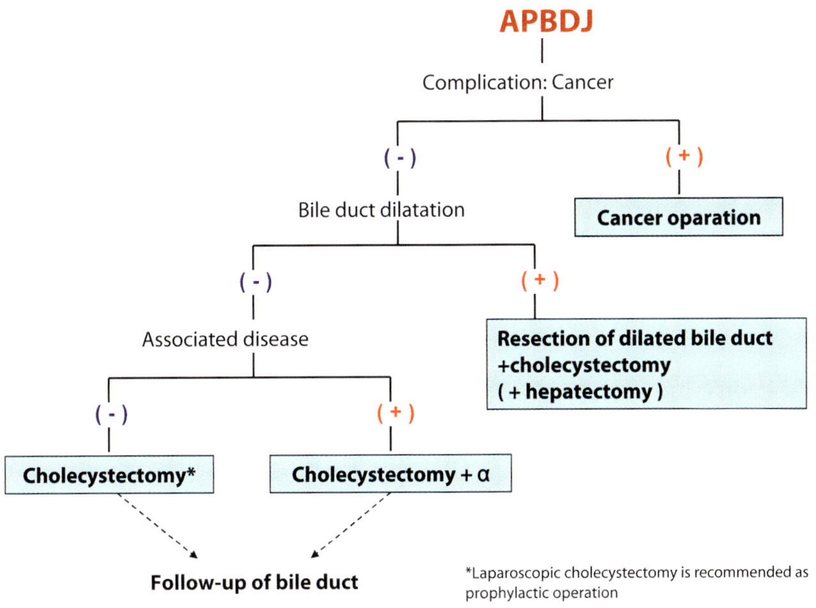

Figure 82.2

Treatment strategy for APBDJ. The treatment strategy for adult APBDJ patients according to the presence or absence of congenital biliary dilatation and/or malignancy

jejunum limits the length from the hepaticojejunostomy to the jejunoduodenostomy (usually 5–10 cm). In this reconstruction method, a physiological stream of bile is achieved, but the reflux of digestive juice occurs readily and causes cholangitis, anastomosis, stenosis, and the formation of intrahepatic stones. Thus, with the Roux-en Y reconstruction, they consider that the length of the jejunum from the hepaticojejunostomy to the Y anastomosis is important to prevent cholangitis and the formation of intrahepatic bile duct stones after bile duct reconstruction. In our Roux-en Y reconstruction technique, the length of the jejunum is usually 40 cm or more.

The management of patients with congenital dilatation of the intrahepatic bile ducts is controversial. Some investigators have shown carcinogenesis and/or gallstone formation in dilated intrahepatic bile ducts after resection of the extrahepatic choledochus [31–43]. Kenmochi et al. also reported that postoperative biliary carcinomas occurred 10 or 20 years after surgery. This suggests that APBDJ patients who undergo surgical treatment develop biliary carcinoma in the prolonged postoperative period. The frequency of postoperative complications was significantly higher for the intrahepatic type as compared to the extrahepatic type. The frequency of cholangitis was particularly high (36.4%). This may be because excision of the bile duct and anastomosis are complicated and difficult procedures for the intrahepatic type and because the stenosis of the intrahepatic bile duct may remain. In order to solve this problem, an extended excision of the bile duct including hepatectomy is proposed. The indications for hepatic resection depend on variations in intrahepatic bile duct dilatation and stenosis. When intrahepatic dilatation, stenosis, and stones are confined to a single hepatic lobe or segment, hepatectomy of the affected lobe or segment may be effective.

Considering the risk of gallstone formation in the intrapancreatic portion of the remnant dilated bile duct after resection of choledochal cysts [44], complete removal of the intrapancreatic portion of the dilated bile duct is also recommended [45]. To prevent injury to the pancreatic duct during manipulation of the intrapancreatic bile duct, intraoperative endoscopy, pancreatography and pancreatic stenting are useful modalities [46]. The indications for pancreaticoduodenectomy depend on the pancreatic pathology. A diagram of the appropriate procedures for APBDJ patients is shown in Fig. 82.2.

References

1. Kimura K (1976) Studies in 28 cases of congenital cystic dilatation of the common bile duct in adults: roentgenological features and a union between the choledochus and the main pancreatic duct (in Japanese) Jpn J Gastroenterol 71:401–414
2. Kimura K, Ohto M, Ono T, et al (1977) Congenital cystic dilatation of the common bile duct: relationship to anomalous pancreaticobiliary ductal union. Am J Roentgenol 128:571–577
3. Komi N, Udaka H, Ikeda N, Kashiwagi Y (1977) Congenital dilatation of the biliary tract: new classification and study with particular reference to anomalous arrangement of the pancreaticobiliary ducts. Gastroenterol Jpn 12:293–304
4. Komi N (1978) Congenital dilatation of the biliary tract (in Japanese). In: Kimoto S (ed) Gendai-Gekagaku-Taikei. Nakayama, Tokyo, pp 245–281
5. Komi N, Takahara H, Miyamoto H, et al (1982) Pathophysiology of pancreaticobiliary maljunction: clinical point of view (in Japanese). J Clin Surg (Tokyo) 37:1775–1780
6. Komi N, Takahara H, Udata H, et al (1983) Surgical treatment of the congenital biliary dilatation (in Japanese). Shujitsu (Tokyo) 37:781–792
7. Komi N (1991) New classification of anomalous arrangement of the pancreaticobiliary ducts (APBD) in choledochal cyst: a proposal of new Komi's classification of APBD (in Japanese). J Jpn Pancr Soc 6:234–244
8. Komi N (1978) Congenital dilatation of the biliary tract (in Japanese). In: Kimoto S (ed) Gendai-Gekagaku-Taikei. Nakayama, Tokyo, p 245–281
9. Komi N, Takahara H, Kunitomo K, et al (1992) Does the type of anomalous arrangement of pancreaticobiliary ducts influence the surgery and prognosis of choledochal cyst? J Pediatr Surg 27:728–731
10. Warshaw AL, Simeone JF, Shapiro RH, et al (1990) Evaluation and treatment of the dominant dorsal duct syndrome (pancreas divisum redefined). Am J Surg 159:59–64
11. Mirsa SP, Dwivedi M (1990) Pancreaticobiliary ductal union. Gut 31:1144–1149
12. Kato O, Hattori K, Suzuki T, et al (1983) Clinical significance of anomalous pancreaticobiliary union. Gastrointest Endosc 29:94–98
13. Kimura K, Ohto M, Saisho H, et al (1989) Association of gallbladder carcinoma and anomalous pancreaticobiliary ductal union. Gastroenterol 89:1258–1265
14. Sugiyama M, Baba M, Atomi Y, et al (1998) Diagnosis of pancreatobiliary junction: value of magnetic resonance cholangiopancreatography. Surgery 123:391–397
15. Mitake M, Nakazawa S, Naitoh Y, et al (1991) Value of endoscopic ultrasonography in the detection of anomalous connections of the pancreatobiliary duct. Endoscopy 3:117–120
16. Yamao K, Nakazawa S, Yoshino J, et al (1992) The diagnosis of the anomalous connection of pancreaticobiliary ducts without biliary dilatation: the usefulness of US/EUS serial examination. Dig Endosc 4:365–375
17. Igarashi H (1991) Imaging features of the gallbladder wall in patients with anomalous arrangement of the pancreaticobiliary ductal system (in Japanese) J Jpn Bil Assoc 5:517–525
18. Irwin ST, Morison JE (1944) Congenital cyst of the common bile duct containing stones and undergoing cancerous change. Br J Surg 32:319–321
19. Flanigan DP (1977) Biliary carcinoma associated with biliary cysts. Cancer 40:880–883
20. Nagorney DM (2000) Bile duct cysts in adults. In: Blumgart LH, Fong Y (eds) Surgery of the Liver and Biliary Tract, 3rd edn. Saunders, London, pp 1229–1244
21. Dayton MT, Longmire WP, Tompkins RK (1983) Caroli's disease: a premalignant condition? Am J Surg 145:44–41
22. Farges O, Menu Y, Benhamou J-P (2000) Non-parasitic cystic diseases of the liver and intrahepatic biliary tree. In: Blumgart LH, Fong Y (eds) Surgery of the Liver and Biliary Tract, 3rd edn. Saunders, London, pp 1245–1260
23. Voyles CR, Smadja C, Shands WC, Blumgart LH (1983) Carcinoma in choledochal cysts. Age-related incidence. Arch Surg 118:986–988
24. Fujiwara Y, Ohizumi T, Kakizaki G (1976) A case of congenital choledochal cyst associated with carcinoma. J Paediatr Surg 11:587–588
25. Flanigan DP (1977) Biliary carcinoma associated with biliary cysts. Cancer 40:880–883
26. Ishibashi T, Kasahara K, Yasuda Y, et al (1997) Malignant change in the biliary tract after excision of choledochal cyst. Br J Surg 84:1687–1691
27. Hopkins NFG, Benjamin IS, Thompson MH, Voyles CR (1990) Complications of choledochal cysts in adulthood. Ann R Coll Surg Engl 72:229–235
28. Abdul MM, Kunitomo K, Komi N (1992) Experimental studies on carcinogenesis in anomalous arrangement of the pancreaticobiliary ducts. Tokushima J Exp Med 39:13–23
29. Abdul MM, Kunitomo K, Wada D, et al (1993) Case report of an anomalous arrangement of the pancreaticobiliary ducts and nuclear DNA ploidy analysis. Surg Today 23 :167–171
30. Qian D, Kinouchi T, Kunitomo K, et al (1993) Mutagenicity of the bile of dogs with an experimental model of an anomalous arrangement of the pancreaticobiliary duct. Carcinogenesis 14:743–747
31. Sheth S, Bedford A, Chopra S (2000) Primary gallbladder cancer: recognition of risk factors and the role of prophylactic cholecystectomy. Am J Gastroenterol 95:1402–1410
32. Sugihara J, Sekita M, Saito Y (1982) Anomalous arrangement of pancreaticobiliary duct and cancer (in Japanese). Tan to Sui 3:487–495
33. Funabiki T, Matsubara T, Ochiai M, et al (1997) Surgical strategy for patients with pancreaticobiliary maljunction without choledochal dilatation. Keio J Med 46:169–172
34. Nakano K, Konomi H, Yamaguchi K et al (2002) Pancreaticobiliary Maljunction in Adults: Clinical Probrems and Surgical Treatment. In: Koyanagi Y and Aoki T (ed) Pancreaticobiliary Maljunction, IGAKU TOSHO, Tokyo, p117–123
35. Babitt DP (1969) Congenital choledochal cyst: new etiological concept based on anomalous relationships of the common bile duct and pancreatic bulb. Ann Radiol (Paris) 12:231–240
36. Kinoshita H, Nagata E, Hirohashi K (1984) Carcinoma of gallbladder with an anomalous connection between the choledochus and pancreatic duct. Cancer 54:762–769
37. Nagata E, Sakai K, Kinoshita H (1986) Choledochal cyst: complication of anomalous connection between choledochus and the pancreatic duct and carcinoma of the biliary tract. World J Surg 10:102–110
38. Komi N, Tamura T, Miyoshi Y, et al (1984) Nationwide survey of cases of choledochal cyst. Analysis of coexistent anomalies, complication and surgical treatment in 645 cases. Surg Gastroenterol 3:69–73

39. Tanaka K, Nishimura A, Yamada K, et al (1993) Cancer of the gallbladder associated with anomalous junction of the pancreaticobiliary duct system without bile duct dilatation. Br J Surg 80:622–624
40. Kenmochi T, Asano T, Miura F et al (2002) Surgical Treatment for Adult. Patients with Pancreaticobiliary Maljunction. In: Koyanagi Y and Aoki T (ed) Pancreaticobiliary Maljunction, IGAKU TOSHO, Tokyo, p367–374
41. Deziel DJ, Rossi RI, Munson JL, et al (1986) Management of bile duct cysts in adults. Arch Surg 121:410–415
42. Gallagher PJ, Millis RR, Mitchinson MJ (1972) Congenital dilatation of the intrahepatic bile ducts with cholangiocarcinoma. J Clin Pathol 25:804–808
43. Ando H, Ito T, Kaneko K, et al (1996) Intrahepatic bile duct stenosis causing intrahepatic calculi formation following excision of a choledochal cyst. J Am Coll Surg 183:56–60
44. Hsu RK, Yu A, Lee JG, Leung JW (2001) Pancreatitis caused by common bile duct stones in a 3-year-old boy with prior surgery for a choledochal cyst. Am J Gastroenterol 96:1919–1921
45. Ando H, Kaneko K, Ito T, et al (1995) Complete excision of the intrapancreatic portion of choledochal cysts. J Am Coll Surg 183:317–321
46. Miyano T, Yamataka A, Kato Y, Kohno S, Fujiwara T (1995) Choledochal cysts: special emphasis on the usefulness of intraoperative endoscopy. J Pediatr Surg 30:482–484

Section 11

Pancreatic Injury

Chapter 83 Pancreatic Trauma: Diagnosis, Treatment, Complications, and Late Outcome *905*
J. M. Mayer, P. Tuncyurek

J. M. Mayer · P. Tuncyurek

Pancreatic Trauma: Diagnosis, Treatment, Complications, and Late Outcome

Pancreatic trauma is a rare, yet severe complication of abdominal injury. In blunt abdominal trauma, pancreatic trauma is noted in 2–4% of all cases [1], while the incidence of a therapeutically relevant lesion to the pancreas is as low as 1% [2]. Typically, these injuries to the pancreas are caused by compression of the organ against the vertebral column, mostly in car- or traffic-related accidents. Blunt trauma to the epigastrium is caused by steering wheels, handlebars, seatbelts, or directly. Other mechanisms of injury include sporting accidents, like directs hits from balls or injuries from horse kicks. While these blunt abdominal traumas are predominant in Europe, centers in the USA and South Africa report extensively on penetrating abdominal traumas caused by shotguns or knives [3, 4].

Due to this, most pancreatic traumas are not isolated injuries but part of frequently complex clinical situations. The decision of when and how to treat a pancreatic injury is therefore part of a differentiated decision-making process. In unstable or very severely injured patients, damage control is a priority over pancreatic reconstruction [5].

In light of this, no one pancreatic injury equals another, and this explains why so few surgeons gather extensive experience in the diagnosis and treatment of these injuries. In this chapter, we hope to give some guidelines rather than set up strict rules.

Classification

The Organ Injury Scaling Committee of the American Association for the Surgery of Trauma has proposed a pancreatic organ injury scale that is widely used and is based on the extent of parenchymal damage as well as the presence or absence of pancreatic duct injury (Table 83.1). Minor contusions or superficial lacerations of the pancreas without duct involvement are classified as grade I injuries. Grade II injuries are major contusions or lacerations without duct disruption. Distal transection of the pancreas or major parenchymal injuries with duct injuries are described as grade III. Grade IV injures are proximal transections or any proximal parenchymal injuries involving the ampulla. Grade V injuries describe massive destructions of the pancreatic head. This classification is especially helpful in clinical decision making and has therefore gained wide acceptance. Typically, two-thirds of all reported pancreatic injuries are without major pancreatic duct involvement (grades I and II), one-fifth are proximal or distal transections of the pancreas including pancreatic duct rupture (grades III and IV). Massive destructions of the pancreatic head occur surprisingly frequently and account for approximately 15% of all pancreatic injuries in blunt abdominal trauma [6].

Table 83.1. Classification of pancreatic injuries

Grade		Description
I°	Hematoma	Minor contusion without duct injury
	Laceration	Superficial laceration without duct injury
II°	Hematoma	Major contusion without duct injury
	Laceration	Major laceration without duct injury
III°	Laceration	Distal transection or parenchymal injury with duct injury
IV°	Laceration	Proximal transection or parenchymal injury involving ampulla
V°	Laceration	Massive disruption of pancreatic head

Diagnosis

Ultrasonography

As most patients with suspected pancreatic trauma will have sustained other injuries, they are treated in emergency rooms with standardized protocols. Usually, an ultrasound examination will be performed that allows even the untrained physician to diagnose free abdominal fluid or gross damage to the liver or spleen. The pancreas is not easily identified and examined in its full extent, therefore pancreatic injuries, parenchymal or ductal, will frequently be missed. However, routine abdominal ultrasound examination in the emergency room will establish the diagnosis of an intra-abdominal injury and therefore establish the need for an urgent explorative laparotomy. To exclude main pancreatic duct injury, especially in penetrating pancreatic trauma, intraoperative ultrasonography has proven to be helpful [7].

Computed Tomography

Many trauma centers use newer-generation helical computed tomography (CT) scanners to quickly achieve an overview of abdominal and skeletal injuries in severely traumatized patients. This "one-stop" examination allows the assessment of complex injuries and substantially speeds up the clinical decision making. In a retrospective analysis, CT of the abdomen, with or without contrast enhancement, also proved to be a useful tool in diagnosing pancreatic injury. While being less sensitive than endoscopic retrograde cholangiopancreatography (ERCP) with regard to revealing disruption of the pancreatic duct, CT allows the additional assessment of the severity and extent of pancreatic tissue damage and concomitant injuries [8]. It is generally accepted that while CT is highly predictive for the presence of pancreatic tissue injury (as well as adjacent injuries), it has a poor correlation with pancreatic injury grade, especially concerning the damage to or disruption of the pancreatic duct. This may be overcome by newer-generation multidetector helical CT scanners [9].

Magnetic Resonance Cholangiopancreatography

While certainly not the first choice in the emergency situation, the imaging of the pancreatic and choledochal ducts as well as the visualization of the extent of pancreatic tissue damage by magnetic resonance imaging/magnetic resonance cholangiopancreatography (MRCP) is an elegant and precise diagnostic tool for assessing pancreatic injury. In particular, in stable patients with suspected (isolated) pancreatic injury, MRCP enables the noninvasive detection or exclusion of pancreatic duct trauma and pancreas-specific complications. It may therefore provide information that can be used to guide management decisions in the further course of these patients [10].

Endoscopic Retrograde Cholangiopancreatography

Like MRCP, ERCP allows the accurate assessment of pancreatic duct injuries and additionally offers the option of therapeutic stent placement in minor ductal lesions. However, ERCP necessitates an experienced examiner and considerable logistics. This may render emergency ERCP almost impossible in the most severely injured or unstable patients. Like MRCP, it as a powerful tool for demonstrating main pancreatic duct injury. In the case of lower-grade leakages of the pancreatic duct, transpapillary stent insertion may seal the injury and stabilize it in a way that eventually leads to a resolution of the leak [11].

Based on ERCP findings, a treatment algorithm has been developed by a Japanese group [12] that allows the allocation of stable trauma patients with a pancreatic injury to a diversified treatment protocol, and thus substantially helps in clinical decision making. In this classification, three grades are distinguished: class 1 patients have radiographically normal ducts. In class 2 patients, branch injuries are noted, with class 2a defined as the absence of contrast leakage from the pancreatic parenchyma, and class 2b having leaks into the retroperitoneal space. Patients with a class 3 injury show an injury or disruption of the main pancreatic duct. The authors of this classification system reported that they were able to treat all class 1 injuries conservatively with no major complication. A nonsurgical approach was also chosen for class 2a patients, while class 2b injuries had to be treated by at least a drainage laparotomy. Interestingly, all class 3 patients eventually underwent laparotomy, including some patients who were initially treated conservatively. Even though this classification seems very promising, it has a major drawback: it may be difficult to perform an emergency ERCP in severely injured trauma patients, and most critically ill or unstable patients would be missed in this classification.

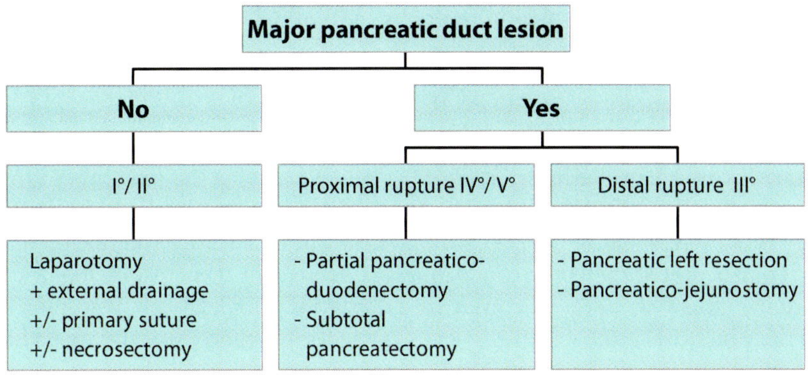

Figure 83.1

Proposed treatment algorithm for the surgical therapy of pancreatic duct injuries

Laboratory Parameters

It has been shown repeatedly that serum amylase is neither a reliable diagnostic nor a significant prognostic parameter in assessing pancreatic injury. The same has been found for lipase, not only in adult patients, but also in pediatric patients. Therefore, while frequently being used as a screening parameter in patients with blunt or penetrating abdominal trauma, the routine day to day measurement of lipase or amylase can not be recommended in the diagnosis of pancreatic injury [13].

Diagnostic Tools in Pediatric Patients

In children, a large portion of pancreatic injuries are missed by either CT scan, ultrasonography, or by laboratory parameters, and are coincidentally found on laparotomy for other intra-abdominal lesions. Due to the nature of pediatric pancreatic injuries, caused predominantly by epigastric blunt trauma, ERCP plays a more important role in the diagnosis, but also in the treatment of pancreatic duct injuries. Reports on the transpapillary stenting of duct lesions are very encouraging and justify the extensive use of ERCP in stable pediatric patients [14].

Therapy

Isolated pancreatic injuries are rare and usually result from a direct trauma to the epigastrium, for example from the handle bar in bicycle accidents or from horse kicks, typically in children or young adolescents. Most patients with pancreatic lesions will present with multiple injuries, some of them hemodynamically unstable, and concomitant abdominal injuries. Therefore, unstable patients may require initial damage control and correct assessment of the extent of pancreatic injury. This usually allows delayed definitive treatment of complex injuries, especially of the head of the pancreas.

Irrespective of this general prerequisite, two major principles apply for the surgical therapy of pancreatic injuries: (1) resection in all pancreatic injuries complicated by a complete duct disruption, and (2) surgical debridement and drainage in the absence of ductal injuries.

We recommend a treatment algorithm based on the presence or absence of a major pancreatic duct lesion (Fig. 83.1). By analogy to the classification system of the Organ Injury Scaling Committee of the American Association for the Surgery of Trauma, four clinical situations that require surgery may be distinguished: (1) pancreatic injury without duct involvement, (2) distal pancreatic injuries with duct involvement, (3) proximal transection or parenchymal injury involving the ampulla, and (4) and massive destruction of the pancreatic head. An approach based on injury grade and location is described below.

Pancreatic Injury Without Duct Involvement

Exploration and external drainage is the treatment of choice for grade I and II injuries. This includes minor lacerations, stabs, or gunshot wounds of the superior or inferior border of the body or tail of the pancreas without visible disruption of the major pancreatic duct. In some cases, debridement, necrosectomy, or suture of the gland may be necessary in addition to the placement of a drainage along the pancreas. The same principle applies to the treatment of stab or gunshot wounds and contusions of the head of the pancreas without major devitalization of pancreatic tissue. These lesions are also best managed by exploration and external drainage. However, associated duodenal injuries may not easily be repaired by direct suture and thus a more complex procedure like partial pancreaticoduodenectomy might be necessary even in minor injuries to the pancreatic head.

Distal Pancreatic Injuries with Duct Involvement

Distal pancreatic injuries with duct involvement include major lacerations or gunshot or stab wounds in the body or tail of the pancreas with an obvious duct injury or a transection of more than half the width of the pancreas. If the clinical condition of the patient allows it, these grade III injuries are best treated by distal pancreatectomy even in the emergency situation. In some cases of complete transection of the pancreatic body from the head, a distal pancreaticojejunostomy and closure of the proximal end of the pancreatic rupture may even become necessary if an organ-preserving approach is attempted. However, the issues of splenectomy and conservative treatment may arise in the individual patient. In a series of 32 grade III patients, Lin et al. [15] treated 19 patients by distal pancreatectomy with splenectomy, 8 by pancreatectomy with preservation of the spleen, and 2 by placing a pancreatic duct stent. The remaining patients were successfully treated nonsurgically by pancreaticojejunostomy or by drainage alone.

Proximal Transection or Parenchymal Injury Involving the Ampulla

Complete transections of the pancreatic head, disruption or complex injuries of the pancreatic head involving the ampulla, or major devitalizing injuries of the pancreatic head and duodenum usually are nonreconstructable injuries. In stable patients, partial pancreaticoduodenectomy is the best definite treatment for these grade IV (or V) injuries. In unstable patients, exploration and placing of an external drainage may be the best choice for damage control. Definitive treatment of the lesion can be achieved later, after the patient has been stabilized.

Massive Destruction of the Pancreatic Head

Typically, patients with grade V injuries will have sustained a very severe trauma and are initially unstable. In these patients, damage control by exploration and drainage may be the only procedure possible. Virtually all patients with a massive destruction of the pancreatic head in whom a definitive treatment is possible are treated by pancreaticoduodenectomy. However, due to the complexity of the sustained injuries in most patients, the morbidity and mortality is very high in this group.

Simple Versus Complex Surgical Treatment

Seemingly, there are two approaches to treating pancreatic injury: a complex repair, including performing a Whipple procedure (partial pancreaticoduodenectomy), versus a simple draining procedure. There is general agreement that internal drainage or complex defunctioning procedures are not useful in the emergency management of pancreatic injuries, and can be avoided without increasing morbidity. Staged laparotomy, debridement of devitalized tissue, and drainage can be successfully applied to wounds of the pancreas in most cases of pancreatic trauma, while temporary exclusion and reoperation can be employed for unstable patients [3, 16]. However, there are situations where a pancreaticoduodenectomy may still become necessary. These indications are massive uncontrollable retropancreatic hemorrhage, massive unreconstructable injury to the head of the pancreas or main pancreatic duct and intrapancreatic portion or distal common bile duct, and massive unreconstructable injury. This procedure is usually performed in grade V injuries – given that the patient is reasonably stable – and results in an acceptable survival rate [17].

Children

The situation is different in children and young adolescents with a higher rate of isolated pancreatic trauma; therefore, a somewhat modified, more conservative treatment is advised in these patients. Most authors report that – unlike in adults – grade I and II injuries (without major injuries to the pancreatic duct) can be treated nonsurgically. If laparotomy is performed, an external drainage can be placed, but this seems to offer no advantage over exploration without external drainage. Distal duct injuries or pancreatic transections (grade III injuries) are best treated by distal pancreatectomy, preferably with preservation of the spleen. Pancreatic duct stenting may allow an initial nonoperative treatment, but typically leads to the formation of pancreatic pseudocysts. These cannot always be treated interventionally and frequently require surgical internal drainage. Therefore, primary resection in distal pancreatic transection (grade III) is favored by most authors. In contrast to this, initial stenting is preferred in proximal pancreatic transection (grade IV injury). Due to the complexity and late morbidity of pancreaticoduodenectomy in children, initial stenting and later drainage of forming pancreatic pseudocysts, or other pancreas-preserving procedures are recommended. [14, 18, 19]

Interventional Treatment by ERCP

As mentioned above, ERCP examination – if possible in the emergency situation – allows an accurate assessment of pancreatic duct involvement in pancreatic trauma. It furthermore offers the possibility of transpapillary stent placement to temporarily seal or bridge a rupture in the major pancreatic duct. This procedure can be used to postpone a definitive surgical repair or to wait for the development of a stable pancreatic pseudocyst that can later be drained interventionally by enteric drainage [20].

Complications and Late Outcome

In general, the complication rate in patients with pancreatic injury is very high; however, most complications are caused or facilitated by the concomitant injury sustained in the initial trauma. It is almost impossible to attribute complications solely to pancreatic injury. In selected cases, a typical complication rate for grade III and grade IV pancreatic injuries would be as high as 60%. One-third to one-half of all patients with grade V injuries will die due to the massive concomitant injuries, about half of them intraoperatively or immediately after surgery [2, 15, 17].

The complication rate of any pancreatic injury is not only associated with concomitant injuries, but also with the severity of the pancreatic injury. As is widely accepted, the grade of pancreatic injury is an independent predictor of both pancreas-associated morbidity and mortality. The American Association for the Surgery of Trauma Organ Injury Score has been shown to predict the development of complications and mortality after pancreatic injury, to identify patients who will require extensive resources and may benefit from transfer to a specialized trauma center [21].

Regarding the overall morbidity and mortality of any abdominal trauma, the presence and severity of pancreatic injury independently of other injuries results in a poorer outcome. In the emergency situation, patients with concomitant pancreatic lesions tend to be more frequently hypothermic, have a higher blood loss and several intra-abdominal organ injuries. Consequently, their rate of infectious complications and sepsis-associated mortality is higher than in patients without pancreatic injury [22].

Other than intra-abdominal abscess formation, typical causes of intermediate and late complications after pancreatic trauma are strictures of the major pancreatic ducts, posttraumatic recurrent pancreatitis and pseudocysts, and pancreatic fistula and biliary fistula. Up to two-thirds of all cases of pancreatic trauma develop one or several of these complications. Interestingly, several authors have noted that delayed diagnosis and/or treatment of severe pancreatic injuries, especially when associated with a disruption of the main pancreatic duct, result in a higher mortality and pancreas-associated morbidity. This is also the case for patients with delayed surgical intervention after an unsuccessful period of observation or a subsequent operation due to undetected injury to the main pancreatic duct. Furthermore, there is a significant risk behind treatment of disruptions of the main pancreatic duct by duct stenting: While this may be used initially in unstable patients or to allow immediate damage control, there is a substantial risk for sepsis in the acute stage and for major duct stricture in the chronic stage of recovery [2, 15, 23].

While deaths in this early stage are typically associated with the severity of the initial trauma and associated parameters, such as hypothermia, blood loss, and injury pattern, late deaths are frequently caused by pancreatic fistula, upper gastrointestinal bleeding, acute respiratory distress syndrome, and serious abdominal infections [24]. If patients survive the initial phase, especially after severe multiple trauma, about one-quarter of them will suffer from pancreas-associated complications. The most frequent complications are late pancreatic abscess, recurrent traumatic pancreatitis, persisting pancreatic fistula with frequent superinfection, and pancreatic pseudocysts. Pancreatic abscesses may be treated interventionally by percutaneous drainage, but are frequently infected by either fungi or multiple resistant bacteria such as methicillin-resistant *Staphylococcus aureus*. This complication significantly prolongs intensive care unit and hospital stays and seriously increases mortality due to recurrent sepsis. Septic complications may also arise from superinfected pancreatic fistulae. This frequent finding after pancreatic exploration – probably associated with an untimely removal of external pancreatic drainages – is difficult to treat, and allowing spontaneous resolution is frequently the treatment of choice. Typically, the treatment of pancreatic pseudocysts poses no major problem to the experienced pancreatic surgeon. As with pseudocysts after acute necrotizing pancreatitis, interventional drainage and sealing, endoscopic gastrocystostomy, or operative enteric drainage are the treatment modalities at hand for this complication of pancreatic trauma [2, 3, 21].

Late outcome is usually better in younger patients, and especially in children. This is partially due to the lower rate of complex multiple injuries in children with pancreatic lesions. However, pancreatic duct injuries are missed more frequently in children, which results in a high rate of pancreatic pseudocyst formation. In children, spontaneous resolution is frequent and interventional drainage frequently successful. If posttraumatic pseudocysts persist, they can easily be managed by internal drainage procedures. Compared to adults, persistent pancreatic fistulae and posttraumatic recurrent pancreatitis occur less frequently in children and usually resolve spontaneously without specific treatment [18].

References

1. Wilson RH, Moorehead RJ (1991) Current management of trauma of the pancreas. Br J Surg 78:1196–1202
2. Mayer JM, Tomczak R, Rau B, Gebhard F, Beger HG (2002) Pancreatic injury in severe trauma: early diagnosis and therapy improve the outcome. Dig Surg 19:291–297
3. Krige JE, Beningfield SJ, Nicol AJ, Navsaria P (2005) The management of complex pancreatic injuries. S Afr J Surg 43:92–102
4. Vasquez JC, Coimbra R, Hoyt DB, Fortlage D (2001) Management of penetrating pancreatic trauma: an 11-year experience of a level-1 trauma center. Injury 32:753–759
5. Chrysos E, Athanasakis E, Xynos E (2002) Pancreatic trauma in the adult: current knowledge in diagnosis and management. Pancreatology 2:365–378
6. Moore EE, Cogbill TH, Malangoni MA, et al (1990) Organ injury scaling, II: Pancreas, duodenum, small bowel, colon, and rectum. J Trauma 30:1427–1429
7. Hikida S, Sakamoto T, Higaki K, Hata H, Maeshiro K, Yamauchi K, Kimura YN, Egawa N, Mizote H, Shirouzu K (2004) Intraoperative ultrasonography is useful for diagnosing pancreatic duct injury and adjacent tissue damage in a patient with penetrating pancreas trauma. J Hepatobiliary Pancreat Surg 11:272–275
8. Bigattini D, Boverie JH, Dondelinger RF (1999) CT of blunt trauma of the pancreas in adults. Eur Radiol 9:244–249
9. Ilahi O, Bochicchio GV, Scalea TM (2002) Efficacy of computed tomography in the diagnosis of pancreatic injury in adult blunt trauma patients: a single-institutional study. Am Surg 68:704–707
10. Fulcher AS, Turner MA, Yelon JA, McClain LC, Broderick T, Ivatury RR, Sugerman HJ (2000) Magnetic resonance cholangiopancreatography (MRCP) in the assessment of pancreatic duct trauma and its sequelae: preliminary findings. J Trauma 48:1001–1007
11. Kim HS, Lee DK, Kim IW, Baik SK, Kwon SO, Park JW, Cho NC, Rhoe BS (2001) The role of endoscopic retrograde pancreatography in the treatment of traumatic pancreatic duct injury. Gastrointest Endosc 54:49–55
12. Takishima T, Hirata M, Kataoka Y, Asari Y, Sato K, Ohwada T, Kakita A (2000) Pancreatographic classification of pancreatic ductal injuries caused by blunt injury to the pancreas. J Trauma 48:745–751
13. Adamson WT, Hebra A, Thomas PB, Wagstaff P, Tagge EP, Othersen HB (2003) Serum amylase and lipase alone are not cost-effective screening methods for pediatric pancreatic trauma. J Pediatr Surg 38:354–357
14. Canty TG Sr, Weinman D (2001) Management of major pancreatic duct injuries in children. J Trauma 50:1001–1007
15. Lin BC, Chen RJ, Fang JF, Hsu YP, Kao YC, Kao JL (2004) Management of blunt major pancreatic injury. J Trauma 56:774–778
16. Rickard MJ, Brohi K, Bautz PC (2005) Pancreatic and duodenal injuries: keep it simple. ANZ J Surg 75:581–586
17. Asensio JA, Petrone P, Roldan G, Kuncir E, Demetriades D (2003) Pancreaticoduodenectomy: a rare procedure for the management of complex pancreaticoduodenal injuries. J Am Coll Surg 197:937–942
18. Jobst MA, Canty TG Sr, Lynch FP (1999) Management of pancreatic injury in pediatric blunt abdominal trauma. J Pediatr Surg 34:818–823
19. Stringer MD (2005) Pancreatic trauma in children. Br J Surg 92:467–470
20. Wolf A, Bernhardt J, Patrzyk M, Heidecke CD (2005) The value of endoscopic diagnosis and the treatment of pancreas injuries following blunt abdominal trauma. Surg Endosc 19:665–669
21. Kao LS, Bulger EM, Parks DL, Byrd GF, Jurkovich GJ (2003) Predictors of morbidity after traumatic pancreatic injury. J Trauma 55:898–905
22. Tyburski JG, Dente CJ, Wilson RF, Shanti C, Steffes CP, Carlin A (2001) Infectious complications following duodenal and/or pancreatic trauma. Am Surg 67:227–230
23. Olah A, Issekutz A, Haulik L, Makay R (2003) Pancreatic transection from blunt abdominal trauma: early versus delayed diagnosis and surgical management. Dig Surg 20:408–414
24. Zhang SH, Wang SM, Li JW (2005) Diagnosis and treatment of pancreatic trauma. Chin J Traumatol 8:303–305

Section 12

Transplantation of the Pancreas

Chapter 84 **Islet Transplantation and Results** *913*
C. Ricordi, A. Pileggi

Chapter 85 **Pancreas Transplantation** *921*
U. T. Hopt

C. Ricordi · A. Pileggi

Islet Transplantation and Results

Intensive treatment with exogenous insulin in combination with diet and exercise in most patients enables good glycemic control and prevents or delays the onset of the dreadful complications associated with chronic unstable glycemia [1]. However, intensive insulin therapy is unable to sustain euglycemia throughout the day and is associated with a threefold increased risk of severe, life-threatening hypoglycemic episodes [1]. Steady progress has been achieved in the recent years in the field of β-cell replacement by transplantation of pancreatic islets to restore insulin production in patients with diabetes [2]. Islet cells sense variations in glycemic values and accordingly synthesize and secrete endocrine hormones (namely, insulin and glucagon) in real time when needed; proper islet function allows for a more physiological glycemic control throughout the day when compared to exogenous insulin. Since the pioneering experiments performed by Ballinger and Lacy in the early 1970s [3], steady progress has been recorded in the fields of human islet isolation and transplantation technology [4–18]. Transplantation of islets of Langerhans can improve metabolic control, normalizing glycemic values, reducing glycated hemoglobin (HbA1c), and preventing the occurrence of severe hypoglycemia when sufficient islet numbers are implanted [4, 6–17]. Similar benefits, including absence of severe hypoglycemia, are observed even after transplantation of suboptimal islet numbers, the patient thus requiring exogenous insulin administration at doses lower than pretransplantation in order to maintain excellent glycemic control [4, 6–17].

Current Indications for Islet Transplantation

The rationale underlying the transplantation of islets holds for several clinical conditions in which β-cell function is lost to autoimmunity, metabolic diseases, or surgery (Table 84.1). Transplantation of allogeneic islets is offered mainly to nonuremic patients with unstable type 1 diabetes (T1DM), hypoglycemia unawareness, and severe hypoglycemia as "islet transplantation alone" (ITA) [4, 8, 10, 11, 13–16], or in patients with end-stage renal disease (ESRD) who are recipients of allogeneic kidney grafts, as either "islet after kidney" (IAK) [7, 9, 11, 15] or "simultaneous islet and kidney" (SIK) [12, 15] transplantation procedures. Transplantation of allogeneic islets is also indicated in patients with diabetes associated with metabolic diseases (i.e., liver cirrhosis, cystic fibrosis, and hemochromatosis) and gastrointestinal defects in combination with other organ grafts [6, 15, 17]. Allogeneic ITA has also been performed with success in the case of T1DM with subcutaneous insulin resistance [19].

Table 84.1. Current indications for islet transplantation

Allogeneic islet transplantation
Type 1 diabetes mellitus
– Islet transplantation alone
– Islet after kidney transplantation
– Simultaneous islet and kidney transplantation
Surgically induced diabetes
– Upper abdominal exenteration in recipients of cluster grafts
– Trauma
– Rescue of pancreatic graft after postoperative complication
Insulin-dependent diabetes associated to metabolic disorders
– Hepatic cirrhosis
– Cystic fibrosis
– Hemochromatosis
Autologous islet transplantation
Surgically induced diabetes
– Chronic pancreatitis
– Benign pancreatic neoplasm
– Trauma

Autologous islet transplantation is indicated for the prevention of iatrogenic diabetes after pancreatectomy for inflammatory diseases (i.e., chronic pancreatitis) [17, 20], benign neoplasm [21], or trauma, and due to the safety of the procedure, it has been performed even in elderly patients and in patients with liver cirrhosis.

Pancreas Procurement

Islets are generally obtained from the pancreas of deceased multiorgan donors (allogeneic islet transplantation). Multiple variables may influence both islet quality and yields obtained from the human pancreas. Implementation of strict donor selection criteria can be of assistance in improving the success rate of the islet isolation process: higher islet yields are generally obtained from adult donors with a high body mass index [22–24].

The pancreas is mobilized and excised following in situ vascular perfusion with chilled organ preservation solution (i.e., UW, University of Wisconsin, USA) and is generally removed en bloc with the duodenum and spleen. Pancreas-harvesting techniques that minimize injury to the gland (i.e., using the nontouch technique) during preparation and perfusion with preservation solution, and excision of the gland before liver procurement allow for higher islet recovery and transplantability rates [22, 25]. Cold-preservation of the pancreas should be maintained within 12 h. The introduction of oxygen-carrying moieties in the preservation solution (two-layer perfluorocarbon, UW/PFC solution (two-layer method, TLM) [26, 27] has enabled higher islet yields from human pancreata, extending cold ischemia time, and utilizing glands from marginal donors (e.g., from the elderly and donation after cardiac death), therefore providing assistance in maximizing the utilization of donor pancreata and expanding the organ donor pool for islet transplantation: it is currently considered the gold standard human pancreas preservation method for islet isolation. The use of living-related pancreas segments for the isolation of islets for transplantation has recently been proposed for selected cases [28], and it is conceivable that this approach will be of assistance in increasing the number of islet transplants in the future. Transplantation of autologous islets represents a viable therapeutic option to prevent the effects of insulinopenia following pancreatectomy for benign diseases of the pancreas [20].

Donor Selection Criteria

Acceptable Donor Organ Criteria

Multiorgan donors of either sex, between 15 and 70 years of age, warm ischemia time <10 min, cold ischemia time <12 h in the absence of UW/PFC

Donor Exclusion Criteria

Preexisting diseases, including T1DM or T2DM (glycated hemoglobin, HbA1c>6.5%), malignancies other than primary brain tumor, septicemia, viral hepatitis, acquired immunodeficiency syndrome, human immunodeficiency virus seropositivity, syphilis, viral encephalitis, Creutzfeldt-Jacob disease, rabies, tuberculosis, periods of relevant hypotension, elevated serum creatinine or abnormal liver function tests, elevation in serum amylase or lipase, history of promiscuous sexual behavior, and intravenous drug use.

Infrastructures

The success of an islet transplant program largely depends on the availability of adequate infrastructures and of a multidisciplinary team. There is the need for constant interactions with organ procurement organizations and for the involvement of medical departments and services, including other organ transplant programs, surgery, radiology, endocrinology, and pathology, amongst others.

Because of the need for pancreas processing, the Food and Drug Administration regulates islet transplantation as an investigational new drug. The islet cell processing facility is therefore organized following General Manufacture Practices, Good Laboratory Practices, and Good Tissue Practices regulations for clinical trials. These requirements aim at ensuring that the highest standards of quality, purity, potency, and safety for medical products for human use are observed. For this reason, the procedures are performed under aseptic conditions in class II biological safety cabinets and in clean rooms with restricted access, designed, tested, and certified to meet International Standards Organization (ISO) class 7 (ISO 14644) standards. Standard Operating Procedures, continuous training, and periodical competency assessment are enforced for all personnel, while both the facility and equipment are inspected periodically to confirm compliance with the required standards. The implementation of centralized regional islet processing centers that isolate and distribute high-quality islets to remote transplant centers represents a viable strat-

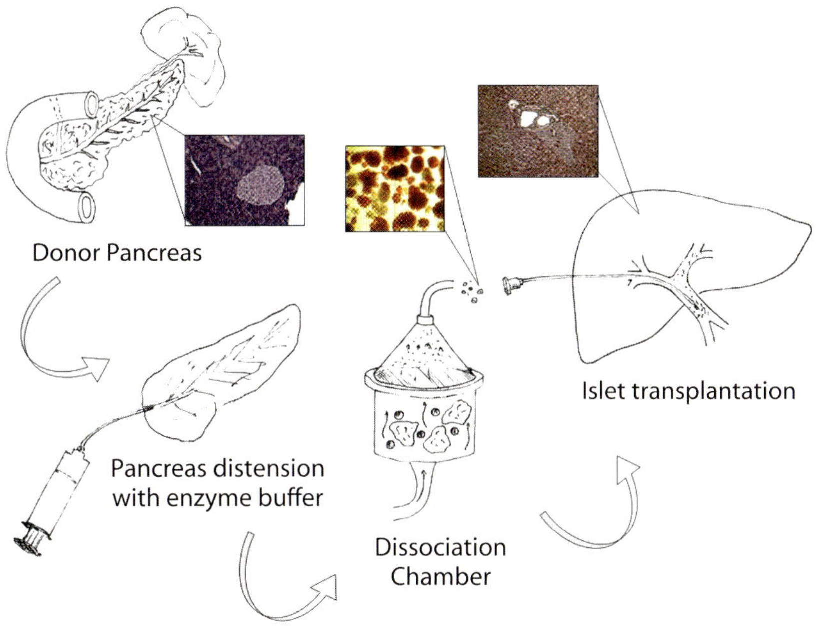

Figure 84.1

Schematic representation of the key steps of islet isolation and transplantation

egy to improve the utilization of cadaveric pancreata, while lowering the costs for islet preparations, therefore contributing to a maximization of the overall success rate of clinical islet transplantation.

Pancreatic Islet Isolation

Islets of Langerhans are endocrine cell clusters that are scattered throughout the pancreas, accounting for approximately ≤2% of the total pancreatic tissue. Complex interactions between islets and the surrounding environment and within the endocrine cells comprising the clusters (α-cells, which produce glucagon, β-cells, which produce insulin, δ-cells, which produce somatostatin, and PP-cells, which produce pancreatic polypeptide) finely regulate glucose metabolism. The goal of the isolation and purification procedures is therefore to release the islets from connective and nonendocrine pancreatic tissues while preserving their structural and functional integrity (Fig. 84.1). The islet isolation procedure consists of two phases aiming at (1) physically dissociating the gland into small fragments using a mechanically enhanced enzymatic digestion (dissociation phase), and (2) obtaining tissue enriched for the endocrine component for transplantation (purification phase) [15].

Dissociation

The pancreas is dissected free from duodenum and surrounding tissues while preserving the integrity of its capsule. At the neck of the gland, two catheters are inserted into the pancreatic duct (toward the head and the tail of the gland, respectively) for the delivery of the dissociation solution containing the enzyme. This is injected manually or using a peristaltic pump until distension of the gland is obtained to enhance the enzymatic digestion. The pancreas is then cut into large pieces and loaded into the dissociation chamber [5], which comprises two portions separated by a removable stainless steel screen: (1) the lower cylindrical chamber with inlet ports and an opening for a temperature sensor, and (2) the upper conical portion with an outlet at the apex. The chamber is part of a circuit through which the dissociation solution is circulated by the means of a peristaltic pump. Along with the pancreas, specially manufactured marbles that serve as digestion enhancers are also loaded into the chamber to contribute to the mechanical disruption of the gland. After sealing the chamber, the circuit is filled with dissociation solution and the temperature increased to enable optimal enzymatic activity. The combination of mechanical (controlled amplitude and frequency shaking enhanced by the marbles) and enzymatic actions result in the release from the digesting pancreas of particles that are continuously removed through the screen (action of the peristaltic flow) to preserve them from further digestion. The progression of the digestion is monitored throughout the process to determine islet integrity and the appearance of acinar tissue. The enzymatic activity is stopped by the means of dilution with serum-enriched cold medium. The pancreatic digest is then concentrated by centrifugation and prepared for the purification phase.

Purification

The goal of the purification step is to enrich in the endocrine component and to reduce the final volume to be transplanted. Islet separation is obtained on density gradients using the semiautomated purification method (computerized centrifuge system COBE 2991), which comprises a centrifuge bowl that accommodates a ring-shaped bag allowing for the separation of large volumes of pancreatic digest in short times. After a short centrifugation, the tissue migrates through the gradient and becomes distributed as a function of its density, allowing its separation according to the characteristics of the clusters: the pellet (mostly acinar tissue) sediments toward the outside and the lower density fractions toward the center of the bag. This allows the collection of different fractions with decreasing islet purity that are assessed and then combined to obtain the best compromise between higher number of islets (≥5,000 IEQ/kg of recipient's body weight) and the final purity of ≥30% in a volume of tissue ≤10 ml for transplantation [15].

Product release criteria include assessment of sterility (negative Gram staining to exclude bacterial contamination, endotoxin ≤5 EU/ml concentrations of final product volume/kg recipient body weight), viability (≥70% by membrane exclusion dyes), and in vitro potency (glucose-stimulated insulin release) of the islet preparation. Islet purity is assessed by dithizone staining to estimate the percentage of endocrine cell clusters and counting of islets in the final preparation. Assessment of the cellular composition of final preparation by immunohistochemistry is also be utilized to further characterize the quality of the transplanted tissue.

Islets can be transplanted immediately after purification or cultured for a short period of time [8, 10, 13, 29].

Recognized advantages of culturing the islets prior to transplant include the possibility of: (1) allowing recovery from the traumatic isolation process (even though a relative loss of islets might be noticed), (2) shipping islets to a distant center, (3) facilitating the logistics for the transplant (i.e., patients living far from the center, pretransplant testing and procedures), and (4) pretreating the recipient (i.e., immunomodulation, immunosuppression, and reduction of inflammation); these factors contribute to maximize both the engraftment and survival of transplanted islets.

Islet Transplantation Techniques

The current gold standard implantation site for islet grafts is the liver (Fig. 84.1). The islets are embolized into the hepatic sinusoids after cannulation of the portal system and infusion by gravity using a closed infusion bag system [30]. This allows the tissue to be maintained in suspension during the procedure, thus preventing undesirable abrupt increases in portal pressure. Heparin is included in the transplant solution in order to prevent thrombosis of the portal tract.

Transhepatic Percutaneous Access

The availability of minimally invasive interventional radiology techniques allows for the transhepatic percutaneous cannulation of the portal vein under ultrasound and angiographic guidance [31]. The portal pressure is constantly monitored using a pressure transducer connected to the catheter. At the end of the procedure, the access tract is sealed using a gel plug and fibrin to prevent bleeding. This outpatient procedure is performed under conscious sedation of the patient and is repeatable on several different occasions, and it is associated with minimal risks and a low incidence of complications.

Laparotomy

In the cases in which the percutaneous approach to the portal system is contraindicated (i.e., use of anticoagulation therapy increasing the risk of hemorrhage, anatomical abnormalities, unavailability of an experienced interventional radiologist, or patient preference), cannulation of a tributary of the portal vein can be obtained under general anesthesia through a laparotomy.

Laparoscopy

A less invasive surgical approach can also be utilized consisting of laparoscopic access to the portal system through the umbilical vein under general anesthesia.

Peritransplant Patient Management

Induction immunosuppression is implemented before the transplantation of allogeneic islets and trough levels should be monitored to ensure achievement of target levels. Prophylactic treatments include antiviral drugs (valgancyclovir daily for the first 3 months after each islet infusion) and trimethroprim-sulfamethoxazole three times a week for the prevention of *Pneumocystitis carinii* pneumonia. The patients are generally maintained on exogenous insulin in the posttransplant period in order to limit the metabolic load on the freshly implanted islets. Glycemic control is closely monitored to prevent hypoglycemia; based on the glycemic control, insulin requirements are adjusted and eventually weaned if sufficient graft function is observed [13].

Posttransplant Monitoring

During the days following islet implantation, hematological and liver function tests are performed to exclude complications related to the transplant procedure.

Graft Function

A variety of metabolic tests is performed before and after islet transplantation to assess graft function (Table 84.2) [9, 13]. Periodical monitoring of pre- and postprandial glycemia, basal c-peptide, and of HbA1c helps evaluating the performance of implanted islets. In addition, in patients requiring exogenous insulin, monitoring of insulin requirements before and after implant may be of assistance in assessing the potency of transplanted islets. Stimulation tests are performed to determine the ability of implanted islets to respond to selected secretagogues (i.e., glucose, arginine, and mixed meal) and therefore monitor whether changes in metabolic function following islet implant (dysfunction or loss of function) occur over time. One limitation of the current tests is the inability to discriminate between loss of graft function due to rejection or consequent to metabolic exhaustion (toxicity of immunosuppressive drugs, increased metabolic demand on an engrafted marginal islet mass, and hyperglycemic microenvironment, amongst others), and the fact that they can not detect loss of graft function early enough to allow prompt implementation of graft-saving treatments.

Table 84.2. Monitoring of graft function. *AIR* Acute insulin release, *ACR* acute c-peptide release, *AUC* area under the curve, *SI* stimulation index, *arg* arginine, *gluc* glucose, *MAGE* mean amplitude of glycemic excursions, *HbA1c* glycated hemoglobin A1c

Standard tests
Insulin requirements
HbA1c
Fasting glucose
Postprandial glucose
MAGE
Basal C-peptide
Stimulation tests
Mixed meal test (AUC_{gluc}, AUC_{ins}, SI)
Intravenous glucose tolerance test (AIR^{gluc}, ACR_{gluc})
Intravenous arginine (AIR_{arg}, ACR_{arg})

Monitoring Immune Response

For allogeneic islet transplantation, the immune response to donor antigens in vitro (mixed lymphocyte reactions), expression of cytotoxic lymphocyte genes (i.e., perforin and granzyme B), and levels of serum levels of autoantibodies (e.g., IA2, GAD-65) are monitored, as they may be of assistance in determining the efficacy of the immunosuppression treatment [13].

Clinical Outcome After Autologous Islet Transplantation

Transplantation of >250,000 unpurified autologous islets generally results in normoglycemia and insulin independence in about 70% of patients with pancreatitis [20]. Successful preservation of β-cell function has been obtained after islet autotransplantation after pancreatectomy for trauma or benign neoplasm, and because of the safety of the procedure it can be considered a viable option for elderly patients and in the case of liver cirrhosis.

Clinical Outcome After Allogeneic Islet Transplantation

A total of 493 allogeneic and 240 autologous grafts were reported to the International Islet Transplant Registry up to 2001 (from 30 centers in Europe, 18 in North America, and 6 centers elsewhere), with insulin independence at 1 year following allogeneic islet transplantation observed in approximately 10% of the cases. The steady improvement in engraftment rates has lead to the report of 100% insulin independence at 1 year following ITA in patients with T1DM using the Edmonton protocol (infusion of freshly isolated islets, induction with daclizumab, maintenance with sirolimus and low doses of tacrolimus) [8]. Numerous clinical trials have followed utilizing similar treatments [4, 10–17]. While the Edmonton protocol has been reproduced in a multicenter ITA trial, the graft outcomes may vary substantially between institutions, and centers with established experience in islet isolation, transplantation, and patient management reported insulin independence in ~80% of the recipients at 1 year posttransplantation, while lower success rates were observed in less experienced centers. Since 2001, a total of 118 patients receiving ITA, 19 IAK, and one islet autograft were reported to the Collaborative Islet Transplant Registry by 19 North American Centers. Insulin independence in 49.1% of the 112 patients who completed a 1-year follow up was reported; 34.8% had detectable c-peptide levels but required insulin, and 13.5% experienced graft loss with undetectable c-peptide.

Islet transplantation can substantially improve glycemic metabolic control even when suboptimal islet masses are transplanted (Table 84.3). Insulin independence is achieved when sufficient numbers of functional islets are transplanted, a goal that is generally attained using more than one islet preparation per recipient as either sequential or combined islet infusions. The immunosuppressive regimens utilized currently are based mainly on the combination of sirolimus and low doses of tacrolimus, with the induction with monoclonal antibodies targeting the interleukin-2 receptor or T-cell depleting antibodies. The treatment is generally well tolerated, although adverse events commonly associated with the use of such drugs may require close follow up and medical interventions (Table 84.4).

The natural history of allogeneic islet transplantation in patients with T1DM using the Edmonton protocol or similar immunosuppressive regimens seems to indicate that approximately 80% of the recipients remain insulin free at 1 year, while a gradual loss of graft function with the need for reintroduction of exogenous insulin at lower doses than pretransplantation to maintain good glycemic control (HbA1c within target ranges) is observed in most of the recipients [11, 13, 14]. Long-term graft survival (the longest follow up of recent trials is 5 years) as a function of de-

Table 84.3. Benefits of islet transplantation

Metabolic control
Reduced insulin requirements/insulin independence
Reduction of MAGE
Reduction of HbA1c
Absence of severe hypoglycemia
Quality of life
Reduced fear of hypoglycemia
Improved diabetes quality of life
Diabetes complications
Improved micro- and macroangiopathy
Improved cardiovascular function
Reduced nephropathy
Stabilization/improvement of neuropathy
Stabilization of retinopathy

Table 84.4. Most frequent adverse events in recipients of allogeneic islet grafts

Procedure-related
Bleedings
Portal thrombosis
Transaminitis
Hematological
Leukopenia (immunosuppression)
Anemia (immunosuppression)
Neutropenia (immunosuppression)
Metabolic
Hyperlipidemia (sirolimus)
Gastrointestinal
Mouth ulcers (sirolimus)
Respiratory Tract
Upper respiratory infection
Neurological
Neurotoxicity (tacrolimus)
Genitourinary
Leg edema (sirolimus)
Nephropathy (tacrolimus, sirolimus)
Ovarian cysts (sirolimus?)

tectable c-peptide is maintained in most of the patients (~80%), while insulin independence is sustained in approximately 10% [14]. One possible explanation for this phenomenon is the suboptimal islet mass engrafting undergoing increasing metabolic stress in the hepatic environment in combination with chronic β-cell toxicity of the immunosuppressive drugs.

Interestingly, prevention of severe hypoglycemia is achieved in these patients, regardless of the reintroduction of exogenous insulin until measurable c-peptide levels are present. It is conceivable that the transplanted islets can, to some extent, restore hypoglycemia hormonal counterregulation [32]. Indeed, reduced anxiety about the symptoms and consequences of hypoglycemia has been recorded in recipients of islet transplants in analysis of health-related quality of life [33, 34], and a sustained positive influence on diabetes quality of life has been observed in recipients of ITA even if experiencing immunosuppression-related side effects [35]. Furthermore, beneficial effects of islet transplantation on diabetic complications have been reported (Table 84.3), including improved renal allograft function, improved diabetic micro- and macroangiopathy, and improved cardiovascular function in IAK recipients, and stabilization of diabetic retinopathy and of diabetic neuropathy in ITA recipients [36–41].

Steady progress has been achieved in the field of islet transplantation. The procedure is safe and has proven efficacy in improving metabolic control, quality of life, and preventing severe hypoglycemia in patients with diabetes. Very encouraging data are emerging from ongoing clinical trials and from translational research studies that justify a cautious optimism for the near future.

Acknowledgements

Supported in part by National Institute of Health, National Institute of Diabetes and Digestive and Kidney Diseases (Immune Tolerance Network), National Center for Research Resources (General Clinical Research Center and Islet Cell Resource Center), Juvenile Diabetes Research Foundation International, American Diabetes Association, and the Diabetes Research Institute Foundation (www.diabetesresearch.org). The Authors are grateful to Dr. Lorenzo Cobianchi for the kind assistance in the preparation of this chapter.

References

1. Diabetes Control and Complications Trial Research Group (1993) The effect of intensive treatment of diabetes on the development and progression of long-term complications in insulin-dependent diabetes mellitus. N Engl J Med 329:977–986
2. Ricordi C (2003) Islet transplantation: a brave new world. Diabetes 52:1595–1603
3. Ballinger WF, Lacy PE (1972) Transplantation of intact pancreatic islets in rats. Surgery 82:175–186
4. Ricordi C, Strom TB (2004) Clinical islet transplantation: advances and immunological challenges. Nat Rev Immunol 4:259–268
5. Ricordi C, Lacy PE, Finke EH, Olack BJ, Scharp DW (1988) Automated method for isolation of human pancreatic islets. Diabetes 37:413–420
6. Tzakis AG, Ricordi C, Alejandro R, Zeng Y, Fung JJ, Todo S, et al (1990) Pancreatic islet transplantation after upper abdominal exenteration and liver replacement. Lancet 336:402–405
7. Alejandro R, Lehmann R, Ricordi C, Kenyon NS, Angelico MC, Burke G, et al (1997) Long-term function (6 years) of islet allografts in type 1 diabetes. Diabetes 46:1983–1989
8. Shapiro AM, Lakey JR, Ryan EA, Korbutt GS, Toth E, Warnock GL, et al (2000) Islet transplantation in seven patients with type 1 diabetes mellitus using a glucocorticoid-free immunosuppressive regimen. N Engl J Med 343:230–238
9. Luzi L, Perseghin G, Brendel MD, Terruzzi I, Battezzati A, Eckhard M, et al (2001) Metabolic effects of restoring partial beta-cell function after islet allotransplantation in type 1 diabetic patients. Diabetes 50:277–282
10. Hering BJ, Kandaswamy R, Harmon JV, Ansite JD, Clemmings SM, Sakai T, et al (2004) Transplantation of cultured islets from two-layer preserved pancreases in type 1 diabetes with anti-CD3 antibody. Am J Transplant 4:390–401
11. Frank A, Deng S, Huang X, Velidedeoglu E, Bae YS, Liu C, et al (2004) Transplantation for type I diabetes: comparison of vascularized whole-organ pancreas with isolated pancreatic islets. Ann Surg 240:631–640; discussion 640–643
12. Lehmann R, Weber M, Berthold P, Zullig R, Pfammatter T, Moritz W, et al (2004) Successful simultaneous islet-kidney transplantation using a steroid-free immunosuppression: two-year follow-up. Am J Transplant 4:1117–1123
13. Froud T, Ricordi C, Baidal DA, Hafiz MM, Ponte G, Cure P, et al (2005) Islet transplantation in type 1 diabetes mellitus using cultured islets and steroid-free immunosuppression: Miami experience. Am J Transplant 5:2037–2046
14. Ryan EA, Paty BW, Senior PA, Bigam D, Alfadhli E, Kneteman NM, et al (2005) Five-year follow-up after clinical islet transplantation. Diabetes 54:2060–2069
15. Pileggi A, Ricordi C, Kenyon NS, Froud T, Baidal DA, Kahn A, et al (2004) Twenty years of clinical islet transplantation at the Diabetes Research Institute – University of Miami. Clin Transpl 2004:177–204
16. Hering BJ, Kandaswamy R, Ansite JD, Eckman PM, Nakano M, Sawada T, et al (2005). Single-donor, marginal-dose islet transplantation in patients with type 1 diabetes. JAMA 293:830–835
17. Matsumoto S, Okitsu T, Iwanaga Y, Noguchi H, Nagata H, Yonekawa Y, et al (2005) Insulin independence after living-donor distal pancreatectomy and islet allotransplantation. Lancet 365:1642–1644

18. Ichii H, Pileggi A, Molano RD, Baidal DA, Khan A, Kuroda Y, et al (2005) Rescue purification maximizes the use of human islet preparations for transplantation. Am J Transplant 5:21–30
19. Gillard P, Ling Z, Lannoo M, Maes B, Maleux G, Pipeleers D, et al (2004) Beta-cell transplantation restores metabolic control and quality of life in a patient with subcutaneous insulin resistance. Diabetes Care 27:2243–2244
20. Robertson RP, Lanz KJ, Sutherland DE, Kendall DM (2001) Prevention of diabetes for up to 13 years by autoislet transplantation after pancreatectomy for chronic pancreatitis. Diabetes 50:47–50
21. Oberholzer J, Mathe Z, Bucher P, Triponez F, Bosco D, Fournier B, et al (2003) Islet autotransplantation after left pancreatectomy for non-enucleable insulinoma. Am J Transplant 3:1302–1307
22. Lakey JR, Warnock GL, Rajotte RV, Suarez-Alamazor ME, Ao Z, Shapiro AM, et al (1996) Variables in organ donors that affect the recovery of human islets of Langerhans. Transplantation 61:1047–1053
23. O'Gorman D, Kin T, Murdoch T, Richer B, McGhee-Wilson D, Ryan EA, et al (2005) The standardization of pancreatic donors for islet isolations. Transplantation 80:801–806
24. Berney T, Buhler LH, Morel P (2005) Pancreas allocation in the era of islet transplantation. Transpl Int 18:763–767
25. Lee TC, Barshes NR, Brunicardi FC, Alejandro R, Ricordi C, Nguyen L, et al (2004) Procurement of the human pancreas for pancreatic islet transplantation. Transplantation 78:481–483
26. Kuroda Y, Kawamura T, Suzuki Y, Fujiwara H, Yamamoto K, Saitoh Y (1988) A new, simple method for cold storage of the pancreas using perfluorochemical. Transplantation 46:457–460
27. Fraker CA, Alejandro R, Ricordi C (2002) Use of oxygenated perfluorocarbon toward making every pancreas count. Transplantation 74:1811–1812
28. Matsumoto S, Okitsu T, Iwanaga Y, Noguchi H, Nagata H, Yonekawa Y, et al (2005) Insulin independence of unstable diabetic patient after single living donor islet transplantation. Transplant Proc 37:3427–3429
29. Goss JA, Goodpastor SE, Brunicardi FC, Barth MH, Soltes GD, Garber AJ, et al (2004) Development of a human pancreatic islet-transplant program through a collaborative relationship with a remote islet-isolation center. Transplantation 77:462–466
30. Baidal DA, Froud T, Ferreira JV, Khan A, Alejandro R, Ricordi C (2003) The bag method for islet cell infusion. Cell Transplant 12:809–813
31. Froud T, Yrizarry JM, Alejandro R, Ricordi C (2004) Use of D-STAT to prevent bleeding following percutaneous transhepatic intraportal islet transplantation. Cell Transplant 13:55–59
32. Rickels MR, Schutta MH, Mueller R, Markmann JF, Barker CF, Naji A, et al (2005) Islet cell hormonal responses to hypoglycemia after human islet transplantation for type 1 diabetes. Diabetes 54:3205–3211
33. Barshes NR, Vanatta JM, Mote A, Lee TC, Schock AP, Balkrishnan R, et al (2005) Health-related quality of life after pancreatic islet transplantation: a longitudinal study. Transplantation 79:1727–1730
34. Johnson JA, Kotovych M, Ryan EA, Shapiro AM (2004) Reduced fear of hypoglycemia in successful islet transplantation. Diabetes Care 27:624–625
35. Poggioli R, Faradji RN, Ponte G, Betancourt A, Messinger S, Baidal D, et al (2006) Quality of life after islet transplantation. Am J Transplant 6:371-378
36. Fiorina P, Folli F, Bertuzzi F, Maffi P, Finzi G, Venturini M, et al (2003) Long-term beneficial effect of islet transplantation on diabetic macro-/microangiopathy in type 1 diabetic kidney-transplanted patients. Diabetes Care 26:1129–1136
37. Fiorina P, Folli F, Maffi P, Placidi C, Venturini M, Finzi G, et al (2003) Islet transplantation improves vascular diabetic complications in patients with diabetes who underwent kidney transplantation: a comparison between kidney-pancreas and kidney-alone transplantation. Transplantation 75:1296-1301
38. Fiorina P, Folli F, Zerbini G, Maffi P, Gremizzi C, Di Carlo V, et al (2003) Islet transplantation is associated with improvement of renal function among uremic patients with type I diabetes mellitus and kidney transplants. J Am Soc Nephrol 14:2150-2158
39. Fiorina P, Gremizzi C, Maffi P, Caldara R, Tavano D, Monti L, et al (2005) Islet transplantation is associated with an improvement of cardiovascular function in type 1 diabetic kidney transplant patients. Diabetes Care 28:1358-1365
40. Fiorina P, Venturini M, Folli F, Losio C, Maffi P, Placidi C, et al (2005) Natural history of kidney graft survival, hypertrophy, and vascular function in end-stage renal disease type 1 diabetic kidney-transplanted patients: beneficial impact of pancreas and successful islet cotransplantation. Diabetes Care 28:1303-1310
41. Lee TC, Barshes NR, O'Mahony CA, Nguyen L, Brunicardi FC, Ricordi C, et al (2005) The effect of pancreatic islet transplantation on progression of diabetic retinopathy and neuropathy. Transplant Proc 37:2263-2265

Chapter 85

Pancreas Transplantation

U.T. Hopt

In healthy people the blood sugar concentration is controlled within very narrow limits by a highly sensitive feedback mechanism. The mainstay of this feedback mechanism is the ß-cell in the islets of Langerhans, which are situated in the pancreas. Within these ß-cells a glucose sensor is continuously active measuring glucose concentration in the blood. Depending on the actual glucose concentration, insulin secretion is either up- or downregulated. In patients with type I diabetes the ß-cells in the islets of Langerhans are completely destroyed by an autoimmune process. Thus, type I diabetics lack the physiological feedback control of blood glucose concentration. They are forced to inject more or less frequently during the day a certain amount of insulin according to the results of a point-to-point measurement of blood glucose. It is clear that exogenous insulin application will never be able to control blood glucose concentration in such a narrow range as is achieved by a normal pancreas. This is also true in patients with intensified insulin therapy. The consequences of such an impaired glucose control are twofold. First, the patients may suffer from severe hypo- or hyperglycemia, which might be life threatening. Much more serious threats for patients with type I diabetes are the secondary diabetic complications. These are the result of an unphysiological and therefore insufficient control of glucose metabolism, especially of the peripheral glucose concentration. As the result, about half of all patients with type I diabetes will ultimately suffer from diabetic nephropathy, retinopathy, and neuropathy. Diabetes mellitus is currently the leading cause of kidney failure and blindness in adults as well as the leading cause of peripheral amputations, impotence, and cardiovascular disease. About one-third of the patients with type I diabetes will progress to end-stage renal disease and the need for dialysis or kidney transplantation. The aforementioned secondary diabetic complications are the main reason for the significantly increased morbidity and the dramatically reduced life expectancy of diabetic patients compared with a healthy population [1].

The key factor in the treatment of type I diabetes is an almost physiological, that means a very tight, control of blood glucose concentration. The diabetes control and complication trial (DCCT) has shown clearly that a very tight control of blood glucose prevents, or at least delays, the onset and progression of secondary complications. However, even with the so-called intensified insulin therapy, blood glucose control is not physiological. In addition, the risk of episodes of hypoglycemia increases significantly. The only possibility of reestablishing a physiological blood glucose control consists at the moment of the transplantation of insulin-secreting tissue. In spite of the enormous developments and advantages related to islet transplantation during the last 3 years, long-term success is still not possible with this kind of therapy [2]. Thus, pancreas transplantation is currently the only possibility for restoring physiological blood glucose control with a high success rate and for a period of more than 10 years in the majority of patients. On the other hand, however, the trade-off for the cure of diabetes relates to the perioperative risk associated with pancreas transplantation and the need for lifelong immunosuppression.

The first pancreas transplantation in combination with kidney transplantation was performed 1966 by Kelly and Lillehei at the University of Minnesota. Endocrine function, however, was sustained for only one week. During the subsequent 15 years the results of the procedure were characterized by a very low success rate and unacceptably high perioperative mortality. Since the introduction of the bladder drainage technique in 1983, however, and due to the use of calcineurin inhibitors, for example cyclosporin A or tacrolimus, as immunosuppressive drugs, pancreas transplantation has regained increasing acceptance. The technical failure rate as well the perioperative morbidity and mortality have decreased dramatically. The 1-year graft survival rates have increased gradually and reached values of more than 80%, especially in cases of simultaneous pancreas-kidney-transplantation [3]. Nowadays the short- and long-term results of simultaneous pancreas-kidney transplantation are comparable with those of other solid organ transplantations such as isolated kidney transplantation or liver transplantation. Meanwhile, the procedure has lost its experimental status and is now accepted therapy. Accordingly, in 1999 simultaneous pancreas-kidney transplantation and pancreas after kidney transplantation was awarded Medicare coverage in the USA. In Germany, too, pancreas transplantations are now covered by all insurances. The number of pancreas transplantations performed is currently 1,500 per year. Most of these transplantations, however, are performed in the USA. The frequency of pancreas transplantations per million inhabitants is still about twice as high in the USA than in most European countries. This is also true for Germany.

Indication for Pancreas Transplantation

More than 90% of patients on the waiting list for a pancreas graft suffer from diabetogenic end-stage renal disease. Thus these patients are candidates for simultaneous pancreas-kidney transplantation from the same donor. Simultaneous pancreas-kidney transplantation is characterized by significantly better long-term results than pancreas after kidney transplantation or pancreas transplantation alone. A major advantage of the procedure is that rejection episodes affecting the pancreas can be diagnosed by monitoring the function of the simultaneously transplanted kidney, since more than 90% of rejections affect both organs. In addition, recipients of a kidney graft need life-long immunosuppression. Thus, additional transplantation of a pancreas imposes on the recipient only the risk of the surgical procedure. It has been shown clearly that the additional transplantation of a pancreas graft does not jeopardize the kidney graft [4, 5].

There is a considerable number of type I diabetic patients who have been transplanted with an isolated cadaveric or living donor kidney graft. If the kidney function is stable with adequate creatinine clearance these patients are candidates for a pancreas after kidney transplantation [6]. The advantages of additional pancreas transplantation are the same as in patients with simultaneous pancreas-kidney transplantation. Detection of rejection of the pancreas graft, however, might be a major problem. Thus, long-term results are not as good as in simultaneous pancreas-kidney transplantation. Nevertheless, the number of pancreas after kidney transplantations is steadily increasing [3].

Pancreas transplantation alone is indicated only in highly selected patients. Patients with hypoglycemia unawareness or hyperlabile diabetes (brittle diabetes), suffering from frequent severe hypoglycemic episodes, and patients with rapidly progressive secondary complications such as neuropathy or proliferative retinopathy might be treated with pancreas transplantation alone. The benefits of a well functioning pancreas have to be balanced with the risks of the surgical procedure and the need for chronic immunosuppression. Pancreas transplantation alone should only be performed in patients with a creatinine clearance of more than 70 ml/min. Otherwise, the risk of progressive deterioration of kidney function due to the nephrotoxic effect of the immunosuppressive therapy is unacceptable high.

Because of the well-known multimorbidity, a thorough preoperative diagnostic work-up of the transplant candidate is mandatory. Considering all organ systems, the patient has to have the ability to withstand a major operation. Because of the prevalence of coronary heart disease, a noninvasive cardiac stress test is performed routinely in all patients. It should be kept in mind that diabetic neuropathy may prevent patients from experiencing typical angina. Patients with symptoms or equivocal stress test should undergo cardiac catheterization. In case of significant coronary heart disease, patients should undergo coronary revascularization with angioplasty/stent or coronary artery bypass before pancreas transplantation. In addition, correction of aortoiliac disease or hemodynamically significant carotid occlusive disease may be necessary before transplantation in order to provide an uncompromised arterial inflow into the transplants as well as to prevent perioperative cerebral complications. The work-up also includes metabolic, neurologic, ophthalmologic, renal, and psychiatric evaluations.

Contraindications include severe uncorrectable cardiovascular disease, the presence of a recent malignancy, chronic therapy-resistant infections, chronic active hepatitis or liver cirrhosis, psychiatric disease, or drug dependency with the consequence of a low patient compliance with respect to, for example, postoperative immunosuppression. Relative contraindications are an age above 55 years; thus it is not the numerical but the biological age that is important. Furthermore, a body mass index above 30 kg/m^2, a generalized severe arterial vascular disease, and a previous severe myocardial infarction are major perioperative risk factors. The decision to perform pancreas transplantation in these patients should only be made after thorough discussion of the patient's situation and after balancing the risks and benefits of the procedure on an individual basis.

In type II diabetic patients pancreas transplantation also effects normalization of blood sugar levels; exogenous insulin application becomes unnecessary. The metabolic syndrome of those patients and all the related problems, however, remain unchanged. Considering the limited number of organs available, extension of pancreas transplantation to type II diabetic patients would result in an exorbitant increase in waiting time for type I diabetic patients. The consequences would be further progression of secondary diabetic complications in these patients. In addition, since the life expectancy of diabetic patients on dialysis is very poor, the mortality of patients on the waiting list for simultaneous pancreas-kidney transplantation would increase dramatically. Thus, at least in the Eurotransplant region, pancreas transplantation is currently only available to type I diabetic patients.

Donor Selection and Management

Donor selection for pancreas transplantation is stricter than for kidney and liver donation. The upper age limit for the donor is about 45 years. It is known that after the age of 55 years the ß-cell mass gradually decreases. There are some hints that postoperative morbidity in the recipient increases with donors over 45 years. For most centers the lower age limit is 8–10 years because of the limited ß-cell mass and the small diameter of vessels in these donors. Since the pancreas is a low-flow organ, the risk of early postoperative graft thrombosis increases significantly with such small grafts. Absolute contraindications for pancreas donation are a history of diabetes mellitus, acute necrotizing pancreatitis, chronic pancreatitis, and severe trauma to the upper abdomen. Relative contraindications are a body mass index of more than 30 kg/m^2, severe arteriosclerosis, severe hypernatremia, treatment on the intensive care unit of more than 7 days, and significant hemodynamic instability. Elevation of amylase, lipase, and glucose concentrations in the serum are not regarded as contraindications since, for example, hyperglycemia can be induced by cerebral trauma and the use of high doses of catecholamines as well as of corticoids, inducing insulin resistance [7]. When deciding on pancreas donation it has to be kept in mind that the medical history of potential donors often is unreliable. Furthermore, most of the aforementioned parameters are not strictly defined. Thus, final assessment of the suitability of an organ for transplantation should always be performed by direct inspection and palpation of the pancreas by an experienced transplant surgeon. The parenchyma of the pancreas should be pliable and without evidence of fibrosis or calcifications, and there should be no fat in the interlobular septa. It is known that the risk of graft pancreatitis and the postoperative morbidity of the recipient will significantly increase when using a fatty pancreas graft.

Allocation of an organ requires only ABO blood group compatibility and a negative cross-match. Contrary to the situation in kidney transplantation, the human leukocyte antigen (HLA) match between donor and recipient does not play a role in pancreas transplantation. Although according to the data of the International Pancreas Transplant Registry pancreas transplantations have been performed successfully with cold ischemia times of more than 25 h, most centers limit cold ischemia time to 12 h in order to reduce the risk of severe ischemia-reperfusion injury and secondary graft pancreatitis. There are several additional absolute contraindications that are valid for any kind of organ donation, such as generalized sepsis and a history of previous or present malignancy or specific infections such as HIV, hepatitis C, and others.

Donor Operation

Pancreas retrieval is usually performed in multiorgan donors. Although the arterial blood supply of the liver and pancreas comes from the same major arteries (celiac axis and superior mesenteric artery), the liver and the pancreas can always be retrieved even in case of anatomical variations. Familiarity with normal and abnormal anatomy in the upper abdomen and gentle and nontraumatizing handling of the pancreas are essential for the donor operation.

The abdomen is opened by a large midline incision from the xiphoid until the symphysis. In the case of heart and lung retrieval, splitting of the sternum is also carried out. The pancreas is inspected after mobilization of the duodenum and opening of the bursa omentalis by division of the gastrocolic ligament. Liver dissection is performed first. It is important to recognize anatomical variations. A right hepatic artery arising from the superior mesenteric artery occurs in about 10% of cases, and a left hepatic artery arising from the left gastric artery in 13%. An anomalous right hepatic artery can easily be identified by palpation of the hepatoduodenal ligament. Such an artery is almost always situated caudal and dorsal to the common bile duct. An atypical left hepatic artery can be found by palpation of the gastrohepatic ligament. The common hepatic artery, the origin of the gastroduodenal artery, and the origin of the splenic and the left gastric arteries are identified. Care is taken not to dissect the hepatic arteries completely because of the danger of vasospasm. The right gastric artery and the coronary vein might be divided at this point. The celiac axis is identified and followed until the aorta is reached. The supraceliac aorta is dissected and looped. The small bowel and the mesenteric root are mobilized from the retroperitoneum. The aorta is encircled just above the bifurcation. The origin of the superior mesenteric artery is dissected free just above the left renal vein. The infrahepatic vena cava is exposed and the origin of the left renal vein is identified.

A gastric tube is advanced into the duodenum and a mixture of betadine, antibiotics, and amphotericin B is instilled into the duodenum. The tube is then withdrawn back into the stomach. After completion of preparation of the liver and in the case of lung and heart retrieval after completion of dissection by the thoracic/cardiac transplant surgeons, 20,000 units of heparin are given intravenously. The aorta is cross-clamped above the origin of the celiac axis and ligated at the bifurcation. A perfusion catheter is introduced into the abdominal aorta and the abdominal organs are perfused with 3–4 l of ice-cold UW solution (Viaspan) or 5–7 l of ice-cold histidine-tryptophan-ketoglutarate solution (HTK; Custadiol). An additional perfusion of the liver via the portal vein does not seem to be necessary. In order to achieve quick and permanent cooling of the pancreas, which at this point of time is still fixed in the retroperitoneum, surface cooling with ice-cold saline solution given via the bursa omentalis is mandatory. This is especially important if the perfusion with UW/HTK is complete and removal of the lung, heart, or liver is held up because of technical reasons. In addition, it is of utmost importance to provide an adequate outflow of the perfusion solution by opening the vena cava supra- or infrahepatically at the time of perfusion; otherwise the pancreas will become edematous and overperfused.

Although the pancreas and liver can be retrieved en bloc and divided outside of the donor, in most cases separation of the liver and pancreas is performed in situ. The gastroduodenal, the left gastric, and the splenic arteries are cut at their origin. The common hepatic artery and the celiac axis are dissected free. The origin of the celiac axis is excised from the aorta with a Carrel patch. The common bile duct and the portal vein are cut near to the pancreas. Care is taken not to dissect the portal vein out of the pancreas in order not to endanger the venous anastomosis of the pancreas graft in the recipient. The infrahepatic and suprahepatic caval vein are dissected and the liver is removed. The right flexure of the colon is mobilized and the right gastroepiploic and midcolic vessels and the inferior mesenteric vein are dissected, ligated, and divided. The head and the lower rim of the pancreas are now completely free. The postpyloric duodenum and the jejunum near the ligament of Treitz are transected with a stapler. It is advisable to transect the mesenteric root also with a stapler; otherwise the vessels will retract into the remainder of the mesenteric root, resulting after reperfusion in significant bleeding and the formation of extensive local hematoma in and around the pancreas graft. It is important that the line of transection is at least 2–3 cm caudally from the processus uncinatus, since in this region the inferior pancreatoduodenal artery originates from the superior mesenteric artery. After ligation of the gastroduodenal artery, arterial perfusion of the pancreatic head is almost completely dependent on this artery. The short gastric vessels are divided in order to separate the stomach from the spleen. The spleen is freed from its retroperitoneal adhesions and used as a handle in order to avoid excessive manipulation of the pancreatic parenchyma. The pancreas is dissected free from the retroperitoneum, the left kidney, and the left adrenal up to the left side of the aorta. The celiac ganglion and the lymphatics around the aorta have to be divided. The superior mesenteric artery is cut at the level of the aorta (a Carrel patch is not needed) and the pancreas is removed (Fig. 85.1).

In case of a right hepatic artery from the superior mesenteric artery, this artery is carefully dissected from the posterior side of the pancreas and followed to its origin from the superior mesenteric artery. Since the origin of the inferior pancreatoduodenal artery is normally 1 or 2 cm distal to the origin of the atypical right hepatic artery, the superior mesenteric artery can be cut between both origins and the atypical hepatic artery can be preserved together with the stump of the superior mesenteric artery and a Carrel patch from the aorta. If the arterial supply of the liver originates completely from the superior mesenteric artery, the diameter of this artery is normally so large that it can be cut at the rim of the pancreas without providing technical problems for reanastomosis in the recipient.

For reconstruction of the arteries of the pancreas it is mandatory that the entire right or left common iliac artery together with its bifurcation into the external and internal iliac artery is procured and shipped together with the pancreas. In order to provide the pos-

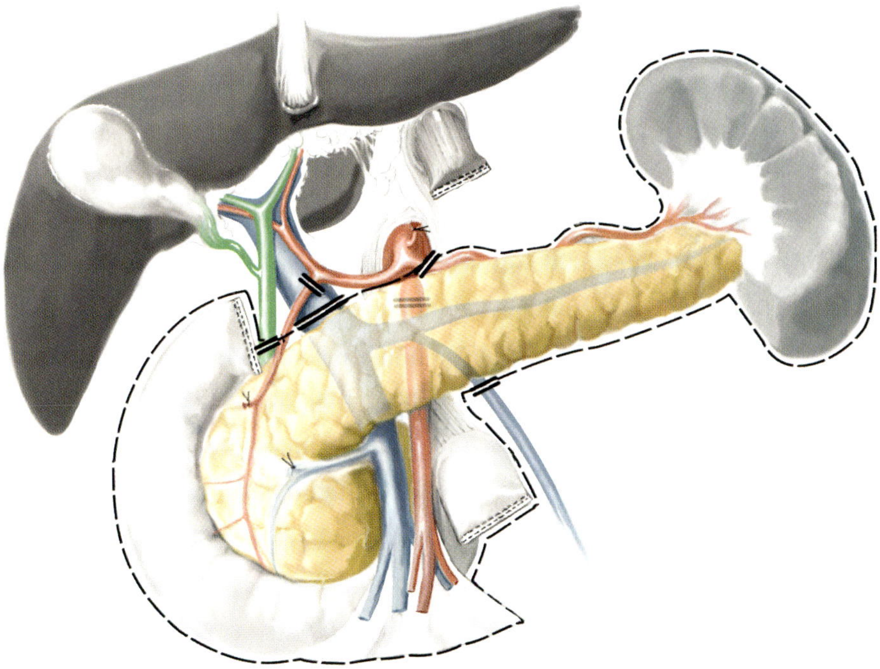

Figure 85.1

sibility of portal venous prolongation of the pancreas graft, the right or left common/external iliac vein of the donor is also included. The pancreas is packed in UW or HTK solution and shipped on ice in a box container to the recipient center.

Back Table Preparation

The spleen is removed, care being taken not to damage the pancreatic tail. The pancreas is cleaned of excessive fat. If enteric drainage of the graft is anticipated, only the distal part of the duodenum has to be resected. The duodenum is closed by a stapler and the staple line is oversewn with single stitches. If the graft will be drained into the bladder, the duodenal segment should be as short as possible (i.e., not longer than 6–8 cm), otherwise the duodenal segment acts in the recipient as a large bladder diverticulum. Thus, the duodenum has to be shortened at the proximal and distal end after identification of the papilla Vateri either by palpation or by insertion of a catheter via the common bile duct into the duodenum. In order to prevent bleeding after reperfusion of the graft, the staple line at the mesenteric root is also secured with several single stitches. The splenic artery and the mesenteric artery are dissected free for about 1 cm. The iliac Y-graft is freed of adherent tissue. The external iliac artery is connected to the stump of the superior mesenteric artery, and the internal iliac artery to the splenic artery via an end-to-end anastomosis using running 6-0 sutures (Fig. 85.2). A series of other reconstruction techniques has been described - for example end-to-side anastomosis of the splenic artery to the mesenteric artery or end-to-end anastomosis of the proximal stump of the splenic artery to the distal stump of superior mesenteric artery. Such reconstruction techniques are important in special anatomic situations; standard reconstruction certainly requires the use of a Y-extension graft. The portal vein is dissected free from the pancreas. A venous extension graft is almost never necessary. If the portal vein is too short, the vein can be prolonged by end-to-end anastomosis between the stump of the portal vein and a segment of the common iliac vein of the donor The gastroepiploic artery and vein coming out from the anterior surface of the pancreas, the stumps of the common bile duct, the gastroduodenal artery, and the inferior mesenteric vein are identified and suture ligated.

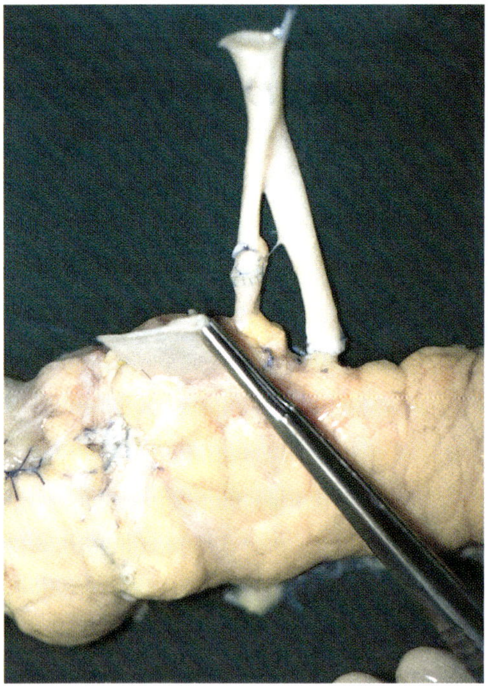

Figure 85.2

Recipient Operation

The vast majority of pancreas transplantations are performed simultaneously with kidney transplantation. In these patients the abdomen is opened by a long midline incision. Because of the poor ischemic tolerance of the pancreas in comparison with the kidney, the pancreas is transplanted first. If there are two operating teams available, the kidney can be transplanted while the second team is doing the back table preparation of the pancreas. Normally, the kidney is connected to the left iliac vessels while the pancreas is placed on the opposite side. Most centers place the pancreas allograft intraperitoneally. In this position exocrine leakage from the graft as well as slight graft pancreatitis seems to be better tolerated. In the case of retroperitoneal placement of the graft, leakage of pancreatic juice might cause extensive retroperitoneal fat necroses, which are very prone to infection. Nevertheless, excellent results have also been published with this technique [8]. While the arterial anastomosis of the pancreas graft is almost always performed with the iliac axis, there are four completely different techniques for venous as well as exocrine drainage of the graft.

Systemic Venous Drainage

The right common or external iliac artery is dissected and the right ureter of the donor is identified. The external/common iliac vein is fully mobilized. Posterior venous branches are divided. Some centers also divide the internal iliac vein in order to make the venous iliac axis more mobile. Such an extensive dissection is not normally necessary. Arterial anastomosis between the graft and the recipient is usually performed by an end-to-side anastomosis of the Y-extension graft at the pancreas and the common or external iliac artery of the recipient. The portal vein is anastomosed to the external or common iliac vein or to the inferior caval vein by a typical end-to-side anastomosis using a running 6-0 monofilament suture. A portal extension graft is almost never necessary. On the contrary, care has to be taken to prevent kinking or twisting of the portal vein of the graft, since small hindrances to the venous outflow might cause early graft thrombosis. Although the frequency of venous graft thrombosis has decreased significantly, it still is one of the major reasons for early pancreatic graft loss. In the case of venous anastomosis to the iliac veins, the pancreas is directed normally with the head toward the pelvis. If the pancreas is placed head up, the portal vein of the graft is normally anastomosed to the inferior vena cava.

Portal Venous Drainage

Systemic venous drainage of the pancreas graft is not physiological, because the blood rich in insulin is not passing through the liver first. Therefore, the so-called "first pass effect" (i.e., hepatic removal of 50% of the insulin from the blood) cannot take place. The consequences are a more or less severe hyperinsulinemia in the systemic circulation [9]. In order to restore the physiological situation completely, the venous outflow of the pancreas graft has to be connected to the portal system of the recipient. Portal venous drainage is currently performed worldwide in only 20% of cases. Nevertheless, since all surgical techniques, which are more physiological than others, have finally succeeded, portal venous drainage might become the gold standard in the future [3].

From a technical point of view, venous anastomosis is performed not directly to the portal vein of the recipient, but to the first tributary of the superior mesenteric vein. Thus, even in the case of local vascular problems, no portal vein thrombosis with extrahepatic portal hypertension must be feared.

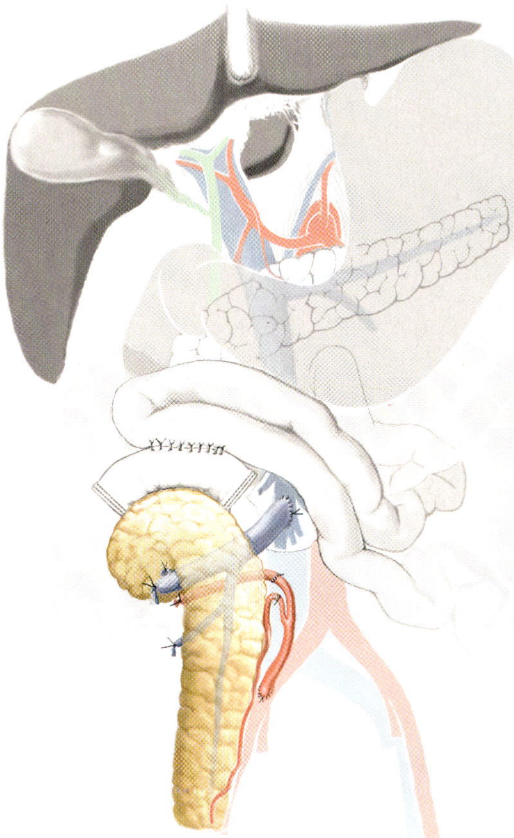

Figure 85.3

In order to perform the venous anastomosis, the mesenteric root is transected at the right side below the transverse mesocolon. The first branch of the superior mesenteric vein is dissected free for about 3 cm. The graft is placed head up right to the mesenteric root. The portal vein of the graft is then anastomosed end-to-side to this venous branch of the superior mesenteric vein by a running 6-0 or 7-0 monofilament suture (Fig. 85.3). The perivascular tissue of the pancreas graft is fixed to the mesenteric root in order to prevent any kinking due to moving of the graft. An adequate length of the portal vein of the graft is of utmost importance. If the vein from the pancreas is too long, the risk of kinking of the donor vein is high. If the portal vein from the graft is too short, kinking of the dissected branch of the superior mesenteric vein might result. After having finished the portal venous anastomosis, the arterial Y-extension graft of the pancreas allograft is pulled through a small whole in the ascending mesocolon and anastomosed as mentioned above to the right common iliac artery.

Urinary Drainage

For about two decades urinary drainage of the exocrine pancreatic secretions has been the gold standard in pancreas transplantation. The technique is simple and safe. The problems of this method, however, are the well-known urological long-term complications (see below) [4]. The bladder drainage technique provides the unique possibility of diagnosing acute rejection of the pancreas graft early after its onset by simply monitoring urinary amylase.

Nowadays, however, the frequency of rejection episodes has dramatically decreased due to new immunosuppressive strategies. In addition, in the case of simultaneous pancreas-kidney transplantation, more than 90% of rejection episodes can be diagnosed by monitoring kidney function and by kidney biopsy sampling. Furthermore, percutaneous or laparoscopic pancreas biopsy procedures have been proven to be safe and effective [10, 11]. Thus, monitoring of urinary amylase is no longer as essential as is was in the early 1980s. Nevertheless, in more than 20% of all pancreas transplantations in the USA the bladder drainage technique is still used [3]. This is especially true in case of pancreas after kidney transplantation or pancreas transplantation alone. In the Eurotransplant region, however, enteric drainage is the generally accepted gold standard.

Exocrine drainage to the bladder is performed by a side-to-side anastomosis between the duodenal segment of the graft and the bladder. The anastomosis can be performed either by a handsewn technique or by stapler. In the case of a handsewn technique, the duodenal segment is opened at the antimesenteric border. The bladder is opened transversely below the dome. Anastomosis is performed by two rows of running sutures using 3-0 polydioxanone sutures (Fig. 85.4).

If a stapler anastomosis is performed, one end of the duodenal segment is opened, while the bladder is opened at the dome. The stapler is introduced into the duodenal segment. The rod of the stapler is pushed through the duodenal wall and the bladder wall. The head of the stapler is connected from within the bladder and a circular anastomosis is performed by firing the stapler. The stapler is removed. The incision in the bladder is closed by suture. The end of the duodenal segment is closed by a linear stapler and reinforced by single stitches.

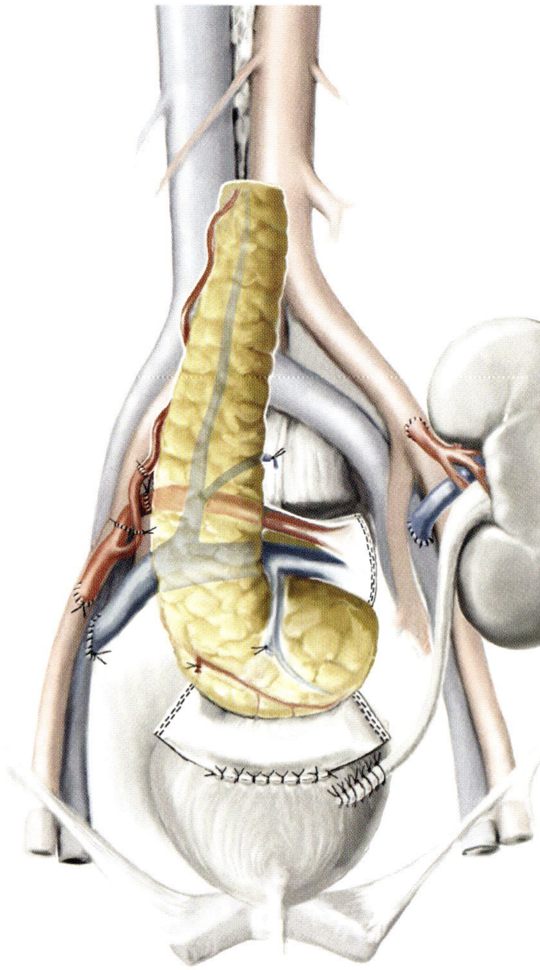

Figure 85.4

Enteric Drainage

The duodenal segment is anastomosed side to side to a loop of the small intestine either by a handsewn anastomosis or by stapler. If the pancreas is directed with the head toward the pelvis, the side-to-side anastomosis normally is performed with a loop of the ileum because of the length of the mesentery (Fig. 85.5). If, on the other hand, the pancreas is directed head up, the anastomosis can be performed with the first loop of jejunum. Irrespective of the technique used for creating the enteric anastomosis, it is important to be sure that there is complete hemostasis at the suture line. Otherwise annoying and sometimes serious gastrointestinal bleeding may result. Direct anastomosis of the duodenal segment to the small bowel is simple and safe. The creation of a separate Roux-loop for anastomosis with the duodenal segment of the graft does not seem to have any advantage.

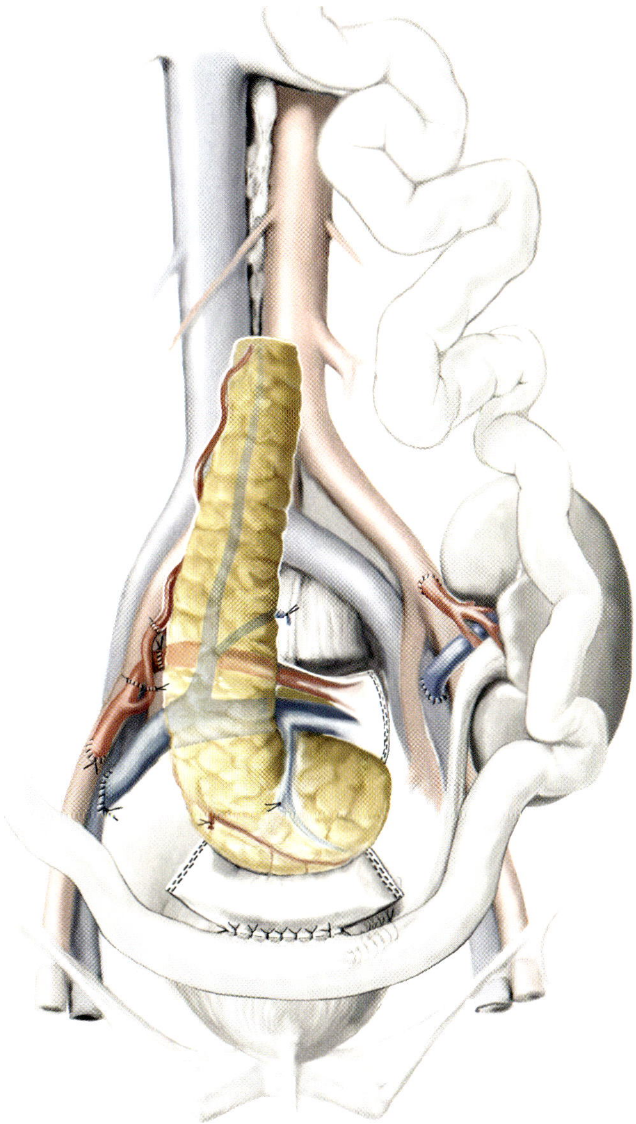

Figure 85.5

Postoperative Management

Anticoagulation

In order to reduce the risk of early postoperative graft thrombosis, most centers use some form of anticoagulation, from one dose of aspirin through low-molecular-weight dextran to intravenous heparin.

Immunosuppression

The pancreas is much more immunogenic than, for example, a kidney or a liver graft. With conventional triple-drug therapy, rejection rates reach 80%. In the last decade, however, early immunological graft loss has decreased dramatically due to the introduction of new immunosuppressive drugs and strategies. Immunological graft loss during the 1st year after simultaneous pancreas-kidney transplantation is currently only 6%. For the time being, standard immunosuppression consists of a quadruple therapy. Induction therapy is done with a T-cell-depleting antibody, such as antithymocyte globulin or with an interleukin (IL)-2 receptor antibody such as daclizumab or basiliximab. The side effects of anti-IL-2 receptor antibodies are few; their immunosuppressive potency, however, seems to be less than that of anti-T-cell antibodies. Almost all patients are treated with a calcineurin inhibitor. Tacrolimus has replaced cyclosporin A in most centers because of a lower incidence of rejection episodes, a better blood pressure profile, and less disturbances of lipid metabolism [12]. Mycophenolate mofetil (MMF), on the other hand, has completely replaced azathioprin. In pancreas transplantation in particular, MMF is much more effective in preventing acute rejection episodes. Most of the patients still receive steroids as the fourth part of their immunosuppressive therapy. Nevertheless, there is increasing interest for rapid tapering or complete steroid-free protocols because of the well-known risks of weight gain, glucose intolerance, dyslipidemia, and bone loss. By using this modern form of quadruple immunosuppressive therapy, the rate of acute rejection episodes within the 1st year could be reduced from 80% to about 20%. This is true in spite of the fact that pancreas transplantation is performed irrespective of the HLA match. Thus, especially in simultaneous pancreas-kidney transplantation, detection and therapy of acute rejection episodes and the risk of immunological graft loss no longer seem to be major problems. Therefore, not stronger immunosuppressive protocols, but immunosuppressive protocols with less side effects are the goal of current research.

Sirolimus, a new target-of-rapamycin inhibitor, is used in addition or instead of one of the aforementioned drugs in some newer immunosuppressive protocols. Contrary to the effect of calcineurin inhibitors, sirolimus does not seem to be nephrotoxic or diabetogenic, and it might be beneficial for the prevention of chronic rejection. Its role in pancreas transplantation, however, remains to be defined.

Surgical Complications

In spite of the improvements in organ conservation, operative techniques and immunosuppressive therapy complication rates after simultaneous pancreas-kidney transplantation is still significantly higher than after isolated kidney transplantation. This is true however, only for the first postoperative year. Later on, the complication rate after simultaneous pancreas-kidney transplantation does not differ from that after isolated kidney transplantation. The most important surgical complications are early postoperative graft thrombosis, graft pancreatitis, leaks of the duodenocystostomy or local bleeding at the duodenojejunostomy, and intra-abdominal infections.

Graft Thrombosis

Pancreas graft thrombosis is the most common cause of early graft loss in pancreas transplantation. The risk has decreased dramatically during the last few years. Nevertheless, with an incidence of 5–8% it is still higher than that for graft loss due to acute rejection [3]. The reasons for the propensity of the pancreas graft for early thrombosis are multifactorial [13]. Unlike the kidney, the pancreas is a low-blood-flow organ. Graft pancreatitis might affect the venous vessels by local inflammation and compression due to local edema. It is known that graft pancreatitis induces a hypercoagulable state, with a dramatic drop in levels of antithrombin 3 and protein C. Prevention of graft thrombosis includes gentle handling of the pancreas, proper orientation vessels, especially prevention of kinking of the veins of the pancreas graft as well as of the recipient, and some form of anticoagulation (see above). Graft thrombosis usually presents with a sudden rise of blood glucose. Serum amylase may or may not be elevated. If it occurs at all, any increase in serum amylase is only transient. The abdominal symptoms are remarkably benign. Diagnosis is achieved with the aid of Doppler ultrasonography or computed tomography (CT)/magnetic resonance imaging (MRI)-angiography, proving a complete stop of perfusion of the pancreas graft. Prompt surgical reexploration is mandatory. In almost every case, graft removal is necessary. Even if graft perfusion can be restored by thrombectomy, a more or less severe graft pancreatitis will result, which might severely endanger the patient. Graft thrombosis occurs most often during the first few days after transplantation. The risk of graft thrombosis is higher after pancreas after kidney transplantation and pancreas transplantation alone than after simultaneous pancreas-kidney transplantation. The well-known uremic thrombopathy might explain this observation.

Graft Pancreatitis

Graft pancreatitis may result from a variety of reasons that ultimately damage the microcirculation within the graft [14]. Prolonged hemodynamic instability and high doses of catecholamines in the donor, excessive manipulation of the graft during procurement, insufficient perfusion of the organ, and a prolonged ischemia time are key factors in this respect. As a result of activation of endothelial cells, release of a variety of inflammatory mediators, and expression of adhesion molecules, the microcirculation will progressively shut down after reperfusion of the graft, resulting in local edema and progressive cell damage. As for genuine pancreatitis, two forms of graft pancreatitis can be differentiated. The edematous form will resolve within a few days without any complications. The necrotizing form, however, might lead to other serious local and systemic complications and often requires removal of the graft. Following the release of active proteases, lipase, and other digestive enzymes, tissue necrosis is induced within the graft as well as in the surrounding mesenteric or preperitoneal fat. Surprisingly, islets and islet function are not affected in the early stage of necrotizing graft pancreatitis. The risk of developing necrotizing graft pancreatitis is clearly correlated to the peak C-reactive protein level within the first 3 days after transplantation. The patients present with abdominal pain and tenderness, prolonged ileus, leukocytosis, hyperamylasemia, and perigraft fluid collections. These fluid collections contain high amounts of pancreatic enzymes such as, for example, amylase. Although in some of the patients necrotizing graft pancreatitis resolves spontaneously, in a high percentage of patients the peripancreatic necrotic tissue and the fluid collections become infected. One or more abdominal explorations with abdominal lavage and debridement of necrotic peripancreatic and intrapancreatic tissue might be required. Percutaneous drainage is, at this stage of transplantation, seldom sufficient, because infection is not confined to a discrete collection or cavity.

Prolonged attempts to treat the peripancreatic infection with antibiotics might lead to fungal peritonitis. Thus, in case of persistent symptoms like fever, leukocytosis, ileus, and peritonitis, the graft should be removed even if the patient is still insulin independent in order to prevent long-term morbidity or mortality. It is certainly a better choice, to attempt a second transplantation (i.e., a pancreas after kidney transplantation) later on.

Anastomotic Leak

An anastomotic leak of the duodenocystostomy or the duodenojejunostomy has to be differentiated from graft pancreatitis. The abdominal signs might be similar. Fluid collections in the perigraft area will also contain high amounts of amylase. In the case of leakage of a duodenojejunostomy or a duodenocystostomy, however, high levels of bilirubin or creatinine, respectively, might also be present. In CT or MRI the pancreas graft by itself seems to be unaffected. While a leak of the duodenocystostomy might be treated by interventional therapy (local drainage of perivesical fluid and long-term catheterization of the bladder), a duodenojejunostomy leak always requires prompt surgical revision. In case of severe local inflammation and peritonitis, the risk of a new suture line breakdown is high and it might be safer for the patient to remove the graft. The incidence of such leaks, however, is very low (i.e., <1%).

Urological Complications

If the bladder drainage technique is used, the early course is surprisingly benign. Late urological complications, however, are rather common. These include hematuria, urinary tract infection, uretritis, and late leaks from the closed stump of the duodenal segment or of the duodenocystostomy. Prolonged irrigation and drainage of the bladder by a transurethral or transcystic catheter and antibiotic therapy might be necessary. In the case of persistent or recurrent symptoms, a conversion from the duodenocystostomy to a duodenoenterostomy is indicated. In the long term, between 20 and 25% of the patients require conversion to enteric drainage [3, 4].

In patients with a bladder-drained pancreas graft, all pancreatic juice is excreted with the urine. Pancreatic juice is alkaline and contains high amounts of bicarbonate. The transplanted kidney is not normally capable of compensating for this massive bicarbonate loss. Thus, patients have to be supplemented with oral bicarbonate in order to prevent severe metabolic acidosis.

Acute Rejection

Diagnosis of acute rejection of the pancreas graft in patients with simultaneous pancreas-kidney transplantation is unproblematic. Since more than 90% of rejection episodes affect the pancreas as well as the kidney, monitoring of kidney function and/or kidney biopsy provides an early and reliable diagnosis. In patients with pancreas after kidney transplantation or pancreas transplantation alone, the diagnosis might be much more difficult. Clinically, the patients may present with fever and tenderness over the graft. Serum amylase and lipase may be moderately elevated. In bladder-drained pancreas grafts, urinary amylase excretion will decrease by more than 50%. Although these findings are relatively sensitive, they are not specific. Graft pancreatitis, for other reasons, will present with the same symptoms. Elevation of blood sugar is not an early sign for a diagnosis of rejection. If blood sugar increases into the pathological region, more than 90% of islets are damaged and in the majority of cases antirejection therapy will no longer be successful. Thus, if pancreas rejection is suspected in those patients, transcystic, percutaneous or open biopsy sampling of the pancreas graft seems to be mandatory. Pancreas biopsy procedures have been proven to be safe and effective [10, 11].

Antirejection therapy consists of corticoid bolus therapy given for 3 days. If this treatment fails, antirejection treatment with anti-T-cell antibodies is indicated. An alternative possibility seems to be rescue therapy with high-dose tacrolimus, increasing the tacrolimus level to 20 ng/ml for 1 week, and/or the use of sirolimus as an additional immunosuppressive drug [15].

Systemic Infections

In addition to peripancreatic sepsis, catheter sepsis, urinary tract infection, and postoperative pneumonia, a variety of other systemic infections might endanger the patient. One of the major risk factors is overimmunosuppression, especially in the case of antirejection therapy. In addition, the typical signs of systemic infections such as, for example, fever, leukocytosis, might be masked by concomitant immunosuppressive therapy. While typical bacterial infections are most common in the early postoperative period, the risk of opportunistic or unconventional infections with cytomegalovirus (CMV), herpes simplex virus, Epstein-Barr virus, *Candida albicans*, aspergillus, cryptococcus, *Pneumocystis carinii*, and nocardia is highest 1–2 months after transplantation. In addition to the well-known systemic sequelae, CMV infection might also affect the pancreas graft and the duodenal segment itself. CMV-induced graft pancreatitis and ulcerations within the duodenal segment, subsequent bleeding, and perforations are well known local complications of CMV infection after pancreas transplantation.

In order to reduce the risk of infection, most patients are treated prophylactically with gancyclovir against CMV, cotrimoxazol against *P. carinii* and some kind of antimycotic drug for 3–6 months after transplantation.

Results

Patient Survival and Pancreas Graft Function Rate

The results of pancreas transplantation worldwide are documented and analyzed annually by the International Pancreas Transplant Registry (IPTR) [3]. The data are reliable since reporting to the registry has been obligatory in the USA since 1987. Up to now, more than 25,000 pancreas transplantations have been performed, and most of them in the USA. The frequency of pancreas transplantation in Germany per million inhabitants is only half of that in the USA. Contrary to the reports of islet transplantation, pancreas grafts are defined as functioning only as long as the recipients are completely insulin independent.

Patient survival and transplant function rates have improved dramatically during the last two decades. The best results can be achieved with simultaneous pancreas-kidney transplantation. In the era from 1999 to 2003, 1-year pancreas survival in the non-USA cases was 89%, kidney graft survival 92%, and patient survival 98%. All survival rates were slightly lower in the combined USA cases [3].

Traditionally, results after pancreas transplantation alone or pancreas after kidney transplantation have been significantly worse. While after simultaneous pancreas-kidney transplantation graft loss for rejection after the first postoperative year is negligible, in pancreas after kidney transplantation or pancreas transplantation alone, the risk of graft loss from rejection remains significant even after the 1st year posttransplant [3, 5]. Nevertheless, the 1-year pancreas function rate in case of pancreas after kidney transplantation is currently 79%, and 76% in cases of pancreas transplantation alone.

Patient survival and pancreas graft survival are identical, irrespective of the duct management technique used. The use of a Roux-loop in enterically drained pancreas grafts did not affect the 1-year results. Whether bladder drainage has some advantages on long-term graft function in case of pancreas after kidney transplantation and pancreas transplantation alone is not yet clear. The technique of vascular venous drainage (i.e., systemic or portal venous drainage) did not have any effect on 1-year graft function rate in simultaneous pancreas-kidney transplantation. Long-term results (up to 10 years), however, are not yet available.

Using multifactorial analysis, several risk factors for pancreas graft loss could be found [16]. These are in the simultaneous pancreas-kidney category: donor age older than 45 years, a prolonged preservation time, and a lack of antibody induction therapy. In the pancreas after kidney category the most important risk factor was the type of duct drainage (enteric drainage worse than bladder drainage). The use of cyclosporin A versus tacrolimus was also associated with lower graft survival rates. HLA-mismatch obviously does not play a role in simultaneous pancreas-kidney transplantation, although it might have some importance in the pancreas transplantation alone category. The risk of graft failure was higher when donor death was caused by cardio- or cerebrovascular events compared with trauma patients. Likewise, while grafts from young donors (20–29 years) have a 1-year graft function rate of 89%, those of older donors from (50–59 years) do significantly worse, reaching only 71%. One of the reasons might be a higher technical failure rate, which more than doubles when using older donors.

Long-term pancreas graft function in simultaneous pancreas-kidney transplantation is excellent, reaching about 65% after 10 years. Unlike the situation for kidney transplantation, chronic rejection does not seem to play a major role in pancreas transplantation. Contrary to the exocrine tissue, the islets of Langerhans seem to be able to compensate somehow for the detrimental effect of progressive vascular damage induced by the chronic rejection process. On the other hand, the endocrine capacity of the graft 1 year after transplantation seems to be important. Insulin-free patients with an impaired oral glucose tolerance test 1 year after transplantation have a significantly lower 10-year graft function rate than patients with a normal glucose tolerance test at that time [17].

Long-Term Effect of Pancreas Transplantation

Glucose Metabolism

Successful pancreas transplantation normalizes glucose metabolism. Endogenous insulin secretion that is responsive to normal feedback control is restored. Patients are completely insulin independent. HbA_{1C} values are normal. Patients do not need to ingest a special diet and are not forced to continuously monitor their blood sugar concentration. When using systemic venous drainage, a significant hyperinsulinemia can be seen in the fasting state as well as after glucose stimulation [9]. In the case of portal drainage of the graft, peripheral insulin concentration is completely normalized. Whether this has any beneficial effect for the patient in the long term with respect to dyslipidemia and progression of arteriosclerosis is still unknown. With respect to the disturbed counterregulation in the case of hypoglycemia, pancreas transplantation normalizes symptom awareness during hypoglycemia and improves both the counterregulatory defects (i.e., the glucagon as well as the epinephrine response) [18].

Long-Term Patient Survival

Several studies from the USA and Europe have shown clearly that 10-year patient survival after simultaneous pancreas-kidney transplantation in type I diabetic patients is significantly better than after isolated kidney transplantation [19, 20]. The 10-year survival rate of diabetic patients with end-stage renal disease reaches about 70% after simultaneous pancreas-kidney transplantation, about 45% after cadaveric kidney transplantation alone, and about 20% without kidney transplantation (i.e., on dialysis). A diabetic patient with well functioning combined pancreas-kidney grafts can expect to live 10 years longer than a diabetic recipient with an isolated cadaveric kidney graft. Thus, pancreas transplantation in the setting of simultaneous pancreas-kidney transplantation is a life-saving procedure in type I diabetic patients with end-stage renal disease. The reason for this beneficial effect might be a reduction of cardio- and cerebrovascular mortality [21].

In spite of these excellent 10-year results with respect to patient survival and pancreas graft function rate, it is obvious that in the late phase after pancreas transplantation death with a functioning graft represents the most frequent cause of graft loss [20]. More than 40% of those patients die from cardio- or cerebrovascular disease. In patients with myocardial infarction before transplantation, 10-year survival after successful simultaneous pancreas-kidney transplantation is drastically reduced, in our own series reaching only 29% in comparison to 75% in the control group. Likewise, the beneficial effect of simultaneous pancreas-kidney transplantation on long-term survival is reduced in patients over 50 years of age. Thus, at least in Europe, pancreas-kidney transplantation is performed too late. It should be done not several years after the beginning of dialysis, but significantly earlier, patients would then not develop such severe secondary diabetic complications that can no longer be halted by normalization of blood sugar. The goal must be to perform a preemptive transplantation in the vast majority of patients (i.e., a simultaneous pancreas-kidney transplantation) well before the onset of dialysis. While in Europe such preemptive transplantations are almost never performed, in the USA large centers such as at the University of Madison transplant more than three-quarters of their patients before the onset of dialysis.

Quality of Life

In patients with chronic disease, quality of life is of central importance. Statistics on graft function rate or short- and long-term mortality will give only an incomplete picture of the therapeutic achievements in this group of patients. Numerous studies have shown that quality of life improves markedly after successful pancreas-kidney transplantation [22, 23]. Freedom from daily insulin injections and the need for frequent blood glucose monitoring, and ending of the strict dietary restrictions appear for many patients almost unbelievable. In addition, metabolic derangements such as severe hypo- or hyperglycemia are completely prevented. Therefore, it is clear that diabetes-related quality of life is significantly improved after successful pancreas transplantation. Fewer restrictions and enhanced capacities lead to an improved sense of well-being and independence. Many report on near-normal activities, physical, social, and psychological well-being, and a self-perception of normality. Although the quality of life of diabetic patients also improves after isolated kidney transplantation, in the long term, patients with an additional pancreas graft seem to experience a significantly better quality of life than those with an isolated kidney graft.

Most patients are convinced that posttransplant immunosuppressive therapy is easier to manage than diabetes. Thus, almost all patients vote for pancreas retransplantation when the graft is lost, despite the perioperative morbidity they might have experienced after the first transplantation and despite of the long-term risks of immunosuppression.

Diabetic Nephropathy

In diabetic patients treated with insulin, diabetic nephropathy can be observed as early as 2 years after kidney transplantation alone. It has been shown by serial biopsy procedures that pancreas transplantation is able to prevent the development of diabetic nephropathy in kidney grafts. Long-term observational studies have shown that pancreas transplantation is able to reverse early diabetic lesions in native kidneys (i.e., the increase in glomerular mesangial volume and the thickness of glomerular basement membrane) after a period of 10 years [24]. Such a beneficial effect could not be demonstrated in the same patients after 5 years, demonstrating again that the effects of pancreas transplantation on secondary diabetic lesions can only be evaluated after rather long study periods. In the case of pancreas transplantation alone, however, this beneficial effect on diabetic nephropathy is counteracted by the nephrotoxic effect of the immunosuppressive drugs.

Diabetic Retinopathy

Many patients receiving a pancreas graft have far advanced diabetic retinopathy. Thus, the point of no return might have been passed. Complete normalization of blood glucose might worsen temporarily in some of the patients the degree of diabetic retinopathy. This has also been described after sudden tight glucose control with intensified insulin therapy. The majority of grafted patients have been treated before transplantation with panretinal laser coagulation, which results in stabilization of the disease. Thus, it is not surprising that during the first 3 years after transplantation, patients with a functioning pancreas graft experience no significant benefit with respect to retinopathy. After that time, however, there was a tendency for better stabilization in patients with a well functioning pancreas graft. Some authors have reported even limited regression of retinopathy in some patients [25]. It has to be kept in mind, however, that due to corticosteroid treatment, almost half of the patients will require cataract surgery after successful pancreas transplantation.

Diabetic Neuropathy

Clinical improvement of neurologic symptoms is a common and relatively early finding after combined pancreas-kidney transplantation. Since polyneuropathy in these patients is caused by uremic as well as diabetic effects, it is rather difficult to differentiate between the beneficial effects of the pancreas and the kidney graft. Nevertheless, recipients with a functioning pancreas-kidney graft in the long term seem to have significantly greater improvements of neuropathy than diabetic patients with a kidney transplantation alone [26]. Motor and sensory nerve conduction velocities improve significantly more after simultaneous pancreas-kidney transplantation than after isolated kidney transplantation. Nevertheless, recovery from diabetic neuropathy is clearly dependent on the severity at the time of transplantation. Thus, even 8 years of perfect glucose control might be not enough in some of the patients to completely reverse preexisting diabetic polyneuropathy.

The effect of successful pancreas transplantation on diabetic autonomic neuropathy is much more controversial. Study results are not consistent because of different severities of dysfunction, study population, and different time points after transplantation. Nevertheless, several studies have reported improvements of gastric, rectal, and bladder function as well as of heart rate variations. It has been reported that diabetic patients with severe autonomic neuropathy have a much higher 5-year survival with a functioning pancreas graft than those without pancreas transplantation or those with early pancreas graft loss.

Macroangiopathy

Most pancreas transplant candidates suffer from macrovascular disease at the time of transplantation. Cardio- and cerebrovascular complications are the main cause of excess mortality in diabetic patients [1]. The risk of a graft recipient of suffering from a vascular complication later on is directly related to the degree of vascular disease that existed before transplantation. Pancreas transplantation has been shown to improve the lipid profile with respect to total cholesterol, high density lipoprotein, cholesterol, and triglycerides. The cause of macrovascular disease, however, is dependent on a variety of other risk factors that are not influenced by pancreas transplantation (e.g., ongoing smoking, hypertension, hyperphosphatemia, excessive body weight, insulin resistance, and genetic predisposition). Nevertheless, it has been reported that carotid intima/media thickness improves 2 years after successful pancreas transplantation [27].

Likewise, a reduced progression of coronary heart disease measured by the mean segment diameter loss on coronary angiography has been reported in patients with functioning pancreas grafts [28]. This is in line with the observation of fewer cardiovascular events in those patients [21]. It is reasonable to assume that these effects are at least in part responsible for the significant prolongation of long-term survival after simultaneous pancreas-kidney transplantation. Considering peripheral vascular disease, the excessive frequency of peripheral amputations will not be reduced after successful pancreas-kidney transplantation. Many of these peripheral amputations are necessary because of peripheral vascular disease. There are, however, a series of other causal factors such as local injury due to severe diabetic neuropathy and local infections induced or aggravated by the immunosuppressive therapy. Taken together, it seems reasonable to assume that macrovascular disease improves in a number of cases after successful pancreas-kidney transplantation. Nevertheless, in many of these patients, the point of no return might have already passed and vascular complications cannot be prevented in the long term in spite of complete normalization of the blood sugar. At the moment the data are certainly inadequate for predicting the risks and beneficial effects of pancreas transplantation in the individual patient.

References

1. Skyler JS (2004) Diabetes mellitus: pathogenesis and natural history. In: Gruessner RWG, Sutherland DER (eds) Transplantation of the Pancreas. Springer, New York pp 11–27
2. Ryan EA, Paty BW, Senior PA, Bigam D, Alfadhli E, Kneteman NM, Lakey JRT, Shapiro AMJ (2005) Five-year follow-up after clinical islet transplantation. Diabetes 54:2060–2069
3. International Pancreas Transplant Registry (2002) Minnesota: University of Minnesota – IPTR. [updated 2004 July 21; cited 2006 March 16] Available from: http://www.iptr.umn.edu/
4. Sollinger HW, Odoric JS, Knechtle S J, D'Alessandro AM, Klayoglu M, Pirsch JD (1998) Experience with 500 simultaneous pancreas-kidney transplants. Ann Surg 228:284–296
5. Sutherland DER, Gruessner RWG, Dunn DL, Matas AJ, Humar A, Kandaswamy R, Mauer SM, Kennedy WR, Goetz FC, Robertson RP, Gruessner AC, Najarian JS (2001) Lessons learned from more than 1,000 pancreas transplants at a single institution. Ann Surg 233:463–501
6. Gruessner RWG, Sutherland DER, Najarian JS, Dunn DL, Gruessner AC (1997) Solitary pancreas transplantation for nonuremic patients with labile insulin-dependent diabetes mellitus. Transplantation 64:1572–1577
7. Shaffer D, Madras PN, Sahyoun A, Simpson MA, Monaco AP (1994) Cadaver donor hyperglycemia does not impair long-term pancreas allograft survival or function. Transplant Proc 26:439–440
8. Boggi U, Vistoli F, Signori S, Del Chiaro M, Campatelli A, Amorese G, Marciano E, Coppelli A, Tregnaghi C, Rizzo G, Marchetti P, Mosca F (2005) A technique for retroperitoneal pancreas transplantation with portal-enteric drainage. Transplantation 79:1137–1142
9. Hopt UT, Drognitz O (2000) Pancreas organ transplantation. Langenbecks Arch Surg 385:379–389
10. Laftavi MR, Gruessner AC, Bland BJ, Foshager M, Walsh JW, Sutherland DE, Gruessner RW (1998) Diagnosis of pancreas rejection. Cystoscopic transduodenal versus percutaneous computed tomography scan-guided biopsy. Transplantation 65:528–532

11. Kayler LK, Merion RM, Rudich SM, Punch JD, Magee JC, Maraschio MA, Leichtman AB, Cibrik DM, Ojo AO, Campbell DA, Arenas JD (2002) Evaluation of pancreatic allograft dysfunction by laparoscopic biopsy. Transplantation 74:1287–1289
12. Bechstein WO, Malaise J, Saudek F, Land W, Fernandez-Cruz L, Margreiter R, Nakache R, Secchi A, Vanrenterghem Y, Tyden G, Van Ophem D, Berney T, Boucek P, Landgraf R, Kahl A, Squifflet JP, EuroSPK Study Group (2004) Efficacy and safety of tacrolimus compared with cyclosporine microemulsion in primary simultaneous pancreas-kidney transplantation:1-year results of a large multicenter trial. Transplantation 77:1221–1228
13. Troppmann C, Gruessner AC, Benedetti E, Papalois BE, Dunn DL, Narjarian JS, Sutherland DE, Gruessner RWG (1996) Vascular graft thrombosis after pancreatic transplantation: univariate and multivariate operative and nonoperative risk factor analysis. J Am Coll Surg 182:285–316
14. Benz S, Bergt S, Obermaier R, Wiessner R, Pfeffer F, Schareck W, Hopt UT (2001) Impairment of microcirculation in the early reperfusion period predicts the degree of graft pancreatitis in clinical pancreas transplantation. Transplantation 71:759–763
15. Rogers J, Ashcraft EE, Emovon OE, Baillie GM, Taber DJ, Marques RG, Baliga PK, Chavin KD, Lin A, Afzal F, Rajagopalan PR (2004) Long-term outcome of sirolimus rescue in kidney-pancreas transplantation. Transplantation 78:619–622
16. Gruessner AC, Sutherland DER (2003) Pancreas transplant outcomes for United States (US) and non-US cases as reported to the United Network for Organ Sharing (UNOS) and the International Pancreas Transplant Registry (IPTR) as of May 2003. Clin Transpl 2003:21–51
17. Pfeffer F, Nauck MA, Drognitz O, Benz S, von Dobschütz E, Hopt UT (2003) Postoperative oral glucose tolerance and stimulated insulin secretion: a predictor of endocrine graft function more than 10 years after pancreas-kidney transplantation. Transplantation 76:1427–1431
18. Kendall DM, Rooney DP, Smets YF, Salazar Bolding L, Robertson RP (1997) Pancreas transplantation restores epinephrine response and symptom recognition during hypoglycemia in patients with long-standing type I diabetes and autonomic neuropathy. Diabetes 46:249–257
19. Becker NB, Brazy PC, Becker YT, Odorico JS, Pintar TJ, Collins BH, Pirsch JD, Leverson GE, Heisey DM, Sollinger HW (2000), Simultaneous pancreas-kidney transplantation reduces excess mortality in type 1 diabetic patients with end-stage renal disease. Kidney Int 57:2129–2135
20. Smets YFC, Westendorp RGJ, van der Pijl JW, de Charro FT, Ringers J, de Jijter JW, Lemkes HHPJ (1999) Effect of simultaneous pancreas-kidney transplantation on mortality on patients with type-1 diabetes mellitus and end-stage renal failure. Lancet 353:1915–1919
21. La Rocca E, Fiorina P, di Carlo V, Astorri E, Rossetti C, Lucignani G, Fazio F, Giudici D, Cristallo M, Bianchi G, Pozza G, Secchi A (2001) Cardiovascular outcomes after kidney-pancreas and kidney-alone transplantation. Kidney Int 60:1964–1971
22. Joseph JT, Baines LS, Morris MC, Jindal RM (2003) Quality of life after kidney and pancreas transplantation: a review. Am J Kidney Dis 42:431–445
23. Drognitz O, Benz S, Pfeffer F, Fischer C, Makowiec F, Schareck W, Hopt UT (2004) Long-term follow-up of 78 simultaneous pancreas-kidney transplantations at a single-center institution in Europe. Transplantation 78:1802–1808
24. Fioretto P, Steffes MW, Sutherland DER, Goetz FC, Mauer M (1998) Reversal of lesions of diabetic nephropathy after pancreas transplantation. N Engl J Med 339:69–75
25. Giannarelli R, Coppelli A, Sartini M, Aragona M, Boggi U, Vistolli F, Rizzo G, Del Prato S, Mosca F, Marchetti P (2005) Effects of pancreas-kidney transplantation on diabetic retinopathy. Transplant Int 18:619–622
26. Navarro X, Sutherland DER, Kennedy WR (1997) Long-term effects of pancreatic transplantation on diabetic neuropathy. Ann Neurol 42:727–736
27. Larsen J, Ratanasuwan T, Burkman T, Colling C, Lynch T, Erickson J, Lyden E, Miller S, Lane J, Mack-Shipman L (2004) Pancreas transplantation improves vascular disease in patients with type 1 diabetes. Diabetes Care 27:1706–1711
28. Jukema J, Smets Y, van der Pijl J, Zwinderman AH, Vliegen HW, Ringers J, Reiber JH, Lemkes HH, van der Wall EE, de Fijter JW (2001) Impact of simultaneous pancreas and kidney transplantation on progression of coronary atherosclerosis in patients with end stage renal failure due to type 1 diabetes. Diabetes Care 25:906–911

Subject Index

A

abscess
- pancreatic 174, 200, 272
- percutaneous therapy, results 276

A-cell 37
achlorhydria syndrome 736
acinar cell 219
- alcohol 387
- carcinoma 506
- cystadenocarcinoma 841

acute pancreatic pseudocyst (APP) 271
acute pancreatitis 107, 138, 771
- acute respiratory distress syndrome 120
- antibiotic prophylaxis 144, 206
- Atlanta classification 173
- biliary 143
- - initial management 144
- - interventions 145
- classification 173
- complications 199
- diagnosis 121
- - CT 195
- - MRI 201
- disseminated intravascular coagulation 121
- enteral feeding 206
- epidemiology 131, 138–140
- ERCP 75, 144
- etiology 132
- - alcohol 133, 136
- - drug-induced 134
- - gallstones 131, 136
- - hereditary 135
- - idiopathic 136
- - metabolic 134
- - traumatic 135
- gallstones 143
- groove 198
- imaging 119, 193
- incidence 138–140
- intensive care 206
- intravascular coagulation 121
- kidney failure 120
- necrosis 120, 174, 225
- nonsurgical management 205
- nutritional support 206
- organ failure 175
- - dynamics 176
- pathogenesis 153, 158
- biliary pancreatitis 154
- pathologic process 193
- pathophysiology 153
- - apoptosis 159
- - colocalization 156, 157
- - cytoskeletal changes 158
- - digestive enzymes 155–157
- - heat shock proteins 159
- - inflammatory 159
- - necrosis 159
- - neural cells 159
- - proteinase-activated receptor-2 159
- - reactive oxygen species 159
- peritoneal pancreatitis 197
- PFCs 271
- physical findings 120
- recurrence 885
- risk factors 119, 203
- segmental 197
- severe (SAP) 121, 173
- - assessment 203
- shock 120
- SIRS 121
- staging 198
- supportive care 205
- symptoms 119
- ultrasonography 194

acute-phase protein 187
ACVR1/2 519
adenocarcinoma
- body and tail 563
- histology 619
- infiltrating ductal 503
- invasive ductal 500
- IPMNs 501
- Kausch-Whipple pancreatectomy 568
- palliation, bypass procedures 666
- pancreas body, symptoms 626
- pancreas head, symptoms 625
- pancreas tail, symptoms 626
- pathology 625
- patient selection 613
- postoperative therapy 675
- prognosis 636, 695
- staging 541, 626
- surgical considerations 613
- survival 695
- symptoms 527
- tumor biology 614
- tumor infiltration 619
- tumor-vessel relationships 614
  vaccines 684

adenoma
- laparoscopic management 653
- mucinous cystic neoplasm 499
- solid serous 498

adenoma-carcinoma sequence 755
adenosquamous carcinoma 505
adjuvant therapy
- chemoradiation 677
- chemotherapy 680
- immunotherapy 680
- radiation 676
- survival 698
- target agents 683
- vaccines 684

advanced chronic pancreatitis 338
AIPDA, see anterior posterior pancreaticoduodenal artery
AIPDV, see anterior superior pancreaticoduodenal vein
AKT2 514, 521
alcohol/alcoholic
- abuse 119
- chronic pancreatitis 111, 122, 311
- consumption
- - pancreatic necrosis 289
- intake 306

allogeneic islet transplantation 918
alpha fetoprotein 866
alpha-inhibin 874
ampulla of Vater 10
ampullary carcinoma 771
amylase 182
- α-amylase 3
- activity, PF 283

anastomosis
- choledochojejunal 575
- pancreatic 575

aneuploid tumor 854
angiogenesis inhibitor 554
antecolic duodenojejunostomy 421
anterior posterior pancreaticoduodenal artery 19
anterior superior pancreaticoduodenal vein 21, 22
antibiotic prophylaxis
- acute pancreatitis 144, 206
- chronic pancreatitis 389
- ERCP 78, 83

– pancreatic duct drainage 389
– total pancreatectomy 640
antigen-presenting cell (APC) 684
antiprotease 186
antrum 454
APACHE II score 173, 175, 176, 204
APBDJ
– anastomosis 898
– cancer, pathogenesis 898
– classification 895
– diagnosis 896
– malignant change 897
– surgical treatment 898
– symptoms 897
APC, see antigen-presenting cell
APP, see acute pancreatic pseudocyst
artery/arterial
– pancreatic 19
– resection
– – pancreaticoduodenectomy 617
ascites, pancreatic 201
aspiration biopsy
– acinar cell carcinoma 92
– biopsy procedure
– – aspiration 88
– – cytology 88
– – histopathology 88
– – immunohistochemical analysis 88
– complications of FNAB
– – pancreatic carcinoma 89
– – risk of acute pancreatitis 88
– CT-guided 85
– ductal adenocarcinoma
– – adenosquamous carcinoma 90
– – undifferentiated (anaplastic) carcinoma 90
– – well-differentiated ductal adenocarcinoma 90
– endocrine tumors 92
– EUS-FNAB 85
– gastrointestinal malignancies 87
– histological diagnosis 87
– inflammatory cells 89
– inflammatory mass caused by autoimmune pancreatitis 87
– intraoperative aspiration 85
– lymph nodes 87
– lymphadenopathy 87
– pancreatic cancer 87
– percutaneous transabdominal aspiration 85
– signet cell carcinoma 92
– small pancreatic cancer 85
– small-cell carcinoma 92
– solid-pseudopapillary tumor 92
Atlanta classification
– acute pancreatitis 173
– modified system 176
– organ failure 175
– shortcomings 174
atypism 839, 840
– epithelial 756
– intestinal 760
– pancreaticobiliary 760
autodigestion 282
autoimmune pancreatitis 123, 198, 296

B

bacterial infection, pancreatitis 174
Balthazar-Ranson CT index 205
B-cell 37
Beckwith-Wiedemann syndrome 841
Beger procedure 415
beta-catenin 840
bevacizumab 554, 555, 684
– survival, metastatic disease 700
bile duct
– cyst 897
– obstruction 121
– resection 809
– stenosis 301
– stricture
– – classification 16
– – definition 15
biliary
– acute pancreatitis
– – nasoenteral feeding 145
– anastomosis 421, 587
– bypass 669
– carcinoma 899
– decompression
– – pancreatic cancer 530
– drainage
– – percutaneous transhepatic 689
– – preoperative 568
– endoprostheses 666
– malignancy, mutagenic substances 12
– obstruction
– – bypass techniques 668
– – chronic pancreatitis 394
– pancreatitis
– – cholecystectomy 145
– – diagnosis 144
– – endoscopic sphincterotomoy 145
– – gallstones 143
– – initial management 144
– stenting, survival 698
– tract, bile duct stricture 15
biliary-enteric bypass 667
biliopancreatic maljunction 895
biochemical
– diagnosis 181, 182
– severity stratification 184
biopsy
– percutaneous 535
– survival 698
– transpapillary 858
bladder drainage 921
blood glucose 186
blunt dissection 417
borderline malignant potential 864
brachytherapy, palliative treatment 692
BRAF 516
Braun anastomosis 804
Brca2 pathway 520
breath test 114, 323
brush cytology 768
bypass procedure
– outcomes 673
– pancreas, carcinoma of the head 665
– postoperative course 672
– preoperative investigation 665
– techniques 668

C

CA19-9 528, 559, 626, 759, 852, 858
calcification 313, 852, 864
Cambridge image severity 414
cancer, see also pancreatic cancer
– adjuvant therapy
– – chemoradiation 677
– – chemotherapy 680
– – immunotherapy 680
– – radiation 676
– APBDJ 897
– – pathogenesis 898
– bevacizumab 554
– body and tail 563
– borderline resectable 682
– Brca2 pathway 520
– chemotherapy 549
– chronic pancreatitis 491
– clinical presentation 625
– cytology 698
– diabetes 491
– diagnosis
– – approach 535
– – laparoscopy 542
– diet 491
– differential diagnosis 536
– EGFR inhibitor 554
– epidemiology 489
– EUS 531, 542
– evaluation 559
– Fanconi anemia 520
– Fbxw7-cyclin E pathway 521
– gemcitabine 549
– gender differences 490
– genetics 492
– hedgehog pathway 522
– imaging 529
– infectious diseases 492
– infiltrating ductal adenocarcinoma 503
– intraoperative staging 546, 562
– laboratory tests 528
– laparoscopy 627, 653
– locally advanced 693
– – survival 699
– MAP kinase pathway 519
– margin assessment 611
– marimastat 553
– MDCT 541
– metastatic 549, 699
– MRI 545
– mTor pathway 521
– new drugs 553
– oncogenes 514

- p53 pathway 517
- palliative treatment 689
- – resection 564
- pancreatectomy, venous resection, conclusions 607
- pancreatic 125
- pathology 497, 625
- percutaneous biopsy 535
- PET 546
- postoperative
- – staging 546
- – therapy 675
- preoperative
- – evaluation 612
- – resectable therapy 681
- – staging 547, 627
- prevention 493
- prognosis 636, 965
- racial factors 490
- rapamycin pathway 521
- Ras
- – inhibitor 554
- – pathway 516
- Rb pathway 517
- resectability 560, 607
- resected prognostic indicators 675
- risk factors 491
- screening 493
- signs 527
- smoking 491
- staging 541, 561, 626
- surgery
- – outcome 493
- – resection, indications 559
- survival 675, 695
- symptoms 527
- target agents 683
- TGF-β superfamily 517
- time trends 490
- tumor biology 614
- tumor markers 528
- tumorigenesis 513
- – epigenetic alterations 513
- tumor-vessel relationships 614
- unresectable, bypass procedures 665
- vaccines 684
- vascular invasion 561
- with immunotherapy 680

CAPAP 186
capecitabine 550
carcinoembroyonic antigen (CEA) 685, 759, 852, 858
carcinoma, see also cancer
- acinar cell 506
- in situ
- – mucinous cystic neoplasm 499
- of the ampulla of Vater 827
- of the pancreas 198
- small-cell 508
- undifferentiated 506

catheter drainage, infected pancreatic necrosis 208
caudal pancreatic artery (CPA) 21
caudate lobectomy 809
CBD 403
- stenosis 403

CCDB, see congenital cystic dilatation of the CBD
CCK, see cholecystokinin
CCNE 514, 521
CDKN2A 515, 517
CEA, see carcinoembroyonic antigen
CECT, see contrast-enhanced computed tomography
celiac
- artery 19
- plexus block 335

central pancreatectomy
- end-to-end 433
- end-to-side 434
- late outcome 438
- left splenopancreatectomy 425
- postoperative morbidity 437

central stellate scar 862
cetuximab 555, 683
- survival, metastatic disease 700

CFTR 363
CHA, see common hepatic artery
chemoradiation 677, 680
- EORTC trial 678
- ESPAC-1 trial 679
- JHH trial 679
- meta-analysis 680
- palliative therapy 690, 692
- RTOG trial 679
- versus chemoradiation 692
- versus radiation 690

chemotherapy 680
- 5-FU 549
- combination 549
- immunotherapy 680
- M.D. Anderson cancer center, results 620
- palliative therapy 692
- versus chemoradiation 692

cholangiopandreatography, endoscopic retrograde (ERCP) 75
cholangitis, endoscopic retrograde cholangiopandreatography (ERCP) 78, 82
cholecystectomy 392
- APBDJ 898
- biliary acute pancreatitis 145

cholecystokinin (CCK) 37, 111
choledochal cyst 897
choledochoduodenostomy 394
choledochojejunal anastomosis 575
choledochojejunostomy 394
cholestasis 108
cholesterin 840
cholesterol stone 143
chronic pancreatitis 295, 301, 311, 334, 439, 885
- acute exacerbation 198
- alcohol consumption 122
- alcoholic 381
- associated problems 393
- autoimmune 122
- cancer 491
- causes 387
- classification 441
- CT 319
- diagnosis 124, 442
- endoscopic retrograde cholangiopandreatography (ERCP) 76
- – calculi 319
- – cysts 319
- – dilatation/obstruction of side branches 319
- – dilatation of main 319
- – stenosis 319
- endotherapy 383
- epidemiology 441
- etiology 441
- hereditary 122
- idiopathic chronic pancreatitis 331
- imaging 388, 442
- interventional procedures 334
- laparoscopic management 653
- late outcome 910
- – alcohol abuse 477
- – cholelithiasis 477
- – comorbidities 483
- – EORTC QLQ-C30 483
- – hereditary pancreatitis 477
- – mortality 481
- – quality of life 483
- medical management 331, 333
- pancreatectomy complications 447
- pancreatic duct drainage 387, 443
- pancreatic resection 444
- patient selection 388
- physical findings 123
- pseudocysts 459, 460
- relapsing pain attacks 331
- surgery 381
- – indications 387, 443, 460
- – procedures 334, 382
- symptoms 122, 441
- ultrasound 319
- weight loss 124

chymotrypsin 3
circumferential incision 791
cisplatin 681, 691
- resectable cancer 682
- with gemcitabine 551

classification
- APBDJ 895
- of postacute pseudocyst 261
- acute pancreatitis 173
- – interstitial-edematous 163
- – necrotizing 163
- – pancreatic abscess 163
- – postacute pancreatic pseudocysts 163

clinical course 164, 165
closed lavage 231, 234, 236
- postoperative complications 237
- results 237

colipase 3
colloid carcinoma 505

colon fistula 286
common
– bile duct 480
– hepatic artery (CHA) 19
– – arterial resection 617
– – variations 21
computed tomography (CT) 119, 194, 323, 906
– acute pancreatitis 194
– – diagnosis 195
– – staging 198
– autoimmune pancreatitis 198
– carcinoma 198
– chronic pancreatitis 119, 198, 388
– contrast-enhanced, helical 529
– groove pancreatitis 198
– minimally invasive necrosectomy 243
– normal pancreas 195
– OPN 271
– pancreatic cancer 529
– – staging 541
– pancreatic necrosis 122
– pancreatic protocol 560
– pancreatic pseusdocyst 200
– preoperative diagnosis 613
– segmental pancreatitis 197
– total pancreatectomy 640
concomitant neoplasm 851
congenital cystic dilatation of the CBD (CCDB) 15
– classification 15
– definition 15
contrast sinogram of pancreatic fistula 283
contrast-enhanced computed tomography (CECT) 283
– angiography 67
– ERCP 67
– Ifs 286
– magnetic resonance imaging (MRI)
– – chemical shift artifacts 70
– – dysfunctions of the sphincter 72
– – gadolinium-enhanced 70
– – magnetic resonance angiography 73
– – malignant obstruction 72
– – MRCP 72
– – periductal structures 72
– – secretin-stimulated dynamic MRCP 72
– – T1 70
– – T2 70
– MRCP 67
– PF 283
– spiral CT
– – arterial phase 70
– – infiltration of vessels 68
– – malignant infiltration 68
CPA, see caudal pancreatic artery
C-peptide 115
creatinine/blood urea nitrogen 185
CRP 187
CT, see computed tomography
Cullen sign 120
cyclin E 521
cyst gastrostomy, sterile pancreatic necrosis 208
cystadenoma 497
– laparoscopic management 653
cystic
– fibrosis 363
– forms of solid pseudopapillary tumor 407
– hamartoma 877
– lesion, solitary cysts 873
– neoplasm
– – exocrine pancreas 497
cystoenterostomy, pancreatic pseudocyst 151
cystogastrostomy
– laparoscopic 149
– pancreatic necrosis 149
cystojejunostomy, pancreatic pseudocyst 151
cytokeratin 874

D
D-cell 37
debridement 232
– necrotizing pancreatitis 220
– – outcome 223
– – postoperative course 223
– – surgical technique 221
delayed gastric emptying 415, 824
dermoid cyst 841, 875
development of the pancreas
– dorsal pancreatic duct 6
– endoderm
– – dorsal pancreatic primordium 3
– – notochord
– – – TGFβ 5
– – – fibroblast growth factor (FGF) family (FGF-2) 5
– – – sonic hedgehog 5
– – – Pdx1 5
– – – insulin-secreting β cells 5
– – – glucagon-producing α cells 5
– – – somatostatin cells 5
– – – PP cells 5
– – primitive gut 3
– – ventral pancreatic primordium 3
– enteric nervous system
– – human islets 7
– – nerve fibers 6
– – neural regulation of secretion 7
– – stage of differentiation 7
– – tubular complexes 7
– lymph nodes develop 6
– neural tube 3
– pancreatic primordia 43
– ventral pancreatic duct 6
DGE 422
diabetes 109, 438
– complications 918
– mellitus 303, 304, 456
– necrosectomy 290
– pancreatic cancer 491
– pancreatic duct drainage 392
– pancreatic resection 289, 449
– total pancreatectomy 650
disconnected duct syndrome 209
distal
– common bile duct carcinoma 776
– half of the bile duct 454
– pancreatic injury with duct involvement 907
diverticulum 10
docetaxel with gemcitabine 552
dorsal
– pancreas 313
– pancreatic artery (DPA) 21
– pancreatic vein (DPV) 22
– wall of the stomach 409
doxorubicin 680, 692
DPA, see dorsal pancreatic artery
DPV, see dorsal pancreatic vein
drainage
– biliary 666
– external 470
– internal pseudocystoenteric 461
– OPN, endoscopic 274
– pancreatic duct 387
– pancreatic necrosis, nonsurgical 272
– PFC 273
– placement 283
– procedure 854
– pseudocystojejunostomy 463
duct mucosa 434
ductal
– adenocarcinoma
– – genetics 504
– – grading 504
– – immunohistochemical labeling 504
– – prognosis 504
– – variants 505
– dilatation 419
– epithelial cell 4
– papillary hyperplasia 860
ductotomy 391
duct-to-mucosa pancreaticojejunostomy 421
ductular
– centroacinar cell 864
– epithelial cell 4
duodenal
– cancer 776, 817
– obstruction 301, 479, 480
– – bypass techniques 668
– – chronic pancreatitis 394
– stenosis 295
– wall cyst 876
duodenectomy
– circular 819
– segmental 818
duodenojejunostomy 415, 588, 804, 813
duodenopancreatectomy, laparoscopic procedure 655
duodenotomy 789

duodenum 312, 454
- fistulas 286
duodenum-preserving pancreatic head resection 336, 408, 892, 893
- biliary anastomosis 411
- early postoperative course 404
- frequency of rehospitalization 406
- gastric emptying 406
- glucose metabolism 406
- head of the pancreas
- - head enlargement 399
- - PMD dilatation 399
- - subtotal resection 400
- long-term outcome after DP-PHR 404
- maintenance of endocrine functions 406
- postoperative morbidity 406
- preservation of the spleen 411
- quality of life 406
duodenum-sparing pancreas head 425
dysplasia 855

E

early severe acute pancreatitis (ESAP) 177
- multiorgan failure 165
- organ failure 165
EBRT, see external-beam radiation therapy
ECOG study 691, 692
EGFR, see epidermal growth factor receptor
elastase, fecal 442
EMR 818
endocarditis
- ERCP 78
endocrine
- dysfunction
- - in CP 108
- - inflammatory 107
- - neoplastic lesions 107
- insufficiency, total pancreatectomy 650
- pancreatic function 303, 478
- pancreatic secretion
- - B-cells 37
- - D-cells 37
- - PP-cells 37
- tumor 47
endodermal stem cell 850
endoscopic
- diagnosis 885
- interventional treatment
- - bile-duct strictures due 377
- - bougienage 374
- - cholangitis 377
- - endoscopic drainage 375
- - endoscopic pancreatic sphincterotomy 374
- - jaundice 377
- - lithotripsy 375
- - long-term outcome 375
- - pancreatic duct endoprosthesis 374
- - pancreatic duct strictures and stones, interstitial pressures 373
- - pancreatic pseudocysts 375
- - removal of stones 374
- minor papilla sphincterectomy, complications 887
- papillectomy 779
- - complications 784
- - recurrence 786
- retrograde cholangiopancreatography (ERCP) 75, 768, 772, 906
- - antibiotic prophylaxis 78, 83
- - APBDJ 896, 897
- - biliary sepsis 144
- - chronic pancreatitis 388, 442
- - complications 78, 82
- - contrast injection 79
- - gallstones 144
- - indications 75
- - instruments 77
- - pancreatic cancer 75, 530
- - pancreaticobiliary drainage 82
- - pancreatitis 75, 76
- - pancreatogram 80
- - PF 284
- - preoperative preparation 77
- - pseudocysts 461
- - radiography 79
- - technique 78
- retrograde pancreatography 324
- stent therapy, pancreatic duct disruption 209
- treatment 885
- - PFC 275
- ultrasound/ultrasonography (EUS) 127, 144, 768, 775, 882
- - abnormalities in the pancreatic duct 325
- - ductular features 326
- - EUS-FNA, pancreatic cancer 532
- - EUS-guided drainage, PFC 273
- - Kausch-Whipple pancreatectomy 567
- - ONYX-015 693
- - pancreatic cancer 531
- - - limitations 534
- - - staging 542
- - preoperative staging 627
- - side branch dilatation 326
- - total pancreatectomy 640
- - tumor resectability 561
endoscopy, pancreatic necrosis 247
endosonography
- acute pancreatitis 121
- chronic pancreatitis 119, 124
endotherapy 335
- chronic pancreatitis 383
enteral feeding, acute pancreatitis 206
enterogenous cyst 875
enucleation, transduondenal 730
EORTC trial 677, 678, 698
epidermal growth factor 314
- receptor (EGFR) 554
- - inhibitor 554
epidural opioid 456
ERBT, resectable cancer 682
ERCP, see endoscopic retrograde cholangiopancreatography
erlotinib 555, 683, 692
- survival, metastatic disease 700
ESAP, see early severe acute pancreatitis
ESPAC-1 698
- trial 677, 679
ESPAC-3 698
- trial 680
estrogen 864
ESWL 334
EUS, see endoscopic ultrasound
exatecan 552
exocrine
- dysfunction
- - in CP 108
- - inflammatory 107
- - neoplastic lesions 107
- insufficiency
- - necrosectomy 290
- - total pancreatectomy 650
- pancreatic function 320
- pancreatic insufficiency 302
experimental models of acute pancreatitis 156
external-beam radiation therapy (EBRT) 677, 691
- palliative treatment 690
extrapancreatic
- cancer 301, 479, 480
- necrosis 167

F

familial adenomatous polyposis (FAP) 765, 772, 779, 820
Fanconi anemia 520
- gene 516
FAP, see familial adenomatous polyposis
FBXW7 515, 521
Fbxw7-cyclin E pathway 521
FDG-PET 97
fecal
- chymotrypsin 362
- elastase 321
- pancreatic-enzyme determination 113
- test 322
fenestration 789
fibrocalculous pancreatic 350
filling defect 844
fine needle aspiration (FNA) 220
- EUS-guided 532
- pancreatic cancer 532
- pancreatic necrosis 220
- resectability 563
fish-egg appearance 858
fistula
- colonic 286

– duodenal 286
– intestinal see Ifs 281
– pancreatic (PF) 281, 447, 448, 635
– small intestine 286
fluid collection
– acute pancreatitis 197
– pancreatic 271, 447
5-fluorouracil (5-FU) 549, 680, 681, 690–692
– pancreatic cancer 549
– radiation therapy 677
– resectable cancer 681
– with gemcitabine 550
FNA, see fine needle aspiration
focal chronic pancreatitis 426
focus control 232
forceps biopsy 768
formation of pancreatic pseudocyst 909
Frey procedure 398, 415
5-FU, see 5-fluorouracil

G

gabexate 82
gallbladder 454
– cancer 12
gallstone 119
– biliary sphincterotomy 209
– diagnosis 144
– prevalence 143
GAP-43 297
Gardner's syndrome 772
gastric emptying 805
gastrinoma 708
– duodenal 729
– MEN-1 729
– triangle 707
gastroduodenal artery (GDA) 19
gastroenteropancreatic cell 850
gastrointestinal factor 42
gastrojejunostomy 667
– palliative 668
GDA, see gastroduodenal artery
gemcitabine 680, 691, 692
– combinations 549, 552
– pancreatic cancer 549
– resectable cancer 682
– survival, metastatic disease 700
– with 5-FU 550
– with oxaliplatin 551
– with platinum 551
– with taxanes 552
– with topoisomerase I inhibitors 551
gene
– genome-maintenance 515
– mutation 315
– tumor-suppressor gene 515
genetic
– BRCA2 492
– clinical applications 522
– counseling 738
– – PRSS1 367
– – SPINK1 367
– ductal adenocarcinoma 504
– factor 351
– functional implications 516
– pancreatic cancer 492, 513
– pancreatoblastoma 507
– PENs 508
– survival 700
– testing 361, 731, 739
G-FLIP 552
giant cell 840
– undifferentiated carcinoma 506
GITSG trial 677, 690, 692, 698
glucagon secretion
– cAMP 44
– hepatocyte membrane 44
– type 1/2 diabetes 44
glucagonoma 707, 709, 737
glucose tolerance 478
glucose-induced insulin secretion 41
glycosylated hemoglobin 115
GPA, see great pancreatic artery
graft survival rate 921
– one-year survival 921
granulous mucosa 857
great pancreatic artery (GPA) 21
Grey-Turner-sign 120
groove pancreatitis 198, 295
GTX 552

H

H_2 blocker 339
HbA1c 115
hedgehog pathway 522
hemangioblastoma 739
hematocrit 185
hemobilia, total pancreatectomy 649
hemoconcentration 203
hemorrhage, total pancreatectomy 649
hepatectomy 809
– APBDJ 899
hepatic diverticulum 10
hepatico-(choledocho)-jejunostomy 669
hepaticojejunostomy 587, 803, 813
hepatobiliary system, embryology 10
hereditary chronic pancreatitis 311
– anionic trypsinogen 361
– cystic fibrosis transmembrane conductance regulator 361
– Kazal type 1 361
– serine protease inhibitor 361
HLA-DR, see human leukocyte antigen DR
honeycomb 839
human leukocyte antigen (HLA) 351
– DR (HLA-DR) 228
hyperamylasemia 194
hypertension, lift-sided portal 201
hypoglycemic attack 456
hypokalemia 736

I

idiopathic pancreatitis 303, 311
IDUS 769, 775
IF, see intestinal fistula
imaging
– acute pancreatitis 193
– chronic pancreatitis 388, 442
– intestinal fistula (IF) 285
– Kausch-Whipple pancreatectomy 567
– pancreatic cancer 529
– pancreatic fistula 283
– percutaneous aspiration 207
– preoperative diagnostic 612
immunization, preoperative 461
immunosuppression 917
immunotherapy with chemoradiation 680
impaired glucose 109
– tolerance 114
IMV, see inferior mesenteric vein
indeterminate category 843
infected
– necrosis 211, 212, 249, 254
– pancreatic necrosis 168, 169
– – bacterial 167
– – fungal infection 167
infection
– pancreas, treatment 207
– pancreatic cancer 492
– pancreatic necrosis 200
– pseudocyst 471
inferior
– mesenteric vein (IMV) 21
– pancreaticoduodenal artery (IPDA) 19
inflammatory mass 311
insufficient bicarbonate secretion 111
insulin 115
– resistance 304
– – C-peptide 42
– synthesis
– – glucagon-like peptide 1 (GLP-1) 40
– – glucose transporter 40
– – glucose-6-phosphate 40
– – incretin effect 42
– – incretin mimetics 43
– – K^+ channel 41
– – MODY 43
– – pulsatile insulin 41
– – type 1 diabetes mellitus 42
– – type 2 diabetes 42
– – typical autoantibodies of type 1 42
insulin-dependent diabetes mellitus 111
insulinoma 707, 708
– carcinoid 47
– clinical case 717
– gastrinoma 47
– glucagonoma 47
– laparoscopic
– – enucleation 716
– – management 653
– – pancreatectomy 716
– laparotomy 715

– malignant 719
– recurrence 719
– somatostatinoma 47
– surgical resection 715
– VIPoma 47
interferon (IFN) 698
– IFNα 680, 698
interleukin (IL) 297
– IL-6 188
– IL-8 188, 297
internal drainage 461
interventional treatment 256
intestinal fistula (IF) 281
– autodigestion 282
– definition 285
– imaging 285
– incidence 285
– management 286
– operative approach 282
– operative technique 282
– pathogenesis 281
intra-abdominal abscess 909
intraductal papillary mucinous
– neoplasm (IPMN) 81, 500, 840, 843, 855
– – branch duct type 840, 854
– – ductectatic 857
– – gastric (null) type 840
– – intestinal type 840
– – main duct type 840, 845
– – minimally invasive 846
– – oncocytic 841
– – pancreatobiliary type 840
– – pancreatogram 81
– – prognosis 501, 861
– tumor (IPMT) 407
intralobular islet 25
– afferent vessels 26
– species differences 26
– vascular connections 26
intraoperative
– duodenoscopy 726
– radiation therapy (IORT) 677
– – palliative treatment 692
– – resectable cancer 682
– – survival 699
– secretin test 727
– selective contact cholangio-pancreatography (ISCCP) 895
ionafarnib 554
IORT, see intraoperative radiation therapy
IPDA, see inferior pancreaticoduodenal artery
IPMN, see intraductal papillary mucinous neoplasm
IPMT, see intraductal papillary mucinous tumor
irinotecan 551
ISCCP, see intraoperative selective contact cholangiopancreatography
islet
– cell tumor 507
– of Langerhans 25
– transplantation
– – allogenic islets 913
– – β-cell replacement by transplantation 913
– – cold preservation 914
– – end-stage renal disease 913
– – HbA1c 913
– – immune response 917
– – living-related pancreas segments 914
– – purification 916
– – transplantation of autologous islets 914

J

jaundice
– biliary decompression 689
– pancreatic cancer 527
jejunojejunostomy 669
John Hopkins hospital (JHH) trial 679
JSBS classification 797

K

Kakita's procedure 803
Kausch-Whipple pancreatectomy, see also Whipple pancreatectomy
– complications 578
– contraindications 568
– EUS 567
– imaging 567
– indications 568
– laparoscopy 568
– long-term outcome 578
– operative approach 569
– PET 568
– postoperative course 576
– preoperative investigation 567
– procedure, variations 575
– rationale 568
– reconstruction 573
– reconstruction, variations 575
Kocher's maneuver 657
– extensive 642
Komi classification 895
K-ras 314, 762
KRAS 514, 516
– KRAS2 839, 841

L

laparoscopy
– anatomy 655
– contraindications 653
– equipment 654
– indication 653
– insulinomas 716
– – enucleation 716
– intraoperative staging 562
– Kausch-Whipple pancreatectomy 568
– multiport technique 628
– pancreatectomy
– – left 660
– – total 662
– pancreatic cancer 627
– – staging 542
– – technique 544
– pancreatic necrosis 246
– pancreatic resection 446
– pancreaticoduodenectomy
– reconstruction 658
– results 660
– technique 656
– port placement 655
– preoperative staging 627
– pseudocyst surgery 470
– rationale 653
– splenectomy 660, 662
– staging 582, 667
– Whipple procedure 659
laparotomy, insulinomas 715
large-duct disease 355
latarjet 809
late outcome of chronic pancreatitis 910
– alcohol abuse 477
– cholelithiasis 477
– comorbidities 483
– EORTC QLQ-C30 483
– hereditary pancreatitis 477
– mortality 481
– quality of life 483
lateral pancreaticojejunostomy 337, 962
leukovorin 550
life expectancy, high-volume centers 696
lipase 3, 182, 339
lobular plexus 23
lobule pancreas 23
longitudinal pancreatic artery 810
loss of exocrine function 111
lower bile duct cancer 831
lumbotomy, pancreatic necrosis 247
Lundh test 113, 322
lymph node
– dissection 797, 860
– involvement 797
– pancreas body and tail 628
lymphadenectomy, survival 697
lymphoepithelial cyst 875

M

M.D. Anderson cancer center 620
macroangiopathy 935
magnetic resonance
– cholangiopancreatography (MRCP) 283, 768, 906
– – APBDJ 897
– – chronic pancreatitis 388, 442
– – pancreatic cancer 530
– – PF 284
– imaging (MRI) 119, 201, 324
– – acute pancreatitis 201
– – chronic pancreatitis 119
– – pancreatic cancer 529, 545
main pancreatic duct (MPD) 80
– narrowing 80
– pancreatogram 80

malabsorption 457
maldigestion 302
malignancy
– extrapancreatic 846
– metachronous 846, 856
– synchronous 846, 856
malignant
– lesion 314
– transformation 767
maljunction, biliopancreatic 895
MAP kinase pathway 519
MAP2K4 515
MAPK 519
margin assessment
– pancreaticoduodenectomy 611
– survival rates 676
marimastat 553
marsupialization of pseudocyst 470
mass lesion 356
matrix metalloproteinaase inhibitor (MMP inhibitor) 553
MCN, see mucinous cystic neoplasm
MCT 850
MDACC trial 691
MDCT 809
– APBDJ 896
– preoperative diagnostics 613
medium-chain triglyceride 339
medullary carcinoma 505
megaduodenum 820
MEN-1 507, 738
– gene 737
mesenchymal stroma 850
metastatic carcinoma 841
microcirculation of the pancreas 22
minimally invasive necrosectomy 241
– laparoscopy 246
– percutaneous
– – complications 246
– – outcome 245
– – postoperative management 245
minor papilla
– cannulation 885
– drainage 887
– endoscopic dilatation 891
– pain relief 891
mitomycin 692
– C 680, 691
– resectable cancer 681
MLH1 516
MMF, see mycophenolate mofetil
MMP inhibitor, see matrix metalloproteinase inhibitor
monitoring of kidney function 931
MPD, see main pancreatic duct
MRCP, see magnetic resonance cholangiopancreatography
MSI phenotype 516
mTor parthway 521
MUC2 501
MUC5AC 501, 876
MUC6 874
mucin excretion 857
mucinous
– cystic neoplasm (MCN) 839, 843
– cystic tumor 407
– fistula 851
– non-neoplastic cyst 876
mucin-secreting 855
multiple endocrine neoplasia type 1 737
mural nodule 844, 846
mutagen, biliary tract cancer 12
mutation rate, genome-maintenance gene 515
MYB 514
mycophenolate mofetil (MMF) 930

N

nasogastric suction 422
natural course
– of acute pancreatitis 163–170, 301
– of pancreatic pseudocyst 260
– of postacute pseudocyst 260
NBT-PAPA test 113
NCOA3 514
necrolytic migrating erythema 709
necrosectomy 231, 234, 236, 249, 251
– closed lavage 250
– closed packing 250
– diabetes 290
– exocrine insufficiency 290
– indication 232
– minimally invasive 241
– open approach 146
– open packing 250
– operative technique 226
– pain 291
– pancreas 146
– pancreatic necrosis
– – indication 225
– – timing 226
– percutaneous 148
– planned staged relaparotomy 250
– postoperative complications 237
– procedure 243
– pseudocyst 290
– quality of life 291
– recurring disease 289
– results 237
necrosis
– pancreatic 120, 174
– pressure 282
necrotizing pancreatitis (NP), see also pancreatic necrosis 219, 249
– management 281
needle aspiration 853
neoadjuvant therapy
– resectable cancer 681
– survival 698
– survival 699
– target agents 683
neoplasm
– endocrine pancreas 507
– exocrine pancreas 497
– intraductal papillary mucinous (IPMN) 500
– metastases to the pancreas 509
– mucinous cystic 498
– – prognosis 499
– pancreatic, laparoscopic management 653
– preoperative staging 653
– solid
– – cystic change 503
– – pseudopapillary 502
neoplastic pancreatic lesion 109
neurogenic inflammation 296
neuron-specific enolase (NSE) 874
NGF 297
– receptor 298
nodal status (N) 827, 831
nonfunctioning PET 708, 709
noninvasive intraductal mucinous 426
non-neoplastic cystic lesion 426
nonsurgical
– approach 906
– management of acute pancreatitis 205
NP, see necrotizing pancreatitis
NSE, see neuron-specific enolase

O

obstruction, pseudocysts 472
obstructive jaundice 771, 776
octreotid 635
– PF management 284
OGTT 304
oligocyst 839
oncogene 514
ONYX-015 693
open packing approach
– pancreatic necrosectomy 146
OPN, see organized pancreatic necrosis
oral
– function test 113
– glucose tplerance 114
– intake 422
organ failure
– acute pancreatitis
– – mortality 205
– – severity 204
– pancreatitis 174
– – dynamics 176
– – severity 175
organized pancreatic necrosis (OPN) 241
– CT 271
– endoscopic drainage 274
– endoscopy 247
– nonsurgical necrosis 272
– percutaneous therapy, results 276
ovarian-type stroma 839, 850
oxaliplatin with gemcitabine 551

P

p16 314
p53 314, 762, 854
– pathway 517
pacemaker 311, 312
paclitaxel 691, 692
PACS 195
pain 304, 332, 456
– chronic pancreatitis 387
– epigastric 527

- extrapancreatic 295
- pancreatic 295
- pancreatic cancer 527
- pancreatic duct drainage 382
- pancreaticojejunostomy 396
- pattern 304
- persistent 396
- upper abdominal 382

palliative
- resection 564
- surgery
- – bypass procedures 666
- – indications 666
- – outcomes 673
- – postoperative course 672
- treatment
- – brachytherapy 692
- – chemoradiation 690, 692
- – chemotherapy 692
- – erlotinib 692
- – IORT 692
- – medical treatment 690
- – nonoperative 689
- – radiation 690
- – surgical interventions 690
- – symptoms-oriented 689
- – targeted agents 692

pancreas divisum 313, 334
- chronic pancreatitis 891
- definition 13
- endoscopic therapy 888
- minor papilla
- – complete forms 881
- – incomplete forms 881
- recurrent pancreatitis 891
- surgical treatment 892
- transduodenal surgical sphincteroplasty 891

pancreas/pancreatic
- abscess 174, 200, 253, 272, 301, 479, 481
- – bacterial spectrum 254
- – clinical presentation 255
- – drainage 251
- – endoscopic therapy, results 275
- adenocarcinoma 97
- anastomosis 419, 575
- anatomy 19
- ascites 201
- branch duct fusion 14
- cancer/carcinoma, see also cancer 198, 307, 479, 480, 489
- – diagnosis 126
- – FDG 97
- – FDG-PET 97
- – history 125
- – increase 307
- – mortality 489
- – of the head, bypass procedure 665
- – pancreatic intraepithelial neoplasia 102
- – physical findings 126
- – risk factors 125
- – ROC curve 100
- – sensitivity 100
- – specificity 100
- – symptoms 125
- CT 195
- D-cell 44
- disease
- – common bile duct dilatation 62
- – main pancreatic dilatation 61
- duct 915
- – change 332
- – communication 284
- – dilatation 81
- – disruption 209, 281
- – drainage 387, 389, 392, 396–398, 443
- – ductotomy 391
- – resection 398
- – stenosis 80
- – stent 208
- elastase-1 184
- embryology 10
- exocrine secretion 3
- – cephalic phase 5
- – nutrient loads 4
- – postprandial 3
- fine-needle aspiration
- – FNA techniques 327
- fistula (PF) 281, 480, 804
- – definition 283
- – diagnosis 283
- – distal pancreatectomy 448
- – imaging 283
- – incidence 283
- – management 284
- – operative approach 282
- – operative technique 282
- – pathogenesis 281
- – spontaneous closure 284
- fluid collection (PFC) 271
- – drainage, indications 272
- – endoscopic therapy, complications 275
- – nonsurgical methods, drainage 273
- – percutaneous therapy 275–277
- – predrainage evaluation 273
- – transmural drainage 273
- focal lesions
- – acute pancreatitis 62
- – chronic pancreatitis 62
- – cystic neoplasms in the pancreas 64
- – early detection of pancreatic cancer with US
- – metastatic pancreatic tumors 63
- – pancreatic cancer 62
- – pancreatic endocrine 63
- head 314
- – chronic pancreatitis 381
- – massive destruction 907, 908
- – massive disruption 905
- – resection 382
- infection 212, 253
- injury without duct involvement 907
- intraepithelial neoplasia 504
- intralobular islets 25
- islet isolation 915
- isoamylase 183
- lobular vascular bed 23
- lymphatic drainage 628
- malignant tumors 75
- microcirculation system 22
- necrosis, see also necrotizing pancreatitis 167, 174, 219
- – acute pancreatitis 199, 204
- – debridement 220
- – endoscopic therapy, results 275
- – extended 177
- – infected 200, 207
- – intensive care 206
- – minimally invasive necrosectomy 243
- – necrosectomy 146, 225, 289
- – nonsurgical necrosis 272
- – operative treatment, complication 228
- – percutaneous drainage 243
- – percutaneous therapy, results 276
- – postoperative course 223
- – postoperative outcome 223
- – preparation for surgery 220
- – pseudocysts 149
- – recurring disease 289
- – sterile, treatment 208
- – surgical technique 221
- nerve 296, 313
- neuropeptide 38
- polypeptide
- – amylin 45
- – islet transplantation 45
- – pancreas 45
- primordium identification 14
- pseudocyst 259, 263, 479
- – cystoenterostomy 151
- – cystogastrostomy 149
- – cystojejunostomy 151
- – diagnostic work-up 263
- – indication for treatment 264, 265
- remnant
- – laparoscopic pancreatic resection 447
- – tail 209
- resection 289
- – carcinoma of the body and tail 628
- – endocrine function 449
- – exocrine function 449
- – laparoscopic approach 446, 447
- – neck transection 633
- – pancreas, mobilization 632
- – postoperative care 635
- – preoperative preparation 628, 629
- – pseudocysts 471
- – somatostatin analogues 635
- – spleen preservation 445

– – splenectomy 445
– – splenic vessels 632
– – subtotal left, operative procedure 630
– – technique 444
– stent 334
– stump 409, 432
– transplantation
– – acute rejection 931
– – anostomotic leak 931
– – antirejection therapy 932
– – diabetic nephropathy 934
– – diabetic neuropathy 934
– – diabetic retinopathy 934
– – donor selection 923
– – enteric drainage 928
– – exocrine drainage to the bladder 927
– – glucose metabolism 933
– – graft pancreatitis 930
– – graft thrombosis 930
– – immunosuppression 929
– – in combination with kidney transplantation 921
– – indication 922
– – long-term pancreas graft function 933
– – long-term patient survival 933
– – monitoring of kidney function 931
– – patient survival 932
– – portal venous drainage 926
– – quality of life 934
– – recipient operation 926
– – systemic infections 932
– – systemic venous drainage, first pass effect 926
– – type I diabetes 921
– – type II diabetic 923
– – urinary drainage 927
– – urological complications 931
– trauma
– – blunt trauma 905
– – distal transection 905
– – grade II–IV injuries 905
– – major contusions 905
– – minor contusions 905
– vein 21
– venous anatomy 21
pancreas-sparing duodenectomy 819, 820
pancreatectomy
– insulinomas, laparoscopic distal 716
– left laparoscopic 660
– postoperative complications 447
– prognosis 636
– pseudocysts 471
– somatostatin analogues 635
– total 383, 639
– – laparoscopic 662
– venous resection 593
– – complications 602
– – conclusions 606
– – contraindications 596
– – indications 596
– – literature review 602
– – personal series 603
– – rationale 594
– – selection citeria 595
– – surgical techniques 597
pancreaticobiliary maljunction (PBM) 9, 895
– anatomical findings 13
– carcinogenesis 12
– clinical aspects 9
– definition 9
– hypothesis 11
– pancreatic juice reflux 13
pancreaticoduodenal artery (PSPDA) 19
pancreaticoduodenectomy 422, 567, 909
– arterial resection 617
– chronic pancreatitis
– – abnormal side branches 414
– – delayed gastric emptying 418
– – main pancreatic duct 414
– – mortality 418
– – PPPD 413
– – pylorus-preserving pancreaticoduodenectomy (PPPD) 413
– – reoperation 418
– – standard pancreaticoduodenectomy (PD) 413
– Kausch-Whipple pancreatectomy 573
– laparoscopy
– – pylorus-preserving 656
– – reconstruction 658
– – results 660
– M.D. Anderson cancer center, results 620
– margin assessment 611
– mesenteric vessels 615
– pathologic assessment 618
– patient selection 613
– pseudocysts 471
– pylorus preservation see PPPD 581
– surgical considerations 613
– survival 697
– tumor biology 614
– tumor-vessel relationships 614
– vascular resection 616
pancreaticogastrostomy 436
pancreaticojejunal anastomosis 392
pancreaticojejunostomosis 382
pancreaticojejunostomy 336, 433, 443, 468, 587, 813
– associated problems 393
– biliary obstruction 394
– diabetes 392
– duodenal obstruction 394
– mucosa-to-mucosa 744
– patient selection 388
– persistent pain 396
– results 392
– retrocolic 586
– small-duct chronic pancreatitis 397
pancreatin
– microsphere 340
– preparation 339
pancreatitis
– acute 75, 119
– – classification 173
– autoimmune 76, 198
– biliary sphincterotomy 209
– chronic 76, 122
– – distal pancreatectomy 441
– – pancreatic duct drainage 387
– – surgery 381
– gallstone 209
– groove 198
– post-ERCP 82
pancreatoblastoma 506, 841, 866
– genetics 507
pancreatoduodenal region
– evaluation 642
– mobilization 642
pancreatoduodenectomy, pylorus-preserving 807
pancreatogram
– ERCP 80
– pancreatic duct drainage 390
pancreatojejunostomy 803
pancreatosplenectomy, antegrade 635
pancreolauryl test 113, 323
papilla of Vater 755
papillary
– excrescence 851, 859
– stenosis 786
parenchymal injury involving the ampulla 908
partial duodenopancreatectomy 336
Partington-Rochelle 468
– modified Puestow procedure 389
– – results 392
pathology
– pancreatic cancers 625
– pancreatic neoplasia 497
– pancreaticoduodenectomy specimens 618
PBM, see pancreaticobiliary maljunction
PEG, see percutaneous endoscopic gastrostomy
pemetrexed 550
PEN
– genetics 508
– well-differentiated 507
Penrose drain 222
percutaneous
– aspiration, pancreatic infection 207
– biopsy, pancreatic cancer 535
– drainage pancreatic necrosis 243
– endoscopic gastrostomy (PEG) 275
periductal
– formation of fibrotic 311
– vascular plexus 26
perigastric lymph node 800
perineural immune cell infiltration 297
peripheral calcification 862

peritoneal pancreatitis 197
persisting pancreatic fistula 909
PET, see positron emission tomography
PF, see pancreatic fistula
PFC, see pancreatic fluid collection
pheochromocytoma 739
phospholipase
– A 3
– A2 188
pigment stone 143
PIPDA, see posterior inferior pancreaticoduodenal artery
PIPDV, see posterior inferior pancreaticoduodenal vein
PMN-elastase 188
polypoid tumor 857
portal vein (PV) 21, 312
– resection 576
– – survival 697
positron emission tomography (PET) 546
– Kausch-Whipple pancreatectomy 568
– pancreatic cancer 546
– PET/CT 97
postacute pseudocyst 262
– clinical symptoms 261, 262
– complication 262
– definition 259
– pathophysiology 260
post ERCP pancreatitis
– prevention 82
– risk factors 82
posterior
– inferior pancreaticoduodenal
– – artery (PIPDA) 19
– – vein (PIPDV) 22
– superior pancreaticoduodenal vein (PSPDV) 22
PP islet 14
PP-cell 37
PPPD 798
– contraindications 581
– indications 581
– intraoperative assessment 582
– postoperative management 589
– randomized clinical trials 589
– reconstruction 585
– surgical technique 582
PPTD 730, 733
preoperative treatment of resectable cancer 681
pressure necrosis, fistula formation 282
procalcitonin 189
progesterone
– immunoreactivity 854
– receptor 864
proinsulin 39
prolactinoma 739
prophylactic antibiotic treatment 211, 212
protein supplementation 350
protuberance 851
proximal transection 905, 907, 908
PRSS1 351
PRSS2 mutation
– autodigestion 365
– mesotrypsin 365
– trypsin 365
– trypsinogen 365
– – activation peptide (TAP) 364
– – autoactivation 365
pruritus, pancreatic cancer 528
pseudoaneurysm 480
– acute pancreatitis 201
pseudocyst 108, 296, 301, 470
– acute pancreatic (APP) 271
– chronic pancreatitis 123, 393
– complications 200, 471
– cystoenterostomy 151
– cystogastrostomy 149
– cystojejunostomy 151
– drainage 393
– – indications 272
– endoscopic therapy, results 275
– external drainage 470
– formation 459
– hemorrhage 471
– infection 471
– necrosectomy 290
– obstruction 472
– pancreatic 200
– – necrosis 149
– – resection 471
– pancreaticojejunostomy 468
– percutaneous therapy, results 276
– postoperative management 472
– pseudocystoduodenostomy 466
– pseudocystogastrostomy 464
– pseudocystojejunostomy 463
– rupture 472
– surgery 459
– – contraindications 460
– – diagnostic work-up 460
– – indications 460
– – laparoscopic approaches 470
– – outcome 473
– – procedures 461
– treatment 459
pseudocystoduodenostomy 466
pseudocystojejunostomy 463, 464
pseudopapillary neoplasm 502
PSPDA, see pancreaticoduodenal artery
PSPDV, see posterior superior pancreaticoduodenal vein
Puestow procedure, Partington-Rochelle-modified 389
PV, see portal vein

Q

quality of life 918

R

R factor 622
– survival rates 676
radiation 676
– palliative treatment 690
– resectable cancer 681
Ranson score 174, 204
rapamycin pathway 521
rapture 865
Ras inhibitor 554
ras pathway 516
Rb pathway 517
recurrent disease
– M.D. Anderson cancer center, results 621
– pancreatic necrosis 289
reflux of pancreatic juice 13
regional pancreatectomy 697
registration 735
resectability
– carcinoma of the body and tail 630
– pancreatectomy, venous resection 595
– pancreatic cancer 560
– tumor invasion 563
resection
– carcinoma of the body and tail 628
– margin assessment 611
– mortality 696
– palliative 564
– pancreatic 289
– procedure 111
– R factor 622
– subtotal left, technique 630
– survival 696, 700
– total pancreatectomy 644
residual disease status (R factor) 611
respiratory distress syndrome 120
retroperitoneal necrosis 167
retropyloric dissection 417
Roux-en-Y jejunal loop 433
RTOG trial 679, 691, 693, 698

S

SAA 187
SAP, see severe acute pancreatitis
SASI test 711, 723, 724
screening 767
SCT
– glycogen-rich 861
– honeycomb 861
– microcystic 861
secretin-pancreozymin (cerulein) test 112, 322
segmental portal hypertension 108
sepsis
– ERCP 78
– ERCP 82
serous cystic
– adenoma 407
– neoplasm 839
serum amylase 173
– levels 194
– pancreatic fistula 283
sessile polyp 857
severe acute pancreatitis (SAP) 173, 193
– complications 173
– early (ESAP) 177
– HLA-DR expression 228

– necrosectomy
– – surgical management 226
– – timing 226
– necrosis 219
– operative treatment, complication 228
– organ failure 175
– pancreatic necrosis 225
– reoperation 227
– surgical source control 227
severe relapsing pain 305
shock syndrome in acute pancreatitis 120
short relapsing pain 305
signet ring cell carcinoma 506
simultaneous pancreas-kidney transplantation 922
sinogram, contrast 283
sirolimus 930
SIRS, see systemic inflammatory response syndrome
skeletonization 800
SMA, see superior mesenteric artery
smad protein 518
– SMAD4 515, 518, 839, 841
small intestinal
– fistulas 286
– transit 6
– – chymotrypsin 6
– – lipase activity 6
– – proteases 6
– – trypsin activity 6
small-cell carcinoma 508
small-duct disease 356
– pancreatic duct drainage 397
SMF 692
smoking, pancreatic cancer 491
SMPV
– confluence 615
– venous resection 617
SMV, see superior mesenteric vein
snare excision 782
solid
– exocrine neoplasm 503
– nodule 851
– pseudopapillary neoplasm 502, 840
– pseudopapillary tumor 864
somatostatin 44, 82
– analogue 711, 739, 745
– – prophylactic 635
– receptor scintigraphy (SRS) 710, 723, 726
somatostatinoma 707, 709, 737
SP 297
sphincterectomy 886
sphincterotomy, biliary 209
SPINK1 351, 363
splanchnicectomy, chemical 668
spleen 454
– mobilization 631, 645
– preservation, pancreatic resection 445, 447
splenectomy
– laparoscopy 660, 662
– pancreatic resection 445
splenic vein (SPV) 21
– thrombosis 480
SPT, metastasized 865
SPV, see splenic vein
SRCV, see superior right colic vein
SRS, see somatostatin receptor scintigraphy
staging 775, 830, 831
– acute pancreatitis 198
– biochemical 181
– intraoperative 546
– laparoscopy 627
– pancreatic cancer 541, 561, 626
– postoperative 546
– preoperative 547, 627
stapler anastomosis 927
steatorrhea 321, 340
– total pancreatectomy 650
stenosis 479, 480
– of the common bile duct 312
stent 784
– biliary decompression 689
– chronic pancreatitis 383
– pancreatic 209
– pancreatic cancer 530
– pancreatic fistula 285
– PPPD, preoperative biliary 588
– small-duct chronic pancreatitis 397
– sterile pancreatic necrosis 208
– survival 698
sterile necrosis 213
stimulation test
– arterial 711
– glucagon 710
– intraoperative 710
– intravenous 710
– secretin 710
STK11 515, 521
stool weight 323
streptozotocin 692
substance P 298
subtotal left resection
– postoperative care 635
– technique 630
sunburst type 862
superior mesenteric artery (SMA) 611, 615
– invasion 668
– margin 611, 619
– – oncologic importance 622
– venous resection 617
superior mesenteric vein (SMV) 21, 615
– venous resection 617
– – pancreatectomy 594
superior right colic vein (SRCV) 21
surgery/surgical 335
– APBDJ 898
– chronic pancreatitis 382, 443
– internal drainage 909
– interventions 249, 509
– laparoscopic 653
– management 214, 215, 253
– palliation, bypass procedures 666
– pancreatic cancer, indications 559
– pancreatic pseudocysts 459
– strategy in pancreatic pseudocyst
– – cystoduodenostomy 266, 267
– – cystogastrostomy 266
– – cystojejunostomy 266
– – external drainage 267
– – internal drainage 265
– – laparoscopic techniques 267, 268
– – open surgery 265
– – pancreatic resection 267
– treatment 257, 335
survival
– adjuvant treatment 698
– biopsy 698
– cytology 698
– factors 695
– genetics 700
– IORT 699
– locally advanced tumors 699
– lymphadenectomy 697
– metastatic disease 699
– neoadjuvant therapy 699
– R factors 700
– rate
– – resected cancer 676
– stents 698
– surgical resection 696
– tumor location 695
– vascular resection 697
– volume effects 696
systemic inflammatory response syndrome (SIRS) 121, 219
– acute pancreatitis 121
– pancreatic necrosis 219

T

TAP 186
teratoma 841
TGFB1/2 519
thick capsule 857
thrombophlebitis in pancreatic cancer 528
thrombosis
– gastrointestinal fistulas 282
– splenic vein 201
– venous resection, complications 602
TIGAR-O 301
timing
– of surgery 214
– of necrosectomy 233
– – pancreatic necrosis 226
tipifarnib 554
TNFerade 693
topoisomerase I inhibitor with gemcitabine 551
total pancreatectomy 337, 860
– complications 649
– contraindications 640
– history 639
– indications 639
– outcome 650
– pancreaticoduodenectomy 453

– postoperative management 648
– preoperative preparation 640
– reconstruction 647
– resection 644
– technique 641
TP53 515, 839, 841
– gene 517
TPA, see transverse pancreatic artery
transabdominal ultrasound 323
– pancreatic cancer 529
transforming growth factor (TGF) 314
– TGF-β superfamily pathway 517
transhepatic percutaneous access 916
transmural drainage 273
transthoracic splanchnicectomy 335
transverse pancreatic artery (TPA) 21
trastuzumab 555
tropical chronic pancreatitis 311
– abdominal pain 352
– abscess 353
– ascites 353
– chronic calcifying pancreatitis 349
– clinical features 351
– cysts 353
– diabetes 352
– – mellitus 352
– ductal strictures 355
– endotherapy 355
– extracorporeal shockwave lithotripsy 355
– food toxins
– – hydrocyanic acid 350
– gastrointestinal bleeding 353
– intractable pain 354
– lithiasis 349
– main pancreatic ductal decompression 355
– malnutrition 350
– micronutrient 350
– obstructive jaundice 352
– pathology 351
– pleural effusion 353
– steatorrhea 352
– weight loss 352
Trousseau's sign 528
trypsin 3
trypsinogen-2 184
T-staging 827
tumor
– abutment 612
– borderline resectable 613
– encasement 612
– invasion, resectability 563
– marker, pancreatic cancer 528
– pancreatic cancer 489
– suppressor gene 515
tumorigenesis 513

U

ultrasound/ultrasonography (US) 61
– acute pancreatitis 194
– APBDJ 896
– transabdominal 529

V

vaccination, preoperative 628, 640
vaccine in adjuvant therapy 684
vanilloid receptor 298
vapreotid 635
vascular
– bed of the pancreas 23
– dissection, multimodality therapy 618
– resection
– – pancreaticoduodenectomy 616
– – survival 697
– thrombosis, gastrointestinal fistulas 282
vasoactive intestinal peptide (VIP) 37
venous resection
– literature review 602
– pancreatectomy
– – complications 602
– – conclusions 606
– – contraindications 596
– – indications 596
– – personal results 603
– – rationale 594
– – resectability 595
– – surgical techniques 597
– pancreaticoduodenectomy 616
ventral pancreas 313
VHL syndrome, see von Hippel-Lindau syndrome
villous
– adenoma 765
– tumor 857
VIP, see vasoactive intestinal peptide
VIPoma 707, 709, 736
von Hippel-Lindau syndrome (VHL syndrome) 498, 737, 738, 839, 874

W

watery diarrhea 736
weight loss in chronic pancreatitis 124
Whipple pancreatectomy, see also Kausch-Whipple pancreatectomy 567
Whipple procedure
– chronic pancreatitis 383
– laparoscopic 659
– pancreaticojejunostomy, persistent pain 396
Wirsung duct 432

Z

ZES, see Zollinger-Ellison syndrome
zinc supplement 739
Zollinger-Ellison syndrome (ZES) 723